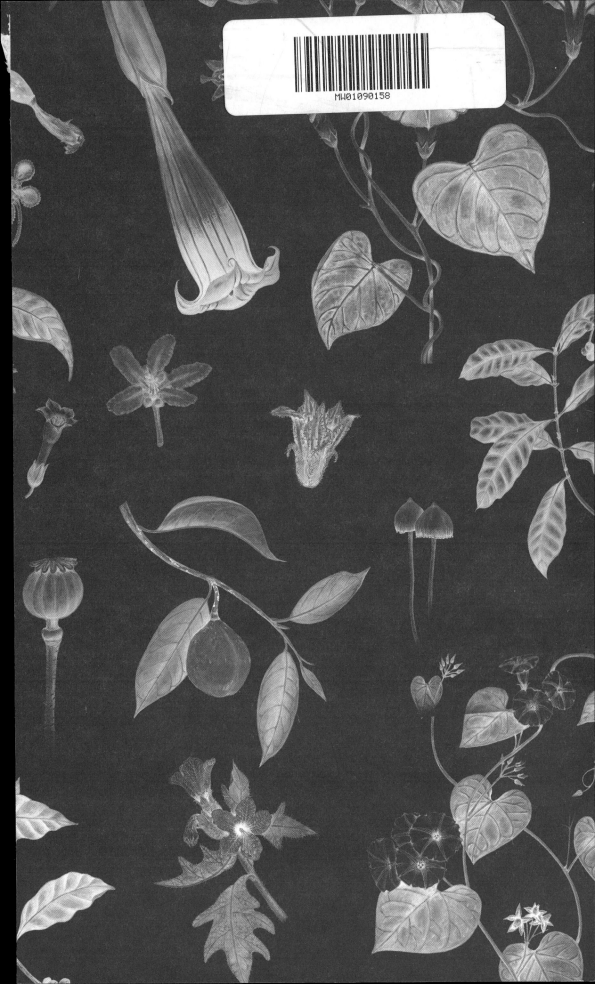

ETHNOPHARMACOLOGIC SEARCH
for PSYCHOACTIVE DRUGS · 1967

Vol. I

This is a digitally remastered facsimile edition
produced from the original publication.

PUBLISHED BY
SYNERGETIC PRESS
Santa Fe | London
In association with the Heffter Research Institute

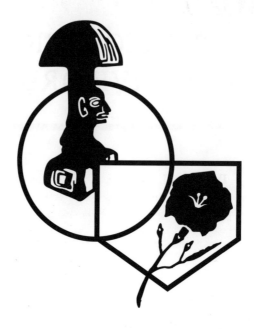

Within the symbolic chemical representation above and
on the cover are shown a view of a mushroom stone of the
Namuth collection and a morning glory blossom. The mushroom stone — early pre-classic, circa B.C. 1000-500 — contains a figure believed to be that of a young woman before a
metate or grinding stone.

Workshop Series of Pharmacology Section, N.I.M.H. Nº 2

Ethnopharmacologic Search for
PSYCHOACTIVE DRUGS

Proceedings of a Symposium held in San Francisco, California
January 28–30, 1967

DANIEL H. EFRON, *Editor-in-Chief,*
National Institute of Mental Health,
Chevy Chase, Maryland

BO HOLMSTEDT, *Co-Editor,*
Karolinska Institutet,
Stockholm, Sweden

NATHAN S. KLINE, *Co-Editor,*
Rockland State Hospital,
Orangeburg, New York

Sponsored by:
Pharmacology Section, Psychopharmacology Research Branch
National Institute of Mental Health   Public Health Service
U.S. DEPARTMENT OF HEALTH, EDUCATION, AND WELFARE

The opinions expressed and any conclusions drawn are those of the participants of the Symposium and are not to be understood as necessarily having the endorsement of, or representing the viewpoints of, the Public Health Service of the U.S. Department of Health, Education, and Welfare.

Public Health Service Publication No. 1645   1967

For sale by the Superintendent of Documents, U.S. Government Printing Office
Washington, D.C. 20402 - Price $4.00

ORGANIZING COMMITTEE

DANIEL H. EFRON   Pharmacology Section, Psychopharmacology Research Branch, National Institute of Mental Health, Chevy Chase, Maryland

SEYMOUR M. FARBER   Continuing Education in Medicine and Health Sciences, San Francisco Medical Center, University of California, San Francisco, California

BO HOLMSTEDT   Department of Toxicology, Swedish Medical Research Council, Karolinska Institute, Stockholm, Sweden

NATHAN S. KLINE   Research Center, Rockland State Hospital, Orangeburg, New York

ROGER H. L. WILSON   Continuing Education in Medicine and Health Sciences, San Francisco Medical Center, University of California, San Francisco, California

CONFERENCE COMMITTEE

Chairman: Seymour M. Farber	Leon Epstein	Chauncey Leake
Virginia Barrelier	Mrs. Bo Holmstedt (Artist)	E. Leong Way
Patricia K. Black	Bo Holmstedt	Florence Webster
Daniel H. Efron	Nathan S. Kline	Roger H. L. Wilson

INVITED PARTICIPANTS

SIRI VON REIS ALTSCHUL

Botanical Museum of Harvard University, Cambridge, Massachusetts

I. I. BREKHMAN

Institute of Biologically Active Substances, Far-Eastern Branch of Siberian Department of Academy of Sciences, U.S.S.R., Vladivostok 22, U.S.S.R.

JOSEPH P. BUCKLEY

Department of Pharmacology, School of Pharmacy, University of Pittsburgh, Pittsburgh, Pennsylvania

GEORG E. CRONHEIM

Riker Laboratories, Inc., Northridge, California

JOHN W. DALY

Laboratory of Chemistry, National Institute of Arthritis and Metabolic Diseases, National Institutes of Health, Bethesda, Maryland

VENANCIO DEULOFEU

Universidad de Buenos Aires, Facultad de Ciencias Exactas y Naturales, Parera 77, Buenos Aires, Argentina

DANIEL H. EFRON

Pharmacology Section, Psychopharmacology Research Branch, National Institute of Mental Health, Chevy Chase, Maryland

CONRAD H. EUGSTER

Department of Organic Chemistry, University of Zurich, Zurich, Switzerland

CLELLAN S. FORD

Department of Anthropology, Yale University, New Haven, Connecticut

DANIEL X. FREEDMAN

Department of Psychiatry, University of Chicago, Chicago, Illinois

CARLETON GAJDUSEK

National Institute of Neurological Diseases and Blindness, National Institutes of Health, Bethesda, Maryland

LOWELL D. HOLMES

Department of Anthropology, Wichita State University, Wichita, Kansas

BO HOLMSTEDT

Department of Toxicology, Swedish Medical Research Council, Karolinska Institutet, Stockholm 60, Sweden

EVAN C. HORNING

Lipid Research Center, Department of Biochemistry, Baylor University College of Medicine, Houston, Texas

HARRIS ISBELL

Department of Medicine, University of Kentucky Medical Center, Lexington, Kentucky

NATHAN S. KLINE

Rockland State Hospital, Orangeburg, New York

MURLE W. KLOHS

Medicinal Chemistry Section, Riker Laboratories, Northridge, California

HANS J. MEYER

Department of Pharmacology, University of Freiburg, Freiburg i. Br., Germany

CLAUDIO NARANJO

Escuela de Medicina, Universidad de Chile, Santiago, Chile

CARL C. PFEIFFER

Section on Neuropharmacology, New Jersey Neuropsychiatric Institute, Princeton, New Jersey

EFRÉN CARLOS DEL POZO

Instituto de Estudios Medicos y Biologicos, Universidad Nacional de Mexico, Mexico D.F., Mexico

THORNTON SARGENT

Donner Laboratory, University of California, Berkeley, California

GEORG J. SEITZ

Köln-Lindenthal, Dürenerstrasse 175, Germany

RICHARD E. SCHULTES

Botanical Museum of Harvard University, Cambridge, Massachusetts

ALEXANDER T. SHULGIN

Department of Pharmacology, University of California, San Francisco Medical Center, San Francisco, California

STEPHEN I. SZARA

Section on Psychopharmacology, Clinical Neuropharmacology Research Center, National Institute of Mental Health, St. Elizabeths Hospital, Washington, District of Columbia

DERMOT TAYLOR

Department of Pharmacology, School of Medicine, Center for Health Sciences, University of California, Los Angeles, California

EDWARD B. TRUITT

Division of Physiology and Pharmacology, Battelle Memorial Institute, Columbus, Ohio

PETER G. WASER

Department of Pharmacology, University of Zurich, Zurich, Switzerland

S. HENRY WASSÉN

Gothenburg Ethnographic Museum, Norra Hamngaten 12, Gothenburg, Sweden

R. GORDON WASSON

Botanical Museum of Harvard University, Cambridge, Massachusetts

ANDREW T. WEIL

Harvard Medical School, Cambridge, Massachusetts (mailing address: 128 Lexington Ave., Cambridge, Massachusetts)

PREFACE

The use of plants or their extracts for medicinal or religious ceremonial purposes is very old—practically as old as the human race. The information about the use of plants as psychotropic agents by man is probably
found in the Bible. The apple that Adam ate (whatever the variety) could
be considered as a psycho-energizer. Was it a stimulator, did it enhance
memory or learning abilities, or did it activiate the desire for acquiring more
information? As with our new psychotropic drugs, I don't know if it brought
happiness and comfort, or new problems, aggravations, and unhappiness.
Another example of early use and knowledge of medicinal plants we find
in the fact that the most ancient medical god of Mesopotamia—Sin—was
also the god of medicinal herbs.

The development of drug chemistry brought: first, isolation from plants
of a number of pharmacologically active substances (e.g. curare, atropine
ouabain, etc.), later, synthesis of these entities and their derivatives; and
finally, creation of completely new molecules, formerly not known, in the
plant or animal kingdom.

We know, also, that in the process of development and worship of chemistry
we somehow forgot about our prime source, the plants. We forgot that we
have used only some of the known substances of plant origin. At the same
time, the intrusions of civilization have been progressively destroying the
sources of our knowledge, as well as the source itself of many plants—plants
which are used either in medicine or in ceremonial and sacred context. Today,
time is running out if we want to save this information, and perhaps use for
medicinal purposes some of the unknown compounds contained in plants.

The idea of acquiring knowledge about these plants and compounds we
have neglected or forgotten was the reason for organizing this symposium.
It was self-evident that this meeting had to be multidisciplinary. We invited
pharmacologists, pharmacists, chemists, biochemists, psychiatrists, anthropologists, etc., etc. We wanted to exchange existing information, confront different points of view, and outline and stimulate research objectives for the
future.

As one of the organizers of this symposium, I am certainly biased, but I
feel that this meeting was very successful. I would like to include here the
opinion of one of the participants.

"This," he remarked, "is the first meeting I have attended that at the end
of the sessions we had as many or even more participants than in the beginning—this is a measure of the interest the meeting has created."

We discovered after the meetings how many scattered researchers in wide
and varied fields could contribute to the knowledge which we seek. This finding alone was one of the very important immediate gains from the symposium. And we hope that in the future we will be able to organize a second

meeting on the same topics, and cover a much broader spectrum of problems in the ethnopharmacologic search for psychoactive drugs.

The meeting was divided into six sessions, all but the first ending in panel discussions. All authors who delivered papers at the session served also as panelists. They discussed different problems among themselves and answered questions from the floor. The discussion after Session IV covered a special topic: "Psychoactive Action of Various Tryptamine Derivatives," and experts in this field were invited. The discussions after Sessions V and VI were merged, and covered, besides specific topics of these sessions, all problems dealt with in the symposium. Speakers from other sessions also participated in this dicussion.

The discussions held after the sessions were recorded *in extenso*, and are printed here following the papers of each session. Because of the multidisciplinary character of the symposium, problems of terminology and the extent of discussion, no restrictions were imposed on participants with regard to nomenclature used, order of material or uniformity of presentation and reference listing. The diversity of form and style of the various presentations was not altered for publication; they remain in their original form.

We extend our deep appreciation and thanks to the local group from the Continuing Education in Medicine and Health Sciences, University of California, San Francisco Medical Center, for their excellent work in organizing this meeting in San Francisco. This group, under the chairmanship of Dean Seymour M. Farber, with the participation of Dr. Roger H. Wilson, and Mesdames Virginia Barrelier, Patricia K. Black, Florence Webster and Matilda Wilson, deserves a great deal of credit for the success of our meeting.

It would be remiss for me not to remark here (and I am doing so with delight) on the contributions of Drs. Bo Holmstedt and Nathan Kline, coeditors of this volume. Without their vision, interest, know-how, persistence and scientific knowledge, this meeting could not have taken place. I would like also to express my thanks to Dr. Albert A. Manian and Mrs. Shirley Maltz from the Pharmacology Section, N.I.M.H., for their help in the preparation of this manuscript.

Finally, many thanks to all speakers, discussants and participants. In final analysis, it was their contributions which made the meeting a success, and helped so much in the stimulation and delineation of new directions in research—directions which may bring us a new arsenal of useful drugs, especially in the field of psychiatry and neurological diseases.

D.H.E.

CONTENTS

GREETINGS

Willard C. Fleming, D.D.S. *Chancellor*
University of California, San Francisco Medical Center,
San Francisco, California

My name is Fleming. I am Chancellor of the San Francisco Medical Center. If you do not know me, I prefer to introduce myself always, because if my friends introduce me I am a little fearful of people I do not know—I do a much better job myself.

I was born some sixty-seven years ago in Sausalito of poor but honest parents. The poverty angle must have been a dominant genetic factor because my daughter has the same problem.

I came here as a student of dentistry in 1918. I became a member of the Dental Faculty in 1923. I became Dean of the Dental School in 1939. After three years of attempting to retire, I took three years to find my successor. I thought this was fine, until one of my "friends" said: "Bill, did it ever occur to you they don't want to make the same mistake twice?"

From there to Dean of Students; and I have since last July been Chancellor of this campus. I have no illusions about why a Chancellor, Mayor or Governor gives introductory speeches. This is for the audience to calm down, chat with one's neighbor, get the identification, and so on.

I will follow the same pattern. After residence here of almost fifty years, you should understand that the local history of this center is of interest to me. History can be a very static chronicle of what has happened; or on the other hand, it can be a very dynamic encounter, and establish a sort of a curve of progress that can be extended as a curve of probability into the future.

I welcome the participants of the symposium entitled, "Ethnopharmacological Search for Psychoactive Drugs." I have a great deal of difficulty with that word. This is really the first time I have gone through it quite smoothly.

If you agree with what I said about history being used as our prediction of events to come, you may agree this campus is historically the logical place to sponsor this idea.

The history of California and in particular the Bay Area, is replete with the part medicine has played in its development. Bear Flag Republic; vigilante movement in San Francisco; the role of California in the years of Civil War; the bubonic plague epidemic; the Golden Gate Park and the health crisis that grew out of the fire and earthquake of 1906; an interesting course of development.

At the start of the very facilities that were in here, now, to give you some idea of how this started: like some medical schools in the early days, this school started with the history of a proprietary school, in other words, a school for profit. Then in the Gold Rush days of '49 and '50, a great many physicians came to California. They were adventurers, charlatans, and also some very highly qualified and respected professional people. They were inclined to be a quarrelsome lot. This is an attribute that has not quite died out yet; and it is hard to think of another group that was so individualistic.

Among them was Dr. Hugh Toland, a well trained and well qualified surgeon. He tried his luck in the gold fields, but like so many others shortly returned to private practice in San Francisco. He was eminently successful both professionally and economically. During the '60's his annual income was reported to be over forty thousand dollars—more than they pay the Chancellor today.

This phenomenal income for those days was accomplished by taking advantage of two situations: The pioneers of those days were subject to many medical conditions and diseases, and of all of these, scurvy and syphilis were high on the morbidity list. Like many physicians of those years, Dr. Toland compounded and dispensed his own drugs, so it is no surprise to learn that in the backroom of Dr. Toland's offices were two barrels. One was labeled "Anti-Syph" and the other, "Anti-Scrof". There were no mail order houses, but there was the Wells Fargo Express throughout the entire west.

Through the dispensing of drugs for treatment of syphilis and scurvy by mail order, Hugh Toland became wealthy. Like so many people of these days, he attempted to memorialize himself by founding a medical school in his name. It is an interesting and intriguing story how, with the aid of Dr. Richard Beverly Cole, his first Dean of the medical school, this pair persuaded Regents of the newly started University of California to take on the Toland Medical School as the medical school of the University of California.

The Regents refused to name it Toland School of the University of California, but they did agree that there should be a physical part or plant with the name of Toland. Thus, today we have in our University of California Hospital a small auditorium known as the Toland Auditorium.

Our Department of Pharmacology has always been strong, as has our School of Pharmacy. Possibly it is our heritage, the fact that our medical center has a strong pharmacological school here, resting on one barrel of Anti-Syph and one barrel of Anti-Scrof.

At any rate, one can see that this symposium and its participants are in a hospitable environment. You are a welcome addition to a long line of predecessors, a fair example of the past and a prologue to the future.

Again I officially welcome you to the opening of this symposium.

INTRODUCTION

The Psychology, Philosophy, Morality and Legislative Control of Drug Usage

NATHAN S. KLINE

Research Center, Rockland State Hospital
Orangeburg, New York

Man's Need for Action

Man is an animal impelled by internal forces to act. Just what form that action will take depends on the sensations experienced, the learned modifications of innate response patterns, and the possible alternatives existing in the immediate environmental situation. Behavior based on purely rational decision, if it exists at all, is certainly rare. Action is usually evoked by the sensual and emotional, or at times by reflex or even motor needs.

Provocations to Action

Each of us is continuously being teased, hoodwinked, wheedled, invaded, bluffed, seduced and assaulted. When such blandishments to action are at the cognitive or even the emotional level the attempts are often obvious enough. More basic and often underriding them are appeals and approaches to primitive patterns of sensation involving incense, drums, drugs, ritualistic postures, idols, pageantry; rhythmic sounds and motions interspersed with abrupt syncopes; vast or close repetitive visual designs, color shock and most of all, movement. There are elusive, lingering, attractive, unidentifiable odors or revolting stenches that stir some troubled layer that lies below consciousness; and the body itself, the skin with its ceaseless prickling, itching, stretching, hotness, coldness never really leaves us alone. Nor do the muscles that protest by making us fidget if they are not moved frequently and then ache if they are exercised too long or too hard; the vague internal stirrings, appetites, "all the nameless feelings that go coursing through our breast." Finally, there is the mind's own place, eternally restless, seeking, peeking, poking, squirming, probing. Quiet and silence is a kind of death, from which we fear we may never be able to rouse ourselves.

The Role of Drugs in Altering Perception: and the Partial Dependence of Such Responses on Environment and Expectation

Evocation and certainly control of these response patterns is still largely "unscientific." Experience and a particular habit of mind are necessary, however, before experience can be decocted into an effective guide through these mazes. Fatigue, hyperexcitement and drugs, by producing dissociation, tend both to heighten such experiences but at the same time to break down sophisticated self-awareness.

The loss of ego integrity with its capacity for reality testing leaves the self wide and uncritically open to prior expectations and environmental influences. How the drug-induced perceptual, kinesthetic or other distortions will be interpreted will therefore vary from culture to culture and even from individual to individual. Occasionally the same drug may induce profound depression, Dionysian ecstasy, terror or bland indifference. Yet if we induce similar expectations and control environment, the response is usually predictable. Duration is yet all too short and side effects still all too great, but we are well along toward recognizing both the circumstances and the agents which will do what we ask of them, by way of temporarily altering the perceived universe.

Society's Moral Attitude

Whether such para-universes lead to improved philosophic or psychologic insights is far from clear. The use of drugs for any thing other than medical therapeutic purposes has always been construed as a threat—even when the purpose was ostensibly religious—few except the in-group would sanction such use. Even at the most simple level there is confusion; "taking drugs" has an immoral connotation despite the fact that the particular drug may be life saving; there is only disapproval of escape from intolerable thoughts, feelings or situations. At times drugs serve to induce actions which would otherwise not be possible; the hope of ex-static (i.e., out of the status quo) movement leads man to seize upon whatever is at hand to try to bring about such alterations. "The desire to take pills" wrote Olser, "is the greatest feature which distinguishes man from the animals."

Why the Increased Interest and Use of Drugs at This Time and Place in History?

Here I repeat what I have written elsewhere:

To varying degrees each of us mortgages the present for the future; we tolerate present discomfort in expectation of eventual relief or even reward. Those parts of the remembered past which make us queasy are usually justified as contributing to some useful purpose yet to be realized. In the process we create a cultural as well as a personal history involving the whence and hence of existence.

On rare and glorious occasions some individual or group floods through time with an epic tide and in sheer admiration we are all swept along. More frequently the individual narrative thread is thin and frayed. In place of the grand patterned fabric we see only the thrums of existence. The whole business becomes a drag. Bugged by what we trail along and hung up on what is yet to come, we seek temporary or semipermanent escapes.

Today we lack any viable universally accepted dramatic plot. The success (not the failure) of nineteenth century rationalism has left us at least momentarily without a denouement. Not that those dated objectives of adequate food, housing and racial equality for everyone have been attained but, as in the stock market, their achievement has been "discounted" since it is obvious that within another few hundred years they will be substantially achieved. The sense of great purpose and broad adventure which these goals engendered has vanished. Instead of singing down the high road we are looking at our sore feet. It requires solid stupidity, bland carelessness or extraordinary courage to disregard signposts which say "To Nowhere." The road is studded with squatters who block those who would pass. The gatherings at the campfires are not for counsels or imaginative planning but to titillate with pointless ghost stories.

Curiosity and action are thus directed inward. Drugs that help sever the tenuous ties with the outside world become highly prized since they both assist and justify the disregard for external realities. . . .

In the search for new values to give rise to a new narrative the towering, probing mystics of the past have sought to recapture the UR-experience upon which every Establishment originally drew strength until it became formalized. This invariably demanded the shattering of the idols or the escape from the Concept. Visions, iconoclasm, transcendence took place as the inevitable realization of a whole life's agon. Smashing a few clay figures or experiencing visual hallucinations does not produce an Abraham or a St. Theresa. Every great mystic has had experiences dissociated from the time and culture in which he lived—but the dissociation arose out of inner necessity. Conversion in turn is facilitated by the ecstasy of dance, ritual death, drugs. Dissociation per se has no value and can become meaningful only as it is integrated into a conceptual framework. This incorporation can be strongly directed from outside. . . .

The dissociation can also produce panic if the attempt is made to retain dissolving ego controls. Once these are surrendered a para-infantile acceptance of the universe is experienced in which there are no clear ego boundaries so that the One-ness with the All comes about. Whether this feeling (or any other) has important value depends entirely on how it alters the organization and action of the organism.

Can We Legislate Control?

Pharmaceuticals, like firearms, in themselves can be described only by such terms as potent or precise. Not their effectiveness but their application determines whether they are "good" or "bad". We probably should not, and in any case *can* not effectively, legislate against exploration of these other worlds. But we must protect ourselves by knowledge of what to expect and by attempting to control who may use these agents and for what purposes. There will obviously be wide differences of opinion on this score. Past epidemics of opiate or of cocaine usage finally required legal restrictions which did serve some useful purpose. Attending, or reading the records of, the present sessions is an act of affirmation in that they lead to increased understanding. We push back the darkness a bit; the darkness of the mysterious world of drugs and the equally dark and mysterious realms of self-knowledge and self-control.

In addition to moralizing, proselytizing, speculating; new legislation has and will continue to emerge in an attempt to influence the natural history of this uniquely human venture in which man deliberately alters his experiences of the world. As to how effective or desirable such legislation has been or will be, I can best end with a comment of Ambrose Bierce about Satan:

Satan made himself multifariously objectionable and was finally expelled from Heaven. Half way in his descent he paused, bent his head in thought a moment and at last went back. "There is one favor that I should like to ask," he said.

"Name it."

"Man, I understand, is about to be created. He will need laws."

"What, wretch! You his appointed adversary, charged from the dawn of eternity with hatred of his soul—you ask the right to make his laws?"

"Pardon; what I have to ask is that he be permitted to make them himself."

LETTER

FROM Albert Hofmann, Ph. D., Pharm. D., H.C.
Deputy Director Sandoz A. G.,
Basel, Switzerland*

January 19, 1967

Mr. Chairman, dear Colleagues,

While it is undoubtedly possible, with the aid of psychoactive drugs, to span both time and space, this method of overcoming these factors is unfortunately possible only psychically and not physically. Would the latter be possible, you may rest assured that I would now have taken the appropriate dosage of LSD or psilocybin so as to be transported on the flying carpet to San Francisco, for the purpose of participating in the symposium on psychoactive drugs.

I very much regret the fact that, for reasons of company policy, it was impossible for me to actively participate in this Congress. It is nonetheless my desire to convey from here in Basel, to the numerous prominent research workers in the field of psychoactive drugs attending this conference, my best wishes and the expression of the hope that the exchange of ideas will be fruitful.

The investigations of the lysergic acid derivatives, from which LSD resulted, have continued uninterruptedly in a variety of directions in the Sandoz research laboratories.

Thus, for example, it was possible, in pursuing the serotonin antagonistic activity first observed in LSD, to develop new lysergic acid derivatives in which a specific serotonin antagonistic activity is of prime importance. One of these highly active compounds has been introduced into therapy for the interim treatment of migraine.

In a particular field of research closely related to the theme of this congress and initiated by the discovery of LSD, our investigations on psychotomimetic drugs have been pursued. In using the experiences gained with LSD as the foundation, the problem of the so-called Mexican magic mushrooms, which has been studied ethnomycologically by Gordon Wasson and botanically by Roger Heim, was solved from a chemical point of view. The active ingredients, psilocybine and psilocine have been synthesised and made available for psychiatric research. The magic mushrooms in turn led us to a further important Mexican magic drug, namely Ololiuqui. In the Ololiuqui seeds, provided us by Wasson, we found the active ingredients to be lysergic acid derivatives, the main components of which are lysergic acid amide and lysergic acid hydroxyethylamide.

It would have given me great pleasure had I been able, at this symposium, to discuss in detail this most unusual, one can almost say magic circle of research which, starting from lysergic acid amides, namely lysergic acid

---

*Dr. Hofmann was unable to attend this meeting and his letter was read to the audience by Dr. N. Kline.

diethylamide (LSD), proceeded via two Mexican magic drugs—the sacred mushroom "Teonanacatl" and the Morning Glory seeds "Ololiuqui" and led back to the lysergic acid amides. I sincerely hope that I shall be able to satisfy this desire at the next symposium on psychoactive drugs in the not too distant future.

In conclusion I should like to express a few general points of view on psychoactive drugs.

These drugs are of especial importance in the following three fields:

1. In neuro- and brain-chemistry they are useful tools for the investigation of biochemical processes which form the basis of the nervous and psychic functions.

2. In psychiatry they have proved themselves to be compounds which, upon sensible administration, are becoming ever more important medical aids in psychoanalysis and psychotherapy.

3. From a epistemological point of view we must face the consequences resulting from the fact that it is possible, with the aid of mere traces of a compound, to radically affect the psychic processes and mental functions. This finding may throw new light on the age-old problem of the relationship and interrelationship of body and soul, or more generally, of mind and matter.

To a large extent the non-medical, partially legitimate, partially illegitimate, interest in and use of hallucinogenics or psychedelics is as a result of the possibilities mentioned under 3 above, namely of attaining a profound transformation of the conscious with the aid of these drugs.

It is in fact this very general interest in psychedelics, which has unfortunately, in some cases, led to dangerous misuse, that behooves scientists to continue research in the field of psychoactive compounds in all directions as quickly as possible, so as to elucidate the possibilities of these potent drugs in order that they may be used for the benefit of mankind.

It is my fervent wish that, in this respect also, this congress will be successful.

Yours

Albert Hofmann

SESSION I

AN OVERVIEW OF ETHNOPHARMACOLOGY

Chauncey D. Leake, *Chairman*

Chairman's Introduction

CHAUNCEY D. LEAKE
Department of Pharmacology, University of California
San Francisco Medical Center, San Francisco, California

Following the example set by Chancellor Fleming, I suppose I should introduce myself. I am Chauncey Leake, and I have little idea exactly why I should be honored by being asked to be the Chairman of this first session. I have had some contact with psychoactive drugs, largely through the association with the late Gordon Alles, who died unfortunately in 1963 at the age of sixty-two. He did a great deal of the work on the amphetamines and the extraordinary hallucinogenic agents that had been developed in the amphetamines in the old pharmacological laboratory that we had over here.

I did some work on the bufotenine, which, when it is injected, is a tough drug to handle. It is difficult to get into solution. I have reported on mushrooms, but they were not hallucinogenic, although it was stated they did cause peculiar feeling, but this was due to the agaric acid in them, which has a local irritant.

I am thrilled to see you here, even in the face of the rain. I understand pharmacologists are tough and I think psychopharmacologists are especially tough, they seem to like this type of weather. It has been this way all across the country last week where the pharmacologists have been meeting.

Our session this afternoon is going to be a good one, and we start appropriately with a consideration of the historical survey of the field of ethnopharmacology by Dr. Bo Holmstedt.

Historical Survey[*]

Bo Holmstedt

Department of Toxicology, Swedish Medical Research Council
Karolinska Institutet, Stockholm, Sweden

The most fascinating part of ethnopharmacology is perhaps that dealing with man's use of intoxicating compounds. A few—not too many—books have been written encompassing this subject, the most prominent being Louis Lewin's "Fantastica" (Lewin 1924).[1] The story of the use of these drugs is as old as man himself. Many people have for example speculated over what drugs and arrow poisons are mentioned in the Iliad and the Odyssey. There is not much need for speculation on this matter since the possible alternatives have been thoroughly discussed in the light of the 19th century achievement in pharmacology by two such authorities as Oswald Schmiedeberg and Louis Lewin. (Schmiedeberg 1918, Lewin 1920). Likewise, the toxic substances used during the middle ages and particularly during the witch trials have been much discussed. There is no need to go into this here.

This review is supposed to cover ethnopharmacology, and there was no ethnopharmacology before there was pharmacology. With some exaggeration it can be said that pharmacology started during the nineteenth century independently in three places.[2] One was Paris where the work of Magendie and his successors paved the way, the second was Edinburgh, where Sir Robert Christison among other things investigated ordeal poisons and coca, and advocated the rapid withdrawal in opium addiction. The third place was Dorpat, later called Jurjew and Tartu, in Estonia, where pharmacology as an academic science started around the middle of the 19th century. Of particular interest to the ethnopharmacology of psycho-active agents are Paris and Dorpat. This review will deal with some of the men who worked at these places.

Taking for granted that no ethnopharmacology can exist without true pharmacology it is appropriate to start this review at the beginning of the 19th century. At that time, the knowledge of foreign people, their habits, food and drugs in Europe and USA was generally speaking negligible. A spearhead thrust into this ignorance was Napoleon's ill-fated adventure in Egypt.

Napoleon was a remarkable general in many respects, in this specific case because he took with him to Egypt a library and 175 learned men who observed, wrote down, sketched and collected information about languages,

[*]This investigation was supported by Grant MH–12007 from the National Institute of Mental Health, U.S. Public Health Service, Chevy Chase, Md.
[1] A new print of the original English edition has recently appeared : Phantastica, Narcotic and Stimulating Drugs ; Their Use and Abuse, by Louis Lewin, Routledge & Kegan Paul Ltd., London, 1964.
[2] Those interested in the history of pharmacology are referred to Readings in Pharmacology by Holmstedt and Liljestrand, Pergamon Press 1963.

3

archeology and folk lore. This ultimately resulted in the publication of 24 volumes (Description de l'Egypte) printed between 1809–1813. These books stimulated enormously the interest in the Orient and led to a series of travels to Egypt, Asia Minor and Africa. Many people published travel accounts, such as the French poet and statesman A. de Lamartine (1790–1851), and the interpreter of the hieroglyphs, J. F. Champollion (1790–1832). Champollion made his expedition to Egypt 1828–1829.

Of particular importance to psychopharmacology is, however, the travel in this part of the world of J. J. Moreau (de Tours), a French psychiatrist whose work unfortunately is much forgotten. Moreau and Champollion apparently had the same guide or dragoman as it was called at the time (Moreau 1841).

Moreau was the first medical man to work systematically with centrally acting compounds. It is therefore appropriate to go into some detail about his life and works.

Jacques-Joseph Moreau (de Tours) was born at Montrésor (Indre-et Loire) June 3, 1804. (Baruk 1962. Collet 1962, Ritti 1887).

His father, a soldier in the armies of the Republic and the Emperor, traversed the whole of Europe, taking part in most of the battles and was finally awarded the cross of the Legion of Honour. He resigned only after the battle of Waterloo, and spent the rest of his life in Belgium, where he devoted all his time to mathematics, for which science he had a great passion.

While the father carried on this turbulent life, the son began his studies of the Classics at the college of Chinon, later terminating them at the college of Tours. Thanks to profound and brilliant studies he passed with success his matriculation examination.

Moreau then continued his studies at the Medical School, where he was characterised as: A zealous and industrious student with a tremendous appetite for learning. The Medical School of the public hospital of Tours at that time was run by one of the most famous medical men of the period, Bretonneau. Moreau was fortunate in hearing the lectures of this teacher.

After a stay of two years with this master, Moreau went to Paris to complete his studies and to take his degree. We are not aware of the circumstances around his application for the position as assistant physician at the Charenton mental hospital, but there is no doubt that on July 6, 1826, the date of his nomination, he found the mission of his life to which he would devote himself as profit for science.

At that time the psychiatrist Esquirol had recently become head of the mental hospital, and thanks to him a number of useful reformations had been introduced for the benefit of the patient. Besides his great intelligence Esquirol was no less great as far as his character was concerned. The following maxim is ascribed to him "One must love the mentally ill in order to be worthy and capable of being of service to him."

Among the various methods of treatment for the mentally sick—travels—had been prescribed even as far back as ancient Greece. Esquirol had a great number of clients— people came from all parts of France and even from abroad to consult him. Among them were rich persons to whom he could prescribe long travels; he entrusted them to the intelligent care of his young assistants. Also Moreau was commissioned with such a task, and visited Switzerland and Italy with a patient.

Travel then became a necessity for Moreau. He had nothing to keep him in France; he was young and had no desire to settle down. He longed to see foreign countries. Esquirol entrusted him with the care of a new patient, this time for a very long absence: An absence of three years and a journey to the Orient. To visit the Orient! What a dream for a young man! And this at a time when eyes were turned towards these sunny countries from where came since ten years the most extraordinary news. Each stage of the journey would lead him to places where classic events faded in comparison with

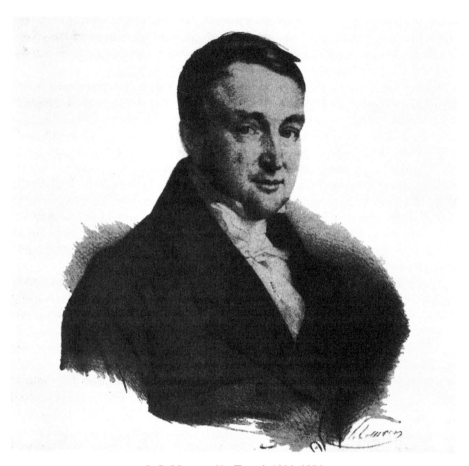

J. J. Moreau (de Tours) 1804–1884

the more recent ones. One hardly thought of the Pharaohs when setting foot on the soil of Egypt, governed by the famous Mohammed Ali. When passing through Asia Minor interest was less lively for the rapid campaign of Alexander the Great than for the exploits of Ibraham-Pasha and his 30,000 Egyptians, the victories of whom had disturbed the Sultan's power.

The young and enthusiastic Moreau wished to learn and profit as much as possible from what he saw and heard, and for this reason he adopted the dress and the customs of the countries he passed through. He wrote down what he experienced, and it is much to be regretted that he never published his observations. Some of them are, however, contained in his medical books.

It is striking that in the Orient the mentally ill appear to be fewer than in Europe. Is this marked difference to be explained by climate, race, or by the political and religious institutions? Moreau adhered to the opinion of Montesquieu, who admitted the joint responsibility of these various causes:

The heat of the climate can be so excessive that all strength leaves the body. The lack of strength passes on to the spirit—no curiosity, no noble sentiments, no generous feelings . . . . laziness is happiness . . . . resignation. . . .

Immediately upon his return to Paris, Moreau hastened to renew his old acquaintances and acquire new ones. He met Esquirol again and his circle

5

of disciples among whom he counted numerous friends. The master received him with open arms; he bestowed on this dear pupil the tokens of his affectionate benevolence, and eased for him his first entry into the medical career, always difficult in Paris.

During his stay in the Orient, Moreau had noted the common use of hashish, especially among the Arabs. He must also have tried it himself since in his travel reports he writes rather lyrically about "pleasures impossible to interpret" which this "marvellous substance" brings about, and which "would be impossible to describe to anybody who had not experienced it". Thanks to a mysterious legend and particularly to the imagination of poets and novelists, only the wonderful effects of this substance were known. Moreau wished to contrast poetry with observation and experience, and his experimental research into the psychopharmacological actions of the extract of Indian hemp permitted him to throw light on psychological phenomena which had previously been obscure. They inspired him also with ingenious ideas on the nature of insanity.

No criticism can be made of his investigative procedures. Moreau took hashish himself. Thanks to the singular property of the substance to keep intact "consciousness and the innermost feeling" of the user, he could analyze all his impressions and in a way be aware of the disorganization of all his mental faculties. In order to complete this internal observation of himself, he also commissioned the persons surrounding him to note carefully his words, acts, gestures and the expression of his face. The results were very characteristic. They fully justified the name of "fantasia" which the Oriental imagination gives to the intoxication with Kief, one of the many names for hashish. Moreau desired, moreover, "controls with other people." He turned to his pupils and with enthusiastic curiosity they lent themselves to experiments with hashish in the most varying doses, giving exact accounts of what they experienced. Moreau observed with scrupulous care every (external) symptom during the course of intoxication. The two series were compared and full conformity was proved.

The effect of the hashish reveals itself by a series of intellectual disturbances, Moreau described all the sensations with meticulous care.

In 1845 Moreau published his extensive book of more than 400 pages entitled Du Hachich et de l'aliénation mentale (Hashish and mental illness). Its detailed accounts of the hashish intoxication aroused the interest of numerous physicians and the curiosity of many writers, and was followed by a great deal of personal experimentation. Moreau's book gave rise to the modern researches regarding the effects of hashish, and can also be held responsible for its use in certain Paris circles in the middle of the 19th century. However, it never became a true epidemic in all parts of Europe, confining itself mainly to the Near and Middle East.

Such factors as origin, education and environment as well as the atmosphere in which hashish is consumed, affects individuals in different ways. Due to the great number and varying nature of the *psychic effects* of the hashish intoxication, these cannot be outlined in the same way as the

6

physical effects. However, Moreau enumerated eight main groups of symptoms. They are:

(1) General feeling of pleasure.
(2) Increased excitement combined with a heightening of all senses.
(3) Distortion of the dimension of space and time (generally a magnification of the actual dimensions: Minutes are changed into days or years, inches into feet, etc.).
(4) A keener hearing combined with a great susceptibility to music and the phenomenon that ordinary noise is enjoyed as though it sounded sweet.
(5) There often arise persistent ideas on the verge of persecution mania.
(6) Disturbances of the emotions, mostly in the form of an increase of already existing feeling.
(7) Irresistible impulses.
(8) Illusions and hallucinations of which evidently only the first named are related to objects of the exterior world.

Moreau pointed out that psychiatry could profit from these experiments by comparing the symptoms to those in mentally ill people. The illusions produced by the hashish—are they not attacks of insanity? These attacks will take on all the characteristics of violent insanity if only the dose of the toxic agent is increased. Moreau had the occasion of sadly experiencing this. His assistant in pharmacy wished to see the effects of the Indian hemp when taken in a larger quantity, and swallowed 16 grams of the extract.

A very intense delirium broke out, followed by agitation, incoherence and hallucinations of all kinds. Three days passed before the young man regained his ordinary calmness and the entire use of his power of reasoning. During the course of the attack he maintained, however, some idea of what was happening to him.

Moreau postulated that there exists in insanity a primary factor which is the source of all symptoms; i.e., excitation, which is the primitive generative power. He attached special importance to this hypothesis, and considered it as equal to other great scientific laws. Moreau also compared insanity with dreams. The hypothesis is not new; it already preoccupied Aristotle. The learned philosopher from Stagira writes in his books on "Dreams" that "the reason why we, even awake, deceive ourselves in certain illnesses is the same which produces in us, in our sleep, an impression of a dream." The favorite formula of Moreau was: "Insanity is the dream of the man who is awake."

Even though Moreau cannot be said to be dependent on his countryman the French materialist and medical man La Mettrie (1709–1751) who said: "Man is what he eats", he still considered a range of causes for insanity. With regard to the conception of an organic origin he writes: "I am not against the conceptions of organic damage but I require to see the lesion: I only believe in damages which are proven, not in those that are supposed

DU HACHISCH

ET DE

L'ALIÉNATION MENTALE

ÉTUDES PSYCHOLOGIQUES

PAR

J. MOREAU ✠

(DE TOURS),

Médecin de l'hospice de Bicêtre, Membre de la Société
orientale de Paris.

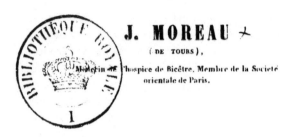

PARIS.

LIBRAIRIE DE FORTIN, MASSON ET Cie.

PLACE DE L'ÉCOLE-DE-MÉDECINE, 1.

Même maison, chez Léopold Michelsen, à Leipzig.

1845.

to exist." This certainly was a very wise position to take. Even in our days, organic or biochemical lesions in mental illness have been difficult to prove.

Moreau loved art in all its forms. He gladly sought the company of writers and artists. His works on hashish had put him in contact with numerous poets and novelists and he was well acquainted with Balzac, Gérard de Nerval and Théophile Gautier. The author of "la comédie humaine" wrote him the day after a "fantasia" about an idea that he had had for twenty years: "To make a new brain in an idiot (with the aid of hashish) in order to see if the mind could be expanded by development of the rudiments." It has a familiar ring.

Moreau passed away June 26, 1884, at the age of 80 after a short illness. He was undoubtedly the first psychiatrist with interest in psychopharmacology. It seems that during his life time he was never recognized as he should have been. Among those who did not understand his qualities was regretfully François Magendie (Collet 1962). On the other hand, Claude Bernard once called hashish a psychopharmacological counterpart of curare. Up to recent years, however, with regard to hashish people have been mostly interested in the literary feats of Théophile Gautier and Charles Baudelaire, and "Le Club des Haschischins" with its strange meeting in the old hotel on Ile St. Louis in Paris. It is perhaps typical that a very recent collection of papers around the subject hashish only mentions Moreau in passing. (Solomon Ed. 1966.)

Unlike Moreau *Ernst von Bibra* (1806–1878), was the prototype of a wealthy, private scientist. Although he acquired academic degrees he performed a good deal of his research in his own house.

Bibra was born in Unterfranken, studied in Würzburg, where he became M.D. and Ph. D. and later partly in Nürnberg living on his estate Schwebheim. He was mostly interested in chemistry, but also was a geographer and a numismatologist (Günther 1901). Of special importance to this account is his trip to South America 1849–1850. He was more or less forced to leave for political reasons, because of his liberal attitude during the revolution in 1848.

The most important result of this journey—except for his travel account ("Reise in Süd-Amerika, B. Mannheim, 1854") which is well worth reading—is the book "Die narkotischen Genussmittel und der Mensch" (Nürnberg 1855). The book was undoubtedly prompted by his South American trip, and is the first of its kind to summarize the effect of centrally acting compounds, in all seventeen. He devotes chapters both to compounds such as coffee and tea, and also to *Amanita Muscaria*, opium, hashish and coca, the chewing of which he had rich opportunities to observe during his trip to South America. Due to the fact that comparatively little was known about these drugs at the time, Bibra's book created quite a sensation. He did not pursue this line of research, but devoted the rest of his life to his private hobbies, such as numismatics and writing of novels.

There were other people who were to make such compilations during the nineteenth century. One of them was *Georg Noël Dragendorff* (1836–1898).

Dragendorff was born in Rostock, Germany, as the son of a medical man, studied chemistry in Heidelberg and learned the trade of pharmacy in his home town (Hartwich 1897–1898). His main interest was chemistry. The famous Witte pharmacy in his home town soon expanded into a house of medicinal chemistry and Dragendorff became employed there. He heard lectures by Bunsen, Kirchhoff, Helmholtz and Erlenmeyer, but it is said that he never had an opportunity to hear a lecture in pharmacognosy either in Rostock or Heidelberg. The first one he ever heard was the one he had to give himself when he had become professor in Dorpat.

In 1862 Dragendorff was called to St. Petersburg to help organize the editing of a journal of pharmacy. He learned to speak Russian and also helped organize the pharmacies in Russia. From St. Petersburg he was called to become professor of pharmacy and director of the Pharmaceutical Institute of Dorpat, 1864. Dorpat came to be his home for 30 years, and when he finally resigned his chair in 1894 he returned to his home town of Rostock, where he organized a private laboratory and carried on research until his death.

Dragendorff's work dealt with two things: one, relevant to the present account, was the chemical investigation of plants; the other was toxicological analysis. He was particularly interested in the medicinal plants used by foreign people, and had acquired collections from far off countries in his institute at Dorpat. His most famous work and a summary of his activities in the field, was published shortly after his death and is now a rare book: "Die Heilpflanzen der verschiedenen Völker und Zeiten", 1898.[3] With regard to his chemical activities we only have to point out that he had numerous pupils from many countries, and that no reputable phytochemist is unfamiliar with Dragendorff's reagent for alkaloids.

Another German pharmacist who perhaps accumulated even greater knowledge in one field of ethno-pharmacology was *Carl Hartwich* (1851–1917). (Schröter 1917.)

Hartwich was born in Tangermünde where his father had a pharmacy, the management of which the son took over in 1879. He was, however, so interested in scientific activities that he sold the pharmacy and moved to Braunschweig. From there he went to Bern in order to take his doctor's degree and then again to Braunschweig to become university lecturer in pharmacy and pharmacognosy. A few weeks afterwards (also in Hartwich's case before he had given one single lecture) he accepted a call to the Swiss Polytechnical Institute in Zürich. He began his service in the autumn of 1892 and stayed for 24 years, as professor and head of the Pharmacology Department.

Hartwich published a multitude of papers dealing with numerous drugs and stimulants. In these studies the historical and ethnographical questions are strongly emphasized. Of a particularly historical interest is "Die Bedeutung der Entdeckung von Amerika für die Drogenkunde" (1892).

Hartwich's most important publication, however, is "Die menschlichen Genussmittel", 877 pages with 24 tables and 168 pictures in the text (1911). He worked on this monumental volume during a decade, with considerable joy and even with the passion of a fanatic collector. The gigantic quantity of material is astounding and includes drawings, photographs, observations of his own, and literary notes from the most remote sources. The physical, historical, ethnographical and commercial and ethical aspects of the compounds are treated with the same love. The richly decorated book is a true gold mine of information that was previously widely dispersed.

In addition to these voluminous collections of ethno-pharmacological and ethno-botanical material there arose during the second part of the 19th century the science of psychology. The pioneers in this field were *Hermann v. Helmholtz* (1821–1894), *Gustav Theodor Fechner* (1801–1887) and *Wilhelm M. W. Wundt* (1832–1920).

The foremost service of W. Wundt to psychology was the introduction of laboratory investigation. Before his time experimental research in psychology had been mainly individual. He gathered around him enthusiastic

---

[3] At the time of writing a reprint of the original has been issued.

Georg Dragendorff, Die Heilpflanzen der verschiedenen Völker and Zeiten, Neudruck der Ausgabe Stuttgart 1898. Antiquariat Fritsch, Postach 1043, 79/Ulm/ Do. Germany.

students and assistants whom he trained in the methods of exact experimentation. The first real institute for psychological studies was erected by Wundt in Leipzig 1879 (Kraepelin 1920). It consisted of two rooms and some tables with equipment, some of which was Wundt's personal property. No grant for equipment·was available and Kraepelin tells how it had to be made by hand from wood, tin, strings and cardboard. They had, however, accumulators and chronoscopes. In spite of the obvious poverty the new institute was filled with a pioneering spirit and enthusiasm.

Wundt had never had near contact with psychiatry or drug research even though he had to do with it now and then. One of his first pupils was *Emil Kraepelin* (1856–1926).

Kraepelin was born in Neu-Strelitz (Mecklenburg-Strelitz), studied in Leipzig and Würzburg with the intention at the very start to become a psychiatrist. He graduated in 1878 and came to the Munich Mental Hospital. In 1882 he became assistant of Flechsig in Leipzig, but soon left in order to work in the Institute of Wundt. At the start working with experimental psychology, he later turned wholly to clinical psychiatry which he endeavored to put on a new basis that brought world-wide fame to his Munich Clinic.

Kraepelin published the first account on the use of the new psychological methods in clinical pharmacology which he undertook during his tenure of a professorship in Dorpat (1886–1890). In that remarkable university at this time worked also not only Dragendorff but Rudolf Kobert, who held the chair in pharmacology. Obviously, Kobert was the one who interested Kraepelin in applying his psychological tools to the study of drug effects in man (Jelliffe 1931). Among the drugs he studied were morphine and alcohol, and after he had left Dorpat this resulted in the first real monograph of psycho-pharmacology where the new methods were applied: "Ueber die Beeinflüssung einfacher psychischer Vorgänge durch einige Arzneimittel—Jena, 1892."

Kraepelin maintained a lifelong interest in the pharmacology of alcohol. In his hospital he introduced variously colored lemonades immediately christened "Kraepelin liquors" (Kolle 1956).

Kobert's association with the clinic of psychiatry in the meantime had resulted in the publication of another epoch-making paper, written together with one of Kraepelin's co-workers (Kobert R. and A. Sohrt: "Ueber die Wirkung des salzauren Hyoscin," 1887.).

Rudolf Kobert (1854–1918) started his medical career in Halle under Theodor Weber and spent many years as assistant to Schmiedeberg before he was called upon to become H. H. Meyer's successor at the famous department of pharmacology in Dorpat (Sieburg 1919). He remained in Dorpat until 1897. The title of his chair was Pharmacology and Physiological Chemistry; he was also a teacher in History of Medicine and Pharmacy. In 1899 Kobert became professor at the university of Rostock where he remained until his death.

From Kobert's hand originate a great many publications concerning pharmacodynamics and toxicology. He wrote a textbook in toxicology which has had a considerable influence on many fields including forensic medicine. He was one of the two great toxicologists of the nineteenth century, the other being Louis Lewin. The great learning and wide scope of his interest is witnessed among other things by the issue during his time in Dorpat of "Historische Studien aus dem Pharmakologischen Institut". This work in five volumes is an invaluable source, among other things for information to early research of drugs, also to research of drugs affecting the central nervous system.

The above mentioned paper by Kobert and Sohrt is of considerable psycho-pharmacological interest. For the first time here, dissimilarities and sim-

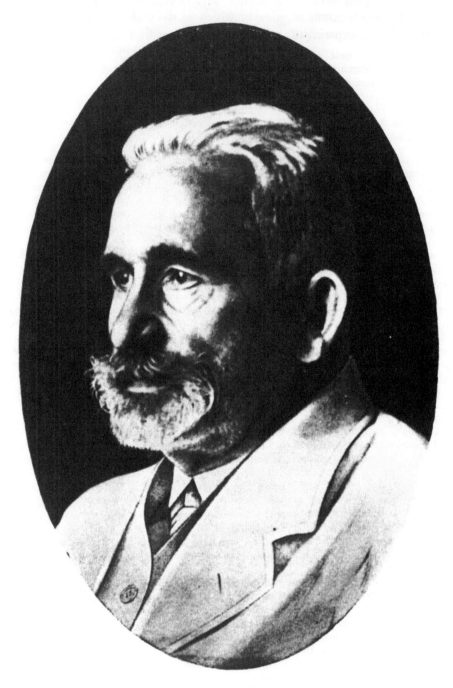

Emil Kraepelin 1856–1926

ilarities between atropine and scopolamine are pointed out, the latter compound at this time called hyoscine. Kobert and Sohrt in their carefully conducted investigation demonstrated the sedative action of the latter compound. The experiments were made both on animals and man, and included a series of self-experiments. Kobert writes the following:

... During the past autumn vacation I had the opportunity to arrange at the Department of Psychiatry in Dorpat and supervise directly an investigation of the actions of a pharmacological agent. This investigation, which lasted several months, was undertaken because work on animals is of value if it is extended to man. The pharmacological agent involved was hyoscine.

... Mr. Sohrt, the assistant in the Department of Psychiatry, wrote up these experiments at my instigation for his inaugural thesis. In view of its limited circulation I wish to present here the following account taken from the thesis:

... Sohrt gave himself at 10.04 p.m. an injection of 0.5 mg hyoscine hydrochloride. The pulse rate before injection was 64 per minute. After a latent period of 10 minutes Sohrt observed as the first symptom a ptosis which made it difficult for him to keep his eyes open. Gradually a feeling of heaviness without headache occurred. His head tended to drop to his shoulders and it became difficult to keep the head upright. His limbs felt as if they were lumps of lead attached to the body. There was a marked tiredness.

Throughout this period S. was fully conscious and able to give an account of everything and to answer questions speedily. He was able to read his own writing without much difficulty and did not feel sick. At 11.25 p.m. he stood up, but his walk was unsteady. He went to bed, therefore, and at once fell asleep. He had a quiet sleep without dreams. On the following morning S. woke up at 9 a.m., instead of at 5 or 6 a.m., which was his usual time. His head felt slightly numb, but this symptom disappeared after breakfast.

These experiments show that hyoscine, 0.5 to 1 mg, given subcutaneously, produces in healthy man dryness of the mouth, dilation of the pupils, marked sleepiness and tiredness, but is devoid of other special actions.

... In nearly all those cases of illness which are associated with a state of excitation hyoscine produced sleep promptly or at the very least induced sedation, even when all other drugs used for this purpose failed to produce an effect.

By far the most interesting personality of all psychopharmacologists of this time was *Louis Lewin* (1850–1929).

Lewin was born in the small town of Tuchel in Western Prussia. In 1854 he came to Berlin where he remained more or less until the end of his life. He graduated from the University of Berlin. In 1875 as an M.D., he studied for a while with Pettenkofer and Voit in Munich, and became "Privatdozent" in pharmacology in Berlin in 1881. In 1894 he became titular professor at the University of Berlin but held no full academic position. Only as late as 1919 did he become permanent honorary professor at the Technical Academy. There has been much speculation about the reasons why Lewin did not advance academically in pharmacology and toxicology, and it has been said that he could have become head of the greatest pharmacology department in Germany had he renounced his Jewish faith and consented to become baptized. Whatever truth there may be in this, he established his own private laboratory and lecture hall in No. 3 Ziegelstrasse in an old tenement house in the centre of the medical district of Berlin. He preferred to teach and to do his research with his own means in these surroundings. Financially, he was partly enabled to do so through the fact that although he had no official position, the courts preferred him to all other experts in Germany in toxicology and industrial hygiene.

Lewin's way of lecturing was extraordinary and held the audiences spellbound. It has been said that he expounded facts with a contagious enthusiasm and performed his

Ueber die Beeinflussung

einfacher psychischer Vorgänge

durch einige Arzneimittel.

Experimentelle Untersuchungen

von

Dr. Emil Kraepelin,
Professor der Psychiatrie in Heidelberg.

Mit einer Curventafel.

Jena,
Verlag von Gustav Fischer.
1892.

experiments with loving care. Any narrow specialization was foreign to him. He could quote flawlessly in foreign languages, and marshal facts from all four corners of the world and all periods of history. Classical and contemporary authors were all familiar to him. Many famous men who visited his lectures were deeply influenced by him. Among them was J. J. Abel who has been called the father of American pharmacology. Lewin's outstanding wide general knowledge meant that he had many friends among scholars in other faculties.

14

Among Lewin's personal acquaintances were the explorer Georg Schweinfurth, and Albert Einstein. In history, geography and anthropology his knowledge was enormous; he showed special interest in travel and topography. It is said that scarcely a travel book of importance was unknown to him. His own travelling included visits, among other places, to the United States, Switzerland and Italy.

When surveying Lewin's works one is greatly helped by a list he compiled himself before his death. The list includes 248 major publications in the years 1874–1929. From the list are excluded book reviews, printed discussions and other minor communications of his which were also numerous. Among the publications there are about a dozen books and monographs. Lewin himself claimed that by 1880 he had already decided to devote most of his time to the side effects of drugs.

Lewin's first major work, in 1881, "Nebenwirkungen der Arzneimittel", Pharmakologisch-klin. Handbuch (Berlin, A. Hirschwald), dealt with this topic and became a classic and the first of its kind. This book had two more editions and was translated into three languages, including English. Notable among the other books are his outstanding textbook in toxicology, a summary of all available knowledge of arrow poisons, two volumes on the effects of drugs on the eye, and another work in which he gives the world's history as seen by a toxicologist, "Die Gifte in der Weltgeschichte" (J. Springer, Berlin 1920).

It is not possible here to summarize all the fields of interest to which Lewin made original contributions, but it is appropriate to dwell on his activities in psychopharmacology, a topic in which he published some 20 articles. His own contributions to the field occurred mostly in the 1880's. Then he more or less left this field, but in 1924 summarized admirably his own work and those of others in the first edition of his book "Phantastica". The long delay certainly did not mean that he remained unfamiliar with the progress in the field; on the contrary, the books show that he kept up to date with all achievements made.

Lewin's first publication, in 1874, was a study of chronic morphinism, which he was one of the first to investigate scientifically. In 1886 there appeared his monograph on *Piper methysticum* (Kawa Kawa): "Ueber Piper methysticum (Kawa)." (Monographie. Berlin. A. Hirschwald). This is a very comprehensive review of all aspects of the use of *Piper methysticum* and current research on its constituents and their chemistry, pharmacology and clinical effects. This admirable monograph is now understandably much out of date in its chemistry and pharmacology, but it was a pioneering work, and the period following its appearance saw the first real progress being made in the chemistry of kaava. In 1889 appeared another similar monograph: "Ueber Areca Catechu, Chavica Betle und das Betelkauen." (Monographie. Stuttgart. F. Enke) an equally comprehensive review.

Before that, however, Lewin had had occasion to get into polemics with Sigmund Freud about coca and cocaine. This strange episode in the history of science runs as follows:

A century ago the height of nationalistic pride was to have a man-of-war circumnavigate the globe. Austria, a sea power in those days, planned to send the Novara on such a trip. Prof. Wöhler of Göttingen just before departure requested the naturalists on the expedition to bring him back a sufficient quantity of coca leaves to carry out a thorough investigation. Dr. Scherzer, one of the scientists, did manage to get some 30 lbs. of leaves to

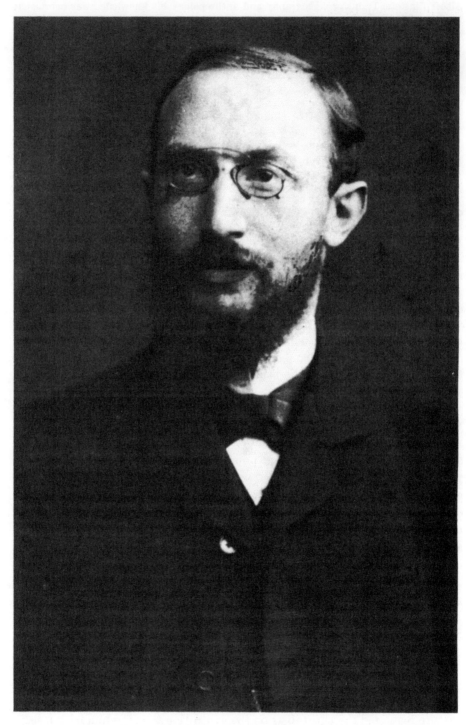

Louis Lewin (1850–1929). Picture taken about the time of his trip to the United States.

Prof. Wöhler. His assistant, Niemann, succeeded in isolating an unusual crystalline organic base.

The first description of cocaine occurs in Tagesber. allgem. med. Zentral-Zeitung, 25 April 1860, p. 262–263. It is noted that, "It would seem that Coca will be of great use to the medicine of the future. . . . It has the remarkable action on the nerves of the tongue that after a few moments the place of contact becomes anaesthetized and almost insensitive". In 1859 Paolo Mantegazza's description of the therapeutic versatility of coca aroused much interest but little confidence, although subsequently his reports have been largely verified. However, early investigations in Austria, Germany and England were largely negative in their findings, and by the 1870s there was general disillusionment.

A military surgeon, Aschenbrandt, in 1883 claimed a remarkable effect of cocaine upon Bavarian soldiers enabling them to better endure hunger, strain, fatigue and heavy burdens. He anticipated a demand of today's purists in experimental design by adding the cocaine to the drinking water and not telling the soldiers. Unfortunately the use of control subjects was overlooked and Aschenbrandt was anything but unbiased. Palmer (1880) in the Louisville Medical News, and Bentley in the Detroit Therapeutic Gazette (1880), had described the use of coca in the treatment of morphinism. The Louisville Medical News said in its editorial comment "one feels like trying coca with or without the opium habit. A harmless remedy for the blues is imperial."

In 1884 Sigmund Freud wrote to his fiancée that he had been experimenting with "a magical drug". After dazzling success in treatment of a case of gastric catarrh he continues "If it goes well I will write an essay on it and I expect it will win its place in therapeutics by the side of morphium, and superior to it. . . . I take very small does of it regularly against depression and against indigestion, and with the most brilliant success." He urged his fiancée, his sisters, his colleagues, and his friends to try it (Jones 1956). That same year he published an article "Über Coca" which among other virtues extolled the drug as a safe exhilarant which he himself used and recommended as a treatment for morphine addiction. For emphasis he stated, in italics, that "Inebriate asylums can be entirely dispensed with" and a cure effected in 10 days. That same fateful year he used it for this purpose in treating his close friend, Ernst Fleischl. For a while the treatment succeeded but increasingly larger doses were needed. Freud spent one frightful night nursing Fleischl through an episode of cocaine psychosis and thereafter was bitterly against drugs, rarely permitting them even for himself during operations for the painful carcinoma of the jaw which finally killed him.

Freud's paper on Coca was subjected to a severe criticism by Louis Lewin (1885). Among other things, he said:

I want to state explicitly that according to all available evidence coca is no substitute for morphine and that a morphine addiction cannot be cured by the use of coca. . . .

I am convinced that coca cannot be a substitute for morphine for any length of time since the real morphine addict wants the specific morphine effect and since he can very well distinguish the euphoria of other substances. Such an exchange does not suit his

17

Ueber

PIPER METHYSTICUM
(KAWA).

Untersuchungen

von

Dr. L. Lewin,

Docent der Pharmakologie an der Universität Berlin.

Mit 1 lithographirten Tafel.

Berlin 1886.

Verlag von August Hirschwald.

NW. Unter den Linden 68.

special needs. The morphinist wants more than the euphoria which can be brought about in normal man and which Freud experienced himself when taking 0.05–0.1 gr. cocaine hydrochloride.

However, even if it were possible to treat a morphine addict for a time exclusively with cocaine and even if he were given very large doses producing hallucinations and a pleasant sopor, there would very likely occur a case of what I would like to call double addiction. The man in question would use cocaine in addition to morphine in the same way as many morphine addicts use chloroform, chloralhydrate, ether, etc.

18

Lewin's clear perception of this question was corroborated by A. Erlenmeyer slightly afterwards, and also by others. Lewin never understood Sigmund Freud, especially not his psychoanalytical works, and used to refer to him as "Joseph der Traumdeuter" ("Joseph, the dream interpreter").

In 1887 Lewin made a cross country trip in the US and Canada. According to some lines in his travel account he had thought about emigration. He traveled together with one Mr. John Warburg whom he called uncle. His wife had grown up in the Warburg family in Hamburg. Other members of this family were famous botanists. Lewin's trip across the country resulted in a hand-written manuscript of more than 300 pages with numerous photos, illustrations and cuttings glued into it. It is a family property never printed and not intended to be.[4] It was written as a gift to his wife and given to her upon his return to Berlin. The manuscript is a treasure of wealth of information about the US about 1880. Lewin's itinerary took him also into Canada, to the big lakes, to San Francisco, Detroit, Washington and back His determined way of travelling is well borne out in what he says about his stay in San Francisco:

My main purpose in visiting San Francisco had been to see for myself "Chinatown", as the Chinese quarter is called, and especially the smoking of opium. In our hotel we asked for a guide. It appeared that we could get one for 10 dollars—40 mark. What an insolent overcharge! We asked in a ticket-office—the same charge, but with a reduction to half the price for a guided tour in the daytime. But during the day there is nothing to see there and everybody can then walk through the quarter and the shops. I decided to show those swindling yankees that we were able to find the right way by ourselves. We asked a policeman what to do to get a policeman as guide. He directed us to the main police-station. There I explained my request after having shown my card. When the captain began long deliberations with someone else I showed him the legitimation I had received from Washington. This proved effective. We were to meet our police-guide at 9 o'clock in the evening at the station. We told this to Mr. H. who wanted to see Chinatown too. Strange to say—the better society of San Francisco does not know it. On the way we passed the stock-exchange and went in. After a few paces we meet the strapping policeman, our companion for the excursion. After a short time we arrived. How many different impressions do I bring home from this visit! From the moment we entered this quarter in which approximately 30,000 Chinese live till we left it, an unpleasant odour did not leave us. It is impossible to describe it, it is so repugnant that even uncle was, at the beginning, somewhat repelled and disgusted. The streets were repulsively dirty and filthy. People throw everything in the streets to let it rot there. It is impossible to use the so-called sidewalks, partly because they are full of baskets and boxes, partly because there yawn everywhere cellar-holes one might easily fall into. I had to roll up my trousers. What a contrast to this filth, when we entered the first shop, a barber-shop! There two Chinese were sitting, under the hands of the barbers. They had just finished shaving the hair from the forehead to the top, and were occupied in tidying the ears and the noses of their clients with very small knives—not wider than a straw—and very fine sponges with handles. The barbers removed all hair and other substances. On the other side of the street there was a food-shop.

The streets are dark, lighted only by the shops and by candles burning in the street in front of the houses. Every few paces 6–8 wax-candles are stuck into the ground. These candles burn down very quickly, but their long stem consists of incense, so that there are hundreds of incense-candles fuming in the streets. Asia in America! What a contrast of customs and habits! But that was not yet the worst by far. We entered a

[4] The author wishes to express his gratitude to Mrs. Irene Sachs, N.Y., for permission to publish part of the travel account and to Mrs. Hertha Jaffé and Mr. Mordechai Yaffé, Israel, for help with the translation.

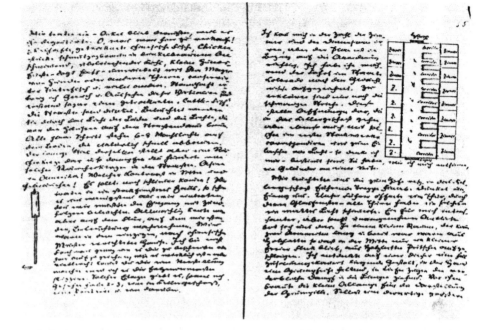

Pages from Louis Lewin's travel account related to visit to Chinatown in San Francisco.

pitch-dark house—or so it appeared to us as we went in, for we had to light up the entrance with matches. By and by we could see some light in the passage we were standing in. We were in the only house built in Chinese fashion. I am not expert enough to describe it to you as it really is or to make a drawing of it. Perhaps you will get some idea? I sketch it as follows. As far as I could see there are 2–3 such stories, a cellar-story, the groundfloor and one above. I might be mistaken as to dimensions and numbers of rooms but the arrangement in the plan is correct. I sketched it from memory while travelling through the State of Colorado. I must explain the broad dark areas. These are apertures leading to the cellar. There are corresponding apertures in the first story, I think for illumination. If I remember right, there is a banister on one side.

We lighted our way down the stairs leading to the courtyard and to the cellar-story. Darkness enveloped us. Our guide opened a door with a glass-window—all the doors have a window like this—through which a faint light was glimmering. What we could see was interesting to me, but in general an unpleasant view. In a small room, less than two arm-lengths long and wide, we saw plank-beds all around leaving only very little free space in the center of the room. On one of these I discovered a crouching figure holding an opium pipe and inhaling deeply the pernicious fume. Before him burned the small oil-lamp for the preparation of the opium-pill. Such a pill, even a bigger one, is, as I saw, enough for 2–3 draughts, seldom four. The extract of opium has an almost honeylike consistence. With a very fine metal-spatula—I have a similar one—he takes a small amount of the extract and puts it somewhere at the clay-top of his pipe. He then again takes the opium up, this time with the needle-like other end of the spatula, passes it lightly through the flame to condense it and make it more malleable and tries by turning the needle round and round to give the opium pill a cylindrical form. After passing the material another two or three times through the flame the desired form is achieved. He sticks the needle into the aperture of the pipebowl and, while drawing it back, he presses the small cylinder of opium into the aperture of the bowl with his index-finger.

20

Now he puts his mouth to the pipe-stem and sucks deeply, deeply, while letting the opium-cylinder evaporate near the lamp—it looks for all the world like a thirsty man putting his pint-glass to his lips and emptying it in deep endless draughts. After approximately half a minute he exhales the fumes which in the meantime have been partly absorbed through the mucous membranes of the lungs. This same procedure occurs 6, 8, 10 times and even more until the gratification of the opium-visions provide the compensation for the troublesome preparations. He feels himself transplanted from his wretched surroundings. He sees palaces, riches, opulent repasts, splendid garments, beautiful amorous women and perhaps officies, titles and decorations descending upon him. In the morning he awakes—on a straw-mat or a heap of rags in a lightless hole filled with pestilential air. Again he trudges by daylight to the hole where he lives. Who can blame this human being—with his low grade of education, deprived of moral support—if he returns again and again to the pleasurable world of the opium-vision at night?

Again we enter a house, going along what seem still narrower passages. You feel your heart beating at the thought of a sudden conflagration. Not the most precipitous point of the Canadian Pacific Railway gave me so much fright: The feeling of being shut-in in these passages nearly choked me!

Lewin also managed during the same trip to visit the stockmarket, Chinese restaurants and theatres, the house of the Salvation army, and another house from which he fled in Victorian dismay.

However interested Lewin may have been in San Francisco's China Town and the smoking of opium, the city he really longed to visit was Detroit. He arrived there on September 16, 1887:

My first errand was, of course, a visit to Parke Davis. We drove along a splendid wide avenue bordered by residences with beautiful gardens. Soon we were marvelling at a grand extensive building adorned with sand-stone. This building which belongs to the company, is not yet fully finished. We enter the office where there work well over fifty book-keepers, male and female, cashiers, clerks, stenographers etc. Mr. Wetzell showed us round the factory and the printing-shop—I had not expected such a magnitude and such a skilled exactitude of workmanship. It is impossible to enumerate all particulars to you. Summing up, I can only tell you that the different departments are exemplary, from the preparation of juices and extract, the extraction of drugs, bottling, labeling, the homogenization of plants to the manufacture of pilular mass, sugaring and coating of pills etc., etc. .... In short, the manufacture of pharmaceutical preparations is worthy of the American genius for machinery and for exactitude and cleanliness of use. Whatever I received—preparations drugs etc.—you will see for yourself when everything arrives in Berlin.

Among these things he carried back with him to Berlin from Parke Davis Co. was Peyotl, the "Mescal buttons". We know this exactly because he has stated himself that he got it from the Parke Davis and Co. during his American trip. He was not long in investigating its properties and there appeared in Schmiedeberg's archives and the Detroit Therapeutic Gazette the first accounts of the pharmacologic properties of Peyotl (Lewin 1888). He says in his summary:

It has been proven for the first time that a cactus can possess an extraordinarily high toxicity. It will now be appropriate to elucidate the chemistry of this Anhalonium and then go further with the investigation of other species of Anhalonium. One must, however, also investigate to what purpose and to what extent these Múscal buttons (Sic!) are used as stimulants. In a not too distant future I hope to be able to give evidence about this.

For some reason he never did, although he wrote in 1894 a second long article on what was then called "Anhalonium Lewinii and other cactea" (Lewin 1894). By then, however, Arthur Heffter had already started his work on the active principles in the mescaline cactus.

Arthur Heffter (1860–1925) was born in Leipzig and representative of the old German school of pharmacologists with a thorough chemical background and a medical training. (Straub 1924, Heubner 1925, Joachimoglu 1960). He worked for some years in agricultural chemistry and then switched to study medicine in Leipzig, at the same time working in the laboratory of R. Böhm. His habilitation took place in 1892, after which he for some time worked under Schmiedeberg in Strassburg. Later he held positions in various universities, Leipzig, Bern, Marburg, and finally in 1908 became Liebreich's successor at the department of pharmacology, University of Berlin, where he held the chair until his death.

Heffter's research activities covered a wide scope of topics. As lecturer he was, however, to say the least, mediocre.

Lewin did not like Heffter and Heffter did not like him. They had very different opinions on many things—this concerned particularly Anhalonium Lewinii (Peyotl) on which Heffter also had done work. It was a priority competition between the two. I don't remember it exactly, but I have the feeling that it was something of the sort. Lewin was more the artist and interested in the social implications of these substances. Heffter was not very verbal, awkward, frankly in the presentation of his material. On the other hand, here was this tremendously stimulating, flamboyant orator Lewin who carried away his audience with his enthusiasm. The atmosphere fused into the most extraordinary experience every time we went to that place to listen to his lecture, and you did that in spite of the fact that you didn't have to—it was enough had you followed only Heffter's lectures. I went to Heffter's lectures, of course, and I was bored. Lewin lectured the first time and I was captured—I went there every time. (Krayer 1963).

Heffter proceeded systematically to find the psychoactive principle in Peyotl by working it up into chemical fractions and testing these on himself in heroic self experiments, much the same way as Albert Hofmann later did with psilocybine. It is psycho-pharmacologically interesting to see what kind of wonderful visions an obviously dry man like Heffter got out of mescaline. Here is his account of the first experiment carried out with pure mescaline in man, in 1897:

Violet and green spots appear on the paper during reading. When the eyes are kept shut the following visions occur. At first there are violet and green spots which are not well defined, then come visions of carpet patterns, ribbed vaulting, etc. From time to time single dots with the most brilliant colours float across the field of vision. The phenomena are generally not as clear as those in the two preceding experiments. Later on landscapes, halls, achitectural scenes (*e.g.* pillars decorated with flowers) also appear. The visions can be observed until about 5:30 p.m. Nausea and dizziness are at times very distressing. The appreciation of time is reduced during the first hours of the afternoon. In the evening well-being and appetite are undisturbed and there is no sign of sleeplessness.

The results described above show that mescaline is exclusively responsible for the major symptoms of peyote (mescal) poisoning. This applies especially to the unique visions. The experiment performed on 23rd November shows that mescaline hydrochloride, 0.15 g, produces a pattern of symptoms which differs in only a few respects from the one obtained with the drug. Both mescaline and the crude drug produced bradycardia, pupillary dilatation, headache, dizziness, clumsiness of limb movements, loss of appreciation of time, and, what is most important, characteristic visions.

An attempt to discuss the action of mescaline in detail would not accomplish anything in view of the limited number of experimental data, but physiologists and experimental psychologists should find work in this field rewarding. It is very likely that we are dealing with an action on the central nervous system, although excitation of the peripheral visual apparatus can not be excluded. In this connection I would like to mention that Privatdocent Dr. Krückmann, the first assistant to the Ophthalmological Department in Leipzig, kindly examined me when I carried out the experiment on November 23. He was unable to find any reduction of the visual field either in general or in relation to colours.

At the present moment I would like to leave open the question of whether or not any of the peyote (mescal) alkaloids has a therapeutic value. As far as mescaline is concerned the answer is probably no. Weir-Mitchell and Ellis believe that peyote (mescal) will also become popular amongst cultured people as an intoxicating drug. I think that this is unlikely because the results which I obtained on myself show that the side-effects are so pronounced that they considerably spoil the appreciation of the beautiful visions.

The discoveries of Lewin and Heffter excited a lively interest in the application of the drug in man. Lewin's pupil, Beringer, carried out numerous experiments in man with mescaline.

Kurt Beringer (1893–1949) was born in Uehlingen (Schwarzwald) as the son in a peasant family (Jung 1949, Ruffin 1950). In 1911–1914 he studied medicine in Heidelberg, and in 1918 he took part in the war as assistant doctor. In 1921 he became attached to the Heidelberg Psychiatric and Neurological Clinic of Wilmanns, where he stayed for 12 years. In 1928 he took part in an expedition to Mongolia. In 1934 he came to Freiburg, where he stayed for the rest of his life.

Among many papers, Beringer published one regarding hashish intoxication: "Zur Klinik des Haschischrausches" (1932), and two papers on superstition: "Hexen- und Aberglauben im Schwarzwald" (1938), and "Formen des Aberglaubens in Schwarzwald" (1938). These papers bear witness to his interest in ethno-pharmacology. His *magnum opus*, however, is "Der Meskalinrausch" (1927), translated into Spanish but never into English. This book is to mescaline what Moreau's book is to hashish. It gives a clear cut description of the psychic and somatic symptoms, and should be consulted by whoever is interested in the actions of mescaline.

A renewed interest in psychopharmacology was awakened in Germany around 1928. It was at this time that Lewin and others became interested in the properties of the South American vine *Banisteria Caapi*.

On the 13th of February, 1929, Louis Lewin and Paul Schuster gave a paper at the Berlin Medical Association. They described the action of Banisterin prepared from Banisteria and later proved to be identical to harmine in experiments both in animals and man (Lewin and Schuster 1929). At this time they had only 1.2 g of the drug, of which they had given 0.02–0.04 g to 18 cases of Parkinsonism. The side-effects were reported to be a slight nausea, paleness, tremor and bradycardia. A quarter of an hour after the injection the patients had a feeling of being able to move more easily, even in difficult cases with contractures. An improvement was reported of, among other things, swallowing, chewing, speech, eating, movements of the arms and

Beiträge zur Giftkunde

Herausgegeben von
Professor Dr. Louis Lewin

Heft 3

.

Banisteria Caapi
ein neues Rauschgift und
Heilmittel

von

Prof. Dr. Louis Lewin

Mit 2 Karten

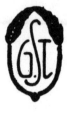

1929

Verlag von Georg Stilke / Berlin

24

walking. They observed a lessening of muscular rigidity. The improvement lasted 2–6 hours, occasionally seven days.

It is remarkable that at this time a film of the action of the drug in three patients was shown. This undoubtedly constitutes the first documentation of the action of monoamineoxidase inhibitors. Lewin pointed out that the drug always affected the ability to move, and seemed inactive psychically. Their demonstration raised a tremendous interest, and the popular press took up the question of this so called "magic drug". Louis Lewin, sick and old at the time, managed to complete a monograph on the subject before he passed away: "Banisteria Caapi, ein neues Rauschgift und Heilmittel" (1929).

In the same year Beringer gave a review of the clinical papers where harmine had been used up till then. He also had occasion to comment upon its pharmacodynamics, and deplored the inaccurate knowledge of how the drug worked. The following sentences are perhaps prophetic:

First of all it is necessary to find out how it affects the central nervous system; whether this is due to a direct action upon certain centers of the brain or indirectly through the autonomic nervous system through a change of metabolism. Many things speak in favour of the latter explanation.

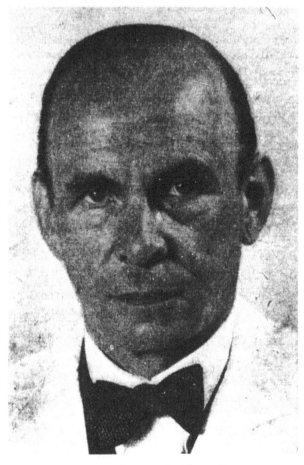

Kurt Beringer (1893–1949)

25

Beringer also commented that new experiments in his clinic showed that the action was not limited to the extrapyramidal system. In his review he pointed out that no differences could be found between banisterine and harmine. It seems at this time that all research workers considered harmine as a new drug for the symptomatic treatment of certain extrapyramidal diseases, and that in many cases it did more than previously known drugs. It proved useful, especially, in the cases of postencephalitic Parkinsonim that were prevalent at the time. Some patients had been on the medication continually for more than a year without decrease in drug effect. The treatment was in no way incompatible with previously used drugs, such as scopolamine.

The most remarkable account from this time is perhaps the description of the self experiments by *L. Halpern* (1930 a and b). Dr. Halpern gave herself doses of up to 0.04 g per os and 0.03 g subcutaneously. The action was sudden, and she had an immediate impression of excitement, with difficulty remaining in one place to continue her intellectual labor. Unrest was the dominant symptom at smaller doses. All actions were felt as if they were more easily done. No euphoria and no clouding of the senses was observed. These symptoms Dr. Halpern explained as stimulation of the cortex:

In all probability, harmine acts upon the motor system as a central cortico-motor regulation as a stimulating agent acts upon the motor neurons, physiologically to increase excitation. By higher doses, this excitation was increased even in a belligerent way: The author, who normally is not belligerent, has herself experienced this discharge of the motor functions. The subject started a fight with a man in the street, where she was the one who attacked, even though according to the circumstances the prospect for the attacker was very unfavorable.

The consciousness was in no way influenced and in no way abnormal, but the impression was felt as if the consciousness was packed in ether. An increased concentration of observance was felt. When lying on a sofa, the lightness increased to a feeling of a fleeting sensation, and the weight of the body was subjectively less. These clinical observations should be compared to the state of levitation frequently reported to occur with the crude drug *ayahuasca* or *caapi*.

Dr. Halpern continued her studies in Parkinson patients, and pointed out the differences in action between scopolamine and harmine and the duality of Parkinson's disease. As is now well known, the monoamineoxidase inhibiting property of the harmala alkaloid was found as late as 1958 by Udenfriend.

The enthusiasm for the harmala alkaloids vanished temporarily during the thirties, as did much of the interest in ethnopharmacology. A few people, however, worked remotely and undisturbed by the rising tide of synthetic chemicals and the general lack of interest in exotic poisons. Among them was Blasius Paul Reko, more commonly known as Blas Pablo Reko.

Blas Pablo Reko (1876–1953) was born in Prerau, Austria (Cook de Leonard 1955–1956). His mother came from Czechoslovakia. Under the influence of his grandfather he decided to study medicine at the University of Vienna, where he graduated in 1901. From the year 1903 he dwelled in America, first in Chicago, in 1907 in Guayaquil Ecuador, and finally in Mexico City. It would seem that he came to Mexico in 1911. He lived no less than 15 years in Oaxaca where he worked professionally for some mining companies. It was during this time that he became interested in the local flora, especially medicinal plants. His interest in this field was combined with ethnographical and etymological studies. He published many articles in "El México Antiguo" about the flora of Oaxaca. He became interested in astromythology through his interest in ethno-botanics.

Reko said himself that he published his papers only to satisfy his personal taste. This concerns perhaps mostly his numerological work. To the present reader, his ethno-botanical papers seem to be of special importance. He was a good botanical observer and had a large collection of indigenous plants, among them the magic mushroom used by the Mazatecs. His studies were summarized in "Mitobotánica Zapoteca", México, 1945.

In Jan. 1937 Reko wrote the following letter to Henry Wassén, anthropologist and curator of the ethnographical museum, Gothenburg, Sweden:

Jan. 31, 1937.
Gelati 15, Tacubaya, D.F., Mexico

Mr. Henry Wassén
Göteborgs Museum
Göteborg, Sweden
My dear Mr. Wassén:

. . . Apparently you confound me with my cousin Victor A. Reko, the author of "Magische Gifte", a journalistic piece of work, by the way, which you need not to take very seriously, since its author is neither a botanist nor has he any personal experience with the drugs described, most of which he has not even seen and would not recognize if he saw them. It is a cleverly made up *mixtum compositum* of compiled facts and wild inventions of his own fancy, intended for popular consumption.

I have deep interest in the work of Prof. Santesson and would like to come in touch with him, as I can furnish him some very important botanical materials, awaiting the solution of their mystery by a competent chemist. I am forwarding to your direction a sample of the "Piule" seed, together with an article of mine on this topic (published in 1920 and reprinted in El. Mex. Ant. 1934) in the hope that Prof. Santesson might get interested in the problem and conduct some experiments in that line.

Very likely I get this year also specimen of the Teonanacatl, still used for religious rites in some secluded places, but so far never identified . . .

> With best regards
> Yours truly

Dr. B. P. Reko.

Both the Piule-Ololiuqui and the Teonanacatl did arrive.

Carl Gustaf Santesson (1862–1939) definitely has a place in ethno-pharmacology. He was professor of pharmocology in Stockholm from 1895 to 1927, and had studied both with Böhm in Leipzig and with Schmiedeberg in Strassburg. (Liljestrand 1939). These teachers influenced his interest in, among other things, the study of compounds such as strychnine, strophanthine and curare. He published about 20 papers on arrow poisons, collected from all parts of the world. Especially important, however, is the work he carried out after retirement. The Mexican drugs he obtained were investigated and the results published in journals that are not easily found nowadays (Santesson 1937, 1938). Among them were Ololiuqui and Teonanacatl, the magic mushroom of Mexico, subsequently investigated by Wasson, Heim and Hofmann. Santesson did not have much of the latter, but succeeded in carrying out animal experiments with Ololiuqui. It is to the credit of

Santesson that he was able to notice the central action of this drug in animals, and that in his paper he writes:

In some way the animals had lost their initiative. It seems to me that there is a a partial paralysis of the brain, a kind of narcosis . . . in these animals there is a certain central depression without any other obvious symptoms.

He concludes his paper by saying:

The drug deserves a thorough investigation which can only be done with a larger supply of material.

With Santesson's papers expire the old pre-World War II activities in the ethno-pharmacologic search for psychoactive drugs. The revival was to come about ten years later.

Acknowledgment

This work has been supported by a grant from the National Institute of Mental Health, Bethesda, USA (MH 12007) and by a grant from the Swedish Medical Research Council.

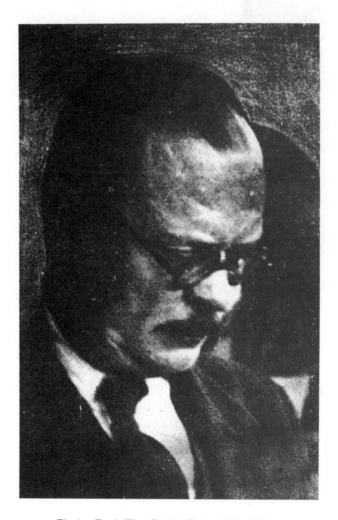

Plasius Paul (Blas Pablo) Reko 1876–1953.

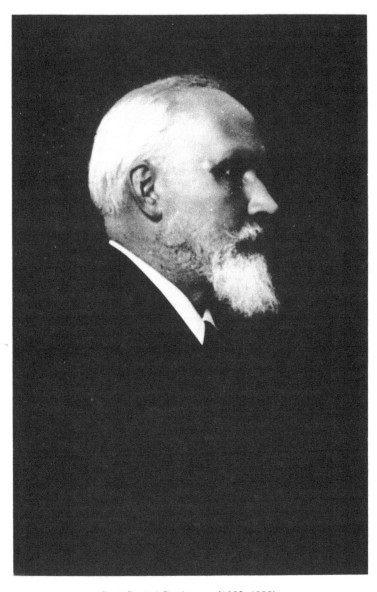

Carl Gustaf Santesson (1862–1939)

REFERENCES

ASCHENBRANDT, T. "Die physiologische Wirkung und die Bedeutung des Cocain muriat. auf den menschlichen Organismus." Deutsche Medizinische Wochenschrift, pp. 730–732, Dez. 12, 1883.

BARUK, *H*. "La vie et l'oeuvre de Moreau de Tours." Paris, Annales Moreau de Tours. Presses Universitaires de France. 1962.

BENTLEY, W. H. "Erythoxylon Coca in the Opium and Alcohol Habits." Detroit Therapeutic Gazette, pp. 253–254, 1880.

BERINGER, K. "Der Meskalinrausch, seine Geschichte and Erscheinungsweise." Monographien aus dem Gesamtegebiete der Neurologie und Psychiatrie, 49: 35–89, 119–315, 1927.

BERINGER, K. "Uber ein neues, auf das extrapyramidal-motorische System wirkendes Alkaloid (Banisterin)." Der Nervenarzt, 1 : 265–275, 1928.

BERINGER, K. "Zur Banisterin- und Harminfrage." Der Nervenarzt, 2: 548–549, 1929 (Sept.)

BERINGER, K., W. v. BAEYER und H. MARX. "Zur Klinik des Haschischrausches." Der Nervenarzt, 5 : 337–350, 1932.

BERINGER, K. "Hexen- und Aberglauben im Schwarzwald." Z. Neur., 161: 535, 1938.

BERINGER, K. "Formen des Aberglaubens im Schwarzwald." Arch. f. Psychiatr., 108 : 228, 1938.

BIBRA, ERNST FREIHERRN VON. "Die Narkotischen Genussmittel und der Mensch." Nürnberg, Verlag von Wilhelm Schmid, 1855.

COLLET, C.-G. "Candidature de Joseph Moreau (de Tours) au Prix Montyon de l'Académie des Sciences en 1846." Paris, Annales Moreau de Tours. Presses Universitaires de France, 1962.

COOK DE LEONARD CARMEN. "Obituary on Dr. Blas Pablo Reko." "El México Antiguo" Vol. 8, 1955, págs. IX–XIV, México, D.F. 1956.

DRAGENDORFF, GEORG. "Die Heilpflanzen der verschiedenen Völker und Zeiten." Neudruck der Ausgabe Stuttgart, 1898. Antiquariat Fritsch, Postfach 1043, 79/Ulm/ Do. Germany.

FREUD, S. "Ueber Coca." Centralblatt f.d. ges. Therapie, pp. 289–314, 1884 (Juli).

GÜNTHER, S. "Ernst v. Bibra." Nürnberg, Naturhist. Ges. Säcular-Feier 1801–1901. Festschrift 1901.

HALPERN, L. "Der Wirkungsmechanismus des Harmins und die Pathophysiologie der Parkinsonchen Krankheit." Deut. Med. Wochenschr. 56 : 651–655, 1930a.

HALPERN, L. "Ueber die Harminwirkung im Selbstversuch." Deut. Med. Wochenschr., 56 : 1252–1254, 1930b.

HARTWICH, C. "Die Bedeutung der Entdeckung von Amerika für die Drogenkunde." Berlin, Springer Verlag, 1892.

HARTWICH, C. "Georg Dragendorff." Ber. Deutsch. Pharmaceut. Ges. 7–8: 297–320, 1897–98.

HARTWICH, C. "Die menschlichen Genussmittel, ihre Herkunft, Verbreitung, Geschichte, Anwendung, Bestandteile und Wirkung." Leipzig, Tauchnitz, 1911.

HEFFTER, A. "Ueber Pellote." Arch. exp. Path. Pharmakol. 40: 418–425, 1897.

HEUBNER, W. "Nachruf auf Arthur Heffter." Gew. Hyg. N.F., 2: 101–103, 1925.

HOLMSTEDT, B. and G. LILJESTRAND. "Readings in pharmacology." Pergamon Press Ltd., 1963.

JELLIFFE, S. E. "Emil Kraepelin, the Man and his Work." Transactions of the American Neurological Association. Boston, 57th Annual Meeting, May 1931. Ed. Dr. Theodore H. Weisenburg, Philadelphia.

JOACHIMOGLU, G. "Eröffnungsansprache." Arch. exp. Path. Pharmak. 238: 6–7, 1960.

JONES, E. "The Life and Work of Sigmund Freud." 1–3. New York, Basic Books Inc. Chapter VI, Vol. 1, 1956.

JUNG, R. "Kurt Beringer." Archiv f. Psych. und Zeitschr. Neurol. 183: 293–301, 1949.

KOBERT, R. and A. SOHRT. "Ueber die Wirkung des salzauren Hyoscin." Arch. exp. Path. Pharmak. 22: 396–429, 1887.

KOLLE, K. "Emil Kraepelin (1856–1926)." Stuttgart, Grosse Nervenärzte, Georg Thieme Verlag, 1956. pp. 175–186.

KRAEPELIN, E. "Ueber die Beeinflussung einfacher psychischer Vorgänge durch einige Arzneimittel." Jena, Verlag von Gustav Fischer, 1892.

KRAEPELIN, E. "Wilhelm Wundt." Zeitschrift f. Neurologic und Psychiatrie. pp. 35–362, Vol. 61, 1920.

KRAYER, O. Personal communication, 1963.

LEWIN, L. "Nebenwirkungen der Arzneimittel." Berlin, Pharmakologisch-klin. Handbuch, A. Hirschwald. 1881.

LEWIN, L. "Referat: Pharmakologie und Toxikologie." Berliner Klinischer Wochenschrift, XXII: 321–322, 1885.

30

Lewin, L. "Ueber Piper Methysticum (KAWA)." Berlin, Verlag von August Hirschwald, 1886.

Lewin, L. "Ueber Anhalonium Lewinii." Arch. exper. Path. u. Pharmakol. 24 : 401–411, 1888.

Lewin, L. : "Anhalonium Lewinii." The Therapeutic Gazette. *IV*, No. 4, April 16, 1888.

Lewin, L. "Ueber Areca Catechu, Chavica Betle und das Betelkauen." Monographie. Stuttgart, F. Enke, 1889.

Lewin, L. "Uber Anhalonium Lewinii und andere Cacteen." Arch. f. exp. Path. u. Pharm. 34 : 374–391, 1. u. 2. Heft, 1894.

Lewin, L. "Die Gifte in der Weltgeschichte." Berlin, J. Springer, 1929.

Lewin, L. "Heilmittel und Gifte bei Homer." Münch. med. Wschr. 67 : 966, 1920.

Lewin, L. "Phantastica." Die Betäubenden und Erregenden Genussmittel, Für Ärzte und Nichtärzte. Berlin, Georg Stilke, 1924.

Lewin, L. "Untersuchungen über Banisteria Caapi Spr." Arch. exper. Path. u. Pharmakol. 129 : 133–149, 1928.

Lewin, L. "Banisteria Caapi, ein neues Rauschgift und Heilmittel." Beiträge zur Giftkunde, herausgegeben von Professor Dr. Louis Lewin. Berlin, Verlag von Georg Stilke, 1929.

Lewin, L. und P. Schuster. "Ergebnisse von Banisterinversuchen an Kranken." Deut. Med. Wochenschr. 55 : 419, 1929. Literatur- und Verhandlungsberichte, 8 März 1929. S. 419, Berlin, Medizinische Gesellschaft, 13.II. 1929.

Lewin, L. "Phantastica, Narcotic and Stimulating Drugs, Foreword by Bo Holmstedt." London, Routledge & Kegan, 1964.

Liljestrand, G., C. G. Santesson. "Skandinavisches Archiv für Physiologie." 83. Band. 1 bis 3 Heft. Berlin, Walter de Gruyter & Co., 1939.

Moreau, J. J. (de Tours). "Mémoire sur le traitement des Hallucinations par la Datura Stramonium." Gazette Médicale de Paris IX, 1841, No. 41, 9.10. 1841.

Moreau, J. J. (de Tours). "Mémoire sur le Traitement des Hallucinations par le Datura Stramonium—Suite—Voir" 1° No. 41. Gazette Médicale de Paris IX, 1841. No. 43, 23.10. 1841.

Moreau, J. "Mémoire sur le traitement des hallucinations par le Datura Stramonium." La Librairie des Sciences Médicales du Just Bouvier, Paris 1841.

Moreau, J. "Du hachisch et de l'aliénation mentale." Etudes psychologiques. Paris, Librairie de Fortin, Masson et C^{le}, 1845.

Palmer, E. R. "Erythroxylon Coca as an Antidote to the Opium Habit." The Therapeutic Gazette, 1, new series, p. 172, 1880. Vol. IV—whole series.

Reko, B. P. "Mitobotanica Zapoteca." Tacubaya, D. F., 1945.

Reko,, V. A. "Magische Gifte." Rausche- und Betäubungsmittel der Neuen Welt. Stuttgart, Ferdinand Enke Verlag, 1949.

Ritti, M. "Eloge de J. Moreau (de Tours)." Annales Médico-Psychologiques, Paris 1887. 7ème Serie, Tome Sixième, 45th year. Paris, G. Masson.

Ruffin, H. "Kurt Beringer." Deutsche Zeitschrift für Nervenheilkunde, 164 : 199–208. 1950.

Santesson, C. G. "Notiz über Piule, eine mexikanische Rauschdroge." Ethnological Studies, 4, 1937.

Santesson, C. G. "Piule, eine mexikanische Rauschdroge." Archiv der Pharmazie und Berichte der deutschen Pharmazeutischen Gesellschaft. Berlin W 35, Verlag Chemie GMBH, 1937.

Santesson, C. G. "Noch eine Mexikanische 'Piule'-Droge Semina Rynchosiae Phaseoloidis DC." Ethnological Studies, 6, 1938.

Santesson, C. G. "Einige mexikanische Rauschdrogen." Archiv für Botanik—K. Sv. Vetenskapsakad. 29 A, No. 12, 1939.

Schmiedeberg, O. "Uber die Pharmaka in der Ilias und Odyssee." Schriften d. wiss. Gesellsch. Strassburg. Strassburg, 1918, Heft 36.

SCHRÖTER, C. "Prof. Dr. C. Hartwich." Schweizerische Apotheker-Zeitung No. 10, Jahrg. 55, Zürich, March 8, 1917.

SIEBURG, E. "Rudolf Kobert." Ber. Dtsch. Pharm. Ges. 29: 285–299, 1919.

SOLOMON, D., *Ed.* The Marihuana Papers, New York. The Bobbs-Merrill Company, Inc., 1966.

STRAUB, W. "Arthur Heffter." Arch. exp. Path. Pharmakol. 105: 1–4, 1924.

The Place of Ethnobotany in the Ethnopharmacologic Search for Psychotomimetic Drugs

Richard Evans Schultes

Botanical Museum of Harvard University, Cambridge, Massachusetts

Introduction

The very descriptive word *ethnobotany* has been defined in sundry ways in the 70 years since it was created and first used by Harshberger (*23*). Although Harshberger indicated how ethnobotanical investigation could be integrated into overall research, he failed to offer a definition of his new term.

Years earlier, in 1874, Powers (*38*) had used the term *aboriginal botany* to refer to a study of "all the forms of the vegetable world which the aborigines used for medicine, food, textile, fabrics, ornaments, etc."

It was, apparently, not until 1916 that a truly broad concept emerged that went beyond mere identification and cataloguing of plants used by primitive peoples. This broad definition of the term *ethnobotany*, now rather widely held, was promulgated by Robbins, Harrington and Freire-Marreco (*42*), and, in effect, attributes to this discipline a study and evaluation of the knowledge of all phases of plant life amongst primitive societies, and of the effects of the vegetal environment upon the life, customs, beliefs and history of the peoples of such societies.

Jones (*27*) has offered the following precise definition: "the study of the interrelations of primitive man and plants." It is interesting to note that Jones and others (*9*) prefer to restrict *ethnobotany* to man in primitive states of culture. While this premise may and probably does almost always obtain, there is really no reason to circumscribe the term in this way. Vestal and Schultes (*62*) looked upon ethnobotany as a part of *economic botany*. Since I do not hold that ethnobotany need be limited exclusively to man in primitive society, my own definition (*46*) circumscribes *ethnobotany* as "a study of the relationships between man and his ambient vegetation."

Ethnobotany and the Search for New Drugs

It is natural that an interdisciplinary field such as ethnobotany be replete with problems for investigation. These are and have been not only numerous but varied as well, and the burgeoning nomenclature bears witness to this variation. In recent years, such terms as *archaeoethnobotany, ethnomycology, ethnoecology* and *ethnopharmacology* have been proposed and have come into use.

Nowhere perhaps have the potentialities of ethnobotanical investigation been more scintillating than in the search for new psychotomimetic drugs (*57*). These potentialities have been realized in the case of a number of new and previously known hallucinogens that are now relatively well understood: the narcotic mushrooms and morning glories of Mexico; the ayahuasca-caapi-yajé complex of South America; the intoxicating snuffs of the Orinoco and Amazon basins. They remain to tantalise us, however, in the case of several narcotics known vaguely from common names or from sketchy reports of travellers and missionaries: several South American snuffs; the marari of lowland Bolivia; an intoxicating "tree-fungus" of the Yurimagua Indians of eastern Peru; the yurema root infusion of the Pankararú of Brazil; the magic woi of the Yekwana of southern Venezuela. Furthermore, they challenge us to find, through ethnobotanical avenues, new psychotropic plants that most certainly are still in use, but which have never been seen nor reported by the prying inquisitiveness of man outside of the culture that employs the narcotics.

I cannot help thinking that Linneaus himself must have had ethnobotany in mind, at least in part, when he in 1754 wrote in a museum catalogue the following philosophy: "Man, ever desirous of knowledge, has already explored many things; but more and greater still remain concealed; perhaps reserved for distant generations, who shall . . . make many discoveries for the pleasure and convenience of life. Prosperity shall see its increasing Musuems, and the knowledge of the Divine Wisdom, flourish together; and at the same time all the practical sciences . . . shall be enriched; for we cannot avoid thinking, that what we know of the Divine works are much fewer than those of which we are ignorant."

In the search for new hallucinogens, we have much to do and little time in which to do it. Peoples in primitive societies, because they live most intimately with their immediate vegetational environment, *do* possess a valuable understanding of the properties of plants, even though their knowledge of plants has sometimes been optimistically exaggerated by both lay enthusiasts and ethnopharmacological zealots. The aborigines' knowledge and understanding, furthermore, is probably everywhere far from complete. It, therefore, behooves all of us interested in a search for new psychotomimetic drugs to carry out our investigations along several avenues of approach, not following the ethnobotanical avenue to the exclusion of others (*52*). It is, however, the place of ethnobotany in this search that I shall here discuss, and I want merely, at the very start, to put it thus into proper perspective.

34

Civilization is closing in on many, if not on most, parts of the world still sacred to the less advanced cultures. It has long been pressing in, but its pace is now accelerated as the result of geographically extensive wars, extended commercial interests, increased missionary activity, widening tourism. Modern methods of travel and penetration have given civilisation the tools for this accomplishment. Road-building programmes in Latin America provide us with but one example of how fast this penetration of the hinterlands is proceeding.

Our great concern lies in the progressive divorcement of man in primitive societies from dependence upon his immediate environment. I have often stated that perhaps the greatest enemy or, at least, competitor, of ethnopharmachological research is the arrival and cheap availability of the aspirin pill. More than once this has initiated an astonishingly rapid disintegration of native medical lore. I doubt that social scientists are fully aware of the rapidity of this disintegration, but the ethnobotanist cannot fail to see it. That the aspirin (meaning, of course, modern medicines in general) may be more beneficial than herbs and magic is not ours to consider here. What does interest us academically and practically is how to salvage some of the medico-botanical lore of primitive cultures before it shall have been forever entombed with the culture that gave it birth (51).

In considering the ethnobotanical approach in our search for new drugs we must constantly bear in mind the widespread exaggeration of the usefulness of ethnobotanical data. Although we cannot afford to pre-judge reports of aboriginal uses of plants simply because they seem to fall beyond the limits of credence, we must nevertheless ever keep in mind that there is no reason to presume that, because man in primitive living does have knowledge as yet unknown to us, he may possess anything more than a limited intuition into the properties of plants.

Although now at long last there is more agreement concerning the larger aims of ethnopharmacological investigations, the field has suffered—as has ethnobotany in general—from lack of orientation and integration. Ethnobotanical research has often, of necessity, been done as a sideline by botanists untrained in ethnology; by anthropologists lacking any knowledge of biology; or even by laymen, dedicated enough, but devoid of preparation in both biology and anthropology. And in more recent years, the training commensurate with thorough ethnobotanical investigations has enlarged its scope to include some familiarity with topics such as chemotaxonomy, which once would never have been considered germane. As a result of this checkered history, ethnobotanical research, its purposes and its potentialities has too often suffered from smug depreciation at the hands of specialists in disciplines that have been academically more clearly delimited.

The potentialities of ethnobotanical research into folk medicine are far too extensive for proper treatment in a short lecture, but certain salient points may and should be made, and these points may be supported by specific examples. In delving into the medicine of primitive societies, we must never lose sight of the vast difference between "medicine" in our sense and that in primitive societies. In almost all, if not all, primitive cultures, the concept of sickness and even of death from natural causes is unknown or incomprehensible. Instead—and we must here over-simplify the problem for our purposes—supernatural spirits or forces of evil work in sundry ways to bring about the impairment of health or cessation of life. We should realize that hexing and witchcraft were widely accepted as recently as three centuries ago in what was, in many respects, the advanced culture of Europe. Amongst the members of primitive cultures to-day, treatment usually comprises various kinds of exorcism; and diagnosis, and often treatment itself, must be carried out through communication with the spirit or supernatural world. Many ways of communicating have been developed, but the employment of vision-producing narcotics or hallucinogens of plant origin seems to have been widespread in both time and space, and to have occurred in many wholly unrelated cultures.

We do not know exactly how many species of plants there are. There may be as many as 800,000. Estimates for the Angiosperms alone vary from the usually cited 200,000 to about half a million (55).

It is interesting to compare the number of species of plants that man has found valuable for nutrition with those that he has employed to induce hallucinations. Of this vast assemblage of Angiosperms, only about 3000 are known to have been used directly as human food. The number of species that actually feed mankind is, however, very small. Only about 150 Angiosperms are important enough as foods to enter the world's commerce. Of these, only 12 or 13 stand, in effect, between the world's population and starvation, and these dozen or so plants are all cultivated species (55).

We find, likewise, that the number of species providing man with narcotic agents is very small. Between four and five thousand species are now known to be alkaloidal,[1] and we must realise that constituents other than alkaloids—glycosides, resins, essential oils and others—may also be responsible for narcotic activity. Probably no more than 60 species, including Cryptogams and Phanerogams, are employed in primitive and advanced cultures for their intoxicating effects. Of these, only about 20 may be considered of major importance. What is even more significant is that so few—coca, opium poppy, hemp, tobacco—are numbered amongst the world's commercially important cultivated plants. Four of these five, if not all five, species are cultigens, unknown in the wild state. This bespeaks long association with man and his agricultural practices (55).

It may likewise be of significance that, whether because of cultural differences or floristic peculiarities or for some other as yet unappreciated reason, the New World is much richer in narcotic plants than the Old. These statistics, naturally, relate merely to those plants the narcotic properties of which man has discovered in his trial and error experimentation during the course of human history. The longer I consider this question, the more I am convinced that there may exist in the world's flora an appreciable number of such plants not yet uncovered by the experimenting natives and still to be found by the enquiring phytochemist. This is an aspect of the problem in which ethnobotanical approaches cannot help, but even though our ethno-

---

[1] R. F. Raffauf, personal communication.

botanical research into narcotic plants is still embryonic, we know enough to realise that both the Old and the New Worlds offer rich fields for potential discoveries.

Where do some of the ethnopharmacological problems in connexion with our search for new and interesting psychotomimetic agents lie? Let us contemplate some of the hints that might guide such research in the future.

Geographically, the problems may be found almost throughout the globe, concentrated, to be sure, in areas where primitive societies still hold sway unmolested by the inroads of modern civilisation.

Consideration of Pressing Problems

Some of the most interesting enigmas lurk in the desert stretches of northern Mexico, where what we might term the "prototype" of the New World hallucinogens—peyote or *Lophophora Williamsii*—has long been the centre of religious and curative rites in the Tarahumare and Huichol country. Peyote, of course, is well known from many aspects, and 13 alkaloids have thus far been isolated from it (*33*). The explorer Carl Lumholtz (*32*) mentioned, however, other narcotic cactus plants, some of which are as yet not even botanically identified. "High mental qualities," he wrote, "are ascribed especially to all species of *Mammilaria* and *Echinocactus*, small cacti, for which a regular cult is instituted. The Tarahumares designate several as *hikuli*, though the name belongs properly only to the kind most commonly used by them . . . The principal kinds are . . . *Lophophora Williamsii*. The Tarahumares speak of them as the superior *hikuli* (hikuli wanamé) . . . Besides hikuli wanamé . . . , the Tarahumares know and worship the following varieties: 1. *Mulato* (*Mammilari micromeris*). This is believed to make the eyes large and clear to see sorcerers, to prolong life and to give speed to the runners. 2. *Rosapara*. This is only a more advanced vegetative stage of the preceding species—though it looks quite different, being white and spiny. 3. *Sunami*. (*Mammilari fissurata*). It is rare, but it is believed to be even more powerful than wanamé and is used in the same way as the latter; the drink produced from it is also strongly intoxicating. . . . 4. *Hikuli walula saeliami*. This is the greatest of all, and the name means 'hikuli great authority.' It is extremely rare among the Tahahumares, and I have not seen any specimen of it, but it was described to me as growing in clusters of from eight to twelve inches in diameter, resembling wanamé with many young ones around it. . . . All these various species are considered good, as coming from Tata Dios, and well disposed toward the people. But there are some kinds of hikuli believed to come from the Devil. One of these, with long white spines, is called *ocoyome*. It is very rarely used, and only for evil purposes."

Several of these narcotic hukuli plants are still unidentified. They are obviously all cactuses. Several species of *Mammilaria* have yielded alkaloids of undetermined identity, but the genus, which is not far removed from *Lophophora*, might be expected to contain active principles. The same may

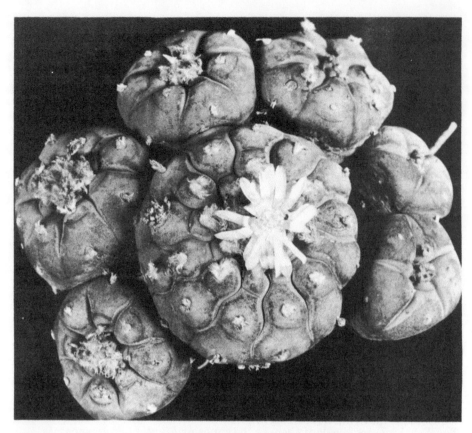

Flowering head of the peyote cactus, *Lophophora Williamsii*, the "prototype" of the New World hallucinogens. Photograph by R. E. Schultes.

be said of *Echinocactus*. In this connexion, it is well known that in Mexico a number of species in seven other genera of the *Cactaceae—Ariocarpus, Astrophytum, Aztekium, Dolichothele, Obregonia, Pelecyphora* and *Solisia*—are popularly classed as peyote, perhaps because they bear some resemblance to the true peyote, *Lophophora*, or perhaps because they have similar toxic effects and may be employed with *Lophophora* or as a substitute for it (*45*). There is much, indeed, that needs ethnobotanical clarification in this whole picture; and it would seem to be a promising problem (*16*). All that we know is that, of these last seven genera mentioned, three—*Ariocarpus, Astrophytum* and *Dolichothele*—have yielded alkaloids (*65*).

Witch doctors in northern Peru (in Piura, Lambayeque and La Libertad) prepare an hallucinogenic drink called *cimora* from at least six plants (*13*). Several of the ingredients are said to be members of the *Cactaceae*. There is indirect evidence of great age for the use of this narcotic drink which is concerned with moon rites of the region. It is taken for therapeutic effects, for diagnosis and divination, and to make oneself owner of another's identity. This intoxicating brew must be potent if the plant ingredients, identified apparently without voucher specimens, are correctly indicated. The principal ingredient is said to be *San Pedro*, a cactus, *Trichocereus Pachanoi*, from

38

which the hallucinogenic alkaloid mescaline has been isolated (*21*). Other cactaceous ingredients—a member of the genus *Cactus* and *Neoraimondia macrostibas* (*Cereus macrostibas*)—likewise enter the preparation of the brew. A further addition is the campanulaceous *Isotoma longiflora*, known to contain the alkaloid lobeline. *Pedilanthus titimaloides* of the Euphorbiaceae is said also to be added. *Datura Stramonium* is furthermore cited as one of the plants in the formula, and this alone, of course, would provide a potent vision-producing base for the drink. With the apparent lack of voucher specimens, however, there is no way at present to verify the determination of these ingredients. An indication that there may be discrepancies in the determinations is that the chief ingredient was at first erroneously determined as *Opuntica cylindrica* (*12*). It has recently, however, been shown, on the basis of botanical collections, to represent *Trichocereus Pachanoi*, and has been ethnobotanically indicated as being a "magic and dangerous" plant (*18*). Whether or not the common name *San Pedro* applies to both *Opuntia cylindrica* and to *Trichocereus Pachanoi*, very dissimilar plants, has not been verified.

This problem is further complicated by a recent citation of the "magic and dangerous" *timora* of Huancabamba, Peru, as a species of *Iresine* of the Amaranthaceae (*18*). Is this *timora* perhaps the same word as *cimora*? We cannot tell at the present time. While several amaranthaceous genera contain alkaloids, no such constituents have been reported from *Iresine*. It is of interest to point out, however, that some of the Indians of southern Colombia are said to employ *Iresine* as an admixture in preparing their strongly hallucinogenic yajé drink (*Banisteriopsis* spp.) to increase its psychotomimetic potency (*49*). Here is one of the most challenging problems in the ethnobotany of hallucinogenic plants, and one which would not be difficult to investigate thoroughly.

In the late 17th and early 18th Centuries, Jesuit missionaries working amongst the Yurimagua Indians in the uppermost Amazon basin found the natives drinking a strongly intoxicating beverage prepared from a "tree fungus" "... the Yurimaguas mix mushrooms that grow on fallen trees with a kind of reddish film that is found usually attached to rotting trunks. This film is very hot to the taste. No person who drinks this brew fails to fall under its effects after three draughts of it, since it is so strong or, more correctly, so toxic" (*10*). Field work in the area has, up to the present time, not yet disclosed any practice of this kind, but it is a culture trait little likely to disappear spontaneously, at least without leaving traces, and the region is still inhabited by tribes in relatively primitive conditions of culture. It has been tentatively suggested that the tree fungus might be the known hallucinogenic *Psilocybe yungensis*,[2] but what might be the reddish film? Here certainly is a most challenging problem in ethnopharmacology.

The Mojo Indians, an Arawakan tribe living in eastern Bolivia, employ an unknown narcotic called *marari* (*34*). It has been reported that "whenever ... the medicine-men had to interview the spirits, they drank a decoction prepared from a plant called marari, similar to our verbena, which caused

---

[2] R. G. Wasson, personal communication.

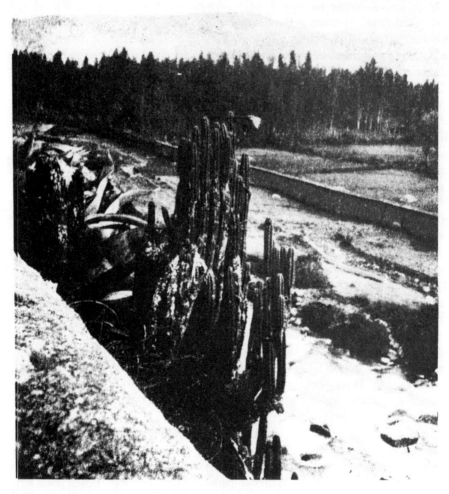

Trichocereus Pachanoi growing on the side of a cliff on the outskirts of Cuenca, Ecuador. Photograph by G. Rose. From Britton & Rose: *The Cactaceae* 2 (1920) fig. 196.

for 24 hours a general condition of excitement characterized by insomnia and pain" (*34*). According to reports, the medicine men try to avoid drinking marari whenever they "could operate without the narcotic." This may be interpreted as an indication of great potency or toxicity of the drug. By likening marari to "our verbena," the French ethnologist Métraux undoubtedly meant *Verbena officinalis*, a well known folk medicine of Europe. The marari might well represent one of the many South American verbenaceous species, but only direct field observation can clear up this enigma.

Oftentimes, no clear distinction has been made between stimulants and narcotics in the writings of early missionaries and other travellers. *Guayusa* is a case in point. Reports of a strongly stimulating plant of the westernmost Amazon, widely known as guayusa, place its use in the westernmost Amazon of Colombia, Ecuador and Peru. The earliest report of guayusa dates from 1682 and comprises a missionary reference that pointed to a use surrounded by superstition in the region of the upper Marañon in Peru.[3] Amongst the several references to guayusa, perhaps the most important is that of Richard Spruce, who reported it to be a species of *Ilex* allied to *I. paraguariensis* "but with much larger leaves" and to be a tonic which, in strong infusions such as those prepared by the Jibaros, may be "positively emetic" (*59*).

The recent writings of Karsten (*28*) seem to indicate that guayusa may have narcotic properties as well, for he states that "just as the Jibaros take certain narcotic drinks when they are preparing for war, to see whether they will be lucky or not in the undertaking, so they also understand a kind of divination in regard to hunting. The drink then used is prepared of the guayusa (*Ilex* sp.), the leaves of which are boiled in water for the purpose. The guayusa is not a real narcotic but a tonic, to which the Indians ascribe magical purifying effects. The Jibaros, however, seem to believe that the drink produces dreams of divinatory significance or, more strictly speaking, what they call 'small dreams,' especially such as have reference to hunting." Other "supernatural virtues" or magical powers are ascribed to guayusa by the Jibaros.

Even though guayusa may not belong strictly to the category of psycho-tomimetic plants, it would be advantageous to know more concerning its curious effects—these "little dreams"—that the Jibaros ascribe to the infusion. Are these effects wholly imaginary, or may perhaps some other plant be occasionally boiled with the guayusa when the "little dreams" are experienced?

And then, what precisely is guayusa? Spruce noted that it was an *Ilex* and reported seeing a group of guayusa trees ... over 300 years old ... "that were not unlike old holly trees in England, except that the shining leaves were much larger, thinner and unarmed." A collection of *Ilex* from eastern Peru was described as *Ilex Guayusa* by Loessener, but it is sterile. Sterile material of a guayusa was gathered recently by one of my students in eastern Peru and represents undoubtedly an *Ilex*. It is not wholly improbable that this widely disseminated vernacular name may refer to a number of different plants with marked physiological action. The guayusa problem is certainly one that might occupy the attention of ethnobotanists interested in native narcotics and stimulants. It is rather disquieting that even the identity of such a plant should, after some three centuries, still be uncertain.

Another interesting reference concerning a plant with marked physiological activity which may or may not be narcotic in character reports the use by the Kakusi Indians of British Guiana of "peppers as a stimulant and excitant" (*43*). Even though the "peppers" were definitely identified as belonging to *Capsicum*, this report should be carefully checked by further field observations.

There is an interesting and very potent narcotic drink used in eastern Brazil that merits much more investigation. The Karirí (*30*) and Pankararú (*31*) Indians along the São Francisco River in Pernambuco have an ancient

---

[3] V. Patiño, personal communication.

cult, still practiced, connected with a root known as *yurema*. Groups of warriors or strong young men are given a gourdful of the yurema root infusion by an elderly chieftain. With bowed heads, the celebrants see "glorious visions of the spirit land, with flowers and birds. They might catch a glimpse of the clashing rocks that destroy the souls of the dead journeying to their goal, or see the Thunderbird shooting lightning from a huge tuft on his head and producing claps of thunder by running about." The yurema rite was formerly much more widespread than at present, for it is known to have been practiced by at least three other tribes (the Guegue, Acroa and Pimenteira) of the general region. The ceremony exists also amongst the Tusha Indians, neighbours of the Pancararús.

There is reason to believe that the yurema-drink is the same narcotic as the intoxicating beverage of the Pankararús which has been reported under the Portuguese name *vinho de Jurema*. This drink is reportedly prepared from the roots of the leguminous tree *Mimosa hostilis* (*20*). Chemically, this plant is extremely interesting because of its close relationship to *Anadenanthera peregrina*, from the seeds of which the hallucinogenic yopo snuff of the Orinoco River basin is prepared. In 1946, an alkaloid was isolated from the bark of the roots of *Mimosa hostilis* (*20*) and was called nigerine, but recent chemical investigation has established the identity of nigerine and N, N-dimethyltryptamine, the same constituent found in yopo seeds from *Anadenanthera peregrina* (*36*).

In a remote tributary of the Apaporis River in Amazonian Colombia, the Peritomé-Tanimukas make use of an as yet unidentified plant to prepare a vision-producing drink employed in the adolescent initiation rites of boys (*57*). It is taken much as is the well known yajé or caapi of the same region prepared from *Banisteriopsis Caapi*, but the Tanimukas, who employ also this malpighiaceous vine, are quick to distinguish the two. The bark of the root of an extensive lacticiferous forest liana, without the admixture of any other plant material, is subjected to long boiling in order to prepare the drink. I was not able to see the vine nor to take the drug during my short stay amongst the Tanimukas, but all information pursuant to my questioning was constant. This liana, reported to be rich in latex, might represent an apocynaceous species, but the problem cannot be solved until extended field work is carried out with these isolated Indians.

There is evidence that natives of the New World have found psychotropic activity in plants introduced from the Old World. It has, for example, recently been reported that Yaquí medicine men from northern Mexico employ *Genista canariensis*, the genista of florists, for the purpose of inducing hallucinations (*17*), a property that has been experimentally substantiated. The genus *Genista* and the closely related *Cytisus*, in which *Genista canariensis* is sometimes included, are extremely rich in alkaloids. Cytisine, an alkaloid that formed the basis for the former hallucinogenic use amongst some North American Plains Indians of seeds of the leguminous *Sophora secundiflora* (*53*), has been isolated from leaves and beans of *Genista canariensis*.

42

Other Old World plants that may have hallucinogenic uses amongst New World natives are several species of the labiate genus *Coleus*. Concurrent to the recent discovery by Wasson in the Mazatec Indian country of Oaxaca, Mexico, of the utilization of the leaves of *Salvia divinorum* as a narcotic (*63*), a similar employment of *Coleus pumila* and *C. Blumei*, both introductions from the Old World, was reported. The hallucinogenic effects of the *Salvia* have been experimentally substantiated, and it has been postulated that perhaps this plant, native to Mexico, might represent the ancient *pipiltzin-tzintli* of the Aztecs. Chemical examination of *Salvia divinorum* has not as yet disclosed a psychotropic constituent, and analysis of these two species of

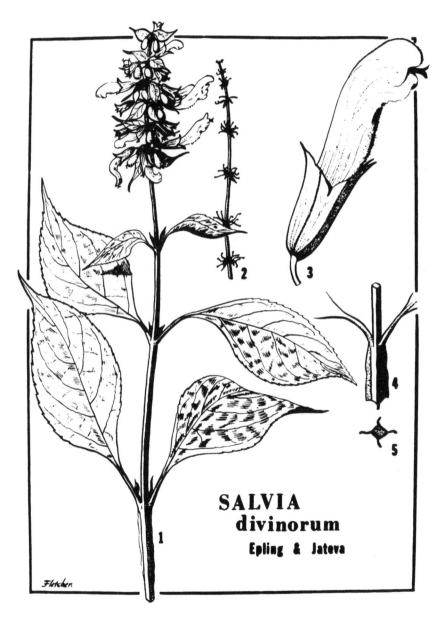

SALVIA
divinorum
Epling & Jateva

Coleus, at least on the basis of the reputedly hallucinogenic material growing in southern Mexico, has apparently not been carried out. Other species of *Coleus* that are employed in the Old World as folk medicines have, however, been studied chemically, but no hallucinogenic substances have been reported from them. There is in Turkestan, nevertheless, another reputedly intoxicating mint—*Lagochilus inebrians* (*7*). The leaves are crushed and mixed with honey or sugar for ingestion. A physiologically active crystalline principle, lagochiline—a polyhydric alcohol—has been reported from this species (*1, 61*).

Without any doubt, one of the most fascinating and promising possibilities of adding to our list of hallucinogens has recently been brought to my attention by one of my former students, Prof. Melvin L. Bristol of the University of Hawaii, who spent more than a year in ethnobotanical field work in southern Colombia. It concerns the solanaceous genus *Brunfelsia* in South America (*57*). A tropical New World genus of about 25 species, *Brunfelsia* plays an important role in aboriginal folk medicine in equatorial America. The fluid extract of one species—*Brunfelsia Hopeana*—is employed pharmaceutically in Brazil as an antidiuretic and antirheumatic. Although atropine-type alkaloids—brunfelsine, manacine and mandragorine—have been reported for *Brunfelsia Hopeana*, little if anything is known of the chemistry of other species (*65*). The aglycone scopoletine, a coumarine derivative found in a number of plant families, has also been isolated from *Brunfelsia*. Consequently, we know that this genus does possess active constituents of very definite physiological activity.

Evidence for the narcotic use of *Brunfelsia* is quite real, but it is not yet corroborated by a good body of field observation. Herbarium records are very helpful in this instance. There are two collections that indicate the use of *Brunfelsia* as a narcotic. One—*Tessmann 3243* from eastern Peru—reports simply that the plant is "a narcotic." The other—*Bristol 1364* from the Colombia Putumayo—states that the plant is a narcotic and medicinal cultivated in Kofán Indian houseyards. Other collections of this genus from Bolivia, Brazil, Colombia, Eucador and Peru indicate a broad spectrum of therapeutic uses ranging from treatment of "yellow fever" to snake bite. Its commonest use in folk medicine seems to be to relieve "rheumatism." Several collections indicate that *Brunfelsia* is toxic. In fact, in the vicinity of Leticia, a Colombian town on the Amazon River, *Brunfelsia maritima* (*Schultes, Raffauf & Soejarto 24108*), escaped from cultivation at an abandoned Indian site on the upper Amazon in Colombia, has been responsible for serious cattle poisoning. The plant is here referred to as *sanango*, which seems to be a somewhat general term applied in the upper Amazon to several plants with medicinal or toxic properties.

The Kofán Indians of the westernmost part of the Amazon of Colombia and Ecuador grow *Brunfelsia* extensively as an ornamental. They know the plant as *borrachera*, a vernacular term in Spanish applied to almost any kind of intoxicating plant, especially to the species of tree-Daturas, in Colombia. The Kofán indicate that they become very cold after taking an infusion of the scraped bark of *Brunfelsia*. This characteristic of the in-

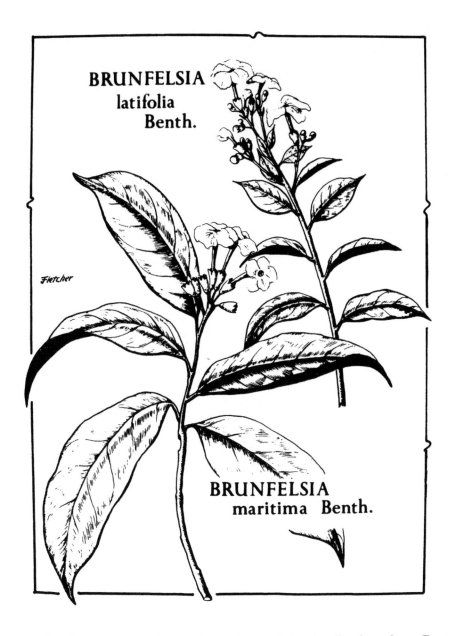

BRUNFELSIA
latifolia
Benth.

Fletcher

BRUNFELSIA
maritima Benth.

toxication has been reported on herbarium labels of collections from Peru, and may well explain the wide use of the plant as a supposed febrifuge. One of my graduate students, Mr. Homer V. Pinkley, who has spent a year living with the Kofán, reports these medicinal applications of *Brunfelsia*, but found no direct evidence that could be interpreted as indicative of its use as an hallucinogen.

Intensive field work may still uncover a former use of *Brunfelsia* as an hallucinogenic agent in the western Amazon or on the eastern slopes of the Andes of Colombia, Eucador or Peru. But *Brunfelsia* is a genus that needs botanical revision and phytochemical investigation. A thorough study could

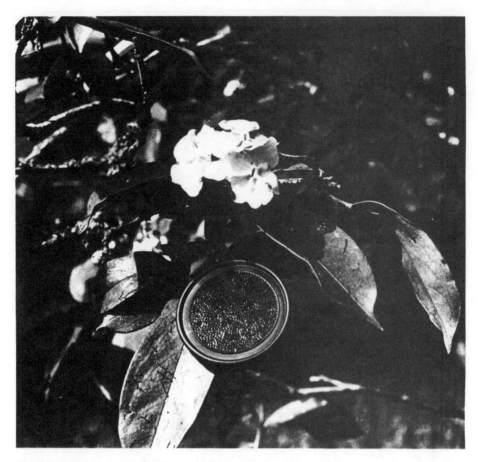

Flowering branch of *Brunfelsia maritima,* a medicinal and ornamental plant common in the western Amazon of Colombia and Ecuador. Río Aguarico, Ecuador. Photograph by H. V. Pinkley.

reward us with a clearer picture of this possible aboriginal American hallucinogen. Might its use as an hallucinogen have disappeared? We should realise that the disappearance of the use of a plant in a given area is not unknown. A century ago, for example, the sapindaceous caffeine-stimulant guaraná, *Paullinia Cupana,* was reported by Spruce as cultivated all the way up the Rio Negro of Amazonian Brazil and into southern Venezuela (*59*). I found that it has now almost completely vanished from cultivation in this region, and the use of the vine as the source of a stimulant is unknown along the Rio Negro at the present time. Might not the same fate have happened to the solanaceous genus *Brunfelsia?*

One of the most interesting enigmas in South America concerns the question of whether or not the apocynaceous genus *Prestonia* is or has ever been used narcotically. The literature is rich in reports, most of them uncritical and unfounded in field work, that *Prestonia amazonica (Haemadictyon amazonicum)* is the source of the hallucinogen known as *yajé*. All manner of confusion has attended this information. Although we believe that we

46

are warranted in asserting that *Prestonia* is not employed as a narcotic, there remains enough doubt to justify further field investigation (*58*). What, precisely, is the problem?

It is well established that a strongly hallucinogenic drink known variously, according to geographic area, as *ayahuasca, caapi and yajé* is prepared from one or more species of the malpighiaceous genus *Banisteriopsis*. Spruce in

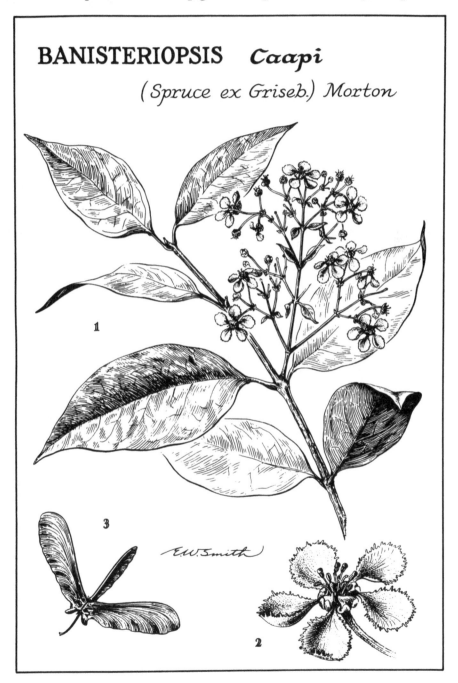

BANISTERIOPSIS *Caapi*
(Spruce ex Griseb.) Morton

1851 first identified the botanical source of this narcotic beverage. He discovered the natives along the upper Rio Negro in Brazil preparing it from a liana which he called *Banisteria Caapi*. It is now more appropriately accommodated in a related genus and bears the name *Banisteriopsis Caapi*. Several years later, he quite correctly identified a similar drink of the western Amazon of Ecuador, where it was called *ayahuasca*, as coming from the same species as caapi.

When he discovered caapi in northwestern Brazil and identified it correctly as a malpighiaceous narcotic, he also meticulously observed that another kind of caapi, known locally as *caapi-pinima* or "painted caapi," might be made from "an apocynaceous twiner of the genus *Haemadictyon*," but he saw "only young shoots without flowers." "The leaves," he writes, "are of a shining green, painted with the strong blood-red veins. It is possibly the same species . . . distributed by Mr. Bentham under the name *Haemadictyon amazonicum*. It may be the caapi-pinima which gives the nauseous taste to the caapi . . . and it is probably poisonous, but it is not essential to the narcotic effect of *Banisteria* . . ." (*59*). I have consulted Spruce's unpublished handwritten field notes at the Royal Botanic Gardens at Kew and find his statement that the caapi drink is made from the lower parts of the stems of *Banisteriopsis Caapi* "beaten in a mortar with the addition of water and a small quantity of the slender roots of the Apocynac (apparently a *Haemadictyon*) called *caapi-pinima* . . . ." "May not be the peculiar effects of the caapi," he queried, "be owing rather to the roots of the *Haemadictyon* than to the stems of the *Banisteria?* The Indians, however, consider the latter the prime agent, at the same time admitting that the former is an essential ingredient."

Spruce presumed that this apocynaceous admixture might play a role in caapi intoxication, but he was not certain. Nor did he make any definite assertions, pointing out cautiously that the malpighiaceous vine alone produces hallucinogenic effects. It was the French anthropologist Reinberg who, in 1921, without the benefit of voucher botanical specimens, tentatively suggested the possibility that yajé might be prepared from *Prestonia* or a related genus (*41*). Unfortunately, this suggestion has been taken up, its tentative nature forgotten or ignored, and is being propagated in technical papers.

While we know that ayahuasca, caapi and yajé are different local names for the same narcotic drink prepared from the same malpighiaceous plants, we cannot too lightly dismiss from further ethnobotanical and phytochemical study this interesting apocynaceous genus *Prestonia*, a tropical American group of some 30 species. It is curious that so little is known about the chemistry of *Prestonia*, a member of one of the phytochemically most assiduously studied families of plants (*39*). No alkaloids have as yet apparently been isolated from *Prestonia*. N, N-dimethyl tryptamine has been reported from "*Prestonia amazonica*" (*25*), but there is every probability that this analysis, for which no voucher specimen is available, was made on leaves of a species of *Banisteriopsis* mistakenly identified through the vernacular name yajé as *Prestonia amazonica* (*58*). The possibility that this alleg-

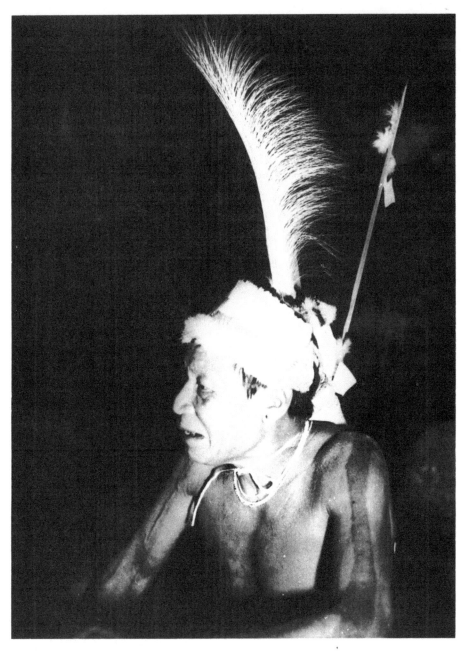

Makuna Indian witch doctor under the influence of caapi (*Banisteriopsis Caapi*). Río Popeyaká, Amazonas, Colombia. Photograph by J. Cabo O.

edly poisonous genus may be the source of an hallucinogenic drug makes the solution of the problem one of both academic and practical urgency.

That there remains much to learn concerning the ayahuasca-capi-yajé complex was recently emphasised by the discovery of the narcotic use of a new species of a genus allied to *Banisteriopsis: Tetrapterys methystica* (*47*).

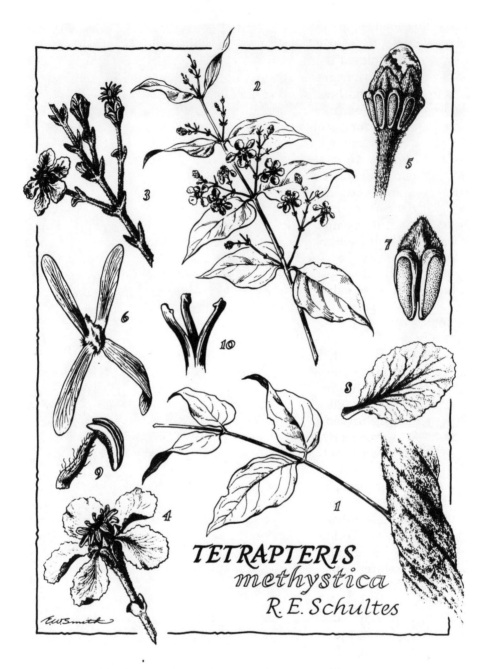

TETRAPTERIS
methystica
R. E. Schultes

It was my good fortune in 1948 to witness the preparation of and take a narcotic drink amongst nomadic Makú Indians along the Rio Tikié in the Brazilian Amazon. The extremely bitter beverage prepared from this plant had strong hallucinogenic effects, was yellowish, unlike the coffee-brown *Banisteriopsis* preparations. It may represent one of the other "kinds" of caapi that Spruce reported.

The identification of various admixtures utilized with *Banisteriopsis* in preparing the narcotic drink represents an interesting and still poorly understood ethnobotanical problem (*19*). In addition to *Prestonia*, which may possibly be added to caapi during preparation of the drink, other plants are known to be employed in this way in sundry areas, and some of these species belong to families and genera that have physiologically active constitutents. It is to be supposed, therefore, that they may alter, sometimes significantly, the flavour and effects of the narcotic preparation. The Siona of the Colombian Putumayo, for example, add what is probably *Datura suaveolens* to *Banisteriopsis* in making yajé (*15*). The Ingano Indians of the same area are said to value *Alternanthera Lehmannii* as an admixture (*49*). I found that Makuna medicine men of the Río Popeyaká in eastern Colombia occasionally use a few crushed leaves of the apocynaceous *Malouetia Tamaquarina* (*49*). One of my graduate students has recently identified a species of *Psychotria* similarly employed by the Kofán Indians of Amazonian Ecuador. A most interesting anthropological report has recently appeared that enumerates five lianas, the barks of which are added to caapi by the Tukano Indians of the Brazilian part of the Rio Vaupés; unfortunately, these plants are as yet identified only by native names (*3*). How many other plants may be used as admixtures throughout the range of use of the South American malpighiaceous narcotics?

Now, what about the possibility of new hallucinogens in the Old World flora? Up to this point, we have concentrated our attention on plants employed in primitive cultures of the New World. As I have already mentioned, the New World seems to be far richer in known hallucinogenic plants than the Old. The argument that the New World flora might be richer in plants possessing psychotomimetic principles would be acceptable probably to few chemotaxonomists, including me. There may be several reasons for this real discrepancy, but most certainly one might be that Old World cultures as a whole seem, at least upon superficial examination, to be much less narcotic-conscious, to feel much less the "need" for these agents in magico-religious rites and in the practice of medicine—and this notwithstanding the great antiquity and probably original basic significance of narcotics to many Old World religious systems.

There must be an appreciable number of problems in the ethnopharmacological search for new hallucinogens in sundry parts of Africa and Asia, but I must content myself with a brief discussion of only a few potentialities.

What is the famous *kanna* or *channa* reported, more than 225 years ago, as a vision-inducing narcotic of the Hottentots who chewed it and held it in the mouth, much as the natives of South America employ coca? The intoxication is interesting, for "their animal spirits were awakened, their eyes sparkled and their faces manifested laughter and gaiety. Thousands of delightsome ideas appeared, and a pleasant jollity which enabled them to be amused by the simplest jests. By taking the substance to excess, they lost consciousness and fell into a delirium" (*29*). The name *kanna* designates, at the present time, in South Africa, various species of the aizoaceous genus *Mesembryanthemum*. While several species of *Mesembryanthemum* are known to be alkaloidal and to induce a state of torpor when ingested, at least one investigator (*29*) doubts that they could produce such startling effects.

51

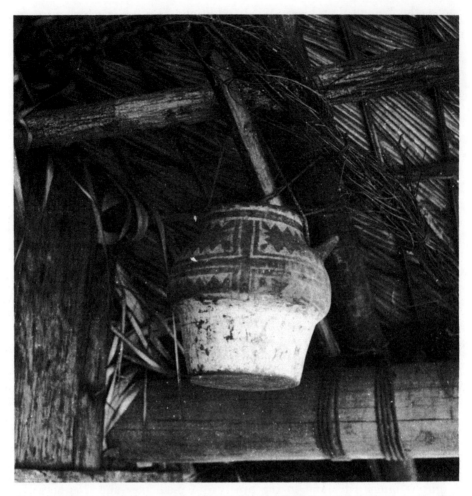

The ceremonial clay pot in which caapi is prepared and from which it is served. The pot must hang always under the eaves at the left front corner of the house. Barasana Indians, Río Piraparana, Vaupés, Colombia. Photograph by R. E. Schultes.

He has suggested that the plant in question might have been *Cannabis sativa*, pointing out, the while, that other plants, like the anacardiaceous *Sclerocarya Caffra*, are employed in South Africa for their intoxicating effects. Here is an area where, because the inroads of civilisation have not been unduly drastic, ethnobotanical field investigation might be extremely productive.

Another Old World genus employed for its narcotic properties is the rubiaceous *Mitragyna*. *Mitragyna speciosa* seems to be the species most commonly used in southeastern Asia, especially in Siam, where the leaves are chewed alone or mixed with the betel quid or else prepared for smoking like opium (*26*). It was first reported as a substitute for opium apparently in 1836, and has cropped up constantly in the literature since that time (*8*). The use of *Mitragyna* is said now to be legally proscribed in Siam.

So much chemical attention has been given to *Mitragyna* in recent years (*5, 40*) that the problems and potentialities offered by this genus are well known. It might, however, be extremely helpful if we knew as much about its use amongst the natives.

Passing mention should further be made of two Old World plants known to possess hallucinogenic principles, but the narcotic use of which by native peoples for intoxication is not well documented. One of these is *Peganum Harmala* (*14*), a rather enigmatic plant that has been placed in the Rutaceae, although now it seems more properly located in the Zygophyllaceae. This species, native in North Africa, the Balkans and from Asia Minor west to China and India, is known to be toxic (*6*), to contain the alkaloids harmaline and harmine (the same constituents found in *Banisteriopsis*), and may have, in addition, a "narcotic hasheesh-like alkaloid" (*6*). Although the seeds of *Peganum Harmala* have proven narcotic properties and figure extensively in folk medicine, going back to the time of Dioscorides, I find no direct references to its religious or hedonistic use as an hallucinogen (*37*). That it may be so employed in Asia or Africa should not be ruled out of our thinking.

Another similarly interesting narcotic is *iboga* of the wet tropical forests of West Africa, especially of the Congo—the apocynaceous *Tabernanthe Iboga* (*61*). Its chemistry is relatively well known, with at least 12 active alkaloids reported, the principal one of which—ibogaine—has effects similar to that of cocaine (*60*). In high doses, it causes nervous excitement, mental confusion, a general state of drunkenness and is a true hallucinogenic agent (*44*). While it has been valued as a medicine and possibly also as an hallucinogen in primitive societies of West Africa, it is not clear that its use as a vision-inducing narcotic was extensive. Ethnobotanical field work is once again indicated.

There have been vague references to the zingiberaceous *Kaempferia Galanga*, to which the natives of several parts of New Guinea attribute hallucinogenic properties (*4*). We know, in fact, nothing about the psychotomimetic use of this genus, nor of its chemical constituents.

The role of mushrooms in the so-called "mushroom madness" of the Kuma people of the Wagti Valley in New Guinea has been, and still is, puzzling. A species of *Russula* has been suggested as the psychotropic agent that suddenly causes individuals or groups to go berserk. Even though the "natives attributed their extraordinary behaviors to mushrooms, several species of *Boletus*, *Russula* and *Heimiella*—or at least most of them—do not seem to cause physiological effects leading to madness." (*24*). I am convinced that much more field work must be done in this fascinating part of the world.

Undoubtedly the greatest enigma in the field of the hallucinogens has been the identity of *soma* (*61*). Some 3,500 years ago, a people who called themselves Aryans, who were the first so to style themselves and who had a right to the name, swept down from the north into the Indus Valley of India. They brought with them the cult of a sacred plant, called soma. They deified the plant and worshipped it, extracting its juice and drinking it. They composed more than one thousand hymns about it, and these have come down to us intact.

What was *soma?* No one knows at the present time. For more than two thousand years, its identity has been clouded in a mystery. For some unexplained reason, the Aryans abandoned the original plant soon after they arrived in their new home, and its identity was forgotten. Other plants took its place as substitutes—plants chosen for reasons other than the psychic effects which, in the case of the substitutes, seem to have been non-existent.

Western civilization discovered the enigma of soma about a century and a half ago when it began to learn about the cultural wealth that India had to offer to the world. Since then, more than a hundred species have been suggested as the source of the original soma, but none of the suggestions has won acceptance. Amongst these, the principal contenders were numerous species of *Ephedra, Periploca* and *Sarcostemma*: the first genus a gymnosperm; the last two asclepiadaceous genera; but all similar in being vine-like, fleshy, leafless or almost leafless desert plants.

For some years now, Wasson has devoted full time to a deep study of the historical, literary and ethnobotanical records concerning soma. He has spent several years in the Far East and much time in European university centers and libraries. We are justified in stating, I believe, that never has greater thoroughness and meticulous scholarship gone into the enigma of soma, for Wasson's avenues of ethnobotanical research have been ingeniously devious and complex. "When I first approached the problem in 1963," he (*63*) wrote, "I could hardly believe what I found . . . a clear-cut botanical question—a psychotropic plant that calls for identification. The clews should be in the Vedic hymns . . . True, the poems contain no botanical description . . . for those remote singers were not modern botanists . . . they were writing for contemporaries . . . and their imagery and terms often elude our understanding . . . But the hymns are all shot through with soma, and about 120 of them are entirely devoted to the plant-god. Was it possible that so much could have been written about a plant, over centuries . . . and its identity not revealed? It was no secret for the poet-priests. How extraordinary it would have been if all of them . . . had withheld from their verses the revealing descriptive terms, the tell-tale metaphors, that the trained reader today needs to spot the plant! But this did not happen. All that has happened is that no ethnobotanist with an interest in psychotropic plants has applied himself to an examination of the texts."

To this age-old enigma, Wasson has suggested a solution: that the true soma was a mushroom, the fly agaric, *Amanita muscaria*, the same mushroom used narcotically today by certain natives in Siberia. All of the many intricately interlocking pieces of indirect evidence gleaned from the Vedic hymns seems to fit in with this clever suggestion so well that Wasson has asked: "Could any key unlock this combination save the fly agaric?" He is now engaged in writing his conclusions and, in view of his contributions to our knowledge of the sacred Mexican mushrooms, of the narcotic morning glories and of the new hallucinogenic *Salvia* of Mexico, we await the completion of his fascinating study with great anticipation.

Guidelines for the Future

The ethnobotanist, especially in his ethnopharmacologic search for hallucinogenic plants, is confronted with these and many more problems throughout the world. Faced with the ever more rapid disintegration of primitive societies and an extraordinary dearth of trained ethnobotanists, science would seem to be doomed to lose. The outlook, however, may not be so dour. Specialists in those fields upon which ethnobotany impinges are experiencing a growing realization of the potentialities of the interdisciplinary approach that ethnobotany affords. There is growing interest in ethnobotanical research amongst younger men going into botanical, anthropological and pharmacological fields. Some of the most startling scientific advances of the past twenty years have been made in various branches of ethnobotany. The future should, therefore, solidly be ours, and our trust must be to prevent its slipping from us.

It might here be appropriate to end with the words of Harshberger, author of the term *ethnobotany*, who wrote: "It is of importance . . . to seek out these primitive races and ascertain the plants which they have found available in their economic life, in order that perchance the valuable properties they have utilized in their wild life may fill some vacant niche in our own."

BIBLIOGRAPHY

(1) ABRAMOV, M. M. "The isolation of lagochilin" [English transl.] Journ. Appl. Chem. USSR, 30 (1957) 691.

(2) ACKERKNECHT, ERWIN H. "Medical practices" in *Handbook of South American Indians*, Bur. Am. Ethnol. Bull. 143, Vol. 5 (1949) 621.

(3) ALVES DA SILVA, ALCIONILIO BRÜZZI. "A civilizacão indigena do Uaupés" (1962) 228.

(4) BARRAU, JACQUES. "Observations et travaux récents sur les végétaux hallucinogènes de la Nouvelle-Guinée" Journ. Agr. Trop. Bot. Appl. 9 (1962) 245.

(5) BECKETT, A. H., E. J. SHELLARD, J. D. PHILLIPSON and C. M. LEE. "Alkaloids from *Mitragyna speciosa* (Korth.)" Journ. Pharm. Pharmacol. 17 (1965) 753.

(6) BLACK, W. L. and K. W. PARKER. "Toxicity tests on African rue (*Peganum harmala* L.)" N. Mex. Arg. Expt. Sta. Bull. 240 (1936).

(7) BUNGE, A. "Beitrag zur Kenntniss der Flor Russlands und der Steppen Central-Asiens" Mem. Sav. Etr. Petersb. 7 (1847) 438.

(8) BURKHILL, I. H. "A dictionary of the economic products of the Malay Peninsula" 2 (1935) 1480.

(9) CASTETTER, EDWARD F. "The domain of ethnobiology" Am. Nat. 78 (1944) 158.

(10) CHANTRE Y HERRERA, JOSÉ. "Historia de las misiones de la Compañía de Jesus en el Marañon español . . . 1637–1737" (1901) 85.

(11) COOPER, JOHN M. "Stimulants and narcotics" in *Handbook of South American Indians*, Bur. Am. Ethnol. Bull. 143, Vol. 5 (1949) 525.

(12) CRUZ SÁNCHEZ, G. "Farmacología de *Opuntia cylindrica*" Rev. Farm. Med Exper. 1 (1948) 143.

(13) CRUZ SÁNCHEZ, G. "Aplicaciones populares de la cimora en el norte del Perú" Rev. Farm. Med Exper. 1 (1948) 253.

(14) DAYTON, WILLAM A. "Notes on harmel or 'Syrian rue'" Journ. Wash. Acad. Sci. 27 (1937) 349.

(15) DE CALELLA, PLÁCIDO. "Apuntes sobre los indios Sionas del Putumayo" Anthropos 35–35 (1944) 749.

(16) DER MARDEROSIAN, ARA. "Current status of hallucinogens in the Cactaceae" Am. Journ. Pharm. 138 (1966) 1.

(17) FADIMAN, J. "Genista canariensis—a minor psychedelic" Econ. Bot. 19 (1965) 383.

(18) FRIEDBERG, CLAUDINE. "Rapport sommaire sur une mission au Péru" Journ. Agric. Trop. Bot. Appl. 6 (1959) 439.

(19) FRIEDBERG, CLAUDINE. "Des Banisteriopsis utilisés comme drogue en Amérique du Sud." Journ. Agr: Trop. Bot. Appl. 12 (1965) 403–437, 550–594, 729–780.

(20) GONÇALVES DE LIMA, OSWALDO. "Observacões sôbre o 'vinho de Jurema' utilizado pelos índios Pancarú de Tacaratú (Pernambuco)" Arqu. Instit. Pesqu. Agron. 4 (1946) 45.

(21) GUTIÉRREZ-NORIEGA, CARLOS. "Area de mescalinismo en el Perú" America Ind. 10 (1950) 215.

(22) GUTIÉRREZ-NORIEGA and G. CRUZ SÁNCHEZ. "Alteraciones mentales producidas por la Opuntia cylindrica" Rev. Neuro-Psiqu. 10 (1947) 422.

(23) HARSHBERGER, J. W. "The purposes of ethno-botany" Bot. Gaz. 21 (1896) 146.

(24) HEIM, ROGER and R. GORDON WASSON. "The 'mushroom madness' of the Kuma" Bot. Mus. Leafl., Harvard Univ. 21 (1965) 1.

(25) HOCHSTEIN, F. A. and A. M. PARADIES. "Alkaloids of Banisteria caapi and Prestonia amazonica" Journ. Am. Chem. Soc. 79 (1957) 5735.

(26) HOOPER, D. "The anti-opium leaf" Pharm. Journ. 78 (1907) 453.

(27) JONES, VOLNEY H. "The nature and status of ethnobotany" Chron. Bot. 6 (1941) 219.

(28) KARSTEN, R. "Headhunters of eastern Ecuador" (1935) 174, 380.

(29) LEWIN, LOUIS. "Phantastica—die betäubenden und erregenden Genussmittel" (1924).

(30) LOWIE, ROBERT H. "The Cariri" in Handbook of South American Indians, Bur. Am. Ethnol. Bull. 143, Vol. 1 (1946) 558.

(31) LOWIE, ROBERT H. "The Pancararú" in Handbook of South American Indians, Bur. Am. Ethnol. Bull. 143, Vol. 1 (1946) 561.

(32) LUMHOLTZ, CARL. "Unknown Mexico" (1902) 356.

(33) McLAUGHLIN, J. J. and A. G. PAUL. "The cactus alkaloids I. Identification of N-methylated tyramine derivatives in Lophophora Williamsii" Lloydia 29 (1966) 315.

(34) MÉTRAUX, ALFRED. "The social organization and religion of the Mojo and Manasi" Prim. Man 16 (1943) 1.

(35) MÉTRAUX, ALFRED. "Tribes of eastern Bolivia and the Madeira headwaters" in Handbook of South American Indians, Bur. Am. Ethnol, Bull. 143, Vol. 3 (1948) 423.

(36) PACHTER, I. J., D. E. ZACHARIAS and O. RIBEIRO, "Indole alkaloids of Acer saccharinum . . ., Dictyoloma incanescens, Piptadenia colubrina and Mimosa hostilis" Journ. Org. Chem. 24 (1959) 1285.

(37) PORTER, DUNCAN M. "The taxonomic and economic uses of Peganum (Zygophyllaceae)" Unpubl. ms. (1962).

(38) POWERS, STEPHEN. Cal. Acad. Sci. Proc. 5 (1873–74) 373.

(39) RAFFAUF, ROBERT F. and M. B. FLAGLER. "Alkaloids of the Apocynaceae" Econ. Bot. 14 (1960) 37.

(40) RAYMOND-HAMET and L. MILLAT. "Les 'Mitragyna' et leurs alcoloides" Bull. Sci. Pharmacol. 40 (1933) 593.

(41) REINBURG, P. "Contribution à l'étude des boissons toxiques des indiens du Nord-ouest de l'Amazone, l'ayahuasca, le yajé, le huanto" Journ. Soc. Amer. Paris, n.s., 13 (1921) 25–54, 197–216.

(42) ROBBINS, W. W., J. P. HARRINGTON and B. FREIRE-MARRECO. Bur. Am. Ethnol. Bull. No. 55 (1916) 1.

(*43*) Roth, E. E. "An introductory study of the arts, crafts and customs of the Guiana Indians" 38th Ann. Rept. Bur. Am. Ethnol. 1916–17 (1924) 25.

(*44*) Schneider, J. A. and E. B. Sigg. "Neuropharmacological studies on ibogaine, an indole alkaloid with central stimulant properties" Ann. N.Y. Acad. Sci. 66 (1957) 765.

(*45*) Schultes, Richard Evans. "Peyote (*Lophophora Williamsii*) and plants confused with it" Bot. Mus. Leafl., Harvard Univ. 5 (1937) 61.

(*46*) Schultes, Richard Evans. "La etnobotánica : su alcance y sus objetos" Caldasia No. 3 (1941) 7.

(*47*) Schultes, Richard Evans. "Plantae Austro-Americanae IX. Plantarum novarum vel notabilium notae diversae" Bot. Mus. Leafl., Harvard Univ. 16 (1954) 202.

(*48*) Schultes, Richard Evans. "A new narcotic snuff from the northwest Amazon" Bot. Mus. Leafl., Harvard Univ. 16 (1954) 241.

(*49*) Schultes, Richard Evans. "The identity of the malpighiaceous narcotics of South America" Bot. Mus. Leafl., Harvard Univ. 18 (1957) 1.

(*50*) Schultes, Richard Evans. "Native narcotics of the New World" Texas Journ. Pharm. 2 (1961) 141.

(*51*) Schultes, Richard Evans. "Tapping our heritage of ethnobotanical lore" Chem. Dig. 20 (1961) 10 ; Econ. Bot. 14 (1961) 257.

(*52*) Schultes, Richard Evans. "The role of the ethnobotanist in the search for new medicinal plants" Lloydia 25 (1962) 257.

(*53*) Schultes, Richard Evans. "Botanical sources of the New World narcotics" Psyched. Rev. 1 (1963) 145.

(*54*) Schultes, Richard Evans. "Hallucinogenic plants of the New World" Harvard Rev. 1 (1963) 18.

(*55*) Schultes, Richard Evans. "The widening panorama in medical botany" Rhodora 65 (1963) 97.

(*56*) Schultes, Richard Evans. "Ein halbes Jahrhundert Ethnobotanik amerikanescher Halluzinogene" Planta Medica 13 (1965) 125.

(*57*) Schultes, Richard Evans. "The search for new natural hallucinogens" Lloydia 29 (1966) 293.

(*58*) Schultes, Richard Evans and Robert F. Raffauf. "Prestonia—an Amazon narcotic or not?" Bot. Mus. Leafl., Harvard Univ. 19 (1960) 109–122.

(*59*) Spruce, Richard. "Notes of a botanist on the Amazon and Andes" Ed. A. R. Wallace 2 (1908) 413 ff. The MacMillon Company, London.

(*60*) Steinmetz, E. F. "Tabernanthe Iboga radix" Quart. Journ. Crude Drug Res. 1 (1961) 30.

(*61*) Tyler, Varro E., Jr. "The physiological properties and chemical constituents of some habit-forming plants" Lloydia 29 (1966) 275.

(*62*) Vestal, Paul A. and Richard Evans Schultes. "The economic botany of the Kiowa Indians as it relates to the history of the tribe" (1939).

(*63*) Wasson, R. Gordon. "A new Mexican psychotropic drug from the Mint Family" Bot. Mus. Leafl., Harvard Univ. 20 (1962) 77.

(*64*) Wasson, R. Gordon. "Soma : divine mushroom of immortality" Unpubl. ms. (1966). Address presented at Peabody Museum Centennial Symposium, Yale Univ., July 14, 1966.

(*65*) Willaman, J. J. and Bernice G. Schubert. "Alkaloid-bearing plants and their contained alkaloids" Tecn. Bull. No. 1234, U.S.D.A. (1961).

Empiricism and Magic in Aztec Pharmacology

EFRÉN C. DEL POZO
Instituto de Estudios Médicos y Biológicos
National University of Mexico

Indigenous pharmacology is always based on empiricism; however, magic procedures and religious ceremonies are often mixed in medical use. When a plant has been found to produce marked physiological effects it is likely than an explanation for those properties is to be looked for according to the substratum culture of the particular ethnic group.

That has been the case for *coca*, "the divine plant of the Incas"; for *peyotl*, "divine messenger"; *teonanacatl*, "God's flesh." These examples show that the magic or religious associations could not be taken as evidence of lack of empirical knowledge. Many times a plant used by medicine-men or priests has been found to be an active pharmaco.

However, the astronomical number of plants, minerals and animals used in popular medicine prescribed by all sorts of medicine men, herb-vendors, magicians, shamen, or used directly by the people, prevents an indiscriminate study of all this materia medica.

An ethnoiatric study (*1*) from the standpoints of social, historical, religious and philosophical contexts, is required for the evaluation of the medical uses of a community. Moreover, even for pharmacology, an extensive knowledge of the socio-cultural background and environment of a tribe is needed for understanding the orientation and purposes in the use of a drug.

The case of Azetc pharmacology is a very peculiar one. A brief history of Aztec civilization will help to evaluate the problem:

The Aztecs were a nomadic and primitive group that arrived in the Mexican Valley only two hundred years before the Spanish Conquest. They had been conducted and governed by a witch called *Malinalxochitl*, and later on by a warrior, *Huitzilopochtli*. They encountered in the Valley of Mexico human groups, the *Nahuas*, of much higher cultural development and with a religion based on spiritual values inspired by the great *Quetzalcoatl*, a god or perhaps a man full of wisdom, who gave to the *Toltecs* codes of ethics and love for art and science. All the *Nahua* groups settled in the Valley of Mexico, inheritors of the old *Toltec* civilization already disappeared, had a great veneration for *Quetzalcoatl*, god and man, father of knowledge and morals. Human sacrifices, the horror of Aztec Society, were not practiced among the *Nahuas* before the Aztec arrival (*2*).

The incongruity of a well-advanced culture with high moral principles as taught by the *Calmecac* or Aztec College, and brutal ritual butcheries, are to be explained by the merger of two different thoughts. One, the Toltec, spiritual and learned; the other, the original Aztec, magical, bellicose and

59

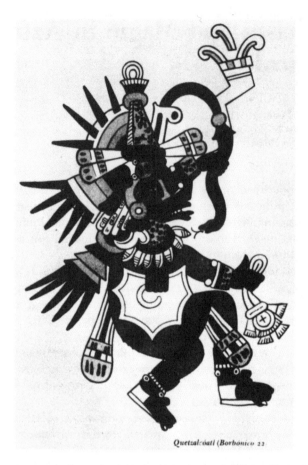

Quetzalcóatl (Borbónico 22

One of the multiple representations of *Quetzalcoatl* (Codex Borbonicus).

imperialistic. The Aztecs brought under their command all the *Nahuatl* groups through wars, treachery and terror, but took advantage of all the knowledge and cultural development of the conquered nations. They adopted the *Quetzalcoatl* title for their highest priest, paid devotion to *Quetzalcoatl* teachings and myths, and kept great respect for Toltec traditions (*3*).

Sahagún, the most eminent Spanish priest who studied the Mexican culture in the XVI Century, said with regard to the Toltecs: "They had great experience and knowledge: They knew the quality and virtues of the herbs, and they left marked and known those that nowadays are used for healing, because they were also physicians and essentially the first in this art. . . . They were the first inventors of medicine . . . So able were they in natural astrology . . . that they were the first to count the number of days in a year . . . They invented the art of interpretation of dreams, and were so learned and wise that they knew the stars of the sky, had named them and knew their influences and qualities. They also knew the movements of the skies through knowledge of the stars . . . The said Toltecs were good men and lovers of virtue . . . " (*4*).

When in 1519 the Spanish Conquerors arrived in Mexico they found a large number of nations or tribes under the tyrannical rule of *Tenochtitlan* Emperor. They were forced to pay heavy and growing tributes, and very often to provide human beings for the continuous sacrificial ceremonies at the Aztec capital. These sacrifices sometimes reached the incredible number of several tens of thousands of human beings, according to several Spanish chroniclers. No wonder that Cortes and their men easily found allies among those subjugated people, who candidly thought they would obtain their freedom.

The fall of the Aztec empire to a handful of Spanish adventurers was also helped by the magic-minded Moctezuma, who had a series of dreams and other warnings about the imminent return of *Quetzalcoatl*.

The complexity of Mexican culture was greatly increased by the arrival of the Spaniards who brought about movements of tribes, displacement of towns, mixtures of people, and emigrations. Terrible wars, destructions of cultural centers, persecution of all people representative of old beliefs and religious and magical practices, were systematically carried out in order to annihilate the influence of the devils. The new religion and the European concept of the world were enforced.

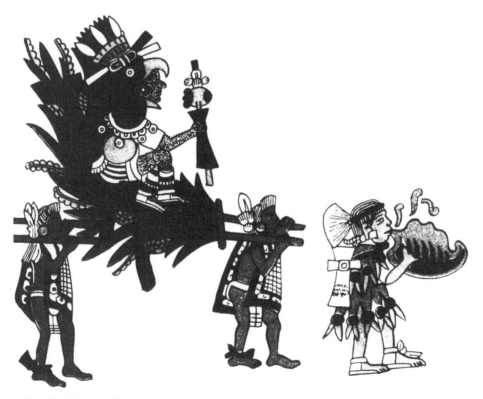

Xochipilli (Magliabechi 23)

Representation of Xochipilli, god of flowers, joy and love (Codex Magliabechi).

61

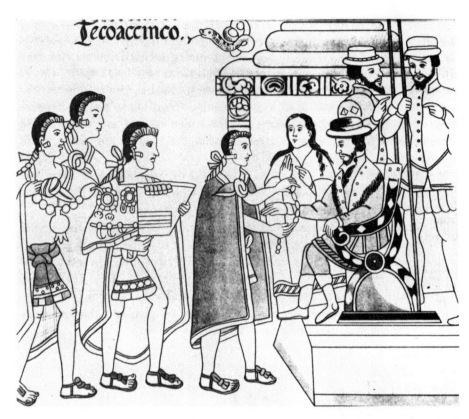

Hommage to Cortés, the Spanish Conqueror, at the time of his arrival. (Lienzo Tlaxcala).

Aztec medicine, as every other field of that culture, was shaken by the arrival of the European conquerors. The most distinguished people who ordinarily set the standards and regulations for the practice of any profession, were killed or removed. The Aztec priests, the most learned people trained at the *Calmacac*, were also killed or prosecuted, and the officers and distinguished representatives of every civilian activity were deposed. All people practicing medicine or any art of healing had to work at their maximal capacity trying to help the thousands and thousands of wounded, injured and sick all over the destroyed towns. Devastating epidemics followed the fall of the Aztec civilization. All books containing their knowledge and tradition in every field were systematically burnt.

Fortunately, the most learned Spanish priests who came to evangelize, had a great need of knowledge of the indigenous "superstitions" to enable themselves to prosecute evil and indoctrinate in the new faith. They went deep into a thorough study of indigenous rites, gods, religions, history, knowledge and morals of the newly conquered people. They learned the native languages and wrote dictionaries and grammars to assist the ordinary priests in their catechization work.

Some of them became seriously interested in the real value of mexican civilization, and developed extensive studies to obtain data and information

62

about every aspect of those cultures. The most distinguished of them, Fray Bernardino de Sahagun, was a true pioneer in the use of scientific methods for ethnological research. He obtained reports from groups of well-selected informers, specialists in every field, and kept protocols in Nahuatl of their statements. He wrote his well-known "General History of Things of New Spain" (4) based on that data. However, only recently have his protocols received attention, and are being translated from Nahuatl into Spanish (5) and English (6).

Another important fact to be mentioned in order to evaluate the information that has reached us is the establishment in 1536 of the Colegio of Santa Cruz de *Tlatelolco*, which was founded with the purpose of indoctrination in European culture of the potentially dangerous youngsters descending from the previously ruling class. These students became very valuable assistants to Father Sahagun and other priests, and even reached positions as lecturers in their own College. We certainly know that one of them, Juan Badiano, was a teacher of Latin and translated the only book of medicine we have that was written directly by an Aztec physician, Martin de la Cruz.

It is evident that Aztec pharmacology at the beginning of the XVI Century had reached an important degree of development: The multiple and well-kept botanical gardens mainly devoted to growing medicinal plants were known and admired not only by Cortes and his soldiers, but by botanists and physicians. Francisco Hernandez, physician to Philip II, collected, described and assayed, numerous plants from those gardens, particularly from the one at Oaxtepec (7).

The discovery of the medicinal properties of those plants was undoubtedly empirical. Contemporaneous chroniclers report that at those botanical gardens the plants were given free to the patients, under the condition that they would inform about the results. In addition to this example of institutional research, we have evidence that the professions of physician and

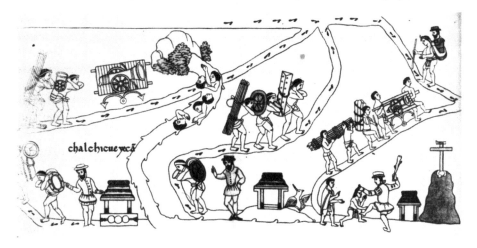

The conquerors receive assistance from local indians for the transportation of all sort of materials, At right lower angle is shown an example of the means used to obtain cooperation (Lienzo de Tlaxcala).

herb-vendor were practiced by individuals other than those devoted to sorcery, magic, witchcraft and religion. We are aware that active plants, mainly those with hallucinatory properties, were used by sorcerers and priests together with their own paraphernalia.

It is a difficult matter to say what part is played by the pharmacodynamic action of a drug, and what is due to suggestion, when psychological procedures are added. The test of healing has always been poor evidence of efficacy. However, in a long run, a conclusion based on repeated experience may be reached.

The plants used in Aztec medicine are mentioned in several chronicles, but ordinarily only the names are given and these in the Nahuatl language. In the case of the Cruz-Badiano manuscript, wonderful color illustrations were added in order to help the European people identify the plants, but even with this data, botanical identification has been difficult. After four and a half Centuries many of the plants contained in the materia medica of the Aztecs remain unknown.

Some authors (8) have thought that Sahagun and other chroniclers gave a too rationalistic idea of Aztec medicine because they tried with the European rationalistic mind to adjust what they saw to what they knew. However, remember that we have the almost *verbatim* protocols recorded in Nahuatl by Sahagun and his mexican assistants, which in this matter coincide with his writings. We believe that these protocols contain an almost literal transcription of the answers given by the informants because, written in Nahuatl, they maintain the peculiar repetitive structure of that language. Series of adjectives, verbs or phrases, one after another, make clear or emphasize the concepts. That style appears in the protocols but not in Sahagun History.

In order to have examples of XVI century European "rationality" in this matter, a few quotations may be useful:

"Thieves knew very well of enchantement, with which they used to deaden or made to faint the dwellers of a house, and then stole everything to be found, and even with his enchantments took out the barn and carried it on his back . . . " (Sahagun) (4).

The enchantments and carrying of barns do not appear in the informants texts, which means that this data is the responsibility of the writer.

"I was called to confess an indian woman . . . because she was dying from a flux of blood by mouth. . . . I had a piece of bone of the Saint and Venerable Gregorio López . . . in a spoon of water I gave her to drink a little of the bone . . . and as soon as she drank it, she felt relief. . . ." (de la Serna) (9).

"There are also some stones called *eztetl* which means stone of blood . . . I had experience of the virtue of this stone because I have one as big as a fist or a little less . . . in this year of 1576 during this pestilence it has given life to many whose blood and life were going out from his nose. Taking it (the stone) in their hand and having it for some time the bleeding stopped and they recovered from this disease from which many have died and are dying in all this New Spain. There are many witnesses in this town of Tlatilulco of St. James" (Sahagun) (4).

Undoubtedly in order to judge the Aztec medicine in its entirety it is required to try to understand the cultural and religious atmosphere of that people living under exceptional conditions of anguish. Their own blood was required to keep the sun shining, everything was under the influence of exacting gods and thousands of major and minor priests were interpreters of the holy designs. Diseases, particularly when chronic, grave or epidemic, were considered as divine punishments for the group or the individual because of deviations from the strict rules of behaviour.

But religious, magical and other psychological methods were also used in order to solve ailments that had not responded to ordinary treatments. Under the circumstances described by Sahagun, one is inclined to believe in the effectiveness of his large stone *eztetl*, to stop epistaxis when that exceptional mineral was held into the tightly closed hand of the patient. The emotional liberation of epinephrine could explain that effect.

Sorcerers and priests used to give to patients and drink themselves *ololiuhqui* and mushrooms to produce hallucinations which would give them leads about the origin of a disease and the way to cure it.

All these facts could give the impression of an impenetrable mixture of magic, religion and empiricism in Aztec therapeutics, but that would be the case if we put together all the resources that present day people many times put in action when they suffer a grave or incurable disease.

Sometimes it is very difficult to decide if a practice is rational or magic, because there is interaction of procedures and influences. The use of amulets, stones, relics, conjures, is not magic any more when they are heavily charged of psychological meaning or had established conditioned reflexes.

Even the classical magician technics based on the use of music (melotherapy), odors (osmotherapy), colors (chromotherapy), dances, cabalistic words and phrases (versotherapy), are not to be disregarded as baseless. Those methods represent sensorial stimulations that could provoke favourable neuro-endocrine reactions.

If we fix our attention to pharmacology the problem has to be envisioned in a different way. It does not matter if a pharmaco has been used by a physician, a sorcerer, a witch or a medicine-man, if we have some evidence of a definite effect.

We know that Aztec pharmacology was based mainly in the use of plants selected by a long empirical testing. Present day laboratory assay has confirmed the activity of many of them. We are now interested in psycoactive drugs. The Aztecs gave us *teonanacatl*, *peyotl*, *ololiuhqui*, *piecetl*, *toloatzin*, already attested in their activity. There are others that have to be studied. We need no proofs that the action of those plants was discovered by empiricism. We would be magic minded if we would suggest that they had reached the hands of the sorcerers by supranatural inspiration. We have no reason for any doubt on what the XVI Century chroniclers tell us about the well trained Aztec physicians with an extensive knowledge of medicinal plants and long experience in diagnosis and treatments. Sahagun said very clearly that they would not use sorcery and gives names of every one of the members of the group that he selected as informants for the chapters on medicine and related subjects of his History: "This relation given above of the medicinal herbs and the other medicinal things above contained was given by the physicians of *Tlatilulco*, James, old and very experienced in those things of Medicine; all of them are in general practice. The names of them and of the amanuensis that wrote it are the following, who, because they did not know how to write, begged the amanuensis to put their names: Gaspar Matías, neighbour of Concepción, Pedro de Santiago, neighbour of Santa Inés, Francisco Simón and Miguel Damián, neighbours of Saint Toribio, Felipe Hernández neighbour of Santa Ana; Pedro de Requena, neighbour of Concepción, Miguel García, neighbour of Saint Toribio, and Miguel Motolina, neighbour of Santa Inés".

It is surprising that Martín de la Cruz was not among them. He was the physician at Santa Cruz de Tlatelolco, Sahagun's beloved College; he wrote the book on the medicinal herbs of the Indians that was translated into latin by Juan Badiano. He could have been absent or dead, but we can not explain the fact that Sahagun does not mention the exceptional and wonderful book written on a subject he was studying at that time and when he refers *in extenso* to that School.

In a study of mine included in our recent edition of the Martín de la Cruz and Juan Badiano book, I discussed this strange fact and arrived at the conclusion that Sahagun might have considered Martín de la Cruz already under the influence of European medicine. In fact, many signs could be found of that contamination, mainly the names of diseases, the pharmaceutical mixtures and even the presence of a reference to Pliny (*10*).

It is a pity that the only book on medicinal plants written by an Aztec physician has to be read with a critical eye, because of European influences. It is interesting to note that *ololiuhqui*, *peyotl* and *teonanacatl* do not appear in the book, either because the use of them was exclusive for sorcerers or because of church censorship. On the other hand, many prescriptions that seem magical because they contain strange substances, now known inert, only means pharmacological mistakes. Lack of activity does not show absence of rationality in the use. Magic implies the performance of acts, pronunciation of words in presence of particular objects, from which only the magician or wizard is capable of managing to produce the effect (*1*). Nothing of that sort appears in the book: medicines could be used by anybody without devices or spells for supernatural powers (*11*).

Magical practices in Aztec society had their own fields and practitioners: sorcerers, necromancers, witches and magicians. However, there are no records of true shamans as defined by Mircea Eliade (*12*), that is with techniques for ecstasy and initiation ceremonies as practiced in Siberia.

Sahagun had left us the description of several of those professions: "The *naoalli* is properly called sorcerer; he frightens men and sucks blood from children during the night" (*4*). "The necromantic (*tlacateculutl*) has a pact with devil; he transforms himself into different animals, and because

MARTÍN DE LA CRUZ

LIBELLUS DE MEDICINALIBUS INDORUM HERBIS

MANUSCRITO AZTECA DE 1552

Según traducción latina de
JUAN BADIANO

VERSIÓN ESPAÑOLA CON ESTUDIOS
Y COMENTARIOS POR DIVERSOS AUTORES

INSTITUTO MEXICANO DEL SEGURO SOCIAL
MÉXICO
1964

Title page of the recent edition of Martín de la Cruz' book (Instituto Mexicano del Seguro Social, México, 1964).

of hatred wishes death for others, using sorcery and many charms against them." (*4*).

The same Sahagun refers to the *ticitl* or physicain in a very different way: "The physician (*ticitl*) used to cure diseases and restore health; the good physician is a knower of herbs, stones, trees and roots, experienced in

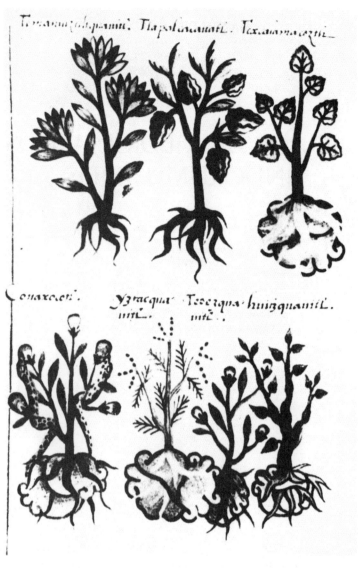

Folio 38 v. of Martín de la Cruz manuscript. Notice the Aztec representation of stone *"tetl"* in the roots of five of these plants.

cures. He also has the profession of knowing how to set bones of people, to purge them, bleed them, to make incisions in them, to sew the wounds and to free people from the doors of death. The bad physician because he is not able, in place of curing the patients, worsens them with his potions. At times he uses sorceries and superstitions to make believe that he makes good cures" (4).

All precolumbian codices were intentionally destroyed, but we should remember that because of the lack of a true written language those documents were only guides for learned people, usually trained at the *Calmecac* who memorized the traditions, history and knowledge of that people. The destruction of that material, temples, sculptures, and every testimony of that culture, was thoroughly carried out for many years with all the zeal of the most fanatical epoch in the history of Spain. The Holy Inquisition soon was prosecuting any man denounced because of keeping in his house objects corresponding to superstition, witchcraft, rites, gods, idolatries and other uses of gentilism (13).

After the Conquest everything related to Aztec culture went underground and declined. When the leading representatives of pre-hispanic medicine were dead or had disappeared, it is natural to suppose that the standards of general practice would deteriorate. XVII Century descriptions of medical practices do not correspond to what had been said a Century before.

This shows the fundamental mistake of people who pretend to draw conclusions about Aztec pharmacology by studying the practices of present day indian communities. Today, Nahuatl groups live in extreme poverty in "refuge localities" far away from civilization; they live in ignorance and poor health. These degenerated vestiges of the Aztecs retain no inheritance from their glorious ancestors. Four centuries of isolation and neglect have left the people without most of the values of their culture; even their physical condition has been affected.

Nobody could expect to obtain from them astronomical or mathematical data, nor to find the marvelous sculptors and architects that left us impressive evidence of their inspiration. However there are investigators who pretend to judge Aztec medicine or pharmacology from the present practices in these deteriorated groups.

Ethnopharmacologic research in Mexico has a great work ahead for exploration of the Nahuatl knowledge and experience with plants. Many writings have not been studied thoroughly. There are documents that have not been translated or interpreted. A great number of plants described under Nahuatl names have not been botanically identified. Some of them, painted with colors in the Cruz-Badiano manuscript, have escaped classification.

Botanical knowledge was advanced among the Aztecs. They had made groups of plants according to morphology, size, structure, fruits and their uses (14). Medicinal plants was one of those groups, but the system allowed having many different plants with the same name. Hernandez used to add to the Nahuatl name of the plant the name of the nearest town where that specimen had been collected (7). The color paintings obtained by Hernandez would have helped for identification, but they were lost in the fire of the Escorial library in 1671. The drawings published in black in the Lincei edition of the New Spain Thesaurus (15) were redrawn from the originals (16). These figures were used again for our recent first complete edition of Hernandez Natural History (7).

A great many of the plants described by Hernandez have not been identified, and now collecting expeditions are planned in order to follow Hernandez' routes in Mexico. It is expected that fresh specimens will allow identification of some of the species described by the Spanish physician in the XVI Century.

FRANCISCO HERNÁNDEZ

Protomédico e Historiador del Rey de España,
Don Felipe II, en las Indias Occidentales,
Islas y Tierra Firme del Mar Océano

OBRAS COMPLETAS
TOMO II

*

HISTORIA NATURAL DE NUEVA ESPAÑA

VOLUMEN I

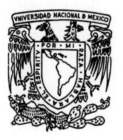

UNIVERSIDAD NACIONAL DE MÉXICO

1959

Title page of Volume 1 of the recent edition of Hernandez "Natural History of New Spain"
(Universidad Nacional de México, México 1959).

Looking for an orientation to pick out active plants used in Aztec medicine we compared different reliable reports. We thought correlation would indicate reputation or general use of the plant. However the results did not justify our premises:

Sahagun mentions in his History 123 medicinal plants and only 86 of them appear in the texts of his informants. This means that he made a rigorous selection and that he used other sources of information that we do not know. The comparison of his protocols kept in Madrid and Florence libraries, showed only 78 plants in common. Of a total of 225 different plants in those texts, 163 appear in the first and 140 in the second. This is new proof of the differences between both manuscripts (10).

When we compared the botanical content of the materia medica in the Cruz-Badiano book, we discovered the surprising fact that among 251 plants mentioned there are only 15 of those included by Sahagun in his History. However, 14 more appear in the Informants' texts. We could speculate about the already mentioned possibility of basic discrepancies between the professional training and methods of Martin de la Cruz, physician at the Spanish College of Tlatelolco, and the Indian physicians put together by Sahagun, who were general practitioners among his folk.

Furthermore the plants that are mentioned in both documents sometimes appear with different therapeutic indications or they are not granted similar interest: *tlatlancuaye* (plants of the genus IRESINE) appear 17 times in Martin de la Cruz, only once in the texts of Sahagun informants, and none in his History.

With regard to Francisco Hernandez Natural History, we should remember that he was an European physician, representative of the medical and philosophical ideas of "humors" and qualities of diseases, and for the "contraries" or medicines. In that way Hernandez described 3076 plants and gives the "dryness" or "humidity", "warmness" or "coldness" degrees of every one of them. According to those European doctrines any plant could be useful in medicine if its qualities were contrary to the nature of disease. Once he says how bewildered he was at the use by the Indians of warm plants against fever.

We know that Hernandez was sent to New Spain to study the medicinal plants in the newly conquered land but he, as a naturalist, devoted himself to a wider field. During seven years, disregarding the royal and urgent requests, he kept collecting and assaying plants and writing his Natural History, instead of obeying the orders for sending his manuscripts. The large extension of his final report and his wider scope perhaps were the origin for the king's decision to entrust somebody else to make an abstract of his writings. That commission given to Recchi was greatly resented by Hernandez.

The difference between the approaches of the writings I have mentioned are evident: Martin de la Cruz wrote about the plants used by him and his kindred Indian physicians; Sahagun strived to obtain uncontaminated information about the pre-hispanic uses of plants by the best known physicians, uses that he described independently of the practices by sorcerers, wizards and soothsayers; Hernandez worked as a naturalist collecting specimens by himself and obtaining information on the spot about the popular uses of the

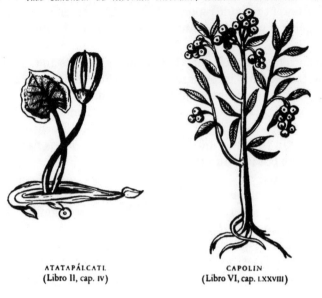

ATATAPÁLCATL
(Libro II, cap. IV)

CAPOLIN
(Libro VI, cap. LXXVIII)

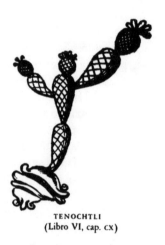

TENOCHTLI
(Libro VI, cap. CX)

Nieremberg figures taken from Hernandez' originals that were kept at the Escorial library. Note the Aztec hieroglyphs for water (*atl*) under *Atatapalcatl* and for stone (*tetl*) under *tenochtli*.

plants. No wonder the reports differ. But they complement themselves if one analyzes the meaning of the data by keeping in mind the wide distance between the standpoints of view.

We have talked about only three of the most reliable sources, but there are many other important chronicles and writings, contemporaneous and posterior. Sometimes late reports relative to cultural and living conditions of

72

TRATADO

DE LAS

SUPERSTICIONES Y COSTUMBRES GENTILICAS

QUE OY VIUEN

ENTRE LOS INDIOS NATURALES

DESTA NUEUA ESPAÑA.

ESCRITO EN MEXICO

POR EL BR. HERNANDO RUIZ DE ALARCON.

AÑO 1629.

PRIMERA EDICIÓN.

MÉXICO.
IMPRENTA DEL MUSEO NACIONAL.
—
1892

Title page of the 1892 edition of Ruiz de Alarcon book written in 1629.

MANUAL

DE

MINISTROS DE INDIOS

PARA EL CONOCIMIENTO

DE SUS IDOLATRIAS, Y EXTIRPACION DE ELLAS.

DEDICADO

AL ILLMO. SR. DR. D. MATHEO DE ZAGA DE BUGUEIRO,

Colegial del de Fonseca en Santiago de Galicia,
y del Mayor de Santa Cruz de Valladolid, su Rector, Cathedratico de letras humanas en la Vniversidad de Compostela,
en la de Valladolid de las Cathedras de Philosophia de Durando y de Prima de Sagrada Escritura,
Canonigo de la Santa Iglesia de Astorga,
Magistral de la Imperial de Toledo,
Arzobispo de la Santa Iglesia Metropolitana de Mexico, del Consejo de S. M.

COMPUESTO

POR EL DR. JACINTO DE LA SERNA,

NATURAL DE MEXICO,
Rector dos veces del Colegio Viejo de Todos Santos,
Dr. Theologo de esta Imperial Vniversidad, Rector tres veces de ella,
Cura mas antiguo del Sagrario de esta Santa Iglesia,
Visitador General
de los Señores Arzobispos D. Francisco Manso, y D. Juan de Mañosca, y Examinador Sinodal
de los mismos Goviernos.

PRIMERA EDICIÓN.

MÉXICO.
IMPRENTA DEL MUSEO NACIONAL.
—
1892

Title page of the la Serna book.

74

the Indian population at the time of the observation, try to refer to the prehispanic society. That error is evident in XVII and XVIII Centuries writings when the old ruling class had disappeared and the Indians, deprived of their land, had been distributed as slave workers to the new owners. New religion and magic, new medicine and superstitions had been imported, and African rites and witchcraft had arrived with the African slaves brought by the Spaniards.

Ruíz de Alarcón, who in 1629 wrote one of the best known treatises on native idolatries (13) recognizes those facts and mentions that the Indians were dying at a fast rate because of bad health and drunkenness a vice not allowed in Aztec society.

Present research requires most careful analysis of data. No doubt we could still find valuable information, but great patience and comprehension have to be used in order to overcome the natural distrust of people that have been subjected to exploitation during Centuries.

Documents on magic are difficult to study. Translations and interpretations are full of problems because of the esoteric language (*Nahuatlatolli*). Literal translations refer to "the nine times beaten" for tobacco, the "red chichimec" for copper, the "red woman" for blood, "one water" for wood, "seven caves" for mouth, "snake" for pain (9). Most of these imaginative expressions have not been explained and many others have not been interpreted. As we say before, magic and its language represent very old myths and such study is full of obstacles.

The scientific study of Aztec pharmacology is very recent and has already given important discoveries. Many more will come if capable people from different fields work together. The personal work of Gordon Wasson and the valuable contributions from people inspired by him, is a good example of what has to be done (17). This symposium on an even wider scope, internationally oriented, is a promising step for closer collaboration.

REFERENCES

(1) SCARPA, A., "Nozioni di Etnoiatrica," Stamperia Valdonega, Verona, 1962.
(2) SÉJOURNEÉ, L., "Burning Water. Thought and Religion in Ancient Mexico," Thames and Hudson, London, 1956.
(3) CASO, A., "El Pueblo del Sol," Fondo de Cultura Económica, México, 1962.
(4) SAHAGÚN, B. DE, "Historia General de las Cosas de Nueva España," Porrúa, México, 1956.
(5) GARIBAY, A. M. and LEÓN PORTILLA, M., "Fuentes Indígenas de la Cultura Náhuatl. Informantes de Sahagún," Universidad Nacional de México, I, 1958; II, 1958; III, 1961.
(6) ANDERSON, A. J. O. and DIBBLE, C. E., "Florentine Codex." School of American Research and University of Utah, Sante Fe, New Mexico, II, 1950; III, 1951; IV, 1952; V–VI, 1957; VIII, 1953; IX, 1954; X, 1959; XI, 1961; XII, 1963; XIII, 1955.
(7) HERNÁNDEZ, F., "Historia Natural de Nueva España," Obras Completas. Universidad Nacional de México, 1959.
(8) AGUIRRE BELTRÁN, G., "Medicina y Magia." Instituto Nacional Indigenista, México, 1963.

(9) DE LA SERNA, J., "Manual de Ministros de Indios, escrito en 1656." Imprenta del Museo Nacional, México, 1892.

(10) DEL POZO, E. C., "Valor médico y documental del manuscrito." In de la Cruz, M., Libellus de Medicinalibus Indorum Herbis, Ms., 1552, Instituto Mexicano del Seguro Social, México, 1964.

(11) DE LA CRUZ, M., "Libellus de Medicinalibus Indorum Herbis," Ms., 1552, Instituto Mexicano del Seguro Social, México, 1964.

(12) ELIADE, M., "El Chamanismo," Fondo de Cultura Económica, México, 1960.

(13) RUIZ DE ALARCÓN, H., "Tratado de las supersticiones y costumbres gentilicas que oy viven entre los indios naturales desta Nueva España," Imprenta del Museo Nacional, México, 1892.

(14) DEL POZO, E. C., "La Botánica Medicinal Indígena de México." Estudios de Cultura Náhuatl, Vol. 5, México, 1965.

(15) RECCHO, N. A., "Rerum medicarum Novae Hispanie Thesaurus seu plantarum, animalium, mineralium mexicanorum historia ex Francisi Hernandez . . .," Tipografia Vitalis Mascardi, Roma, 1651.

(16) DEL PASO Y TRONCOSO, F., "Estudios sobre la historia de la medicina en México. I. La botánica entre los aztecas." Anales del Museo Nacional de México, 3: 137–235, 1886.

(17) WASSON, G., "Notes on the present status of *ololiuhqui* and the other hallucinogens of Mexico," Botanical Museum Leaflets, 20: 161–212, 1963.

Perspectives on the Use and Abuse of Psychedelic Drugs

Daniel X. Freedman

Department of Psychiatry, University of Chicago, Chicago, Illinois

Introduction

It has been remarked that tradition-bound scientists will predictably conclude that the proper use of hallucinogens is for research and medical application; the illicit abuse is for kicks and cults (*69*). Our puritanical ethics are said to prohibit us from even exploring whether the use of hallucinogens could improve the healthy, or possibly transform Western society into a Zen elysium.

Whatever scientists may think, history does indeed record our unceasing urge to transcend limits and escape dreary reality or anxiety with the aid of magic, drugs, drama, festival rites, and (with biological regularity) through dreams. Even though we could doubt that drugs produce pleasure without the risk of harm, and wonder if man is built to sustain and to manage more than a brief chemically-induced glimpse of paradise, we must still examine the data of ethnology, pop culture, and clinical use for real evidence. Do such data indicate that there are drugs which specifically enhance these varied transcendent purposes? If so, how do they, why and how exclusively or to what extent do they work and at what cost? These questions will require

77

more explicit answers and more extensive research than we can presently report.

To discriminate and analyze drug effects, quite imperfect tools will have to be borrowed from a variety of disciplines and contexts: from the social psychology of religion, of deviant behavior generally, of recreation, of social change and self-help movements, as well as the social psychology of aesthetics, pleasure and euphoria, and that of groups and of altered mental states.

We should recognize that analysis of these problems occurs in the context of prevailing prejudices and publicity untempered by rational scrutiny. It already seems clear that whatever the motive for their use, the consequences of these drugs range from isolated awe or benign or even bored surprise, to reported shifts of values to transient or occasionally long-term psychoses, to varieties of religious or aesthetic experience, and to clique formation and ritual. There are now conflicting reports of therapeutic efficacy in alcoholism, depression, character disorders and severe neurosis (2, 12, 19, 57, 62, 66, 73, 79, 80, 82, 87). There is also a mushrooming psychedelic culture. This underlies the tribal motions (or brownian movements) of groups of long haired, barefooted dropouts, and the paraphernalia of fringe fashions, music and art—the trappings and trippings commercialized as psychedelic " go-go." Some serious theologians as well as our peripatetic prophets now seek the drugs as a promoter of love, of religious or self-enhancement (8, 21, 44, 83, 91). Some are sincere and private in these pursuits, some provocative and evangelistic.

We are in any event presented with a barrage of elaborately literate (though not thereby the more accurate) claims. Of course, prophets, seers, gentle and ferocious reformers, acting for good or evil, have often held that special visions were not only their inspiration but their guide. They promise salvation. They also threaten misery to those who do not accurately assess (i.e., agree with) the efficacy of such claims. Truly dispassionate assessment—the exercise of judgment—may, as the elect warn, deprive one of access to the mysteries revealed in special states; thus if one is "in," there may be no way out! The only answer to such dilemmas posed by any cult is exposure to experience, to knowledge and assessment over time—i.e., perspective.

Thus these drugs are often used for a variety of purposes more complex than the simple pursuit of pleasure. In any event, hedonistic kicks can be achieved far more reliably with other chemicals or activities. If we take LSD as a prototype, I believe that in their extreme and most potent form we are examining drugs which influence that complex psychological machinery with which we establish meaning and communion with others. There are few drugs which can so unhinge us from the constancies which regulate daily life, or so clearly present us with data from the "inside world" and from the many normally "inutile" perceptions potentially available to us. Surely, it is tempting to snatch some good from this. It also can do us little harm to place such experiences in the continuum of other states in

78

which a range of sensory impressions and insights revealed to the self are regarded with awe or claimed as therapeutic, or as personality if not world-transforming events (1, 3, 5, 10, 56, 57, 67, 80, 86, 88). Given an ample smorgasbord of effects, claims and usages, we can eventually best gain perspective by concentrating on what—if anything—is common to all of these varied drug effects.

The Drug Mystique

The young—who are being importuned by "friendly" advocates (and the young always have such friends) or lured by dire warnings—are entitled to what facts we now know about these problems. We in turn might learn from their interest, from not uncommon tragedies (of which we are seeing an increase) and ponder the adequacy of our responses to their probings and needs. My own patchwork impression of the growing use of marijuana and, to a lesser extent LSD, in intellectual groups is that these are *by and large* more socially interesting (or irritating) than socially important phenomena. Rather, a drug mystique has been welded to the underlyingly serious shifts and strains inherently experienced by the most potentially unstable group of any society—the adolescent and young adult. That our society and our youth have problems is not at issue. Nor can we determine here whether indeed this generation is a "now" group, tending to confrontations, valuing honesty, love, direct and uncomplicated action, and avoiding ideologies in favor of simple justice; these values—however germane to the LSD experience—were not born from the drugged mind. What *is* clear is that an ideology couched in the language of drugs or pseudo-zen philosophy has been insinuated into youth culture, and by a band of quite articulate writers and vagrant psychologists. These have replaced the old medicine show of yesteryear with an updated campus version complete with readings and alluring arguments, if not pills to sell: "drop out, tune in, turn on." Thus, this mystique has been generated by frenetic advertisements for themselves by the fad and fashion makers and idea mongers, and the press has been ready to exploit each sensation.

The philosophical arguments of the advocates are carefully dissociated from the social consequences of their publications. They insist they have the civil right to take any agent which "does not harm others." Such claims gained their real momentum when a few psychologists who peddled the drug resented the notion that scientific and medical—or at least nurse's—training were required for responsible drug administration; the requirement for such institutionalized "know-how" was viewed as a plot of a smug establishment. This argument, if carried to its extreme, would counsel a case requiring cardiac surgery to refuse care from a trained expert who votes Republican—and to do so, if necessary, on trumped up religious grounds. It seems ridiculous to have to state that while each of us in our infant development has attempted to assert the right to do what we want when and where we want it, every society has shaped some constraints—ranging from some form of toilet training to traffic control—constraints impinging on our private views of our capacities, rights and bodily urges. Such is the uncivil level to which "debates" about the drugs lead! It is, of course, hardly a private matter (and it *is* a civil matter) when such proselytizing leads to a number of drug-related cases requiring medical and psychiatric care for brief or longer periods of time.

The irresponsibility of the psychedelic gurus is demonstrated in the fact that while they advertise the drug as only a part of *their* version of a way of life, they are not in a position to manage the consequences of their ideological schemes. Can they really be innocently surprised if the drug per se is more alluring and interesting to the immature than their philosophical preachings? They may reach certain segments of our youth far more readily than most conventional authorities, but nothing in their performance to date shows they know how to manage or anticipate what they so blithely initiate. Psychiatrists who have worked intensively in private institutions with young borderline or schizophrenic patients are quite familiar with some of the tribal behaviors, excesses, philosophizing, and "freak outs" similar to those which occur in psychedelic cults. "Wild analysis" and "psyching"—probing into one another's supposedly unconscious motives—characterized youth of previous generations, as did self-experiments with hypnosis even in the 19th century.

Scope of Contemporary Problems

The increasing problem of drug abuse in most countries is alcohol, followed by barbiturates, amphetamines, opiates and mild tranquilizers. As I see it, the consequences to national health and social welfare of these drugs are not as yet startling—either in terms of the utility of LSD *or* its harm. Debates about whether to use or not to use LSD are hardly as consequential as the use of "The Pill" in our society. The agent most frequently used by youth for illicit purposes and with lethal effect is the automobile; and the most faithful monitor of the scope of such social problems is the prevailing high insurance rates for young males. I know of no rate changes for medical, psychiatric or mortician's coverage which have been instituted by this actuarial superego of our society in response to these chemicals. This is an interesting generation but they have not yet gone completely to pot! On the campus scene, *interest* in these drugs clearly flies high, but not in the majority of students. "Acid" commentaries are, if not more abundant, more influential than trips. While in the large picture, the scope and pattern of hallucinogenic drug use in our society must be said to be more sensational than consequential, the development of cults and a sharp increase in drug-taking behavior in relatively small, often elite or fringe segments of our society warrants investigation.

Inherent Problems in the Study of Abuse

For opiate use and abuse and for the abusive potential in marijuana (*4, 6, 13, 15, 16, 40, 60, 61, 63, 68*), excellent studies have been done. Designs for the study of LSD abuse could profit from these. It is clear that the motives for experimenting with a drug, for trying a drug, for interpreting the subjective effects of a drug (*81*), and for continuing drug usage and for seriously maintaining it can be quite different. The ability of the habituated to control their intake also varies; e.g., many people have the alcohol habit but control their intake in accord with their social obligations. It is also clear that the population of users shifts; e.g., cannabis users have shifted throughout history even in countries such as India, and before 1910, middle class women were frequently represented among our opiate addicted population. The response of society to drugs differs, often mecurially and rarely in response to sober judgments. For example, over 30 years ago, the Federal Narcotics Bureau saw no harm in marijuana and within 2 years—and with no more objective data—decided there was a menace. The complexities of the drug-taking, drug selling and drug policing groups (who form subsocieties "needing" each other), should be noted. When underworld vendors specialize in one class of illicit imports, they may also market others. Thus heroin and marijuana are occasionally though not usually sold by the same peddlers. This association is a social consequence of prohibition and policing—not an actual or pharmacological link of the drugs. Marijuana users, psychedelic drug or opiate users, "goofball" or amphetamine abusers, are not commonly the same population (although there is overlap), nor has the illicit supply of psychedelics yet been merged with that of heroin.

For the nonaddicting but so-called hallucinogenic drugs, we have much yet to learn about current practices. Only a minute fraction of persons who have taken these drugs could be said to constitute a reliable base for study of long-term users; groups of persons who drift in and out of the category of users are not easy to identify, and are hardly reliable reporters since some are always first discovering the drug while others are experiencing disillusion or worse. Indeed, over the past ten years we have been greeted with fresh pronouncements of new discovery of the effects of a synthetic compound (LSD) which has recurrently startled its takers since it was first known— well over 20 years ago. Scrutiny of the response to the mescaline-containing peyote—known since the last century—similarly reveals cycles of startled amazement as several new groups or persons came to learn of it and adapt to it; e.g., Havelock Ellis and William James (who did not, incidentally, form cults in 1902) (*28, 30*).

Complications for research arise from the current publicity. Selling and propaganda create a bandwagon effect and complicate a sober assessment of the extent and nature of drug use. The hucksters gain attention, audiences and monetary support as they threaten the establishment with love and— long before the fact of truly increased drug usage—announce that hordes of young people are, if not their followers, then independently dedicated drug users. The establishment, on the other hand, must react with irritation or even fright at the announced threat. The head of the Food and Drug Administration has a political hide which can be at stake since he must answer to readily alarmed legislators—not to research scientists. Accordingly, those scientists studying the effects of drugs on brain chemistry and behavior in animals have clear-cut procedures for obtaining and accounting for supplies of narcotics but not of psychotomimetics (in spite of the promise by the FDA in May of 1966 to set up machinery and explicit guidelines). Finally, as the advertising escalates and the empirical problem grows, the young and their parents must enter the debate and assess the claims of value. Physicians hysterically crying alarm rather than pointing rationally to danger join the melee. The use of these drugs in experimental psychiatry to study altered states or the genesis of symptoms or new learning or the nature of brain mechanisms related to altered perception (10, 29, 48, 52, 58, 72, 93) proceeds with National Institute of Mental Health support, but not without severe problems of sanction contingent upon sensationalism and fear in the bureaucracy.

Physicians who make headlines with reports of dire results both lure the susceptible and generate their clientele who are latently worried about what they are doing. Sober medical assessment would be *more* effective—and honest—as a deterrent. It is also most important to sort out the various factors which might complicate the picture the physician sees when patients are brought by drugged friends or in other disorganized circumstances to hospitals for one or another indication. The possibility of complicated drug-taking patterns in such patients, of prior instability if not mental disorder, is to be investigated. In brief, the fact that the drug is a precipitant or concommitant of an ongoing disorder must very clearly be distinguished before we determine anything really definitive about long-term effects (22, 23, 24, 31, 32, 42, 45, 64, 77, 92). If we recall the reaction of the medical community to the psychotogenic effect of steroids, and if we take cognizance now of the fact that these disorders still occur, the difference is that we now know what the steroid psychoses portend; we can predict with more confidence what the results will be and accordingly (even though attending physicians are often uncomfortable) there is little scare literature presenting unevaluated snapshots of steroid psychoses in cross-section, so to speak. As a general public we are gullible, vulnerable to sensationalism and to over-reactions on any side of the issues involving behavior active drugs. This is true also not only of the press, of poets genuine and manqué, but of legislators, bureaucrats, and physicians.

Inherent Problems in Ethnopsychopharmacology

We react with similar responses to a variety of drug-induced experiences, but there are characteristic behavioral patterns and social uses which cluster around one or another drug; e.g., opiates probably do differ not only pharmacologically and psychologically but in terms of patterns of social use from LSD or peyote. Research is required both at the psychopharmacological and ethnological levels to be certain. A major problem exists anytime we study the varieties of so-called irrational behavior. This is that there is nothing intrinsic to the training and practice of a wide number of professionals which equips them knowledgeably to handle and interpret either the irrational itself or themselves when dealing with it. What little knowledge resides within the experienec of psychiatry has not been made sufficiently explicit to be extensively applied by others. If a historian documented the distractions inherent in trying to understand or deal with schizophrenia, with hypnosis, with dreams, or with such questions as religious conversion— and certainly with cannabis and LSD—we would see that it has not been easy for men to comport themselves with the best of rational, let alone scientific skill in these areas. Judgments and assertions, then, have to be continuously assessed.

The sorting of the intrinsic patterns of drug effects from their varied elaborations presents difficulties. For example, the social use of a drug cannot tell us infallibly about the basic pattern of its effects. What Barron, Jarvick and Bunnell (5) called "drug-induced ego disruptions" refers to a wide range of substances which can provide a change of scene, a moment of being out of it, a holiday from the constrictions of reality. A wide variety of agents can shift our normal engagement with the world, producing an altered state. This state *in intself* may promote the release of effects and be welcomed for its novelty value as a remarkable trip from reality. Etched upon it may be a specific pattern of the drug. I believe that LSD extends and accents this primary ego state in a salient and sustained way.

A second complication is that sufficiently strong motives can capture any opportune occasion in order to generate uninhibited or cultist behavior. Thirdly, in case a cultural pattern of drug effects seems at first glance invariant, the powerful role of set and setting should be assessed; for example, the exclusive "Mexican-ness" of Hoffman's visions when he first ingested psilocybin (derived from a Mexican mushroom) is hardly ascribable to a specific chemical action.

Pharmacological factors such as dose, route and dosage schedule, and the form and preparation of the active agent are also critical. For brevity, cannabis can be taken as an example: by and large, the more potent the preparation—the more concentrated the form of the resin—the more psychedelic or psychotomimetic the effects. Panic states, temporary psychosis and paranoid episodes similar to those observed currently with LSD, occur more freqeuntly with the more potent preparations illicitly available in India (16, 17) and the Near East (7). Many abusers in Morocco and India are found in settings not unlike our alcoholic skid rows. The weaker marijuana used here has drastically fewer such effects. Inhalation or ingestion alters the intensity of effects (69).

The pattern of use of LSD is determined in part by the dose-dependent tolerance induced (39, 47, 95). Three or four days are required for its full development or its full loss: daily dosage leads to dramatically diminished effects unless the dose is considerably increased. "Cyclicity" in tolerance (53) is seen with higher daily dosages; e.g., tolerance is lost and regained with every eighth or ninth consecutive daily dose. After a single dose there is "psychological satiation," as McGlothlin calls it, which is characteristic for any single LSD experience: one dose is emotionally sufficient, if not exhausting, for most people for quite a period—days, or weeks, or years.

If we wish to discern some universally basic pattern of effects (37), we also have to consider at what level drug effects on behavior can intrinsically be analysed. Dubos (27), expressed the fundamental notion that even a highly selective drug would react with some structure other than the one for which it was designed; absolute selectivity for effects is a chemical impossibility. This does not mean that there are not intrinsically discrete chemical controls or that chemical reactions within cells are not under exquisite feedback regulations, but the control of integrated sequences of behavior remains a complex problem. Yet, in view of the surprising associations and dissociations of which the nervous system is capable (for example, phenothiazine-induced sedation in the presence of motor excitation) it is not inconceivable that chemicals exist which can produce desirable modifications in components of the pattern of effects of a drug such as LSD. The fact that the indole and catechol derivatives which are psychotomimetic induce a response in brain (altering brain serotonin metabolism and probably increasing the utilization of norepinephrine (33, 34, 35, 36, 38, 43), that most of these show cross tolerance, and that agents—such as atropine or Ditran—producing a deleriod type of response (33, 58, 93, 94), affect brain acetylcholine indicates that we are dealing with agents for which some exquisite biological specificity exists; indeed this is the basic reason for scientific interest in the mode of action of the drug, a search that could lead to critical neurochemical mechanisms. Each of the brain monoamines appears to be lawfully related to specific, largely polysynaptic neural systems and it is not unlikely that with autoradiography (90), and fluorescence and electron microscopy that our knowledge of the involved neural systems and chemical changes induced by these drugs can be more finely specified (33, 38).

Finally it will be noted that most of the drugs mentioned in this conference have had multiple therapeutic usages, from carbuncles to mania. The Navaho clearly seek the cure of all manner of both physical and psychic ailments with peyote. This fact means that the ethnologist must be wary of the extent to which reported effects are specifically drug related. The distinction between symptoms of organic dysfunction and those of bodily discomfort in various psychic states is never easy. We see this confusion in small children; there are quite probably differences in social classes, personalities, and cultures in the extent to which the body becomes a "sentient referent" for the consequences of social and personal anguish. This surely could lead to confounding reports of drug effects.

Apparently where drugs can disrupt normal ego functions they can comprise a polytherapeutics for the so-called functional factor in illness. How this is accomplished is not clear; perhaps through an ultimate shift of attention as in hypnosis; or through the effects of powerful wishes for cure—which observably dampen anxiety. Something as nebulous and as potent as faith and confidence is involved. When we ingest a drug because of anxiety or weakness, there is a monotonous regularity in the "non-empirical" interpretations which may be evoked; psychologically, the drug is seen as a power, either one evoking terror (poison or devils) or one producing sexual, physical or spiritual strength leading to salvation or healing. Accordingly, in reviewing the folk usages of drugs for therapeutic clues and in obtaining discriminative information on the effects of drugs on patterns of behavior, we have to distinguish the general range of effects of ego disruption *and* what is commonly called the power of suggestion. Doing so, we can more confidently focus on what is *specific* about the so-called hallucinogenic drugs, including the ways in which they do and do not enhance suggestion.

The Definition of a "Psychedelic" Dimension

Comparative psychopharmacological studies of the various potent drugs would lead to a better appreciation of the fundamental dimensions of behavior, of the ground out of which complex but related behaviors emerge. That element contributed by *specific drug* effects to the entire picture of drug usage will require more focus. Given such reservations, it seems that the recurrent theme in historical records is that certain drugs are compellingly related to learning, to self-revelation, and that they are involved in some mystical, often ritual, use. McGlothlin notes that the American Indian often states that "peyote teaches." He does not find this major theme running through accounts of marijuana usage (*69*). Again the potent preparations of cannabis are an exception and the milder preparations have been used to enhance contemplative states as well as for a "high". Apparently, there is a continuum of effects along the dimension of self-revealing and ritual usages.

To the extent that there are classes of agents which starkly reveal something about the depths or the dimensions of the mind—exposing these dimensions to our attention—we can say that both use and abuse stem from our amazed response to the subjective experience revealed by these drug states. If this is what Humphrey Osmond meant by the term "psychedelic" or "mind manifesting" for drugs such as LSD, it is an apt though not novel description. There is a wide range of contexts—including clinical disorder in which states of heightened awareness with varying degrees of mental clarity occur, and a variety of initiating causes. The mode of functioning and experiencing called psychedelic reflects an innate capacity (like the dream) of which the human mind, in a general sense, is capable (*10*). The fact that a certain class of drugs so sharply compels this level of function is what so intrigues the behavioral scientist.

A rather famous and wordy Harvard professor noted that drug-induced intoxication "expands, unites and says yes . . . it makes . . . (man) for the moment . . . one with truth." William James (*49*) went on to write that parted from normal consciousness " . . . by the flimsiest of screens, there lie potential forms of consciousness entirely different . . . apply the requisite stimulus and at a touch they are there in all their completeness . . . somewhere (they) have their field of application and adaptation. . . . How to regard them is the question . . . *they may determine attitudes through they cannot furnish formulas and open a region though they fail to give a map.*" (Italic mine.)

Many authors have stressed that the human mind is apparently built with mechanisms for constancy with which to structure and use these fluid and irrational components. Indeed in the most systematic series of neuropsychological drug studies extant—those of Heinrich Klüver (52) with mescaline—the author concludes with speculations about the drug's differential action on those subcortical areas of brain which are characterized by emotionality and variability and those anchoring sensory-motor systems which aid in constancy. The question perhaps is not so much expanding the mind—it is expanded enough—but to see if there are drugs which can enhance a better and more creative coordination among these so-called regions.

The Drug State and its Consequences

So whether we set out on a personal or on a scientific research effort to discover and explicate this order of the mind, whether we examine it by introspection or examine its effects on natives, patients and others, we embark on a search which is intrinsically difficult and fraught with misunderstanding. One can expect nothing else if we attempt to deal with the irrational. In any event, we shall try to describe a multipotential state which, in its most general sense, can underwrite a variety of outcomes: religious feeling and conversions, states of hyper-perception leading to inspirational insights, to psychosis, to exalted states or to behavior or value change.

The more we can grasp some of the intrinsic features of this state, the more we will be able to understand some of its variable outcomes. So if we had little experience with drugs, we might still be able to predict their consequences and understand, for example, why these drugs might be properly called, among other ascriptions, "cultogenic agents." Some of the modes of experience—the styles—which characterize the drug experience seem frequently to be linked to the outcome or to the style of life commonly centered around drug taking: whether this "hang-over" of drug effects is learning or reinforcement of the ongoing trend of goals and adaptions, or based on more complex variables and mechanisms is not known.

Some Features of the Drug State

The sequence of effects following the usual doses has been described elsewhere (48, 78). During the first four and half hours there is generally a clear cut self recognition of effects—an internal "T.V. show" which is followed by another four or five hour period in which a subjective sense of change is not marked but during which heightened self centeredness, ideas of reference and a certain "apartness" are observed. At 12–48 hours after drug ingestion there may or may not be some let-down and slight fatigue. There is no craving for a drug to relieve this if it occurs and no true physiological withdrawal, as is the case with opiates, alcohol, sedatives, and certain tranquilizers.

It is the intense experience without clouded consciousness—the heightened "spectator ego" witnessing the excitement, which is characteristic for these drugs in usual dosages. Thus there is a split of the self—a portion of which is a relatively passive monitor rather than an active, focusing and initiating force—and a portion of which receives vivid experiences. Some people seem to repeat this long after the drug state; standing apart from life or relying on the group to direct events, they turn away from the prosaic world—or else are turned away by society, as well as turned on by the drug. They may find a clique or a group which tolerates this disposition.

During the drug state, awareness becomes intensely vivid while self-control over input is remarkably diminished; thus there is the lurking threat of loss of inner control—loss of control of integral stability—of the "dying of the ego" so often reported in bad trips or in phases of mystical experiences with the drug. In the drug state, customary boundaries become fluid and the familiar becomes novel and portentous. Events take on a trajectory of their own; qualities become intense and gain a life of their own; redness is more interesting than the object which is red; meaningfulness more important than what is specifically meant; connotations balloon into cosmic allusiveness; the limits of sobriety are lost. The very definition of the importance of the external world shifts when most mental activity is absorbed either in monitoring the novelty of experience or in maintaining the integrity of the self. And, after the drug state, we may find more tolerance for ambiguity and a diminished readiness for the quick answer; we also can find an associated inability to decide, to discriminate, to make commitments. Spindler reported the latter as a Rorschach pattern in certain Indian peyote users (89). Such a tendency to avoid distinctions could lead to alienation and retreatism, even if these were not pre-existing traits (as they often are). A certain isolation, or sense of it, tends to occur as a trait in many drug experimenters; the after-effects may emphasize the pre-existing traits. For many the drug experience may represent a beginning which without luck or expertise, cannot easily come to a useful conclusion; neurotic acts also have been viewed as misguided attempts at self cure. Thus many reported immediate after effects of LSD—both good and bad—could depend largely on the motive for taking the drug and in fact could be transient rather than transforming.

In any event, when portentous implications and hidden meanings perpetually contaminate the response to the explicit signs and conventions of everyday life, "focus" and goal directed efficiency are usually impaired. Since judgment is not enhanced *during* the drug state and since isolation or apartness (even when sanctioned by a minority group) bring their own problems, it is clear that persons who continually overvalue the modes of experience of the drug state could develop patterns of poor practical judgment. The consequences of long-term and frequent use of the drug—involving probably 5–15 percent of those experimenting with LSD—would probably have to be evaluated in this context.

Immediacy, Novelty and Creativity

In the drug state, the experience of compelling immediacy diminishes the normal importance of past and future. One's organized anticipation of time dissolves (which may incidentally be why, when properly given, the drug can replace narcotics in dying cancer patients). It also is related to the overvaluation of "nowness," the fickle pursuit of the novel apparent in certain youth subcultures (76, 84). The ability to see old and familiar events in a new light is a facet of the shift in organized anticipations and equally a facet in the poorly understood processes related to creativity. The impairment of goal directed efficiency also carries with it the impairment of integrative and synthetic functions and abilities. Thus the mere mergings of sensory objects (the synesthesias, the plastic rearrangements or the clear focusing upon fine details or usually disregarded elements) is hardly the same as an organized building and arrangement in which "boundaries" are, at some juncture, essential. Creativity requires some use of the drug-induced facility for seeing new meanings; but there is nothing about the drug effect which specifically enhances this synthetic and organizing facility. Indeed as we shall stress, the need for synthesis—not the ability to synthesize—is what is enhanced in the drug state.

"Cultogenic" Actions

An important feature of the state is an enhanced dependence upon the environment for structure and support as well as enhanced vulnerability to the surrounding milieu. With the loss of boundaries, persons or a group are used for such elemental functions as control—for helping one to know what is inside and what is outside, for comfort and for binding and balancing the fragmenting world (10). When one is absorbed either in monitoring the novelty of experience or in maintaining self integrity the major changes in the external world will be overlooked or slight changes will assume a critical role. Persons or objects in the environment have positive or negative value in terms of quite elemental functions: e.g. as threats or as anchors in maintaining control (quite as in the so-called psychotic transference). Persons are self-centeredly seen as objects—not to be related with nor evaluated in their own right—but either to be clung to or to be contemplated in terms of what essentially is a self centered, esthetic or ideologic frame of reference. At best this narcissistic reworking of one's relationship to others and to one's own ambitions can lead to outcomes which are socially valued—wisdom, humor, perspective—but such internal syntheses never guarantee socially pleasant behavior (e.g., non-competitive behavior or conduct which takes an ideal regard for others into account (54). In other words, the claims for a different perspective have to be evaluated both in terms of how this is integrated in the life and in the internal rearrangements of values of the user; one need not argue with the asserted shift in values (although even this can be monitored (72)), but the consequences of this can be assessed.

Thus with the dissolving boundaries of self and outside, with the fusion of self and surroundings some of the strain between harsh authority and personal strivings can for the moment be transcended or dissolved. At the same time there is a leaning on others for structure and control and hence, when the drugs are taken in a group setting, the breach with reality represented by the drugs can be filled by the directive mystique and support of the group. This is, in part, why I have termed these drugs "cultogenic."

"Model Psychosis" in the Drug Experience

The elements of a model psychosis are present. By model we do not mean identity; rather we mean an approach to certain processes which are present to some extent both in the drug state and psychoses; the conditions for either state have similarities and obvious differences (just as do dreams and psychosis (41)). For example, what is impinging on an ongoing perception is a vivid memory of what has *just* been perceived; these co-existing images can compete for attention and thus give rise to illusions. These can be immaginatively elaborated into hallucinations. Similarly, past memories can emerge vividly, competing for the status of current reality. The failure to suppress the prior perception or memory or thought characterizes what Bleuler called "double registration" in schizophrenia or what, in Rorschach parlance, is called contamination. Similarly the failure of identities and categories to be maintained underlies most of the descriptions of paralogic in schizophrenia. The capacity to direct one's focus is impaired; allocation of the source of a feeling, a sound, a sight, or a thought becomes difficult since inside and outside become fused. Accordingly there are frequent "projections" or misconceptions of motives. This tendency is reinforced when one must exercise energy to account for slight changes in the environment. It of course bears upon our thinking about any psychosis to recognize that primary or secondary shifts in the elemental ego functions of discrimination underlie a range of symptoms.

Similarly effects can be enhanced under the drug state but are difficult to specify since several contrary feelings co-exist or fluctuate—reminiscent of ambivalence. Thus euphoria mixed with tension may be seen. Laughing and/ or crying in the first three hours are not uncommon. Subjects later refer to the total state as a pleasant-unpleasant experience. However these experiences are represented, they are evolved from a ground work entailing a co-existence, heightening, and fragmenting of component urges and feelings. With care, one observes that preceeding this there is a primary need for elemental tension-discharge—a welling up which requires laughing or crying for relief. Subjects have to laugh or cry and they then seem to find the appropriate setting to rationalize this; the cognitive and structural aspects of affect seem to follow the need for discharge.

Thus the enhanced value and intense attention placed on the self, the "double registrations" the ambivalence, heightened tension and diminished control all can represent the primary symptoms of a psychosis. The appearance of peak experiences (or acute psychedelic experiences) in psychosis has long been documented (*10, 49, 67*). Thus we have with these drugs at least a tool with which to study the genesis and sequence of a number of familiar phenomena in psychiatry. Whether this can lead us to a better sorting and description of the varied elements which are present in the range of clinical disorders is yet an unanswered question; it is for example, obvious that differences in outcome of LSD states depend upon specific prior strengths as well as varying circumstances. These various elements may also be relevant in the phenomena and outcomes we encounter in clinical psychiatry.

Adaptations in the Drug Experience

Some persons endure all this without evident harm. The spectator ego can simply be interested in the reversal of figure and ground, the visual tricks, or—with higher doses—the spectator is entranced or totally absorbed. The experiencing ego can—especially with increasing dosage—be overwhelmed. At any level, defensiveness can appear; the spectator shuts his eyes and a blind struggle for control may dominate. There are different modes of coping with the drug state which could be called protective. One protection is *not* to fight the experiences during the drug state. An upsurge of the traditional defensive operations may lead to temporary panic even in relatively stable people. This has been reported both in the LSD and peyote cults, and has been observed by medical therapists.

Most people working with the drug (either licitly or illicitly) note that unstable surroundings or confused motives may lead to "bad trips." The attitudes under which the drug is taken are important. The Indians of the Native American Church emphasize sincerity, and the desire to learn, and they link bad peyote experiences with the presence of aggression and competition rather than the setting of sincerity and brotherly love and a willingness to learn. It is striking that when self examination or confrontation with internal problems is the motive for drug-taking, effects are sometimes bad. When problems are aptly externalized or shared there is less panic and subsequent upset. Thus a certain yielding and surrender of ambition and personal autonomy helps some individuals to have a good experience, but this requires if not group support a certain personal strength, or at least a facility. *It also requires stable groups.*

Some people achieve an overall stability by a disposition to react with an astounded pleasure to the whole flux of events. Others are encouraged or equipped to transcend the fragmented disparate elements, letting them flow into the sway of a mystique, or letting them be steered by latent guiding interests or memories. Thus all that occurs is given a tone—or a very diffuse direction. With higher dosages and the increasing loss of the capacity for detailed focusing, the importance of guiding "sets" (music, mystique, affective expectations such as the doctrine of boundless love) is enhanced.

The drug experience is compelling and hard to convey but incredibly vivid, and the extent to which the experience of a specific "trip" is related to outcome requires finer study. So too does the fact that one good trip does not predict a second. Nevertheless the primary changes are the background state from which a number of outcomes and adaptations ensue—adaptations *both* during and after the drug experience. No doubt the rearrangements of reality which occur during this state produce a memorable experience, but one is reminded of Sidney Cohen's remark that most people get what they deserve or what they are equipped at the time to experience as modified by set, equipment and setting (*21*).

The Need for Synthesis

Anyone who has experienced this intense episode must come to deal with it. Our dreams also are an episode in a sequence of states which we usually can somehow integrate into the normal fabric of living; similarly something must now be done with the total drug experience—nightmare, illusion or ecstasy. Some borrow stability from ready-made explanations. Still others will decide that the sense of cosmic comprehension is equivalent to mastery. They will tend to deny the anxiety about the loss or potential loss of control. In any event, when such a profound breach with normal functioning occurs, there is some need to synthesize and integrate this experience, to represent and to cope with it in some way.

Some individuals will isolate it; some will set it aside in an attempt to master it and still others, lacking any other means of mastery, will be compelled repeatedly and unexpectedly, to confront what was experienced. We see this in students who come in for help weeks after a trip.

In others the breakdown of those constancies and habits which normally smooth over the disparate details of our perceptions and actions can persist in benign ways. One scientist experienced his peripheral vision to be enhanced during the drug state; it is not uncommon that there is an equivalence of value for what is at the periphery and what is normally perceived at the center of the visual field. He commuted daily, reading during the trip. For months after the drug, he was bothered by the telephone poles which flashed by his train window. He could no longer suppress what normally is background rather than a compelling figure. Similarly, the unconscious "background" to thoughts and feelings can emerge. (There are numerous anticipatory sets or constancies which operate to keep the body oriented in space and ready to meet the environment as we expect to experience it; the mind provides constancy wherever the sense organs deal with variability. We anticipate or correct for the images on our retina to keep the world stable and ordered; the hand stretched 8 inches before one, may appear small though on the retina or camera it is large. Coming off a boat one may still waddle anticipating the roll of the ship.) LSD appears to affect such perceptual anticipations and more complex regulatory systems. It rearranges our ideas of order. It is striking that prior to psychedelic ideology and experiments with self-therapy, mescaline produced more "perceptual" than self-revealing experiences, but the *mode* of breakdown of constancies is similar whether the self or perceptions are a referent.

The intensity of the drug experience manifest in the change of constancies can lead to a number of repetitive behaviors. Gordon Allport noted that, once the vividly religious state is experienced, one seeks throughout life to recapture its inspiration (*3*). The search for synthesis may take the form of attempts to re-experience the intensity of elements within the drug experience in order to master it. The classic example, of course, is the traumatic neurosis in which, following a traumatic episode in the trenches, the soldier recurrently dreams the nightmare—apparently in order to master it. This has been noted in every major theory of psychopathology since the 19th century. The hypnoid state described by Breuer was one of two causes which he and Freud offered for mental symptoms. Put simply, in a state of altered consciousness where control over awareness is diminished, there is no way to bind the intensities experienced and symptoms may ensue. Similarly, in growth and development, many bits and pieces of impressions, many intense experiences—experiences which for the child are intense— have to be organized in the ongoing stream of developing psychological control, and often this fails.

Repetitive symptoms—such as acting out—may be viewed as misguided attempts to give structure to these pre-verbal impressions and intensities— to restore or find constancies and boundaries. Some experience a "loss" manifest by depression and an urge to recapture the illusionary world of the drug. We know that people may produce vivid consequences or experiences in order to see them in a new light. These are experiences which are presented to consciousness, but what often is lacking is the element of guidance, correction, reflection and structure which leads to authentic self-mastery; this may be the chief source of danger of LSD—the lack of structure and autonomy and the traumatic and potent intensity!

Thus acting out behavior with or without a drug often compels control, correction and guidance, and appears as a provocative accusation against authority. The young do not merely "turn on" themselves but seem to display great anger at the guides whom they feel failed them (indeed the prophets counsel students to "turn on" their parents—one of their metaphors which is most likely *not* to be concretely interpreted). Displacing the total experience and the anxieties inherent in it by attacks upon the establishment, they thereby keep a link—and a very strong one—to the very strictures which had previously absorbed them (just as a misbehaving child is tied to his parents by evoking their involved irritation or punishment). Others show delayed panic, depression or anxiety, and seek out friends for help, and still others aggressively talk about their experience as if they were trying to put it together. Some kind of continuity with the gap in reality is sought for. The bridge may be a book as it was with Huxley, a silent synthesis or change of values and tastes, or the understanding of a group or person. In the Native American Church, the Indian utilizes all these elements—religious explanation and adherence, specific ceremonies and the group with its ideology—to integrate the experience which serves a purpose in the total fabric of his life. It has been speculated that during the ceremonies, by borrowing the strength of "father peyote" and experiencing an enhancement of self, he transcends personal anxiety and inadequacy. Some sects are tutored to ignore the visions and disparate elements of the drug state to achieve this higher cosmic state. The Indian does not accordingly seek a simple "high" or thrill with the drug (*1, 55, 86*).

For some, denial of inadequacy and enhanced omnipotence—delusional autonomy—may lead to various outcomes: that of the benevolent and foolish prophet, or the defensive, alienated therapist, angry at those who prevent his curing the rest of the world. Indeed we must seriously wonder why those who find salvation are so generous and so ready to proselytize and advertise! Implied are unsolved problems with authority figures. In any event it appears that salvation often involves renunciation of previous ties and that those who are saved must repetitively convince others in order to diminish their own doubt, isolation and guilt. At best, they may do this in order to reachieve union with those with whom they have been separated by their unique vision and experience, and to synthesize these breaches with important others.

The Role of Groups in Synthesis

We have referred to the strain between the exertion of personal strivings for autonomy (i.e., needs to order reality and influence the world) and internal authority (the voice of conscience). Certain groups seem built to absorb this strain. Many successful self-help groups appear to be peer groups. With such arrangements the distance between authority and the miscreant (reminiscent of that between parent and child) is diminished and so too is the inner tension. The cost is a surrender of certain order of autonomy to the group and dependence upon it. It may be less painful to drop pretense and to permit less masking of inadequacy in the presence of uncritical and non-threatening peers. Of course there may also be a tendency to externalize the conflict with authority, a tendency reinforced by peer-grouping. Still this can permit authentic self involvement at a level which is realistically available to the persons involved.

Ideally, autonomy and involvement might mean not to be distracted by arguments with authority; such terms should connote putting oneself in the place of authority—not imitatively—but in terms of real commitments involving risk, initiative and responsibility. To some extent self-help groups can aid members to move in these directions. Yet, such adjustments mean relying heavily on the concrete presence and reinforcement of a sane group which shares the burdens of initiative. This is not always achieved. In some chronic users one sees a bland impulsiveness—an indifference to the habitual and customary which may border on a supercilious posture of superiority. The elect of many cults either assume the attitude or the outsider *feels* this to be the attitude of those who know something he does not. This posture has also been remarked upon in the American Indian peyote users, although they, too (as with the Navaho), are often subcultures not infrequently at odds with established groups and leaders (*1*).

Group sanctioning of the drug state can diminish the intensity and isolation; the group mystique tends to give integration through a credible rendition, if not sanction to events which by their very nature cannot easily be translated into public language. The mystique may not be more descriptive of the drug state but simply apparently precise and sufficiently allusive to serve as a representation of and compensation for the breach with reality.

Mystical or religious representations also are remarkably apt for synthesizing the experience. Religion relates man to his limits while taking account of his boundlessness which occurs in all aspects of this realm of the mind. It may be that religious symbolism aptly represents the transformations characteristic of this latent part of the mind. Against fragmentation and directionlessness something coherent lends continuity to experience. Against dread, transcendent love can prevail; loving like redness can apparently be enhanced and is remembered. The "lovingness" and "strongness" of a parent can be parted from the particular persons and transcendentally represented in various forms of power ascribed to deities.

Use and Abuse of Conversion

There are, then, a number of features of this multipotential state related to its intensity, its novelty, its boundlessness which account for some of the expectable occurrences within it and some of the expectable—and observed—dangers and outcomes. There are observations about the uses and abuses of religous conversion which are not dissimilar from what we can describe in the current drug scene.

In Clark's topology (20), the outcomes can be: a sudden change of role—he calls this abrupt conversion. Another outcome entails an allegiance to values rather than a behavior change; e.g., adolescents who are converted to their parents' religion. Similarly there are student LSD users who talk like psychedelicists but continue to be headed for a career of suburbia and the office. Gradual conversion entails what Clark calls role assimilation (and this is reminiscent of the more protracted therapies). There are clearly various levels of personality which can be involved either in the drug experience or in conversion experience. Classifications of pathological outcomes of conversion (including irresponsibility and omniscience) startlingly resemble patterns we see with LSD (20, 88).

Even the conversion experience, if we follow Christiansen's description (18), is not dissimilar from that described by therapists who have worked with LSD. He notes a pre-conversion conflict which reaches a peak, a moment of "giving up" (an intention to cease the struggle) which can be followed by an opportunity to come up with a new solution. The conflict must become sufficiently accessible to that part of the mind which can organize and synthesize it in religious terms. If this did not happen there might be a confrontation of old intensities and strivings and continuing struggle rather than yielding and reworking (very much as we described in the instance of acting out behavior). Such struggles in which past experience must be disowned yield pathologically defensive behavior, and symptoms easily ensue; there would be a lack of coherence of the personality which the conversion experience might achieve.

94

LSD in Psychiatry

There are a number of psychotherapists who have attempted to use the loosening of associations *and* the intense experiencing produced by the drug in order to influence behavior change. Yet the history of LSD therapy by physicians represents a picture of both use and abuse. In the late 1950's many physicians were not only struck by the drug-induced phenomena, but apparently addled by them. Perhaps they were simply jealous of the subject when they insisted upon taking the drug concurrently with him. They certainly discovered a reality of the mind, but it was a region of mental activity about which they were supposed to be expert prior to the advent of these drugs. When a therapist in our culture has little sense of intellectual control over the events he is monitoring, we are dealing with a healing cult; what is rational about therapy is our obligation to study and control that with which we work. Critical observation and empathy have led us as far as we are in our present dealing with schizophrenia; there is no evidence that any further progress has been made by those therapists who insisted on being drugged themselves.

There are a number of ongoing controlled projects in this country and a long history of experience with the use of LSD in therapy. Two major modes of treatment prevail. The treatment employed by many European workers (often called "psycholytic") represents a method by which certain defenses are breached. With a strong drug-enhanced tie to the therapist, feelings and memories are allowed to emerge vividly and unforgetably before the eye of consciousness and their strength discharged. The events are later worked over with care. Dosages are regulated in part by the capacity of the patient to steer a course between being utterly lost on the one hand or overly constrained by habitual defenses on the other. A kind of active participation in the presence of a general loosening is sought. The need for a certain autonomy and directiveness, a certain inner capacity to integrate and pull together at least a part of the experience is recognized. The integration which follows is a collaborative venture requiring the active participation and the output of the patient (2). Yet how to reinforce any shifts in attitude which occur with the drug without running the risk of often repeated drug sessions is a largely unstudied issue.

In the so-called psychedelic therapies as they are now being tested, there is an awareness of an immense amount of preparation, of salesmanship with an evangelical tone in which the patient is confronted with hope and positive displays of it, before he has his one great experience with very high doses of drug. The experience is structured by music and by confident good feelings. With the support of the positive therapist throughout this experience, the patient is encouraged to see his life in a new light, to think of his future accordingly. There now tends to be a rather long period of follow-up and support before the patient is discharged. An earlier mode of intervention attempted to avoid the tangled problems of relationship between therapist and patient with one single high dose drug session as the chief therapeutic contact; the current approach is more explicitly ritualized (in the model of nativistic movements), and the person and attitude of the therapist tends not to be analyzed but incorporated. It is speculated that the egocentric problems of the alcoholic may be specifically tailored for this ego-dissolving, ego-building technique. Other approaches lie somewhere between these two. It is interesting that peyote cultures also report cures of alcoholics, but the effects may not persist without sustained group support and leadership. The efficacy and selectivity of current therapies is far from settled and research is still ongoing (2). Obviously careful follow-up is essential, since the immediate glow which occurs with drug-induced personality change can be deceptive.

Abuse of LSD

I have noted my current opinion that the chief abuse of LSD is irresponsible, alluring and provocative advertising. We are surely at an advanced enough stage of our culture to identify folly and even to study it. Professor McClelland at Harvard (44) noted some of the effects upon the research of the psychedelic fanatics at the height of their proselytising in the early 1960's. He documented certain features of their research which appeared to be related to the drug state. Of course whether poor research is to be considered a drug abuse is a moot point, but some of the features noted were a high opinion of their own profundity; dissociation and detachment—a feeling of being above and beyond the normal world of social reality; interpersonal insensitivity; omniscience and philosophical naivete—a simplistic satisfaction in visions. Finally he noted impulsivity which might be seen as intolerance of any limits, questions or skepticism, let alone inability to predict the consequences of irresponsible, provocative actions. These consequences of drug taking observed in the very home of transcendentalism have been observed in other settings; perhaps we are delineating one intrinsic pattern of outcome of extensive, repeated LSD use. While such descriptions may give us a guide for future research, conclusive and analytical studies simply are not available.

In a few current illicit self-help groups the drugs surprisingly are used reportedly to achieve a conventional outcome. A group of ex-convicts— allegedly—require that members have an honest job before becoming part of the LSD-taking religious group. Similarly one group of homosexuals are reported to use illicit LSD to enhance heterosexual behavior. Several groups, recognizing that overly frequent use might have insidious and profound effects on judgment and that careless use can lead to dangerous panic, have set up agencies to be phoned when required. We seem to be living in an era when many practices (half-way houses, group therapies, "cathartic" therapy) built into the fabric of psychiatric work are imitated by self-help groups. If these lay LSD groups learn from experience, they will do so with even less guidance and self critical checks than the professionals have had in coping with adolescent confusion and turmoil and even the more serious dysfunctions. It is the patient who pays for such experimentation by the gurus. On the other hand, other organizations such as Alcoholics Anonymous have continued to evolve patterns of response to the problems with which they are concerned without damage to their adherents; members are free to get whatever professional help they need. The discipline of abstention and the general reality orientation of this group is important.

From the evidence available, it appears that users who end up in hospitals with prolonged and serious psychoses are initially a quite unstable group. They are, in any event, a small group. More frequently one sees a transient panic occurring during the drug state, from which recovery is generally rapid. Others who have come to the attention of physicians do not require hospitalization but often seek treatment because they are nervous or concerned about having taken the drug, or about some of their thoughts and experiences during the drug state. And a few others as noted may have non-drug induced panics some weeks after the drug state very much as a bad dream recurs. It is somewhat easier within a college population to get some gauge on the prior adjustment of the students. Certainly there are a group of students, even some of the repeaters, who appear relatively stable (9, 51, 65, 71, 74, 75).

Motives for Use

The motives for LSD use are varied. Sociologists refer to problems of commitment and alienation and at least add thereby to the younger generation's verbal mythology. A "need to feel"—to gain access to themselves and others—a pervasive sense of being constricted, seems to characterize some of the college takers I have studied. In a recent report (9) of a group in which Rorschach and other studies were available, this theme dominated even though outcomes sharply differed: these ranged from psychosis, to instability, to a reaction of bemused enlightenment. Some college students clearly tried the drug as a part of clique activity; thanks in part to sustained advertising, drugs and drug talk are a part of a student's vocabulary. Taking the drug puts the student one-up—he has "been there". This is a challenge evoking interest among friends and can provide the basis for a loose group cohesion. Others sincerely feel they should confront an experience advertised to be so important. They see the drug as an emotional fitness test, somewhat analogous to physical fitness. The issue for many is "control". They experiment with the right to drink and test their ability to stop. At this age they are doing the same, often, with cigarette smoking or with masturbation. In general they are rehearsing their strength and autonomy at a time when their lives are largely unwritten. Many behaviors of this age constitute a probing for consequences—an attempt to come to grips with life and to seize the fruits and risks promised in the future, the threshold of which is now visible. This underlies many of the grimmer statistics of the 18–25 age group, including accidents and suicide. One wonders if these represent the inevitable costs of learning the lesson of consequences, of limits, of mortality.

Summary View of the Value of Psychedelic Drugs

In psychiatry we know something about how to use drugs to cope with grossly inadequate functioning and to compensate for deficit states. With respect to the LSD experience, we know that many serious persons have reported some transient or even long-term value in it. They say their æsthetic appreciation is enhanced, and McGlothlin indeed has some evidence for a slight shift of this sort in some but not all of a group of normal subjects (70). If though, we search for major productions of art, letters, music or visionary insight, few clear cut monuments to the drug are available. Related to creativity, the effects of the drug do not seem to have compelled it. Huxley's greatest output preceded his mescaline states; he thereafter, as I read him, tended to write *about* drugs, not to create with them. If we ask whether there have been cultures which have eradicated mental disorders and disease with these drugs, or groups which have seen the dissolution of deviant behavior or even deviant drug-linked behaviors (for example, alcoholism), we find some slight association but no clear cut overall differences that I know of in the general titre of human misery. In fact the use of these drugs is often associated with some form of psychosocial deprivation—or (equally) with marked privilege (as in Brahmins and college students). That private satisfactions might have been achieved, that groups with the presence of these plants could have attained some spiritual equilibrium seems apparent, but whether the plants and their effects are both necessary and sufficient to get such results— whether no alternative means exist within a culture—is another question.

We should not forget to assess the cost of sustained euphoria or pleasure states; we have to wonder whether the mind of man is built to accommodate an excess either of pleasure or of over-rationality. We do not know whether or not there are individuals with sufficient strength to take these drugs for growth or pleasure within the social order without enhanced and credulous alienation from it. Is a stable person really under sufficient control of his motives and shifting circumstance, let alone the dosage, to take these drugs as a civil right for whatever personal reasons he wishes? If so, who has to care for the consequences of his misjudgments? Some side effects cannot be avoided if we are correct about the way the mind is built, and if we learn from the effects of drugs on much simpler biological systems. How can the stability of religious custom protect drug takers who have little authentic orientation to religion and unstable groups and barely reliable leaders upon whom to lean?

Thus etched upon the variabilities of culture and personality are drugs with a certain skew toward that mystical realm of the mind which knows both psychosis and religion, both heightened and useful self insight, and impaired and distorted judgment about the everyday world. Perhaps similarities and differences of these various plants and their effects could—if analyzed—reveal means for finer control of these experiences—at least in terms of their intensities. Some research should point towards elucidation of critical neurochemical mechanisms.

In general, it seems to me that we have been more awed than aided by our experience with these drugs. They still remain agents which reveal but do not chart the mental regions; to do that we must employ our mental faculties available in the undrugged state. Accordingly we should do better than repeat the ontogeny of past encounters with mind revealing drugs. We should strive to make distinctions so that—at some future date—if we knew how the elements of mind really were related, we could specify for the chemist the designs he should seek in nature. But to begin with we have to learn to analyze how behavior is organized, and to see what nature can teach us about the ways in which the chemical organization of the brain is related to the dimensions of mind.

REFERENCES

(1) ABERLE, DAVID F., "The Peyote Religion Among the Navaho," Chicago: Aldine Publishing Company, 1966.

(2) ABRAMSON, H. A. (ed.), "The Use of LSD in Psychotherapy and Alcoholism," Indianapolis: Bobbs Merrill, 1967.

(3) ALLPORT, GORDON, W., "The Individual and His Religion," New York: Macmillan, 1950.

(4) AMES, F., "A Clinical and Metabolic Study of Acute Intoxication with Cannabis Savita and Its Role in the Model Psychoses", J. Mental Sci 104: 972–999, 1958.

(5) BARRON, F., JARVIK, M. E. and BUNNELL, S., Jr., "Hallucinogenic Drugs", Scientific American 210: 29–37, 1964.

(6) BECKER, H. S., "Becoming a Marihuana User", Amer. J. of Sociol. 59: 235–242, 1953.

(7) BENABUD, A., "Psycho-pathological Aspects of the Cannabis Situation in Morocco: Statistical Data for 1956", Bulletin on Narcotics, 9: No. 4, 1–16, 1957.

(8) BLUM, R., (ed.), "Utopiates, the Use and Users of LSD-25, New York: Atherton Press, 1964.

(9) BOWERS, M., CHIPMAN, A., SCHWARTZ, A., and DANN, O. T. "Dynamics of Psychedelic Drug Abuse—A Clinical Study", Archives of General Psychiatry 1967 (in press).

(10) BOWERS, M. B. and FREEDMAN, D. X., " 'Psychedelic' Experiences in Acute Psychoses", American Medical Association Archives of General Psychiatry 15: No. 3, 240, 1966.

(11) BOWERS, M. B., HARTMANN, E. L. and FREEDMAN, D. X., "Sleep Deprivation and Brain Acetylocholine", Science 153: No. 3742, 1416, 1966.

(12) CHANDLER, A. L. and HARTMAN, M. A., "Lysergic Acid Diethylamide (LSD-25) as a Facilitating Agent in Psychotherapy", Archives of General Psychiatry 2: 286–299, 1960.

(13) CHAREN, S. and PERELMAN, L., "Personality Studies of Marihuana Addicts", American Journal of Psychiatry 102: 674–682, 1946.

(14) CHEEK, FRANCES E., "Exploratory Study of Drugs and Social Interaction", Archives of General Psychiatry 9: 566–574, 1963.

(15) CHEIN, I., GERARD, D. L., LEE, R. S. and ROSENFELD, E., "The Road to H", New York: Basic Books, 1964.

(16) CHOPRA, I. C. and CHOPRA, R. N., "The Use of Cannabis Drugs in India", Bulletin on Narcotics 9: No. 1, 4–29, 1957.

(17) CHOPRA, R. N. and CHOPRA, I. C., "Treatment of Drug Addiction: Experience in India", Bulletin on Narcotics 9: No. 4, 21–33, 1957.

(18) CHRISTIANSEN, C. W., "Religions Conversion", American Medical Association Archives of General Psychiatry 9: 207, 1963.

(19) CHWELOS, N., BLEWETT, D. B., SMITH, C. M. and HOFFER, A., "Use of D-Lysergic Acid Diethylamide in the Treatment of Alcoholism", Quart. J. Stud. Alcohol. 20: 577–590, 1959.

(20) CLARK, W. H., "The Psychology of Religion," New York: Macmillian, 1958.

(21) COHEN, S., "The Beyond Within," New York: Atheneum, 1964.
(22) COHEN, S. and DITMAN, K. S., "Complications Associated With Lysergic Acid Diethylamide (LSD-25)", Journal of American Medical Association 181: 161-162, 1962.
(23) COHEN, S. and DITMAN, K. S., "Prolonged Adverse Reactions to Lysergic Acid Diethylamide", Archives of General Psychiatry 8: 475-480, 1963.
(24) COLE, J. O. and KATZ, M. M., "The Psychotominetic Drugs, An Overview", Journal of American Medical Association 187: 758-761, 1964.
(25) DEIKMAN, A. J., "Experimental Meditation", Journal of Nervous and Mental Disease 136: 329-343, 1963.
(26) DOZIER, EDWARD P., "Problem Drinking Among American Indians", Quart. J. Stud. Alcohol. 27: No. 1, 72-87, 1966.
(27) DUBOS, R., "On the Present Limitations of Drug Research", Drugs in Our Society edited by Paul Talalay, Baltimore, Maryland: The Johns Hopkins Press, 1964.
(28) Editorial, "Paradise or Inferno?", British Med. J., 1898, p. 390.
(29) EGGERT, D. C and SHAGASS, C., "Clinical Prediction of Insightful Response to a Single Large Dose of LSD", Psychopharmacologia (Berl.) 9: 340-346, 1966.
(30) ELLIS, H., "Mescal: A New Artificial Paradise", Contemporary Rev. 73: 130-141, 1898.
(31) FINK, M., SIMEON, J., HAQUE, W. and ITIL, T., "Prolonged Adverse Reactions to LSD in Psychotic Subjects", Archives of General Psychiatry 15: 450-454, 1966.
(32) FINK, P. J., GOLDMAN, M. J. and LYONS, I., "Morning Glory Seed Psychosis", Archives of General Psychiatry 15: 1966.
(33) FREEDMAN, D. X., "Aspects of the Biochemical Pharmacology of Psychotropic Drugs", Psychiatric Drugs, p. 32, P. Solomon (ed.), New York: Grune and Stratton, Inc., 1966.
(34) FREEDMAN, D. X., "Effects of LSD-25 on Brain Serotonin", J. Pharmacol. Exptl. Therap. 134: 160, 1961.
(35) FREEDMAN, D. X., "LSD-25 and Brain Serotonin in Reserpinized Rat", Fed. Proc. 19: 266, 1960.
(36) FREEDMAN, D. X., "Psychotomimetic Drugs and Brain Biogenic Amines", American Journal of Psychiatry 119: 843, 1963.
(37) FREEDMAN, D. X., "Toward A Systematic Psychopharmacology", Internat. J. Psychiat. 2: No. 6, 666-670, 1966.
(38) FREEDMAN, D. X., and AGHAJANIAN, G. K., "Approaches to the Pharmacology of LSD-25", Llyodia 29: No. 4, 309, 1966.
(39) FREEDMAN, D. X., AGHAJANIAN, G. K., ORNITZ, E. M. and ROSNER, B. S.,, "Patterns of Tolerance to Lysergic Acid Diethylamide", Science 127: 1173, 1958.
(40) FREEDMAN, H. L. and ROCKMORE, M. J., "Marihuana, Factor in Personality Evaluation and Army Maladjustment", J. Clin. Psychopathology 7 & 8: 765-782 & 221-236, 1946.
(41) FREUD, S., "An Outline of Psychoanalysis," New York: W. W. Norton & Co., Inc., 1949.
(42) FROSCH, W. A., ROBBINS, E. S. and STERN, M., "Untoward Reactions of Lysergic Acid Diethylamide (LSD) Resulting in Hospitalization", New. Eng. J. Med. 273: 1235-1239, 1965.
(43) GIARMAN, N. J. and FREEDMAN, D. X., "Biochemical Aspects of the Actions of Psychotomimetic Drugs", Pharmacol. Rev. 17: 1, 1965.
(44) GORDON, NOAH, "The Hallucinogenic Drug Cult", The Reporter, August 15, 1963.
(45) GRINKER, R. R., "Bootlegged Ecstasy", Journal of American Medical Association, 187: 768, 1964.
(46) HUXLEY, A., "The Doors of Perception," New York: Harper Brothers, 1954.
(47) ISBELL, H. et al., "Cross Tolerance Between LSD and Psilocybin", Psychopharmacologia 2: 147-159, 1961.
(48) ISBELL, H. et al., "Studies on Lysergic Acid Diethylamide (LSD-25)", Arch. Neurol. Psychiat. 76: 468-478, 1956.

(49) JAMES, W., "Varieties of Religious Experience", New York: Longmans, Green and Company, 1916.

(50) KENISTON, K., "The Uncommitted", New York: Harcourt, Brace & World, Inc., 1960.

(51) KLEBER, H. D., "Student Use of Hallucinogens", Journal of American College Health Association 14: 109–117, 1965.

(52) KLÜVER, HEINRICH, "Mescal and Mechanisms of Hallucinations", Chicago: The University of Chicago Press, 1966.

(53) KOELLA, W. P., BEAULIEU, R. F. and BERGEN, J. R., "Stereotyped Behavior Cyclic Changes in Response Produced by LSD in Goats", International Journal of Neuropharmacology 3: 397–403, 1964.

(54) KOHUT, HEINZ, "Forms and Transformations of Narcissism", Journal of the American Psychoanalytic Association 14: No. 2, 1966.

(55) LABARRE, W., "Twenty Years of Peyote Studies", Current Anthropology 1: 45–60, 1960.

(56) LAING, R. D., "Transcendental Experience in Relation to Religion and Psychosis", Psychedelic Review 6: 7–15, 1965.

(57) LEARY, T. and ALPERT, R., "The Politics of Consciousness Expansion", The Harvard Review 1: No. 4, 33–37, 1963.

(58) LEBOVITS, B., VISOTSKY, H. M. and OSTFED, A. M., "LSD and JB318: A Comparison of Two Hallucinogens. Part III", American Medical Association Archives of General Psychiatry 7: 39–45, 1962.

(59) LENNARD, H., "Lysergic Acid Diethylamide (LSD-25): XII. A Preliminary State-ment of Its Effects Upon Interpersonal Communication", Journal of Psychology 41: 186–198, 1956.

(60) LINDESMITH, A. R., "The Addict and the Law," Bloomington: Bloomington Indiana University Press, 1965.

(61) LINDESMITH, A. R. and GAGNON, J. H., "Anomie and Drug Addiction", Anomie and Deviant Behavior, pp. 158–188, M. B. Clinard (ed.), New York: The Free Press, 1964.

(62) LING, T. M. and BUCKMAN, J., "Lysergic Acid and Ritalin in the Treatment of Neurosis," London: Lambarde Press, 1963.

(63) LIVINGSTON, R. B., "Symposium on the History of Narcotic Drug Addiction Prob-lems", National Institute of Mental Health, Bethesda, Maryland, 1963.

(64) LOURIA, D. B. et al., "The Dangerous Drug Problem", New York Medicine 22: No. 9, May 5, 1966.

(65) LUDWIG, A. M. and LEVINE, J., "Patterns of Hallucinogenic Drug Abuse", Journal of American Medical Association 191: 104–108, January 11, 1965.

(66) MACLEAN, J. R. et al, "The Use of LSD-25 in the Treatment of Alcoholism and Other Psychiatric Problems", Quart. J. Stud. Alcohol 22: 34–45, 1961.

(67) MASLOW, A. H., Toward a Psychology of Being, New York: D. Van Nostrand Co., Inc., 1962.

(68) Mayor's Committee on Marihuana, New York City: Cattell Press, Lancaster, Pa., 1944.

(69) MCGLOTHLIN, W. H., "Hallucinogenic Drugs: A Perspective With Special Refer-ence to Peyote and Cannabis", Psychedelic Review 6: 16–57, 1965.

(70) MCGLOTHLIN, W. H., COHEN, S. and MCGLOTHLIN, M. S., "Long Lasting Effects of LSD on Normals", Arch. Gen. Psy. 17: 1967 (in press).

(71) MCGLOTHLIN, W. H. and COHEN, S., "The Use of Hallucinogenic Drugs Among College Students", American Journal of Psychiatry 122: 572–574, 1965.

(72) MCGLOTHLIN, W. H., COHEN, S. and MCGLOTHLIN, M. S., "Short-Term Effects of LSD on Anxiety, Attitudes and Performance", J. Nerv. Ment. Dis. (in press, 1967).

(73) O'REILLY, P. O. and REICH, G., "Lysergic Acid and the Alcoholic", Dis. Nerv. Syst. 23: 331–334, 1962.

101

(74) PEARLMAN, S. J., "Drug Experiences and Attitudes Among Seniors in a Liberal Arts College", Unpublished Manuscript, Brooklyn College of the City University of New York, 1966.

(75) PHILIP, A. F., "Drugs on Campus", Presented at Twentieth Anniversary Meetings, Group for the Advancement of Psychiatry. Philadelphia, Pa., November 12, 1966.

(76) POLSKY, NED, "The Village Beat Scene; Summer 1960", Dissent 8: No. 1, 339–359, 1961.

(77) ROSENTHAL, S. N., "Persistent Hallucinosis Following Repeated Administration of Hallucinogenic Drugs", American Journal of Psychiatry 121: 238–243, 1964.

(78) SALVATORE, S. and HYDE, R. W., "Progression of Effects of LSD", Arch. Neurol. Psychiat. 76: 50–59, 1956.

(79) SANDISON, R. A., SPENCER, A. M. and WHITELAW, J. D. A., "The Therapeutic Value of Lysergic Acid Diethylamide in Mental Illness", J. Ment. Sci. 100: 491–507, 1954.

(80) SAVAGE, C., TERRILL, J. and JACKSON, D. D., "LSD, Transcedence and the New Beginning", J. Nerv. Ment. Dis. 135: 425–439, 1962.

(81) SCHACTER, S., "Interaction of Cognitive and Physiological Determinants of Emotional State", Psychobiological Approaches to Social Behavior, Liederman, H. and Shapiro, D. (eds.), Palo Alto, California: Stanford University Press, 1964.

(82) SHORVON, H. M., "Abreaction and Brain", Hallucinogenic Drugs and Their Psychotherapeutic Use: Proceedings of the Royal Medico-Psychological Association, pp. 74–78, Croket, R., et al. (eds.), London: H. K. Lewis & Co., Ltd., 1963.

(83) SIEGEL, J., "The New Sound: Tune In, Turn On, and Take Over", The Village Voice, November 7, 1966.

(84) SIMMONS, J. I. and WINOGRAD, B., "It's Happening", Santa Barbara: MarcLaird Publications, 1967.

(85) SLATER, P. E., Morimoto, K., and Hyde, R. W., "The Effects of LSD Upon Group Interaction", Archives of General Psychiatry 8: 564–571, 1963.

(86) SLOTKIN, J. S., "The Peyote Religion", Glencoe: The Free Press, 1956.

(87) SMITH, C. M., "A New Adjunct to the Treatment of Alcoholism: the Hallucinogenic Drugs", Quart. J. Stud. Alcohol 19: 406–417, 1958.

(88) SOUTHARD, S., "Conversion and Christian Character", Nashville, Broadman Press, 1965.

(89) SPINDLER, G., "Personality of Peyotism in Menomini Indian Acculturation", Psychiatry 15: 151–159, 1952.

(90) STUMPF, W. E. and ROTH, L. J., "Dry-Mounting High-Resolution Autoradiography", Isotopes in Experimental Pharmacalogy, pp. 133–143, Roth, L. J. (ed.), Chicago: The University of Chicago Press, 1965.

(91) UNGER, S. M., "Mescaline, LSD, Psilocybin, and Personality Change", Psychiatry 26: 111–125, 1963.

(92) UNGERLEIDER, J. T., FISHER, D. D. and FULLER, M., "The Dangers of LSD", Journal of American Medical Association 197: 389–392, 1966.

(93) WILSON, R. E., and SHAGASS, C., "Comparison of Two Drugs with Psychotomimetic Effects (LSD and Ditran)", J. Nerv. Ment. Dis. 138: No. 3, 1964.

(94) WOLBACH, A. B., MINER, E. J. and ISBELL, H., "Comparison of Psilocin With Pslio-cybin, Mescaline and LSD-25", Psychopharmacologia 3: 219–223, 1962.

(95) WOLBACH, A. B., Jr., ISBELL, H. and MINER, E. J., "Cross-Tolerance Between Mescaline and LSD-25", Psychopharmacologia 3: 1–14, 1962.

SESSION II

PIPER METHYSTICUM (KAVA)

Georg E. Cronheim, *Chairman*

Chairman's Introduction

GEORG E. CRONHEIM

Riker Laboratories, Northbridge, California

The first session of this conference dealing with a particular plant, is devoted to Kawa or Kava-Kava or Piper methysticum, which is indigenous to many islands of the South Pacific.

The use of Kawa in certain parts of Oceania is apparently very old. It has been described already by early travelers, for instance by James Cook in 1768. It is important to remember that the Kawa drink is mentioned not only quite early, but also repeatedly by a number of observers. The descriptions uniformly indicated that the Kawa experience is apparently pleasant, and free from hangover or other side- or after-effects. Many travelers, and also such scientific investigators as L. Lewin, have reported that Kawa can induce a form of euphoria, described as a happy state of complete comfort and peace, with ease of conversation and increased perceptivity, followed by restful sleep.

In many areas, the use of Kawa was connected with religious cults and ceremonies. Thus, it is not surprising that missionaries tried to suppress the drinking of Kawa. In some islands, this campaign was very successful, especially when it coincided with the introduction of alcoholic beverages. This replacement of Kawa by alcohol may have some significance, which I hope will be discussed by some of the speakers. Could it be that enough people preferred the effects induced by alcohol over those of Kawa? Otherwise the change-over would not have taken place as rapidly or as completely as was apparently the case in many islands. Also, the preference for alcoholic beverages is—if not an absolute proof—at least a good indication that the Kawa drink did not contain or simulate alcohol.

The first major scientific examination of Kawa was published by L. Lewin in 1886. Subsequently, other investigators in Europe and in this country studied the chemical constituents and the pharmacological properties of Kawa and of its components. However, the number of people interested in this plant was always relatively small. Kawa did not become the subject of more wide-spread use (or mis-use), or of numerous scientific investigations. Perhaps our colleagues in anthropology and sociology can tell us whether this is purely coincidental or whether there is some specific reason that in spite of the sudden interest and cult-like fadism related to substances with hallucinogenic or euphoria-producing properties, Kawa remained, outside of the South Pacific Islands, a relatively little known drug. Moreover, the fact that Kawa did not gain any popularity may have another explanation. In more recent references to the Kawa Ceremony and present-day Kawa use, none of the previously described effects on the central nervous system were mentioned. This represented always a great puzzle. How could one explain numerous detailed eye-witness accounts of unmistakable central effects of Kawa when taken by natives or by white people, travelers or settlers? Even addiction has been described for these groups. Also, Kawa was an article of commerce. Still more important, it was not just collected as a wild plant, but was regularly cultivated. In other words, Kawa represented something which native people in the South Pacific Islands wanted and for which they were willing to pay in the form of money or physical labor. Doesn't it seem reasonable to assume that they derived some pleasure from Kawa? And wouldn't this explain that drinking of Kawa—both for ceremonial and social purposes—is still practiced?

Pharmacological studies of Kawa and certain of its constituents have shown some rather remarkable properties, which will be discussed in the course of this program. Studies in our laboratories were in fact so promising that we carried out the necessary chronic toxicity studies in animals, in order to permit an evaluation in human volunteers and in patients. Unfortunately, the results were not very striking. Some anti-epileptic activity was seen in patients, but none of the "tranquilizing" effects that had been described. At the same time, signs of skin reactions became apparent, which precluded further chronic administration.

So here we have some obvious discrepancies, for which I am sure there must be some explanation. It is the purpose of the present conference to present such discrepancies and questions to groups composed of anthropologists, botanists, chemists, clinicians and pharmacologists, because the complementary approach evolving from an interdisciplinary discussion has the best chance of solving some of the existing problems.

We are fortunate that the group of speakers in this Kawa symposium includes three investigators who have had extensive first-hand knowledge of the use of Kawa in various island groups of the South Pacific. This information will be supplemented by some clinical observations in patients, as well as special investigations of central nervous system effects of Kawa and some of its constituents in human volunteers. The pharmacological properties of these substances and the chemistry of Kawa will also be presented in adequate detail. All in all, a fairly comprehensive picture of Kawa should emerge. It is my hope that the combined knowledge of the seven speakers, each a specialist in his field, may provide some of the missing answers to the Kawa problem.

The Function of Kava in Modern Samoan Culture

LOWELL D. HOLMES
Department of Anthropology, Wichita State University, Wichita, Kansas

In the Manu'a island group of American Samoa no formal or informal meeting of chiefs would be complete without the distribution of the traditional Polynesian beverage kava. This drink known locally as *'ava*, is prepared by steeping the pulverized roots of the *Piper methysticum* plant in a prescribed amount of water until a cloudy, khaki-colored liquid is produced.

Kava is in no way alcoholic, but much has been made of its narcotic properties. Early missionaries maintained that the concoction partially paralyzed the lower extremities, making it difficult to walk. More recent partakers of kava, including the author, have experienced no debilitating effect which could be attributed to consumption of the drink. Instead they have found it a refreshing, astringent drink which produces nothing more than a tingling sensation in the mucous membrane of the mouth and a short-lived numbness of the tongue. The partial paralysis of the lower limbs is not caused by the kava but by sitting cross-legged for hours while the kava ceremony is in process. Samoans who find the sitting posture a more natural one do not complain of any impairment to walking. Missionary V. A. Barradale, writing in 1907 stated, "I have heard it said that if people drink too much [kava], it makes them drunk in their legs; it paralyzes their lower limbs, and they have to sit where they are till the effect wears off. But it would certainly need a very large quantity to affect a man in that way, and I never saw or heard of any one in that condition"(2).

Although Beaglehole (3) reports rare cases of kava addiction in Pangai, Tonga, such a phenomenon was not personally observed in Samoa. The author's informants did on one occasion refer to one recently deceased chief whom they believed drank kava in excess because he had it prepared every morning so that he could partake throughout the day. They also felt this excessive use of kava was the cause of his death. Actually he had died at the age of seventy-five from cancer of the stomach. Another claim made by native informants is that over-indulgence of the drink can result in skin diseases and eye ailments. The literature produced by early missionaries contains numerous references to a scaly skin condition being attributable to kava drinking. These claims were not corroborated by the author. One European observer believed that the consumption of kava had the effect of preventing the Samoans from developing a taste for alcoholic liquors. The author has not observed this phenomenon either.

Krämer reports that he observed the addition of *Capsicum* pepper pods to the kava concoction and believes this strengthened its stimulating effect thereby rendering kava the equivalent in its use to *Piper betle* in Indonesia.

He tells of having broken open a *Capsicum* pod and accidentally having touched his face with his soiled hands. He complains of having "endured severe pain for a long time; thus the pepper affects even the epidermis." (*6*).

The addition of this pepper to the kava mixture was not observed in contemporary Samoa, and the extent of its use in earlier days is not known. Kramer is the only 19th century observed to record its use.

Kava is often drunk by Europeans, who upon acquiring the taste, find it very refreshing. Many urban centers in the South Seas boast kava saloons where local businessmen—native and European—take a kava break during the mid-morning hours. Some government offices have kava prepared in the morning for the comfort and enjoyment of their employees.

The relative importance of kava varies from island group to island group. Kava drinking in Polynesia is primarily a phenomenon of the cultures in the west, such as Tonga, Fiji and Samoa. The plant does not grow on the atolls of the Tokelaus. Beaglehole (*3*) reports universal use of the beverage in Tonga, but maintains that accompanying ritual is almost totally absent in villages inhabited by commoners. Hawaii and Tahiti had the drink at one time but it has practically disappeared in recent years. The Cook Island cultures formerly used the plant for drinking purposes also, but many of the Bernice P. Bishop Museum monographs on the cultures of this region do not even mention kava. The Maori did not drink kava although a variety of the plant which could have been used for such purposes was indigenous to New Zealand. Aitken (*1*) reports that in the Australs the occasional and somewhat unimportant practice of kava drinking was abolished by missionaries in 1822. New Caledonian Polynesian populations are described by Leenhardt (*7*) as ignoring the plant altogether.

Other centers of kava drinking in Oceania are Ponape in the Carolines, the Marind District of West New Guinea, the New Hebrides and the Wallis and Futuna islands. In Melanesia the drink is described as being made from fresh roots, and the concoction is said to have the effect of rapidly inducing deep sleep. Chronic drinkers in this area are said to suffer from a state of depression accompanied by a permanent decrease in appetite. Malnutrition is also said to be observed among some addicts. The difference in effect between this area and western Polynesia is possibly attributable to the state of the kava root at the time of production of the beverage. The dried roots used in Polynesia apparently do not produce as strong a drink as that concocted from fresh ones.

In Samoa it appears that kava drinking and its attendant ceremonies has a long history, the practice being intimately related to indigenous religious practices and village social and political organization. Mythology relates how kava drinking was given to mortals by the first high chief, Tagaloa Ui, and prescribes the form for modern kava ceremonies. The myth which provides these sanctions was recorded in Manu'a as follows:

Not far from the village of Fitiuta there is a place where the rising sun is first seen in Samoa. This place is called *Saua*. Long ago there was a custom that one day a year one of the families of Fitiuta must sacrifice the daughter to the sun. On the day of the "celebration of the sun" a daughter from the family of Matainaumati went to Samoa

108

to be sacrificed. The girl's name was Ui. When the sun came for the girl he saw that she was very beautiful and instead of eating her he decided to take her as his wife. He took the girl to live with him in the sky. After a time she became pregnant and wanted to go home so that her first child could be born in her family's village, and she wanted to show her parents that she had not been killed.

While journeying home, Ui had a miscarriage, and the fetus floated away upon the waters where it was found by the hermit crab, the plover and the shrike. By manipulating the fetus and breathing life into it the animals created the first Samoan chief, Tagaloa Ui.

After his creation Tagaloa Ui made a kilt for himself out of *ti* leaves and started to walk toward the village of Fitiuta. On his way he walked through a grove of kava plants and discovered the house of the mortal, Pava. Pava invited the chief to enter his house and there the first kava ceremony involving mortal men was held.

When Tagaloa Ui entered the house he took a place at the end of the house (today the seat of honor), and Pava sat in the front of the house (the traditional place for talking chiefs) and began to prepare the kava. Pava chewed and spit the kava into a taro leaf (*laupula'a*) which served as the kava bowl. Cups consisted of *tautava* leaves, and Pava used his fingers to wring the kava as no strainer was then known.

While Pava·was wringing the kava, his son, Fa'alafi, laughed and played near the bowl. Tagaloa Ui instructed Pava to make the boy sit down and be quiet, but nothing was done about the irreverent boy. After several unheeded warnings, Tagaloa Ui picked up a coconut frond, formed it into a knife, and cut Pava's son into two pieces. Then Tagaloa Ui said to Pava, "This is the food for the kava. This is your part and this is mine." Pava mourned and could not drink the kava.

Then Tagaloa Ui said, "Let us have a new kava ceremony." The kava and the leaf bowl and cups were thrown away and Tagaloa Ui told two of Pava's sons to go to the highest mountain, the house of Tagaloa Lagi, and bring down a wooden kava bowl, coconut cups, a hibiscus strainer and a new kind of kava, *latasi*, a single branch kava tree. These things were brought, and a second kava ceremony was started. Again Pava served as the kava wringer, and when the kava was ready, Tagaloa Ui said, "Bring me my cup first." Tagaloa Ui did not drink the kava but poured it onto his piece of the dead son of Pava and then onto Pava's piece. Then he said, "*Soifua*" (life). The two parts came together and the boy lived. Pava was so happy he clapped his hands. Pava drank his cup of kava and Tagaloa Ui gave the following orders: "Pava, do not let children stand and talk while kava is being prepared for high chiefs, for the things belonging to the high chiefs are sacred."

A number of ritual details of the modern Samoan kava ceremony seem to relate directly to this myth. They are:

1. The seating arrangement of the chiefs and the talking chiefs.
2. Prohibitions against children, or indeed any unauthorized untitled persons, attending the ceremony.
3. The solemn atmosphere which must prevail.
4. The proper equipment for the production and distribution of kava— a carved wooden kava bowl, a hibiscus strainer, a coconut cup, and a certain type of kava.
5. The order of drinking—high chiefs first, talking chiefs second.
6. The pouring of a bit of kava from the cup onto the mat.
7. The concept of food for the kava.
8. The use of the term "*Soifua*."
9. The clapping of hands when the kava is ready.
10. The duty of talking chiefs to direct the kava ceremony.

The importance of the above is indicated by the fact that although short-cuts are often taken in the modern kava ceremony the features listed are seldom if ever altered.

Kava in contemporary Samoan society has been likened by Keesing (5) to the European cocktail or highball, in that it produces a relaxed and friendly atmosphere conducive to social cooperation.

Every chief is expected to keep a stock of dried kava on hand for his own use and for the many demands made upon him by the protocol of hospitality. Whenever any elite visitor enters the village, the welcoming ceremony requires that each of the host chiefs present him with a dried kava root.

The kava ceremony is invariably the initial act of any meeting of the village council (*fono*), and is therefore a definite part of formal discussion and decision making. It is also an essential part of all ceremonies associated with births, marriages, deaths and title installations. No bonito canoe or house is ever constructed without the labor being prefaced by the kava ceremony wherein the carpenter is served first kava in the name of Sao (a name which people claim was given to the first carpenter by the god Tagaloa). The ceremony is said to insure successful work.

Kava drinking is without doubt the most important element of the *aiavā*, the ceremony of greeting for visiting parties (*malaga*), and therefore carries much of the burden of Samoan hospitality.

In earlier, less peaceful days kava was consumed by warriors prior to battle. On such occasions, the ceremony was referred to as *'ava mua au*. Fe'epulea'i Ripley (7) reported observing such a ceremony wherein the chiefs lined up along each side of the road and set up the kava bowl in the middle of it.

Aside from its ceremonial use, kava is reported to have certain medicinal uses. It is often consumed in an attempt to counteract the chills which accompany filariasis. Some Samoans believe that kava chewed in large quantities will cause abortion. It is also claimed to be a cure for gonorrhea, and it is a matter of record that German drug houses at one time imported small quantities of the plant for this purpose.

Although the kava ceremony is considered the exclusive property of titled men there are certain ceremonial occasions, such as the entertainment of a visiting party, when the society of untitled men (*aumaga*) or the wives of the village chiefs (Woman's Committee) conduct their own social kava ritual. On such occasions the order of drinking is determined by one's relationship to the title holders of the village. Having a father or husband who is the village paramount chief entitles one to be honored with first kava.

Some regional variations in kava ritual may be observed from village to village, and even in a given village the ceremony is not always performed in the same way. Certain parts may be abbreviated or eliminated altogether, and perhaps the ceremony to be described in this paper is closer to the ideal than to the real. However, all the steps described herein have been observed frequently on occasions of high ceremony. Regional variations include differences in who may wring kava, the number of attendants involved in serving the kava, and in some cases, the status and sex of those served. In some villages only men are permitted to wring kava, but in others the ceremonial village maiden (*taupou*) may do the honors. On the island of Tutuila it is not uncommon for women to hold *matai* titles and serve on the village council. They are, therefore, as titled individuals, qualified to participate in the kava cere-

110

mony. In Manu'a women neither hold *matai* titles nor partake in the drinking of kava at formal ceremonies where chiefs are present. The one exception to this was the female sovereign Tuimanu'a Makelita.

The Modern Kava Ceremony

In preparing for the modern Manu'an kava ceremony the talking chief who will later direct the kava distribution selects a piece of kava root. This part of the kava plant is called the Brother Roots (*'ava uso*). The name drives from a myth which recounts how two brothers, the sons of Tagaloa, found a piece of floating wood while swimming west from the Manu'a Group. They divided the wood and used the two pieces as floats. One of the brothers returned to Fitiuta where many similar plants were observed to be growing already, while the other brother swam on to Western Samoa where kava was unknown. Here he planted his piece of wood and thereby introduced kava drinking in this area.

After the initial selection of a piece of kava root, the society of untitled men (*aumaga*) takes over and the root is cut into still smaller pieces by one of their members. In this form kava is known as *una o le i' a sā*, scales of the sacred or forbidden fish. This term alludes the fact that like many other sacred or taboo foods kava is reserved for the exclusive use of the chiefs.

While the pieces of kava were formerly chewed, final processing today involves pulverizing in a crude stone mortar (*ma'a tu'i'ava*). Other preparations for the ceremony include washing the kava bowl and bringing water in coconut shell containers (sometimes a galvanized bucket is substituted today).

A full inventory of the ceremonial paraphernalia includes a carved bowl, eighteen inches in diameter, which traditionally had four legs but now may have as many as twenty-four, a strainer made of shredded hibiscus bast, and a polished coconut cup.

Village kava ceremonies are usually held in the house which serves as the meeting place of the village council. As the chiefs enter the council house an attitude of reverence prevails. Nothing may be worn above the waist, and body ornaments of all types must be laid aside. The men speak in whispers and refrain from smoking as the kava ceremony begins.

At a place near the back of the house three untitled men, members of the village *aumaga*, station themselves at the kava bowl while a fourth remains outside to clean the hibiscus strainer of kava fibers when it is periodically thrown to him by the wringer. The man who is to wring the kava sits immediately behind the bowl with a water pourer to his right, and to his left, the man who will carry the cups of liquid to the assembled chiefs. Several taboos must be observed by the wringer. These include never wearing a flower necklace, a ring, a shirt or any other clothing except a wrap-around (*lavalava*). *Lavalavas* of all untitled men involved in the ceremony must be worn so they do not extend below the knees. The wringing of the kava must be done correctly and with precision. Untitled men take pride in their ability in this art. There are a number of specific steps in the preparation of the liquid, and each has a traditional name. They are:

1. *Fa'apulou*—Covering the kava in the bottom of the bowl with the strainer.
2. *Vau*—Pressing down on the strainer with the heels of the hands and with the fingers.
3. *Aōga*—Collecting pieces of kava fiber in the strainer by drawing it toward the back of the bowl.
4. *Tatau*—Wringing the kava. The strainer is lifted from the bowl and wrung three times only. It is grasped in both hands like one would grip a baseball bat. At the end of each wringing stroke the clenched hands are bent forward so the liquid will not run down the arms.
5. *Mapā*—Cleaning the strainer. After the above steps have been carried out three times the strainer is passed under the right knee of the wringer and thrown back, with a side arm motion, to the untitled person outside the house who catches it in his right hand and removes the kava particles in it by snapping it three or four times. The hibiscus strainer is then thrown back underhand and caught by the wringer in his right hand.

The above process is continued until the bowl is free of pieces of kava root. When this has been accomplished and the kava is ready for drinking, the wringer wipes the rim of the bowl, cleans the strainer himself by snapping, forms it into a ball, and plunges it into the kava, and lifts it above the bowl with both hands, allowing the stream of liquid to fall into the bowl. This final gesture, known as *sila alofi*, permits the chiefs to see whether the kava requires more water. It is said that the correct mixture is judged by the sound of the kava splashing into the bowl as well as by its color.

If the talking chief serving as kava announcer does not call for more water the hibiscus strainer is wrung out and placed on the rim of the bowl. The kava wringer then places his hands on the sides of the bowl, his right covering the strainer. He remains in that position until the kava has been distributed.

It is the responsibility of the talking chief directing the ceremony to watch the progress of the wringing from his position behind and to the right of the bowl. When the kava is nearly clear of fiber particles, he must commence the verbal part of the ceremony with a poetic recitation (*solo*) which recounts the mythical origin of the kava or particular kava ceremonies of importance held by the ancient Samoan gods. A typical *solo* is as follows:

Si'i le faiva e to'alua
Papa ma Lotulotua
Aumai se i'a setasi
Le Manini mai le Sami
Telemu ma Telea'i
O mai lua te taufetuli ile lagi
Fati mai se la tasi
Se la o le la 'ava o tu felata'i

Gaugau ma sasa
Gaugau ma falava

Translation

Two people went fishing
Papa and Lotulotua (members of the Tagaloa family)
They brought one fish
The Manini, from the sea.
Telemu and Telea'i (two brothers of the Tagaloa family)
Were sent to run to the heaven
To bring a branch of kava
They broke and hit the kava
They broke and hit the fierce kava

Many *solos* are traditional, but clever talking chiefs may and do compose their own. It will be noted that the example given above is composed of rhyming couplets. There is, however, little concern for rhythm. The *solo* is timed to be finished the moment the kava is completely clear of fibers, whereupon the kava announcer states, "*Ua usi le alofi*" (The kava is already cleaned). The color and consistency of the mixture is then analyzed and if pronounced acceptable, the assembled chiefs respond by clapping their hands several times. Informants state that this act of clapping corresponds to the clapping of Pava when his sons was returned to life through the action of Tagaloa Ui at the first kava ceremony.

The distribution of kava begins by calling the cup title of the high chief who, because of his rank, is permitted to drink first. It must be understood that the cup title is not the family title of the chief. For example, in Si'ufaga village High Chief Lefiti (Lefiti is the family title) has the cup title *Lupe lele talitali lau ipu* (The pigeon who flies, receive your cup). Only high chiefs have cup titles. Talking chiefs receive their cup after the announcement of their family title and the words "*Lau 'ava*" (your kava). Chiefs of secondary rank receive the cup after their family title and the word "*Taumafa*" (drink) is pronounced.

The order of drinking is of the utmost importance as it signifies the relative rank of the drinker. The chief of highest rank in the village receives first kava; the highest talking chief, second; second highest chief, third; second highest talking chief, fourth; and so on down the ranks of chiefs and talking chiefs. In some villages this procedure is altered, and certain divisions of chiefs, or certain sections of the village, drink before others. To drink last kava is as prestigeful as to drink first.

Drinking etiquette, which varies according to rank, is as follows: When the high chief receives the cup he does so with both hands. Before drinking he pours a few drops onto the floor mat and says, "*Ia fa'atasi le Atua ma i tatou i lenei aso*" (May God be with us today) or "*Ia ta'ita'i le Atua i lenei aso*" (May God be our leader for today). Smith (*8*) records a typical prayer as, "Let the god drink kava that this gathering may be pleasant."

Following this prayer the high chief raises his cup, says *"Soifua"* or *"Manuia,"* and drinks what is contained in the cup. If the high chief says *"Soifua"* the other chiefs respond with *"Manuia."* If the latter word is pronounced by the drinker the chiefs reply with *"Soifua."* Informants point out the connection between this aspect of the modern kava ceremony and the action of Tagaloa Ui in the first kava ceremony. The pouring of kava onto the mat represents the pouring of the liquid onto the two parts of the dead son of Pava, and the word *"Soifua,"* which may be translated "Life" or "May you live," alludes to the command given by Tagaloa Ui when he performed the miracle of returning the boy to life. The word *"Manuia"* may be translated "Blessings" or "May the gods bless you," and perhaps relates to an expression of gratitude by Pava. It is also contended by informants that the right of the high chief to drink first kava and to sit in the end of the house is sanctioned by the Tagaloa Ui myth.

The drinking etiquette to be observed by a high talking chief varies somewhat in that he receives the kava cup with two hands if high chiefs are occupying both ends of the house, but if only one high chief is seated to the high talking chief's right, the cup must be received with the left hand to avoid showing the high chief the back of the hand. Of course the cup will be taken with the right hand if the high chief is seated to the talking chief's left. A high talking chief usually does not pour any kava onto the floor mat although he may say "Soifua" or "Manuia" before drinking.

Chiefs and talking chiefs of secondary rank do not pour kava onto the mat, nor do they say anything before drinking. Furthermore, they are not expected to respect the position of the high chief by receiving the cup with any particular hand.

Some Samoans do not care for kava and they "drink" symbolically by merely touching the bottom of the cup as it is passed to them. The cup may also be raised in a form of salutation and then returned to the cup bearer, with the kava untouched. On rare occasions a chief may take the liquid into his mouth, swish it about and then turn and spit it out onto the apron of the house outside. All these actions represent acceptable etiquette for the non-drinker.

When many chiefs are assembled there is often not enough kava to serve everyone. In such cases it is important for the kava announcer to judge when but a single cup of kava remains and then to announce rapidly the names of those who are entitled to drink. Following the recitation of this list of titles the announcer calls the cup title of the high chief who is then honored by drinking last kava, and the final cup is served to him. When talking chiefs of secondary rank are aware that there is not sufficient kava to go around they will often interrupt the announcer and call, "I will drink with my chief." When this occurs the lesser talking chief's title is not announced but the cup is taken to him immediately after the high chief of his family has been served.

Partially consumed kava must be cast away and the cup returned empty. It may be handed or thrown back to the server. If the cup is thrown to the server it is done to test his alertness.

114

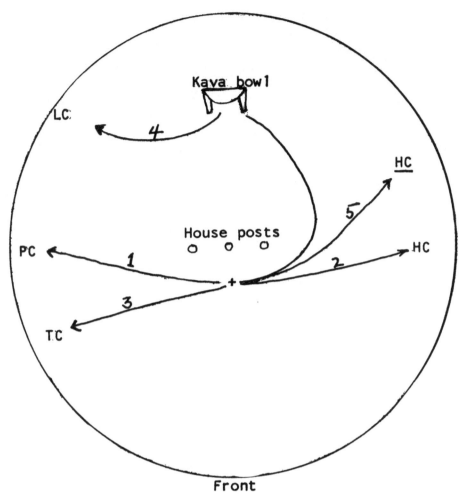

Front

1=Serving route to paramount high chief (PC); 2=Serving route to high chief (HC) 3=Serving route to talking chiefs (TC); 4=Serving route to lesser chiefs and talking chiefs (LC); 5=Serving route to high chief who will receive last kava (HC); +=Point at which the kava server stops before approaching chiefs of high rank.

All *aumaga* members who expect to take part in the kava ceremonies must master the etiquette of serving kava. Each rank of chief or talking chief must be served in a special and distinct manner. Respect is paid to the half of the house in which the paramount chief is seated, and the kava server must walk in this area as little as possible in making his rounds to the drinkers.

When serving a high chief the kava distributor dips the coconut cup into the kava and carries it with the thumbs and index fingers at the level of his waist to the center of the house where he stops, raises it to his forehead and walks in the direction of the high chief. About four feet from the chief, the server lowers his right hand and with his left, places the cup on his upturned right palm. The left hand is placed behind the back, and the cup is handed to the high chief chest high. The young man then walks to the

115

center of the house where he stands at attention until the chief has finished drinking.

Lower ranking chiefs are served kava with the right hand, but in the case of these lesser personages the cup is held by the edge with the thumb inside, thus showing the palm of the hand to the chiefs as it is presented to them.

In serving a high talking chief, the cup is held by the edge with the thumb, index and middle finger of the right hand. As it is carried from the bowl it is held just above the left shoulder. When in front of the high talking chief, the kava server swings the cup forward and down, presenting it with the back of his hand toward the talking chief. The kava cup for lower ranking talking chiefs is carried in the right hand, waist high, but is presented with the left. As in the case of high talking chiefs, the cup is held by the edge and the back of the hand is shown to the drinker.

After delivering the kava the server returns to the center post of the house and stands facing front while the kava is consumed. In rare cases he may return to a position in front of the kava bowl and face the front of the house.

When all of the assembled chiefs and talking chiefs have drunk or have been acknowledged as having the right to drink, the kava announcer concludes the ceremony with *"Ua moto le alofi"* (The kava is finished). *"Ale le fau ma le ipu e tautau"* (The bowl will hang with the *fau* (strainer) and the cup). Perhaps a more traditional closing is that recorded by Smith (*9*) as *"Le 'ava 'au motu"* (The kava is broken off). *"Ua matefa le fau"* (The strainer is poor). *"Ua pa'u le alofi"* (The company of chiefs has fallen down).

The assembled chiefs respond to these final words of the kava announcer with an expression of thanks, *"malo fa'asoasoa."* At the conclusion of the kava drinking ceremony there is always the *fono o le 'ava* (food for the kava ceremony). According to the Tagaloa Ui myth the food for the first ceremony was the son of Pava and the food for the second was the sacred fish Manini and *talofa'afana* (recooked taro). Today the *Manini* and *talofa'afana* remain the traditional foods for the kava ceremony but there are frequent substitutions of rice, tinned beef, or other prestige foods.

The present day kava ceremony contains a number of elements which can be traced to older religious concepts of Samoan culture. The pouring of a bit of kava onto the mat not only relates to ancient mythology, but a number of scholars feel that it is a ritual reenactment of an ancient religious custom of pouring an evening offering to family or village gods. Steubel records in *Samoanische texte* (1895) that the typical prayer accompanying this act was "O the kava to drink of thy highness Sepo. Be lovingly disposed. Bless this village." (Sepo was primarily a war god, but in many villages served as a household god.)

Mead (*8*) suggested that the casting away of unconsumed kava may be related to ancient ceremonies wherein kava was entreated to depart and take all misfortune with it. On the other hand it may be related to precautions about unconsumed food or drink which might be used for purposes of sorcery. Certainly the sanctity of the mixing bowl and gear, the air of solemnity and respect which accompany the entire ceremony, and the inclusion of poetic recitations which always allude to ancient Samoan gods, testify to the religious nature of the ancient ceremony.

Although the kava ceremony contains these unmistakable references to pre-Christian religion there seems to have been no great problem in fitting it into the Christian context. Bits of Christian prayer frequently accompany the pouring of kava onto the mat prior to drinking, and it is not uncommon to see local pastors included in the kava circle. On such occasions the village pastor (*faife'au*) drinks first kava, thus being accorded honors even greater than those shown to the village paramount chief. Since village pastors do not hold titles, their privileged position of drinking indicates their exalted status within the social structure of the village. Samoan medical practitioners and village school teachers are accorded similar honor by being served kava second only to the highest village chiefs.

Neither the church nor the American government has attempted to do away with the kava ceremony, and it is not unusual to see chiefs partake in a communion service in church, and then go home and conduct a kava ceremony while waiting for the midday meal. All visiting dignitaries in American Samoa, including President Lyndon B. Johnson in 1966, are honored with a kava ceremony by the paramount chiefs of the territory.

It has been said that while other Polynesian people worshipped gods, Samoans worshipped their village and social organization. The kava ceremony would seem to be a part of this veneration. The detailed etiquette of serving, the prescribed order of drinking, the use of special honorific cup names, and the insistence that the beverage be prepared and served only by specially qualified persons, have been tremendously important in dramatizing the whole system of Samoan rank and prestige. When the kava ceremony is completed there is little doubt of the status of those present and of the rights and privileges of their respective offices. Through continual ceremonial exercise, social relationships are reiterated and Samoan values are intensified. The result of this seems to be an unusual stability and resistance to change which is found among few other Polynesian peoples. In an attempt to explain this remarkable resistance to change, John Copp has commented, "Samoan custom now serves as a 'refuge' from the conflict of choice and judgment resulting from Western contacts." (*11*). Perhaps it has been the stabilizing influence of the kava ceremony and other rituals that has allowed the Samoans to make satisfactory adjustments to European influences. Traditional aspects of Samoan culture such as the kava ceremony are, in a manner of speaking, bits of solid ground on which to anchor in a changing world.

It is believed that the influence of the kava ceremony is one of the explanations for the amazing stability of a people who, as Douglas Oliver puts it, have survived "the strong impact of western civilization without losing their numbers, their strength, their dignity, or their zest for a good fight." (*9*).

BIBLIOGRAPHY

(*1*) AITKEN, ROBERT T. "Ethnology of Tubuai." Honolulu, Bishop Museum Bulletin No. 70, 1930.

(*2*) BARRADALE, V. A. "Pearls of the Pacific." London, London Missionary Society, 1907.

(*3*) BEAGLEHOLE, ERNEST and PEARL. "Pangai: Village in Tonga." Wellington, Polynesian Society, Memoir Vol. 18, 1941.

(*4*) BUCK, SIR PETER. "Samoan Material Culture." Honolulu, Bishop Museum Bulletin No. 75, 1930.

(*5*) KEESING, FELIX. "Elite Communication in Samoa." Stanford, Stanford University Press, 1956.

(*6*) KRÄMER, AUGUSTIN. "Die Samoa-Inseln," Stuttgart, 1902.

(*7*) LEENHARDT, MAURICE. "Gens de la Grande Terre." Paris, 1937.

(*8*) MEAD, MARGARET. "Social Organization of Manua." Honolulu, Bishop Museum Bulletin No. 76, 1930.

(*9*) OLIVER, DOUGLAS. "The Pacific Islands." Cambridge, Harvard University Press, 1951.

(*10*) SMITH, S. PERCY. "Kava Drinking Ceremonies among the Samoans and a Boat Voyage round 'Opulu Island, Samoa." Journal of Polynesian Society Supplement, 1920.

(*11*) STANNER, W. E. H. "The South Seas in Transition." Sydney, Australasian Publishing Co., 1953.

Recent Observations on the Use of Kava in the New Hebrides

D. Carleton Gajdusek
National Institute of Neurological Diseases and Blindness, N.I.H.
Bethesda, Maryland

Of all the Pacific islands on which kava is still used today, Tongariki is the one on which its use has attained maximum frequency and intensity. I have had occasion to be resident, with Professors Jean Guiart and Robert Kirk, on this small island of the Sandwich group in the New Hebrides, for several weeks in two periods during the past three years, while working on an intensive study of human adaptability in isolated populations. Quite apart from our medical and genetic studies, we were soon aware that the entire social life, mood and spirit of the island villages changed nightly at dusk to a more subdued, whispering and cautious quiet than we had seen in native villages elsewhere in the Pacific. This restrained atmosphere we found to be caused by kava drinking: nightly, most of the men were drinking fresh kava.

Whereas on most Pacific islands kava prepared by the ancient technique of premastication (particularly of the fresh, undried root) has been abandoned in favor of a much less pharmacologically potent beverage made by grating or pounding the root, usually dried, here on Tongariki the current extensive nonceremonial drinking of kava makes use of the "green", freshly harvested, locally-grown root and of mastication and salivary digestion of the pulp by the adolescent and young men. Fresh cold water is used with hand mixing and wringing through a sieve of cocoanut fiber to extract the active ingredients from the chewed pulp. The many variations of this procedure have been described exhaustively since the earliest reports from Captain Cook's voyages, and similarities in minute details of the kava ceremony have been used to suggest affinities between peoples on different islands. On Tongariki the procedures are now relatively unformalized and thus subject to considerable variation. Kava drinking on this island is unusual, furthermore, in that its extent and pattern is a relatively recent phenomenon, and in that it has reached faddish proportions in terms of the number of kava drinkers and the frequency of their use of kava, which in both cases exceeds that of pre-European contact.

This resurgence of kava drinking suggests the extensive revival of kava usage on the southern New Hebridean island of Tanna in the early 1940's as a ritual of a flourishing cargo cult which repudiated much of the missionary teaching. Jean Guiart, in his study of this cargo cult, believed that the fierce battle the Presbyterian Church had waged against kava drinking had focused undue attention onto the traditional use of the beverage; this served to endow its new prohibition-defying use with such psychological import that the renewal of kava drinking became an important part of this anti-missionary movement, which appeared on the island during World War II and has not yet subsided. Early in the cargo movement (called the John Frum movement after a neomythical man of that name) there was an anarchical use of the drink, without respect for the ancient ceremonial and age-group restrictions on its use; even adolescents drank it; the drinking took place in small informal groups at odd times of the day and in unappointed places, as was never permitted in pagan times.

Tongariki has a population of about 500 living in four small villages; it has not had a full-blown cargo cult or Messianic movement, but the resurgence of the use of kava has been associated with a reluctance to become involved in Protestant mission or government-instigated activities, an increased clannishness, and a withdrawal from outside contacts. No European missionary has ever been resident on Tongariki, but native missionaries from other islands have been sent there by the Presbyterian Church. In spite of attempts to suppress it, the use of kava here was never fully stopped; in recent years most adult male members of the population turn each night to kava. Moreover, only the fresh root and not the dry variety is usually employed. The users still attend Sunday church services on the island, and do not associate their use of kava with a revolt against the church such as occurred on Tanna.

Kava drinking on Tongariki is a relatively relaxed and unceremonious affair, without the strict adherence to prescribed etiquette characteristic of kava drinking in much of the Pacific. It is prepared entirely by chewing, never by the use of mortars, graters, or other mechanical aids. Boys from pre-adolescent age to young adulthood usually do the chewing for their kinsmen or guests, or out of courtesy for others. Older youths or young men mix, wash, and wring the kava from the chewed pulp. Girls and women may occasionally participate in the chewing, whereas this was not so in the past. Adolescents and, more rarely, women may drink kava without censure. It is drunk in various places within the village proper, usually in a quiet house, and strict exclusion of children and women from the proximity and view of the proceedings has lapsed. Thus, the current kava drinking on Tongariki is more like that of the early John Frum movement on Tanna in its lack of formality and restraints. On Tanna, however, by the 1950's kava usage had returned essentially to the old traditional ceremonially controlled forms.

Usually, half of a cocoanut shell or a bowl of the same capacity is used to prepare the kava and the full contents—about 100 ml.—drunk slowly in one draught. Sometimes twice this quantity is drunk. A kava drinker usually eats immediately after taking the kava; the kava is prepared while the evening meal is being cooked. The effects come on in a half hour or less, and the drinking is thus usually postponed until food is ready. Those who have drunk the kava find a comfortable place to sit, often beside a dying fire in the dark house, where they remain hunched over and avoiding light and sound disturbances of all sorts. Conversation ceases, and slowly they fall into a kava-induced stupor, which is not true sleep. This stage occurs about an hour after drinking. From it they can be aroused by being addressed or gently shaken, but this ruins the effect they are seeking from the kava. A

120

few hours after they have drunk kava they arise and walk to their own houses to fall asleep promptly again; others remain where they have first "fallen". In early morning they appear fresh and without any "hangover"-like sequelae. Those whom we have seen walking a few hours after the drinking are usually somewhat ataxic, photophobic, and slowed in their reactions. A few who have had a higher dose are extremely ataxic and could return to their homes only with assistance from the children or myself. There is no belligerency or irritability—only a quiet and friendly somnolence associated with the weakness of the lower limbs and the accompanying ataxia.

The drinkers reply rationally and are well oriented in time, place, and person; they respond intelligently, even sometimes quickly, to complex questions. Bright or moving lights, noise or other sound, touch, and even the subdued bustle of nearby activity annoy them, and the villagers of all ages have extreme respect for this. In discussions the kava users refer to a heaviness and weakness of their extremities, particularly of the feet and legs, and to an earlier paresthesia ascending from their feet to their trunk and described with such words as "numbness", "tingling", and "coldness". They demonstrate a tactful avoidance of the disturbance my questioning produces, a very subdued annoyance at my "breaking" their kava. I have taken pulse rates and blood pressure measurements on a number of kava drinkers at varying intervals from one to three hours after drinking and found no significant change in either from that observed on the same subjects during examinations in the daytime, when they had had no kava for the preceeding eighteen hours or more. Respiration is shallow and regular; deep tendon reflexes remain intact.

Of interest to us in our genetic studies has been the effects that kava might have on fertility, since it is quite evident that kava drinkers rarely engage in sexual activity on the nights when they drink. Interviews with the women substantiate this. There is no dearth of children on Tongariki, but the population is not increasing explosively as it is in some parts of the Pacific, and kava drinking may serve as an interesting means of birth control for the small island, which could be easily over-populated.

Dam-Bakker, DeGroot and Luyken have suspected the use of wati, as kava is called in southwest New Guinea, as a possible cause of the infertility in the Marind-Anim people. Their studies on chronic kava administration to rats, however, failed to demonstrate any impaired fertility, but they admit that they hardly reproduced essential features of kava use in the human community in their rat experiments.

Jean Guiart and I have occasionally taken kava with the natives, and have noticed subjectively little difference in the sequence of symptoms and reactions from those reported by many Pacific voyagers since Captain Cook's days. A few peculiar paresthesiae of the face, legs and arms—especially of the legs—a slight feeling of numbness, tingling, coldness and then weakness, accompanied early by shorter flashes of warmth or flush, occurred during the first half hour after ingestion. We have boorishly "broken" our kava at times, and walked off to engage in other activities without noticeable impairment of motor or sensory function. This has been after rather low doses. There is, with higher doses, a pleasant, relaxing, paresthesia-enjoying, refreshing state of somnolence without mental dulling which eventually leads to sleep. At times, members of our team have taken large doses—a large cocoanut shell full—and real weakness, even a paresis making walking impossible, has been present for several hours after ingestion. Such an over-dose left one of us slightly ataxic with a persistent feeling of weakness in the lower limbs on into the next morning.

Several recent accounts report little or no pharmacological action from kava prepared from grated or pounded dried kava root and used socially or ceremonially on Fiji and Samoa. My own experience in drinking such kava in Fijian villages is the same lack of effect. It is this dried kava root that has entered commerce, particularly on Fiji, and I wonder whether it is not this product that has been used in the pharmacological and chemical laboratories. The freshly harvested root, prepared by chewing, appears to result in the more potent preparation, the effects of which I have described. The stronger physiological actions of the kava used on Tongariki and Tanna may well be from the use of freshly harvested root rather than dried root, but there is also the possibility that the chewing and salivary digestion that is used to break up the fibers and emulsify the ingredients may be responsible for the pharmacologically more potent product. It is also likely that a higher dose of active ingredients is taken on Tongariki, since a considerably more concentrated extract appears to be prepared; far more root is used per individual drinker than on Fiji or Samoa.

APPENDIX

Historical and Ethnographic Accounts of Kava Usage

AITKEN, R. T. "Ethnology of Tubuai." Bernice P. Bishop Museum, No. 70, (Bayard Dominick Expedition, publication no. 19), Honolulu, Hawaii, 42, 1930.

BEAGLEHOLE, E. and P. "Ethnology of Pukapuka." Bernice P. Bishop Museum, No. 150, Honolulu, Hawaii, 25, 1938.

BEARDMORE, E. "The natives of Mowat, Daudai, New Guinea." Journal of the Anthropological Institute of Great Britain and Ireland, 19: 460, 1889-90.

BEVAN, T. F. "Toil, travel, and discovery in British New Guinea." London, 258, 1890.

BIRO, S. L. "Neu-Guinea (Astrolabe Bai)." Ethnografische Sammlung des Ungarischer Museums, 3: (Budapest), 102, 1901.

BOURGAREL, A. "Des races de l'Océanie Française de celles de la Nouvelle-Calidonie. In particulier, seconde partie." Memoirs de la Societe d'Anthropologie de Paris, 2: 403, 1865.

BUCK, P. H. "Samoan material culture." Bernice P. Bishop Museum, Honolulu, Hawaii, No. 75, 92, 140, 147-164, 545, 548, 641, 679, 1930.

——— "Ethnology of Tongareva." Bernice P. Bishop Museum, No. 92, Honolulu, Hawaii, 81, 119-121, (April) 1932.

——— "Ethnology of Manihiki-Rakanga." By Te Rangi Hiroa. Bernice P. Bishop, Museum No. 99, Honolulu, Hawaii, 1932.

——— "Mangaian society." Bernice P. Bishop Museum, No. 122, Honolulu, Hawaii, 1934.

——— "Ethnology of Mangareva." Bernice P. Bishop Museum, No. 157, Honolulu, Hawaii, 1938.

——— "Arts and crafts of the Cook Islands." Bernice P. Bishop Museum No. 179, Honolulu, Hawaii, 18-20, 1944.

BÜHLER, A. "Versuch einer Bevölkerungs-und Kulturanalyse auf den Admiralitätsinseln." Zeitschrift für Ethnologie, 67: 1–32, 1935.

BURROWS, E. G. "Ethnology of Futuna." Bernice P. Bishop Museum, No. 138, Honolulu, Hawaii, 200–204, 1936.

—— "Ethnology of Uvea (Wallis Island)." Bernice P. Bishop Museum, No. 145, Honolulu, Hawaii, 75–76, 139–143, 1937.

CHRISTIAN, F. W. "The Caroline Islands." London, 86, 87, 100, 188–193, 211, 1899.

CHURCHILL, W. "Samoan kava custom." Holmes Anniversary Volume, Washington, 53–64, 1916.

CHURCHWARD, W. B. "My consulate in Samoa." London, 47–59, 313, 347, 348, 1887.

COLLOCOTT, E. E. V. "Kava ceremonial in Tonga." Journal of the Polynesian Society, 36: 21–47, 1927.

COOK, J. "A voyage to the Pacific Ocean." 3 Volumes, London, vol. 2; 145, 155–56, 1784–1785.

CORNEY, B. C. "The quest and occupation of Tahiti by emissaries of Spain in 1772–76"; 3 volumes, The Hakluyt Society, London. Second Series, Nos. 32, 36, 43. II: 85n, 130, 159, 168, 208, 218, 281, 472; III: 6, 51, 52, 59, 1913–19.

CUMMING, CONSTANCE F. G. "At home in Fiji." Edinburgh, 50–51, 1882.

D'ALBERTIS, L. M. "New Guinea, what I did and what I saw." 2 volumes, London; II: 197, 1880.

DAM-BAKKER, A. W. I. VAN, DEGROOT, A. P. and LUYKEN, R. "Influence of wati (Piper methysticum) on the fertility of the male rats." Tropical and Geographical Medicine, 10: 68–70, 1958.

DEIHL, J. R. "Kava and kava-drinking." Primitive Man, 5: 4, 61–68, 1932.

—— "Position of women in Samoan culture." Primitive Man, 5: 2 and 3, 25, 1932.

DILLION, P. "Narrative of the discovery of the fate of La Pérouse's expedition." 2 volumes, London, II: 42–52, 1829.

DURRAD, W. J. "Notes on Torres Islands." Oceania, 10: 389–403, 1940.

EILERS, ANNELIESE. "Inseln um Ponape." Ergebnisse der Sudsee Expedition 1908–10. G. Thilenius, ed., Hamburg, Friederichsen, de Gruyter and Co., II, B–8, 103, 1934.

ELLIS, W. "Polynesian researches." J. & J. Harper, New York, IV: 277–278, 1833.

EMERSON, O. P. "The Awa habit of the Hawaiians." The Hawaiian Annual, Honolulu, Hawaii, 130–140, 1903.

FINSCH, O. "Samoafahrten." Leipzig, 61, 1888.

—— "Südseearbeiten (Abhandlungen des Hambergischen Kolonialinstituts)," 14: 1–605, Hamburg, 1914.

FIRTH, R. W. "Primitive economics of the New Zealand Maori." New York, E. P. Dutton, 1929.

FORNANDER, A. "Hawaiian antiquities and folk-lore." Editor T. G. Thrum, Memoirs of the Bernice P. Bishop Museum, Honolulu, Hawaii, VI: 72, 110, 112, 258, 260, 405, 471, 505, 540, 1919–20.

FOSTER, G. A voyage round the world in his Britannic Majesty's sloop, Resolution. Two volumes, London, 1777.

FOX, C. E. "The Threshold of the Pacific." London and New York, 44, 67, 216, 1924.

GIFFORD, E. W. "Tongan society." Bernice P. Bishop Museum, No. 61, Honolulu, Hawaii, 156–170, 1929.

GUIART, J. "Un siècle et demi de Contacts Culturels à Tanna, Nouvelles-Hébrides." Publication de la Société des Océanistes, No. 5. Musée de l'Homme, Paris 15–16, 246–254, 1956.

HADDON, A. C. "Kava drinking in New Guinea." Man, 16: 145–152, (Oct.) 1916.

HAMBRUCH, P. "Die Kawa auf Ponape." Studien und Forschungen zur Menschen- und Völkerkunde, Stuttgart, 14: 107–115, 1917.

HAMBRUCH, P., and EILERS, ANNALIESE. "Ponape." Ergebnisse der Südsee Expedition 1908–10, 231–246, 1936.

HANDY, E. S. C. "The native culture in the Marquesas." Bernice P. Bishop Museum, No. 9 (Bayard Dominick Expedition, Publication No. 9), Honolulu, Hawaii, 202–203, 1923.

HANDY, E. S. C. "Polynesian religion." Bernice P. Bishop Museum, Honolulu, Hawaii, No. 34, 46, 136, 162–163, 173, 219, 322, 327–328, 1927.
—— "History and culture in the Society Islands." Bernice P. Bishop Museum, Honolulu, Hawaii, No. 79, 20–21, 1930.
—— "History and culture in the Society Islands." Bernice P. Bishop Museum, No. 79, Honolulu, Hawaii, 1931.
HAWKESWORTH, J., Editor. "An account of the voyages undertaken by the Order of His B. Majesty for discoveries," II : 200, 1773.
HENRY, T. "Ancient Tahiti." Bernice P. Bishop Museum, Honolulu, Hawaii, No. 48, 531, 538, 539, 562, 583, 587, 1928.
HOCART, A. M. "Lau Islands, Fiji." Bernice P. Bishop Museum, Honolulu, Hawaii, No. 62, 59–70, 108, 1929.
HOUGH, W. "Kava drinking as practiced by the Papuans and Polynesians." Smithsonian Miscellaneous Collection, 2: 85–92 (Aug. 6), 1904, Quarterly Issue, Washington, D.C., 1905.
HUMPHREYS, C. B. "The southern New Hebrides. An ethnological record." Cambridge, 1926.
KING, J. "A voyage to the Pacific Ocean." Second edition, 3 volumes, London, 3: 126–127, 1785.
KRÄMER, A. "Die Samoa-Insel." Stuttgart, 1902.
LEDYARD, J. "John Ledyard's journal of Captain Cook's last voyage." Munford, J. K., ed., with introduction by Hitchings, S. H. Oregon State University Press, Corvallis, Oregon, August 1777, Customs of Otaheite, 51, 1963.
LESTER, R. M. "Kava drinking in Vitilevu, Fiji." Oceania, 12:2, 97–121, 1941; 12:3, 226–254, 1942.
LEWIN, L. "Über Piper Methysticum (Kawa)." A. Hirschwald, Berlin, 60 pp., 1886.
—— "Phantastica : narcotic and stimulating drugs; their use and abuse." K. Paul, Trench, Trubner and Co., London, 215–225, 1931.
LING SHUN-SHENG. "A comparative study of kava drinking in the Pacific regions." Bulletin of the Institute of Ethnology, Academia Sinica, 5: 77–96, 1958.
LINTON, R. "The material culture of the Marquesas Islands." Memoirs of the Bernice P. Bishop Museum, Honolulu, Hawaii, VIII: 5, 366, 1923.
LLOYD, C. G. "The use of kava by the Samoan Islanders." Pharmaceutical Review, 18: (June), 261–266, 1900.
LOEB, E. M. "History and traditions of Niue." Bernice P. Bishop Museum, No. 32, Honolulu, Hawaii, 172, 1926.
MACGREGOR, G. "Ethnology of Tokelau." Bernice P. Bishop Museum, No. 146, Honolulu, Hawaii, 151, 1937.
MACGREGOR, W. "British New Guinea." Journal of the Anthropological Institute of Great Britain and Ireland, XXI: 76, 204, 1891–92.
—— "British New Guinea: country and people." London, 73, 75, 1897.
MARINER, W. "An account of the natives of the Tonga Islands." 2 Volumes, London, 1817.
McFARLANE, S. "Among the cannibals of New Guinea." 126, 1888.
MELVILLE, H. "TYPEE: a peep at Polynesian life. During a four months' residence in a valley of the Marquesas." New York, 194–195, 1857.
MÉTRAUX, A. "Ethnology of Easter Island." Bernice P. Bishop Museum, No. 160, Honolulu, Hawaii, 159, 1940.
MIKLUKHO-MACLAY, N. VON. Bulletin of the Imperial Russian Geographical Society X: ii, 1874.
—— "Ethnologische Bemerkungen ueber die Papuas der Maclay-Küste in Neu-Guinea.' Natuurkundig Tijdschrift voor Nederlandsch Indie, 35: 71, 1875.
NEVERMANN, H. "Admiralitäts-Inseln." Ergebnisse der Südsee Expedition 1908–10, II–A3 Hamburg, 40, 1934.
—— "Kawa auf Neuguinea." Ethnos, 3: 179–192, 1938.
PARKINSON, R. "Dreissig Jahre in der Südsee." Stuttgart, 373, 1907.

124

PARKINSON, S. "A journal of a voyage to the South Seas, in His Majesty's ship, The Endeavour (1768)," London, 37, 1784.

PORTER, D. "A voyage to the South Seas." London, 95, 1823.

PRATT, M. A. R. "A kava ceremony in Tonga." Journal of the Polynesian Society, 31: 198–201, 1922.

PUKUI, MARY K. (WIGGIN). Translations in the Bernice P. Bishop Museum, Honolulu, Hawaii: 1) "Against Awa (Ka Elele)," 2) "The evils of Awa (Ke Au Okoa)," 3) "On Awa drinking (Ko Hawaii Ponoi)."

RIESENBERG, S. H. "The cultural position of Ponape in Oceania." Dissertation for Ph. D., University of California, Berkeley, 1949.

───── "The Ponapean aboriginal political structure." Smithsonian Institution, Washington, D.C., 1967.

RIVERS, W. H. R. "The history of Melanesian society." 2 Volumes, Cambridge, 1914.

SARASIN, F. "Ethnolgoie der Neu-Caledonier und Loyalty-Insulaner." 2 Volumes, München, 1929.

SARFERT, E. "Kusaie." Ergebnisse der Südsee Expedition 1908–10, Hamburg, II–B–XII, 410–412, 1919.

SMITH, S. P. "Uea; or Wallis Island and its people." Journal of the Polynesian Society, Wellington, 1: 112, 115, 116, 1892.

───── "Kava drinking ceremonies among the Samoans and a boat voyage round Opulu Island, Samoa." Journal of the Polynesian Society, supplement, 1920.

SPEISER, F. "Ethnographische Materialien aus den Neuen Hebriden und der Banks-Inseln." Berlin, 162–164, 1923.

STEINMETZ, E. F. "Piper methysticum: kava, kawa, yagona; famous drug plant of the South Sea islands. Amsterdam, 46 pp., 1960.

THOMPSON, LAURA M. "Southern Lau, Fiji: an ethnography." Bernice P. Bishop Museum, No. 162, Honolulu, Hawaii, 68–72, 97, 109, 168, 1940.

THOMSON, B. "Savage Island, an account of a sojourn in Niué and Tonga." London, 95, 97, 1902.

───── "The Fijians: A study of the decay of custom." London, 1908.

TITCOMB, MARGARET. "Kava in Hawaii." Journal of the Polynesian Society, 57: (June), 105–171, 1948.

TRUE, R. H. "Kava-kava." Pharmaceutical Review, Milwaukee, 14: 2, 28–32, 1896.

TYERMAN, D. and BENNET, G. "Journal of voyages and travels (compiled by James Montgomery)." 3 volumes, 2: 43, Boston, 1832 (from London edition 1831).

VANCOUVER, G. "A voyage of discovery to the North Pacific Ocean, and round the world." 3 volumes, London, 1: 116, 1798.

WILLIAMSON, R. W. and PIDDINGTON, R. "Essays in Polynesian ethnology." Cambridge, 1939.

Chemistry of Kava

Murle W. Klohs

Riker Laboratories, Northridge, California

Kava (*1*) is one of the popular names for the intoxicating drink prepared from the roots of the plant *Piper methysticum* Forst. by the inhabitants of the South Pacific Islands. The interesting tranquilizing properties ascribed to this romantic brew has prompted numerous chemical investigations over the last century, in the search for the physiologically active principles. These investigations have resulted in the isolation of a series of closely related substituted 5,6-dihydro-α-pyrones (Fig. 1), members of which have been shown to possess some of the actions on the central nervous system exhibited by the Kava extract, and a series of substituted α-pyrones (Figs. 2 and 3) which are relatively inactive in the test system employed.

The first of the compounds to be isolated in the 5,6-dihydro-α-pyrone series, methysticin, was reported by Cuzent in 1861, followed in turn by Winzheimers isolation of dihydromethysticin in 1908. The most extensive investigation of this plant, however, was carried out by Borsche and coworkers, who reported their findings in a series of fourteen papers published between 1914 and 1933. This work covered the isolation of Kawain and dihydrokawain, and their structural elucidation along with that of methysticin and dihydromethysticin. (Figure 1)

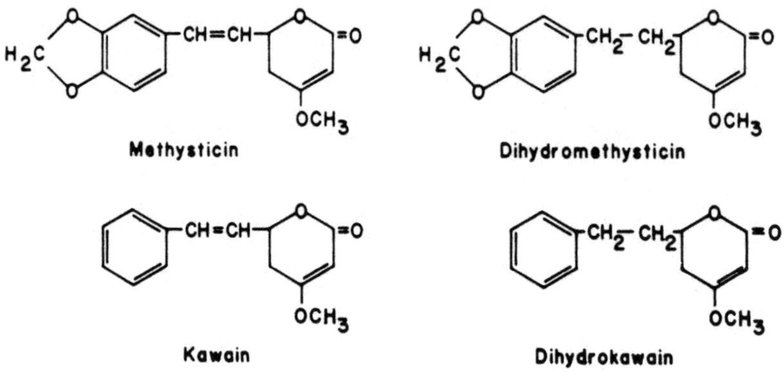

Methysticin   Dihydromethysticin

Kawain   Dihydrokawain

Fig. 1

Yangonin (Figure 2) was isolated by Reidel in 1904, and the γ-pyrone structure (I) was proposed by Borsche. This stood as the only naturally occurring 2-methoxy-γ-pyrone derivative until 1958 when Chmielewska, on the basis of spectral data, revised the structure to that of an α-pyrone (II). Secure support for these spectroscopic deductions has now been established by the unambiguous synthesis of yangonin by Bu'Lock and Smith.

126

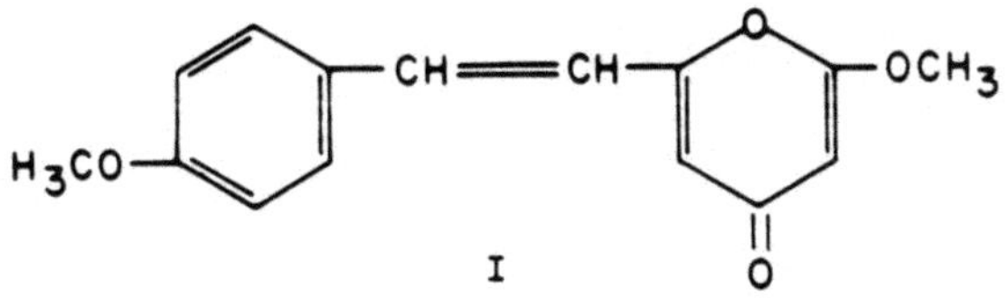

FIG. 2

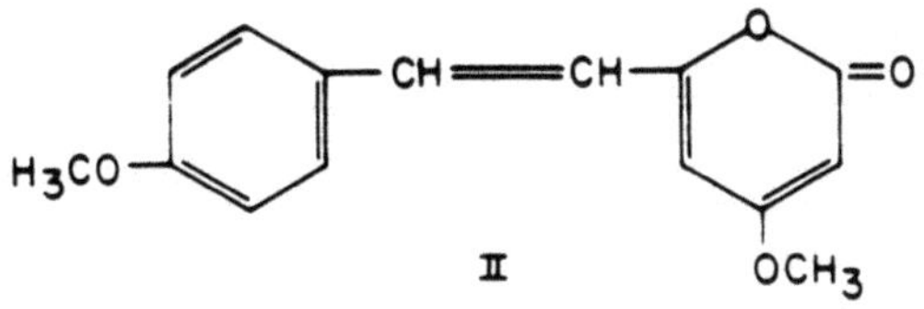

In more recent times subsequent investigators have added four new compounds to the α-pyrone series, with the isolation of 5,6-dehydromethysticin, desmethoxyyangonin, 11-methoxyyangonin and 11-methoxynoryangonin (2) (Figure 3). The Structures of these compounds have been confirmed by synthesis.

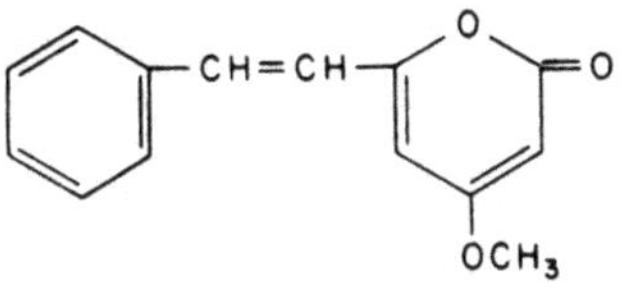

Desmethoxyyangonin

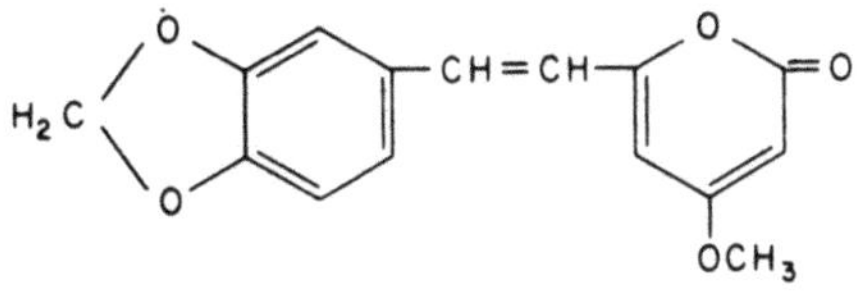

5,6-Dehydromethysticin

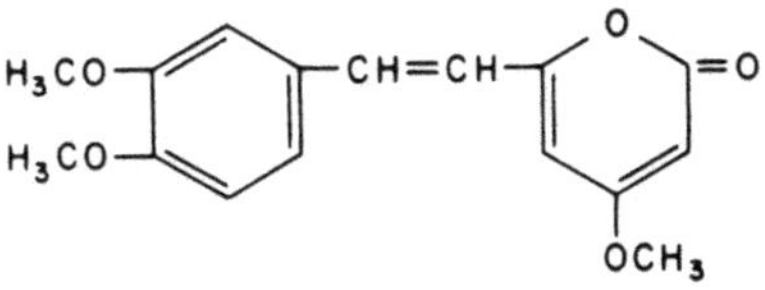

11-Methoxyyangonin

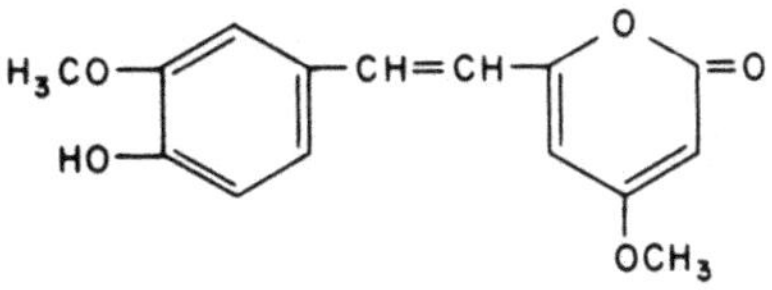

11-Methoxy-nor-yangonin

FIG. 3

With the structures of a physiologically active series of natural products established and the synthesis of analogues feasible, it is only natural for the medicinal chemist and pharmacologist to turn next to a molecular modification program to seek an optimum relationship between structure and activity. In studies with this objective in mind, which were carried out in our laboratory some twelve years ago, the physiological activities of the naturally occurring compounds (Table I) that had been isolated at that time were used as the base line for comparison with the activities of the synthetic analogues. In these experiments the compounds were administered orally to mice in a 10% Tween suspension, and screened initially for their effect on the central nervous system as determined by their ability to antagonize strychnine induced convulsions and death, cause fall out in the roller cage experiments, and potentiate sodium pentobarbital induced sleeping time.

Compound	Strychnine $ED_{50} + 95\%$ C. L. mg/Kg	Roller cage dose mg/Kg result	Sleeping time dose in % mg/Kg controls
Dihydrokawain	340 (270 – 430)	300 no effect	160 150
Yangonin	no protection at 1,000	300 no effect	160 150
Kawain	215 (160 – 290)	300 no effect	160 235
Desmethoxyyangonin	no protection at 200	300 no effect	160 130
Methysticin	160 (110 – 232)	300 no effect	160 250
Dihydromethysticin	115 (97 – 152)	300 no effect	60 413
Chloroform extract	140 (121 – 162)	300 12/18	160 340
Ground root	1,700 (1,400 – 2,100)	10,000 12/18	10,000 400

TABLE I

On the basis of these results it can be seen that the crude extract, methysticin and dihydromethysticin were particularly effective in affording protection against the lethal effects of strychnine. Using "fall-out" from revolving cages as an index, none of the crystalline compounds had significant activity which is in sharp contrast to the ground root and the crude extract. On the basis of this latter test it would seem reasonable to say that there are compounds present in the extract possessing this activity which have not as yet been isolated. Dihydromethysticin proved to be the most potent agent in increasing the pentobarbital-induced sleeping time, showing good activity at 60 mg/kg whereas the other compounds were only slightly or moderately active at 160 mg/kg.

The physiological activity observed with methysticin and dihydromethysticin as compared to yangonin and desmethoxyyangonin, indicated the importance of the 5,6-dihydro-α-pyrone ring to overall activity, and this was corroborated further by the complete loss of activity observed in the three test systems on opening the lactone ring of methysticin to yield methysticic acid (Figure 4).

With this knowledge on hand a number of C_6 substituted 5,6-dihydro-α-pyrone derivatives were prepared (3) by the Reformatsky condensation of the appropriate aldehyde and methyl-γ-bromo-β-methoxycrotonate, using the conditions as previously employed in our synthesis of dl-methysticin (Figure 5).

128

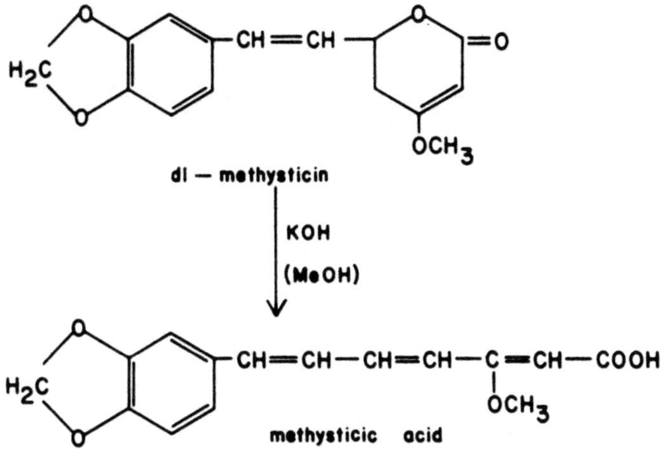

dl — methysticin

KOH

(MeOH)

methysticic acid

Fig. 4

3, 4 — methylenedioxy –
cinnamaldehyde

γ—bromo – β – methoxy –
methylcrotonate

THF — Zn
reflux

dl—methysticin

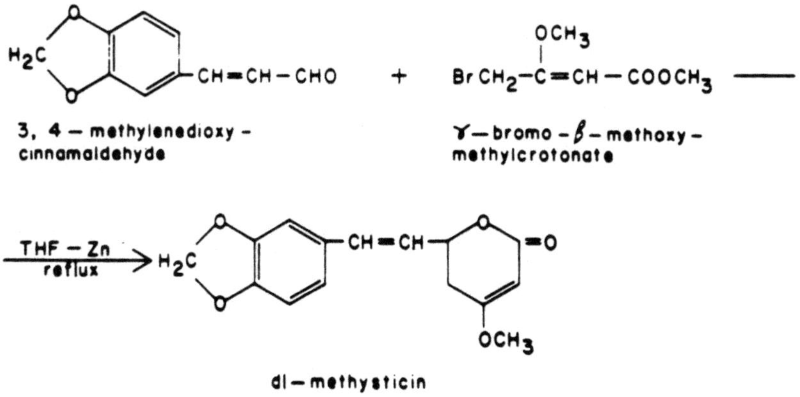

Fig. 5

In the first series of analogues (Table II), the ethylene bridge of dihydromethysticin was omitted as represented by compound 2, and methoxyl groups were substituted in place of the ethylenedioxy group as shown by compounds 3 and 4. These screening results would indicate that the methylenedioxy group is the preferred substituent and that the loss of the ethylene group causes a decrease in activity over dihydromethysticin as measured by its ability to inhibit strychnine convulsions and potentiate barbiturate sleep time. There is an indication, however, of activity in the roller cage where dihydromethysticin is inactive.

The effect of varying the ethylene bridge on activity is shown in Table III. The first and second compounds, where the bridge has been lengthened to butylene and butadienyl respectively, showed little activity with the exception of sleep time potentiation with the butylene analogue. The third com-

129

Table II — structure: R—(pyranone ring)=O with OCH_3; R substituents shown per row.

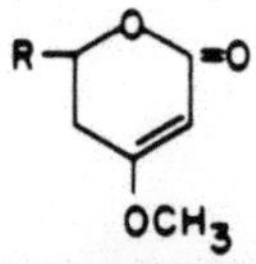 R	Strychnine $ED_{50} \pm 95\%$ C L mg/Kg	Roller cage dose mg/Kg	result	Sleeping time dose mg/Kg	in % controls
1. 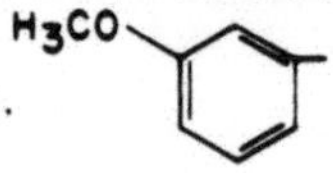 H_3CO— (benzene)	470 (375–590)	300	7/18	160	240
2. 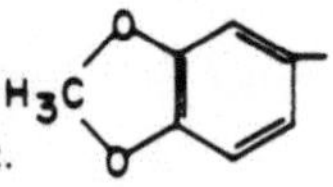 methylenedioxy (H_3C, O–O) benzene	260 (210–320)	300	5/18	160	472
3. 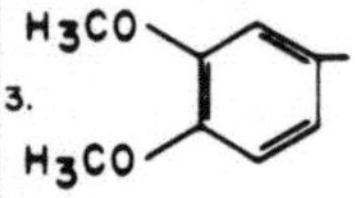 H_3CO, H_3CO benzene	950 (680–1480)	300	5/18	160	152
4. 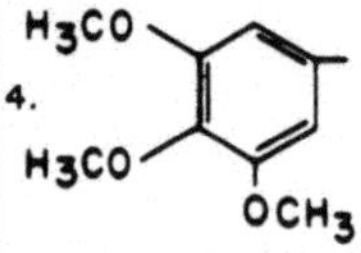 H_3CO, H_3CO, OCH_3 benzene	no protection at 500	300	3/18	160	165

TABLE II

Table III — structure: R—(pyranone ring)=O with OCH_3; R substituents shown per row.

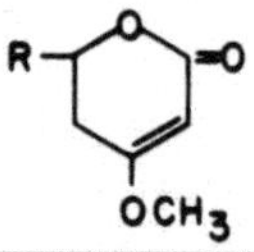 R	Strychnine mg/Kg	Roller cage dose mg/Kg	result	Sleeping time dose mg/Kg	in % controls
1. 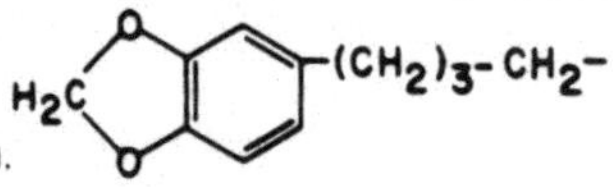 H_2C(O–O)benzene—$(CH_2)_3$–CH_2–	no protection at 500	300	1/18	160	536
2. H_2C(O–O)benzene—$(CH{=}CH)_2$– 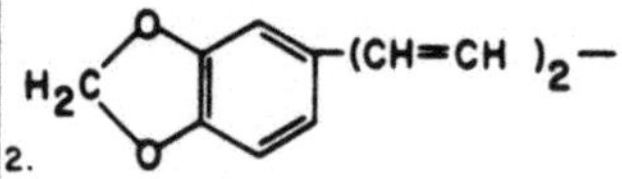	50% protection at 500	300	0/18	160	115
3. 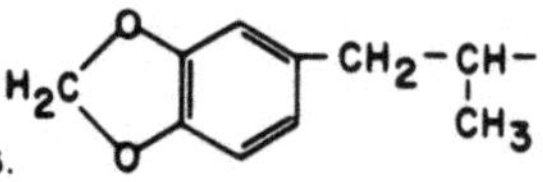 H_2C(O–O)benzene—CH_2–CH–CH_3	no protection	300	3/18	20	283
4. 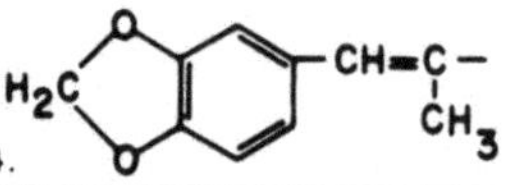 H_2C(O–O)benzene—$CH{=}C$–CH_3	60% protection	300	10/18	60	304

TABLE III

130

pound, in which a methyl group has been introduced on the carbon adjacent to the pyrone ring of dihydromethysticin, gave no protection at 500 mg/kg against strychnine, slight activity in the roller cage, and the highest activity of all the compounds in the potentiation of sleep time. The last compound, which is the corresponding analogue of methysticin, evidenced some activity in protecting against the effects of strychnine at 500 mg/kg, but good activity was observed in the roller cage and the potentiation of sleep time.

The last series of compounds (Table IV) represent a more radical departure from the structure of dihydromethysticin. In the first compound, where R is 3,4-methylenedioxyphenylethyl and R^1 is methyl, there was no protection obtained at 500 mg/kg against strychnine, moderate activity in the roller cage, and activity exceeding that of dihydromethysticin in the potentiation of sleep time. In the second compound where R is phenyl and R^1 is methyl, there was again no protection afforded against strychnine at 500 mg/kg, there was good activity in the roller cage and moderate activity in sleep time potentiation. In the last compound, where both R and R^1 are phenyl, no significant activity was observed in the first two tests and moderate activity was realized in the potentiation of sleep time.

All of the above synthetic compounds including dl-methysticin and dl-dihydromethysticin, with the exception of compounds 1 and 2 in Table III, were then screened against supramaximal electroshock at an oral dose of 770 mg/kg. At this dose range only compound 1 in Table II, compounds 3 and 4 in Table III, and dl-methysticin and dl-dihydromethysticin, showed significant activity, giving 50% protection or better.

On reviewing the structure activity relationship observed in this series of compounds it is apparent that the 5,6-dihydro-4-methoxy-α-pyrone ring plays

		Strychnine mg/Kg	Roller cage 300 mg/Kg	Sleeping time dose in % mg/Kg controls
R	R'			
1. H_2C (3,4-methylenedioxyphenyl) $-CH_2-CH_2-$	$-CH_3$	no protection at 500	5/18	20 250
2. (phenyl)	$-CH_3$	no protection at 500	10/18	160 266
3. (phenyl)	(phenyl)	no protection at 500	3/18	160 331

TABLE IV

a key role in the physiological activities as evidenced by the loss of activity realized on opening of the lactone ring, or by the introduction of unsaturation in the C_5–C_6 position. Rigid overall specificity for drug receptor interaction in this series is discounted, however, by the variations of substituents which can be substituted at C_6 while retaining activity in one or more of the test systems employed.

REFERENCES

(1) References to the work covered in this paper may be found, unless otherwise cited, in three recent reviews: (a) Keller, F., and M. W. Klohs, Lloydia, 26: 1–15 (1963) ; (b) Mors, W. B., M. T. Magalhaes and O. R. Gottlieb. In L. Zechmeister Progress in the Chemistry of Organic Natural Products, Vol. 20, Wien, Springer Verlag pp 131–164; (c) Hänsel, R., Deut. Apoteka ztg. 104 (15) : 459–64 (1964) and 104 (16) : 496–501 (1964).

(2) HÄNSEL, R., H. SAUER and H. RIMPLER, Arch. Pharm. 299 : 507–511 (1966).

(3) TANABE, M., J. BOLGER, F. J. PETRACEK, F. KELLER, M. W. KLOHS and G. E. CRONHEIM, Unpublished work from these laboratories.

Pharmacology of Kava

HANS J. MEYER

Department of Pharmacology, University of Freiburg, Germany

Pursuant to a continuing study of the pharmacological properties of the Kava rhizome (Piper methysticum Forst), the six C_6-aryl-substituted alpha-pyrones kawain (K), dihydrokawain (DHK), methysticin (M), dihydromethysticin (DHM), yangonin (Y), and desmethoxyyangonin (DMY) isolated from the rootstock, were further investigated in attempts to bring the central nervous and peripheral effects observed in man after consumption of Kava preparations (Forbes 1875, Kesteven 1882, Thomson 1908, Deihl 1932, Leclerc 1937, Van Esveld 1937, Van Veen 1938, Titcomb 1948, Frater 1958) in relation to adequately characterized constituents of the plant. Major interest was attributed to the question, in how far these substances can be regarded as the active principles of the drug.

Because of low water solubility the pyrones were dissolved in peanut oil for the intraperitoneal and oral route of application. For intravenous injections and on isolated organs polyethylene glycol (Carbowax) 300 was employed.

As is shown in FIG. 1, the absorption of K and DHK from the gastrointestinal tract was remarkably rapid. The time of peak effect in mice

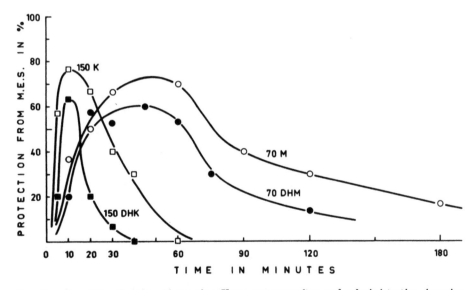

FIG. 1.—*Duration of action of genuine Kava pyrones after oral administration in mice.* Prevention of the tonic extensor component of maximal electroshock seizure (MES test). Corneal electrodes; square impulses of 50 mA, 60 Hz, 0.3 sec, 1 msec. Each point represents the mean of 15 animals. Doses employed: 150 mg/kg of kawain (K) and dihydrokawain (DHK), 70 mg/kg of methysticin (M) and dihydromethysticin (DHM). Notice the rapid onset of K and DHK action as compared to that of M and DHM, the latter being about twice as effective when given orally.

133

proved to be 10 min as judged by the MES test. M and DHM have a longer induction period (30–45 min) and an appreciably longer duration of action in equieffective doses.

The most characteristic central nervous action of all Kava pyrones, including Y and DMY, was shown to be their ability to produce a mephenesin-like muscular relaxation in all species of laboratory animals. According to Meyer and Kretzschmar (1966), who were the first to recognize this mechanism of action, Kava pyrones represent a new group of potent centrally acting skeletal muscle relaxants, the first of natural origin. Larger doses of the pyrones, with the exception of Y and DMY, produce ataxia and an ascending paralysis without loss of consciousness, followed by complete recovery. Pyrones were most effective when given intravenously (10–30 mg/ kg); the oral median paralyzing dose is some 10 times higher. In doses causing muscular relaxation and paralysis Kava pyrones did not possess a curare-like action on the myoneural junction (Meyer 1966). Death after large oral or intraperitoneal doses is the result of respiratory failure.

Kava pyrones were found to depress polysynaptic responses such as the flexor, crossed extensor, skin twitch, pinna—prior to corneal—and linguo-mandibular reflexes in unanaesthetized animals. Effective doses ranged from 20–40 mg/kg iv., whereas in anaesthetized animals corresponding doses were found to be 5–10 times smaller. An example is presented in FIG. 2, showing the depressant effect of 5 and 10 mg/kg of Y and DHM on the crossed extensor reflex in the anaesthetized guinea-pig. The normal knee jerk was aside from a transient increase in reflex magnitude little or not affected. Most sensitive to the pyrones proved to be the tonic stretch reflex (Meyer and Kretzschmar 1966). Thus, in unanaesthetized rabbits and guinea-pigs the tonic responses of alpha montoneurons to muscle stretch were either

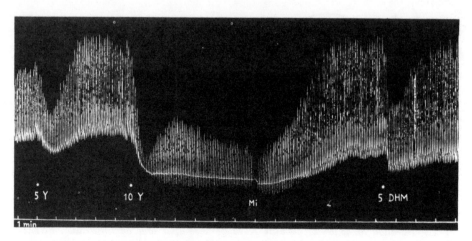

FIG. 2.—*Effect of yangonin (Y) 5 and 10 mg/kg and dihydromethysticin (DHM) 5 mg/kg on the crossed extensor reflex.* Guinea-pig, male, 740g. Urethane 1.0 g/kg intraperitoneally. Reflex elicited every 5 sec. Pyrones given intravenously in 30 sec. Stimulation of the afferent stump of sciatic nerve: 5.4 mA, 1 msec duration. Notice equipotency of Y and DHM relaxation of the quadriceps muscle indicated by the lowering of base line, and slower onset of Y action compared to that of DHM. Mi=miction.

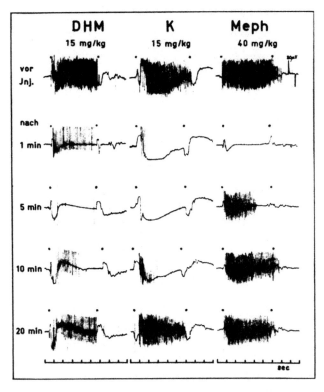

Fig. 3.—*Inhibition of the tonic stretch reflex by dihydromethysticin (DHM), kawain (K), and mephenesin (Meph)*. Rabbit, male, 3.1 kg, unanaesthetized. Electromyograms of the quadriceps muscle, before and 1, 5, 10, and 20 min after injection. The injections were given intravenously with 2 hours interval. Time of stretch is indicated by points.

abolished or restricted to an initial phasic response by 15 mg/kg of K or DHM intravenously. The action of mephenesin was about 3 times weaker and much shorter in duration (FIG. 3). Doses which produce decrease or block of spinal reflexes had little effect on the electroencephalogram (FIG. 4), and left EEG arousal from stimulation of the midbrain reticular formation unimpaired.

In protecting mice from convulsions and death caused by toxic doses of strychnine Kava pyrones proved to be considerably more effective than mephenesin. Thus, complete protection from 4 mg/kg strychnine sulf. sc. was afforded by the intraperitoneal dose of 50 mg/kg of M, the most effective of the pyrones, whereas mephenesin was ineffective in antagonizing this degree of intoxication independent of the dose employed. With high doses of the pyrones (from 120 mg/kg intraperitoneally upwards) there was a seizure syndrome of long periods of generalized clonic convulsions (15–17/sec) similar to that observed after barbiturates or meprobamate (Loewe 1958; Simon 1959). In addition, all six Kava pyrones were effective in depressing or abolishing the maximal tonic seizure induced by electroshock in mice. At the time of peak effect the following ED_{50} values (in mg/kg) were found after oral administration: 70 K, 98 DHK, 44.5 M,

135

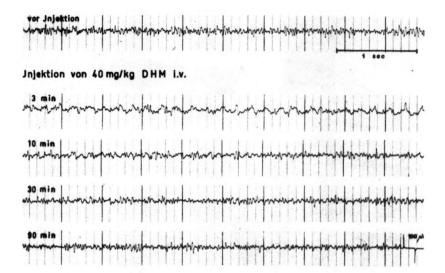

Fig. 4.—*Spontaneous cerebral cortex electrical activity in the unanaesthetized rabbit before and after injection of 40 mg/kg of dihydromethysticin (DHM) intravenously.* Duration of injection 100 sec. The dose produced complete paralysis. Bipolar electrodes on sensomotor cortex. The records cover experimental periods of 5 sec each, obtained 3, 10, 30, and 90 min after injection.

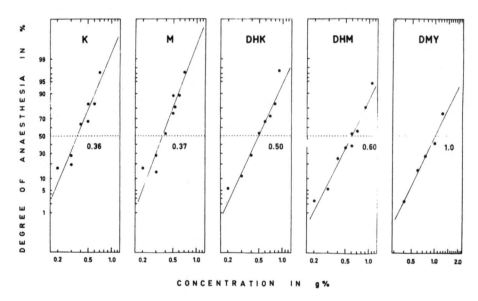

Fig. 5.—*Local anaesthetic activity of genuine Kava pyrones.* Mean effective concentrations as established by the intracutaneous wheal method in guinea-pigs. The graph shows the relation between the concentration of the various pyrones (abscissae, logarithmic scale) and the average response from 6 animals for each concentration (ordinates). The dose was always injected in 0.25 ml of peanut oil, which proved to be inert. The response was tested 6 times in succession 1 min after injection.

136

50.5 DHM, 420 DMY, and 740 Y; by intravenous injection these figures were: 6.0 K, 6.1 DHK, 6.2 M, 8.1 DHM, 6.25 DMY, 11.5 Y, respectively, showing the striking difference in Y and DMY potency with the route of administration. Pyrone anticonvulsant activity and time course of action after intravenous administration were intermediate between mephenesin and procaine HCl with maximum effects 1 min after injection, made in 15 sec. The effect produced by 10 mg/kg most commonly had worn off after 20 min.

In addition to inducing changes in motor function, reflex irritability and seizure threshold and pattern (Meyer 1964), Kava pyrones reduced the edema produced by formalin, serotonin, dextran, or carrageenin. Their anti-pyretic action is mild. Contractions of isolated ileum or uterus produced by histamine, barium, acetylcholine, bradykinin, 5-HT, or nicotine were in-hibited by the pyrones in concentrations of 1:1.000.000 to 1:100.000. This ap-plies to all pyrones, including DMY and Y. Kava pyrones posses local anaesthetic properties. Median anaesthetic concentrations as established by the intracutaneous wheal method in guinea-pigs (FIG. 5) increase in the following sequence: K 0.36%, M 0.37%, DHK 0.50%, DHM 0.60%, DMY 1.0%, and Y>1.0%. Comparable values of procaine HCl, benzocaine and mephenesin were found to be 0.10%, 0.34% and 0.36%, respectively. In sur-face anaesthesia K was shown to be equipotent to cocaine HCl, when con-centrations of 0.5% were employed. Its duration of action was markedly longer than that of benzococaine (FIG. 6). Further details concerning the antiinflammatory, spasmolytic and local anaesthetic properties of the Kava pyrones were previously described (Meyer 1965a,b; Meyer and May 1964).

As can be seen in FIG. 7, rapid intravenous injection of 10–30 mg/kg DHM causes a transient drop in blood pressure which depends on speed of injection and which was stronger in anaesthetized than in unanaesthetized rabbits. The mechanism underlying this action appears to be primarily the result of peripheral vasodilatation. In intact cats, rabbits and mice the blood pressure fall after DHM was followed by a characteristic bradycardia lasting several hours with a maximum reduction of heart rate by 40%. This effect was not observed in anaesthetized animals and was almost completely prevented by previous injection of atropine or bilateral vagotomy. No intravascular hemolysis was obtained in cats with solutions containing 20 mg/ml DHM or pyrone mixture. Oral or intraperitoneal administration of Kava pyrones had little or no effect on cardiovascular functions.

It has been established that Y and DMY possess only weak central nervous activity when given orally or intraperitoneally. On intravenous injection and in experiments on isolated organs, however, the potency of both pyrones was shown to be of the same order of magnitude as observed with the other pyrones of the kavaroot, indicating poor absorption from the gut resp. peritoneum and/or rapid elimination of these materials. In further experi-ments it was found that the activity of orally or intraperitoneally admin-istered Y or DMY is markedly increased when given in combination with other pyrones. Both Y and DMY proved to be synergistic with all other

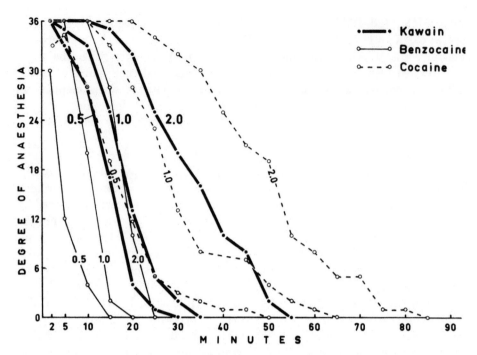

FIG. 6.—*Surface anaesthetic action produced by kawain, benzocaine and cocaine HCl in the cornea of the rabbit.* Concentrations tested were 0.5, 1.0, and 2.0%, respectively. Abscissa is time in minutes after instillation and ordinate is degree of anaesthesia in the range between zero and maximum possible effect (=36). Each point represents the mean of 6 animals. The corneal reflex was tested 6 times in succession at 5 min intervals until anaesthesia had worn off. Kawain and benzocaine were instilled in 0.25 ml of peanut oil, cocaine HCl in saline.

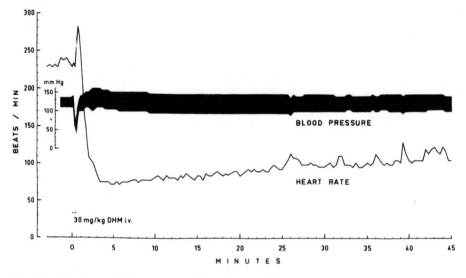

FIG. 7.—*Responses of heart rate and femoral arterial pressure to the intravenous injection of 30 mg/kg dihydromethysticin (DHM).* Rabbit, female, 2.7 kg, unanesthetized. The injection was given in 30 sec. Systolic and diastolic blood pressure obtained before injection are indicated throughout the whole experiment by the broken lines showing the increment in amplitude under DHM.

138

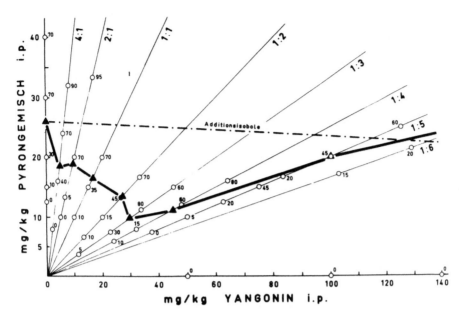

Fig. 8.—*Isobologram of combined yangonin-pyrone mixture effects in protecting mice from electrically induced convulsions (MES test)*. Abscissae: dose scale of yangonin (Y), ordinates: dose scale of pyrone mixture (PM) consisting of methysticin, dihydromethysticin, kawain, and dihydrokawain in equal parts. All injections were given intraperitoneally, Y and PM at the same time. Ratios of PM:Y tested were 4:1 to 1:6. Open circles indicate percentage of protected animals, triangles the mean effective doses (ED$_{50}$). The isobole of combined doses having the same anticonvulsant effect (ED$_{50}$) is represented by the line connecting the triangles. Rectilinear connection between ED$_{50}$ of PM (26 mg/kg) and ED$_{50}$ of Y (1.000 mg/kg) = isobole of addition. Y was without any effect when given alone in doses up to 300 mg/kg ip.

pyrones studied in producing muscular relaxation, hypothermia or preventing mice from MES (Meyer et al.). This potentiation could be demonstrated in isobolometric experiments; an example is presented in FIG. 8. The greatly arcuate course of the isobole of median anticonvulsive doses running far below the rectilinear isobole of addition is characteristic of an effect more than additive. On the other hand, 5, 6-hydrogenated pyrones, behaved additive when given in combination.

The experiments have shown that all the six known pyrones of the Kava rootstock are pharmacologically effective, differences in action being largely quantitative in nature. The finding that Y as well as DMY, contrary to all previous reports on this matter since the beginning of Kava investigation, represent biologically active principles especially on combined administration with the other pyrones, is of particular interest in view of the relatively high amount of these two compounds in the kavaroot which is reported to be one quarter to one third of total pyrone content (Hänsel and Beiersdorff, 1959; Klohs et al., 1959). The synergism between Y and the other pyrones may provide an explanation for the high activity of a chloroform extract and of the crude root, reported by Klohs et al. (1959), which according to the authors was not evidenced by any of the pure isolated materials. The central nervous and peripheral activities of the pyrones as reported herein further substantiate the idea that the various ethnopharmacological phenomena ascribed to Piper methysticum are due to the pyrone content of the plant.

REFERENCES

DIEHL, J. R.: Primitive Man, 5, 61 (1932).

FORBES, L.: "Two Years in Fiji," London 1875, p. 190–195, 235–236.

FRATER, A. S.: Trans. Proc. Fiji Soc. Sci. Ind., 5, 31 (1958).

HANSEL, R., and BEIERSDORFF, H. U.: Arzneimittelforsch., 9, 581 (1959).

KESTEVEN, L.: Practitioner (London), 199–201 (1882).

KLOHS, M. W., KELLER, F., WILLIAMS, R. E., TOEKES, M. I., and CRONHEIM, G E.: J. med. pharmaceut. chem., 1, 95 (1959).

LELERC, H.: Presse médicale, No. 9, 164 (1937).

LOEWE, S.: Arch. int. Pharmacodyn., 114, 451 (1958).

MEYER, H. J.: Arch. int. Pharmacodyn., 150, 118 (1964).

MEYER, H. J., and MAY, H. U.: Klin. Wschr., 42, 407 (1964).

MEYER, H. J.: Arch. int. Pharmacodyn., 154, 449 (1965a).

MEYER, H. J.: Klin. Wschr., 43, 469 (1965b).

MEYER, H. J.: "Pharmakologie der Kawa-Droge- Zugleich ein Beitrag zum Problem des Kawa-Trinkens," Habilit, Schrift, Freiburg 1966.

MEYER, H. J., and KRETZSCHMAR, R.: Klin. Wschr., 44, 902 (1966).

MEYER, H. J., et al.: In press.

SIMON, I.: Proc. I. int. congr. neuropharmacol., Elsevier 1959, p. 414.

THOMSON, B.: "The Fijians. A Study of the Decay of Custom," London 1908, p. 213, 341–351.

TITCOMB, M.: J. Polynes, Soc., 57, 105 (1948).

VAN ESVELD, L. W.: Ned. T. Geneesk., 81, 3961 (1937).

VAN VEEN, A. G.: Geneesk. T. Nederl. Ind., 78, 1941 (1938).

Pharmacology of Kava [1]

Joseph P. Buckley, Angelo R. Furgiuele,
and Maureen J. O'Hara

Department of Pharmacology, School of Pharmacy
University of Pittsburgh, Pittsburgh, Pennsylvania

Piper methysticum Forst. (Piperaceae) is a perennial shrub indigenous to many islands of the South Pacific. Roots of this plant have been used by inhabitants of these islands to prepare a beverage known as Kava, Kawa, or Awa, which has been reported to allay anxiety and reduce fatigue *(1, 2)*. The pure crystalline alpha-pyrones, isolated from the roots of the plant which possess sedative-type activity, are soluble in the usual fat solvents but insoluble in water. Three of these, methysticin, dihydromethysticin, and dihydrokawain, possess sedative activity similar to that of the whole root *(3–6)*. Since Professor Meyer and his colleagues have worked extensively on the pharmacology of these water-insoluble α-pyrones, this present report will be concerned primarily with the pharmacological activity of water-soluble fractions of Kava.

Experimental

The plant material used was obtained from S. B. Penick Company, New York, New York, and consisted of finely pulverized root of *P. methysticum* (Piperaceae).

Steam Extraction

One hundred grams of the finely pulverized root was mixed with approximately 100 ml of distilled water giving a slurry having a volume of approximately 200 ml. The slurry was steam distilled and the first 100 ml of distillate collected, filtered, and lyophilized. The yield for each extraction was approximately 50 mg of a yellow-white powder designated LE–1. When this fraction was reconstituted in a concentration of 10 mg/ml in distilled water, some of the material was insoluble and formed a fine suspension. Since preliminary studies on the spontaneous activity of mice indicated that both the filtrate and suspension possessed depressant activity, the following procedure was used to prepare subfractions. LE–1 was suspended in distilled water in a concentration of 20 mg/ml, shaken for 3 minutes. The mixture was then filtered through Whatman #1 filter paper, the filtrate shaken with two equivalent volumes of chloroform, the remaining aqueous solution lyophilized, and the resulting amorphous solid labeled F_1. The residue from the initial filtration was washed from the filter paper and made up to 15 ml

[1] This investigation was supported by a P.H.S. research grant MH–03029 from the National Institute of Mental Health.

141

with distilled water, shaken for 3 minutes, and filtered. The filtrate was collected and the remaining minute residue discarded. This filtrate was also washed with two equivalent volumes of chloroform and the resulting aqueous solution lyophilized and the amorphous solids labeled F_2.

Pharmacological Studies

Spontaneous and Forced Motor Activity Studies.—The effects of LE–1, F_1, and F_2, on spontaneous motor activity of male albino Swiss-Webster mice were evaluated in photocell activity cages as described by Furgiuele et al. (7). Fifty to 60 minutes after receiving an intraperitoneal injection of one of the fractions or saline, 1 hour prior to testing. Maximum per-activity cages (Actophotometer, Metro Industries, New York) and a 15 minute count taken 10 minutes later. Each fraction was tested at 4 dose levels using 4 to 6 groups of 5 mice per group. The effects of the fractions on forced motor activity were investigated using the rotarod (8, 9). Each group was trained to walk a 1.5 inch diameter hardwood rod rotating at 15 rpm or a 1 inch diameter rod rotating at 29 rpm (10, 11). The mice were trained to walk the rotating rod and on test days received i.p. injections of either one of the fractions or saline, 1 hour prior to testing. Maximum per-formance time was set at 120 seconds for the 1 inch rod and 180 seconds for the 1½ inch rod.

Septal Rats.—LE–1 was investigated for possible antagonism of the exaggerated irritability and aggressiveness of rats having lesions in the septal area (12). Three to four days following production of the lesions behavioral abnormalities were scored as described by Schallek et al. (13). This involved scoring the responses obtained by (a) a puff of air on the back, (b) gently touching the whiskers with a probe, (c) gently prodding the animal's back with a probe, and (d) approaching the rat with a gloved hand. Each test was rated on a scale ranging from 0 for no response to 6 for the most violent response. Different groups of 5 rats were tested, 0.5, 1, and 2 hours following intraperitoneal injection of fraction LE–1. Since chlordiazepoxide has also been reported (12) to be particularly effective in this preparation, it was compared to the activity of LE–1. The ED_{50} was determined graphically using the method of Miller and Tainter (14).

Conditioned Avoidance Response.—The rat pole climbing procedure of Cook and Weidley (15) was modified for these tests (10). Each cycle con-sisted of 15 seconds of tone followed by a maximum of 30 seconds of shock, at 2.75 minute intervals and the number of times the animal responded to either tone or shock was recorded. Each animal was subjected to 2 to 3 ten-cycle training sessions. Trained groups of 6 male albino Wistar rats received i.p. injections of either LE–1, 50, 100, and 200 mg/kg; chlordia-zepoxide, 10, 20, and 40 mg/kg; or saline, 0.1 ml, one hour prior to a 10 cycle session. The number of times that the rat failed to respond to tone but did respond to shock was a measure of the inhibition of the conditioned response.

142

Electroencephalographic Studies.—Cats with chronically implanted cortical and subcortical electrodes were prepared as described by Horovitz and Chow (*16*). Bipolar electrodes were implanted into the amygdala (AP=13, L=9, H=5), hippocampus (AP=5, L=12.5, H=1.5), and pontine reticular formation (AP=35 mm anterior to F=0, L=0, H=32 mm at an angle of 25 degrees) according to the atlas of Jasper and Ajmone-Marsan (*17*) and into the posterior hypothalamus (AP=9, L=0.5, H=2.5) according to the atlas of Bleier (*18*). Monopolar electrodes were placed over appropriate cortical areas, 5 to 10 mm apart. Simultaneous recordings were obtained from three different leads onto a Grass polygraph. A Grass square-wave stimulator was used to stimulate the posterior hypothalamus or brain stem reticular formation for a period of 15 seconds with pulses of 100 c.p.s. having a duration of 5 msec and at 0.5 to 8.5 volts. The animals were placed in a semi-soundproof constant environment chamber fitted with a one-way glass window and a small light. The animals were fed, placed into individual chambers, and allowed a period of one hour to acclimatize. Control recordings were obtained and the threshhold for EEG arousal determined following the electrical, visual (blinking lights) or auditory (clap) stimulation. A desynchronization of the resting EEG for a period of approximately twice the duration of the stimulus or longer was taken as the arousal response. The posterior hypothalamus of two cats and the brain stem reticular formation of two other cats were stimulated and cortical and subcortical activity recorded. After control recordings, the cats were removed from the chambers, and an aqueous solution of either LE–1 or chlordiazepoxide administered intraperitoneally. The effects on spontaneous EEG activity and upon arousal were observed 30, 60, 120, and 180 minutes following administration. An interval of at least 5 days was permitted between injections to insure recovery of the test animals. At the termination of the study, the animals were sacrificed, the brains perfused with 10% formalin and location of the electrodes verified.

Antiserotonin Activity.—A rat uterine horn obtained from virgin rats (Wistar) in the estrus stage, as determined by microscopic examination of vaginal smears, was suspended in a 10 ml tissue bath containing modified deJalon's solution (19), containing calcium chloride, 20 mg/1, and oxygenated with 95% O_2 and 5% CO_2 at a temperature of 37.5°. Uterine contractions were recorded on a smoked kymograph drum via a muscle lever so that the magnification was approximately 3×. All test substances were added in volumes not exceeding 0.15 ml and the α-pyrones investigated were administered in a suspension of 1% methylcellulose, 1500 cps. Maximal contraction of the uterine horn was induced by serotonin creatinine sulfate, 0.5 to 1.0 mcg/10 ml bathing solution. The dose producing maximal contraction was added to the bath every fourth minute; following the contraction the tissue was washed with fresh deJalon's solution. After two equivalent responses to serotonin were obtained, a given quantity of one of the α-pyrones or subfraction F_1 or F_2 was added to the bath, 30 seconds prior to the next dose of serotonin. Additional doses of the antagonists were not added until the serotonin response had returned to normal. Equivalent volumes of 1% methylcellulose did not affect the response of the uterine horn to serotonin.

143

Effects on Brain Serotonin Content.—Dihydromethysticin, 100 mg/kg, F_1, 100 mg/kg, F_2, 100 mg/kg, chlordiazepoxide, 5 mg/kg, and reserpine phosphate, 1.25 mg/kg were each administered to 5 mice. The animals were sacrificed one hour following i.p. administration by stunning and exsanguination. The brains were removed intact, weighed, and transferred to a glass homogenization tube containing sufficient 0.1 N HCl to make a total volume of 3.0 ml. The tissue was homogenized with a motor driven teflon homogenizer and the homogenate rinsed with 7.0 ml of glass distilled water and transferred to a 30 ml centrifuge tube containing 3.0 ml of borate buffer. Serotonin was extracted using the method of Bogdanski et al. (*20*) as modified by Aprison et al. (*21*) and serotonin concentration determined with a Turner fluorometer (*22*).

Results

Physical-Chemical Characteristics of Subfractions F_1 and F_2.—Subfraction F_1 was found to be 16 times more soluble in water than F_2. The physical-chemical characteristics and average yield of F_1 and F_2 are summarized in Table 1. Nitrogen could not be detected in either fraction and aldehydes and/or ketones were detected in F_2 only.

TABLE 1.—*Some physical and chemical characteristics of subfractions F_1 and F_2 from the lyophilized steam distillate of Kava*

Property	F_1	F_2
Physical state	Amorphous solid	Amorphous solid
Color	Amber	Yellowish white
Odor	Aromatic	Aromatic
Sodium Fusion	Nitrogen absent	Nitrogen absent
Ignition	Burned with a sooty flame, small residue	Burned with a sooty flame, no residue
Solubility	8 mg/ml	0.5 mg/ml
Av. yield	60 mg/200 mg LE–1	18 mg/200 mg LE–1
2,4-Dinitrophenylhy-drazine	No dinitrophenylhydrazone formed	Red needle shaped crystals of insoluble dinitrophenyl-hydrazone formed

Spontaneous and Forced Motor Activity.—The effects of the aqueous fractions from Kava on spontaneous motor activity of mice are summarized in Table 2. LE–1, F_1, and F_2 depressed spontaneous motor activity in a dose-related manner. The estimated ED_{50} for F_1 being 31.6 mg/kg and F_2 5.4 mg/kg. Loss of righting reflex was not observed even at those doses which almost completely abolished spontaneous motor activity. Doses of the fractions showing marked inhibition of spontaneous motor activity did not alter the forced motor activity of mice placed on the rotarod.

Septal Rats.—The effects of LE–1 and chlordiazepoxide on the hyper-irritability of septal rats are summarized in Table 3. LE–1 was approxi-

144

Fraction	I.P. Dose (mg/kg)	N[a]	Percentage Inhibition Photocell Activity
LE–1	42	6	67
	84	6	77
	120	6	89
	240	6	91
F_1	5	4	14
	10	4	28
	25	4	35
	50	4	67
F_2	5	4	47
	10	4	59
	25	4	84
	50	4	92

[a] Number of groups, 5 mice/group.

mately one-tenth as effective as chlordiazepoxide in reducing the hyper-irritability of these animals; however, even the 50 mg/kg dose significantly affected the experimental animals and ataxia was not observed in those animals receiving doses as high as 200 mg/kg of LE–1 whereas moderate to marked ataxia occurred at the 20 and 40 mg/kg doses of chlordiazepoxide.

Conditioned Avoidance Response.—LE–1 in doses ranging from 50 to 400 mg/kg i.p. produced a significant inhibition of the CAR which was dose dependent. The ED_{50} for LE–1 was 82 mg/kg and for chlordiazepoxide 21 mg/kg. (see table 4). LE–1 did not inhibit the shock response whereas chlordiazepoxide, 40 mg/kg, did produce a significant reduction in shock responses.

Electroencephalographic Studies.—The effects of LE–1 on the duration of the arousal response after threshold stimulus are summarized in Table 5.

TABLE 3.—*Effects of LE-1 and chlordiazepoxde on the rage score of septal rats*

Drug	N[a]	Dose (mg/kg, i.p.)	Mean Score ± S.E.	ED $_{50}$ ± percent S.E. (mg/kg)
Control	20		62 ± 3	
LE–1	5	50	47 ± 6[b]	
	5	100	37 ± 6[b]	170 ± 19
	5	200	26 ± 6[b]	
Chlordiazepoxide	5	10	48 ± 3[b]	
	5	20	26 ± 12[b]	17 ± 20
	5	40	14 ± 2[b]	

[a] N, number of rats tested.
[b] Significantly different from controls (p<0.05).

145

TABLE 4.—*Effects of* LE–1 *and chlordiazepoxide on the rat conditioned avoidance response* (*CAR*)

Drug	N[a]	i.p. (mg/kg)	Percent Inhibition of CAR	ICR$_{50}$ ± percent S.E. (mg/kg)
Control	24	---------	8	--------------
LE–1	6	50	[b] 48	--------------
	6	100	[b] 65	82 ± 31
	6	200	[b] 70	--------------
	6	400	[b] 92	--------------
Chlordiazepoxide	6	10	[b] 26	--------------
	6	20	[b] 37	21 ± 14
	6	30	[b] 64	--------------
	6	40	100	--------------

[a] N, number of rats tested.
[b] Significantly different from controls (p<0.05).

TABLE 5.—*Effects of* LE–1 *on duration of arousal following threshold stimulation in cats*

Cat No.	i.p. (mg/kg)	Area Stimulated	Area Recorded	Duration of Arousal, Seconds				
				0 hr [a]	0.5 hr	1 hr	2 hr	3 hr
4	50	Ret. Form.	P. Sigmoid	32	20	15	30	------
			A. Suprasyl.	32	20	15	30	------
			P. Hypothal.	32	20	15	30	------
3	50	P. Hypothal.	P. Sigmoid	25	13	9	22	------
			A. Suprasyl.	25	13	9	22	------
			Amygdala	25	13	9	22	------
2	50	P. Hypothal.	A. Sigmoid	40	30	21	35	------
			P. Sigmoid	40	30	24	35	------
			Amygdala	40	30	21	35	------
1	100	Ret. Form	P. Sigmoid	29	0	0	16	22
			A. Suprasyl.	29	0	0	16	22
			P. Hypothal.	26	0	0	10	29
4	100	Ret. Form.	P. Sigmoid	42	10	0	0	36
			A. Suprasyl.	42	10	0	0	39
			P. Hypothal.	48	10	0	0	48
4	150	Ret. Form.	P. Sigmoid	60	0	0	0	[b] 0
			A. Suprasyl.	50	10	0	0	[b] 37
			P. Hypothal.	50	2	0	0	[b] 0
2	150	P. Hypothal.	A. Sigmoid	37	(c)	10	0	12
			P. Sigmoid	37	(c)	10	0	11
			Hippocampus	37	(c)	10	0	12

[a] Predrug.
[b] Recovery in 4 hours.
[c] Unable to record.

The lowest dose of LE–1 shortened the duration of the arousal response for approximately one hour. Although this effect was observed in recordings from both cortical and subcortical sites, no significant changes in the EEG activity were evident. The larger doses of 100 and 150 mg/kg effectively blocked EEG arousal and caused a slowing of spontaneous cortical and subcortical activity. Mild to marked ataxia occurred following the 100 and 150 mg/kg doses, respectively. The duration of the arousal response after auditory stimulation was unaffected at the 50 mg/kg dose and shortened after 100 mg/kg and completely abolished following the 150 mg/kg dose of LE–1. The EEG arousal induced by visual stimulation was unaffected at the 50 mg/kg dose, shortened somewhat following 100 mg/kg, and blocked for more than 2 hours following the 150 mg/kg administration of LE–1. Moderate ataxia was observed in those cats receiving 150 mg/kg and was still evident 12 to 14 hours after drug administration.

Chlordiazepoxide effectively reduced cortical and subcortical arousal in doses ranging from 5 to 15 mg/ kg, i.p. In two cats, chlordiazepoxide induced a period of excitation of sufficient intensity that recording was prevented.

Antiserotonin Activity.—Desmethoxy-yangonin, dihydromethysticin, kawain, and F_2 antagonized the serotonin induced contractions of the isolated rat uterus whereas F_1 did not alter the serotonin activity in doses ranging from 100 to 400 mcg/10 ml bath (Fig. 1). The ED_{50} (dose per 10 ml bathing

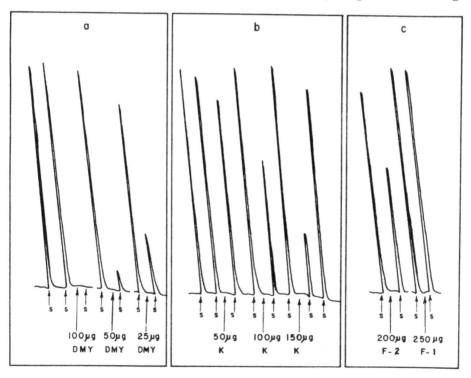

F<small>IG</small>. 1.—Kymograph tracings showing the effects of (a) desmethoxy-yangonin (DMY), (b) Kawain (K) and (c) F_1 and F_2 on serotonin induced contractions of the isolated rat uterus (from O'Hara, M. J., Kinnard, W. J., and Buckley, J. P., J. Pharm. Sci. *54*, 1021, (1965).

fluid inhibiting serotonin response by 50%) for desmethoxy-yangonin was 32 mcg, kawain 100 mcg, dihydromethysticin 75 mcg, and F_2 225 mcg. This antagonism of the α-pyrones to the serotonin induced contraction of the isolated rat uterus appears to be specific since dihydromethysticin failed to alter the contraction induced by either bradykinin or acetylcholine (see Table 6 and Fig. 2).

TABLE 6.—*Responses of an isolated rat uterus to dihydromethysticin showing specificity of antagonism to serotonin*

Serotonin (mcg/10 ml)	Acetylcholine (mcg/10 ml)	Bradykinin (ng[a]/10 ml)	DHM (mcg/10 ml)	Contraction (cm)
1. 0	0. 0	0	0	4. 5
1. 0	0. 0	0	100	1. 4
0. 0	5. 0	0	0	7. 2
0. 0	5. 0	0	100	7. 2
0. 0	0. 0	400	0	7. 8
0. 0	0. 0	400	100	7. 8

[a] ng., nanogram.

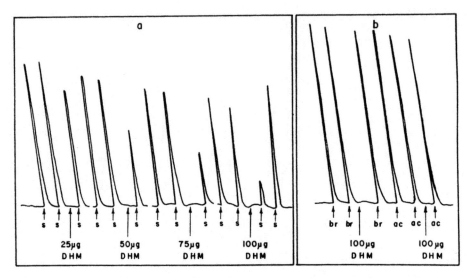

FIG. 2.—Kymograph tracings showing the effects of dihydromethysticin (DHM) on (a) serotonin, and (b) bradykinin (br) and acetylcholine (ac) induced contraction of the isolated rat uterus (from O'Hara, M. J., Kinnard, W. J., and Buckley, J. P., J. Pharm. Sci. *54*, 1021, (1965).

Brain Serotonin.—Brain levels of endogenous serotonin were not altered 1 hour after the i.p. administration of dihydromethysticin, F_1, F_2 and chlordiazepoxide. Reserpine reduced brain serotonium levels by 27%.

148

Discussion

LE–1, a lyophilized steam distillate of *Piper methysticum* Forst., and the two water soluble apparently distinctive subfractions of the distillate produced marked depression of spontaneous motor activity of mice without altering the rotarod performance. Chromatographic data indicated that the pharmacological actions of this fraction were due to substances other than the known α-pyrones (*10*). LE–1 reduced the behavior abnormalities of septal rats in a manner similar to that of chlordiazepoxide in doses which exerted a specific blockade of the conditioned avoidance response. King and Meyer (*23*) have postulated that in the rat the septal area normally acts to dampen hypothalamic output, associated with an emotional state, whereas the amygdala may facilitate this hypothalamic activity. Destruction of the septal areas should remove its restraining influence and result in a hyperirritable animal. Schallek et al. (*13*) theorized that the reduced activity in the amygdala is related to the psychodepressant effects of chlordiazepoxide.

LE–1 caused moderate slowing of cortical, hypothalamic, and hippocampal activity with concomitant ataxia and motor deficiency. After cortical activity had returned to pretreatment levels, subcortical (hypothalamic and hippocampal) activity was still reduced, evidenced by the absence of EEG arousal. Although return of the arousal pattern generally marked the end of an experiment, ataxia and uncoordinated movements were still present, an indication that LE–1 was exerting a skeletal muscle relaxant effect. Ataxia was one of the most consistent responses obtained with LE–1 in mice and rats (with the exception of septal rats) also suggesting skeletal muscle relaxant activity. A single intravenous dose of 20 mg/kg of LE–1 completely blocked the flexor reflex for approximately 3 hours in two cats. It appears that at least part of the altered behavioral effects observed in mice and rats as well as cats could be due to blockade of the spinal interneurons, with progressive weaker depressant effects on the reticular formation, subcortex, and cortex respectively. Certain of the α-pyrones exhibited a dose-related antagonism of the serotonin-induced contraction of the rat uterus and exhibited potency comparable to N-(β-dimethylaminoethyl) cinnamamide (*24*). The α-pyrones isolated from Kava possessing this antiserotonin activity have a cinnamoyl moiety which may be responsible for this particular pharmacological action. Antiserotonin studies further substantiated the difference in activity between F_1 and F_2 in that F_1 did not affect the serotonin response whereas F_2 was antagonistic to it. Subfraction F_1 was a much weaker depressant on a weight-weight basis than subfraction F_2. Since thin-layer chromatograms demonstrated that F_1 is absolutely free of known α-pyrones (Fig. 3) and since the overall pharmacological profile may be quite different than that of F_2, studies are currently being undertaken to isolate the pharmacologically active constituents in this more water soluble subfraction.

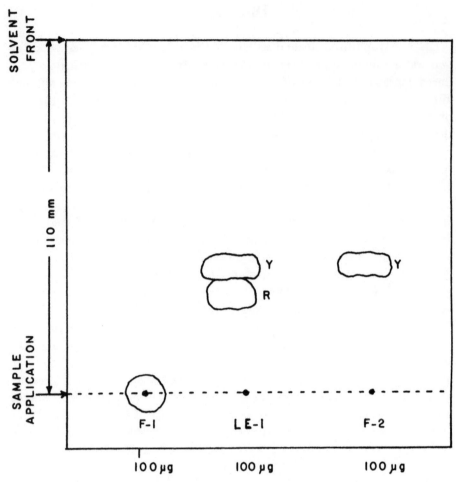

Fig. 3.—Thin layer chromatogram of certain aqueous fractions of Kava (from O'Hara, M. J., Kinnard, W. J., and Buckley, J. P. J. Pharm. Sci. *54*, 1021, (1965).

REFERENCES

(*1*) SCHUBEL, K., J. Soc. Chem. Ind. 43, 766 (1924).

(*2*) VAN VEEN, A. G., Rec. Trav. Chim. 58, 521 (1939).

(*3*) VAN VEEN, A. G., Tijdschr. Nederland India 78, 1941 (1938).

(*4*) KLOHS, M. W., KELLER, F., WILLIAMS, R. E., TOKES, M. I., and CRONHEIM, G. E., J. Med. Pharm. Chem. 1, 95 (1959).

(*5*) MEYER, H. J., Arch. Int. Pharmacodyn, 116, 45 (1958).

(*6*) KELLER, F. and KLOHS, M. W., Lloydia 26, 1 (1963).

(*7*) FURGIUELE, A. R., KINNARD, W. J., and BUCKLEY, J. P., J. Pharmacol. Exp. Therap. 137, 356 (1962).

(*8*) KINNARD, W. J. and CARR, C. J., J. Pharmacol. Exp. Therap. 121, 354 (1957).

(*9*) WATZMAN, N., BARRY, H., BUCKLEY, J. P., and KINNARD, W. J., J. Pharm, Sci. 53, 1429 (1964).

(*10*) FURGIUELE, A. R., KINNARD, W. J., ACETO, M. D., and BUCKLEY, J. P., J. Pharm. Sci. 54, 247 (1965).

150

(11) O'HARA, M. J., KINNARD, W. J. and BUCKLEY, J. P., J. Pharm. Sci. 54, 1021 (1965).

(12) RANDALL, L. O., SCHALLEK, W., HEISE, G. A., KEITH, E. F., and BAGDON, R. E., J. Pharmacol. Exp. Therap. 129, 163 (1960).

(13) SCHALLEK, W., KUEHN, D., and JEW, N., Ann. N.Y. Acad. Sci. 96, 303 (1962).

(14) MILLER, C. L. and TAINTER, M. L., Proc. Soc. Exp. Biol. Med. 57, 261 (1944).

(15) COOK, L. and WEIDLEY, E., Ann. N.Y. Acad. Sci. 66, 740 (1957).

(16) HOROVITZ, Z. P. and CHOW, M., J. Pharm. Sci. 52, 198 (1963).

(17) JASPER, H. H. and AJMONE-MARSAN, C., "A Stereotaxic Atlas of the Diencephalon of the Cat", The National Research Council of Canada (1960).

(18) BLEIER, R., "The Hypothalmus of the Cat", The Johns Hopkins Press, Baltimore (1961).

(19) BURN, J. A., "Practical Pharmacology", Blackwell Scientific Publications, Oxford, England, p. 13 (1952).

(20) BOGDANSKI, D. F., PLETSCHER, A., BRODIE, B. B., and UDENFRIEND, S., J. Pharmacol. Exp. Therap. 117, 82 (1956).

(21) APRISON, M. H., WOLF, M. A., POULOS, G. L., and FOLKERTH, T. L., J. Neurochem. 9, 575 (1962).

(22) UDENFRIEND, S., WEISSBACH, H., and BRODIE, B. B., "Methods of Biochemical Analyses", D. Glick (ed.), Academic Press, Inc., New York, N.Y. p. 105 (1958).

(23) KING, F. A. and MEYER, P. M., Science 128, 655 (1958).

(24) DOMBRO, R. S. and WOOLLEY, D. W., Biochem. Pharmacol. 13, 569 (1964).

Electropharmacological and Behavioral Actions of Kava

AMEDEO S. MARRAZZI
Department of Pharmacology, University of Minnesota Medical School, Minneapolis, Minnesota

This compound in interesting for its consistencies, and I also want to make a point illustrating a concept of a potential mechanism of tranquilizer action. We first got interested in 1959, because of the descriptions and because of the confirmation of these descriptions by Dr. Franck of the American Medical Association Editorial Staff.

I simply wanted to show you two slides, and I need to show you two older slides for reference. (*Fig. 1*)

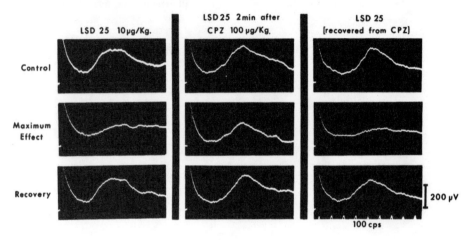

FIG. 1

In the first of these slides showing evoked cortical potentials in a cat, you see that a tranquilizer, in this case chlorpromazine (CPZ), prevents (2nd column) the cerebral synaptic inhibitory effect of LSD (1st column). It controls LSD. After the chlorpromazine has been dissipated, there is recovery (3rd column) and LSD again produces its cerebral action. This is one of the typical actions of a psychotogen, and we think that tranquilizers have a similar but weaker action. The data actually then lend themselves to the notion—and we have further data supporting it—that they have the same kind of action as the psychotogens, illustrated by LSD, but weaker, and therefore are able to compete for the same receptor.

It seemed interesting to see what Kava would do under similar circumstances. A preliminary water extract proved quite potent, and three-tenths of a cc given intracarotidly, elicited an affect very similar to that of LSD. (*Fig. 2*)

152

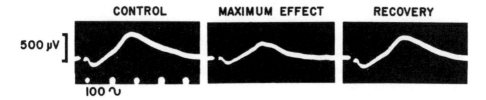

CONTROL   MAXIMUM EFFECT   RECOVERY

500 μV]

100 ∿

FIG. 2

Obviously we are interested in the relation of an electrical effect in anesthetized animals to the behavior that the nervous system controls. *Fig. 3* is interesting in this connection.

This happens to be a rat conditioned approach experiment, in which the response latency to the signal tone is indicated by the length of the upright lines. The effect of LSD is a prolongation of the response time. This would be expected from the synaptic inhibitory action. Inhibition of inhibition, i.e. disinhibition or a release phenomenon, occurs at smaller doses but is here masked by the over-riding over-all inhibition. I won't go into the chlorpromazine protection at the moment.

This (*Fig. 4*) is the same kind of an experiment with Kava. There is a great prolongation in the response time. The sharp cut-off at the top is simply because the equipment turns off after twenty seconds without a response.

It then seems interesting, in the first place, that this material is quite active, because that amount of synaptic inhibition is the equivalent of forty micrograms of serotonin.

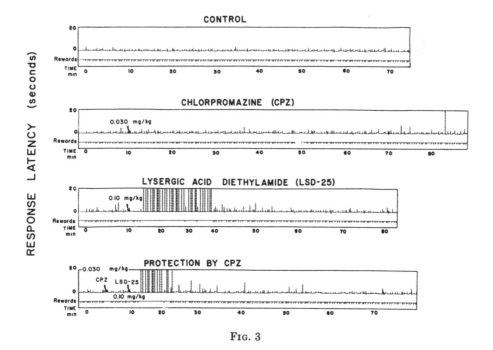

FIG. 3

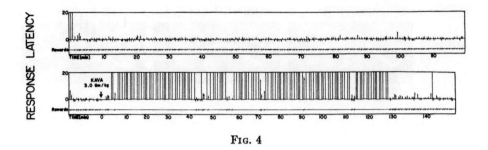

F_{IG}. 4

In the second place, it acts like LSD on synaptic transmission and behaviorally, and you heard rather an extensive follow-up from Dr. Buckley and related data from Dr. Meyer.

The point that I was trying to bring out is the possibility that a tranquilizer is, in fact, a weak psychotogen, and this has very definite implications for the method of looking for new tranquilizers. Thank you.

Effect of Kava in Normal Subjects and Patients

CARL C. PFEIFFER, HENRY B. MURPHREE AND LEONIDE GOLDSTEIN
Section on Neuropharmacology
New Jersey Institute, Princeton, New Jersey

Those of you who watched the television news last October saw that the Samoans offered cups of Kava to President and Mrs. Johnson. The New York Times (10–19–65) reported the incident as follows: (*1*)

Mrs. Lyndon B. Johnson is the first woman ever offered the royal Kava drink, the highest honor Samoan chiefs can bestow on a visitor. She drank it, too.

Samoans who turned out from every corner of the island to welcome the Johnsons yesterday applauded delightedly as the First Lady sipped the bitter juice from a coconut cup. The President only touched his lips to the cup.

Later Mrs. Johnson said the drink tasted a little like the milk of coconuts—watered down—with a slightly medicinal taste.

Drinking the brew, made from the pulverized root of the Kava tree, bound Mrs. Johnson in fellowship with the chiefs. Both she and her husband also made the traditional gesture of pouring a bit of the juice on the ground to get rid of evil spirits.

Subsequently President Johnson, the abstainer, needed two surgical operations while Mrs. Johnson's health has remained excellent! What is in this obviously marvelous brew made from the root of the Kava tree? This conference allows us to review data on Kava gathered in animals and man over the period 1954–1962. The data vary in their accuracy from global clinical impressions to objective double blind studies using quantitative amplitude analysis of the EEG.

In 1954 we made various extracts of the powdered Kava root and obtained brown gums which, while insoluble in water, could be easily suspended in gum tragacanth. The alcohol extracted gum appeared to be the most active in mice, particularly against strychnine convulsions.

One of the active ingredients, dihydrokawain, was compared to mephenesin and found to be effective but very fleeting in its anti-strychnine effect (*2, 3*) Table 2. The testing in mice was perforce done in the first 30 minutes after oral dosing in order to see the characteristic anti-strychnine effect. The very short acting drug mephenesin had a comparable effect to that of dihydrokawain.

Our interest next turned to the two compounds which the Riker Laboratory Scientists found to be very active in their animal tests (*4*). These were dl-methysticin and dl-ethysticin. The methyl congener occurs in Kava while the ethyl congener was prepared synthetically. Both compounds are optically active so that synthesis provides the racemate while the natural compound is an optically active enantiomer.

We studied in two groups of six normal subjects at the Atlanta Federal Penitentiary both dl-ethysticin and dl-methysticin in single oral doses of

155

TABLE 1.—*Anticonvulsant effect of Kava Kava in mice*

[All tests at 1 hour after oral dose]

Compound	Dose/kgm	Metrazol ratio		Strychnine ratio	
		FT	PC	PC	% Surv.
Crude Root	2. 0 gm	*1. 6	*1. 6	2. 1	50%
Hot Alc Extr.	150 mg	1. 4	1. 2	1. 7	28%
CH Cl₃ Ext.	150 mg	1. 2	1. 1	1. 8	35%
Alc. Extr.	150 mg	1. 5	1. 2	2. 2	32%
Control Mice		1. 0	1. 0	1. 0	0

FT=first twitch.
PC=persistent convulsion.
N=14 mice/group.
*Read 1.6 times the control group of mice.

800 mgm. This dose was chosen because therapeutic trials in epileptics showed some degree of seizure control. No significant changes in blood pressure, pulse rate, grip strength, hand steadiness, or pupil size occurred. The subjective responses were equally divided between stimulant, placebo and sedative reports. We conclude that these two congeners were not sufficiently active to be recognized by our crew of drug sophisticated tasters.

When the crude root was given to 9 selected, uncontrolled epileptics (5) in doses up to 6 grams per day a better degree of seizure control was obtained. The same degree of control was provided by an alcoholic extract of the root in a dose of 1.0 gm/day. However, continued therapy for several weeks produced a lemon tinted skin and sclera which was apparently owing to a chemical pigment and is seen characteristically in the Samoans who take Kava regularly. Because of this skin reaction the use of root and extract was discontinued in favor of the study of the pure, more active and uncolored principles of the root.

TABLE 2.—*Anticonvulsant effect of dihydrokawain*

	Dose	Test time	Metrazol		Strychnine, P.C.
			F.T.	P.C.	
DHDK	200	10″			*1.6
	400	10″	1.5	1.1	2.0
	400	30″	1.3	1.1	
	400	60″	1.1	0.9	1.1
Meph.	200	10″			1.2
	400	10″			2.0

Min. Atax. Does=250 mg/kg.
F.T.=first twitch.
P.C.=persistent convulsion.
*Read 1.6 times the control group of mice. 12 mice/group.

156

Of the available congeners dl-dihydromethysticin is the most active in animals. This compound became available for clinical trial in 1956 as Riker Laboratories #532, and was used in doses up to 1200 mgm/day to control epileptic seizures. The anti-epileptic effect was characterized by fewer grand mal seizures but no change in petit mal seizure activity. However, after one month of continuous therapy some patients showed conjunctival and circumorbital erythema, vomiting and diarrhea. These symptoms were considered to be drug induced so that dl-dihydromethysticin was discontinued.

Saunders and Kline (6) treated schizophrenics with this drug using doses of 800 mgm/day. After 3 months, 14 or 15 patients developed typical drug induced skin rashes of the groin and axillae. The reaction disappeared 10 to 20 days after the drug was stopped, but reappeared when the drug was again given to selected patients. The drug had no antipsychotic effect in the schizophrenic patients.

EEG Studies in Normal Volunteers

The quantitative EEG technique provides an accurate method to measure CNS stimulation, sedation or sleep. Quantitation of the EEG was performed with an electronic integrator. This device, the operation of which has been fully described elsewhere (7), transforms the complex EEG signals into pulses inscribed directly and concomitantly with the direct tracings. The number of pulses, for any given time period, is directly proportional to the cumulated electrical energy. Calibration is by the application of known energy constants. The values obtained therefore can be related to fixed standards. The basic time-unit chosen for data analysis was 20 seconds, that is, 2 pages of standard EEG recording. Thus any 10-minute recording run yielded 30 successive measurements.

All the corresponding values from each predrug and postdrug run, as obtained from all the subjects involved in each particular study, were averaged, and mean energy contents (MEC) for the group were thus determined. The statistical significance of the changes was ascertained with the t-test.

Besides these measurements of the level of electrical energy, a careful analysis of variability was performed for each time period. We find that this parameter of quantitated EEG data is highly informative, not only for the detection and characterization of drug effects, but also for baseline features. For example, we have found that male schizophrenic patients have much less EEG variability than nonpsychotics. In the Tables, the values of the standard deviation are computed from the "between subjects, within drug" covariance values. Statistical significance of the differences in variability was based on F-ratios. For convenience, the covariance levels are expressed as the coefficient of variation (CV). Table 3 summarizes our objective findings using this technique.

The subjective reaction of these normal subjects was that the Kava principles produced mild sedation or sleepiness. This would be in accord with the quantitative EEG findings of the most effective congener, namely

TABLE 3.—*Quantitative electroencephalographic studies in normal volunteers given Kava type chemicals*

Drug	Oral dose, mgm	N		C	Hours following admin.					
					1	2	3	4	5	6
Dihydrokawain	200	5	MEC	100	105	101	99	112	117	114
			CV	20	20	22	20	19	19	16
dl-dihydromethy-sticin	160	10	MEC	100	99	103	110	104	101	105
			CV	20	27	31	30	17	23	25
d-dihydromethy-sticin	160	10	MEC	100	108	108	108	103	106	101
			CV	21	26	26	28	*39	*40	*51
Placebo		11	MEC	100	100	107	102	110	102	94
			CV	20	20	19	19	20	20	20
Meprobamate	800	10	MEC	100	96	*71	*77	88	89	107
			CV	19	*29	*32	*38	*46	*56	*39

*Significant at the 1 in 20 level of confidence.

160 mgm of d-dihydromethysticin. This is evident in the increase in the coefficient of variation at the 4, 5 and 6th hours after the oral dose.

Computer analysis of the EEG after 160 mg of dl-dihydromethysticin revealed that there were significant increases in total electrical energy without significant increases in variability. These increases affected all frequencies and were maximal two to three hours after dosage. The increases were more evident in low-alpha records. When very prominent alpha was present, little or no change occurred in total energy or in energy in the alpha band, but significant increases occurred in the low frequency portion of the electroencephalographic spectrum, again without any significant change in variability.

Discussion

We have found that dihydrokawain is very similar to mephenesin in its effect on the strychnine thresholds of mice. Meyer (8) and Meyer and Kretzschmar (9) find a close similarity in the pharmacological action of the Kavapyrones and mephenesin when tested on the reflexes of guinea pigs. The chemical structures are similar in that both can be described as blocking compounds of simple oxygen functions.

If more were known about the physiological deposition of the Kavapyrones a second analogy might be made to the diketone *griseofulvin* which is also a mild CNS sedative, and is known to exert its antifungal effect by deposition in the skin, hair, and nails. This fungicide however is well tolerated by the human skin while the Kava-pyrones are not. If Samoan groups can be found who imbibe Kava only during a ceremonial week one would expect to find some degree of yellow banding of their finger and toe nails if the Kava-pyrones are deposited in keratin.

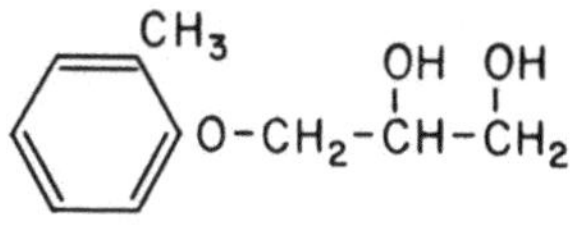

Mephenesin 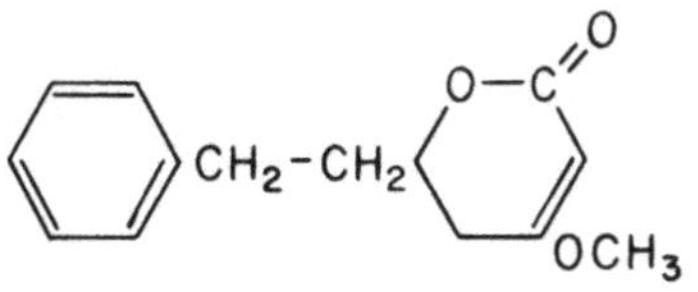 Dihydrokawain

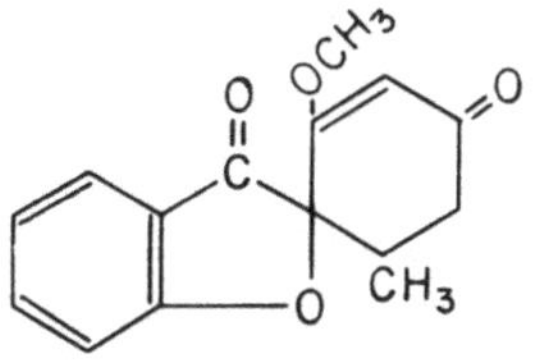

Griseofulvin 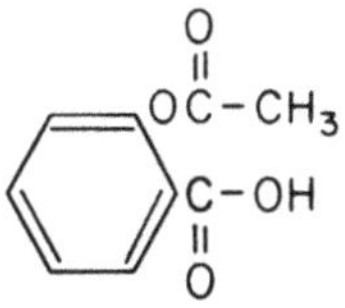 Aspirin

FIG. 1.—The Kava ketopyrones are blocking compounds of three oxygen and a methyl functional groups. Other molecules which have a similar sedative effect are griseofulvin and aspirin.

Perhaps the simplest chemical which is a blocking compound containing 3 oxygens and a methyl functional group is aspirin. This has not been studied in animals for its central relaxant action. Quite independently of the Kava study we have determined recently the effect of aspirin and other mild analgesics on the quantitative EEG of man. Aspirin is the only small analgesic which has a typical sedative or antianxiety effect on the human brain. One wonders then if aspirin is not a mild type of Kava which has been developed in modern society and used without ceremony by the tons (as long as the recommended dose on the label does not exceed two tablets).

TABLE 4.—Comparison of meprobamate and buffered aspirin by the quantitative EEG technique

Drug	Mgm dose	N		C	1	2	3	4	5	6
Meprobamate	800	10	MEC	100	96	*71	*77	88	89	107
			CV	19	*29	*32	*38	*46	*56	*39
Placebo		30	MEC	100	101	100	101	102	103	104
			CV	19	20	17	17	26	18	19
Buffered asprin	1000	20	MEC	100	90	*83	*75	*85	*85	*83
			CV	26	*37	*40	*42	*39	*40	*34

*Significant at the 1 in 20 level of confidence.

159

Conversely one might ask if the Samoans use Kava as a "pain-killer". I have been told that the plains Indians have in times past used peyote as a pain killing drug.

We have heard the chemists describe the active Kava-pyrones which can be found in the Kava plant. We have studied one minor synthetic modification of a Kava principle, namely Ethysticin. We have not had reported today any serious attempt to synthesize more complex Kava pyrones with more adequate blocking groups. Thus in dihydrokawain the synthesis of a methylene bis compound would be of interest, as also would be a benzohydryl kawain. One should keep in mind that as the molecule becomes larger and more effective as a blocking moiety, the structure and perhaps the pharmacological effect will approach that of dihydrocannabinol another oxygen-containing molecule. Also the main physical characteristic of these Kava principles, that of poor water solubility and good lipid solubility, will always result in a preponderance of pharmacological action on the brain and skin i.e. ectodermal tissues. This selectivity should be put to good use in the transport of a properly tailored and more active molecule.

Finally the study of the Samoans and their Kava ceremony remains the best and possibly the last area of scientific interest insofar as the intoxicating effect of Kava is concerned.

Summary

We have studied in animals and man various extracts, extracted chemicals and congeners of piper methysticum (Kava Kava). The main pharmacological action is like that of central relaxants of the mephenesin-type as shown by a specific antagonism to strychnine infusion. Compared to modern synthetic central relaxants all of the Kava congeners are relatively inactive. The most active congener appears to be dihydromethysticin, but this compound when given to man in the dosage range of 800 to 1200 mgm daily produces side effects and allergic skin reactions. The crude root and extract produces a yellowing of the skin similar to that reported in the Kava drinkers of Samoa. From the data now available, further study of Kava as a modern medicinal agent would not appear to be needed.

REFERENCES

(1) New York Times October 19, 1966.
(2) ORLOFF, M. J., WILLIAMS, H. L. and PFEIFFER, C. C. Proc. Soc. Exp. Biol. 70: 25 257 (1949). Timed Intravenous Infusion of Metrazol and Strychnine for testing anticonvulsant drugs.
(3) JENNEY, E. H. and C. C. PFEIFFER. Annals N.Y. Acad. Sci., 64: 679–89 (1956). The Predictable Value of Anticonvulsant Indices.
(4) KELLER, F. and KLOHS, M. W. Lloydia 26: 1–15 (1963). A Review of the Chemistry and Pharmacology of the Constituents of Piper Methysticum.
(5) PFEIFFER, C. C. Unpublished data this laboratory.
(6) CRONHEIM, G. Report of N. Kline to Riker Labs.
(7) PFEIFFER, C. C., GOLDSTEIN, L., MURPHREE, H. B. and JENNEY, E. H. Arch. Gen. Psych. 10: 446–453 (1964). Electroencephalographic Assay of Anti-Anxiety Drugs.

(8) MEYER, H. J. Arch. int. Pharmacodyn. 150: 118–131 (1964). Untersochungen Uber Den Antikonvulsiven Wirkungstyp Der Kawa-Pyrone Dihydromethysticin Mit Hilfe Chemisch Induzierter Krampfe.

(9) MEYER, H. J. and KRETZSCHMAR. Klin. Woch. 44/15, 902–903, 1966. Kawa-Pyrone eine nenartige substansgruppe zentraler Muskelrelaxantien vom Typ des Mephenesins.

Ethnographical Aspects of Kava

CLELLAN S. FORD

Department of Anthropology, Yale University, New Haven, Connecticut

The Polynesian term *kava* is generally used in English to specify the shrub *Piper methysticum* (Forster), its root, and a beverage made from it. With slight variation, this is the term used in western Polynesia, including Tonga. In Samoa the form is *'ava*, in Tahiti *ava*. In Hawaii it is *awa*. The Maori took with them to New Zealand tales concerning the use of kava but did not find the plant in their new home. They found another plant, *Piper excelsum*, which they did not make into a beverage, but which they named *kawakawa*. The term kava or its equivalent in Polynesia is also an adjective designating various properties of food and drink. In Hawaii it means bitter, sour, sharp, pungent. In the Marquesas it signifies bitter, sour, sharp. In Tahiti the range is broad, including bitter, sour, acid, acrid, salt, sharp, and pungent (Churchill p. 56).

The use of *Piper methysticum* is not confined to Polynesia. In Micronesia it is found in the Caroline Islands. It is found in many places in eastern Melanesia: in New Britain, New Ireland, the Admiralties, the Banks and Torres Islands, the New Hebrides, and in Fiji. In Melanesia its use is of spotty distribution. In some instances islands only a few miles apart differ from one another in regard to the use of kava. For example the people of Ambrym in the New Hebrides look down upon their neighbors on Pentecost Island, only seven miles away, because they drink the beverage. Sometimes, as in the case of Tikopia (a Polynesian outlyer in Melanesia), betel chewing and kava are found together. On Tikopia, interestingly enough, the beverage is not drunk but is poured on the ground as a libation to the gods.

Since our personal experience with kava and its uses is for the most part confined to Fiji and Tonga, the remainder of this discussion will relate to those islands. My wife and I have visited most of the major islands in Tonga, the islands of central and southern Lau, the Yasawas, Kandavu, Taveuni, Ovalau, and a number of villages on Viti Levu and on Vanua Levu. In practically all of these places we have participated in kava ceremonies of one sort or another, and I must admit that this has been an enjoyable experience.

The Fijian term for the plant, the root, and the beverage made from it is *Yaqona*. This term is apparently without parallel outside the archipelago, in either Melanesia or Polynesia. The word does not appear to be used in an adjectival form. Lester, however, reports that a word *Qona* is used on the northwest coast of Viti Levu to denote both "beverage" and "bitter." He suggests that this may indicate that it was to this part of Fiji that kava was first brought and that these were the people who supplied the name Yaqona, which is now universally used throughout the archipelago. More commonly in Fiji "bitter" is *gaga*, which also means "*poisonous*."

Our first introduction to kava was on the island of Naviti in the Yasawas off the northwest coast of Viti Levu. We had been taken there by a small copra vessel and dropped off on the reef in the early hours of the morning. We were met by a number of Fijians who carried us and our luggage ashore and who escorted us to the house of Roko, Ratu Filimone Kama, in the village of Kese.

It was, for us, an awkward situation. The Fijians on the island of Naviti had an English vocabulary of scarcely more than "quite," "rather," and "hello," and our Fijian was nil. We were in age approximately twenty-five and quite unaccustomed to the South Pacific. Of course we had read a good bit about the Fiji Islands and the indigenous customs, including kava drinking. We had, for example, been able to read about kava in the *Encyclopaedia Britannica*—you can still read it there—and I quote:

KAVA . . . an intoxicating, but non alcoholic beverage, produced principally in the islands of the south Pacific, from the roots of leaves of a variety of the pepper plant (*Piper latifolium* or *P. methysticum*). The preparation is peculiar. The roots or leaves are first chewed by young girls or boys, care being taken that only those possessing sound teeth and excellent general health shall take part in this operation. The chewed material is then placed in a bowl, and water or coco-nut milk is poured over it, the whole is well stirred, and subsequently the woody matter is removed by an ingenious but simple mechanical manipulation. The resulting liquid, which has a muddy or *café-au-lait* appearance or is of a greenish hue if made from leaves, is now ready for consumption. The taste of the liquid is at first sweet, and then pungent and acrid. The usual dose corresponds to about two mouthfuls of the root. Intoxication (but this apparently only applies to those not inured to the use of the liquor) follows in about 20 minutes. The drunkenness produced by kava is of a melancholy, silent and drowsy character. Excessive drinking is said to lead to skin and other diseases, but *per contra* many medicinal virtues are ascribed to the preparation. . . . [Anonymous].

We also had read various colorful reports about kava and its use written by earlier visitors to Fiji, as in the following examples:

In their devotion they have a kind of sacrament, using the root called on the Sandwich islands *ava*, but *angooner* in this country. In the first place they wash the root clean, and then chew it, and put it into a large plantain leaf, which is as big as a small tea table, which they lay in a hole in the ground, and then pour a small quantity of water to it, and rinse the substance out. This liquor the Rombetty serves out in small plantain leaves to his people, and as each one receives it, they all clap their hands and say *mannor angooner*, which is returning thanks to God in their way. After partaking of this they think they are happy, its effect being similar to that of laudanum [Patterson p. 90].

The great token of hospitality, when one enters a native house, and especially that of a chief, is the preparing and presenting to the guests the native drink, called kava, an article never lacking in tipling Fiji, as we were often convinced, to our sorrow. So we are not surprised that Patioli should call for kava the moment the conversation waned. In Samoa it is considered very rude to refuse to drink the beverage, but that is a punishment we can hardly inflict upon ourselves; so we will allow some pressing engagement to call us away. . . . Kava has medicinal qualities of not a little power. Drunk to excess, it acts like opium, and the habit once formed cannot easily be broken. There are white men, on some of the islands in the South Seas, who live almost entirely upon the baleful preparation. To them it is as much a necessity as is the morning dram to an inebriate in other lands. To the inexperienced, the very thought of drinking the stuff is repelling, but if he can summon courage to try it, he will find a cup of it refreshing and somewhat nutritive. The natives very justly attribute some of their ailments to an inordinate use of it. The habitual kava drinker may be recognized by his fishy-looking eyes and the scaly appearance of his skin [Adams pp. 117–20].

I had tasted it on several occasions, this *kava* of the other islands, without enjoyment. But I recalled a warning from several old-timers I had met that one could not more grievously offend a Fijian than by refusing this beverage, whose serving is everywhere such a ceremonial, prescribed by such rigid custom. . . . "Will this go to my head?" I asked Sakobi, remembering the waiting boat.

"No. No go to head," he assured me. And *kava*, as a matter of fact, is not an alcoholic intoxicant. Rather it might be described as a mildly stimulating drug. A brownish murky fluid, slightly pungent and acrid, it is usually obnoxious to the novice, but Europeans in the islands often acquire a taste for it, and business men frequently keep it in the office for an occasional swig with their customers. Its constant and immoderate use over a long period of years is sometimes injurious to the eyes, so that old *kava*-topers often become nearly blind, but taken moderately or even in large quantity from time to time it is of acknowledged medicinal value, to such extent that the most zealous missionaries do not combat the native custom. And, not being an intoxicant, it does *not* go to one's head; one can drink any amount of it and remain clear minded. The funny thing about it, however, is that it *does* go to one's legs. Sakobi, answering my query literally, had neglected to tell me this. But I discovered it for myself when, bidding my hosts adieu at midnight, I felt my knees wobble and slid like a fireman down the slippery pole that led across the moat. At the moment, I attributed the mishap to the stiffness resultant from sitting cross-legged all evening in an unaccustomed posture. But when we started out across the maze of roads and tracks toward the wharf, where the skipper was conscientiously sounding the promised fog-horn as a summons to hasten, there was no question but that something was wrong with the legs themselves.

"Come here, Sakobi. Give me a hand."

He locked his arm through mine. But *his* legs were just as bad. For a quarter-mile we made progress, leaning against each other as our feet gravitated toward the center. Then, despite all efforts at control, his started for the left and mine for the right, and we both sat down heavily [Foster pp. 238–40].

These and many of the other early missionary and travel reports were equally disturbing, and it was with no little apprehension that we sat in the Roko's hut while the Yaqona was being prepared for our welcome reception. To our relief, the root had been pulverized with a mortar and pestle rather than chewed. But there were other sources of concern. We had been schooled to beware of water unless it had been boiled. And here was a stalwart Fijian plunging his brown hands and wrists into a wooden bowl to knead the mixture while another poured water over the powdered root. What risks were we taking: drunkenness, disease, polluted water, unclean hands? The boat had left, not to return for six months, and there was no other way off the island, not even by outrigger. And the only medical assistance on the island was said to be a Fijian "doctor" with one year's training in first aid. To drink or not to drink was the question.

We had been told by Europeans in Suva that it was imperative that we accept what we were offered, including kava, when we were in a Fijian village. Furthermore, we had been told that the brew was not as bad as it was made out to be and that the best thing to do was to drink it down rapidly—that if we sipped it we would be lost and never finish the cupful, which would be really bad mannered of us. So when the cupbearer, glistening with coconut oil, brought a cupful to me and then to my wife we downed it without hesitation. To me it tasted like the smell of a cedar lead pencil when it is sharpened, and aside from a slight numbing sensation at the base of the tongue and in the throat, there was nothing out of the ordinary about the experience. In fact when we struck lights to our cigarettes after having had our first taste of kava, they seemed to be especially satisfying.

During the year that we spent in Fiji on that field trip in 1935–36 we drank a great deal of kava, probably as much if not more than many of the Fijians. We became quite fond of it and never experienced, insofar as we could detect, any of the ill effects attributed to the drink. Nor did we ever, during that trip or subsequent shorter trips to the islands of the South Pacific, see a native "drunk" from kava drinking. Exhausted, yes. Some of the all-night three- and four-day-long festivities that we attended could not fail to wear people out, but I am convinced that the kava did little to cause what could more accurately be described as a state of being "punch-drunk" with fatigue.

Apparently the early inhabitants of Fiji brought the kava plant with them from Indonesia. From Fiji it was probably introduced somewhat later to Tonga and to Samoa. In Fiji, as far as can be determined it appears that the root was originally grated on mushroom coral or pounded with stones before it was mixed with water to prepare the beverage. The practice of chewing (*mama*) the root seems to have been introduced to Fiji by Tongans or Samoans, although there is a possibility that it may have come to them from other parts of Melanesia. The custom of chewing kava was observed by early travelers and missionaries in the eastern islands of Lau and in the coastal settlements on Viti Levu. Young men chewed the root and deposited it in a bowl to form the basis of the kava mixture. But chewing the root was never practiced in much of the interior of Viti Levu or Vanua Levu. The church and the government discouraged the practice, and today the root is either brayed between two stones or pulverized in a wooden mortar with a pestle. An oft-repeated story justifying the discouragement of chewing kava as a method of preparation relates that in the 1870s a Dr. Macgregor weighed six ounces of the root, which was then chewed in the usual manner. When deposited in the bowl it weighed seventeen ounces (Gordon-Cumming p. 51).

There is some evidence to indicate that the beverage was at one time prepared in an earthen pit lined with leaves, constructed much like an earth oven. The development of pottery in Fiji took place quite early, however, and pottery bowls took precedence and were used in many parts of the islands for kava mixing. Very crude wooden bowls resembling the pottery ones were used elsewhere. At least four to five hundred years ago the modern wooden bowls came into general use and for the most part replaced the pottery bowls. As far as is known, these wooden bowls were made only on Kambara in Lau, and were thence disseminated to the rest of Fiji and to Tonga. Whether the design for the bowl originated in Kambara or was introduced there from Samoa and/or Tonga is not known, but since the term by which the bowl is known in Fiji, *tanoa*, is a Polynesian word, it seems likely that the bowls are of Polynesian origin. In any case, the tanoa has been in use throughout most of Fiji for the past few centuries.

The kava bowl varies in size and shape, but it is generally round, from one to three feet in diameter, and with four legs (occasionally more) all made from one piece of wood, vesi (*Afzelia bijuga*). The front of the bowl has a triangular suspension lug with two holes, to which sennit braid is attached to provide a means of hanging the bowl on the wall. Today all chiefly kava bowls have white cowrie shells attached to the end of the cord. The lug and its attached braid are important parts of the kava bowl and play a major role in the kava ceremonial, as will be described below. The tanoa is never used for any other purpose than that of mixing kava, and after a long period of use its interior surface collects a blue-green patina.

The most usual cups for serving kava are the pointed halves of coconut shells, scraped thin and highly polished. Most cups are about two inches in diameter, but some are much larger. We have one that was presented to me which measures six inches across and holds well over two cupfuls of liquid. It is very old and, like the older kava bowls, it has an interior patina.

When the time comes for the kava to be mixed, the pounded or grated root is placed in the bowl. To this is added water, which is kneaded together with the powdered root. More water is added and the mixing progresses. A strainer of *vau* (hibiscus fiber) is used at the end of the mixing to strain out the woody particles from the drink. As the strainer collects fibers, it is wrung out and taken out of the bowl so that the particles can be shaken out. This process is repeated several times until the liquid is relatively clear. If the mixture appears to be too concentrated, more water is added. Then the kava is ready for serving.

It is believed that the kava ceremony in Fiji was formerly a predominately religious rite, carried out by priests. The purpose was to establish communion with the supernatural. Through the kava ceremony the priests were believed to reach the gods and ensure their assistance in life here and hereafter. Rivalry existed between these religious leaders and the political leaders. As the latter grew in strength by virtue of consolidating more and more territory under their control, they ousted the priestly class from their position of power. Coincidentally, the missionaries came in to take over the all-important function of cementing the relationship between the people and the supernatural. The political leaders took over the kava ceremony, and from that time on it has been more socio-political than religious, though much of the ritual can be traced back to usages in the past that were strictly religious in character. This change in emphasis apparently occurred early in the eighteenth century, and the formal kava ceremony has remained much the same ever since.

In placing the current kava ceremony in perspective it is important to note that Fijian and Tongan society was and still is highly conscious of differences in rank or status. Persons are arranged according to inheritance in a hierarchy from kings to high chiefs, to lesser chiefs, and to commoners. One of the major functions of the kava ceremony is clearly to reaffirm (or establish) status. When visiting dignitaries arrive, this is the means by which strangers are accorded their position in the village or district to which they have come. Among a people whose inter-island and inter-district relationships were more often than not of a warlike nature, this was a respected medium through which rapport could be established, at least a temporary truce declared, and a modicum of trade relations ensured.

Formal kava ceremonies, *yaqona vakaturaga*, are imbedded in a large complex of activities. Much has to be done in preparation, for many days in advance. When the participants have gathered and are properly seated, the ceremony begins with the formal presentation of offerings: kava roots, whales' teeth,[1] tobacco, food, and articles such as pandanus mats and tapa cloth. Then comes the kava mixing and drinking. After this solemnity there may be dances and songs. In any case there follows, perhaps an hour or two later, the distribution of the feast foods and all those assembled proceed to eat.

The seating of the participants during the presentation of offerings and the kava ceremony is most important. The kava bowl is located in the middle of the meeting place. Behind it is seated the kava mixer. At his side, both to the right and the left are what might be termed helpers. Behind the kava mixer and the bowl are seated a number of men who will form the chorus for the chanting which accompanies various parts of the ritual. The *wa ni tanoa*, the sennit braid with its white cowries, is stretched out directly away from the mixer pointing toward the most important personage present, the chief of the district or a visiting dignitary. The first cup of kava will be presented to him. To his left and slightly forward sits his talking chief. To his right sit a selected number of lesser chiefs, all slightly forward toward the bowl.

The significance in Tonga of the suspensary lug and its cord has been vividly described by Sir Peter Buck, himself part Polynesian (Maori):

The following incident illustrates the method of indirection dearly loved by the Polynesians. After the death of the last Tui Tonga, two of the greatest supporting chiefs of the Tui Tonga dynasty came to George Tubou, who had been gathering the reins of temporal power into his hands, and informed him that they wished to make kava for him. They conducted him into the guest house and, seating themselves behind the kava bowl, proceeded to prepare the kava. George Tubou sat down opposite and waited. He looked casually across at his companions and saw what must have been a soul-stirring sight. The suspensory lug of the bowl was pointing at him. The chiefs had not spoken, but the speechless bowl was announcing a king [Buck p. 299].

The precise seating arrangement and the form of the ceremonial differs slightly from one island and district to another, and there is no need to describe these in detail here.

However, it may be useful to attempt a generalized description so that some picture of such an occasion is before us. Imagine then, the chiefs sitting

---

[1] The *tabua*, or whale's tooth, is the ceremonial currency of Fiji. Holes are bored in each end of the tooth, to which is attached a cord of sennit braid or pandanus. A proper cord is made of four-ply braid, known as *sui ni gata* or "bones of the snake." Interestingly enough, the tabua is not just a whale's tooth; it must be old, oiled and polished, and it must have an acceptable cord. What was employed in its place before whales' teeth were available is not known. Stones shaped much like whales' teeth have been found dating back to early times. Wooden tabuas have been known to be used. A suggestion has been made that originally the human collar bone was used. Be this as it may, for many generations the tabua has been the most important possession of any Fijian, and generally speaking they are predominantly in the custody of high ranking chieftains. With the presentation of a tabua at a proper kava ceremony, one may obtain from a chief almost anything one is desirous of having.

167

facing the bowl and the proceedings about to begin. The occasion is that of a visiting chief from another village. All of the actual participants are in colorful costume: some with yellow pandanus kilts, some with green leaf *sulus*, some garbed with colorful tapa, the native bark cloth. All are glistening with coconut oil.

On both sides, at a short distance away from the circle of those participating, may be several hundred men, women, and children—observers only. Suddenly there is a hush of voices, and then complete silence. From this point on none of the participants, seated cross-legged in fixed position, will make any movement that is not a part of the prescribed ritual. There is no talking, no smoking, no uncrossing of the legs, no extraneous movements of the arms or head. All attention is focused on those who are performing their roles in accordance with traditional rules.

The visiting chief moves into the center of the circle, crawling on his knees. He carries with him in his hands the root of the kava plant, or perhaps a tabua. Now comes the presentation: *ai sevu sevu*. With cupped hands he claps three times and addresses the host chief. He says then in effect "here is a small offering . . . " The host's talking chief, or master of ceremonies and the chief himself interrupt to say "a great thing, a great thing," and an interchange of deprecatory remarks on the part of the visitor followed by complimentary comments by the host continues for a short time. Finally the master of ceremonies says "let it be presented." At this point the participants clap their hands in unison.

The master of ceremonies, with his hands lightly resting on the offering, announces in stylized form the acceptance. This concluded, the kava mixer tilts the bowl toward the host chief, to show him that the powdered root is ready. In response, the master of ceremonies says *"lomba"* which means "proceed to mix." An attendant pours water in the bowl and the kneading process takes place. After several minutes the kava mixer holds the strainer above the bowl, allowing some of the beverage to pour into it. If the master of ceremonies thinks the drink is too strong he calls out in effect "More water!" Water is added and the procedure repeated until the master of ceremonies, satisfied, says "Enough water, strain it." At this point the men behind the bowl begin to chant, and this will continue until the kava is served to the chief.

When the kava maker considers the beverage properly strained he strikes a pose with hands together and, looking into the bowl, murmurs that "the kava is ready to be served." Hearing this, the master of ceremonies says loudly *"Cobo*—i.e. Clap," whereupon the kava mixer and his attendants, one on either side of him, clap with cupped hands three times. The cupbearer, whose face is usually blackened and whose arms and legs bear circlets of leaves, appears at the bowl. The kava mixer lifts his strainer and allows the beverage to trickle into the cup which the cupbearer holds out for him. In time with the chanting the cupbearer, now partly upright with knees bent, sways and moves forward in graceful movements until he is quite near the chief. At this point the chanting stops. The cupbearer crouches down low, holding his cupful of kava in both hands with arms outstretched toward the chief. The master of ceremonies says "Go ahead, rise up" and the cupbearer stands up and walks to the chief, to whom he gives the cup of kava. The chief now drinks the kava. As soon as the master of ceremonies sees that the chief has finished drinking (in some instances the chief may spin the empty bowl in the center of the mat) he signals again for the participants to clap three times.

The master of ceremonies receives a cup of kava from the cupbearer, and perhaps the visiting chief and his talking chief. This ends the formal part of the ceremony, and this is announced by the master of ceremonies who proclaims that the "chiefly kava is dry." The *wa ni tanoa* is pulled back out of sight. The kava mixer and his attendants clap three times. From then on the formalities are slackened. It is now permissible to talk and to smoke while the other chiefs are being served their kava. This may last from one half hour to more than two hours, until the bowl is emptied. Never is a kava bowl left containing unused beverage. Following this comes the division of feast foods and then the feast itself.

Good descriptive accounts much more elaborate than the sketch provided above are available in the literature (cf. Hocart, Lester, and Mariner). The important things to note here are, first, that throughout the entire proceeding the arrangement of participants and their behavior, including the chanting and the movements of the cupbearer who serves the kava, are rigidly prescribed by custom and, second, that the occasion is a very solemn affair. In the not-too-distant past, the entire village was compelled to be silent while kava was being prepared in formal fashion, and if anyone, even a child, made any noticeable noise, he was clubbed. We have a recording of a formal kava ceremony held at Naviti in the Yasawas in 1960 that was performed especially for the purpose of getting it on record. The tape recorded the ceremony clearly, and despite the fact that there was an audience of more than two hundred men, women, and children, no noise extraneous to the performance is to be heard except for the occasional cackling and crowing of the native fowl.

Apart from the Yaqona *vakaturaga*, the formal kava ceremony with which we have been concerned, kava drinking takes place in Fiji quite informally. It is frequently drunk in casual fashion by all inhabitants, including Europeans. Children do not drink kava, and at what age they begin to participate is difficult to determine. In native schools they are taught the ceremonial, using plain water as a substitute for kava and wooden tabuas. In Suva, kava is available in most stores and shops for the customer who wishes a cup. A large bowl of kava is always available at the Tourist Bureau, where, to please American tourists, there is usually a lump of ice floating in the drink to keep it cool—to my taste, definitely not an improvement. Among the Fijians, kava seems to be holding its own against the importation of alcoholic beverages and soft drinks. An interesting story concerning Ratu Sekuna relates that upon going to Oxford for his LL.D., he was concerned that he would not find kava there. So he had many bowls prepared, placed them in the sun, and took with him to Oxford the residue, "instant kava," which he could then simply mix with water when he desired.

It is clear that after one gets used to its peculiar odor and flavor, kava does provide a pleasurable sensation. Added to this fact is the long tradition of kava drinking as a part of a large and important complex of activities, including gift exchange, chanting, dancing, and feasting. Drinking kava is considered appropriate to a wide variety of occasions, from birth through marriage and death. It is the only chiefly way to welcome an important visitor. Sharing a bowl of kava tends to foster socializing and friendship, and to the Fijian it is unthinkable that kava should not be a part of commemorating any important event. Kava is never, to my knowledge, drunk alone. The practice is solidly imbedded in social and political context.

The complex of the customs surrounding kava, which has been briefly described above, is unique to those islands in the South Pacific where it has been traditional for generations. It is impossible to find precise parallels in other parts of the world. On the other hand, if one concentrates upon one particular aspect of the complex at a time, it is possible to examine somewhat similar phenomena for comparative purposes. It is important to remember, however, that such parallels as may exist in other parts of the world rarely imply any direct historical connection.

If one singles out the practice of chewing the root as a method of preparing the beverage, which was widely practiced in western Polynesia, one can find many parallels elsewhere. Throughout southern Asia there are customs of premasticating rice or other grains to produce fermented drinks or wines. South American *chicha*, a fermented drink, is prepared in similar fashion from premasticated maize or sweet cassava. Despite the similarity between the preparation of these fermented drinks and the method of preparing kava in some parts of the South Pacific, there seems to be little justification for going further than to point out that premastication has its uses as a means of producing chemical changes in the substances chewed. And the premastication of food by mothers to feed their infants is such a universal custom that the probability of independent inventions using this method for the preparation of beverages is extremely high. There certainly does not appear to be any support for the notion, implied by Ling Shun-sheng (pp. 84–86), for example, that there is a specific historical connection between the practice of premasticating grains for fermented beverages in Asia and in South America and the chewing of kava in the South Pacific.

If one concentrates on kava itself, no direct equivalent is available. But a related plant, *Piper betel*, is used throughout a wide area to the west of the kava drinkers, including western Melanesia, Indonesia, Formosa, and much of Asia. In these areas, people chew a mixture of betel leaf or seed together with lime and the nut of the areca or other palm tree. The effects of chewing this mixture are said to be much like drinking kava, only more so. Betel chewing has its social connotations, and in many places, sharing the betel mixture, either before or after mastication, plays an important

170

role in establishing friendships, in courtship, and in marriage. But there the resemblance to the kava complex comes to an end.

As to other aspects of the kava ceremonial and its associated practices, there are many parallels elsewhere and many of these it might be interesting to examine, but it does not seem appropriate to do so here. For example, the attention paid to the precise seating arrangements has much in common with formalized gatherings in most societies that are conscious of status differences, including official dinners in Washingon, D.C. The sharing of food and drink as a means of declaring a temporary truce or ensuring protection through the establishment of a mutual bond has many parallels, extending from "breaking bread" to the establishment of "blood brotherhood." In its religious aspects, some of the rituals associated with kava drinking have parallels that come readily to mind, including certain aspects of Christian ritual.

Although certain aspects of the complex may be related functionally to practices in other parts of the world, it is clear that the kava ceremony and its associated practices as known in the South Pacific have become an institution which is unique in the part it plays in the life of the people.

There still remains the basic question: To what can the all-pervasive role of kava be attributed? Is it due to the physiological effects of the beverage itself? Are these so powerful that they in a sense demand recognition and that from this flows the development of the involved social, political, and ceremonial practices which surround its usage? Are the accounts of early travelers and missionaries to be trusted? If so, how is their evidence to be reconciled with our experiences?

It has been suggested that the accounts of the effects of drinking kava are simply erroneous fabrications by the early missionaries, which have been perpetuated throughout the decades (Churchill pp. 57–59). In this connection it is interesting to note that some of the early descriptive phrases continue to be repeated verbatim in later accounts, usually without any reference to an earlier source. At the same time, it is difficult to dismiss without consideration personal experiences reported by a trained observer, such as that related by Hocart (p. 59), who writes:

The intoxication caused by kava is called *mateni*, meaning death from or illness from. The expression *mate ni yanggona* is also used. To recover is *mbula* (to live). This intoxication dulls the countenance. As I experienced it, it gives a pleasant, warm, and cheerful, but lazy feeling, sociable, though not hilarious or loquacious; the reason is not obscured. In time a certain dullness settles on the company, in which the kava and the late hour probably both have a part. Once after heavy drinking I felt miserable and found it difficult to walk straight; on turning into bed, I felt sick and could not get to sleep. Such intoxication is rare because in Lau the kava is so diluted and served in such small cups that many rounds can be drunk with impunity. Habitual drinkers are said to become intoxicated more quickly than occasional ones. Kava has no unpleasant reaction next morning, other than indolence and lack of appetite. Habitual drinkers can be noted by their watery and bleary eyes, their dull skins, which in bad cases become scaly.

On the other hand it will be noted that the latter part of his statement carries the usual description of the effects of drinking kava without any substantiation from personal experience. His illness might easily have

171

been from some other cause, since he does not indicate that on other occasions he was similarly affected.

One matter which has not been stressed but which might conceivably be important is that social kava drinking commonly takes place inside of a *bure*, or native house. The drinking may last for hours. During this time quantities of strong native tobacco are smoked. And if the doors are closed, as is the case in relatively cool weather, the atmosphere can become pretty thick with smoke. Several times this happened to us and the effects were not pleasant. The atmosphere, coupled with sitting cross-legged for such a long time, can easily produce some unsteadiness which, I suppose, could be attributed to the drinking of kava if one were predisposed to think so.

Of course it is possible that the experiences we have had are not comparable to those of earlier times. The drink may have been much stronger than that which we have been accustomed to. Kava prepared by premastication, which we have never had, may, through the action of saliva, have quite different properties. However, those who have drunk both remark merely that kava prepared by premastication is a smoother and more pleasant drink than that prepared by pounding and grating.

With the evidence available, it seems that early reports on the physiological effects of kava drinking were greatly exaggerated. That kava does have some rather noticeable reactions, including the slight numbing of the tongue and throat, is clear, and it is certain also that a desire for the odor, taste, and sensation provided by drinking kava can be acquired. But this seems hardly sufficient by itself to account for the part which kava plays in the socio-political and ceremonial life of the people.

It seems more likely that in considerable measure the importance of kava to the people of western Polynesia and Fiji is derived from the part it plays in their life rather than from whatever physiological effects it may have. Kava has become the focus of importance in so much of their lifetime activities that they have come to treasure it far more than seems warranted by its intrinsic properties. Kava drinking has become part of the traditional way of life. As the Fijian puts it kava is *vaka viti*—Fijian custom.

REFERENCES

ADAMS, EMMA H. "Jottings from the Pacific. Life and incidents in the Fijian and Samoan islands." Oakland, Pacific Press Publishing Company, 1890.

ANONYMOUS. "KAVA (Cava or Ava)." Encyclopaedia Britannica 13: 299. Chicago Encyclopaedia Britannica, Inc., 1944.

BUCK, PETER H. "Vikings of the sunrise." New York, Frederick A. Stokes Company, 1938

CHURCHILL, WILLIAM. "Samoan kava custom." Holmes Anniversary Volume, pp. 56–66 Washington, 1916.

FOSTER, HARRY L. "A vagabond in Fiji." New York, Dodd, Mead and Company, 1927.

GORDON-CUMMING, CONSTANCE FREDERICA. "At home in Fiji." New York, A. C. Armstrong and Son, 1882.

HOCART, ARTHUR MAURICE. "Lau Islands, Fiji." Bernice P. Bishop Museum Bulletin 62 Honolulu, 1929.

LESTER, R. H. "Kava drinking in Vitilevu, Fiji." Oceania 12: 97–121, 226–254, 1941–1942

LING SHUN-SHENG. "A comparative study of kava-drinking in the Pacific regions (summary)." Bulletin of the Institute of Ethnology, Academia Sinica 5: 77–96, 1958.

MARINER, WILLIAM. "An account of the natives of the Tonga Islands, in the South Pacific Ocean." Compiled and arranged from the extensive communications of Mr. William Mariner, several years resident in the islands. By John Martin. 2 vols. London, printed for the author, 1817.

PATTERSON, SAMUEL. Narrative of the adventures and sufferings of Samuel Patterson. Compiled by Ezekiel Terry. Palmer, Mass., from the press in Palmer, 1817.

Discussion

Chairman—GEORG E. CRONHEIM
Members of the Panel—JOSEPH P. BUCKLEY
CLELLAN S. FORD
CARLETON GAJDUSEK
LOWELL D. HOLMES
MURLE W. KLOHS
HANS J. MEYER
CARL C. PFEIFFER

CHAIRMAN DR. CRONHEIM: Perhaps we can start with some of the written questions. I also want to make it plain that if any participant wants to ask a question of, please feel free to do so.

Here is a question that we may direct to either Dr. Holmes or Dr. Ford, or to both of them, and it reads as follows: "Several of the speakers have stated that, while Kava drinking produces ataxia and physical weakness, it leaves the intellect clear. Is there any corroboration for this other than introspective reports?"

DR. HOLMES: I might start with this. I would point out that much of the analysis of Kava drinking that I have done has been after the fact. In other words, this symposium came into view about two and a half years ago, and by that time I had already made a study of Kava drinking. It is one of the foremost institutions found in the area, and you can't help but notice it and write down all of the details, but I don't have any quantitative data.

I do have a few ideas that might relate to this: For example, the drinking of Kava by the young men very frequently is followed by very active dancing. It is a very energetic and physical sort of dancing, and if there were any problems with the legs I doubt if they could do it, because a lot of time it involves going down very slowly, that is to say, bending the knees very slowly until they almost touch the ground, and then raising up again. If there were any muscular problems, I doubt if they could do this sort of thing.

As far as keeping the intellect clear, I can recall one occasion when I was in the islands by myself—my wife was on another island teaching nurses. I found things kind of boring, having nobody to talk to for a portion of the day. I would have the boys prepare Kava, and I would sit there and work up my notes and drink Kava constantly.

I will admit I didn't get up very much. I was sitting there typing, but I was thinking and reasoning out certain things that I had observed, and as far as I am concerned, I did not experience any curtailment of intellectual abilities, nor did I experience any emotional problems.

DR. FORD: I might just add one observation. In Fiji they have meetings of the men who sit around and discuss what the day's activities are going to be, and what their long term, maybe two or three activities are going to be.

such as the building of a house, going on a fishing expedition, or whatever it might be. These meetings are invariably accompanied by a good deal of Kava drinking. It seemed to me that the Fijians were much sharper in their decisions and thoughts how to proceed while they were having Kava, than during other casual conversations.

I never noticed that drinking Kava made the men dull. If it were anything it would be the reverse; they would be more aware of what was going on after having had Kava than before.

CHAIRMAN DR. CRONHEIM: Maybe we can turn to a question on a completely different aspect. Here is a question directed to Dr. Pfeiffer: "Will you please describe the effect of alcohol on the mean energy content and coefficient of variance, and compare these effects with those of Kava Kava?"

DR. PFEIFFER: The effect of alcohol in a relatviely low dose, that of an ounce and a half of bourbon, or similarly diluted laboratory alcohol, is that of an anti-anxiety drug, meaning a depression in mean energy content and an increase in variability.

I would like to add that in the early days of mephenesin testing we had a ten percent suspension of mephenesin; this could be ingested at about the teaspoonful level and produce everything that has been described as happening with Kava. I wonder if there is any emulsifying agent in the natural Kava that would suspend some of the substances that we consider not water soluble but which have a definite effect?

CHAIRMAN DR. CRONHEIM: Does anybody want to comment on this last question from Dr. Pfeiffer?

MR. KLOHS: I would suspect in regard to the compounds we worked with, the d-pyrones, where water solubility is negligible, that mastication may result in a sort of an emulsion being formed where the particles are suspended in the water, and in that way you could get some of the physiological effects. That is the only thing that I could suggest.

DR. FORD: The Kava is stirred before each cup is provided.

MR. KLOHS: You would get suspended material here.

CHAIRMAN DR. CRONHEIM: I have a question here for Dr. Gajdusek: "What is the cargo cult," you spoke of?

DR. GAJDUSEK: Cargo cults form the subject of detailed studies by professional anthropologists for each area in New Guinea or the Islands. In the particular cult on Tanna, there was a gradual disenchantment of the people on the Island with the European planters, and the missionary people. There was a turning back to traditional ceremonies and the traditional way of life, with the addition of many of new features taken from the missionary teaching but re-interpreted in the way the people themselves wanted to interpret them.

This was definitely associated with a request that all Europeans leave the Island and that the Government not bother them. A great deal of mythology sprang up around it. There is a whole French book on it, published in Paris, devoted to the cults and myths associated with this movement, or "cargocult".

Kava came into the matter in that it became a part of the whole cult. Women and children occasionally drank, but all of the adult males were drinking a great deal of Kava made from the fresh root. It is only on Tanna that a fully fledged cargo cult of that sort has developed in the New Hebrides.

Tongariki, where the observations I was reporting were made, is an isolated island with a very clannish community that has never really accepted any residents from Europe, British administrative people or missionaries on the island. We have good evidence that our own sojourn was the first that had been spent overnight.

CHAIRMAN DR. CRONHEIM: One question that I only want to mention because there is apparently some misunderstanding, says: "What is known of the chemistry or pharmacology of Kava Kava as distinct from Kava?" They are two terms for the same plant and the same material.

The next question is directed to Drs. Meyer, Pfeiffer and Buckley: "Dr. Pfeiffer dound dl-dihydromethysticin effective for only major sezures. Dr. Meyer, on the other hand, found it to behave like the diazopans, which are more effective in all but major seizures?"

DR. MEYER: I think there must be a mistake here, since I never quoted on the anticonvulsive effectiveness of the benzodiazepines which is indeed not very strong, at any rate much weaker than is found with the Kava pyrones. What I compared, however, was the muscular relaxant activity of both groups of drugs which is produced likewise by a central, most likely supraspinal mechanism of action.

DR. BUCKLEY: None of our work has been done on this problem, and the only finding we have to corroborate the work of Dr. Meyer is that the water soluble material that we are working with is a very potent muscle relaxant.

DR. PFEIFFER: If one compares in animals the effect of chlordiazepoxide against the Kava principles, the Kava has an anti-strychnine effect, and the chlordiazepoxide is barbiturate-like and has an anti-Metrazol effect. One can use both of them in epileptic seizures since the patients who are not responding to classical anti-epilepsy therapy have usually mixed epilepsy, and one can get a variety of beneficial effects. Our sample was at the most twelve patients. In these the predominant effect was a decrease of grand mal seizures and no change in their minor seizures. Had we had a larger sample, and had we done a careful comparison with chlordiazepoxide, we might have found different results.

CHAIRMAN DR. CRONHEIM: Here is another question: "Why is the characteristic Easter Island wooden statue of a man called Moa Kava Kava?" Maybe Dr. Holmstedt who sent in this question can provide also the answer.

DR. HOLMSTEDT: No.

CHAIRMAN DR. CRONHEIM: The next question, which perhaps can be answered by our anthropologist friends, who have seen the effects of Kava, is as follows: "Are cola drinks adequate substitutes for Kava insofar as claimed effects are concerned?"

DR. FORD: I suppose that by cola drink you mean soft drinks such as Coca Cola or Pepsi Cola. All I can say is that in my experience with the Fiji people, men particularly, would rather drink Kava than either a soft drink such as the colas, or beer. That does not mean to say that they won't drink cola, but I am quite certain that there is a distinct preference for Kava, and had if they had to choose one as opposed to the other, they would take their own native drink.

CHAIRMAN DR. CRONHEIM: The next question is to anyone on the panel: "Is there any specific therapeutic use of Kava by natives, or does any occur to you?" This can be answered by anyone on the panel. (No answer was forthcoming.)

DR. PFEIFFER: I have a question, and that is, since griseofulvin is fungicidal and deposits in the skin, I think it would be of interest to determine if there is any fungicidal effect of any of these Kava principles, because we know in this particular area of the world "jungle rot" or fungal infections are very common, so that the incidence of fungal infections might be less in the male than in the female.

I have already brought up the question of whether or not it is a pain killing drug and the consensus seems to be that it is not a pain killing drug in general.

DR. HOLMES: I did mention this morning that it is often taken to relieve the chills of filariasis, but other than that I know of no claims for Kava as a therapeutic drug.

DR. BUCKLEY: I can mention that the preliminary data that we have on the aqueous subfraction F–1 of Kava, indicated by the pharmacologic profiles, would suggest that if we are ever able to isolate the active constituent that it has potential tranquilizing activity, if it is effective orally.

CHAIRMAN DR. CRONHEIM: The next question is directed to Dr. Meyer and Dr. Buckley: "Since Kava ingestion causes a soporific effect, coupled with loss of muscle tone, have any studies been carried out relating the active principles of Kava to the physiological mechanisms of sleep in general, and to REM-sleep in particular?"

DR. BUCKLEY: I will introduce the subject. Data that we have obtained indicate that in the dosages used we get a very marked sedative effect, but not an effect as far as inducing sleep. These animals are very alert, and it appears that the reaction is at the subcortical level rather than the cortex. It is only when we get up to the higher doses that we get a true effect on the spinal cord and on the cerebral cortex.

DR. MEYER: One of the most striking manifestations during sleep revealed by electrophysiological recording is the reduction in the activity of skeletal muscles. In our experiments with Kava constituents of the pyrone group, we found a decrease of the tonic properties of the alpha motoneurones, followed by a loss of muscle tone which may resemble in some respect the reduced muscular activity observed in sleep.

On the other hand, there is no effect, no depressing effect, on the arousal response of the cerebral cortex elicited by electrical stimulation of the midbrain reticular formation, which is in contrast to the depressant action of the barbiturates on this system. We think that this is an appreciable difference between hypnotics and soporific agents like the Kava pyrones, the action of which are apparently more related to the physiological mechanisms of sleep. Moreover, animals put into sleep by Kava pyrones, easily can be aroused at any time of drug action.

177

Investigations with pyrones related to REM-sleep have not been carried out so far.

CHAIRMAN DR. CRONHEIM: I have a question here to Dr. Ford and the rest of the panel: "Would you please expand on the comment you made concerning possible enhancement of mental ability. Do any of the members have anything to add on this subject?"

DR. FORD: Well, all I can say is what I said before, and this is, of course, very tenuous judgment; but it did seem to me that the Fijians were just as alert, if not more alert, while they were drinking Kava, than when they were not.

It may be that other aspects of the situation account for part of this. For example, decision-making and considering future plans of the villagers might help to provide this alertness rather than the Kava itself.

From my own experience, and here again I think there might be individual differences, I never felt that Kava affected my thinking. Our youngest son, who was twenty-three years old at the time, came and spent two months with us in Naviti. The young men of the village sort of challenged him to Kava drinking bouts, much as beer drinking bouts might take place among such young people here. He claims that during the first half hour of such a drinking bout, during which he consumed maybe a quart or so of this diluted Kava, he became quite drowsy and sleepy, but that after this period passed he was well alert and wide awake enough to actually speak Fijian better than he felt he had normally been able to do.

DR. GAJDUSEK: I just never felt this drowsy feeling, and I don't know what the answers to this might be. The Tongarikans obviously are not drinking Kava socially. Often they are drinking alone. They are anxious to get the expected effect, and therefore having taken a large dose and eaten, and if they are not getting the effect, they often go back and have their boys chew more. They are subjectively evaluating what is happening; and if a sufficient reaction is not observed within the first half hour, they drink more; they raise the dose.

Those who are obviously casual drinkers, like myself, are likely to get a half portion, they are a little stingy about the Kava, they don't want to waste it on those who don't enjoy it, and with that half dose I could leave the area, go back to whatever work I was going to do that evening without any noticeable subjective impairment; and my colleagues do the same.

When one pushes the point and tries several doses one does get an effect. It is the effect I described: there is a market paresthesia of the lower extremities, numbness and cooling. It is not real anesthesia; you can still feel sensations with the extremities.

The men describe the same effect and they don't want to be disturbed as they subjectively observe it. They like the feeling and they refer particularly to numbness of their lower extremity up to the waist. They claim, and we find this to certainly be the case, that when one takes enough and tries to get up, one falls on one's face. They still have reflexes at this stage as I looked at them, but there are plenty of men who leave for home at too early a stage,

178

and need assistance to go home. They fall off the trail, but these are people who are concerned about their Kava and are drinking plenty of it.

Two other items which I think pharmacologically ought to be kept in mind. There is a great deal of concern whose Kava one is using, what garden plot it comes from, whether it is too dry, or if it is grown in the wrong soil or in the wrong place. I wonder whether one may not have a variety, depending on growth and hydration of the roots.

CHAIRMAN DR. CRONHEIM: I have a short question to Dr. Pfeiffer, and then one to the panel. The question to Dr. Pfeiffer is: "How would one reconcile the arousal or excessive cerebral activity of schizophrenics with the apparent decrease of synaptic transmission shown in the cat?"

DR. PFEIFFER: This represents two different test preparations, one the pentobarbitalized cat as a model on which to test hallucinogenic drugs. The other represents the natural state of psychosis in unanaesthetized patients. There is such a world of difference that I don't think one can compare the two, except in an average overall sample of brain wave activity. The brain wave of the schizophrenics are those of an over aroused or hyper-regulated type.

In regard to the previous question on performance under Kava, which asked if the mind was more clear, we know of many colleagues who are constantly over-stimulated and do their best when they have a sedative in them, whether it be meprobamate, chlordiazepoxide, or bourbon. I know one very fine author who can only write a book consuming a case of bourbon a week. It is a very fine book and this is the way the man works; he is productive on whiskey but not otherwise productive.

CHAIRMAN DR. CRONHEIM: I have two more questions, both pertaining to the same subject, and I am going to read them and will add to these questions one additional point, and then we will have to stop this discussion because of the time factor.

One question reads: "Will one of the speakers trace the introduction and migration of the beverage throughout the Pacific? Is it used throughout the range of the plant? What cultural modification of the natural range took place in the Pacific?"

The other question reads: "Dr. Ford mentioned parallel distribution and use of Betel and Kava, but cited as an example that in Tikopia, Betel was chewed, whereas Kava was poured on the ground. Parallel distribution of plants occurs in Micronesia, but usage is not parallel. Would Dr. Holmes care to comment on this?" I think in line with this, perhaps the most important, the most interesting question is a kind of summing-up question, namely:

We have heard from Dr. Gajdusek some very definite experiences of Kava effects that he has observed both on himself, on his associates, and also on the natives in the Islands where he worked. We have heard from Dr. Ford and Dr. Holmes that they did not see such effects or did not experience them on themselves; and so to relate it to the questions I just read to you, can the three of you in some way point out the differences, either in the time of the year or the type of the plant? Is it really botanically the same plant, or are there other differences, conceivably other than the question of dosage that Dr. Ford already mentioned? Could you explain this very apparent dichotomy?

Dr. Holmes: I would like to answer that last question, because I would hate to try and trace the distribution in the short time we have. We did attempt to do a bit of this in our papers. But there are a couple of things I would like to say about this last question: I think we ought to resolve these problems, or at least attempt to do so. I would think that part of the answer might rest in the amounts, or concentration. The Kava ceremony that you observed in my film involved about as much Kava as would fill my hand level. I have no measurements of this. It is a very rough estimate. This would be placed in a fairly large bowl about sixteen inches across. I imagine there would be close to a gallon of water in there, because sometimes as many as thirty Chiefs will be served a cup of Kava, and the cup is pretty good sized. It might be that it is much more diluted in some places than in others.

There is the possibility of the saliva factor, and I might comment on this. The Kava that I have seen drunk and have drunk myself was not chewed and therefore did not involve saliva. I did not mention this in my talk this morning, but formerly Kava was prepared by chewing in Samoa also. However, all of my informants told me that the Kava chewers were trained not to get saliva on the Kava. I don't know how you do this, but the attempt was made not to get a big, messy cud and to keep the Kava as dry as possible. Apparently, at least according to my informants, the attempt was made not to get too much saliva in the mixture.

Dr. Ford: A relatively amusing thing happened back in the early 1860's. The missionaries got disturbed about the fact that in parts of Fiji, particularly along the coast, they chewed the Kava root in preparation, and one fellow thought he had clinched things. What he did was to weigh pieces of Kava root before they were chewed and then swipe them from the chewer before he packed them back into the bowl; and from six ounces of Kava root, it increased to seventeen ounces after having been chewed. This was used as a stock example by everybody to justify stamping out this horrible, detestable habit of pre-masticating Kava. I have never tasted Kava that has been pre-masticated and this would seem to be one variable.

Another is the variable of the green versus the dry root.

Another is the variable of maybe different varieties in different soils, and the final one is obviously the tremendous difference in the amount of concentrate.

Dr. Gajdusek: The dosage matter is very important. The quantity of Kava you are describing is less than is used in Tongariki for one man, let alone for thirty Chiefs. A large quantity sufficient for six young men is made, and I suspect this amount of root is more than you are using for your whole ceremony. This is one person's production.

From the Floor: Did the chewers get a Kava effect?

Dr. Gajdusek: The young men that are chewing the Kava have a thoroughly anaesthetized mouth. They claim that they cannot taste anything for the rest of the evening. They also have a stiff mouth and claim they have difficulty in articulating.

DR. LEAKE: We should always remember that the active principles in any plant vary enormously with respect to the soils in which they may grow. This is well known with nicotine and tobacco, or ephedrine. This may be a factor in the variation in Kava, since the soils in those areas do vary greatly.

DR. HOLDER (from the floor): I am an anthropologist from the University of Nebraska. In 1943 on the Northern New Hebrides Islands, I drank Kava and helped prepare it, and in Dr. Gajdusek's comments and other comments this might be worthwhile. The Kava was dried and smoked in the roof timbers, and the preparation was made by taking a piece about twice as large as your thumb and chewing it for about three to four minutes. The natives themselves said it was necessary to get the saliva in to release the active principle.

I had been chosen as a chewer and did chew on many occasions, and I got anaesthetized tongue and the inner lining of my mouth was anaesthetized. This chewed mass was mixed with water in cocoanut cups and from four to five people drank; and it was chewed again. There was a marked diuretic effect; everybody had to leave about every twenty minutes, as in drinking beer. This was social, but the total effect was to loosen tongues and to talk far into the night, and no hangover the next day. There was absolutely none of this depression, and here again, these were small doses.

This was on the Island of Espiritu Santo on the southern slope of Mount Santo, at a village called Batuito at about five thousand feet, and they told me that in the past Kava had been used as part of the sexual ceremony, which was poured over a stone phallus prior to being mixed and drunk.

DR. GAJDUSEK: Jean Guiart, our colleague who worked both in Santo and Malakoa, never himself experienced any reaction from the Kavas on Malakoa.

CHAIRMAN DR. CRONHEIM: We have already exceeded by ten minutes the time allotted to us, so it is with great regret that I have to close the discussion.

I want to thank all the participants for a most enlightening and most stimulating panel.

SESSION III

MYRISTICA FRAGRANS (NUTMEG)

Edward B. Truitt, Jr., *Chairman*

Chairman's Introduction

EDWARD B. TRUITT, JR.
Battelle Memorial Institute, Columbus, Ohio

In this introduction, I would like to formulate several questions which I believe are crucial for this section of the program. The presentations to follow will likely answer very few of these questions. Rather, I think, the juxtaposition of these questions with the scanty information so far collected about the physical and physiological actions of nutmeg will emphasize the real need for further research into the dietary, ritualistic, and drug-seeking habits of man with this spice, and their possible significance.

The uppermost question that plagues the conscious of an investigator in this field is whether, by discussing publicly a substance with a potential for abuse by the lay public, he is inadvertently opening another Pandora's box of human ills. One answer to this question, in the case of nutmeg, appears to be that this substance has enough unpleasant effects mixed with its centrally stimulating actions to discourage misuse by any but the most reckless psychodelic adventurers. This will certainly be borne out by the reports to follow about the toxic effects of human overdose by ground nutmeg in the crude drug form. Whether the same will be true of myristicin or other active components of the volatile fraction will need to be learned, because experience with the purified products is quite meager. A lesson from LSD should be applied here, so that the human risks of nutmeg derivatives, mental as well as organic, will be carefully evaluated by clinical pharmacologists in anticipation of the possibility of widespread misuse.

A second question might appraise the need for further investigation on a substance which appears to be another stimulant to a central adrenergic receptor already affected by mescaline, cocaine, the amphetamines, epinephrine, adrenochrome, and possibly by LSD and other tryptamine-like hallucinogens. An answer to this question certainly lies in the importance of the study of structure and activity variations. Pharmacologists and medicinal chemists are strong advocates of the advisibility of characterizing drug activity in terms of the effects of structural changes in the molecule. Thus, we should look in the session to follow for those clues to variation in the central activity produced by myristicin, which has a slightly different formula from mescaline, as shown in Figure 1.

Myristicin is unique among psychotropic agents in that it lacks a nitrogen atom. This unusual characteristic has led Dr. Shulgin to propose an interesting hypothetical mechanism for its action which I am sure he will find time to discuss.

Another question which can be asked is how the information to be presented here on nutmeg and myristicin can be helpful to a better understanding of the workings of the mind. Since a partial answer to the previous question appears to be that nutmeg intoxication is in some ways different from mescaline

Myristicin (5-allyl-2,3 methylenedioxyphenylmethyl ether or
3-methoxy-4,5-methylenedioxyallylbenzene)

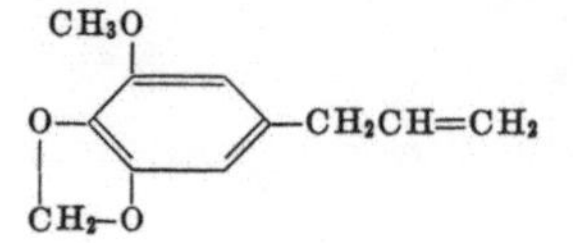

Mescaline (3,4,5-trimethoxyphenylethylamine)

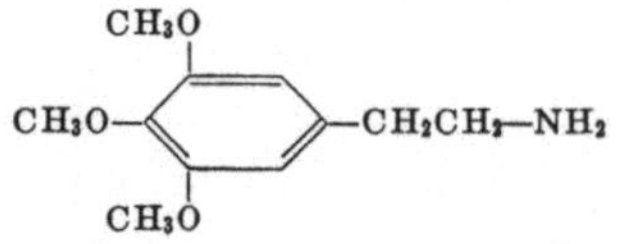

FIGURE 1.—*Structural formulas of myristicin and mescaline.*

and similar drugs, how does this difference contribute to better understanding? What is the relationship between the central feelings of anxiety, detachment, and excitation with somatic effects such as tachycardia, xerostomia, hypothermia, vasomotor lability, pupillary changes, and heaviness of the limbs? The marked degree and variety of peripheral effects prompts the question as to how much of the psychic action is attributable to the centripetal stimuli.

From a therapeutic viewpoint, one might ask whether some aspect of the syndrome induced by nutmeg might have a therapeutic application. This is, indeed, the most central question to the purposes of this conference. However, this goal has not yet been achieved for any of the drugs presently labeled as hallucinogens. Another useful advantage of this discussion could be the recognition of a means of treating nutmeg intoxication which occurs, although infrequently, and may be expected to increase.

The program to follow cannot begin to treat all aspects of nutmeg because extensive communication with other scientists and reviews of the scattered literature did not lead to the finding of experts on the anthropogical and other facets of the spice. It is perhaps appropriate that a pharmacologist, such as myself, inherited the chairmanship of this section. The reason for this is that three of the major early investigators, Arthur Cushny, Sir Henry Dale and George Wallace were all pharmacologists, and venerable ones also.

The first speaker, Mr. Andrew T. Weil, has produced perhaps the most detailed review of the nutmeg literature while essaying his honors thesis in botany. (1) Following this introductory review, Dr. Alexander T. Shulgin will describe research which already has put into practice one of the objectives of this conference. Dr. Shulgin and his associates have used the empirical observations of psychopharmacological activity in nutmeg and mescaline as a starting basis for the synthesis and testing of newer, more active and varied psycho-active drugs. Dr. Shulgin has also surpassed everyone for continued interest and publications on myristicin (2–9). My own interest in the action of nutmeg emerged from Dr. John C. Krantz's scientific curiosity in response to several cases of nutmeg poisoning referred to him by graduates of the University of Maryland Medical School. (10) It was

186

also continued by the then-growing importance of norepinephrine and 5-hydroxytamine in brain function. (*11*) The last speaker, Dr. Enoch Callaway, III, is an authority on nutmeg by reason of personal experience as well as having conducted clinical experimentation with a purified myristicin-containing fraction of oil of nutmeg. (*10*) I believe that his experience with the drug, if widely known, should certainly dissuade public abuse of nutmeg.

BIBLIOGRAPHY

(*1*) WEIL, A. T. "Nutmeg as a Narcotic." Economic Botany, 19: 194, 1965.

(*2*) SHULGIN, A. T., S. BUNNELL, and T. SARGENT, III. "The Psychotomimetic Properties of 3, 4, 5-Trimethoxyamphetamines." Nature (Lond.), 189: 1011, 1961.

(*3*) SHULGIN, A. T. "Composition of the Myristicin Fraction from Oil of Nutmeg." Nature (Lond.), 197: 379, 1963.

(*4*) SHULGIN, A. T. "Psychotomimetic Agents Related to Mescaline." Experientia, 19: 127, 1963.

(*5*) SHULGIN, A. T. "Concerning the Pharmacology of Nutmeg." Mind, 1: 299, 1963.

(*6*) SHULGIN, A. T., and H. O. KERLINGER. "Isolation of Methoxyeugenol and Trans-Isoelemicin from Oil of Nutmeg." Naturwissenschaften, 15: 360, 1964.

(*7*) SHULGIN, A. T. "3-Methoxy-4,5-Methylenedioxyamphetamine, A New Psychotomimetic Agent." Nature, 201: 1120, 1964.

(*8*) SHULGIN, A. T. "Psychotomimetic Amphetamines: Methoxy-3,4-Dialkoxy Amphetamines." Experientia, 20: 366, 1964.

(*9*) SHULGIN, A. T. "Possible Implication of Myristicin as a Psychotropic Substance." Nature (Lond.), 210: 380, 1966.

(*10*) TRUITT, E. B., Jr., E. CALLAWAY, III, M. C. BRAUDE, and J. C. KRANTZ, Jr. "The Pharmacology of Myristicin. A Contribution to the Psychopharmacology of Nutmeg." Journal of Neuropsychiatry, 2: 205, 1961.

(*11*) TRUITT, E. B., Jr., G. DURITZ, and E. M. EBERSBERGER. "Evidence of Monoamine Oxidase Inhibition by Myristicin and Nutmeg." Proceedings of the Society for Experimental Biology and Medicine, 112: 647, 1963.

Nutmeg as a Psychoactive Drug

ANDREW T. WEIL

Harvard Medical School, Boston, Massachusetts

Clearly, nutmeg is unique among the less familiar psychoactive drugs. It is the only one widely known to millions of persons in all countries—albeit for other-than-pharmacological purposes. It is also the only one whose use as a drug may be on the verge of an enormous increase. The aim of this paper is to review the botany, history, and commerce of nutmeg as well as to describe the ways it is used for effects on consciousness.

Two spices—nutmeg and mace—come from the nutmeg tree, *Myristica fragrans* (family Myristicaceae), a handsome tropical tree native to the Banda Islands and other islands of the East Indian archipelago. The genus *Myristica* comprises about 100 species found throughout the torrid zone, especially in the Malayan region; but of these *M. fragrans* alone contains enough of an aromatic essential oil to make it worthy of cultivation. Usually 30 or 40 feet tall, the nutmeg tree has a dark gray bark, spreading branches, and alternate, oblong-ovate leaves that are four inches long, leathery, and glossy green. Normally, the species is dioecious. Flowers, male and female, look like those of the lily-of-the- valley; they are pale yellow, fleshy, and have a strong scent of nutmeg. The fruit is a pendulous, fleshy drupe resembling an apricot (*1,2,3*).

When ripe, the fleshy husk, or pericarp, of this fruit splits open into two halves, revealing a shiny brown seedcoat, or testa. Inside this shell is the seed, which is the nutmeg of commerce. Outside the shell, closely enwrapping it, is a bright crimson network, or arillus, which is the mace. In preparing the spices for export, fieldworkers first remove the pit with its mace from the husk. The aril is then carefully peeled away from the seedcoat. Fresh arils are brilliant red and leathery with a strong flavor of turpentine. The mace may be kept in one piece (called "double blade" in the trade) or separated into two halves ("single blade") before it is flattened by hand or between boards. It is then dried thoroughly in the sun or by artificial heat; during this process it gradually turns orange, then orange-yellow and acquires its characteristic aroma (*3,4*).

The nutmegs, still in their shells, are also dried, frequently over a smouldering fire. When completely dry, the seed rattles in the testa. Usually the shells are then cracked by machine or with wooden mallets and the seeds are removed for export. Sometimes, shelled nutmegs are treated with lime before shipping to protect them from insects. They are then sorted by size and packed. For the spice trade, nutmegs are valued according to size, smoothness, and freedom from adulteration with wild seeds (*2,4*).

The nutmeg tree requires a hot, humid climate. It is widely cultivated in the tropics, particularly on the Spice Islands (the Moluccas, an island group of eastern Indonesia), on Penang and other islands of Malaysia, and in the

Caribbean, notably on Grenada. The tree is slow-growing, taking 15 years to produce full yields. A good specimen produces 1,500–2,000 nuts annually—a weight of ten pounds of nutmeg to one-half pound of mace. The finest mace and the finest nutmegs come from Penang; because of their higher content of volatile oil, the East Indian spices are preferred to the West Indian (4).

Products of M. Fragrans

Nutmeg Husks: The pericarp of the nutmeg fruit may be preserved in sugar, salted and dried as a condiment, or made into jellies. All of these preparations have the flavor of nutmeg and all are reported to be delicious. But they are unknown outside the regions in which the tree is grown (2, 3).

Nutmeg: Whole nutmegs are oval and woody with a ridged or wrinkled, light brown surface. Most are about an inch long, three-quarters of an inch in diameter. On cross section they show a heavy network of dark brown "veins." Ground nutmeg, the familiar kitchen spice is a granular, orange-brown powder with characteristic aroma.

Depending on the variety, whole nutmeg contains from 5 to 15 per cent of a volatile oil that accounts entirely for the aroma and flavor of the spice. Ground nutmeg is subject to rather rapid losses of this component. In addition, dried nutmeg contains 25 to 40 per cent of fixed oil and 5 to 15 per cent ashes. The remainder is moisture, fiber, and starch (5). In the calendar year 1965, the United States imported nearly 5,300,000 pounds of nutmeg worth about $3,800,000. Of this total, nearly 72 per cent came from Indonesia, while 24 per cent came from the Caribbean, with the remainder from a number of smaller ports. Imports over the past ten years have been fairly constant (Table I), but there has been a change in the major source of this spice. Until 1955, the U.S. obtained about half of its annual supply of both nutmeg and mace from the West Indies. In that year, however, a hurricane devastated the island of Grenada, and the nutmeg groves there have still not recovered from the damage (6).

Mace: Mace, another popular spice, is a brownish-yellow or brownish-orange granular powder with a strong aroma closely resembling that of nutmeg. The flavor of mace is somewhat less sweet and less delicate than the flavor of nutmeg. Whole mace contains from 4 to 14 percent of a volatile oil very similar to that found in nutmeg, along with moisture, fat, starch, etc.

TABLE I.—U.S. imports of nutmeg and mace*

[pounds]

	Average 1950–54	Average 1955–59	Average 1960–64	1963	1964	1965
Nutmeg	4, 852, 221	4, 141, 074	4, 151, 480	5, 124, 638	3, 505, 450	5, 271, 524
Mace	658, 193	549, 072	563, 874	558, 541	648, 900	619, 394

*Source: U.S. Department of Commerce, Bureau of the Census Compilation by American Spice Trade Association.

(*5; 7*, Vol V). In 1965, the United States imported 619,000 pounds of mace worth $750,000. Seventy-six percent came from Indonesia, the rest from Malaysia, Hong Kong, Japan, and the Caribbean. As with nutmeg, imports of mace have not varied much over the past ten years (Table I).

Uses of Nutmeg and Mace: Both spices are classified as "baking spices" since they are much used in foods like doughnuts and other sweet doughs. Both have a warm, aromatic, slightly bitter taste. Nutmeg is commonly added to custards, puddings, pies, and eggnog. Mace is used in soups, sauces, and pastries, particularly pound cake. In addition, both spices are important ingredients of frankfurters and other meat products, pickles, tomato ketchup, and similar condiments. The American Spice Trade Association estimates that 55 percent of nutmeg and mace imported into this country is sold through retail stores to home consumers. The rest goes to institutions (hotels, restaurants, bakeries, sausage manufacturers, and other bulk users). Formerly, housewives bought whole nutmegs and grated them at home; today, most of the nutmeg and all of the mace sold for home consumption is ground.

Fixed Oil of Nutmeg: Known also as "nutmeg butter," this vegetable fat is obtained by exposing the nuts to hydraulic pressure and heat. At room temperature, it is an orange, tallowy mass with a pronounced aroma of nutmeg and the consistency of butter. Formerly used in medicine as an external application for rheumatism and sprains, it has some commercial importance today as an ingredient of certain soaps, hair tonics, and perfumes (*2, 3, 5*).

Essential Oils of Nutmeg and Mace: The essential or volatile oils of nutmeg and mace are obtained by steam distillation. Commercial oil of nutmeg is a mobile, pale yellow liquid with an odor and flavor of nutmeg. It is not satisfactory as a substitute for the spice in cooking because it does not exactly reproduce the flavor of whole nutmeg. ("Essences" of nutmeg and mace sold by spice dealers are alcohol extracts not essential oils.) But oil of nutmeg has been widely used in industry as a flavoring agent for perfumes and dentifrices. Chemically, it is a complex mixture of alcohols, esters, and organic acids, including about four percent myristicin, the main pharmacologically active component (*7*, Vol V; *8; 9*).

History of Nutmeg

Nutmeg was unknown to the ancient Greeks and Romans, but probably, Arabian traders began importing it from the East Indies by the first centuries A.D. No definite evidence of Myristica's appearance in Europe is recorded until the 12th Century, and the source of nutmeg was not discovered by the West until the Portuguese reached Banda in 1512. Portugal controlled trade in nutmeg and mace from that year until the beginning of the 17th Century, when most of the Pacific spice-producing territories fell into the hands of the Dutch. In order to keep prices of the spices very high, the Dutch tried to limit cultivation of the nutmeg tree to two islands, but their monopoly was eventually challenged successfully by the French and British. Gradually, commercial development of *M. fragrans* spread throughout the world, reaching Grenada, for example, in 1843 (*3*).

Like most aromatics, nutmeg was as important in early medicine as it was in cooking (*10*). Its therapeutic applications were first catalogued by Arab physicians as early as the 7th Century A.D. Originally, it seems to have been a remedy for disorders of the digestive system, but before long it was considered beneficial in such diverse conditions as kidney disease, pain, and lymphatic ailments; it was even described as an aphrodisiac. Many of these beliefs are preserved in contemporary Arab folk medicine; in fact, Yemenite men still consume it to increase virility.

Similarly, nutmeg was and is a significant item in the Hindu pharmacopeia, where it has been prescribed for fever, consumption, asthma, and heart disease. Traditional Malayan medicine designates nutmeg for madness as well. According to an adviser in the Indian Ministry of Health, nutmeg is still used as an analgesic and sedative by folk practitioners, and is given in small quantities to induce hypnotic effect in irritable children.

Medieval European physicians, who generally followed the precepts of their Arab colleagues, also prescribed nutmeg for a long list of ailments. By the 1700's the spice attained its greatest reputation; thereafter, with the development of modern pharmacy, its importance as a medicine gradually subsided.

Curiously, nutmeg's popularity as a folk remedy had a brief, spectacular resurgence less than one hundred years ago. Near the end of the 1800's, a rumor spread among women in England and America that nutmeg could bring on overdue menstruation and even induce abortion. The origin of this mistaken belief is unclear, but its influence is well documented in dozens of case reports of nutmeg poisoning published in British and American medical journals of the period (*10*). The idea has even persisted into our times: Green in 1959 wrote of a 28-year-old Virginia woman who ate "18.3 Gm. of finely ground nutmeg in an attempt to induce the menses, which had been delayed two days (*11*)."

Reports of nutmeg poisoning date back to the late Middle Ages when several early physicians first wrote down their observations on the stupor-inducing powers of the spice. Doubtless, most of these intoxications resulted from overdoses taken as remedies. A late example comes from *A Treatise on the Materia Medica* written in 1789 by an English physician, William Cullen. He wrote:

I have myself had an accidental occasion of observing its [nutmeg's] soporific and stupefying power. A person by mistake took two drams or a little more of powdered nutmeg; he felt it warm in his stomach, without any uneasiness; but in about an hour after he had taken it, he was seized with a drowsiness, which gradually increased to a complete stupor and insensibility; and not long after, he was found fallen from his chair, lying on the floor of his chamber in the state mentioned. Being laid abed he fell asleep; but waking a little from time to time, he was quite delirious: and he thus continued alternately sleeping and delirious for several hours. By degrees, however, both these symptoms diminished, so that in about six hours from the time of taking the nutmeg he was pretty well recovered from both. Although he still complained of head-ache and some drowsiness, he slept naturally and quietly through the following night, and next day was quite in his ordinary health.

There is no doubt that this was entirely the effect of the nutmeg. . . .

In 1829, the great physiologist J. E. Purkinje conducted self-experiments with nutmeg. Following a dose of three whole nutmegs, he experienced spatial and temporal disorientation similar to that of Cannabis intoxication. He wrote (12):

At half-past six, when it was almost dark, I woke up in order to go to the Royal Theatre at Brueder Street where I lived. The distance was long, but this time I thought it had no end. My movements appeared entirely adequate, but were lost momentarily in dream pictures, from which I had to extricate myself with considerable force in order to keep on walking. My feet did their duty and, since I had to stick to a straight road, there was no danger of going astray. I went forward in this dream, for, if I attempted to orient myself, I could not even recognize the cross streets. Time seemed long, but I got to the opposite side of the place where I was going. During this time dreams and physical activity battled one another. The return journey was good, and I slept well that night and next day.

There is a similar, more dramatic report of mace intoxication from 1848 (13). But as stated earlier, the greatest numbers of people poisoned by Myristica have been English and American women of the late 19th and early 20th Centuries. Summarizing many of these cases in 1962, McCord wrote (14):

. . . patients have consumed from 1 to 3 nutmegs and have experienced restlessness, dizziness, fear of death, coldness of extremities, occasional nausea and vomiting, abdominal pain, and precordial pain or oppression. These patients were found to be extremely agitated, delirious, and dyspneic and have had weak, rapid pulses and de-creased body temperature. On several occasions patients were found unconscious. Oc-casionally there was flushing of the face while at other times pallor with cyanosis of the lips and nails predominated.

He attributed these intoxications to "a central nervous system depressive effect with periods of stimulation and associated respiratory and cardio-vascular difficulties."

Only one fatality has ever been ascribed to nutmeg ingestion: near the beginning of this century, an eight year old boy ate two whole nutmegs, became comatose, and died less than 24 hours later (15).

Use of Nutmeg as an Intoxicant

The apparent epidemic of nutmeg intoxications around the turn of the century subsided after the First World War. Cases since then have been rare. In 1963, Payne presented one of the only published reports of deliberate ingestion of Myristica for narcotic effects. He described two college students, 19 and 20 years old, who each consumed two tablespoonfuls (about 14 g. or the equivalent of two whole seeds) of powdered nutmeg suspended in milk (16). About five hours later

. . . each had the onset of a significant pharmacologic effect, heralded by a leaden feeling in the extremities and a nonchalant, detached mental state described as 'un-real' or 'dreamlike.' Rapid heart rates and palpitation were noted, and both complained of dry mouth and thirst. Onlookers observed that one student became quite hyperactive and agitated and talked incoherently. It was noted that the faces of both were as 'red as beets.' Nausea, vomiting, and abdominal cramps were absent. . . . One described a sense of impending doom, as if he were 'breaking up inside.'

Extreme drowsiness occurred about seven hours after these symptoms began and continued for the next 24 hours. Recovery was complete, but "both patients stated emphatically that a sense of unreality persisted for 48 to 60 hours from the time of one oral dose of nutmeg."

A history of the use of nutmeg for the express purpose of inducing these bizarre physical and mental effects is hard to piece together simply because reliable data on Myristica narcosis are not available. The medical literature is of no help, for example, because nearly all the reported cases have resulted from accidental ingestions or overdoses taken as remedies. Most of the information on nutmeg as a psychoactive drug is anecdotal, and it has been most difficult to document the anecdotes.

Stories in circulation about nutmeg at the present time develop several recurrent themes. One is that Myristica is used as an intoxicant in certain parts of Asia. Another is that nutmeg is widely consumed by prison inmates in this country. A third is that students and 'beatniks' have adopted the the spice as a new hallucinogen.

For the first story little supporting evidence can be found. A suggestive clue is one of the synonyms for nutmeg used in Ayurveda, an ancient Hindu scripture. Here, nutmeg is called *Mada shaunda* meaning "narcotic fruit." There is reason to believe that nutmeg is, in fact, eaten as an intoxicant even today by some people in India who add it to betel chew. It may also be mixed with tobacco and snuffed in this part of the world. Equally vague is a report that nutmeg is taken as a stimulating snuff by natives in remote regions of Indonesia. Still another unsubstantiated assertion is that nutmeg is often substituted for hashish in Egypt when the hemp product is not available.

It is much easier to confirm rumors of nutmeg use by prison inmates, despite denials by prison officials. One interesting reference occurs in *The Autobiography of Malcolm X* (*17*), in which the late Black Muslim leader describes his incarceration in a Boston prison in 1946. He was then a user of marihuana and other drugs and found himself suddenly cut off from them. He wrote:

I first got high in Charlestown [prison] on nutmeg. My cellmate was among at least a hundred nutmeg men who, for money or cigarettes, bought from kitchen-worker inmates penny matchboxes full of stolen nutmeg. I grabbed a box as though it were a pound of heavy drugs. Stirred into a glass of cold water, a penny matchbox full of nutmeg had the kick of three or four reefers.

A more recent but less accessible reference was a short article on page 22 of the Chicago *Sun-Times* for March 3, 1961. It told of the dismissal of a Cook County Jail guard caught smuggling nutmeg and nose inhalers into the jail.

An officer of the Federal Bureau of Prisons has written (*18*):

We are aware of the narcotic reaction these spices may have when improperly used, and, therefore, it is standard practice in the Federal prisons to maintain careful control of both items [i.e., nutmeg and mace]. Due to this control and also to the fact . . . that few people are aware of their stupor-inducing powers, we have no problems with these items. I have read articles in various publications which imply that the use of nutmeg and mace is widespread in prisons. However I do not know of a single instance in the Federal Prison system where either spice was used by inmates for its narcotic effect.

There is, however, ample confirmation of this rumored use of nutmeg in a study conducted by Weiss at the New Jersey State Prison at Trenton in 1960. Weiss wrote (*19*) :

It is widely believed by inmates of correctional institutions that the drug action of nutmeg produces reactions similar to those of legally prohibited drugs which are considered habit-forming and addicting. Although its illicit application is most certainly not widely known in the extra-mural setting, personal communications by prisoners are to the effect that it is used, not only in the community [i.e., the outside], but was also used in the armed forces in Europe in World War II.

Weiss studied ten male inmates of the prison, most of whom had had previous experiences with marihuana and other drugs. Six of them had learned of the use of nutmeg during their imprisonment; the others had already known about it. The number of times these men had tried *Myristica* was impressive. One had taken nutmeg on 10 different occasions, one 30, one 52, and one 475. The minimum amount of ground nutmeg any man ingested was 2 to 3 tablespoonfuls, and one had once taken two cups of the spice as a single dose (apparently without untoward effects). The drug was always taken orally, usually stirred into hot liquids.

Weiss noted no uniformity of time of onset of action, which ranged from 10 minutes to four hours. Duration of action ranged from four to 24 hours. Most of the subjects compared nutmeg to marihuana, although some also likened it to heroin and alcohol. Most experienced a sense of being transported aloft, along with drowsiness in some cases and excitement in others. In all instances thirst was increased, but hunger was not stimulated. Reported side effects included nausea, abdominal spasm, vomiting, constipation, tachycardia, insomnia, and drowsiness.

Two cases of acute brain syndrome, with psychotic reaction due to nutmeg intoxication, were reported. Each of the two subjects had chronically ingested powdered nutmeg over a long period. . . . Aside from these cases of poisoning, the hallucinogenic effects reported were transitory and of brief duration.

Consumption of nutmeg was an important aspect of life in the prison. Weiss has added (*20*) :

Inmates would carry little matchboxes in which they would store a supply of nutmeg (equivalent to one dose). They could then take the dose along with them to the shops in which they worked during the day. Users consider themselves to be more lively and cheerful. Thus, they feel they have dispelled their inner gloom. However, drug users seldom take nutmeg once they leave the prison since they consider its effects to be inferior to those of heroin or marihuana, whatever may be the similarity between them.

Shortly after Weiss's article appeared, nutmeg was banned from the New Jersey State Prison kitchen.

I have received information from several former prison inmates, suggesting the practice to be common. One correspondent writes: "During 16 months in a Massachusetts correctional institution, I knew three individ-

194

uals who on occasion did use nutmeg as a snuff for 'kicks.' It was done on weekends and widely dispersed as to time." Another, from California, writes: "I can tell you that nutmeg is a commonly used high within prison walls—so much so that it is frequently locked up apart from the other normally used spices. . . . Convicts, because of the nature of their environment, have rarely any alternative high."

A final reference is this line from William Burroughs's *Naked Lunch* (*21*): "Convicts and sailors sometimes have recourse to nutmeg. About a tablespoon is swallowed with water. Result vaguely similar to marihuana with side effects of headache and nausea."

Like prisoners, jazz musicians are said to have long used nutmeg as a substitute for other drugs, especially marihuana. Confirmation is hard to come by. The only clear reference I have been able to find is a 1962 biography of the late Charlie Parker, known as "Bird." The leader of the band in which Parker made his recording debut in 1942 is quoted as reminiscing (*22*):

Bird introduced this nutmeg to the guys. It was a cheap and legal high. You can take it in milk or Coca Cola. The grocer across the street came over to the club owner and said, "I know you do all this baking because I sell from 8 to 10 nutmegs a day." And the owner came back and looked at the bandstand and there was a whole pile of nutmeg boxes.

To summarize thus far: The toxic properties of nutmeg have been recognized for hundreds of years, probably ever since the spice was first prescribed medicinally in large doses. Published reports of Myristica narcosis were most frequent around the turn of the last century when many women took nutmeg as an emmenagogue or abortifacient. Some evidence suggests that nutmeg may have long been used as an intoxicant in certain parts of Asia. In our century, for at least the past thirty years, prisoners, jazz musicians, sailors, and probably others have used nutmeg as a substitute for marihuana or other drugs. They either eat or snuff it in variable amounts and commonly experience symptoms much more like those of the familiar hallucinogens than those described in the old reports of nutmeg poisoning.

Use by Students

In our own society the fastest-growing group of drug-takers is not the prison population or jazz world but rather students and "student-types." I do not care to add another guess to the many published estimates of what percentage of college youth experiments with hallucinogens. I will simply point out that most observers find that significant numbers of students now try marihuana and stronger drugs like LSD. It is especially noteworthy that many of these people would never have indulged in such activities even five years ago. I doubt, for example, that more than a handful of law students, medical students, or divinity students had experienced the effects of Cannabis before 1963, when hallucinogens first came to the full attention of the national press. But today many occasional marihuana smokers come from these groups. Students have also been the initiators of drug fads in recent years. The flurry of excitement over morning-glory seeds in 1963 and 1964 was generated largely by college undergraduates and high school pupils. One would expect that nutmeg, because of its frequent use by other groups as an alternative hallucinogen, might also be included in the student's or beatnik's index of psychoactive substances.

I have been particularly interested in this possibility because I first learned of Myristica's psychopharmacological potential through an invitation to a "mace party" given by several undergraduates at Haverford College near Philadelphia in 1961. The students said they and many of their classmates had been introduced to the spice by a visiting beatnik from Baltimore, who had sponsored several mace parties on campus.

Only one case of this sort has appeared in the medical literature—Payne's report of 1963, mentioned earlier. His two students had gotten the idea of taking nutmeg from a "beatnik acquaintance," who told them it would provide "a mental state somewhat akin to ethanol intoxication without requiring the use of alcohol" (16). I have been able to find only one other published account—an article titled "Nutmeg Jag" in the summer, 1964 issue of a University of Mississippi student magazine. It described a nutmeg party attended by eight persons. One participant—a young man who consumed a whole standard-size can of the ground spice (nearly 40 g. or 1.5 oz.)—recalled afterward (23):

> I felt as if I were in an echo chamber . . . my voice sounded vague and distant . . . it was like being drunk without the ordinary alcoholic effects. . . . Two friends of mine had told me about the 30-cents, three-day drunk they had after taking nutmeg, so I tried it out of sheer disbelief.

Over the past six months I have been in touch with officials of student health services at representative universities throughout the country in an attempt to collect additional reports of Myristica intoxications. Significantly, most of the responding physicians were unaware of nutmeg's non-culinary uses. Only two university clinics had cases on record. Dr. Henry B. Bruyn of the University of California at Berkeley student health service notes two instances of intoxication. In October, 1963, two days after an issue of the *Ladies Home Journal* appeared with a reference to nutmeg in a story on hallucinogenic drugs, a 20-year-old female student was admitted to the hospital with a chief complaint of abdominal cramps. The night before she had taken 4 teaspoons of ground nutmeg because a friend had told her it would get her high. Her roommate joined her in this ingestion. The next morning she awoke drowsy and fainted in the bathroom. Physical examination was normal except for orthostatic hypotension, and she was recovered the day after admission. She told a physician she had taken the spice because she "felt she needed something to do."

In January, 1965, a second female Berkeley student was admitted, age 17, again with abdominal cramps. Four hours previously she had eaten 2½ teaspoons of nutmeg because she had heard it would give her hallucinations. She, too, recovered quickly.

Dr. B. W. Murphy of the University of Maryland contributes one other case. He writes that he knows of a male student who induces dreamy hallucinatory states by ingesting a whole can of ground nutmeg.

Does the scarcity of reported cases indicate a low frequency of nutmeg use by students? Probably not—just because students are reluctant to present themselves for medical treatment of drug intoxications, even when they suffer alarming symptoms. Relying solely on health services records, one would conclude that marihuana is also very little used by college students.

To get a more accurate idea of the extent of experimentation with nutmeg on college campuses, I placed advertisements requesting information on the spice in several student newspapers and also interviewed students from many areas of the country. By these methods, I easily collected a number of accounts of nutmeg narcosis. I have selected some of these to illustrate typical patterns of use.

Case #1 (college sophomore)—

I heard about the effects of mace from a beatnik who visited our campus and induced students to "turn on" with two teaspoons of this spice stirred into fruit juice. I didn't try it at the time, but a few months later five of us held a mace party in my apartment. To the disappointment of all, we felt just the same three hours after drinking down the mace. Convinced that the alleged hallucinogenic properties of mace were imaginary, we separated and I went to bed. I remember feeling somewhat lightheaded and having vague stomach pains before falling asleep, but I had no other sypmtoms until I woke up the next morning with a splitting headache, a burning thirst, and malaise. I later learned the other four had felt much the same on arising.

Case #2 (college juniors)—

Five of us tried to get high by eating two whole nutmegs each. They are terrible things to try to chew up and swallow. We all had warm feelings in our stomachs immediately afterward and began sweating more than usual. One of us eventually had a pronounced reaction, but the rest of us noticed nothing unusual and gave up after two hours. The next morning we all had headaches, extreme dryness of mouth and throat, creaking joints and dizziness.

One of us had a different experience. He went back to his room to read, and exactly four hours after taking the nutmeg he was suddenly overcome by a drowsiness so profound that he could hardly get up to turn off the light. As he fell into bed he had impressions of 'strange shapes floating' around him. He then sank into a heavy sleep. When he woke up seven hours later, he could barely move. He was very dizzy and staggered when he tried to walk; also, he could not see clearly for several minutes. His mouth and throat were parched, and water did not relieve the dryness. Two hours after he got up he again became drowsy and "sank into a sort of trance state." At this time he had a vivid impression that he was floating with his limbs separated from his body. Eight hours later he was fully recovered.

Case #3 (an ex-student in San Francisco)—

I have had completely negative results from nutmeg, perhaps partly precipitated by the environment and definitely partly by the nauseating effects of the drug. I ate three ounces, which may well have been too much. About two hours later I drank four beers. Then about three-quarters of an hour after the beer I began noticing unusual effects. I was in an unfamiliar night club and started to become disoriented. I talked continuously and repetitively, but it seemed as though another person were talking. I seem to have been wandering around in a daze, unaware of my surroundings. I was then ejected from the club. Paranoid delusions set in. I believed the owners of the club had drugged me. I forced my way back in, which resulted in my being jailed for drunk and disorderly conduct. The day I spent in jail was one of total confusion. In fact, it was a full day before I realized I was in jail. I was very belligerent, a condition apparently precipitated by the belief that I was going to be executed. I became ill and vomited. I imagined the other prisoners were Nazis who were guarding me. One day in jail finally restored my reason, and I was released. No hallucinations occurred as far as I can recall.

Case #4 (college junior)—

I drank one ounce of nutmeg in water. Four hours later I began feeling feverish and delirious. These sensations continued for several hours and left me with a bad hangover. I would not repeat the experience.

Case #5 (21-year-old female secretary for a student newspaper)—

I took one teaspoon of nutmeg in water after reading about it in Malcolm X's autobiography. Nothing happened.

Case #6 (college junior)—

I took a whole can of nutmeg mixed with water. I had no effects at all from it.

Case #7 (medical student)—

When I was a junior in college at the University of Colorado, I got to know a group of nutmeg-takers because the leader of it had been a close high-school friend. In 1963, I went to his apartment for drinks, and he told me to take a matchboxful of ground nutmeg, packed into gelatin capsules. The method of these people was to take the nutmeg before they went to bed so that they would wake up high and avoid the nausea nutmeg often caused. Most said the effects were different from both morning-glory seeds and marihuana. Some experienced floating feelings. They took nutmeg occasionally for kicks, but did not attach too much importance to it. I do not know where they first learned of this habit, but my friend had worked as a volunteer in a prison before 1963 and may have been told about it there.

Case #8 (college sophomore)—

One evening my roommate and I each took a tablespoon of nutmeg in water after reading about it in Malcolm X's book. Nothing happened, so I went to bed. I woke up the next morning with incredible malaise and tachycardia. These symptoms eventually subsided but have recurred about once a week accompanied by severe anxiety for the past year. This reaction occurs spontaneously but also is brought on by eating anything containing more than a minute amount of nutmeg. One doctor has suggested that it may be an allergic reaction. My roommate had no effects except that he still cannot eat anything with nutmeg without experiencing an overpowering taste of the spice.

Case #9 (college junior)—

A friend told me about nutmeg and came over to show me how to do it. He mixed a drink of about half coffee and half nutmeg, which my roommate and I drank. Nothing happened to us in an hour, so we went to bed. Next morning I found myself on the floor with the worst hangover of my life. My roommate felt as bad. To this day neither of us can eat anything with nutmeg—we can't bear the taste.

Case #10 (a 42-year-old Berkeley woman who describes herself as "eccentric" with a "terrible fear of marihuana" and other drugs. After reading of nutmeg in a "manual of hallucinogenic drugs" she decided to try it since it was "cheap, legal, and available." She took nutmeg on several occasions and wrote extensively about her experiences. Here is one description.)—

I drank about five grams of nutmeg in a glass of fruit juice at about 9:30 a.m. An hour later I felt a surge of happiness when a freight train whistled. I closed my eyes in search of hallucinations, but none came. A certain diuretic effect and pungent scent in my urine were evidence that the drug had already taken effect. I read the morning paper until 11:30 when there came a pleasant drowsiness. I closed my eyes and saw: silver spears of grass waving across an azure sky, silver waves of poplar trees swaying and dancing in the sun. I arose to walk and staggered. The light was flickering and dim as if I were partially blind, so I lay down on a couch in the kitchen. Closing my eyes again, I was overwhelmed by visions: golden spangles and rings of light on moving water, dancing moons and stars, everywhere a predominance of gold and silver images. . . .

About 12:30 I opened my eyes and noticed that the stove was far, far away; the very walls had receded; the kitchen was cathedral-like in its dimensions. I stood up to look at myself, and I was unusually tall. My feet were small and far away; it was like looking through the wrong end of binoculars. I thought to myself, "This must be what marihuana is like."

The effect continued several hours until she fell asleep. There were no aftereffects.

Conclusions

From these and other cases I draw the following conclusions:

1. Significant numbers of students and persons living in student communities attempt to induce hallucinations with Myristica.

2. Unlike prisoners or musicians, who resort to nutmeg when their supplies of standard drugs are cut off, students often take nutmeg as a first experience before they try Cannabis or other substances. Nutmeg and mace are cheap, legal, and available at the nearest grocery store.

3. Typically, the young nutmeg-eater first learns of the spice's psychoactivity from a friend or from a published reference.

4. Doses range from one teaspoon to a whole can of ground nutmeg. Almost always, the spice is drunk in a glass of juice or water.

5. Onset of action is commonly 2 to 5 or more hours after ingestion. Most neophytes are not aware of the delay. In a very common pattern of intoxication, a person takes an adequate dose of nutmeg in the evening, goes to bed after several hours of waiting in vain for effects, and wakes up the next morning with many of the physical symptoms of toxicity: malaise, headache, dry mouth, tachycardia, dizziness.

6. Some of the reported reactions to nutmeg must be purely psychological. A dose of one teaspoon is probably insufficient to cause true symptoms. Similarly, hallucinations or mental changes that come on within thirty minutes of ingestion are likely to be factitious.

7. Reactions to nutmeg vary from no mental changes at all to full-blown hallucinogenic experiences like those caused by hashish or LSD. There is no apparent correlation between dose and psychoactive effect. Might this extreme variability represent differences in pharmacological potency of different batches of nutmeg? Or do people vary greatly in their sensitivity to the active principle?

8. Visual hallucinations are rather less frequent with nutmeg than with drugs like LSD or mescaline, but distortions of time and space perception

with feelings of unreality are common, as with Cannabis. Sensations of floating, being transported aloft, or having one's limbs separated from the body are frequently reported.

9. Effects of a single dose of nutmeg usually subside within 12 to 48 hours An intriguing aftereffect occasionally mentioned is persistent sensitization to the taste of the spice.

10. Most young people who try nutmeg take it once or twice but do not use it habitually. Those who regularly smoke marihuana regard nutmeg as an inferior hallucinogen, largely because of the unpleasant side effects.

11. Ignorance of the psychoactive properties of nutmeg is unquestionably the most important factor limiting extent of its use as a drug.

I want to emphasize the last point. I began this general review by indicating the differences between nutmeg and other hallucinogens. From a public health viewpoint, the crucial difference is that most persons in the country have not yet heard that nutmeg is intoxicating. Not only is nutmeg cheap, legal, and available, it is also familiar, which makes it seem safe and inviting to those looking for a first hallucinogenic experience. These considerations lead to one inference: as publicity is accorded the psychopharmacological properties of Myristica, use of nutmeg and mace as intoxicants will certainly increase. Hopefully, we will soon have the knowledge to determine the dangers and potential values of this modern use of an ancient spice.

BIBLIOGRAPHY

(1) FERGUSON, A. M. and J. FERGUSON. "All About Spices." Colombo, Ceylon, 1889.

(2) RIDLEY, HENRY N. "Spices." London, 1912.

(3) WARBURG O. "Die Muskatnuss." Leipzig, 1897.

(4) "What You Should Know About Nutmeg and Mace." New York, American Spice Trade Association, 1966.

(5) REDGROVE, H. STANLEY. "Spices and Condiments." London, 1933.

(6) U.S. Department of Commerce, Bureau of the Census figures complied by American Spice Trade Association, New York.

(7) GUENTHER, E. "The Essential Oils." New York, 1952.

(8) "The Pharmacopoeia of the United States of America." XV, Easton, Pa., 1955.

(9) POWER, F. B. and A. H. SALWAY. "The constituents of the essential oil of nutmeg." J. Chem. Soc., 91 : 2037–2058, 1907.

(10) WEIL, ANDREW T. "Nutmeg as a Narcotic." Econ. Bot., 19 : 194–217, 1965.

(11) GREEN, ROBERT C., Jr. "Nutmeg Poisoning." J. Amer. Med. Assoc., 171 : 1342–1344, 1959.

(12) PURKINJE, J. E. "Einige Beitraege zur physiologischen Pharmakologie." Neue Breslauer Sammlungen aus dem Gebiete der Heilkunde. 1 : 423–443, 1829; quoted in Hanzlik, "P. J. Purkinje's pioneer self-experiments in psychopharmacology." Calif. and Western Med., 49 : July and Aug., 1938.

(13) WATSON, G. C. "Symptoms of poisoning after eating a quantity of mace." Prov. Med. Surg. J., Jan. 26, 1848.

(14) McCORD, J. A. and L. P. JERVEY. "Nutmeg (myristicin) poisoning." J. S. Carolina Med. Assoc., 58 : 436–438, 1962.

(15) CUSHNY, A. R. "Nutmeg poisoning." Proc. Royal Soc. Med., 1908–I : 39.

(16) PAYNE, ROBERT B. "Nutmeg intoxication." New Eng. J. Med., 269 : 36–38, 1963. (Mention of this article was made a few weeks later in the "Medicine" section of TIME Magazine.)

(*17*) X, MALCOLM with ALEX HALEY. "The Autobiography of Malcolm X." New York, Grove Press, 1964.

(*18*) ALLDREDGE, NOAH L., Deputy Assistant Director, U.S. Bureau of Prisons. Personal communication, April 6, 1964.

(*19*) WEISS, GEORGE. "Hallucinogenic and narcotic-like effects of powdered myristica (nutmeg)." Psychiat. Quart., 34 : 346–356, 1960.

(*20*) WEISS, GEORGE. Personal communication, April 18, 1964.

(*21*) BURROUGHS, WILLIAM. "Naked Lunch." New York, Grove Press, 1959.

(*22*) REISNER, ROBERT GEORGE. "Bird: The Legend of Charlie Parker." New York, Citadel Press, 1962.

(*23*) ANDRE, SIGRID. "Nutmeg jag." Mississippi Mag., 4 : 18, 1964.

The Chemistry and Psychopharmacology of Nutmeg and of Several Related Phenylisopropylamines

ALEXANDER T. SHULGIN
Department of Pharmacology, University of California
San Francisco Medical Center, San Francisco, California

THORNTON SARGENT* AND CLAUDIA NARANJO
Centro de Estudios de Antropologia Medica
Universidad de Chile, Santiago, Chile

Our report today has been divided into two separate portions. The discussion of nutmeg and its composition, and of the possible involvement of its chemical components. The psychotropic intoxication has a natural division into two areas of presentation. The first is a brief description of the plant; a presentation of the methods and procedures for the isolation and the identification of the many components in the oil from the plant, and a careful definition of those components that are most probably involved in the intoxicative syndrome.

The extension of these components in to the corresponding amphetamines, their effectiveness in humans, and the likelihood of their being an acceptable explanation of the effects of the total nutmeg, will constitute the latter part of this report. In the previous paper there was presented some of the history of nutmeg, and a description of the style and extent of its usage in various cultures. In the reports that will follow, specific descriptions of the human syndrome of intoxication, and some of the pharmacological ramifications of its study, will be presented.

At this point we would like to present a factual description of the various chemical materials that have been found to make up the volatile (and presumed active) fraction of nutmeg. On the hypothesis that one or more components may be appropriately assigned the responsible role for the nutmeg intoxication, there is a need for an exact chemical definition of nutmeg. But even before this, we must define in botanical terms just what is meant by the name nutmeg.

Properly the nutmeg tree is any plant found in the Genus *Myristica*. Two species are known to be native to India. *M. malabarica* produces a seed some four centimeters long and elliptically shaped, and *M. canarica* produces a small spherical seed about two centimeters across. Both contain primarily fats and myristic acid, and being virtually without odor or volatile oil have achieved no position of importance. In the East Indies the seeds of *M. succedanea*, known as "Pala Maba" in the Indonesian areas, are also small and quite elongate in shape, but they have proven valuable as rich sources of the nutmeg essential oils. Another species, *M. argentea*, has actually been used

---

*Present address: Donner Laboratory, University of California, Berkeley, California.

in the spice trade under the name of "New Guinea Nutmegs" or "Long Nutmegs". However the quantity and quality of the volatiles from its seeds are quite low. The plant that has achieved the widest study and commercial exploitation, and which is the subject of this portion of this symposium, is *M. fragrans*. This species originated in the Mollucas and has been propagated throughout the adjoining Indonesian islands, giving rise to the so-called East Indian nutmeg of commerce.

A little over a hundred years ago, the tree was introduced into the Carribean area and since the end of World War II has led to the establishment of a major industry. Grenada, of the windward islands, now supplies a major portion of the world's needs. The West Indian nutmeg is generally conceded as being of a somewhat lower quality than its East Indian forebears; the best grade of mace still comes from Asia.

The tree has also been translocated into Ceylon, and much of the early analytical work on the composition of the natural extracts was conducted on nutmegs from this source. It is no longer possible to obtain commercial samples with this designation however, and it must be assumed that any product from this area has been absorbed into the East Indian category.

The three areas of the plant *M. fragrans* that have received any analytical attention are the leaf, the arillode (which lies within the husk but outside of the shell of the seed, and which is known as mace), and the kernel of the seed itself, the nutmeg. The leaves have received only a cursory examination, which has indicated that although there is only a small amount of steam-distillable material present (about 1.5% of the dry weight) its composition is substantially the same as that of the plant parts associated with the seed (*1*). The studies that concern the volatile oils of mace are best presented later in direct comparison with the analysis of nutmeg itself. As it is only the nutmegs that are invested with the reputation of psychotropic efficacy, they have served as the primary focal point of our analysis.

The actual nutmeg, when removed from its hard brown shell or testa is a spherical kernel that weighs about five grams. The thorough work of Power and Salway (*2*) must serve as a definitive study of the composition of the entire nutmeg. There are two classical ways of extracting the potentially interesting materials from the whole fruit.

Figure 1 shows the approximate distribution to be expected with the employment of these methods. The process of expression, or the extraction with an organic solvent, provides about a third of the total original weight. This fraction is known as the fixed oils, and has also been called Nutmeg Butter or "Oleum Myristicae expressum". This fraction is substantially free of volatiles, and is composed primarily of triglycerides. Myristic acid is the principle compound here, although both oleic acid and linoleic acid are also found. This fraction has been used as a source of trimyristin (*3*). The small non-fat remainder is composed of unsaponifiable compounds, primarily oxygenated polyterpenes and phytosterols.

The subjection of the total crushed seed to distillation with live steam removes some 10 to 15% of the weight, known as the volatile oil fraction. The small overlap that is shown with the expression fraction is due to the

CHEMICAL GROUP DISTRIBUTION IN NUTMEG

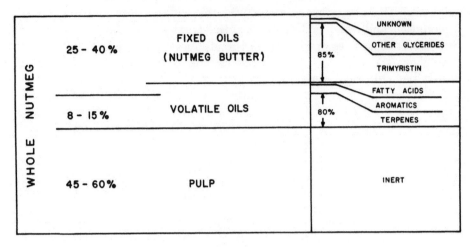

FIG. 1

fact that some of the volatile components are removed in the solvent extraction and are held tightly by the fixed components present. This volatile fraction is composed primarily of terpenes, which make up some 80% of its total weight. The remainder is the aromatic fraction, composed of ethers and phenolic bodies.

The residue that remains after the expression of the solubles and the distillation of the volatiles constitutes some 50% of the original mass of the nutmeg. It is presumably a cellulose-like pulp, and it remains totally unexplored as far as any chemical analysis is concerned.

It must be stated here, in anticipation of later discussions on the pharmacology of nutmeg, that no definitive evaluation of these fractions (fats and pulp) have been made. It has, however, been generally accepted that it is the volatile oil fraction to which one must look for the effective agents of nutmeg, and it is this "Oil of Nutmeg" that has been admitted to the U.S. Pharmacopeia as a medicinal. This oil comprises between an eighth and a twelfth of the entire fruit, and it serves as the object of the present study.

An exacting analysis of this volatile fraction has been performed. To this end a five pound sample of West Indian Oil of Nutmeg (from the George Lueders Company, New York) was subjected to fractional distillation employing a 70 tray Oldershaw column. Fractions were collected in a continuous sequence and each of these was in turn analysed and further fractionated employing a preparative gas liquid chromatographic procedure. Identity of each component was established by direct isolation, (employing a Varian A–700 Autoprep) and spectral comparison to reference samples (through infra-red and high resolution mass spectroscopy). Quantitative measurements were achieved employing a Varian Aerographer 1200 with a flame detector, and peak areas were established with an Aerograph 475 Integration System.

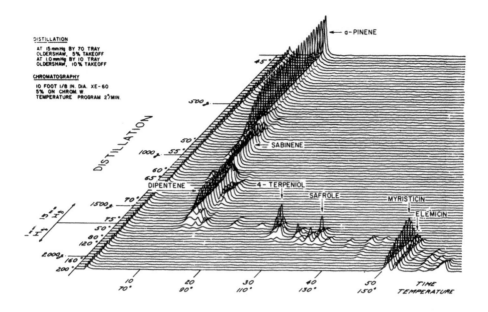

CHROMATOGRAPHY

FIG. 2

Figure 2 shows what might well be called a fingerprint of the oil of nutmeg. On the z-axis is shown the results of the distillation. This was continued on the 70 tray column at 15 mm/Hg until the aromatic fraction was reached. Then the distillation was completed at 1 mm/Hg through a shorter column. Although the actual fractions collected were not exactly of 25 grams as is presented in the figure, the weights have been normalized to this amount, and each horizontal line thus represents an equal weight of distillate.

The x-axis represents the progress of gas liquid chromatographic separation. The time required for desorbtion of each of the peaks is shown, and as the system has been programmed for a rise of 2°/min., this also represents the temperature of desorbtion.

The y-axis is peak height and, as it is characteristic of temperature programmed GLC spectra to display a constant peak half-width, this height is proportional to peak area.

Several peaks (components) are obvious that would be superimposed by one of the techniques alone (GLC or distillation), but are readily separated by applying the other.

The long ridge down the left hand side of the presentation, parallel to the z-axis, represents the similar terpenes α-pinene, sabinine, and dipentene, and this is separated in a natural division from the second and smaller group, the aromatics.

The preponderance of α-pinene has been mentioned, but both sabinine and γ-terpinene (1, 4-menthadiene) warrant special note as neither has been observed in nutmeg before. The terpenyl alcohols have been included in this

205

group as are the two aromatic hydrocarbons cymene and the previously undetected toluene. On the other hand both cineole and camphor have been recently reported to be present to the extent of a percent or two, and citronellol and citronellal have been reported in trace amounts (4); none of these were present in the sample we investigated. d-Borneol, which had originally been assigned to nutmeg on indirect evidence (5) was not present in our sample.

The second and smaller group, the aromatic ether fraction, is the more interesting and as will be shown later is the more likely to be implicated in the psychopharmacology of nutmeg. In Table I are shown the nine aromatics that have definitely been established as being present in nutmeg, and it also shows the extent of their contribution to the sample analysed.

The three major components, myristicin, elemicin, and safrole constitute nearly 9/10 of the group. In the previously reported studies of nutmeg, myristicin has always been recognized as a major component, and has thus often been thought to be responsible for the psychopharmacological activity of the total extract. In the thorough study conducted on the Ceylonese Oil of Nutmeg (5) safrole was found only in very small quantities, but recently its identity as a significant component of East Indian oils has been reported, (6) although it appeared to be absent in the West Indian varieties.

COMPOSITION OF OIL OF NUTMEG
LUEDERS WEST INDIAN

TERPENIC FRACTION	%	AROMATIC FRACTION	%
α-PINENE	36.16	SAFROLE	1.29
β-PINENE	6.16	METHYLEUGENOL	0.62
CAMPHENE	2.97	EUGENOL	0.17
SABINENE	12.75	METHYLISOEUGENOL	0.36
1,4-p-MENTHADIENE	3.47	ISOEUGENOL	0.19
1,4(8)-p-MENTHADIENE	1.12	MYRISTICIN	7.04
1,8-p-MENTHADIENE	12.78	ELEMICIN	2.36
TOLUENE	0.10	ISOELEMICIN	0.11
p-CYMENE	1.82	METHOXYEUGENOL	0.25
1-MENTHENE-4-OL	2.93		
1-MENTHENE-8-OL	0.41	OTHERS	
LINALOOL	0.15	MYRISTIC ACID	2.87
GERANYL ACETATE	0.20	UNIDENTIFIED	3.72

TABLE I.

206

DISTRIBUTION OF THE PRINCIPLE AROMATICS IN VARIOUS _MYRISTICA_ OILS

	L. WI. NUTMEG	F. WI. NUTMEG	L. EI. NUTMEG	F. EI. NUTMEG	D. ? NUTMEG	L. ? MACE	F. EI. MACE	D. ? MACE
SAFROLE	1.29	1.43	1.09	2.69	1.38	0.53	3.42	1.41
MYRISTICIN	7.04	5.58	8.08	8.48	5.62	3.86	12.78	5.53
ELEMICIN	2.36	0.02	0.48	0.02	0.99	2.07	0.05	0.69
% OF TOTAL OIL THAT IS AROMATIC	12.7	7.5	10.7	12.5	8.2	7.2	18.2	8.1
·% OF TOTAL AROMATIC THAT IS ACCOUNTED FOR ABOVE	84	94	90	90	94	90	89	95

TABLE II.

We have made a comparative study of the aromatic fraction of several samples of Oil of Nutmeg from different geographical origins, and of Oil of Mace as well. These results are shown in Table II. Here the surprisingly wide variation that can occur between these principle components is apparent. The single consistent item is the presence of myristicin as a major component. In the figure the F found at the heads of the columns represents the source, Fritzsche Bros., New York. Similarly, L stands for Lueders Co. and D for Dreyers Co. The WI represents West Indian sources, and EI East Indian. The question marks refer to samples whose origin was undesignated. Safrole has been found in both East and West Indian oils and appears, in this analysis, to be present in an amount from 15–30% of the myristicin present. The amount of elemicin present is most erratic. It has been found to vary from over 2% in the Lueders West Indian Oil of Nutmeg, to only trace amounts in the Fritzsche samples. The various oils of mace show neither consistency nor correlation with the nutmeg samples, except that again, myristicin appears as the principle component.

The assignment of the chemical structures of these compounds is a direct and simple matter when compared to the task of assigning responsibility for the intoxicating and psychotropic properties of nutmeg. The kernel itself is the only component of the tree that is invested with the reputation for biological activity. Further, it may be asserted that the psychoactive compound or compounds probably reside in the volitale oil fraction of the nutmeg, for this fraction has been shown in animal toxicology studies to carry the effectiveness of the entire seed. Human experiments with ground nutmeg depleted of its volatiles have failed to show psychopharmacological responses (7).

207

With the satisfactory assignment of the identities of the various conspicuous components to be found in nutmeg, one must examine how each of these
individually, or more likely in concert, may achieve a role in a reasonable
explanation of the activity of the entire seed. Here there are two groups of
compounds to consider, the terpenes and the aromatic eithers. It is tempting
to dismiss the terpenes out of hand. Although they constitute by far the
larger portion of the volatile fraction, the terpene hydrocarbons are generally
held to be of biological effectiveness mainly as irritants. Turpentine has a
composition quite similar in make-up to this terpene fraction; it has been
widely used in many home remedies, but it has certainly not commanded
reputation as an intoxicant. It may, however, have some function in assisting
in the absorption of the various aromatic compounds through the gut.

The aromatic fraction, then, would seem to be the most likely source of
the psychotropic activity of nutmeg. Table III shows the structure of each of
the compounds we have found in the aromatic fraction. Also shown is the
amount in milligrams of each of these components that would be present in 20
g. of the whole nutmeg, 20 g. being assumed to be that required to produce

AROMATIC FRACTION OF OIL OF NUTMEG

STRUCTURE	NAME	AMOUNT TO BE FOUND IN 20 GRAMS TOTAL NUTMEG (IN MILLIGRAMS)
	SAFROLE	39
	METHYLEUGENOL	18
	EUGENOL	5
	METHYLISOEUGENOL	11
	ISOEUGENOL	6
	MYRISTICIN	210
	ELEMICIN	70
	ISOELEMICIN	3
	METHOXYEUGENOL	8

TABLE III.

208

psychotropic effects. As stated earlier, safrole, myristicin, and elemicin account for some 84% of the aromatic fraction, and thus are the primary materials that we will consider. The possibility must always be kept in mind that one of the minor components could have an unusually high potency and thus contribute to the activity.

Of the primary constitutents, myristicin is by far the most abundant, and for this reason was tested specifically for psychotropic activity by Truitt, et al (7). Doses of 400 mg. myristicin, almost twice the amount present in 20 g. of typical nutmeg, were given to human volunteers and the observed symptoms were at least suggestive of psychotropic effects in 6 out of 10 subjects. It will be seen later that those effects which might be expected from myristicin may be rather subtle, and so may require some synergistic activity of some of the other aromatic compounds to produce the full nutmeg syndrome.

Safrole is also a component of other natural oils and spices, the most notable being the Oil of Sassafras which contains some 80%. Both the oil and the derived sassafras tea have enjoyed wide use, modestly as a flavoring, and in larger amounts as an internal medicament; yet neither has a reputation for psychotropic activity as does nutmeg.

Elemicin is unusual in that among the flavoring oils and spices, it occurs in appreciable amounts only in nutmeg. Further, as mentioned earlier, even in nutmeg the amount of elemicin is highly variable and depends upon the source of the extract. It also occurs in several obscure essential oils, none of which have been reported to have been used pharmacologically. It is, further, not separable from myristicin by fractional distillation. The myristicin employed in all earlier pharmacology (including the human studies mentioned) was obtained by distillation from oil of nutmeg, and was taken to be the single substance myristicin. It thus may or may not have contained elemicin as well, depending on the origin of the oil. The variability of elemicin may account for the apparently highly variable degree of reported psychoactive effects of nutmeg, which in turn implies that elemicin may indeed be an active component. Of the aromatic components present in lesser amounts, only eugenol and isoeugenol have found use either as flavoring agents or as medicinals. They comprise about 80% of the Oil of Cloves for example, but again search of the literature on such natural products for some reputation for abuse as an intoxicant has been futile.

There are thus several possibilities by which one or more of the aromatic components might be implicated as psychotropic agents;

1. One of the compounds that is present only in very small amounts may have unusually high potency,

2. Elemicin may be a major contributor of activity, or

3. A combination of two or more of the aromatics present may be involved. The three most abundant ones, myristicin, elemicin and safrole may be sufficient to account for the total activity.

It is worth noting that nutmeg is the only plant source within which these three compounds have been reported as occuring together in any appreciable quantity, and as will be seen later, each may contribute slightly different aspects to the total psychotropic effect.

With the exception of myristicin none of the individual components of the aromatic fraction have been evaluated specifically as to their psychological effects. The ring substitution patterns of these compounds are notable in that several of them, specifically myristicin, elemicin and safrole, are identical to the ring structures of materials of established psychotogenic activity. The allylic side chain is amenable to chemical modification, as shown is Fig. 3, which could convert the naturally occuring compounds into ones of known psychotropic activity. It has been suggested (8) that the *in vivo* addition of ammonia to the olefinic site in either the allyl or the propenyl isomer would yield amphetamines directly. To speak of amphetamines as a chemical class is not strictly correct, but we use it to refer to variously methoxylated phenyl-isopropylamines. The "RO" in the figure indicates the presence of any variety of ether groups on the ring, and thus would include all of the aromatic ethers in the oil of nutmeg and in many other natural oils as well. The possible mechanisms of such an *in vivo* transformation have been elaborated upon, and are plausible to the extent that each of the reactions has been achieved *in vitro*. Support for this transformation occurring *in vivo* has been obtained by Barfknecht (9), who found evidence for the production of amphetamine in rats after feeding them allylbenzene. This corresponds to ammonia addition in Fig. 3 without the "RO" ether groups.

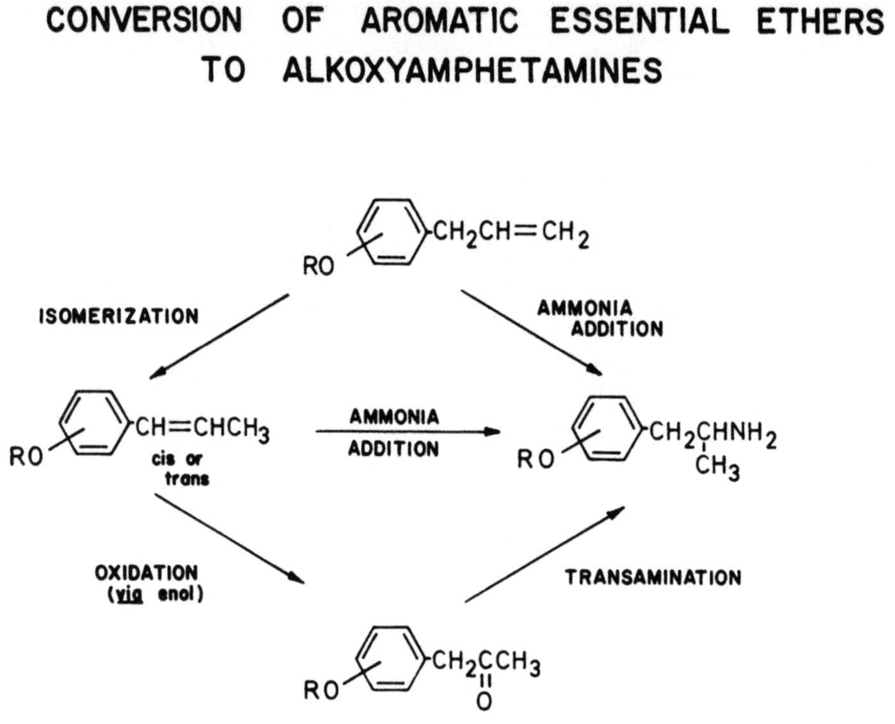

CONVERSION OF AROMATIC ESSENTIAL ETHERS TO ALKOXYAMPHETAMINES

FIG. 3.

Throughout the general area of spices and of essential oils from plant sources there is about a score of substituted phenylpropenes, all of which are characterized by ring substitution of either methoxy groups or a methylenedioxy group (or both) and by the allyl or the propenyl side chain mentioned above. Of these a total of eleven different ring substitution patterns have been reported as occuring; the balance of the twenty known aromatics consists of isomeric variations of the side chain. The addition of an amine to this olefinic system might be extremely sensitive to substitutions near it, that is, whether the side chain be allyl, *cis*-propenyl or *trans*-propenyl. It may thus be in turn a determining factor in the psychotropic activity of any such substance under consideration.

In the preparation for the study of this possible *in vivo* amination of these ring-substituted natural oils, a series of amphetamines that would be the result of such an addition has been completed. These are tabulated in Table IV, showing the principle natural source of each of the natural oils, the common name as they occur in the allyl (A) or propenyl (P) form, the orientation of the ring substituents, the code letter abbreviation of the resulting base, the cogent physical and chemical data, and the potency of the compound in mescaline units. The latter measure is defined as the quotient of the effective dose of mescaline (assumed to be 3.75 mg/Kg as the base) divided by the effective dose of the substance in question, as determined by human titration. This ratio permits a direct comparison of relative potencies, based on mescaline equaling one. Mescaline has a ring substitution pattern identical with number 6, TMA, except that the side chain has only two carbons instead of three.

It will be noted that several of the possible amphetamine derivatives of the components of the aromatic fraction of nutmeg do not appear here:

AMPHETAMINES RELATED TO THE NATURAL ESSENTIAL OILS

$$RO\text{---}\bigcirc\text{---}CH_2CHNH_2\cdot HCl$$
$$\overset{|}{CH_3}$$

	COMMON NAME	PRINCIPLE SOURCE	RING ORIENTATION	CODE	SYNTHETIC ROUTE	M.P.°C	YIELD	POTENCY MESCALINE=1
1.	ESTRAGOLE (A)	O. OF ANISE	4-OCH$_3$	MA	A	211	60	?
2.	NOTHOSMYRNOL (P)	O. OF N.JAPANICUM	2,4-(OCH$_3$)	2,4 DMA	A	147	90	?
3.	METHYLEUGENOL (A)	O. OF CITRONELLA	3,4-(OCH$_3$)	DMA	A	147	76	?
4.	SAFROLE (A)	O. OF SASSAFRAS	3,4-(OCH$_2$O)	MDA	A	186	29	2
5.	ASARONE (P)	O. OF CALAMUS	2,4,5-(OCH$_3$)	TMA-2	B	181	60	18
6.	ELEMICIN (A)	O. OF ELEMI	3,4,5-(OCH$_3$)	TMA	A	209	63	2
7.	CROWEACIN (A)	O. OF E.CROWEI	2-OCH$_3$-3,4-(OCH$_2$O)	MMDA-3a	A	154	59	18
8.	MYRISTICIN (A)	O. OF NUTMEG	3-OCH$_3$-4,5-(OCH$_2$O)	MMDA	B	191	60	3
9.	— (A)	O. OF PARSLEY SEED	2,3,4,5-(OCH$_3$)$_4$	Tetra MA	C	136	13	?
10.	DILLAPIOLE (A)	O. OF DILL	2,3-(OCH$_3$)$_2$-4,5-(OCH$_2$O)	DMMDA-2	C	130	94	?
11.	APIOLE (A)	O. OF PARSLEY SEED	2,5-(OCH$_3$)$_2$-3,4-(OCH$_2$O)	DMMDA	B	175	64	?

A: VIA BENZALDEHYDE, NITROETHANE, LiAlH$_4$.
B: VIA CLAISEN REARRANGEMENT, METHYLATION, ISOMERIZATION, C(NO$_2$)$_4$, LiAlH$_4$.
C: VIA NATURAL ALLYL COMPOUND, ISOMERIZATION, C(NO$_2$)$_4$, LiAlH$_4$.

TABLE IV.

namely those which contain an OH substituent in addition to the methoxyl groups. These comprise some 5% of the aromatic fraction, and still remain to be explored in the human subject, either as purified components themselves, or as their amphetamine extensions. Should the free hydroxyl group of any of these several materials confer an unusually high psychotropic potency on any of these compounds or on the corresponding amphetamines, this would contribute to the nutmeg intoxication beyond the explanations considered here. Eugenol itself has had some known medical uses however, and it would seem reasonable to expect that its psychotropic activity would have been noted had it existed.

Published detail has appeared on the psychotropic effects in normal human subjects for the four compounds that are trisubstituted, numbers 5, 6, 7 and 8 (10). In every case the compounds had a greater potency than that of the reference substance mescaline.

The base that corresponds to safrole, number 4, is 3,4-methylenedioxyamphetamine, or MDA. This was first described pharmacologically by Gordon Alles (11) who reported visual effects at some 120 mg. Subsequent experience (12) on a more extensive number of subjects has shown modest, if any, distortion or change of either visual or auditory perception, but rather a pronounced increase in emotional effect, which has proved to be of considerable value in psychotherapy.

The base that would be the result of the addition of ammonia to myristicin, number 8, is 3-methoxy-4,5-methylenedioxyamphetamine, or MMDA. A complete description of the animal and human pharmacology and psychopharmacology of this compound is forthcoming (13). With regard to the work mentioned earlier in which 400 mg. of myristicin was tested in human subjects, the experience with MMDA indicates that the effects although identifiable in a psychotherapeutic setting, or in subjects trained to identify psychotropic effects, are rather subtle and may not have been detected by the psychological tests used in the study. The psychotropic effects of MMDA are rather similar to those of MDA, but in addition some 30% of the subjects reported rather vivid and well structured visual images appearing when the eyes are closed, although there are virtually no changes in eyes-open perception. The possibility that myristicin in the amounts present in nutmeg may contribute to the total effects of nutmeg, cannot at this point be discarded.

The base that corresponds to number 6 is 3,4,5-trimethoxyamphetamine, TMA. This has been known as a psychotropic agent for some time (14, 10a). It has variously been described as having potent hallucinatory effects and as leading to apparently hostile reactions. More extensive appraisal of this compound in psychotherapeutic settings has confirmed the eyes-opened distortions and occasional hallucinatory phenomena, and strongly suggests that its characteristic property is one of causing projection, in the psychological sense, by the subject. This can produce visual distortions, delusions (alterations in social perceptions), and sometimes apparently hostile projections which, however, have never led to any overt actions.

212

The analogous bases that correspond to the eugenols have not yet been evaluated, and as mentioned earlier represent another group of compounds that could contribute to the activity of nutmeg.

There are two ways in which further investigations might be pursued; namely human evaluation of the individual compounds of the aromatic fraction of the oil of nutmeg, preferably synthetically derived to avoid contamination, and secondly, the further evaluation of the effects of the amine derivitives. It is entirely possible that the combination of the amines derivable from the essential oil aromatics could produce the psychological effects of nutmeg, while the clearly toxic effects could be due to the terpene fraction. Human evaluation of a mixture of these amines, in the proportions found in nutmeg, would explore the possibility of any synergistic amplification of the activity of these compounds. A corollary study would involve the chemical investigation of the metabolic fate of both the essential oils and the derived amines, on administration to human subjects, and may clarify whether or not these oils are in fact converted to amines *in vivo*. From the results of these studies, it is hoped that the interrelationship between the complex composition, and the yet more complex psychopharmacological structure of nutmeg, can be resolved.

REFERENCES

(1) "Essential Oil from the Leaves of Nutmeg (*Myristica fragrans* Houtt.)", Th. M. Meyer. Ing. Nederland.-Indie 8 No. 1 VII 7–8 (1941). (CA 35: 4549⁴).

(2) "The Constituents of the Expressed Oil of Nutmeg", F. B. Power and A. H. Salway, J. Chem. Soc., 93: 1653 (1908).

(3) "Trimyristin", O. D. Beal, Org. Syn., Coll. Vol. I., Second Edition p. 538 (1941).

(4) "Application of Gas Chromatography to a Study of Nutmeg Oil Flavor", G. D. Lee, F. L. Kauffman, J. W. Harlan and W. Niezabitowski, Intern. Gas Chrom. Symp., I.S.A. Proc. 301 (1961).

(5) "The Constituents of the Essential Oil of Nutmeg", F. B. Power and A. W. Salway, J. Chem. Soc., 91: 2037 (1907).

(6) "Gas Chromatographic Analysis of Oil of Nutmeg", E. A. Bejnarowicz and E. F. Kirch, J. Pharm. Sci., 53: 988 (1963).

(7) "The Pharmacology of Myristicin, A Contribution to the Psychopharmacology of Nutmeg", E. B. Truitt, Jr., E. Callaway III, M. C. Braude, and J. C. Krantz, Jr., J. Neuropsych. 2: 205 (1961).

(8) "Possible Implication of Myristicin as a Psychotropic Substance", A. T. Shulgin, Nature 210: 380 (1966).

(9) C. F. Barfknecht, University of Idaho (personal communication).

(10) a. "The Psychotomimetic Properties of 3,4,5-Trimethoxyamphetamine", A. T. Shulgin, S. Bunnell and T. Sargent, Nature, 189: 1011 (1961); b. "3-Methoxy-4, 5-Methylenedioxyamphetamine, a New Psychotomimetic Agent", A. T. Shulgin, Nature 201: 1120 (1964); c. "Psychotomimetic Amphetamines; Methoxy 3,4-dialkoxyamphetamines", Experientia 20: 366 (1964).

(11) "Some Relations between Chemical Structures and Physiological Action of Mescaline and Related Compounds." G. A. Alles, in Neuropharmacology, The Josiah Macy Jr. Foundation, Madison Printing Co., Inc., 1959.

(12) "The Psychological Effects of 3,4-Methylenedioxyamphetamine (MDA) Intoxication." C. Naranjo, T. Sargent and A. T. Shulgin (in preparation).

(*13*) "The Chemistry and Pharmacology of 3-Methoxy-4,5-methylenedioxyamphetamine (MMDA)." A Monograph. C. Naranjo, T. Sargent and A. T. Shulgin (in preparation).

(*14*) "A New Hallucinogen: 3,4,5-Trimethoxyphenyl-β-aminopropane, with notes on the stroboscopic phenomenon." D. I. Peretz, J. R. Smythies and W. C. Gibson, J. Mental Sci., 101: 316 (1955).

The Pharmacology of Myristicin and Nutmeg

EDWARD B. TRUITT, JR.

Battelle Memorial Institute, Columbus, Ohio

The long history of observations concerning the pronounced psychotropic effect of Myristica fragrans (nutmeg) has not gone unnoticed by many distinguished investigators, including some famous pharmacologists. A central problem in the pharmacology of nutmeg has been identification of the active component of the crude drug. As early as 1676, van Leeuwenhoek, the original microscopist noted that a volatile component which evolved from pieces of nutmeg in a glass tube repelled or killed mites. (*1*) Although Warburg, as late as 1897, still expressed doubt (*2*) it was clear by then that the volatile fraction, the oil of nutmeg, was more toxic than the crude drug. The well-known English pharmacologist, Cushny, stated that the residue from which the volatile oil has been removed has no effect upon animals. (*3*) In our early studies at Maryland, we confirmed this observation by human testing of a steam-distilled residue and noted only gastrointestinal effects. (*4*)

Another pharmacologist, George Wallace, used the highest distillate fraction (149°C, 14 mm), which he found to be the most active and easily administered component, and observed that the cat was the most susceptible species among the mammalia to the toxic action of the drug. (*5*) Both Wallace and, a year later, Jurss (*6*) correctly attributed the high toxicity to hepatic fatty degeneration, but the cat is also most sensitive to the central excitation, tremor, salivation, and stupor produced by oil of nutmeg. Sir Henry Dale in 1907 most clearly differentiated the primary psychotropic effect from the secondary hepatic coma causing death in cats. (*7*) Although he noted, as others had, that the oil required a higher myristicin amount than the crude drug in order to produce symptoms, Dale attributed this to absorption difficulties with the purified product. Power and Salway, reexamining the question in 1908, concurred that myristicin was probably responsible for the central effect, but was unfavorable for absorption in the pure state. (*8*)

Pharmacologic interest in nutmeg then subsided for more than 50 years, until renewed by the curiosity of Dr. John C. Krantz at the University of Maryland who was consulted by several former students encountering cases of nutmeg intoxication. (*4*) This study was conducted with a myristicin-containing fraction distilled from oil of nutmeg at 145–155°C and 15 mm Hg pressure. Subsequent gas-chromatographic studies by Shulgin have shown this to be a mixture of myristicin with elemicin and perhaps a small amount of methylisoeugenol. (*9*)

Initial studies on the pharmacologic action of myristicin and nutmeg which were conducted at the University of Maryland sought to answer a variety of questions. (4) Toxicity studies showed that the East Indian spice was more toxic than a West Indian product. Animal toxicity determinations before and after steam distillation also confirmed Cushny's original observation that the volatile fraction was more toxic than the residue (3) In planning for human administration of a dose of the myristicin-elemicin fraction amounting to 400 mg per subject, a chronic study in rats was conducted and showed no growth inhibition at a daily dose of 10 mg/kg.

A stimulant effect of myristicin was demonstrated by a shortening effect of the oil fraction on barbiburate sleeping time. These data are shown in Table 1.

TABLE 1.—*The effect of myristicin on the sleeping time induced by phenobarbital in the rat*

Group	Mean sleeping time	Standard error	p value
Phenobarbital 120 mg/kg I. P.	162 min	± 5. 31	
Phenobarbital 120 mg/kg I. P. plus 100 mg/kg myristicin I. P.	144 min	± 2. 27	< 0. 01

The intravenous injection of large doses in the order 50–76 mg/kg to dogs, monkeys, and cats confirmed the feline species toxicity and showed clearly that tranquilization of wildness is not produced in the jungle-bred monkey. It is of interest that the product was hypotensive in the dog as are other monamine oxidase inhibitors. These intravenous injections were suspensions of the oily substance in acacia solution. More recently a stable emulsion has been achieved having the following composition:

	Percent
Myristicin	1.0
Pluronic F-68	0.3
Dextrose	4.2
Ethyl alcohol	1.0
Distilled water qs	100.0

Using this formula, mice were injected into the dorsal tail vein with doses of 100 mg/kg. Within 1 to 2 minutes, loss of righting reflex and apparent sedation appeared.

One contribution to the metabolism of myristicin has recently evolved from interest in its synergistic effect upon other insecticides. Casida and his associates have shown that the methylenedioxy bridge is the initial point of metabolic attack by hepatic microsomes and requires $NADPH_2$ (10). This reaction is shown in Figure 1. This metabolic transformation increases the chemical similarity of myristicin to the catecholamines.

The structural resemblences of myristicin to mescaline and epinephrine prompted studies directed at measuring competitive inhibition of myristicin to other monoamine oxidase substrates. The method of Tedeschi et al, (11) was employed for estimation of monoamine oxidase (MAO) inhibition by potentiation of the central convulsant action of tryptamine HCl. A 0.5%

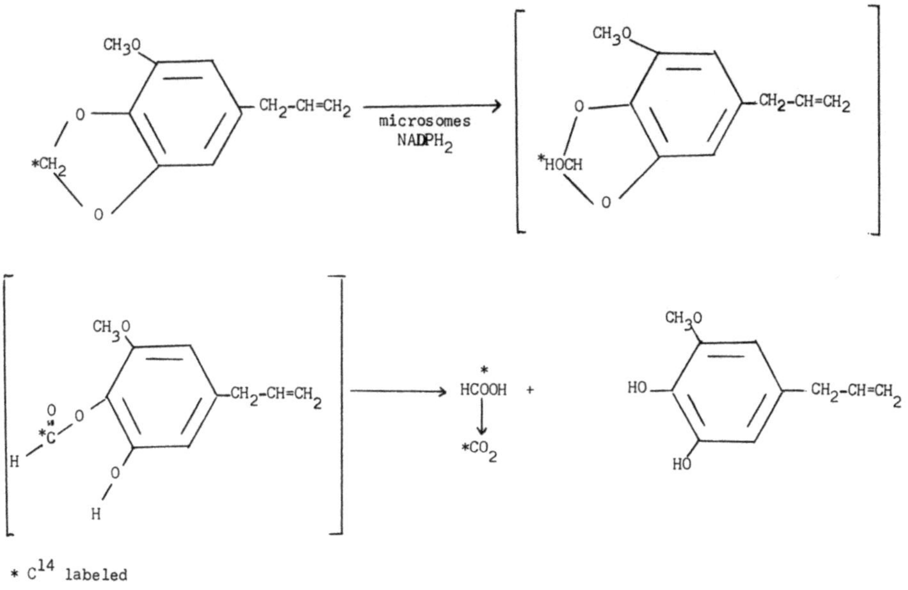

* C^{14} labeled

FIG. 1.—Major metabolic pathway for methylene C^{14} dioxyphenyl labeled myristicin in liver microsomal systems of the mouse. (Modified from Casida, et al. (10).)

solution was injected intravenously into 10 mice per dose level. Three seconds or more of clonic jerking, tremors, and/or side-to-side head movements were the endpoint criteria used to calculate the CD_{50} from dose-response lines by the method of Rubin et al. (13) in rats, scoring both eyes on a 5-point scale. Cerebral 5-hydroxytryptamine was measured by the Mead and Finger modification (14) of the method of Bogdanski et al. (15)

Results

No apparent effect was evident from the drug vehicles on the CD_{50} of tryptamine (Table 2). When given orally 18 hours in advance, East Indian ground nutmeg gave some evidence of tryptamine potentiation (Figure 2). The optimum dose was 500 mg/kg. However, a much larger dose, 1000 mg/kg showed reversal of the activity.

Several samples of synthetic myristicin [1] were tested by the tryptamine potentiation test 18 hours after their oral administration. These results are shown in Figure 3. Both of these preparations showed considerable activity when the sample was fresh and lemon yellow in color. Later tests (not shown) after the liquid had turned to a light amber color consistently showed a considerable decline in tryptamine potentiation. These deteriorated solutions when studied by gas chromatography showed the appearance of an unknown component in addition to the myristicin.

The distilled concentrate of oil of nutmeg was much less active than the synthetic myristicin and, like ground nutmeg, reversed its activity with a

---

[1] Synthetic myristicin was kindly made available by Dr. Carl D. Lunsford, A. H. Robins Company, Richmond, Virginia.

TABLE 2.—*Tryptamine convulsion test for monoamine oxidase inhibition* in vivo. *Summary of control tests*

Species	No.	Vehicle-18 hr prior, cc/kg	CD_{50}, mg/kg	95% confidence limits, mg/kg
Mouse	40	None	25.0	15.4–40.5
"	21	"	17.3	12.1–24.7
"	28	Liq. pet.	24.5	19.9–30.1
"	38	" "	28.0	18.4–42.6
"	37	Acacia-2%	25.8	18.3–36.3
Avg	164		25.0	21.6–29.0
Rat	54	None	18.6	13.6–25.5

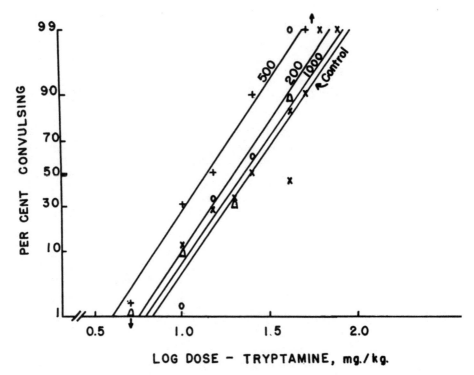

FIG. 2.—Effect of ground nutmeg on tryptamine convulsive threshold in mice when given orally in acacia suspension 18 hr before test: X——X Control, CD_{50} mg/kg (±95% confidence limits) 25.0 (15.2–41.0); O——200——O 200 mg/kg nutmeg, 20.0 (14.2–28.2); +—500—+ 500 mg/kg nutmeg, 14.0 (10.1–19.5); △——1000——△ 1000 mg/kg nutmeg, 23.0 (16.1–32.9).

large dose (Figure 3). Gas-chromatographic analysis of this oil showed the presence of volatile components similar to ground nutmeg, but no increased concentration of the myristicin, as expected from the selected distillation temperature.[2]

[2] These analyses and supplies of ground nutmeg were kindly furnished by Dr. William K. Stahl, McCormick and Company, Baltimore, Maryland.

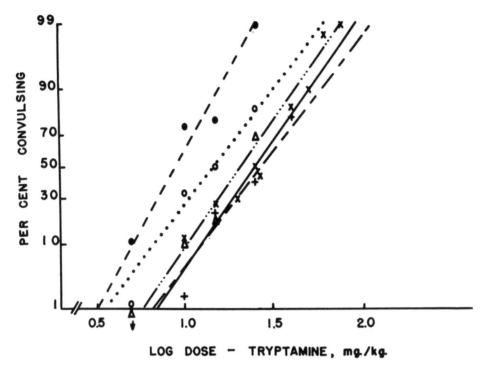

F<small>IG.</small> 3.—Effect of synthetic myristicin samples and oil of nutmeg concentrate on tryptamine convulsive threshold in mice when given orally in acacia suspension 18 hr before
test: X— — —X Control, CD_{50} mg/kg ($\pm 95\%$ confidence limits) 25.0 (15.2–41.0);
○——○ Myristicin sample 1 at 500 mg/kg, 8.7 (5.7–13.4); ○— . . . ○ myristicin
sample 2 at 500 mg/kg, 14.0 (9.3–21.0); . . . . . oil of nutmeg concentrate 500
mg/kg, 20.5 (14.5–28.9); +— — —+ oil of nutmeg concentrate — 1000 mg/kg, 27.0
(19.9–36.7).

In Figure 4 the slope and activity of the best tryptamine assay for myois-
ticin is compared to tranylcypromine and iproniazid. All three drugs were
administered orally 18 hours before the test. It may be seen that myristicin
is less potent but parallel to the comparative drugs. Safrole, isoborneol, and
geraniol, which are other volatile components of nutmeg, did not cause potentiation of tryptamine in doses up to 1 g/kg despite obvious signs of hyperactivity and excitement in the mice.

In Figure 5 the antagonism of reserpine ptosis in rats was used to study
variations in dose and time for myristicin activity. Myristicin appears
to be less active in the rat. Comparable activity to other MAO inhibitors was
obtained only with the largest dose 17 hours after oral administration.

Myristicin treatment of six rats increased brain 5-hydroxytrptamine from
control values averaging 0.48 ($\pm$ 0.05) μg/g to 0.82 ($\pm$ 0.03) μg/g when
given in an oral dose of 1 g/kg; the difference was statistically significant
($p < 0.001$). Lower doses were not significantly active.

A further test of an hypothesis of monoamine oxidase inhibition was conducted using the kynuramine disappearance rate in brain homogenates as

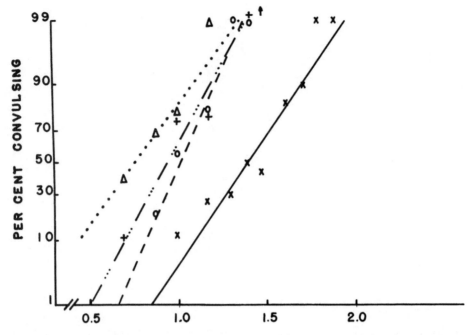

FIG. 4.—Effect of monoamine oxidase inhibitors and synthetic myristicin on tryptamine convulsive thresholds in mice when given orally in acacia suspension 18 hr before test: X———X Control, CD_{50} mg/kg ($\pm 95\%$ confidence limits) 25.0 (15.2–41.0); O———O 150 mg/kg iproniazid, 10.4 (8.8–12.2); $\triangle$. . . .$\triangle$ 4 mg/kg tranyleypromine, 5.8 (4.4–7.7); +− . . . + 500 mg/kg, 8.7 (5.7–13.4).

described by Weissbach et al. (*16*) The results of this test are shown in Table 3. Slight inhibition was found in the mouse but not in the rat-brain preparation. One year after these data were obtained, the same ground-nutmeg source was completely inactive in the mouse as well, and the declining activity was attributed to a loss of volatile components owing to a nearby heater.

Discussion

Although the myristicin fraction from oil of nutmeg originally used in these experiments might not represent 100 percent myristicin, both this and elemicin most likely produce similar actions. The potency of myristicin is not adequate in most of these tests to account for the full action of nutmeg. The insufficiency is present with intravenous doses and therefore poor absorption is not a likely explanation. More rapid biodegradation of purified myristicin in contrast to its slow release from nutmeg might suggest a greater efficiency of the crude drug.

These data demonstrate a mild degree of monoamine oxidase inhibition by a variety of tests. The low potency of myristicin in comparison to tranylcypromine, a potent inhibitor, is in keeping with the large doses required for *in vivo* activity. The tryptamine potentiation test, although indirect, has been

220

shown to correlate with other *in vivo* assays. (*17*) It is quite likely that although myristicin displaces kynuramine from MAO with difficulty, it still may show inhibiting activity.

The main virtue of these data may be to reawaken interest in myristicin and its activity. Low activity of a prolonged nature, such as that shown by nutmeg, is sometimes a more useful drug attribute than high potency and rapid onset. An important question remains to determine if the myristicin stimulation is inevitably followed by depressed feelings, even upon continued intake. Work is indicated to improve absorption, and further pharmacologic studies are needed to define a proper course of treatment for nutmeg intoxication.

Summary

A myristicin-elemicin fraction of oil of nutmeg produces many of the characteristics of crude ground nutmeg, but lacks adequate potency to explain the nutmeg intoxication syndrome on a quantitative basis. Nutmeg and

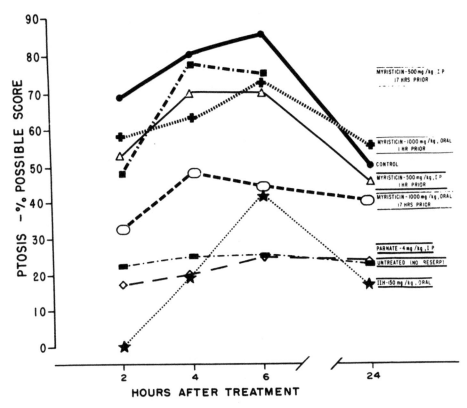

FIG. 5.—Effect of monoamine oxidase inhibitors and various schedules of myristicin on reserpine ptosis in rats. Ptosis score: 0=Eyelid fully open—5=Eyelid fully closed. Maximum score = 10/rat (both eyes). Group ptosis score (%)

$$= \frac{\text{No. rats/group} \times \text{Max score/rat}}{\text{Sum of group eyelid scores}} \times 100.$$

TABLE 3.—*The effect of ground West Indian nutmeg on brain monoamine oxidase (MAO) activity in mice and rats measured by the kynuramine (Kyn) method of Weissbach, et al. (16)*

Species	No.	μM-ynK/mg/hr x 10^{-3a}	No.	Nutmeg treated [b] percent of control
Mouse	14	3. 64±0. 013	10	78. 0±4. 2%
Rat	6	4. 74±0. 18	5	104. 0±5. 5%

[a] Micromoles of kynuramine/mg of brain (wet weight)/hour x 10^{-3}.
[b] 18 hours after 500 mg/kg—mice or 1000 mg/kg—rat, P.O.

the synthetically made myristicin demonstrate a mild degree of monoamine oxidase inhibiting activity by *in vitro* and *in vivo* tests. Activity of this synthetic product declines with aging accompanied by color change. Monoamine oxidase inhibition and other actions of crude extracts depend upon the volatile component.

BIBLIOGRAPHY

(1) HANZLIK, P. J., "Purkinje's Pioneer Self-experiments in Psychopharmacology," California and Western Medicine, 44 : 1, July–August, 1938.

(2) WARBURG, O. "Die Muskatnuss" Leipzig, 1897.

(3) CUSHNY, A. R., "Nutmeg Poisoning." Proceedings of the Royal Society of Medicine 39 : I (3), 1908.

(4) TRUITT, E. B., Jr. E. CALLAWAY, III, M. C. BRAUDE, and J. C. KRANTZ Jr., Journal of Neuropsychiatry, 2 : 205, 1961.

(5) WALLACE, G. B., In Contributions to Medical Research, Vaughn, Ann Arbor, Michigan, 1903, pp. 351–364.

(6) JURSS, F., "On Myristicin and Some Closely Related Substances," Berichte, Schimmel & Company, Leipzig, 1904.

(7) DALE, H. H., Proceedings of the Royal Society of Medicine, 23 : 69, 1909.

(8) POWER, F. B. and A. H. SALWAY, American Journal of Pharmacology, 80, 563–580, 1908.

(9) SHULGIN, A. T., Nature (Lond.), 197 : 379, 1963.

(10) CASIDA, J. E., J. L. ENGEL, F. G. ESAAC, F. X. KAMIEUSKI, AND KUWATSUDA. Science, 153 : 1130–1133, 1966.

(11) TEDESCHI, D. H., R. E. TEDESCHI, E. J. FELLOWS, Journal Pharmacology and Experimental Therapeutics, 126 : 223, 1959.

(12) LITCHFIELD, J. T., AND F. WILCOXON. ibid., 96 : 99, 1949.

(13) RUBIN, R., M. H. MALONE, M. H. WAUGH, and J. C. BURKE. 120 : 125, 1957.

(14) MEAD, J. A. R., and K. F. FINGER, Biochemical Pharmacology, 6 : 52, 1961.

(15) BOGDANSKI, D. F., A. PLETSCHER, B. B. BRODIE, and S. UDENFRIEND. Journal of Pharmacology and Experimental Therapeutics, 117 : 82, 1956.

(16) WEISSBACH, H. V. T. E. SMITH, J. W. DALY, B. WITKOP, and S. UDENFRIEND. Journal of Biological Chemistry, 235 : 1160–1163, 1950.

(17) MAXWELL, D. R., W. R., GRAY, and E. M. TAYLOR. British Journal of Pharmacology, 17 : 310, 1961.

Discussion

Chairman—EDWARD B. TRUITT, JR.
Members of the Panel—CLAUDIO NARANJO
THORNTON SARGENT
ALEXANDER T. SHULGIN
ANDRER T. WEIL

CHAIRMAN DR. TRUITT: We might begin with a comment. One of the guests found that there is a whole state in our fifty in the Union that has a reputation for nutmeg, and perhaps he would like to make his comment again, which was quite interesting: that of a psychotogenic substance identifying a state.

DR. PHILLIPS (from the floor): I am a psychiatrist. I understand that Connecticut is known as the Nutmeg State, and I remember when I was in college about twenty years ago there was some reference to the fact that people in Connecticut acted awfully crazy, because they ate so much nutmeg.

MR. WEIL: I am afraid the origin of Connecticut's nickname is somewhat less romatic. In colonial times, Connecticut traders often palmed off carved wooden nutmegs as the real thing. This practice was considered a fine example of Yankee shrewdness in business; consequently, Connecticut acquired the name "Nutmeg State".

CHAIRMAN DR. TRUITT: I wonder if Dr. Naranjo would like to discuss the activity of the compound he is engaged in testing?

DR. NARANJO: This amphetamine substituted with the methylenedioxy group is the first that was tested. The subjective reactions had been described by Gordon Alles from experimentation on himself. It was first used in a group of subjects under the assumption that this would be a hallucinogen, as suggested by Dr. Alles. This did not appear to be quite the case, for the drug produced only enhancement in feelings. In the face of this, it was suggested that it could be used as facilitating agent in psychotherapy. It is not something to be used as an antidepressant, but only to increase communication during a therapeutic session.

When we used this compound on patients with psychoneurotic symptoms, we saw that the effects were sometimes very dramatic in an unexpected way. I have tried several drugs to facilitate psychotherapy, including the more widely known hallucinogens, and never as with this compound has there been such a frequency of reminiscence of childhood events, in a very dramatic and spontaneous way, completely unexpected by the subjects.

This has been described in therapy with LSD and mescaline, but in my own experience has occurred spontaneously only once in approximately fifty experiences with LSD (though I understand that if a therapist searches for this, it could be precipitated). On the other hand, about half of the persons who in a therapeutic setting took this compound, (MDA), had this kind of experience an experience with almost no symbolic content, without

223

the aesthetic or mystical overtones that is so characteristic of most hallucinogens.

This was quite rare and, in turn, there was the experience of reminiscence. It is notable that in many of the subjects there was amnesia after it, and this was very much like the similar events that take place sometimes in the hypnotic trance. In two instances out of thirty, at least, the effects were those of a delirium, and in one of these there was erratic behavior, none of which was remembered afterwards.

Now with the trimethoxy substituted compound, which has been previously described as evoking hostile reactions when we used this in a therapeutic setting, this did not occur overtly; but the compound was remarkable in that the delusional content was more frequent that with any of the others that I know. This delusional content was very often paranoid.

CHAIRMAN DR. TRUITT: Could I ask if there were any color effects, which are characteristic of mescaline, seen with it?

DR. NARANJO: This produces the greatest incidence of color effects, whereas the previously mentioned one, (MDA), is notable for the absence of distortions and color effects.

The 3-methoxy-4,5 methylenedioxyamphetamine, (MMDA), has a methylenedioxy bridge in common with MDA, but has the oxygen substitution pattern of TMA. MMDA produces the qualities of both, and what is typical of this substance is that the experience, which has mostly a personal quality, enhancement of feeling, warmth, but very little symbolic content, makes it different from mescaline.

CHAIRMAN DR. TRUITT: There is one point, I think, that many people have possibly underestimated, and that is the theoretical importance of this aspect, which is pointed out by one question from Dr. Waser: "What is the evidence for direct amination of the olefinic side chain of myristicin in the body?"

DR. SHULGIN: Dr. Sargent mentioned one experiment where the formation of amphetamine in rats was actually observed. Administration of allylbenzene led to chromatographically distinct spots, with the strong implication that these spots were amphetamine. Although allylbenzene may be converted to propenylbenzene first, the simple addition of ammonia to the allyl double bond would be the most direct route. I don't know if it has any validity.

CHAIRMAN DR. TRUITT: We have a related question: "Could the transformation of a non-saturated aromatic side chain to a carbonyl group be possible?"

DR. SHULGIN: I don't know of this specific transformation having occurred. Certainly the double bond can participate in oxidation reactions, and substitution isomers have been converted to their corresponding acids in the body. Therefore the double bond is capable of being oxidized, or at least partially oxidized.

CHAIRMAN DR. TRUITT: We have two questions apparently directed to Mr. Weil, and I wonder if he would like to read them and comment.

224

Mr. WEIL: The first one is, "What are the comparative psychoactivating potencies of nutmeg and mace?"

They are the same, but mystiques about the uses of the two spices have sprung up. It is interesting, for example, that at Haverford College students believed they could only get "high" with mace, even though they knew nutmeg to be very similar in taste. Other groups use nutmeg only, and are unaware of mace as an intoxicant.

The second question is, "Do other kitchen spices have any psychoactive properties?"

Who knows? Perhaps in five years we will have a symposium just on spices. I have received scattered reports on the use of cinnamon for these effects: One bit of information is that cinnamon sticks are smoked by certain Indian tribes of Mexico. I have no documentation for this report.

People who are avid for experimenting with possibly active substances often try spices. In fact, a distant friend writes that anything in the spice cabinet except monosodium glutamate will get you "high". Ginger, paprika, cinnamon and pepper have all been said to have effects on the mind, but we have no reliable evidence on them.

CHAIRMAN DR. TRUITT: We really must resolve the action of somatic input on the gastrointestinal tract, and other sources on the psychic effects before we accept them, too.

I am a little chary of the next two questions. I have an antagonistic question from Dr. Efron, and a protagonistic question from Dr. Kline.

DR. EFRON (from the floor): Being a pharmacologist, I would like to comment on the pharmacology of the tested compounds. Dr. Truitt has really done an excellent pharmacological job but I have some small objections.

First, in my opinion the psychopharmacology testing is such a difficult one that we never can use one or two tests. One has to use a battery of tests, and even then, often we are not sure what they mean.

In this case, you have put all your chips on the monoamine oxidase inhibition. If this would be really the only action of these drugs, then we should forget about them, because we have much more potent reversible and irreversible monoamine oxidase inhibitors that we can use.

Further about the test that you used: the antagonism to reserpine, we all now agree that it is not valid as an antidepressant activity measurement. It was used for tricyclic types of drugs, and even then there was a question as to its validity. Is there a correlation between this test and the activity of nutmeg?

The other problem I would like to comment on is that I really don't know why everybody is working with myristicin, the compound represented mostly in this large mixture of compounds found in nutmeg extracts. There might be a possibility that one of the other compounds present in a very small amount may be much more potent.

The next thing that would be very interesting would be to elucidate for structural-activity relationship, and to see the activity of all the compounds in some battery of tests. Then we really could see how the location of one

225

methyl group, adding another methyl group or taking one off, affects the activity of the compounds.

CHAIRMAN DR. TRUITT: Thank you very much, Dr. Efron. I fully agree with your comments.

DR. KLINE: Dr. Efron's remarks are as a pharmacologist; mine are as a psychiatrist.

The anti-reserpine part of the story is the one I am protagonizing for you. A very curious cycle is involved, because every drug which has been useful in the treatment of schizophrenia or the major psychoses has produced Parkinsonism as one of its side effects. Another part of the curious business is that the monoamine oxidase inhibitors or other antidepressants, if given in large enough doses, will produce hallucinations, delusions and uncontrolled euphoria.

All this would seem to tie somewhere into the extrapyramidal system. We reviewed this problem a few years ago with Mettler, and although there is a lot of presumptive evidence, one cannot yet draw a comprehensive picture. At a meeting which Dr. Efron chaired last year, it was pointed out that tricyclic antidepressants reduce the frequency of extrapyramidal side effects from phenothiazines and reserpine. The rats and mice who developed reserpine depression were given much higher doses per kilogram than we use on humans. When asked how one judges if depression is present in rats and mice, the answer was that this is judged upon the basis of reduced activity and reduced "sociability"; i.e. they didn't go poking around at each other. Then I asked: "What about Parkinsonism in the rats and mice?"— and I discovered to my amazement that the animals were barely able to move because they were so Parkinsonized. What was called depression might simply be the fact that the animals couldn't get to sniff their neighbors. The monoamine inhibitors, and perhaps the tricycle antidepressants, act as anti-Parkinsonian agents. Professor Holmstedt mentioned yesterday that Lewin has found harmine, a monoamine oxidase inhibitor, useful in the treatment of Parkinsonism.

CHAIRMAN DR. TRUITT: I heartily agree with you, Dr. Kline, because you recognize our problems in the laboratory. We have a great deal of difficulty in defining these parameters, isolating them, and analyzing them. Certainly I would be the first to disclaim that we can extrapolate easily this way from a test to the whole animal. When we speak of the appearance of tremor and absence of tremor or antagonism of tremor, we are dealing with a fairly precise parameter. When we are speaking of emotional effects rising and falling, we are speaking of a complex set of behavior changes that we have a healthy respect for.

A couple of other related questions that might follow Dr. Kline's. This is from Dr. Buckley: "Does myristicin have anticholinergic activity?"

Only in the respect that generally anticholinergic activity in the CNS is in some ways similar to potentiation of adrenergic activity. We have not specifically tested this in any respect.

"Does myristicin inhibit adrenergic reuptake of norepinephrine by the nerve endings?"

This is postulated as the mechanism of action for the tricyclic antidepressants. This hypothesis is too new for our consideration. If it is, perhaps a combination of a weak monoamine oxidase inhibitor, such as nutmeg, and the trycyclic agents, might be of interest.

Going to the more physical aspects, we have a question from Dr. Beavers, concerning the effects of nutmeg on blood pressure in human subjects, and asking whether we have any evidence of monoamine oxidase inhibitors either increasing or decreasing effects of nutmeg in humans. We certainly need to know more about this. Dr. Naranjo, have you done blood pressure examinations with the compound?

DR. NARANJO: There is slight variation in blood pressure. There is occasionally an increase but this is not consistent, and it is hard to evaluate to what extent the observed changes are secondary to the emotional states, for sometimes anxiety is a prominent component of the induced reaction.

No lowering of blood pressure has been observed. This is in contradiction to the observations on some persons who experienced intoxication with nutmeg.

CHAIRMAN DR. TRUITT: Dr. Leake has a question.

DR. LEAKE: I want to amplify a point made by Dr. Efron. This concerns the systematic investigation of all of the phenyl amines. This actually was Dr. Gordon Alles' undertaking, as you know. One extremely important feature of it I would recommend to all workers in the field. It bears on some of the reports that were made today. Even though chemical compounds in a series are very close, insofar as their molecular weights are concerned, Gordon Alles insisted on using equal molecular concentrations so as to compare each drug with the other on a molecular basis. This is important, particular when there is any significant difference in molecular weight.

Alles had an enormous amount of material that has never been published, and I don't know whether it will be. He made a methylenedioxy derivative of an amphetamine, in which he found extraordinary enhancement of auditory sensation. This he did describe informally at one of the Macy Conferences. This compound produced another remarkable effect: if he were to strike his finger, he could see the strike, and feel it afterwards by a definitive period of time.

DR. SHULGIN: That was the methylenedioxyamphetamine compound that we called MDA earlier.

DR. LEAKE: He made similar observations of this sort on other compounds. Since he had them all on an equal molecular basis, and since he did most of the experimentation on himself as one subject, at least his findings had that comparative validity.

DR. MARRAZZI (from the floor): In line with what is being said, and the comparison with mescaline, I thought you might be interested in the comparison that we have been making of methoxyphenylethyl amines, using cortical synaptic inhibition. At the moment it looks like mescaline (a trimethoxy compound), would have a potency of 1, the dimethoxyphenylethylamine of 1.8, while the demethylated or dihydroxyphenylethylamine, dopamine, would have a potency of 10.

This is reminiscent of the old work of Gunn, which showed that the methoxylation has a muzzeling action, decreasing activity. Apparently in preliminary data it seems to decrease cortical inhibitory activity.

CHAIRMAN DR. TRUITT: How much do you think this variation in activity is due to rate of transfer across the blood-brain-barrier, and how much to the differences in actual potency?

DR. MARRAZZI: I am not able to answer that. These are closearterial injections, and the latency of beginning action is approximately the same. It should be measured more carefully than I have done so far, but there is no remarkable difference, which would suggest that it is not a difference in passing through the blood-brain-barrier.

CHAIRMAN DR. TRUITT: We have a question directed to Dr. Shulgin and Dr. Sargent: "Could you describe your human bioassay methods further?"

DR. SHULGIN: The human bioassay follows a preliminary pharmacological and pharmacodynamic analysis of the investigated material on animals. Generally, three species, the mouse, the rat and the dog, are used. Most of the cardiovascular work is done on the dog. The compounds were then assayed within our experimental group. The human threshhold level was established by successively increasing the dose in small increments until this level was reached. This testing and the subsequent psychopharmacologic comparisons of the several compounds were done essentially by the "double conscious" method of Alles. (see our reference *10*).

DR. SARGENT: I would like to comment on the remarks of Dr. Efron and Dr. Leake, as far as the structure-activity relationship studies go.

Actually this was originally Dr. Shulgin's and my interest in investigating these compounds, and we could perhaps elaborate a little bit on one of the slides in which two other substituted phenylisopropylamines are mentioned, the precursors of which are not present in nutmeg. They were tested specifically to measure the effect of the orientation of these methoxy groups.

Our scale in mescaline units is the same as Dr. Leake's. However, we assign some of the numbers a little differently from his. We grade LSD as 3000 in mescaline units, the effect dose being a tenth of a milligram.

DR. LEAKE: You understand that my grading was off the cuff.

DR. SARGENT: I might mention in regard to the previous discussion of Parkinson effects of harmine and harmaline, these compounds are also hallucinogenic. To get back to the structure-activity relationships of these methoxy-substituted amphetamines, which are summarized in our figure 7, note that when the structure of TMA with the 3,4,5-methoxy substitutions is changed to 2,4,5-, or TMA-2, the activity in humans of the compounds is increased tenfold. Again, when the structure of the 3-methoxy-4,5-methylenedioxy compound, MMDA, is changed to 2-methoxy-3,4-methylenedioxy or MMDA-3a, the activity is again increased, this time by a factor of 6. In both cases, the change of a methoxy group from a meta- to an ortho-position markedly increased the potency of the compound. The more active compounds are derived from croweacin and asarone, which occur in natural oils but not oil of nutmeg.

228

CHAIRMAN DR. TRUITT: We have one last question that I would like to direct to Mr. Weil: "What significance would you give to hypothermia observed after nutmeg intake?"

MR. WEIL: In the acute intoxications that have come to clinical attention—and there have been few—a number of symptoms suggestive of vasomotor instability has been noted. I suspect that many of the constituents of nutmeg might have effects on the autonomic nervous system and on general homeostasis that we have not spelled out very well: possibly, this fall in temperature is one of them.

CHAIRMAN DR. TRUITT: This is the end of our time for this afternoon. I thank you again for your indulgence.

SESSION IV

SOUTH AMERICAN SNUFFS

Bo Holmstedt, *Chairman*

Anthropological Survey of the Use of South American Snuffs

S. Henry Wassen

Gothenburg Ethnographic Museum, Gothenburg, Sweden

Early Reports and Archeological Evidence from the West Indies and the Contents

Introductory Remarks

The first contacts between Amerindians and Columbus and his men were established in the West Indies. It is also from the Antilles and the surrounding mainland that we have our first information about the Indians' use of what we now understand to have been a psychotomimetic snuff. Although this early information is limited, and not until our days has it been really considered to its full worth, it is of outstanding importance. Thus, at least some evidence has been saved in the reports of the chroniclers from the Circum-Caribbean culture area, for, as stated about the tribes referred to as Circum-Caribbean, "whether insular or on the mainland, they were readily accessible from the coast, and were quickly overrun by the Spanish conquerors. The great majority of them have long been extinct culturally if not racially." [1]

The difficulty in defining what plant material an early description refers to must be considered in any serious study. In my opinion we cannot, as Jerome E. Brooks has done in his work on tobacco (1937),[2] take it for granted that observations by Amerigo Vespucci during his voyage with Alonso de Ojeda and Juan de la Cosa (May, 1499–June, 1500), bear on tobacco chewing—even though many kinds of American tobacco later have been observed. These observations related, supposedly, at least, to natives of Margarita Island, off the coast of Venezuela.

According to Brooks (1937: 189), Vespucci's notice in his letter of 1504 to his friend, Piero Soderini, "was the first published which relates to a

---

[1] Steward, Julian H. 1948 : 1.
[2] Brooks, Jerome E. 1937 : 189.

262-016 O—67——17

habit we know to have been tobacco chewing." I quote the following from Vespucci's description in the rendering presented by Brooks:

> The customs and manners of this tribe are of this sort: In looks and behavior they were very repulsive, and each had his cheeks bulging with a certain green herb which they chewed like cattle, so that they could scarcely speak, and each carried hanging from his neck two dried gourds, one of which was full of the very herb he kept in his mouth; the other full of a certain white flour like powdered chalk. Frequently each put a certain small stick (which had been moistened and chewed in his mouth) into the gourd filled with flour. Each then drew it forth and put it in both sides of his cheeks, thus mixing the flour with the herb which their mouths contained. This they did very frequently a little at a time.

From the continuation of the description, we deduct that the European observers believed that the natives "carried the herb and flour in their mouths in order to relieve their thirst", and, also, "that the women did not themselves indulge in the habit" (Brooks 1937: 191).

If we now should give a description of how e.g. the actual Kogi (or Ká-gabba) Indians of Sierra Nevada de Santa Marta in Colombia use their *poporo* (bottle-shaped gourd for lime) and chew their coca (*hayo*), a process that I myself have observed many times, we could word for word repeat the description quoted from Vespucci. As a matter of fact his words can as well refer to the habit of coca chewing. Such an eminent Americanist as Erland Nordenskiöld of Gothenburg considered Vespucci's words as clearly referring to coca,[3] and Cooper (1949: 549) has included the Cumaná area of Venezuela among the regions from which "early historical sources report coca chewing and/or ritual use of coca leaves as prevalent." To this must be added also the observation by Vespucci that "the women did not themselves indulge in the habit." No rule is without an exception, but just as an addition, I wish to add that "more commonly, coca chewing is a masculine rather than a feminine habit" (Cooper 1949: 552).

The Cohoba Snuff and Its Paraphernalia

The *cohoba* snuff used by the Taino of the West Indies has, as we know, caused much discussion which I previously tried to summarize in two papers.[4] We must note that Columbus himself observed the use of a powder, though he does not mention it by name. During his second voyage, 1493–1496, Columbus not only commissioned the Friar Ramon Pane to undertake what we now call anthropological field work among the aboriginal population of Española ("to collect all their ceremonies and antiquities," Bourne 1906: 4), but he himself made valuable observations presented in his narrative of the second voyage.[5] As has been pointed out by Bourne, we possess this narrative "only in the abridgment of Las Casas and Ferdinand Columbus." The original is lost,[6] but both Las Casas and Ferdinand Columbus "in

---

[3] Nordenskiöld, Erland, 1919 : 14.

[4] Wassén, S. Henry and Bo Holmstedt. 1963 : 27–35; Wassén, S. Henry. 1964 : 97–120.

[5] Bourne, Edward Gaylord. 1906 : 3, quite correctly has credited Christopher Columbus as the person who "set on foot the first systematic study of American primitive custom, religion and folklore ever undertaken."

[6] Bourne. 1906 : 4, "The original Spanish text of these documents is no longer extant and, like the *Historie* which contains them, they are known in full only in the Italian translation of that work published in Venice in 1571 by Alfonso Ulloa."

condensing the original, incorporated passages in the exact words of the Admiral. It is from such a passage in Ferdinand's abridgment that we derive the Admiral's account of the religion in primitive Hayti" (Bourne 1906: 4). Ferdinand Columbus says that he recorded "the very words of the Admiral", and we can now, in Bourne's translation (p. 4–6), find the following information of a powder which evidently must be the same as that mentioned by Ramon Pane as *cohoba:*

I was able to discover neither idolatry nor any other sect among them, although all their kings, who are many, not only in Española but also in all the other islands and on the mainland,[7] each have a house apart from the village, in which there is nothing except some wooden images carved in relief which are called *cemis;*[8] nor is there anything done in such a house for any other object or service except for these *cemis*, by means of a kind of ceremony and prayer which they go to make in it as we go to churches. In this house they have a finely wrought table, round like a wooden dish in which is some powder which is placed by them on the heads of these *cemis* in performing a certain ceremony; then with a cane that has two branches which they place in their nostrils, they snuff up this dust. The words that they say none of our people understand. With this powder they lose consciousness and become like drunken men.

In addition to the secluded *cemi* houses for snuffing ceremonies, Columbus mentions two paraphernalia, namely a "finely wrought table" for the powder, and a "cane that has two branches" to snuff up this dust. Both are of immediate interest.

In a paper from 1964 dealing with the Neo-Indian epoch, Irving Rouse has referred to the statement that the Arawak in the West Indies placed the powder on top of *cemis*, adding that "many of the statues found in caves have a platform on top for this purpose."[9] In this connection Rouse has republished the 66 cm. high wooden British Museum *cemi*, in the shape of a bird standing on what seems to be a turtle. This figure, originally published by Joyce,[10] was republished also by Wassén 1965: fig. 4. A kneeling stone figure from Puerto Rico, published by Palmatary,[11] may also be taken into account as such a West Indian *cemi* with platform on top. I have in my work from 1965 (pp. 30–31, figs. 5 and 53), pointed out that we still find a South American ethnographic parallel to this in the ceremonially used tabletops for snuff, and snuffing paraphernalia used among the tribes of the rivers Branco and Colorado in western Brazil. These tabletops are carefully made and polished, but according to Franz Caspar's observations among the Tupari, the table has no special function beyond its mechanical use during the snuffing seances.[12] We can observe that the snuffing ceremony among the Tupari takes place inside the house. When used, the tabletop is supported by three wooden legs on which it is loosely placed. The tabletops are irregularly square-shaped and provided with a handle. They are

---

[7] According to Bourne, Cuba, which Columbus believed to be the mainland.

[8] Bourne. 1906: 5, footnote. "Ulloa in his Italian gives this word in various forms e.g. *cemi, cimi, cimini* and *cimiche*. The correct form is *cemi*, with the accent on the last syllable. Las Casas says, "Estas—llamaban *cemi,* la ultima silaba luenga y aguda.""

[9] Rouse, Irving. 1964: 510–511.

[10] Joyce, Thomas A. 1916, pl. 21.

[11] Palmatary, Helen C. 1960, pl. 120 *d,* and text on p. 92.

[12] The photo published in Wassén, 1965, fig. 5, was taken by Dr. Franz Caspar among the Tupari, during his second expedition to this tribe in 1955.

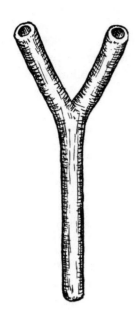

FIG. 1.—Y-shaped snuffing tube from Haiti. After Oviedo.

cut from the wood of flat supporting roots of a tree. Dr. Franz Caspar considers them as particular for the tribes of the Branco and Colorado Rivers.

If we now turn to the "cane that has two branches", Columbus evidently was observing the use of Y-shaped snuffing tubes, of which there were finely worked ones used by the chiefs and principal men, and others made of reeds for those who could not afford the finer ones. The "poor hermit" Ramon Pane apparently does not refer to a forked tube when he says that "the *Cogioba* is a certain powder which they take sometimes to purge themselves, and for other effects which you will hear of later. They take it with a cane about a foot long and put one end in the nose and the other in the powder, and in this manner they draw it into themselves through the nose and this purges them thoroughly" (Bourne 1906: 17; cf. Lovén 1935: 393).

In Wassén 1964 (pp. 102–103), there is a discussion of the West Indian snuffing instruments according to the sources, and I here again republish the tube from Haiti (Fig. 1) which we find in the work by Oviedo,[13] who also has stated that it was the Y-shaped snuffing instrument, and not the plant, which was called *tabaco* by the Indians (vol. I: 131). The famous Bishop and Historian, Bartolomé de las Casas, also described the West Indian snuffers, "made in the size of a small flute, all hollow as is a flute." To make his readers understand the Y-shaped form of the instrument, he uses the picture of the fingers in an out-stretched hand.[14]

Even if we accept the occurrence in the West Indies of Y-shaped snuffing tubes as an obvious parallel to tubes of the same type found in South America,

---

[13] The original is found in volume I, pl. I: 7, of Oviedo's *Historia general*, etc. (1851). The corresponding text on p. 130.

[14] Las Casas, Bartolomé de. 1909: 445. ". . .; la hechura de aquel instrumento era del tamaño de una pequeña flauta, de los tercios de la cual en adelante se abría por dos cañutos huecos, de la manera que abrimos los dos dedos del medio, sacado el pulgar, cuando extendemos la mano."

we must also note the observation made by Lovén (1935:393), that "the Tainos differ from the whole South America in that their forked snuff-tubes were not made from bones, and certainly not from those of birds, as in the Orinoco and Cayary-Uaupés regions. Suitable bones for tubes were not accessible on Española; other material had to be sought there." [15]

We find another parallel between Haiti and the northern South American mainland, in the round trays for snuff now found among the Indians of the Orinoco region (see Wassén 1965, fig. 1, p. 21), and the fine and polished round trays described by Las Casas from the island. He says that the snuffing instrument was made of the same kind of dark wood as the tray.[16]

That the snuffing tubes of wood used on Haiti in some cases were fine pieces of sculpture is clearly understood from the specimen found at La Gonâve (Fig. 2), first published in 1941 by Mangones and Maximilien, later also by Rouse and Wassén.[17] Dr. Grete Mostny of Santiago, Chile, has in a paper from 1958 [18] compared the elaborate tube from Haiti with specimens of finely sculptured straight snuffing tubes from the Atacaman region, where the Y-shaped tubes do not seem to exist. As the description of the tube from Haiti is very poor in the work by the two Haitian authors, it is fortunate that Mostny has been able to quote a letter from Louis Maximilien (Febr. 11, 1956). In this, some particulars are given regarding the motif on the specimen found in the Picmi cave on the island of Gonâve, namely a kneeling man crowned by a bird's head.

Further Details about the Cohoba Powder

At the end of his report from the second voyage, Christopher Columbus refers to an account he had ordered from "one Friar Roman (Ramon) who knew their language" (Bourne 1906: 6). As far as we know, through the Admiral's son and other chroniclers, who know Pane's text, "to this day our most authentic record of the religion and folk-lore of the long since extinct Tainos, the aboriginal inhabitants of Hayti" (Bourne 1906: 4), we meet in it not only the name of a certain powder they inhaled, but also most interesting field observations on the psychotomimetic effects of the drug.

Friar Ramon Pane whose text is best read in the careful edition of Bourne,[19] uses two words, *cohoba* and *cogioba*, for a snuff used for special

---

[15] For various types of South American snuffing tubes see Wassén, 1965.

[16] In the text of Las Casas, 1909 : 445, a snuff tray is described as follows : "... plato redondo, no llano, sino un poco algo combado ó hondo, hecho de madera, tan hermoso, liso y lindo, que no fuera muy más hermoso de oro ó de plata ; era cuasi negro y lucio como de azabache."

[17] Rouse. 1964, fig. 18 ; Wassén. 1964, fig. 2, and 1965, fig. 51. The original in Mangones and Maximilien, 1941, pl. 50.

[18] Mostny, G. 1958 : 387–389. I quote from the text of the letter (p. 388) : "Les deux branches supérieures du Calumet se terminaient par des bouts olivaires—afin de rendre aux marines un contact doux —; le point de jonction des trois branches porte le motif sculpté, représentant un homme agenouillé, les bras liés derrière le dos et la poitrine incliné dans une attitude de prière ; le tout surmonté d'une tête d'oiseau d'un haute relief."

[19] Bourne. 1906: 8–9. "To facilitate a study of this material in its earliest record I have translated Ramon's treatise from the Italian, excerpted and collated with it the epitomes of Peter Martyr and Las Casas, and have prepared brief notes, the whole to form so far as may be a critical working text of this source for the folklorist and student of Comparative Religion in America. The proper names in each case are given as in the 1571 edition of the *Historie*."—"At best the spelling of these names offers much perplexity. Ramon wrote down in Spanish the sounds he heard, Ferdinand, unfamiliar with the sounds, copied the names and then still later Ulloa, equally unfamiliar with the originals, copied them into his Italian. In such a process there was inevitably

purposes. We have already referred to the text where it is said that "the *cogioba* is a certain powder which they take sometimes to purge themselves," etc. (Bourne 1906: 17). Later, in this text, we meet the word *cohoba:*

When one is ill they bring the *Buhuitihu* (Bohuti) to him as a physician. The physician is obliged to abstain from food like the sick man himself, to play the part of sick man which is done in this way which you now will hear. He must needs purge himself like the sick man, and to purge himself he takes a certain powder called *cohoba* snuffing it up his nose, which intoxicates them so that they do not know what they do, and in this condition they speak many things incoherently, in which they say they are talking with the *cemis*, and that by them they are informed how the sickness came upon him.

Further on (Bourne 1906: 24), a description of great interest to the psychotomimetic studies follows, which I quote:

And when they want to know if they will be victorious over their enemies they go into a cabin into which no one else goes except the principal men; and their chief is the first who begins to make *cogioba*, and to make a noise; and while he is making *cogioba*, no one of them who is in the company says anything till the chief has finished; but when he has finished his prayer, he stands a while with his head turned (down) and his arms on his knees; then he lifts his head up and looks towards the sky and speaks. Then they all answer him with a loud voice, and when they have all spoken giving thanks, he tells the vision that he has seen, intoxicated with the *cogioba* which he has inhaled through his nose, which goes up to his head. And he says that he has talked with the *cemi* and that they are to have a victory; or that his enemies will fly; or that there shall be a great loss of life, or wars or famine, or some other such things which occur to him who is intoxicated to say. Consider what a state their brains are in, because they say the cabins seem to them to be turned upside down and that men are walking with their feet in the air.

I have had in my hands photographic copies of some pages of "*P. Martyris Angli-mediolanensis opera Legatio babylonica Occeani decas Poemata Epigrammata*," the Gothic edition from Seville 1511, of Peter Martyr's *First Decade*. It is in this text (see Fig. 3, a–b), that the author, who never himself went to the New World, after having seen Pane's manuscript deals with the *cohoba* powder. For a translation I follow MacNutt,[20] however with some corrections and notes.[21]

Translation of the Latin text of 1511 (fvi r. and v):

It is the augurs, called bovites, who encourage these superstitions. These men, who are persistent liars, act as doctors for the ignorant people, which gives them a great prestige, for it is believed that the zemes converse with them and reveal the future to them.

If a sick man recovers the bovites persuade him that he owes his restoration to the intervention of the zemes.

---

some confusion of u and n and u and v, (Spanish b). In the Italian text v is never used, it is always u. In not a few cases the Latin of Peter Martyr and the Spanish of Las Casas give us forms much nearer those used by Ramon than the Italian." It is now clear that both Las Casas and Peter Martyr underestimated the importance of Ramon Pane's work. For this see e.g. Bourne, p. 7.

[20] MacNutt, Francis Augustus. 1912. Vol. I: 172–174. As pointed out by Wassén, 1964: 105, Ramon Pane used *buhuitihu* and *bohuti*. This evidently Island-Arawak word has been latinized into *boitius* (pl. *boviti*) by Pedro Martyr and is written *buhuti* by Oviedo, and *bohique* and *behique* by Las Casas. If we try to connect it with other known words, we are probably safe to do so with the also Island-Arawak *buhio, bohio,* a common word in the Spanish reports for house but sometimes a designation for special houses, very probably also those for medicine-men's cures.

[21] The first printing of Decade One which was authorized by Martyr is that of 1516, in which the plural *boitii* for medicine-men occurs.

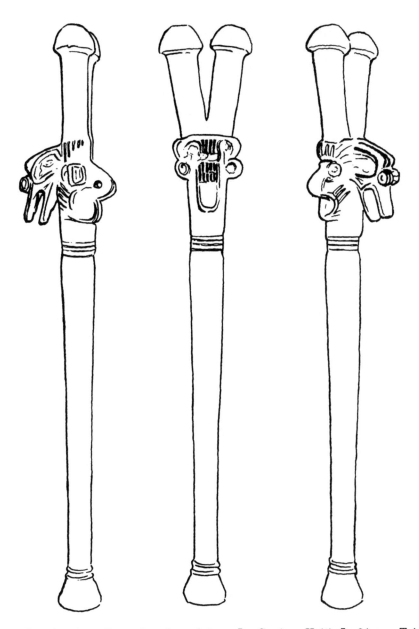

Fɪɢ. 2.—Sculptured snuffing tube of wood from La Gonâve, Haiti. L. 24 cm. Taino Culture. After photographs published by Mangones and Maximilien.

When they undertake to cure a chief, the bovites begin by fasting and taking a purge. There is an intoxicating herb which they pound up and drink,[22] after which they are seized with fury like the maenads, and declare that the zemes confide secrets to them. They visit the sick man, carrying in their mouth a bone, a little stone, a stick, or a piece of meat. After expelling every one save two or three persons designated by the sick person[23] the bovite begins by making wild gestures and passing his hands over

[22] MacNutt translates *drink*. The Latin text has *sorbeo*, absorb.
[23] The Latin says : "from a semicircle," etc.

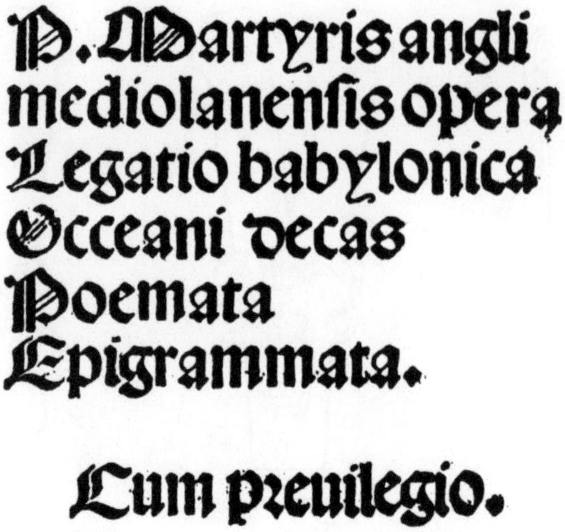

P. Martyris angli mediolanensis opera Legatio babylonica Occeani decas Poemata Epigrammata.

Cum preuilegio.

FIG. 3 a–b.—Title and text, fvi(r.), in Peter Martyr's work from Seville, 1511, in which Ramon Pane's notices of *cohoba* snuffing first appeared. After a copy in "Arents Tobacco Collection," The New York Public Library.

the face, lips, and nose, and breathing on the forehead, temples, and neck, and drawing in the sick man's breath. Thus he pretends to seek the fever in the veins of the sufferer. Afterwards he rubs the shoulders, the hips, and the legs, and opens the hands; if the hands are clenched he pulls them wide open, exposing the palm, shaking them vigorously, after which he affirms that he has driven off the sickness and that the patient is out of danger. Finally he removes the piece of meat he was carrying in his mouth like a juggler, and begins to cry, "This is what you have eaten in excess of your wants; now you will get well because I have relieved you of that which you ate."

If the doctor percieves that the patient gets worse, he ascribes this to the zemes, who, he declares, are angry because they have not had a house constructed for them, or have not been treated with proper respect, or have not received their share of the products of the field. Should the sick man die, his relatives indulge in magical incantations to make him declare whether he is the victim of fate or the carelessness of the doctor, who failed to fast properly or gave the wrong remedy. If the man died through the fault of the doctor, the relatives take vengeance on the latter. Whenever the women succeed in obtaining the piece of meat (*erroneous transl.*)[24] which the bovites hold in their mouths, they wrap it with great respect in cloths and carefully preserve it, esteeming it to be a talisman of great efficacy in time of childbirth, and honouring it as though it were a zeme.

The islanders pay homage to numerous zemes, each person having his own. Some are of wood, because it is amongst the trees and in the darkness of night they have received the message of the gods.[25] Others, who have heard the voice amongst the rocks, make their zemes of stone; while others, who heard the revelation while they were cultivating their ages—that kind of cereal I have already mentioned,—make theirs of root.[26]

Perhaps they think that these last watch over their breadmaking. It was thus that the ancients believed that the dryads, hamadryads, satyrs, pans, nereids, watched over the fountains, forests, and seas, attributing to each force in nature a presiding divinity.

---

[24] This passage has evidently been wrongly translated by MacNutt. The women could hardly keep the pieces of meat. From the Latin, *"de lapillis aut ossibus quos ore gestasse bouijtus aliquis putatur: se femine,"* etc., it is clear that the women collected the stones and the pieces of bones for the said purpose.

[25] In the original *visionibus*, "visions", are mentioned.

[26] "That kind of cereal" for *genus panis* has in the Argentine edition of 1944 been translated as *"clase de alimento."* In the Latin text of 1516 it says *genus edulii.*

240

En illuſtriſſime princeps omni preconio dignā maris originem:nec ab eis parui cū
fieri putes:qui hec illis recitare didicerit.Aiunt deinde fratres hos iaie metu tā diu
per diuerſa fuiſſe vagatos:vt fere iam fame perirent:quia nullubi ſiſtere pedem au
debant:hinc quoniā acrius vrgerentur:ad pinſoris domum pulſare ceperunt caza
bi.i.panem petentes pinſor autem in primo igredientem cōſpuiſſe ita acriter fertur:
vt illi ex ictu ſputi exortum ſit turgidiſſimum intercus:quo fere iterierit.Aſt fratruz
conſilio accepto lapide acuto apertum eſt:ex cuius vlcere natam aiunt feminaz:qua
mutuo poſt fratres illi omnes vſi ſunt:atcz ab ea ferunt filios filiaſcz genuiſſe.Iu
cundius aliud aduertito princeps illuſtriſſime.Antruz extat aliud iouanaboina no
mine in cuiuſdam reguli dioceſi:qui Machinnech vocatur.Io religioſius cz co:in
thium quondam aut cyrrham niſamcz greci colunt:ac venerantur:mille varijs or
natum picturis.In huius antri foribus duos habent ſculptos zemes:quorum vnū
bintaitellem.Marobum alterum vocant.Cur tanta ſpecum colerent pietate:inte
rrogati:quia ſol inde lunacz lumē orbi prebituri prodierunt:grauiter ſenſatecz reſ
pondent.Concurſationibus antra veluti nos vrbem ʒ baticanum noſtre religiōis
caput:aut Compoſtellam ʒ Iheruſalem domini ſepulcrum frequentant.Subia
cent ʒ alteri ſuperſticionum generi:mortuos putant noctu vagari:ac veſci guanua
ba (fructu nobis incognito)cotono ſimili:lectiſcz inter viuos verſari aiunt ac deci
pere mulieres:ſumpta namcz virili forma coire velle videntur:aſt quom ad opus p
uenitur euaneſcunt.Si quis autem apud ſe iacere mortuum aliquando ſuſpicatur
(quom quid noui ſenſerit in lecto)vteri attrectatione ſe dubio ſolui balbutit.Cun
cta nācz aiunt mortuos poſſe humana membra ſuſcipere preter vmbilicuz:ſi vmbi
lico igitur mortuum eſſe dignoſcit:tactus illico reſoluitur.Noctu ʒ ſepiſſime(in iti
neribus precipue vijſcz publicis)mortuos occurrere viuis creduntur:contra quos
ſi viator intrepidus ſteterit:diſoluit fantaſma:ſi vero pertimeſcat:illum ita adorien
do perterret:vt ſepius ea formidine multi debilitentur ac ſtupeāt.Interrogati a no
ſtris inſulares vnde ſibi cos ritus inanes tancz contagionem comparauerint:a ma
ioribus hereditarios reſpondent:ritcz miſcz aiūt vltra hominū memoriam:iſta cō
texta quc neminem licet preter regulorum filios edoceri:memorie illa cōmendant ne
cz enim litteras vncz habuere:diebuſcz feſtis(alio pulſante populo)canentes velu
ti ſolemnia ſacra preponunt:inſtrumentum habent vnicum ligneum:concauum:re
boans tantum:cz cōcutitur impaniſ more.His illos imbuunt ſuperſticionibus eor
augures quos bouijtas vocant:ſunt ijdem medici qui plebecule rerum inſcie mi
lle aſtruunt fraudes.Credere cogunt plebem hi augures(quia ſunt apud eam au
ctoritatis eximie)cz zemes ipſos alloquantur futuraſcz predicēt:ʒ ſi quis aduerſa la
borans valitudine conualuerit:ſe dono zemis id aſſecutum perſuadent.Ieiunio ʒ
purgationi ſe obligant bouijte:cz do curaz de primario ſumūt aliquo.Herbamcz
ſumunt inebriāte quā quom puluceream ſorpſerit(veluti menades)in furorez verſi
multa ſe azemibus audiſſe immurmurant.Valitudinarium adeunt oſſe vel lapillo in
os ſumpto aut fruſtulo carnis.Er hemiciclo dicunt omnes preter vnum aut duos
quos ipſemet elegerit.Circuit primarium bouijtus ter aut quater:faciem:labia na
reſcz extorquens ſedis geſtibus:in frontem:in tempora:in collum ſuflat egroti ab
ſorbens aerem:poſt hec ſe morbum ex laborantis venis exhaurire dicit.Per hu
meros deinde ac femora ʒ crura egrotum fricans:cōnexas a pedibus manus dedu
citatcz ſic manibus complexis:ad hoſtium procurrit apertum:ac manus excutit

241

The islanders of Hispaniola even believe that the zemes respond to their wishes when they invoke them. When the cacique wish to consult the zemes, concerning the result of a war, about the harvest, or their health, they enter the houses sacred to them and there absorb the intoxicating herb called *kohobba*, which is the same as that used by the bovites to excite their frenzy.[27] Almost immediately, they believe they see the room turn upside down, and men walking with their heads downwards.

This kohobba powder is so strong that those who take it lose consciousness; when the stupefying actions of the powder begins to wane, the arms and hands become loose and the head droops.[28] After remaining for some time in this attitude, the cacique raises his head, as though he were awakening from sleep, and, lifting his eyes to the heavens, begins to stammer some incoherent words. His chief attendants gather round him (for none of the common people are admitted to these mysteries), raising their voices in thanksgiving that he has so quickly left the zemes and returned to them. They ask him what he has seen, and the cacique declares that he was in conversation with the zemes during the whole time, and as though he were still in a prophetic delirium, he prophesies victory or defeat, if a war is to be undertaken, or whether the crops will be abundant, or the coming disaster, or the enjoyment of health, in a word, whatever first occurs to him.

Bourne (1906: 20) accepted *cohoba* as a word for tobacco, and I have previously (see Wassén, 1964: 102) been inclined to accept the explanation by Friederici[29] that the Taino word *cohoba* probably stood for tobacco, while the word *cogioba* should stand for *Piptadenia*. Brooks (1937: 189), however, has made it perfectly clear that "none of the early commentators on the custom says that the substance inhaled was derived from the tobacco plant," and when taking into account all the forms of the word *cohoba*, such as *cohobba, cahoba, cojoba-cogioba, cojioba, cohiba, coiba*,[30] I am now of the opinion that it is one and the same word, and that *cohoba* as Brooks (1937: 196) expresses it "was employed by the medicine-men chiefly to induce a state of trance." We have every reason to believe that the *cohoba* identification by E. W. Safford and other writers as a snuff prepared from the seeds of *Piptadenia peregrina* is valid.[31] According to Brooks (1937: 197) "this plant, indigenous to certain parts of South America and to some places in the Antilles (including Haiti), still bears the name *cohoba*." Here it is interesting to add that Pittier (1926: 189) has found the word *cojoba* for the tree used in northern Venezuela (cf. Rosenblat, 1965: 272, 344).

In this connection I wish once again to underline the statement of Dr. Siri von Reis Altschul in her botanical thesis of 1964 (p. 42) that the Indians of the West Indies "may have found it easier to plant the trees than to maintain communication with the mainland for their source of supply" (of *cohoba*). It is interesting to add that Oviedo says that the snuff came from an herb (*hierva*), which the Indians valued much, and kept it cultivated.[32] Las Casas mentions that the Indians "had certain powders of certain herbs well dried and finely ground and of the color of cinnamon or powdered henna,

---

[27] The Latin text has it, and this is important, that the *chohobba* was absorbed *per nares*.

[28] In the Latin edition of 1516 there is a small change in the text, ". . . *insania brachiis demisso capite genua complectitur* . . ."

[29] Friederici, Georg. 1925.

[30] Friederici, Georg. 1947 : 198.

[31] Already in 1898, Max Uhle (p. 9) draws the conclusion that "the extreme strength of the powder as described by Petrus Martyr, exceeding that of tobacco, decides its different nature and its Piptadenia character."

[32] Oviedo, *Historia*, etc. 1851 : 131.

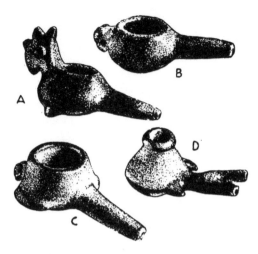

Fig. 4.—Archaeological bird-shaped pottery snuffers from Costa Rica. *A*, Guanacaste, *B–D*, Línea Vieja. Coll. Gothenburg Ethnographic Museum, *64.16*. Length of specimen *C*, 9 cm.

etc.[33] " With Brooks (p. 196) and others, we may assume that the "word *cohoba* may have meant snuff as well as the act of snuffing any powder. Pulverized tobacco seeds may have been mixed with the narcotic snuff inhaled by the medicine-men, and only the nicotian ingredient of this compound recognized by the Spanish observers." The Arawakan Jirara and Caquetio in N.W. Venezuela, tribes which according to Steward (1948: 21) had "certain specific resemblances to the Arawakan Taino of the Antilles," had medicine-men who "practiced divination with tobacco ash and communed with spirits while taking tobacco and a narcotic herb." The mixing of tobacco and *yopo* has been reported from many S. American tribes.

Archaeological Evidence for the Use of Snuff

If we consider the South American origin of the West Indian tribes, it is only natural that the close parallels referring to the snuffing complex in the West Indes should be sought in South America. I believe, however, that also the archaeologically found, often bird-shaped and bifurcated clay snuffers from Costa Rica, (Fig. 4), should be taken into account.[34] These small clay snuffers with one or two tubes were, according to Doris Stone, "probably used for *cojoba* (*Piptadenia* sp.) or tobacco." [35], [36]

As always, the South American influence as far north as in Costa Rica is worth studying. To a possible explanation of the bird motif in the clay snuffers I will return later. Here I, want to refer to Fig. 5, where I, after Dr. Otto Zerries, can show an old bifurcated and nicely carved bird-shaped snuffing tube from South America. This highly interesting old specimen is

[33] Las Casas. 1909 : 445.

[34] See Wassén and Holmstedt, 1963, fig. 6, and p. 24 ; also Wassén, 1965, fig. 2, and pp. 25–26.

[35] Stone, Doris. 1958 : 16. Her figures 19 *a*, *b*. Stone counts "snuffing and the playing of flutes by medicine men" as "southern traits" in Costa Rica's cultures (p. 25).

[36] See Wassén and Holmstedt. 1963 : 24.

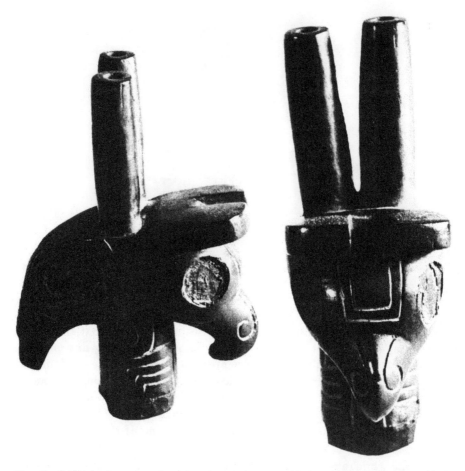

Fig. 5.—Bifurcated snuffing implement of wood. Coll. *Mus. f. Völkerkunde*, Mannheim, "V. Am. No. 1894." According to Zerries, 1965, from Brazilian Guayana. Courtesy Dr. Otto Zerries.

now in the Ethnographical Museum of Mannheim, Germany, where it has been observed and studied by Dr. Zerries, who has attributed it to the region of Brazilian Guyana.[37] The old snuffer in the German museum undoubtedly points to a South American background also for the clay snuffers in Costa Rica.

In spite of many omissions and too hastily drawn conclusions, the study of Max Uhle of the bifurcated snuffing tube of bone that he found in 1895 at Tiahuanaco seems to be one of the first of a comparative interest for the use of snuffs among the South American Indians. A drawing after Uhle's illustration of the tube he found is shown in Fig. 6. According to Uhle (1898: 1), "the tube consists of the wrist or leg bone (*metacarpus* or *metatharsis*) of a

[37] Zerries, Otto. 1965 : 185–193. In the same paper Zerries describes two more, richly decorated wooden objects from the Ethnographical Museum in Mannheim (numbers Am. 1987 and 1988), in the form of jaguars with bowls, which evidently have been receptacles for a powder. In the old museum entry it says *"Gerät zum Schnupfen,"* 'snuffing implement.' Zerries seeks the origin for all three in the lower R. Trombetas region.

young llama-like animal," . . . "and the bone has been cut off at each end, and while at the upper end a part of the shaft has disappeared, at the lower end, bifurcating naturally, only the distal articulations have been cut away and each part bored, so as to communicate with the main tube. The caliber of the former is ¼, and that of the latter 13/32 of an inch."

Uhle reported from Tiahuanaco. Following him it has only slowly and after a long series of attempts at all sorts of more or less fanciful explanations, become evident that the many finds in the region of the former Atacameño in Argentina and Chile of wooden trays and their corresponding tubes, must be classified as paraphernalia connected with the taking of some kind of a snuff. Several earlier references have been mentioned in Wassén 1965 (pp. 34–36 and p. 78) as well as in Wassén and Holmstedt (1963: 24–25); but I can perhaps best refer to the summary of the extensive literature presented in the archaeological thesis by A. M. Salas.[38] For the understand-

---

[38] Salas, Alberto Mario. 1945. Especially pp. 209–226, *"Area de dispersión de tubos y tabletas."*

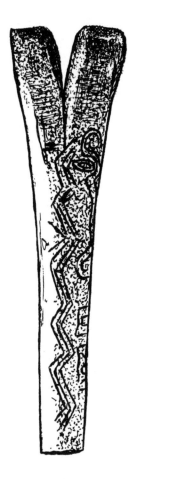 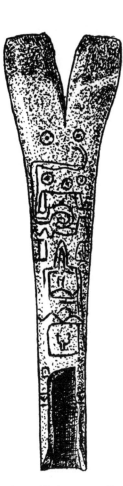

FIG. 6.—Naturally bifurcated snuffing tube of bone from Tiahuanaco. Drawing after Uhle's photographs in his publication from 1898.

245

ing of the snuffing complex in the Atacama region, important publications have recently been published. I want particularly to refer to the classificatory study by Lautaro Nuñez,[39] and the same author's references to the taking of *rapé* during successive cultural periods in northern Chile.[40] A small but interesting contribution is the paper by G. Mostny from 1958, in which she also refers to the tube from La Gonâve, Haiti. Her paper from 1952, in which she offers a recapitulation of the various opinions regarding the finds of *tabletas* and *tubos* in Chile and Argentina, is also of high interest for the description (p. 8) of a grave find of a *paricá* tray with one sculptured and one plain tube. The tray was protected by a surrounding leather wrapping, which when taken away showed the handle in the form of a nicely carved condor. The circumstances prove that the Indians had taken much care in protecting this specimen when the owner got it with him in the grave. The sculptured tube in the same find shows, according to Mostny's description (p. 11), a masked human being.

In a new work from 1965, Father Gustavo Le Paige is also writing about several highly interesting finds of snuffing paraphernalia used in the Atacama region.[41] The list could easily be made much longer, but it was neither here nor in my study from 1965 my intention to present a complete catalogue of all such finds from a given area. My intention has been to underline the importance of archaeologically found snuffing paraphernalia in relation to the ethnographically known details. Scientifically it must be of an overwhelming importance to learn what kind of powder the Indians in the Atacama regions used, and what we can deduct about the ceremonial importance of the habit from the finds.[42] In Fig. 7–10 three wooden tablets and a tube from Chiuchiu and Argentina are shown from material kept in the Museum of the American Indian, New York City. Fig. 11, taken from Fig. 57 in Casanova's paper of 1946, shows interesting Argentine specimens with features often discussed in this work.

---

[39] Nuñez Atencio, Lautaro. 1963 : 148–168.

[40] Nuñez A., Lautaro. 1965. In this study the author has pointed out the use of snuffing tubes of bone among groups with a knowledge of both agriculture and pottery in the period he calls Early (0–700 A.D.), a period still without influence from the Tiahuanaco culture. During a Middle Period (700–1000 A.D.) the snuffing paraphernalia are continuously used, and a strong influence from Tiahuanaco is observed. The use of snuff trays and tubes continues during the Late Period (1000–1450 A.D.), when several local cultures developed after the influence from Tiahuanaco.

[41] Le Paige, Gustavo. 1965. His work from 1964 has been quoted at the end of this paper.

[42] I am most thankful to Dr. Lautaro Nuñez A., Director of the Department of Archaeology of the *Universidad de Chile, Zona Norte*, Antofagasta, for his kindness in sending to me with a letter of October 7, 1966, samples of snuff powder archaeologically found and associated with a snuff tray from a pre-Incaic grave at the coast of Chile, near Iquique (Bajo Molle). The material has been forwarded to Prof. Bo Holmstedt, Stockholm, for analysis. We certainly need qualified analyses of archaeological snuff. Dr. Alberto Mario Salas (1945 : 222) indignantly criticizes Max Uhle, who once found powder associated with a snuff tablet at Calama, and concluded he had found a narcotic powder only from the fact that he and his assistant started sneezing after having blown the powder into the nostrils. Ricardo E. Latcham (1938 : 133–135), started a discussion on which type of powder the Atacameño could have been using. He suggested *Piptadenia macrocarpa,* "common in the subtropical valleys of Tucumán and in the Chaco, and also used by the Calchaquíes," but immediately added that more probably it was some kind of tobacco. The *Piptadenia macrocarpa* should be the same as the Peruvian *vilca*. Latcham rejected the idea, suggested by Dr. A. Oyarzún, that *Piptadenia peregrina* had been used by the Atacameño.

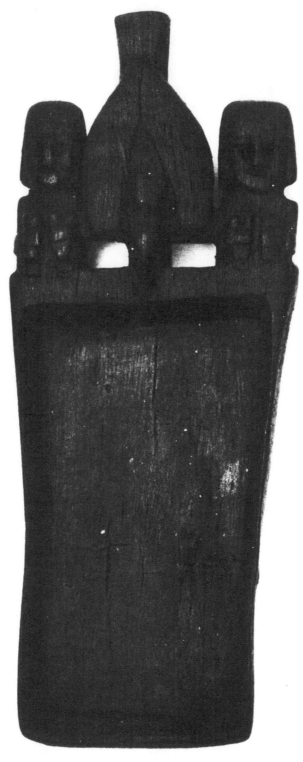

FIG. 7.—Wooden snuff tray with human and condor motifs. Argentina. Photograph courtesy of Museum of the American Indian, Heye Foundation. Specimen No. 13/3658.

247

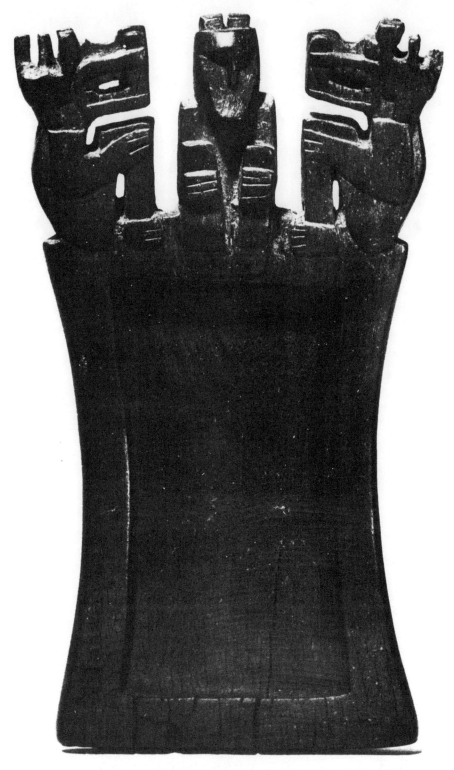

FIG. 8.—Wooden snuff tray with human and feline motifs. Argentina. 3¾'' x 7½'', specimen No. 15/1489. Photograph courtesy of Museum of American Indian, Heye Foundation.

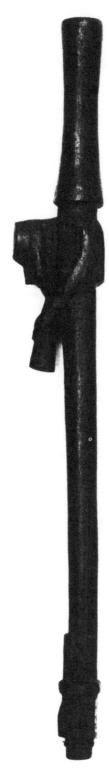

FIG. 9.—Snuff tube from Argentina. Sculptured motif seems to show a man holding a tube. Photograph courtesy of Museum of the American Indian, Heye Foundation. Specimen No. 15/2407.

249

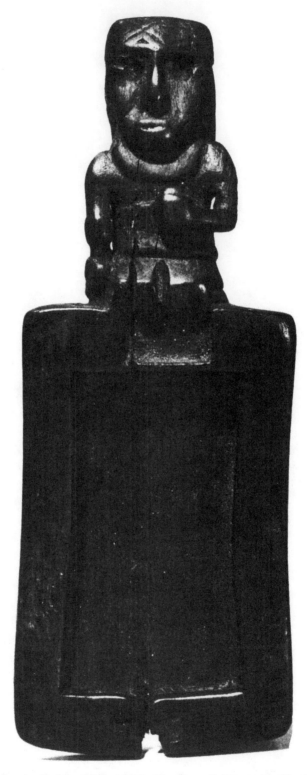

FIG. 10.—Wooden snuff tray, 2⅛″ x 5½″. Handle probably personification of deity. Chiuchiu, Chile. Photograph courtesy of Museum of the American Indian, Heye Foundation. Specimen No. 14/3741.

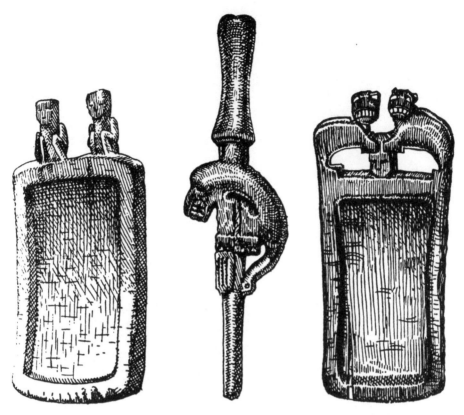

Fig. 11.—Snuffing paraphernalia, tablets and tube of wood decorated with zoomorphic and anthropomorphic figures. After fig. 57 in Casanova, 1946. Originals in Buenos Aires.

In 1885, the Brazilian archaeologist Ladislau Netto when commenting upon the zoomorphic stone figures (often bird-shaped) found in the *sambaquis* (shell middens) of Santa Catarina, Brazil, was long ahead of his time. With reference to the cavities observed in these figures (see Fig. 12), he took them to have served as a deposit for a vegetal powder, of exciting quality and ascribed with supernatural virtues.[43] This aspect is interesting and I must dedicate some time to it.

The so-called *antropolito de Mercedes*, a stone figure from Uruguay in the shape of a human being with a rectangular cavity on its front side (in the style of the Mexican *Chacmool* figures) has been labeled by Serrano (1939) as a *tableta*. This stone figure can be seen as Fig. 4 in the posthumous work by J. I. Muñoa about the prehistoric peoples of Uruguay. The author

---

[43] Netto, Ladislau. 1885 : 516–517. "Uma advertencia cabe-me aqui interpor sobre a palavra vaso que tenho dado a estes ambuletos. Alguns, na verdade, pódem ter este nome, não outros, porém, que são, a bem dizer, fetiches zoomorphos com uma peqñena e mal distincta cavidade no dorso, no ventre ou 'no flánco, onde', ao que presumo, o pó vegetal excitante, a que attribuiam virtudes sobrenaturaes, era depositado e sorvido. Quanto aos vasos fetiches ou zoomorphos, muito é de crer que n'elles fossem depositadas substancias varias com attribuição de eguaes preconceitos, ou que servissem para pulverisar as folhas de alguma planta sagrada ou qualquer outra materia destinada a ceremonias religiosas."

251

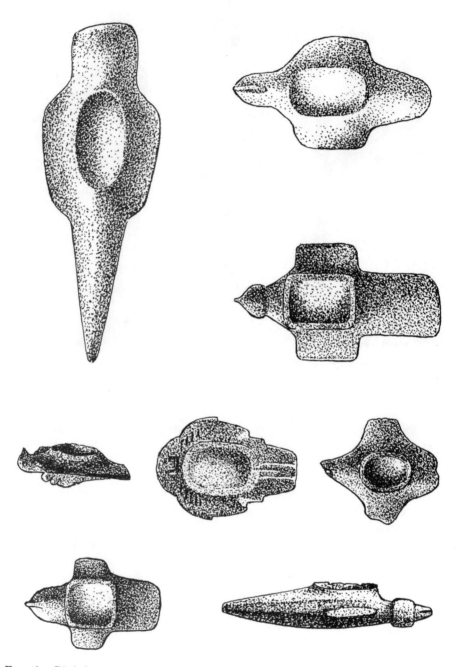

Fig. 12.—Bird-shaped so-called *zooluthos* from *sambaquis* in Santa Catarina, Brazil. Drawings after pl. VI in Netto's publication of 1885.

shows how the nicely sculptured stone specimens (*litos*) in animal form, and often birds ("*que figuran comunmente aves*") belong to a stone-working culture of the (later) Tupi-Guarani region of southern Brazil (Santa Catarina and Rio Grande do Sul) and the eastern parts of Uruguay.[44]

These special stone figures in human or animal form (birds, fishes, etc.) with cavities have been classified by Muñoa (p. 16) as "*tabletas shamánicas para aspirar paricá*", and included in what Serrano used to call the Guayaná Culture, which also goes under the name of the Rio Grande Culture. The Guayaná, according to Métraux (1946: 445), should be counted with the Caingang, a designation for several "non-Guaraní Indians of the States of São Paulo, Paraná, Santa Catarina, and Rio Grande do Sul, who previously were known as Guayaná, Coroado, Bugre, Shokleng, Tupí, Botocudo, etc., but who are all linguistically and culturally related to one another and form the southern branch of the *Ge* family." Nothing, however, seems to indicate that the Caingang were the masters of the stone objects mentioned here. On "Narcotics", Métraux (1946: 469) says only that "a great many stone pipes have been found in the Caingang area—a puzzling fact since smoking has not been observed among the Indians." This, however, was contradicted on the following page, where he says that "the Caingang shaman consults spirits at night, puffing his pipe until he is surrounded by a cloud of smoke."

But, as these *litos* evidently are of interest as possible ceremonial receptacles for snuff, to which culture do they really belong? The question seems open to discussion. Muñoa assigned them to a first wave of Indians in Uruguay, the *Sambaquianos*. Serrano placed the *litos* in a pre-Tiahuanaco period or *Middle Sambiqui* phase.[45] The culture is said to have come from the north. Vidart has on p. 61 of his edition of Muñoa's work dated the culture which left the shamanistic stone tablets ("*las tabletas shamánicas en piedra*") at 3.000 B.C., but no reasons for this very early dating have been given. For my own part I should prefer to consider the *litos* in southern Brazil and eastern Uruguay in some way related to the finds from the Amazon region (the *contas, muiraquitas*, etc. of the "Rio Trombetas," see Wassén, 1965: 34), perhaps so that a specialization in a craftsmanship connected with a ceremonial use of psychotomimetics has some center of origin until now unknown; however, within the Amazon region.

In Wassén, 1965: 34, the *Mercedes* figure from Uruguay has already been mentioned following a presentation of the "*idolo*" or "*conta*" from the Rio Trombetas region with its "Alter ego" motif, and its carefully hollowed out cavity on its back (Fig. 13) as having been used for holding some kind of a psychotomimetic snuff. When publishing this specimen from the Gothenburg Ethnographic Museum, I saw its "beautiful craftsmanship reflected in the snuff boards with animal motifs used by the Cashuena, and earlier also by

---

[44] Muñoa, Juan Ignacio. 1965: 14–19 (edition and notes by Daniel Vidart). I have not said that the Tupí used snuff of the kind discussed here. Alfred Métraux (1948 *a*: 127) has not mentioned the use of *paricá*, but that of tobacco smoking, "one of the favorite pastimes in daily life as well as on ceremonial occasions." He also points out that "stone pipes, found in several points of the Brazilian coast, perhaps belong to another culture anterior to that of the Tupí."

[45] Muñoa, ed. by Vidart. 1965. P. 16 and map on p. 12.

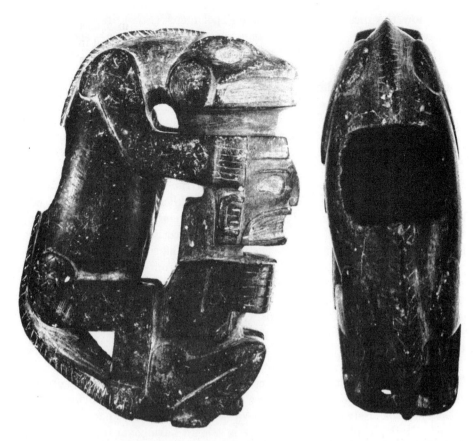

Fig. 13.—Stone figure with cavity. Sucurujú, R. Trombetas, Brazil. Gothenburg Ethnographic Museum, Coll. No. 25.12.1. Height 17.5 cm.

other Amazonian tribes." I could in 1965 also show a direct parallel to its artistic motif, a man being dominated by a jaguar on his back, when referring to a detail of a snuffing tube from Puna de Jujuy published by Ambrosetti in 1908 (see Wassén, 1965, Fig. 7, and this work Fig. 14). The figure shown in Fig. 14 is by no means a single example. In Fig. 15 we see the same motif, that is a jaguar dominating and above a human representation, on a fragment of a wooden snuffing tube found together with a tray with handles in the form of two human figures in an excavation in the Antigal de Ciénega Grande of the Puna de Jujuy, Argentina, and published by Salas (1945: 205–208, Figs. 86–89).

As mentioned in Wassén 1965: 36, Dr. A. A. Gerbrands in 1955 related the carved stone objects from lower R. Trombetas to the Maué Indian sculpture in wood. We can safely connect the *paricá* trays with two human figures found in Argentina and Chile, with the beautiful Tucano *paricá* tray in the Oslo University's Ethnographical Museum analyzed in 1965.[46]

The Jaguar, as a powerful and dangerous animal, has certainly always played a very important part in Indian beliefs as reflected in their ceremonial-

---

[46] Wassén. 1965 : 68–80, and figs. 31–36 and 38–39.

ism. It is thus not without reason that we in the American Museum of Natural History, New York, find the Jaguar repeatedly represented in a series of snuff tablets and tubes originating from the "Gentilar de Caspana", north Chile.

In one special case, the comparison that can be made between ethnographically known snuff tablets in the Amazon region and a wooden snuff tray with feline head archaeologically found in Atacama, Chile, is absolutely surprising. For this I refer to Fig. 22 in this work, with kind permission published from a photo received from the *Museo de Arte Precolombino* in

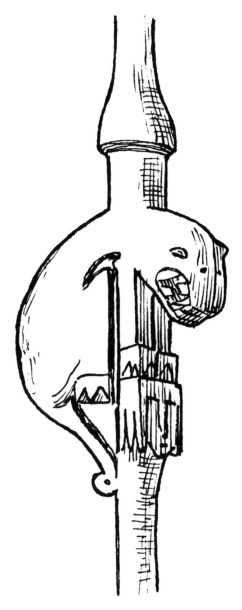

Fig. 14.—Detail of snuff tube from Puna de Jujuy. After Ambrosetti.

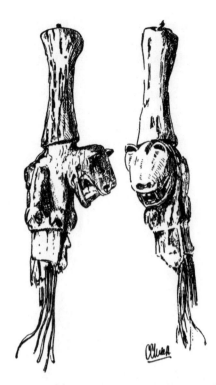

FIG. 15.—Section of snuff tube from Ciénega Grande, Puna de Jujuy, Argentina. After Salas.

Montevideo.[47] I am in this case nearly prepared to accept the Atacaman tray as a direct trade piece from the Amazon region. The late Dr. Stig Rydén, in his work on the archaeology of the Rio Loa region, was specifically interested in the trade relations between the Atacameño and the lowlands in the east.[48]

If we now look for other archaeological finds of snuffing paraphernalia in South America, the snuff tablet and its tube reported by Dr. J. B. Bird from near the Huaca Prieta, Chicama Valley, Peru, is the most interesting, as it appears in a very old culture sequence.[49] According to information received from Dr. Bird following my visit to New York in September, 1966, it is the question of a "snuff tablet of whalebone, Chicama Valley, Peru, near the Huaca Prieta. Test 4, House 3, associated with skeleton 99.1/880, the snuff tube 41.2/4722 a, b., and a broken jet mirror. The burial was made during the period when Guañape pottery was in use. (The oldest pottery known in this area). Estimated Age, c. 1200 B.C.; oldest known tablet (as of 1966)." (Letter of Nov. 2, 1966). See Fig. 23 for this specimen.

Dr. Bird has also had the kindness to inform me about a find of a snuff tray of wood collected by Mr. G. S. Vescelius in 1959, "from a Late Inter-

[47] See plate 38 in *"Arte Precolombino, Colección Matto,"* Museo de Arte Precolombino, Montevideo, 1948.

[48] Rydén, Stig. 1944. See his summary, pp. 206–212, also the discussion of the origin of the material of a leather cuirass made of the skins of alligator and monkey (pp. 115–116). According to Wendell C. Bennett (1946 : 603) the "Atacameño were great traders."

[49] Bird, Junius B. 1948 : 21–28. Also Wassén and Holmstedt, 1963 : 25, and Wassén, 1965 : 79–80.

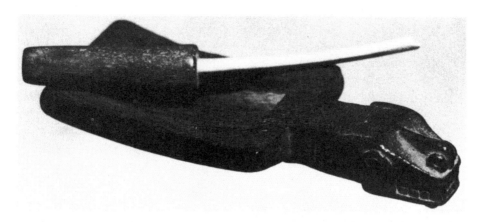

FIG. 16.—Snuff tray with feline motif and corresponding tube. Atacama. Specimen courtesy of the *Museo de Arte Precolombino*, Montevideo.

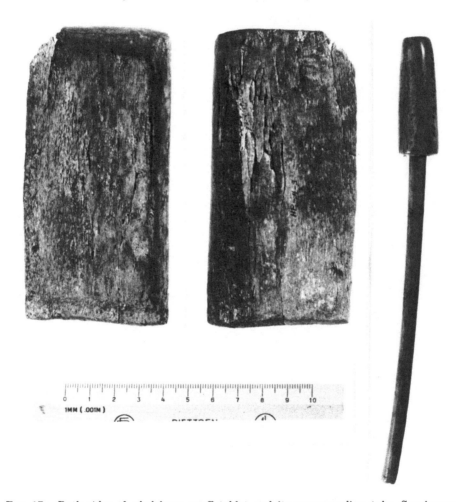

FIG. 17.—Both sides of whalebone snuff tablet and its corresponding tube. Specimens discovered by Dr. Junius B. Bird near the Huaca Prieta, Chicama Valley, Peru. Oldest known tablet (as of 1966). Coll. and courtesy of the American Museum of Natural History, New York. Specimen 41.2/4721 (tray), 41.2./4722 a, b, bird and fox bone snuff tube, found with the tray.

257

mediate burial at Santa María Miramar, a site near Mejía, on the Peruvian coast about 20 kilometers south of Mollendo. There are two phases (one Inca, the other immediately pre-Inca) represented at this site. The burial dates from the earlier, pre-Inca phase. Associated with the snuff tray in the grave were a miniature raft with its paddle, a bagfull of model harpoon foreshafts, and a spindle with rectangular whorl." Various specimens in the collections of the American Museum of Natural History, N.Y., are shown in Figs. 16–21.

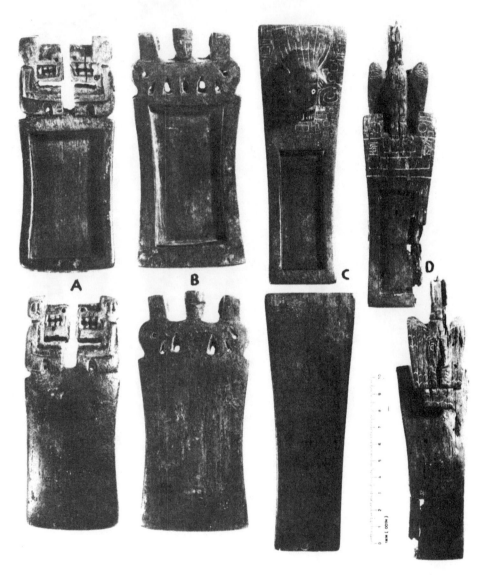

FIG. 18.—Both sides of four snuff tablets of wood in the American Museum of Natural History, New York. Photographs courtesy of A.M.N.H. *A*, 41.0/8754, Cemetery at Chiuchiu, Chuquicamata, Chile; *B*, 41.0/8746, same data; *C*, 41.0/8911, Grave site near San Pedro, Chuquicamata region, North Chile; *D*, 41.0/8912, same data as *C*.

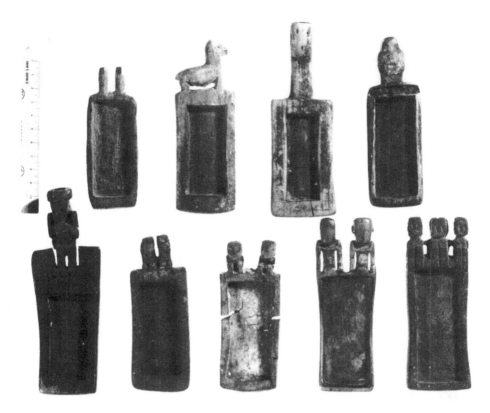

FIG. 19.—Nine snuff trays of wood from Chile. Coll. and courtesy of the American Museum of Natural History, New York. Eight specimens from Cemetery at Chiuchiu, one from Puntas Tetas near Antofagasta (bottom row, third from left).

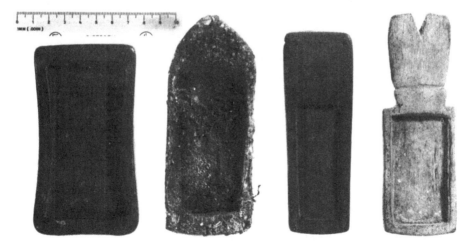

FIG. 20.—Four snuff tablets of wood from Chile. Coll. and courtesy of the American Museum of Natural History, New York. From left: 41.0/8750, Cemetery at Chiuchiu; B/9568, "Taken from child's grave," Juan Lopez Bay, near Antofagasta; 41.0/8964, Cemetery about 3 km. from Chiuchiu, and 41.0/8751, Cemetery at Chiuchiu, Chuquicamata.

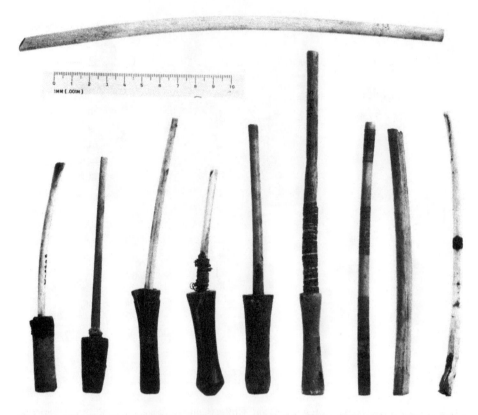

Fig. 21.—Snuff tubes of bird bone and bone and wood. Chile. Coll. and courtesy of the American Museum of Natural History, New York. These specimens come from Chiu-chiu, Cobija and Lasana ruin, near Chuquicamata.

From the Huaca Prieta find, it is evident that snuffing paraphernalia were in early use in the Peruvian high culture area. I have in my book from 1965 (p. 80) referred to W. von Hagen's statement that "there is no doubt that the coastal yuncas, as their contemporaries, the Andean dwellers, had a wide knowledge of drug-yielding plants." Specific trade routes were mentioned: "Huancabamba had extensive trade alliances with the coast people. It was also a trade-axis for the jungle; a route less than sixty miles ran from the mountains about Huancabamba down to Jaen, near to the Rio Marañon, one of the tributaries of the Amazon rivers system." [50] It was, according to von Hagen, the milieu of the widely spread and trading Shuara (or Jívaro). Among various articles traded by these Indians, von Hagen (p. 150) espe-cially mentions several narcotics, among them "*niopo* snuff (which was in-haled into the nose through the shank bone of the Oil-bird.") In this con-nection it is tempting to refer to a painting on a Mochica vessel from Period V (c. 600–700 A.D.) published by Alan R. Sawyer.[51] The vessel, which belongs to the Nathan Cummings Collection in the Metropolitan Museum of Art, New York, shows according to Sawyer an "ornately caparisoned war-

[50] Hagen, Victor W. von. 1965: 149.
[51] Sawyer, Alan R. 1966: 46.

rior-bird" which is "collecting the narcotic fruit of the *ullucho* tree, which grows in the highlands."

Following my publication of the claysnuffers from Costa Rica, Doctors Clifford Evans and Betty J. Meggers of the U.S. National Museum in a letter of March 24, 1966, raised the question if the so-called "pottery spoons from Marajoara Phase" published by them as plate 81 in Bulletin 167 of the Bureau of American Ethnology might be a snuff device. "These were ruled out as smoking pipes because of two factors; one, was position of the hole in all but one, and in that one, there was no indication whatsoever that it had been used for a pipe. Since they don't occur in the culture we use the term that has been used by others, namely pottery spoons. If they are actually used in snuff taking it would move the distribution down to the mouth of the Amazon and at a earlier time zone than the rest of your region." (Letter of March 24, 1966). The possibility that these objects served as some kind of snuffing paraphernalia should perhaps be taken into account. In the general form these clay specimens very much resemble the mortars of fruit shell used for preparing the *paricá* snuff in parts of the Amazon region.[52]

---

[52] Comp. for instance the object, pl. 81*b*, in the publication by Meggers and Evans (1957) with the mortar, fig. 25 (p. 60) in Wassén 1965.

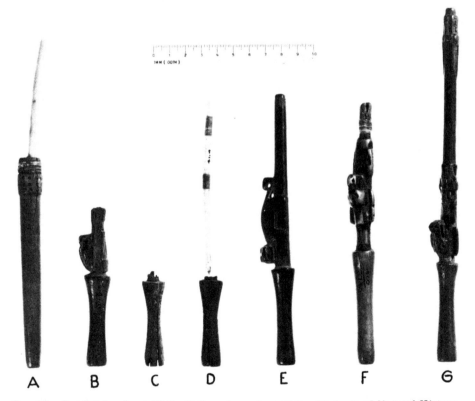

Fig. 22.—Snuff tubes from Chile. Coll. and courtesy of the Museum of Natural History, New York. *A*, B/4452, bone and wood, Arica; *B*, 41.0/8742, wood, Cemetery at Chiuchiu; *C*, 41.0./8994, wood, Chiuchiu; *D*, 41.0./3415, wood, Chiuchiu; *E*, 41.0.8739, wood, Cemetery at Chiuchiu; *F*, 41.0.8740, wood, metal at nd, Cemetery at Chiuchiu; *G*, 41.0.8741, wood, Cemetery at Chiuchiu.

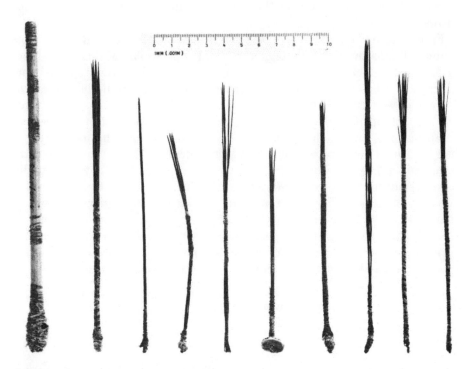

Fɪɢ. 23.—Snuff tube and thorn bundles from snuff tubes. Coll. and courtesy of the American Museum of Natural History, New York. The tube, 41.0/1713 J, from Chiuchiu, Chile. The bundle of seven thorns beside the tube was found in the tube. Wrapping is sinew. The other thorns belong to 41.0/8662, all unassociated with original tubes. Cemetery at Chiuchiu, Chuquicamata, Chile.

The map in Fig. 24 shows the distribution of archaeological finds which definitely, or in some cases possibly, should be related to the taking of psychotomimetic snuffs.

Ethnographical Data About the Use of Snuffs in South America

The first thing prepared for this chapter has been the distribution map in fig. 25 with its legend. In this map tribal names and data about the snuffing of *paricá* or *yopo* as well as *epéna* snuffs as presented in Zerries (1964, map 10, text pp. 85–93) have been incorporated with the ethnographic information presented in the map in Wassén, 1965, p. 13. The data given by Cooper (1949, map 10, pp. 536–537) have also been used, as have some of the information from Colombia presented in the paper by Nestor Uscategui M. (1959). As far as I understand the final result must give a fairly complete picture of the distribution of psychotomimetic snuffing among the South American Indians according to published reports.

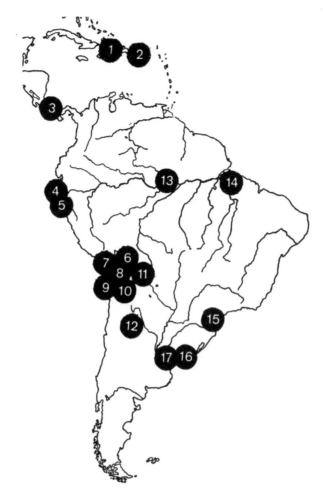

Fig. 24.—Distribution of Archaeological Finds. See Legend.

Legend to Map in Figure 24.

1. Haiti. Finds connected with the use of *cohoba*.
2. Puerto Rico. Stone *cemi* with platform on top.
3. Finds of clay snuffers in Costa Rica.
4. Mochica Culture, N. Peru. Painted motif on a pottery vessel supposed to show the collecting of the narcotic fruit of the *ullucho* tree (?).
5. Whalebone snuff tablet and bone tube. Huaca Prieta, Chicama Valley. Fig. 17.
6. Uhle's snuffing tube of bone from Tiahuanaco. Fig. 6.
7. Pre-Inca phase wooden snuff tray from Santa María Miramar, south of Mollendo.
8. Finds of snuffing paraphernalia at Chiuchiu, Chile.
9. Finds from the Changos, Coast of Antofagasta, Chile.
10. Finds from the Atacama region.
11. Finds from the Puna de Jujuy, Argentina.
12. Province of Córdoba, Argentina.
13. Stone figure (17.5 cm. high) with cavity on its back. Sucurujú, R. Trombetas, Brazil. Gothenburg Ethnographic Museum, Coll. 25.12.1.
14. So-called pottery spoons from the Marajoara Phase. (?)
15. Zoomorphic stone figures (*litos*) from S. Catarina and R. Grande do Sul, Brazil. Fig. 12.
16. Finds of *litos* in Eastern Uruguay.
17. The *antropolito de Mercedes*, Uruguay.

263

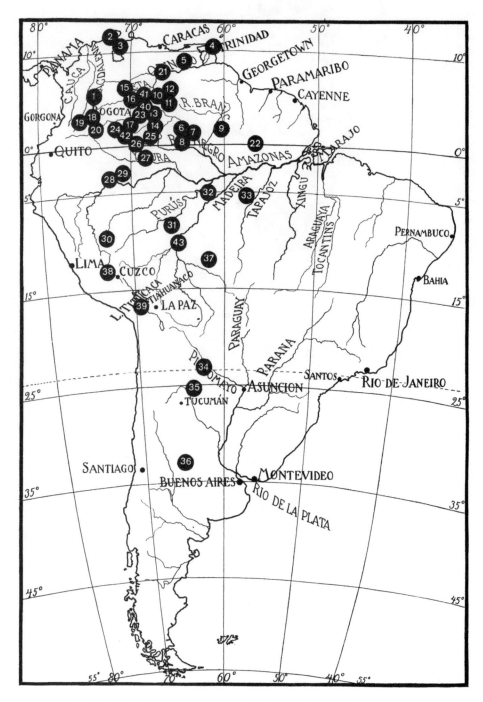

Fig. 25.—Ethnographical data, Distribution Map. See Legend.

1. Highland *Chibcha* and *Tunebo*, Chibcha neighbors on the east. *Piptadenia* snuff, see Cooper, 1949:536. According to Oviedo, *Historia* etc., vol. IV:607 (Madrid 1855), *yop* was a *"yerba de adivinacion, usada por los mojas ó sacerdotes del sol en los valles de Tunja y Bogotá. (Lengua de Nueva Granada)."* A reduced number of *Tunebo* are still found in "the humid jungle regions in the southwestern part of the Comisaria de Arauaca," Colombia (Uscategui, 1959:298–299). Same author, p. 299: "The custom of snuffing *yopo* was acquired probably from their Arawak neighbors in Venezuela and Colombia." A knowledge of nutmeg (at least for trade purposes) existed among the Tunebo of the early 18th century. According to Gumilla (1744:307) "el Padre Pompeo Carcacio, que fué Missionero de los *Tunevos* muchos años, nos asseguró, que en su tiempo traían aquellos Indios *Nuez moscada*, tan parecida en todo á la que traen del Oriente, que no se podian distinguir unas nueces de otras; pero yo no la he visto, ni sé que oy la saquen."

2–3. *Caquetio* and *Jirajara*, extinct tribes. The medicine-men took tobacco and a narcotic herb when they practised divination and communed with the spirits. Cf. Wassén, 1965:105. Probably *Piptadenia* snuffers.

4. *Inyeri*, Arawak Indians of Trinidad, *yopo* snuffers (Zerries, 1964:88, and Cooper, 1949:536, "early Contact Indians of Trinidad." Castellanos, 1950:93: (in "canto cuarto"),"*Uno toma tabaco y otro yopa para poder saber lo venidero.*"

5. *Palenque* and *Pirití*. Two Carib tribes (Zerries, 1964:88). According to Hernández de Alba, 1948:411, "the *Palenque, Pirití* and *Sáliva* shamans also used "yopa" for divination."

6. *Waica, Samatari, Surára, Sanemá* and *Pakidái*, subgroups of the *Yanoama*, southern Venezuela. These Indians use snuff prepared from *Virola* sp., the snuff now internationally known as *epéna* (the Waica name). See information and references in Wassén *and* Holmstedt, 1963:8, and Wassén, 1965:98–99. Also, Holmstedt, 1965. According to Zerries, 1964:85, the *Waica* should also use *Piptadenia peregrina*.

7. *Karimé* (or *Shuári*), Indians culturally related to the Waica. According to G. Salathé, quoted in Wassén, 1965:99, and in Wassén *and* Holmstedt, 1963:14, these Indians prepare a snuff made of leaves from a small plant called *kokoime*. A 30 cm. long straight tube is used. Another person blows into the nostrils.

8. *Araraibo*, Indians at the upper Cauaburi River, an affluent of R. Negro, border region between Venezuela and Brazil. Visited by Georg J. Seitz, see his book from 1960. Information on the powder prepared of material from *Virola* sp. has been summarized in Zerries, 1964:85–86. Evidently closely related to the *Samatari* (Seitz, 1960:306, has published a short "Araraibo-Xamatari Word List"), or a Waica group.

9. *Paravilhana*, Carib Indians. Martius, 1867:631, has reported the use of *paricá* powder from *Mimosa acacioides*. Cf. Zerries, 1964:87.

10. *Yecuaná-Makiritare*, Carib Indians of southern Venezuela. See the translation of Th. Koch-Grünberg's description of the use of the *hakúdufha*, a "bark of tree"-powder from these Indians in Schultes, 1954:245, also quoted in Wassén, 1965:97. According to Schultes, an identification of the unusual narcotic *Virola*-snuff with the powder mentioned by Koch-Grünberg seems almost certain. Dr. Helmuth Fuchs (letter of March 9, 1962, quoted in Wassén, 1965:97), has described *a'ku:duwha* as a snuff powder with ingredients which botanically can be shown to have come from *Piptadenia peregrina*, or another *Piptadenia*. There are also other ingredients from a tree, probably *Virola* sp. See also discussion in Wassén *and* Holmstedt, 1963:10–12. Cf. Zerries, 1964:87–88. Cf. No. 24.

11. *Yabarana*. Carib Indians, related to the Makiritare. Johannes Wilbert, 1963:133, mentions the use of tobacco, *yopo*, and *cápi* among the Yabarana (Wassén, 1965:20). Zerries, 1964:88, quoting a paper by Wilbert from 1959, mentions that the Yabarana should obtain their *yopo* from a liana (?), and a tablet and Y-formed snuff tube are used.

12. *Piaroa*, Indians of the Salivan Family, Orinoco-Ventuari territory, see Wassén, 1965:103. According to Wilbert they use *yopo*, a strong *"tabaco-rapé,"* prepared from the seeds of *Piptadenia* sp. The powder is passed around in a round tray with

265

handle in the form of a fin (of a fish) and Y-shaped tubes of bird bone are used. According to J. J. Wurdack, bark of *Lecythidaceae* is burned and the ash added to the *yopo* of *Piptadenia* seeds. Quotation in Wassén, 1965:103.

13. *Puinave*. Indians at the lower Infrida River, southeast Colombia and adjacent territory of Venezuela. Several quotations in Wassén, 1965:99–100. Dr. R. E. Schultes, 1954:248, has repeatedly observed the preparation of "a violently toxic snuff" among the Puinave. This snuff is prepared from an exudation of *Virola calophylla* and *Virola calophylloidea*.

14. *Kuripako*, Arawak Indians of the Guainía River. Schultes has described a narcotic snuff prepared of *Virola* sp. Quotations in Wassén, 1965:100.

15. *Achagua*, once widely distributed Arawak-speaking Indians in Venezuela and eastern Colombia. Hernández de Alba, 1948:409, says that "the Achagua used a snuff made of the narcotic powder of certain leaves called *"niopa"* or *"yopa."* Two Indians took this snuff simultaneously; with two crossed bird bones, each blew it into the other's nose." Cf. No. 19 in this list. Also Zerries, 1964 : 89. Sven Lovén, 1935:387, says that *yopa* "is an Achaguan name." For a full quotation of the prognostication combined with the taking of *yopo* powder from the relation written by the Jesuit missionary Juan Rivero in 1736, I refer to Wassén, 1965 : 19. "A nasal secretion from the right nostril signified success, from the left meant failure, and from both was an indeterminate sign."

16. *Guahibo, Chiricoa, Saliva*. Several references to these Colombian-Venezuelan Llanos tribes in Wassén, 1965:104. The Guahibo and Chiricoa men "invariably carried a shell or a jaguar bone containing parica. These tribes were said to carry the habit of parica snuffing to extremes not found among the neighboring tribes" (Kirchhoff, 1948:455). Cf. Zerries, 1964:89.

17. *Piapoco*, snuffers of *Piptadenia*. See Cooper, 1949:536.

18. *Guaupé* and *Sáe*, Arawak Indians. Zerries, 1964:89, has quoted Kirchhoff's article on these Indians in vol. 4 of the Handbook of South American Indians (Washington: 1948), p. 385–391, about the taking of "coca (yupa), and tobacco." The probably Arawak Indians once lived "in the southernmost section of the Venezuelan-Colombian llanos," the Guayupé "also in large parts also inhabited the dense rain forests of the Andean sloops" (Kirchhoff, p. 385.)

19. *"Ouitoto"* Indians of the upper Yapurá River. See Zerries, 1964:91, and the discussion of the crossed tubes for snuffing among the "Ouitotos" of Dr. Crevaux in Wassén, 1965:87–90. It is a possibility that hernández de Alba when formulating the statement about the *Achagua* (see No. 15 in this list) has been influenced by the drawing and text in the work of Crevaux. No source is given for the statement about the Achagua. Until such a reliable source has been presented, I prefer to consider the often published drawing in the publications of Dr. Crevaux of two Indians using crossed snuffing tubes, as dubious.

20. *Taiwano*. Indians of the R. Kananari, Comisaria del Uaupés, Colombia (Cerro Isibukurí). According to Schultes, 1954:242, they use a narcotic snuff of *Virola*.

21. *Otomac*. Tribe in the Venezuelan Llanos, between Orinoco, the Apure, and the Meta Rivers. According to Paul Kirchhoff's paper on these Indians in vol. 4 of the Handbook of South American Indians, pp. 439–444 (Washington, 1948), "Otomac shamans, under the influence of ñope, predicted the future." Humbolt was a witness of Otomac snuffing the powder of *Acacia niopo* seeds with lime as an ingredient. As he is one of the very few who really gives a description of the preparing of the snuff, I quote from the *"Personal Narrative"* (Humbolt and Bonpland, 1818–1929, vol. V:661–663): "The Otomacs are a restless turbulent people, with unbridled passions. They are not only fond to excess of the fermented liquors from cassava and maize, and of the palm wine, but they throw themselves into a peculiar state of intoxication, we might almost say of madness, by the use of the pwoder of *niopo*. They gather the long pods of mimosacea, which we have made known by the name of *acacia niopo*, cut them into pieces, moisten them, and cause them to ferment. When the softened seeds begin to grow black, they are kneaded like a paste, mixed with some flour of cassava and lime

procured from the shell of a helix, and the whole mass is exposed to a very brisk fire, on a grate of hard wood. The hardened paste takes the form of small cakes. When it is to be used, it is reduced to a fine powder, and placed on a disk five or six inches wide. The Otomac holds this disk, which has a handle, in his right hand, while he inhales the *niopo* by the nose, through a forked bone of a bird, the two extremities of which are applied to the nostrils. This bone, without which the Otomac believes that he could not take this kind of snuff, is seven inches long: it appeared to me to be the leg bone of a large sort of the plover (*échassier*). 1 sent the *niopo*, and all this singular apparatus, to Mr. de Foucroy at Paris." According to Rosenblat, (1965:272) nothing of all this is now remembered among the *Llanero* population said to be descendants of the Otomac. Also, their language has gone.

22. *Cashuena*. Indians of the Carib Family on the Casuro (Cashorro) River, a tributary of the middle Trombetas River, Brazil. From this tribe Protátasio Frikel has described a *mori* snuff, which can be made "simply of tobacco" or of other ingredients among which *paricá* is mentioned. A full quotation is found in Wassén, 1965:103, and also in Wassén *and* Holmstedt, 1963:21–23. The snuff mentioned by Mr. Gottfried Polykrates seems to originate from *Piptadenia* seeds. Details in Wassén, 1965:103.

23. *Tuyuca* and *Bará*, Tucanoan tribes on the upper Tiquié River. As quoted in Wassén, 1965:100, the use of *paricá* or *niopo* has been mentioned by Whiffen from the Tuyuca, and Zerries, 1964:90, refers to Koch-Grünberg's statement about the use of a snuff from *Mimosa acacioides* Benth. among both tribes.

24. *Cubeo*, one of the Eastern Tucanoan tribes at a section of the Uaupés River. Schultes, 1954:242, describes the Cubeo as users of *Virola* snuff. Cf. Wassén, 1965, about their use of *Banisteriopsis caapi*. According to Goldman, 1948:796, "the shamanistic novice spends a month learning the art from at least two professionals. He obtains tree resin, dupa (*Tucano*), and inhales it in a powdered form for 4 days." Bödiger, 1965:151, refers this to the Cubeo novices, and mentions also Koch-Grünberg's explanation of the word *dúpa* as meaning small white stones used for sorcery. In the meaning tree resin which is inhaled as a powder, the word is of direct interest through the term *hakúdufha*, offered us by Koch-Grünberg from a linguistically mixed region with contact zones between several language families.

25. *Tucano*. In this word an important group of Indians of the Uaupés and Papuri Rivers are included. Schultes has in 1954 reported the use of *Virola* snuff, and Uscategui has in 1959 mentioned a mixture of *Virola* and *Theobroma subincanum* powders. Mr. Georg J. Seitz has photographed a Tucano medicine man grinding the dry crust of evaporated *Virola calophylloidea* exudation to snuff powder with a stone. The photos were taken by him at Tapuruquara, upper R. Negro, Brazil, in 1965 (see Wassén, 1965:100–101, also p. 73). In Wassén, 1965:68–76, it has been demonstrated that the Tucano used very fine sculptured snuff trays in earlier days. Uscategui, 1959:294, remarks that the Tucano commonly use the Tupí-Guaraní loan-word *pa-ree-ká* (*paricá*) for the snuff prepared from "the blood-red resin of certain species of the myristicaceous tree, *Virola*, especially *V. calaphylla* and *V. calophylloidea*."

26. *Barasana, Makuna, Yahuna, Yabahana, Menimehe*. Zerries, 1964:90–91, has mentioned that Koch-Grünberg found the same snuffing paraphernalia among the Tucanoan tribes (or groups) Makuna, Yabahana and Yahuna at the lower Apaporis River, as he had found among the Tuyuca and Bará (No.23) at the upper Tiquié River. Schultes found Barasana and Makuna Indians living together at the R. Piraparaná, both tribes snuffers of *Virola* (see Wassén, 1965:101). This drug seems also to be used among the Yakuna and Yabahana. Whiffen has listed the Arawak Menimehe at the Yapurá River as users of a narcotic snuff. See Zerries, 1964:91.

27. *Pasé, Juri* and *Uainuma*, once important Arawak tribes south of the Yapurá River, noted as *paricá* snuffers and also listed among such tribes by Zerries, 1964:91, as also by Wassén, 1965:66, according to Métraux. The Pasé have been mentioned in Wassén, 1965:68, as one of the Brazilian tribes called "black-faces," as they used a special tribal identification, the so-called *malhas*. They have been reported as excellent wood-carvers.

28. *Omagua*. In Wassén, 1965:83, there is a detailed description of this Tupí tribe through Father Samuel Fritz, who in 1701 had to calm an uprising in the Settlement of San Pablo. Pots with powdered *curupá* were found, "with which to deprive themselves of their senses, so as to carry out any evil deed without compunction." This material was all consumed with fire upon orders given by Father Fritz after his Mass. Métraux has stated that both the Omagua and Cocama, also a Tupí tribe further west, "inhaled powdered *curupá* leaves (*Mimosa acacioides*), to which they ascribed great therapeutic and magical powers." According to Métraux, the *curupá* "was blown into the nose through Y-shaped tubes or, with the help of small rubber syringes, administered as a clyster which provoked agreeable visions." Quotations in Wassén, 1965:83. Zerries, 1964:92, seems to doubt the use among the Cocama. According to La Condamine's *Relation*, etc. from 1778 (quoted in Wassén, 1965:84) the word *curupá* for *Piptadenia* should originate from the language of the Omagua. Monteiro de Noronha, writing in 1768 about the Omagua, which he calls *Umauá* or *Cambébas*, "Flat Heads," criticizes La Condamine for his statement that the *curupá* intoxication should last 24 hours, and corrects it to "apenas dura tres horas" (Monteiro de Noronha, 1862:58). The same author adds that the Cambébas used the juice from the bark of the *manacá*, which has been identified with *Brunfelsia hopeana* Benth. of the *Solanaceae* family.

29. *Tucuna*. As follows from the analysis in Wassén, 1965:82–83, these Indians who now only snuff tobacco, are known to have been using *paricá* snuff in earlier days for their ceremonial snuff called *ka'/vi*. The very important snuff tray found in the Oslo University's Ethnographical Museum and published in Wassén, 1965, fig. 41, has by an ethnographical analysis been shown to come from the Tucuna, and to represent the *prego* monkey demon. See Wassén, 1965:80–86.

30. *Piro*. One of the Arawakan-speaking tribes of the headwaters of the Ucayali and Madeira Rivers, by Julian H. Steward and Alfred Métraux counted as a primitive Montaña subgroup. The use of the seeds of *Acacia niopo* has been reported among the Piro by William Curtis Farabee in 1922. For the hunter and his dog, see Wassén 1965:94. Cf. No. 31 in this list.

31. *Catawishi*, Indians of the river Purús. Spruce has in 1874 reported from these Indians that they used to absorb *paricá* through a bent tube, and also that they administered an injection of *paricá* to dogs, thus a confirmation of that stated from the Piro. Full quotation in Wassén, 1965:96. See also Cooper, 1949:547.

32. *Mura*. For the once much feared Mura Indians of the Madeira River the use of *paricá* must have been of outstanding importance. This is clearly demonstrated in the descriptions quoted in Wassén, 1965:37. The roasted seeds of the *paricá* tree were taken either as a snuff or an enema. The snuff was blown into the nostrils by means of bone tubes. The effects of the drug consumption in this tribe have been drastically described. Schultes has warned that we cannot be absolutely sure that the snuff used by the Mura and Maué was prepared from *Piptadenia*, as a botanical consideration must be kept in mind. Cf. Wassén, 1965:23.

33. *Maué*. These Central Tupí Indians were formerly famous for their *paricá*, which they do not use any more (see Nunes Pereira, 1954:71). *Mimosa acacioides* is given as the source. They have also been carving very nice specimens of snuff trays, now kept in several museums. See the description in Wassén, 1965:39–63.

34. *Mataco*. Indians of the Gran Chaco, among whom the shamans have been reported to use snuff from the seeds of *cebil*, that is *Piptadenia macrocarpa*. Information collected by Métraux has been quoted in Wassén, 1965:29.

35. *Lule*. Extinct Indians in western Chaco, Argentina. Métraux has mentioned the Lule together with the Mataco. An old information from the Lule comes from Pedro Lozano (1733), who states that *cevil* was blown into the nostrils by a small tube in order to provoke rain when necessary for their cultivations. Full quotation in Wassén, 1965:11–12.

36. *Comechingones*. Cooper, 1949:536, has listed the extinct 16th-century Indians around Córdoba, Argentina, among those taking *Piptadenia* powder. See Zerries,

1964:93, for further references to the use of *cebil* and,'or *wilca* in the southern region, where also the *Zanavirones* are reported to have used it. Max Uhle, 1898:9, has quoted vol. II of the "*Relaciones Geográficas de Indias, Perú*", p. 152, from a report dealing with "la Ciudad de Córdoba," where the Indians spoke *comechingona* and *zanavirona*: "*Toman por las narices el sebil, ques una fruta como vilca; hácenla polvos y bébenla por las narices.*" Uhle comments (p. 9): "The curious expression, they drink the powder with the nostrils, means without doubt that the Indians took the powder by means of an instrument like a tube. Concerning the word *sebil*, Napp (The Argentine Republic, 1876, p. 114) tells us that *sebil* is in Argentine the name of the Acacias. Now, the fact that Humboldt originally pointed out the *niopo* tree as a species of Acacia by mistake and von Martius called it *Mimosa acacioides* proves that Piptadenias and Acacias have sometimes been confounded. We know, further, that Piptadenia trees of the variety *niopo* are also common in eastern Bolivia and the Argentine (for instance *Piptadenia macrocarpa*, in the province of Tucuman). As the bark of the *curupau* tree, which from its name and general description may be a *niopo* tree, serves, according to Cardús, to tan hides in eastern Bolivia, so in like manner the bark of *sebil* is used to tan hides, as I noted, in the environs of Tucuman. All this leads to the conclusion that the tree, from whose seeds the powder was made, is related to *niopo*, and a scientific determination may perhaps show it identical with *niopo*. The custom of snuffing *sebil* in the environs of Córdoba was, therefore, derived from another part of the continent, where snuffing *niopo* was practiced." The conclusion by Uhle must be considered as very important also when we take the distribution of paraphernalia into account.

37. *Tupari, Guaratägaje, Amniapä*, and other tribes in western Brazil, in the R. Branco region and on the Mequéns River, affluents of the Guaporé River. Cooper, 1949:536, refers to "the upper Guaporé tribes." Zerries, 1964:91, has, according to a report of Dr. Etta Becker-Donner, Vienna, added the *Aikaná* or *Hauri*, as their medicine-men use a snuff of *Piptadenia peregrina* mixed with bark ashes. Dr. Becker-Donner has also reported the use of such powder among the *Salamay* in the same region, as quoted by Zerries, 1964:91. The most valuable information from the whole Guaporé region as regards snuffing has been given by Dr. Franz Caspar from the Tupari. I refer to his book from 1952, and his manuscript from 1953, both quoted in Wassén, 1965:102, and as regards the snuffing tubes, especially pp. 24–28.

38. *Quichua.* See Discussion in Zerries, 1964:92, for the use of *wilca* (or *vilca*) snuff among the Andean Quichua, according to data given by Safford in 1916 and by O. F. Cook in 1915. Cooper mentions the Highland *Quechua* of Peru among the consumers of *Piptadenia*, and this is also fully reflected in his Map 10 in his work for the *Handbook* (1949), where a solid black covers most of the central part of the western Highland.

39. *Aymara.* Zerries, 1964:95, has listed the Aymara, Tiahuanaco, as *yopo* snuffers and mentions the word *coro* as probably $=curupa=yopo$. His text seems to indicate that the yopo powder should have been known among the Aymara through the old tribes in northwest Argentina. La Barre, however, does not mention *yopo* among the narcotics in his work from 1948, but he has the information from Bertonio, "*Sincantatha:* Tomar tabaco por las narizes. *Thusa thusa* es el tabaco" (La Barre, 1948:66).

Max Uhle (1898) was the first to take up a serious discussion about what kind of snuff really was used in the Highlands. Garcilasso de la Vega's information is clear and refers to tobacco: "The Indians made great use of the herb of plants which they call *Sayri*, and the Spaniards called tobacco. They applied the powder to their noses to clear the head" (Markham, 1869:188). According to Uhle, we learn from this source "that the practice of snuffing must have been nearly general in the Highlands of middle and southern Peru," . . . Uhle here refers only to the snuffing of tobacco.

It is in one of the sources known to him, namely a report from La Paz found in the "*Relaciones Geográficas de Indias, Peru*," vol. II, p. 76 (Madrid, 1885) that we find the word *coro*. "*Hay tambien entre los indios tabaco, que ellos le llaman sayre, de que los negros usan mucho, y los indios de la raíz que llaman coro, y se purgan con ello y lo toman en polvos.*" Uhle (1898 : 17) comments: "There is nothing published which points to the practice of snuffing the powder of *niopo* in Peru, if not in the report of the province of La Paz. In this province two powders were used as snuff—tobacco and *coro*. This *coro*, without any hesitancy, should be declared to be *curupa*, if it had not been reported as being a root. But the use of *niopo* being confirmed from the region of Córdoba, it seems more reasonable to suppose that the writer of the report was mistaken than that there existed a third powder, never elsewhere reported, with a name similar to that of *niopo*, which was taken as snuff in the environs of La Paz."

40. *Desano* and *Tariano*. Two Arawak tribes along the lower part of the Colombian course of the Uaupés River. According to Uscategui, 1959 : 295, they know "and employ *paricá* or *Virola*-snuff as do their Tukanoan neighbors." *Paricá* (*pa-ree-ká*) is a loan-word from the Tucano but of Tupí-Guaraní origin (cf. No. 25). The tribes are also called *Desana* and *Tariana*.

41. *Kuiva, Amorua, Sikuani*, and

42. *Guayaberos*. "Various tribes," according to Uscategui, 1959:299, "located between the Meta and Inirida Rivers, most of which belong to the Arawak and Guahibo linguistic families." He has for these tribes or tribal groups received personal communications from Meden and Schultes. Other tribes mentioned by Uscategui in this context are the Puinave, Piapoco, Saliva, and Kuripako, which already have been listed separately:

"All of these use or were formerly acquainted with *yopo*, especially for purposes of magic. *Yopo*, prepared from the toasted and pulverized seeds of *Piptadenia peregrina*, is normally taken only by men, for there exists a certain taboo which, however, seems no longer so strict as it once was. In the most acculturated of these people, both sexes take it. Snuffing of this violent intoxicant, which looks rather like ground coffee, is carried out with very different kinds of instruments, the most generally used of which is a double Y-shaped tube of bird bones (the arms of the Y being soldered into place with pitch) ending in two hollowed palm-nuts. These nuts are placed at the opening of the nostrils, and the powder is inhaled from the palm of the hand. Another kind is the long V-shaped snuffing tube, one leg of which is inserted into a nostril, the other into the mouth, thus making self-administration possible. There are additional types of snuffing-tubes as well, both of bone and of small bamboo-like grasses. One other primitive type is made of a palm-leaf: the apex of the leaf is cut off truncated, and this funnel-shaped end is placed over the snuff, while the snuffer draws in strongly through the petiole which is bound into a tube. Generally, some kind of wooden mortar and pestle is used to grind the *Piptadenia*-seeds which have previously been roasted in the fire. The powder is kept in a case made of the leg-bone of the jaguar, partly closed with wax and adorned with feathers. The addition of an alkaline admixture may or may not be the practice." This long quotation with its excellent description to which practically nothing could be added has been taken from Uscategui, 1959:299–300.

43. *Caripuna*. A Panoan-speaking tribe referred to by the Austrian naturalist Johann Natterer as having snuffing implements. Natterer himself encountered a Caripuna subgroup, probably the Sinabo, at the Madeira River (quotation from Métraux in Wassén, 1965:47). According to Métraux "the Caripuná provoke a state of trance by taking *paricá* (Piptadenia sp.) in the form of clysters they administer to each other with rubber syringes provided with a bone tube."

The distribution of tobacco snuffing (and other ways of taking tobacco as chewing, drinking, and licking) in many cases covers the same areas (see map 10 in Cooper, 1949, and maps 11–12 in Zerries, 1964). These data, however, have not been considered here, as I have had to limit myself to special powders.[53] The legend to the map in fig. 25 gives the available information in a concentrated form.

What we learn from the map in Fig. 25 is the concentration of the use of psychotomimetic snuff drugs to certain regions of South America with a western and northwestern dominance, if we consider still remaining tribes or such extinct or no longer snuffing tribes from which data have been recorded. What we do not learn from the map, but perhaps may recognize by reading the legend, is how very few good observations there are. This fact is deplorable, as it is obvious that we now face in the Uaupés region a strongly disappearing usage (cf. Wassén, 1965: 16–17).

A scattered information on the use of *paricá* or *yopo*, by which words mostly a snuff prepared from *Piptadenia* seeds seems to be understood, has been saved. When we turn to other kinds of psychoactive drugs such as the snuff prepared of exudates of *Virola* species, the available data is sparse indeed. It is only through the intensive field work of such an eminent botanist as Richard Evans Schultes, the repeated collecting and observations among the Waica of Mr. George J. Seitz of Rio de Janeiro, and scientific research by Prof. Bo Holmstedt, that we now are able to fully grasp the outstanding importance of this drug.

It is in our days mostly impossible to find out merely from vague ethnographical descriptions, which kind of snuff many tribes have been using; if a pure powder or a mixture, and in the latter case which ingredients. It was only through a chain of lucky detective work in the documented museum material in Gothenburg, that I was able to trace back to the Tucuna Indians the perfect and unusual snuff tablet No. 1219 in an 100-year old Brazilian museum collection in Oslo (see Fig. 26, and Wassén, 1965: 80–86 with illustrations). It has also only been possible to consider another of the three snuff trays in Oslo (No. 1169) as probably Tucanoan (see Wassén, 1965: 68–80), through an ethnographical comparative ornamental study in several museum collections. It is this unique specimen with its double human figures as handles (Fig. 27) which especially leads us to look for an origin in the Amazon region also for the snuff trays among the Atacameño. There are many tablets in the Atacaman collections with two human figures as handles, but I use this opportunity to refer specially to a specimen from Calama, Antofagasta, Chile (fig. 27), now in the collection of the Field Museum of Natural History, Chicago. Dr. Carl Schuster of Woodstock, N.Y., who takes an extreme interest in all double-headed figures, writes to me (May 9, 1966) that "the fact that the two-headed snuff tray as a type occurs in N.W. Brazil, N.W. Argentina and Chile is very interesting. Double-headed human figures begin in South America archeologically very early—with the Valdivia Culture in Ecuador; and I know of some ethnological specimens (Caduveo, Mato Grosso), etc."

As already declared, this study is not dealing with the snuffing of tobacco. Such a study has, however, been undertaken by Zerries in his *Waika*-book (1964: 93–95, map 11). Naturally, this Americanist when trying to sum-

---

[53] For the *rapé dos indios* from the *Olmedioperebea sclerophylla* tree, see Schultes, R. E. 1963: 26.

marize the details of both distributions, had the same difficulties everyone must find in the sources, namely that many times we cannot differentiate the two kinds of snuff when reading the reports. For instance, the Guaporé tribes are mixing *yopo* and tobacco powders, and many tribes use both powders. Zerries (1964: 95) exemplifies the latter cases with Waica, Piro, Tupari, etc.

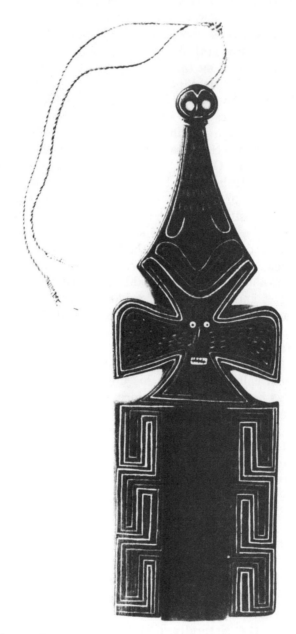

FIG. 26.—Wooden snuff tray representing the prego monkey demon of the Tucuna Indians. Length 25 cm. Coll. and courtesy of the Oslo Univ. Ethnogr. Museum. Specimen No. 1219.

272

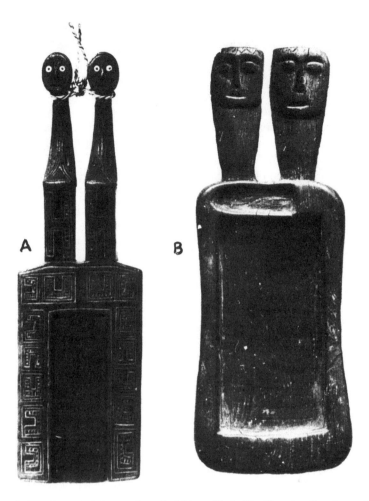

Fig. 27.—*A*, Wooden *paricá* tray, length 20 cm. Probably Tucano. Specimen No. 1169 in the Oslo Univ. Ethnogr. Museum. *B*, Snuff tray of wood, archæological find from Calama, Antofagasta, Chile. Length 15 cm. Coll. Field Museum of Natural History, Chicago.

The distribution of the snuff taking indicates that we have to look upon northern and northwestern South America as the origin area for both powders. Zerries also stresses this fact and points out that we, with such an important exception as the Maué, generally do not find the habit of snuffing among the Central Tupí tribes. According to Zerries (p. 95) Eastern Brazil should not be taken into account at all, as the only statement is dubious. I translate the following from Zerries work (1964: 92): "When Uhle (1898, p. 163/4), following Martyr, wants to credit the Tupi of Eastern Brazil for snuffing *paricá*, this seems *unlikely*." He supports this statement with the information that such a specialist on the Tupí-Guaraní peoples as A. Métraux does not say anything about such a habit among them. This is perfectly correct, and as has been conclusively shown by Métraux in his work on the religion of the Tupinamba (1928: 88), these Indians were blowing smoke of the *petun* plant (tobacco) from a tube for magic and healing purposes. On the other hand an examination of the text in Uhle's paper shows that he (dealing with the *paricá* snuffing) uses the phrase ". . . and has been occasionally ascribed to the Tupis of Eastern Brazil." The reference given by Uhle is the small paper by A. Ernst (1889), but Zerries had been misreading and found the name of Martyr on the line just above. The old chronicler should be omitted in this case, and Ernst on page 135 of his paper, to which Uhle refers, is only mentioning an Old Guarani word *petycui* which has been translated with "*pó* (powder) *de tabaco para ser aspirado.*"

Leaving the Eastern Tupí aside we must, however, keep in mind that the very words *curupá* and *paricá* for the snuff of *Piptadenia* originate in the Tupí-Guaraní languages, and were spread through the *Lingua geral* (Friederici, 1947: 229). Esteban Pinto has written in a paper on the medicine-men among the Tupinamba, that they, in order to get in a state of ecstacy, used "*ilusogénicos o estupefacientes, indicados genéricamente con el nombre de Kurupá* (Pardal)." This plant he identifies with *Piptadenia* species. As a source for the information he gives only "*algunos testimonios.*" [54]

With the Tupí word *curupá* in mind, we must realize that snuff taking does not always follow the language families. Zerries has found how, for instance, several Arawakan tribes north of the Amazon are *yopa* snuffers, while other tribes of the same language stock south of the river take tobacco snuff. Most probably the botanists would be the best equipped to find if such a varying use has its explanation in the distribution of the botanical species. In the following chapter, I am suggesting that the old word *cohoba* from the West Indies and a word *khoba*, now used in the Atacameño region, should be the same, and have spread south via the Arawak and the Andes. This finds a support in the observations by Zerries that we should ascribe the very habit of snuff taking to a sub-Andean stratum of tribes. Here the sub-Andean Arawakan tribes fit, and Zerries finds it probable that the clue to the snuffing should be found among the Arawak, and that the use of *yopo* should be considered as the oldest of the two main classes of snuff.

In my work from 1965 I have treated the same problems, pointing to "a common old tradition in the Amazonian and sub-Andean regions"; equally, I have stressed the fact of "an obvious northern Arawak influence far south into northwestern Argentina" (Wassén, 1965: 77–78).

Comparative Outlooks and Symbolism

Certain living and extinct tribes and certain archaeological and ethnographical objects have been mentioned in this paper in regard to their importance for the whole study. We have first the ceremonially used *cemi*-figures of wood and stone in the West Indies, with platforms on top for the placing of *cohoba*. A mainland ethnographic equivalent to these Antillean *cohoba* "platforms" are the table tops used by the Tupari in Brazil when snuffing ceremonially.

---

[54] Pinto, Esteban. 1944 : 324.

We have through Oviedo's drawing, the descriptions in words and the find in the La Gonâve cave, a fairly good knowledge of the more simple and the more elaborated snuff tubes of wood on the Islands. These specimen have their counterparts in the Y-shaped tubes used among many mainland tribes. We recognize the round snuff trays, which Las Casas describes from the Antilles as perfectly made pieces, when we see the generally much simpler round trays used by the Llanos tribes of northern South America, and certainly also the more unusual round snuff trays found archaelogically in the marginal Atacameño region. For the latter I refer for instance to plate 34 in Le Paige's description of San Pedro de Atacama (1965), where the author refers to a grave for 25 adults, a child's offering and also the offering of snuff trays. Finally, we are certain to look for the origin of the *cohoba* drug itself in the now more and more studied species of plants which botanically belong to the South American mainland. But the very word *cohoba!* Would it be possible to trace it back to some actual situation and still find it used on the mainland? It looks as if it should be possible, and I will return to this problem later in this chapter. I have already mentioned that the word *cojoba* occurs in northern Venezuela.

In this paper I have repeated my opinion from 1965, that the elaborate stone figure from the R. Trombetas region shown in Fig. 13 has been especially sculptured and used to hold a psychotomimetic snuff. The whole character of this famous piece is ceremonial, and we meet in the sculpture a very important South American combination of man and jaguar. It is therefore a small but important piece of information that we have from Dr. Schultes, when he tells us that the Inga and Kamsá Indians in the Valley of Sibundoy, Colombia, called a narcotic prepared from the leaves of *Methysticodendron Amesianum, mits-kway borrachero*, or the "intoxicant of the jaguar." [55] Even if no further explanation has been given as to the nature of the relationship jaguar—intoxicant—we have at least an indication of a connection between the feline and an intoxicant with certain properties for the users. May we guess that the jaguar is thought of as the "owner" of the drug?

The alter-ego sculpture in Fig. 13 is of stone. When we try to get a picture of the archaelogical distribution of snuffing paraphernalia in the Amazon region, we must take into account that very little of perishable material, such as wood, has been saved to our days. As pointed out in Wassén, 1965: 77, an origin in the Highland Tiahuanaco has often been considered for the trays and other snuffing paraphernalia now found in northern Chile and northwestern Argentina. Apart from the fact that snuffing paraphernalia now have been dated in Chile to an earlier epoch than that with an influence from Tiahuanaco, I have for ethnographical reasons considered an origin of the marginal Atacameño snuffing material in the Amazonian and sub-Andean region. I have later found that René Naville, in an article published in Switzerland in 1959, more or less has been of the same opinion; that is, that we should look for the origin of the snuff ceremonialism in the Amazon region, possibly among the Arawak Indians; but that later a cult associated

---

[55] Schultes, R. C. 1955: 10.

with it in the Atacama region and manifested in human offering, had an Andean origin. Mr. Naville's contribution to the whole problem is valuable, and I prefer to quote him here in his language, French:

On peut conclure en disant que si l'absorption d'un narcotique au moyen de tubes et de tablettes semble être originaire d'Amazonie, peut-être arawak, son usage rituel et son association avec le culte rendu à une divinité accompagné de sacrifices humains est très probablement d'origine andine. Il est donc possible que ses deux pratiques se soient conjointes dans le Nord du Chili et le Nord-Ouest de l'Argentine, points d'intersections des grands courants culturels venus du Nord et de l'Est, pour donner naissance aux pièces décrites plus haut.[56]

From what already has been stated in this work, it is with full evidence clear that wooden tablets and tubes for the taking of some kind of a snuff must have been of outstanding importance in the now marginal region where once the Atacameño dominated. According to Bennett (1946: 599), "the term *Atacameño* (*Atacama*, *Kunza*) refers to a people, with a distinctive language and culture, who once occupied the northern Chilean provinces of Tacna, Arica, Tarapacá, Antofagasta, and Atacama, and much of the Northwest Argentine provinces of Los Andes, Salta, and Jujuy." "Today, the few remaining *Atacameño* are located in isolated sections of Chile and the Puna de Jujuy, but culturally and linguistically they have been absorbed by *Aymara* or Spanish."

One may ask if in such a region *anything is remembered about the ancient use of snuffing paraphernalia* among the modern mestizo population?

As the Atacameño were basically agriculturists and herders, my question came after I had read two special articles both dealing with the actual culture of typical parts of the old region.[57] Both authors, Horst Nachtigall (1965) and Ana María Mariscotti (1966) underline the importance of traditionally old offering ceremonies to Pachamama, so-called *señaladas*, during which the offers of llama animals (or part of them), alcohol, chicha, coca leaves, etc. are obligatory and important.

The cultural correspondence with the *samiri* concept among the Aymara and Chipaya Indians of the Highland as studied by the late Alfred Métraux during his expedition in 1930 seems important for a very special reason, namely that it has been suggested by Sven Lovén that we consider the Taino word *cemi* as related to Samiri, because of certain facts, among them that the Arawak had asserted themselves also in the western Highland.[58]

On my written question to authors Nachtigall and Mariscotti both declare that the former use of the *tabletas de rapé*, tubes, etc. now is absolutely unknown to anybody in the actual rural population.[59]

---

[56] Naville, René. 1959 : 3.

[57] Nachtigall, Horst. 1965. Mariscotti, Ana María. 1966.

[58] Wassén, H. 1934 : 633. "Dr. Sven Lovén, at the museum of Gothenburg, has mentioned for me that he for certain reasons—among these the fact that the Arawaks have asserted themselves also in the western highland—considers the constituent *sami* of the word *samiri* to be the same as the Tainan *zemi*."

[59] Mrs. Mariscotti, after four different periods of investigation in the Quebrada de Huamahuaca and Puna de Jujuy can assure "that the use of the *tabletas de rapé* which with such frequency are embodied in the "Puna Complex" of Bennett, is absolutely unknown." (Letter, November 16, 1966).

If we now return to the *señaladas*, both Nachtigall (1965 : 216) and Mariscotti (1966 : 74) report *the burning of leaves of khoa or khoba*, an aromatic plant for which they botanically refer to *Mentha pulegium* (of the Family *Labiatae*). This is said by La Barre to be used also amongst the Highland Aymara.[60] With a letter of December 5th, 1966, Mrs. Ana M. Mariscotti has had the kindness to send me a botanical sample of *khoba* collected during her latest trip to Puna de Jujuy. This botanical sample has been examined by the botanist, Dr. Bo Peterson, chief of the Museum of the Gothenburg University's Botanical Institution. According to Dr. Peterson it is not at all the question of a genus of the *Labiatae* Family, but instead a genus of the Family *Compositae*, namely *Lepidophyllum quadrangulare*. Reference has been given to Angel Lulio Cabrera's "*Sinopsus del genero Lepidophyllum (Compositae)*" in the Boletín de la Sociedad Argentina de Botánica (vol. I : 48–58, La Plata, 1945), where the author also gives the popular names *chacha* and *coba* for this plant.

In accordance with what has been said above regarding a possible relation between the word *samiri* and the Island Arawak *cemi*, it is also interesting to suggest a relationship between the Island Arawak (Taino) word *cohoba* and the *khoba* for an aromatic herb in the former Aracameño region with its influence from the Highland and its trade relations. I would like to suggest that *cohoba* and *khoba* are the same words, even if they now refer to different plant material and are used in two widely separated geographic areas. The word we still meet so far south in the form *khoba* should in that case belong to an old stratum of Arawak influence. Professor Nils M. Holmer, specialist on Amerindian languages, write to me (November 17, 1966) that he is sure that an Andean *khowa* (*khoa*) with a strongly aspirated *kh*-, may have been heard as *cohoba*.

The *señaladas* among the present rural mestizo population in Puna de Atacama and Pune de Jujuy represent offshoots of an old Highland tradition with offering to a deity (Pachamama) principally ruling the agricultural cycle. To the Indians, gods, or spirits, were benevolent or ill-disposed, and the medicine-men or other important tribal functionaries had to face a situation which I described in 1965 as influencing the benevolent ones and to weaken or if possible destroy the ill-disposed ones. I have also said that "we are in our full right to believe that such important goals have been reflected also in the art of the Indians, even if we now mostly lack the mythological or other information explaining the connections" (Wassén, 1965 : 38). As the psychotomimetic snuffs must be considered as a means of contact with the spirit world, it is consequently fully understandable that we find Indian representations of their supernatural beings expressed in the art concerning the snuffing paraphernalia. We can, as an example, mention the jaguar motif in the sculpture on ethnographically known snuff trays from the Cashuena Indians of the Trombetas and Cachorro Rivers, Brazil.[61]

---

[60] La Barre, Weston, 1948 : 184. "The leaves and stems of *qoa* (*Mentha pulegium* Linnaeus) are burned in the fields "to make a good harvest," but it is uncertain if this is done for magical reasons, or for the same sound fertilizing reasons with which they place animal manueres on the field." Cf. same author, p. 56, about the use of *Mentha pulegium* as a condiment.

[61] See Frikel, 1961, describing the *mori* feast. Quoted in Wassén and Holmstedt, 1963 : 21–23.

As the illustration on page 8 in Frikel's paper of 1961 on the *mori* feast among the Cachuena unfortunately is very unsharp, I am glad that, thanks to my friend Dr. Carl Schuster of Woodstock, N.Y., I can publish two photos here (Figs. 28 and 29) of the Cashuena specimens. Fig. 28 corresponds to the illustration on page 8 in Frikel's paper. Among the implement for snuffing *mori*, the "shovel" or tray at the right has two confronted jaguars on its handle. Frikel calls the snuff tray *yará-kukúru*, which in Cashuena means "figure of the mythological onça (jaguar) *yará*". The *yará* are "*bichos do fundo, da agua*," "water-jaguars", conceived as a pair, male and female,[62] a fact also of interest for the principle found in Amazonas that "magical substances are always in pairs, male and female" as discussed in Wassén 1965 (p. 76) in regard to the double-headed *paricá* tray of Tucanoan origin. The Cashuena used to have special songs, *iwarawá-yorêmuru*,

---

[62] Frikel. 1961 : 7–8.

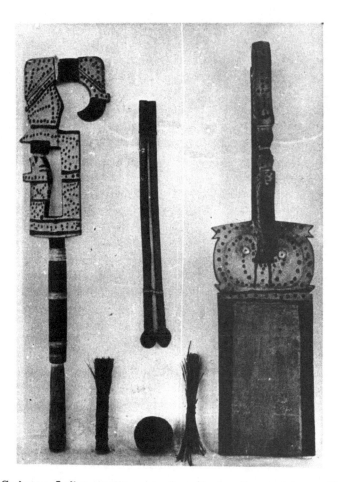

FIG. 28.—Cashuena Indian snuffing paraphernalia for the *mori* feast. Mythological 'water-jaguars' form the handle of the tray. Photo courtesy Dr. Carl Schuster, Woodstock, N.Y. Collection in Brazil.

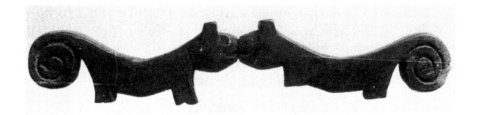

Fig. 29.—Pair of jaguars, one, as of 1954, "three or four generations old" handle of a Cashuena snuff tray. Coll. in Brazil. Photo courtesy Dr. Carl Schuster.

for their snuffing boards. It is deeply regretted that they now are lost (Frikel, 1961: 9) as they probably could have helped to explain the symbolism of the carved motives. As regards the Maué we have the statement by Pereira (1954: 68) that their medicine-men (pagés) used the paricá to get in trance and be able to contact their gods of the waters and the jungle. We are probably save to assume that the "water-jaguars" of the *Cashuena* stand for such deities or spirits.

Dr. Carl Schuster took his photo in Fig. 28 in the Convento dos Franciscanos in Santarem, and the objects were then said to be kept in a Franciscan museum at Ipauarana, Paraiba State. At the same time (November 1954) Schuster also copied a photo of an handle of an old snuff tray from the Cashuena, said to be 3 or 4 generations old, c. 80–100 years. This handle (Fig. 29) has been published in a drawing on page 7 in Frikel's paper from 1961. We see a pair of jaguars, originally with beads in their eyes. Father Frikel informed Dr. Schuster at the time, that a complete tray which he wanted was buried with a shaman. This information confirms my statement from 1965: "If also in former days the carved and ceremonially used snuff trays were placed with the dead this could very well explain their scarcity in collections.[63]

For the tribes of the Uaupés-Caquetá region, Goldman has informed us that "the shaman in the area is generally referred to as a jaguar, and combines the functions of medicine-man and sorcerer. Older shamans assume the guise of the jaguar and are particularly feared. Every jaguar who attacks human beings is assumed to be a shaman, and a shaman who is suspected of such an attack is not infrequently put to death. As the spirit of a murdered shaman enters another jaguar, however, little relief is expected from killing them" (Goldman, 1948: 796). Bödiger (1965: 150) has shown how the names for jaguar and shaman are similar or identical in many of the tribal languages, and how the shaman through this identity in name is considered to have the power of transforming himself into a jaguar—this in a detailed investigation of the Tucano religion.

Again and again we come back to the importance of the jaguar motif for paraphernalia related to snuffing. It is most likely that tribes using jaguar leg-bones as snuff containers do this out of some magical reasons related to the real and magical power of the animal. And, when we find a

---

[63] Wassén. 1965 : 74.

4 cm. long puma figure of stone dominating the snuff tray No. 10718 from Tiahuanaco in the Ethnographical Museum of Buenos Aires (Coll. Debenedetti, 1911), it is really not surprising (Fig. 30).[64] In the *tabletas de rapé* of the Atacameño, the jaguar is seen as a mighty god. Also for this a highly interesting parallel with pure Amazonian ethnographical material can be presented.

In the Ethnographical Museum at Munich we find the so-called Erlangen ceremonial staff, an object which has been studied by Zerries [65] and by him found to be a medicine-man's staff, probably from the Carib *Waríkyana* or *Arikiêna* of the Kachúru (Cachorro) River. Frikel considers the Cashuena, often mentioned in this work, as descendants of the old Waríkyana (see Wassén, 1965: 33), and consequently every old piece of art from that tribe or region must to be of immediate interest also for a study of ceremonially used snuff trays. Zerries found on the Erlangen staff the supernatural vulture, the medicine-man's most important helper, and the figure of a jaguar, "the werwolf of the South American shamans." An anthropomorphic jaguar (or "werwolf" figures) is now seen in Fig. 31 from photos

[64] Photo kindly supplied by Dr. Carl Schuster.
[65] See complete description in Zerries, 1962, and his photo on p. 615.

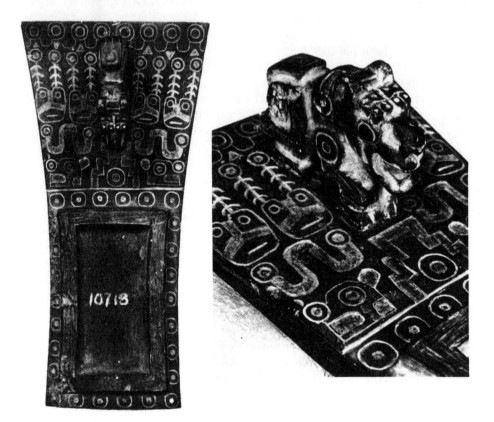

FIG. 30.—Snuff tray with 4 cm. long puma of stone. Tiahuanaco. Coll. No. 10718 (Debenedetti, 1911), *Museo Etnográfico*, Buenos Aires. Photo courtesy Dr. Carl Schuster.

280

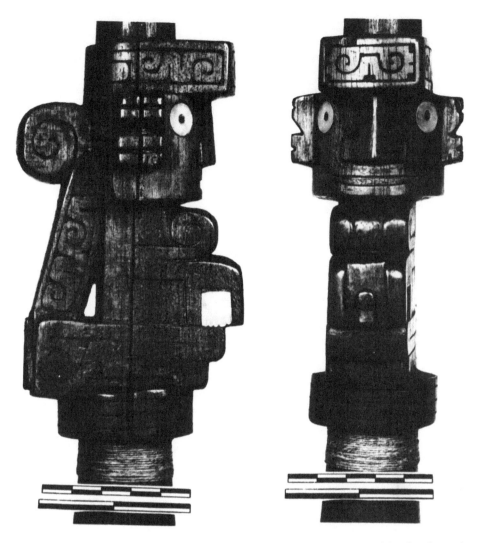

Fɪɢ. 31.—Ornamental detail, anthropomorphic jaguar on a trumpet of hard red wood. Old specimen in the Pitts Rivers Museum (No. 130, J. 44), without provenience but certainly from the Lower Amazon Region, probably the old Waríkyana. Photographs courtesy of Mr. Jeremy P. S. Montagu, London.

which have been kindly supplied by Mr. Jeremy P. S. Montagu, London. The figure shows a "side-blast trumpet made of two semicylindrical pieces of hard red wood." This specimen, now in the Pitt Rivers Museum (entry 130.J.44) came from "the Bodleian" to the University Museum in Oxford, presumably, then transferred to the Pitt Rivers Museum in 1886." It is an old piece of Indian art for which the provenience is lacking, but as far as I understand it should be referred to the same region as the Erlangen staff, that is, the Lower Amazon region and from the old Waríkyana in the art center of the *Rio das contas* (cf. Wassén, 1965 : 34). A similar 123 cm. long trumpet with jaguar motif (his tail curled down) from an old collection

262–016 O–67—20

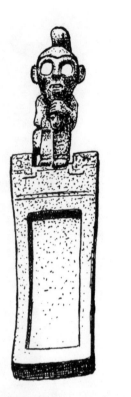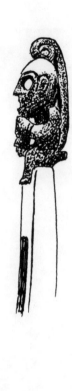

Fig. 32.—Snuff tray from "Quitor 5", San Pedro de Atacama, Chile. Dominating anthropomorphic feline god. Drawing after photographic illustration in Le Paige, 1964.

and the Amazon is found in the Rijksmuseum voor Volkenkunde, Leyden. It belonged originally to "Het Kon. Kabinet van Zeldzaamheden."

An important detail in this jaguar-man on a trumpet is the tail, which goes up on the back and ends in a characteristic curl. The reason I find it important might be understood from Fig. 32, in which the figure on a snuff tray found in "Quitor 5" in the region of San Pedro de Atacama, Chile, by Gustavo Le Paige, has been copied from plate 125 in Le Paige's work of 1964. The snuff tray from Chile is an expression of the same idea of a jaguar (or puma)-man-deity as found on the old trumpet, and the tail is a characteristic of both figures. To me these specimens form another link in a chain of evidence for an early Amazon cultural influence on the Atacaman region. Thanks to a numerous series of snuff tray finds in the dry region, Father Le Paige has been able to demonstrate specific manifestations of magico-religious art in which the taking of a man's head is involved. In snuffing paraphernalia which he found, he can follow a complete series of ceremonies, from the presentation of a condemned man with backbound hands and the executioner with his attribute, an axe, to the priest carrying the head of the victim—in that important moment imitating the sacred puma god by walking on all fours and carrying a puma mask and the wings of a condor.[66]

---

[66] Le Paige, Gustavo. 1964: 61. Mostny (1964) has been able to show such ceremonialism also in the petroglyphs of Angostura, Prov. of Antofagasta, Chile.

282

Gustavo Le Paige and other archaeologists working in the Atacaman region find this richness of evidence thanks to a dry climate. What the anthropologists have found, or may expect to find, in the eternally wet Amazon region, are just a few fragments of a formerly rich ceremonialism in which the taking of psychotomimetic drugs seems to have been integrated.

A group of snuff trays from the Amazon region with an obviously important zoomorphic motif are the Maué specimens said to depict caymans or snakes. Several of these old fine Maué wooden trays have fortunately been saved in museum collections.[67] The specimen in Oslo is shown also here (Fig. 33). Typical for most of the Maué trays, is the fact that they are rectangular in form and have a finely polished depository for the snuff, open on the edge of the board. The other edge of the tray ends in an animal's head, often with an accentuated tongue, a trait typical for representations of snakes but hardly for caymans in which the tongue is not easily observable. It is true that a Maué Indian has once stated that a *paricá* tray owned by him represented a *yacaré*, but as I have said, this label can not be stamped on all snuff trays from this tribe.[68] Anthropological colleagues such as Etta Becker-Donner in Vienna, and Antonio Serrano in Argentina, as well as Otto Zerries in Munich, seem to favor the idea of snakes.[69] The Atacama specimen published in Fig. 22 has, however, *a feline head*. As this archaeological specimen is much older than the 19th century ethnographical objects from the Maué, it is of interest also for the discussion of the Maué pieces. As a matter of fact, some of the Maué tray handles in the form of animal heads may be conceived as conventionalized feline heads, perhaps with some idea of "water-jaguars" behind as in the case with the Cashuena. The outstreatched tongue is accentuated in the feline powder cup published as Fig. 5 in Zerries: 1965. A most interesting snuff tray with two feline heads found in a grave at the Pucará de Lasana (Río Loa, Chile) has been published by Spahni (1964, Fig. 5). His Fig. 4, showing a snuff tray from another grave said to represent an armadillo, most probably also depicts a feline.

Another group of animals which in a particular symbolic and magic way seem to be connected with the use of drugs are birds with very good eyesight, such as eagles, vultures, very often condors, and also such good night-hunting birds as owls (the Cashuena snuff tray in Fig. 28). I have treated this in detail in my work from 1965 (pp. 24–29), and I can reiterate here, that we are entitled to consider birds as patrons for ecstatic intoxication in several Indian societies. I refer, for instance, to snuff trays with condors, bird-shaped snuffers, snuffing tubes which terminate in hollow nuts, often shaped like a bird's head (Fig. 34), and also, to direct explanations by medicine-men that they use feather crowns, etc. so that they may see better into the world of spirits. This connection between the shamans as users of drugs and the world of bird-spirits is a fact. The reason for it is probably to be found in

[67] See figs. 8, 10, 11, 12 and 15 in Wassén 1965.
[68] Wassén. 1965 : 43.
[69] Wassén. 1965 : 43 and 50.

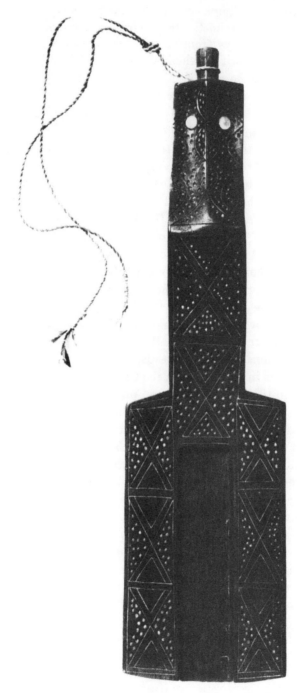

FIG. 33.—Maué Indian snuff tray of wood for *paricá*. Length 28 cm. Coll. and courtesy Oslo Univ. Ethnogr. Museum. Specimen No. 1170.

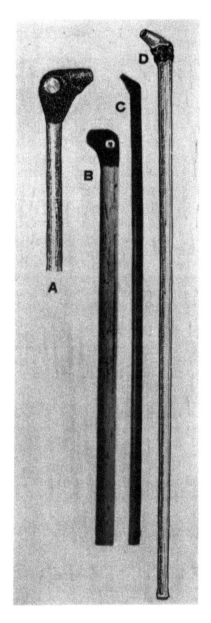

Fig. 34.—Snuff tubes from the Guaporé Territory. *A*, Mondé Indians, after photo by Caspar; *B*, Salamay Indians, coll. *Mus. f. Völkerkunde der Univ.*, Zürich, No. 11307; *C-D*, Tupari Indians, coll. Dr. Franz Caspar in the *Mus. f. Völkerkunde*, Basel, No. 1V C 9052, length 88 cm. (photo and drawing of the same tube).

the drugs,[70] and I point, in passing, to the complex of Siberian shamans being described as of bird-type, who visit the spirits up in the air. This, incidentally, is a contrast to the other type of Siberian shamans, who have their contacts in the world below.[71] The ideas among the Koryak about the Big-Raven and the fly-agaric give a good illustration of this.[72] I hope that later a common component will be found in all this, through the analytical work by experts on the drugs involved.

No specific search has been performed for this paper regarding the possible use of snuff tubes outside America, where they seem to be autochthonous.[73] Dr. Gordon Willey (1966: 22), has counted "the chewing of lime or ashes with some kind of a narcotic" as one of the very ancient traits, possibly the survival of a Palaeolithic heritage, which "are shared by Asia and the New World." Willey naturally refers to the use of betel-nut in Asia and the coca leaf in South America, and he finds a considerable age for the trait in the Americas.

BIBLIOGRAPHY

BENNETT, WENDELL C. (1946). "The Atacameño." Handb. of S. Amer. Indians, 2: 599–618. Bur. of Amer. Ethn., Bull. 143. Washington.

BIRD, JUNIUS B. (1948). "Preceramic Cultures in Chicama and Virú." Pp. 21–28 in Wendell C. Bennett: A Reappraisal of Peruvian Archaeology. Mem. of the Soc. for Amer. Arch. No. 4, Suppl. to Amer. Antiquity 13: 4, pt 2. Menasha, Wisc.

BÖDIGER, UTE. (1965). "Die Religion der Tukano." Kölner Ethnol. Mitteilungen 3. Cologne.

BOURNE, EDWARD GAYLORD. (1906). "Columbus, Ramon Pane and the Beginnings of American Anthropology." Reprinted from the Proc. of the Amer. Ant. Soc., Worcester, Mass.

BROOKS, JEROME E. (1937). "Tobacco." Its History illustrated by the Books, Manuscripts and Engravings in the Library of George Arents, Jr. Vol. I, 1507–1615. New York, The Rosenbach Company.

CASANOVA, EDUARDO. (1946). "The Cultures of the Puna and the Quebrada of Humahuaca." Handb. of S. Amer. Indians, 2: 619–631. Bur. of Amer. Ethn., Bull. 143. Washington.

CASPAR, FRANZ. (1952). "Tupari." Unter Indios im Urwald Brasiliens. Braunschweig.

CASPAR, FRANZ. (1953). MS. "Ein Kulturareal der Hinterland der Flüsse Guaporé und Machado (Westbrasilien), dargestellt nach unveröffentlichten und anderen wenig bekannten Quellen, mit besonderer Berücksichtigung der Nahrungs- und Genussmittel." (Dissertation). Hamburg.

CASTELLANOS, JUAN DE. (1850). "Elegías de Varones Ilustres de Indias." 2nd ed. Bibl. de Autores Españoles, t. IV. Madrid.

[70] Wassén. 1965: 29. I can add that the sensation of being airborne through the taking of *ayahuasca* has been described from the Zaparo already by Manuel Villavicencio in 1858 (p. 372) :" Su accion parece dirijirse á escitar el sistema nervioso ; todos los sentidos se avivan i todas las facultades se despiertan ; sienten vahidos i rodeos de cabeza, luego la sensación de elevarse al aire i comenzar un viaje aéreo ; . . ."

[71] La Barre, Weston. 1964: 121. "En Sibérie, peuve être distingués deux types de chamans : le chaman-oiseau qui visite les esprits dans les airs et règne sur le temps qu'il fait, et le chaman-renne qui visite le monde souterrain et règne sur les esprits des vivants et de morts."

[72] Jochelsen, Waldemar. 1905 : 120.

[73] Prof. B. Holmstedt has drawn my attention to a paper by Chinachoti and Tangchai (1957 : 689), where the U-shaped metal tubes used in Thailand for the nasal absorbtion of a mixed tobacco powder has been treated. A pair of such tubes with the commercial packages of such ingredients as tobacco, quicklime and perfume, are found in the Gothenburg Ethnographic Museum (Coll. 64.25.97–102).

CHINACHOTI, NINART and PRASAN TANGCHAI. (1957). "Pulmonary Alveolar Microlithiasis Associated with the Inhalation of Snuff in Thailand." Diseases of the Chest, vol. 32, No. 1, pp. 687–689.

COOPER, JOHN M. (1949). "Stimulants and Narcotics." Handb. of S. Amer. Indians, 5: 525–558. Bur. of Amer. Ethn., Bull. 143. Washington.

ERNST, A. (1889). "On the etymology of the word tobacco." The Amer. Anthropologist, 2: 2, pp. 133–142. Washington.

FRIEDERICI, GEORG. (1925). (Review). "Sven Lovén, Ueber die Wurzeln der Tainischen Kultur." Göttingische Gelehrte Anzeigen, 187. Jahrg., pp. 32–43. Berlin.

FRIEDERICI, GEORG. (1947). Amerikanistisches Wörterbuch, Hamburg.

FRIKEL, PROTÁSIO. (1961). "Mori—A Festa de Rapé." Boletim do Museu Paraense Emilio Goeldi, Antropologia No. 12, Belém, Pará.

GOLDMAN, IRVING. (1948). "Tribes of the Uaupés-Caquetá Region." Handb. of S. Amer. Indians, 3: 763–798. Bur. of Amer. Ethn., Bull. 143. Washington.

GUMILLA, JOSEPH. (1744). "El Orinoco Ilustrado, y defendido." Historia Natural, Civil, y Geographica de este gran Río, etc., tomo I. Madrid.

HAGEN, VICTOR W. von. (1965). "The Desert Kingdoms of Peru." New York Graphic Soc. publ., Ltd. Greenwich, Conn.

HARRISON, D. F. N. (1964). "Snuff—Its Use and Abuse." British Medical Journal, 1964, 2, 1649–1651.

HERNÁNDEZ DE ALBA, GREGORIO. (1948). "The Achagua and their neighbors." Handb. of S. Amer. Indians, 4: 399–412. Bur. of Amer. Ethn., Bull. 143. Washington.

HOLMSTEDT, B. (1965). "Tryptamine derivatives in epená, an intoxicating snuff used by some South American Indian tribes." Arch. int. Pharmacodyn., 1965, 156, No. 2: 285–305. Brussells, Belgium.

HOLMSTEDT, B. (1966). "Gas Chromatographic Analysis of Some Psychoactive Indole Bases." Amines and Schizophrenia, Pergamon Press, Oxford & Now York, 1966, pp. 151–166.

HUMBOLDT, ALEXANDER VON and AIMÉ BONPLAND. (1818–1829). Personal Narrative of Travels to the Equinoctial Regions of the New Continent during the years 1799–1804, translated by Helen Maria Williams. 7 vols. London.

JOCHELSEN, WALDEMAR. (1905). "Religion and Myths of the Koryak." Mem. of the Amer. Mus. of Nat. Hist. X. New York.

JOYCE, THOMAS A. (1916). Central American and West Indian Archaeology, London.

KIRCHHOFF, PAUL. (1948). "Food-Gathering Tribes of the Venezuelan Llanos." Handb. of S. Amer. Indians, 4: 445–468. Bur. of Amer. Ethn., Bull. 143. Washington.

LA BARRE, WESTON. (1948). "The Aymara Indians of the Lake Titicaca Plateau, Bolivia." Mem. Series of the Amer. Anthrop. Ass., No. 68. Amer. Anthrop., Vol. 50: 1, pt. 2. Menasha, Wisc.

LA BARRE, WESTON. (1964). "Le complexe narcotique de l'Amérique Autochtone." Diogène 48: 120–134. Paris.

LAS CASAS, BARTOLOMÉ DE. (1909). "Apologética historia de las Indias." Historiadores de Indias, I, M. Serrano y Sanz, Ed., Madrid.

LATCHAM, RICARDO E. (1938). "Arqueología de la Región Atacameña." Prensas de la Univ. de Chile.

LE PAIGE, GUSTAVO. (1964). "El precerámico en la Cordillera Atacameña y los cementerios del período agro-alfarero de San Pedro de Atacama." Anales de la Univ. del Nort, Antofagasta: 3. Antofagasta.

LE PAIGE, GUSTAVO. (1965). "San Pedro de Atacama y su zona." Anales de la Univ. del Norte, Antofagasta: 4. Antofagasta.

LOVÉN, SVEN. (1935). Origins of the Tainan Culture, West Indies. Göteborg.

MACNUTT, FRANCIS AUGUSTUS. (1912). "De Orbe Novo. The Eight Decades of Peter Martyr d'Anghera." Transl. from Latin with Notes and Introduction. 1–2. New York and London.

MANGONES, EDMOND and LOUIS MAXIMILIEN. (1941). L'Art Précolombien d'Haïti. Port-au-Prince, Haïti.

287

MARKHAM, CLEMENTS R. (1869). First part of the Royal Commentaries of the Yncas by the Ynca Garcilasso de la Vega. Vol. I. Works issued by the Hakluyt Soc. London.

MARISCOTTI, ANA MARÍA. (1966). "Algunas supervivencias del culto a la Pachamama." El complejo ceremonial del 1°. de Agosto en Jujuy (NO. Argentino) y sus vinculaciones. Zeitschrift f. Ethnologie 91 : 1, pp. 68–99. Braunschweig.

MÁRTIR DE ANGLERÍA, PEDRO. (1944). "Décadas del Nuevo Mundo." Editorial Bajel. Buenos Aires.

MARTIUS, CARL FR. V. (1867). Beiträge zur Ethnographie und Sprachenkunde Amerika's zumal Brasiliens. I. Zur Ethnographie. Leipzig.

MATTO, FRANCISCO. (1964). "Arte Precolombino." Colección Matto. Museo de Arte Precolombino. Montevideo.

MEGGERS, BETTY J. and CLIFFORD EVANS. (1957). "Archaeological Investigations at the Mouth of the Amazon." Bur. of Amer. Ethn., Bull. 167. Washington.

MÉTRAUX, A. (1928). La Réligion des Tupinamba et ses rapports avec celle des autres tribus tupi-guarani. Paris.

MÉTRAUX, A. (1946). "The Caingang." Handb. of S. Amer. Indians, 1: 445–476. Bur. of Amer. Ethn., Bull. 143. Washington.

MÉTRAUX, A. (1948). "The Guarani." Handb. of S. Amer. Indians, 3 : 69–94. Bur. of Amer. Ethn., Bull. 143. Washington.

MÉTRAUX, A. (1948 a). "The Tupinamba." Handb. of S. Amer. Indians, 3 : 95–134. Bur. of Amer. Ethn., Bull. 143. Washington.

MONTEIRO DE NORONHA, JOSÉ. (1862). Roteiro da viagem da Cidade do Pará, até as ultimas colonias do Sertao da Província. Pará.

MOSTNY, G. (1952). "Una tumba de Chiuchiu." Bol. del Museo Nacional de Hist. Nat. 26 : 1. Santiago de Chile.

MOSTNY, G. (1958). "Máscaras, tubos y tabletas para rapé y cabezas trofeos entre los atacameños." Miscellanea Paul Rivet Octogenario Dicata, Vol. II : 379–392. Mexico.

MOSTNY, G. (1964). "Petroglifos de Angostura." Zeitschrift f. Ethnologie, 89 : 1, pp. 51–70. Braunschweig.

MUÑOA, JUAN IGNACIO. (1965). "Los pueblos prehistóricos del Territorio Uruguayo." Ed. Daniel Vidart. Amerindia 3. Montevideo.

NACHTIGALL, HORST. (1965). "Beiträge zur Kultur der indianischen Lamazüchter der Puna de Atacama (Nordwest-Argentiniens)." Zeitschrift f. Ethnologie 90 : 2, pp. 184–218. Braunschweig.

NAVILLE, RENÉ. (1959). "Tablettes et tubes à aspirer du râpé." Bulletin No. 17, Soc. Suisse des Américanistes. Geneva.

NETTO, LADISLAU. (1885). "Investigaçoes sobre a Archeologia Brazileira." Arch. do Museu Nacional, VI : 257–554. Rio de Janeiro.

NORDENSKIÖLD, ERLAND. (1919). "Sydamerika." Kampen om guld och silver 1498–1600. Uppsala.

NUÑEZ A., LAUTARO. (1963). "Problemas en torno a la tableta rapé." Anales de la Univ. del Norte, Antofagasta : 2. Antofagasta.

NUÑEZ A., LAUTARO. (1965). "Desarrollo cultural prehispánico del Norte de Chile." Estudios Arqueológicos No. 1 : 37–115. Univ. de Chile, Antofagasta. Antofagasta.

OVIEDO, GONZALO, FERNANDEZ DE. (1851–1855). "Historia general y natural de las Indias, Islas y Tierra-Firma del Mar Oceáno." Vols. 1–4, Real Acad. de Hist., Madrid.

PALMATARY, HELEN C. (1960). "The Archaeology of the Lower Tapajós Valley, Brazil." Transactions of the Amer. Philosophical Soc., n.s. 50 : 3. Philadelphia, Pa.

PEREIRA, NUNES. (1954). "Os Indios Manés." Coleção "Rex". Rio de Janeiro.

PINTO, ESTEBAN. (1944). "La extraña figura del pagé tupinambá." Actas Ciba 11, La medicina de los tupí-guaraníes, pp. 319–328. Buenos Aires.

PITTIER, H. (1926). Manual de las plantas usuales de Venezuela. Caracas.

REIS ALTSCHUL, SIRI VON. (1964). "A Taxonomic Study of the Genus Anadenanthera." Contr. from the Gray Herbarium of Harv. Univ., No. 193. Cambridge, Mass.

ROSENBLAT, ANGEL. (1965). "Los Otomacos y Taparitas de los Llanos de Venezuela." Anuario I., 1964 : 227–377. Instituto de Antropología e Historia. Caracas.

288

Rouse, Irving. (1964). "Prehistory of the West Indies." Science, vol. 144: 499–513. Washington, D.C., May 1, 1964.

Rydén, Stig. (1944). Contributions to the Archaeology of the Río Loa Region, Göteborg.

Salas, Alberto Mario. (1945). "El antigal de Ciénega Grande (Quebrada de Purmamarca, Prov. de Jujuy)." (Publ. del Mus. Etnográfico de la Fac. de Fil. y Letras, Serie A V. Buenos Aires.

Sawyer, Alan R. (1966). Ancient Peruvian Ceramics. The Nathan Cummings Collection. The Metropolitan Museum of Art. New York.

Schultes, Richard Evans. (1954). A new narcotic snuff from the Northwest Amazon. Bot. Mus. Leaflets, Harv. Univ., vol. 16: 9, pp. 241–260. Cambridge, Mass.

Schultes, Richard Evans. (1955). A new narcotic genus from the Amazon slope of the Colombian Andes. Bot. Mus. Leaflets, Harv. Univ., vol. 17: 1, pp. 1–11. Cambridge, Mass.

Schultes, Richard Evans. (1963). "Hallucinogenic Plants of the New World." The Harvard Review, I: 4, pp. 18–32. Cambridge, Mass.

Seitz, Georg. (1960). "Hinter dem grünen Vorhang." Fahrt zu den nackten Indianern an der Grenze Brasiliens. F. A. Brockhaus, Wiesbaden.

Serrano, Antonio. (1939). "Las tabletas para "paricá" del Museo Nacional de Rio de Janeiro." La Nación, June 4, 1939. Buenos Aires.

Spahni, Jean-Christian. (1964). "Le cimetière atacaménien du Pucará de Lasana, Vallée du Rio Loa (Chili)." Journ. de la Société des Américanistes, vol. 53: 147–179. Paris.

Steward, Julian H. (1948). "The Circum-Caribbean Tribes: An Introduction." Handb. of S. Amer. Indians, 4: 1–41. Bur. of Amer. Ethn., Bull. 143. Washington.

Stone, Doris. (1958). Introduction to the Archaeology of Costa Rica. San José, C.R.

Uhle, Max. (1898). "A Snuffing Tube from Tiahuanaco." Bull. of the Mus. of Science and Art, Univ. of Penna., Vol. I: 4. Phila., Pa.

Uscategui, M., Nestor. (1959). "The present distribution of narcotics and stimulants amongst the Indian tribes of Colombia." Bot. Mus. Leaflets, Harv. Univ., vol. 18: 6, pp. 273–304. Cambridge, Mass.

Wassén, Henry. (1934). "The Frog in Indian Mythology and Imaginative World." Anthropos 29: 613–658. St. Gabriel-Mödling at Vienna.

Wassén, S. Henry. (1964). "Some General Viewpoints in the Study of Native Drugs Especially from the West Indies and South America." Ethnos 1964: 1–2, pp. 97–120. Stockholm.

Wassén, S. Henry. (1965). "The Use of Some Specific Kinds of South American Indian Snuff and Related Paraphernalia." Etnologiska Studier 28: 1–116. Göteberg, Etnografiska Museet.

Wassén, S. Henry and Bo Holmstedt. (1963). "The Use of Paricá, an Ethnological and Pharmacological Review." Ethnos 1963: 1, pp. 5–45. Stockholm.

Villavicencio, Manuel. (1858). Geografía de la República del Ecuador. New York.

Wilbert, Johannes. (1963). "Indios de la Región Orinoco-Ventuari." Monografía No. 8, Fundación La Salle de Ciencias Naturales. Caracas.

Willey, Gordon. (1966). An Introduction to American Archaeology. Vol. I, North and Middle America. Prentice-Hall, Inc., Englewood Cliffs, N.J.

Zerries, Otto. (1962). "Der Zeremonialstab der Erlanger Sammlung aus Brasilien in Staatlichen Mus. f. Völkerkunde" in München. Akten der 34. Internat. Amer. Kongr., Vienna, 1960, pp. 613–620. Vienna.

Zerries, Otto. (1964). "Waika." Die kulturgeschichtliche Stellung der Waikaindianer des oberen Orinoco im Rahmen der Völkerkunde Südamerikas. Klaus Renner Verlag, Munich.

Zerries, Otto. (1965). "Drei unbekannte Holzschnitzarbeiten aus Brasilianisch-Guayana im Museum für Völkerkunde zu Mannheim." Tribus 14: 185–193. Stuttgart.

The Botanical Origins of
South American Snuffs

Richard Evans Schultes

Botanical Museum of Harvard University, Cambridge, Massachusetts

Introduction

Man in primitive societies the world around has found the most ingenious ways of administering narcotics. Intoxicating plants, or products from them, have been chewed in crude form or variously elaborated and consumed. They have been drunk as decoctions or infusions. A few have been prepared in the form of thick syrups or pastes that are licked or smeared on the tongue or gums. Some have been smoked directly, as in pipes, cigars or cigarettes, or the fumes of them have been inhaled in sundry ways. There are those that have been applied to the skin or membranes in the form of ointments or unguents. Several are known to have been taken as an enema. Snuffing has been the preferred method of using a number of these agents.

The verb *to snuff* (and the corresponding German *schupfen* and Skandinavian *snusa*), stems, of course, from the same Germanic root that has given us the English word *to sniff*. There is a significant difference between the two actions. Whereas one *sniffs* an odour or fragrance—that is, a substance such as an essential oil, smoke or ethereal component of the atmosphere—one *snuffs* actually solid substances variously inserted or drawn into the nostrils.

The snuffing of plant materials for narcotic, especially for hallucinogenic, effects seems to be peculiarly New World. To be sure, sternutation induced by various means is a recognized therapeutic practice in many cultures. In the Middle Ages, European medicine recommended sternutation to draw off bad humours. Hellebore, the German *Nieswurz* and English *sneezewort*, was one of the most favoured therapeutic sternutatory powders taken into the nostrils together with marjoram and other plants to cleanse the brain through sneezing. Sternutation was used even for prophesying and in superstition and magic. A person who sneezed on New Year's morning, for example, would not die during the year. *Snuffing* now refers usually to the use of tobacco. This is true in languages other than English. The German *schupfen*, for example, has been more or less restricted to the snuffing of tobacco and other stimulants since the 17th Century.

It does seem probable, however, that the use of narcotics as snuffs is of American origin and that it went to the Old World with tobacco. The custom of snuffing tobacco, widespread apparently in pre-Conquest America, became common and accepted as a recreational practice devoid of therapeutic intent in Spain during the first quarter of the 17th Century. There is evidence that it was imported directly from the New World and that tobacco snuffing, as well as chewing and smoking, represents one of the most significant culture traits passed on to the western civilisation from the American aborigines.

Principal Sources of South American Snuffs

Undoubtedly the most important snuffing material in pre-Conquest America was tobacco. At least two species of tobacco, possibly several additional ones, are known to have been employed as a narcotic (4). These two are *Nicotiana Tabacum* and *N. rustica*. *Nicotiana Tabacum*, from which comes most of the tobacco that is smoked, snuffed and chewed at the present time, was likewise the source of most of the narcotic in pre-Conquest South America, Middle America and the West Indies. Originally a tropical species, it has been cultivated so long that it is not known in the truly wild state. *Nicotiana rustica*, native to North America, where it is still wild in some localities, is a hardier species thought to have originated in Mexico. It is this species that was smoked and probably snuffed by Indians of Mexico and North America before the arrival of the European. Europeans introduced *Nicotiana Tabacum* from the Old World to North America long after the Conquest, and until this introduction, it was apparently unknown in most of the territory now included in the United States and Canada (9).

Although there are indirect evidences that tobacco may have been taken as snuff in Mexico and other parts of North America, there can be no doubt that in much of South America this was the most widespread method of utilizing the narcotic, especially in the wet, tropical lowland areas, such as the Amazon Valley. So many observations attest to this fact that there would seem to be little if any need for a discussion of the custom, were it not that perhaps confusion as to the source of a number of snuff preparations may have led to the assumption that tobacco snuffing, though widespread, might have been even more widespread than it actually was. Yet botanists and anthropologists have consistently warned against such generalisations. Mason, for example, stated (13) that "the snuff taken throughout . . . most of the Amazon and West Indies . . . is more frequently made from other plants than tobacco." And Cooper owned (4) that "tobacco snuffing . . ." is "not always distinguishable in our sources from *Piptadenia* snuffing."

Garcilaso de la Vega (8) reported that the Inca did not cultivate tobacco or *sayri*, but they are thought to have utilised several varieties native to the Andes, the roots of which were pulverised and used medicinally and as a snuff (15).

Botanists are understandably wont to be somewhat more conservative in ethnobotanical generalisations than are anthropologists. Goodspeed, for example, in his classic work (*9*) on the genus *Nicotiana*, wrote that "presumably *N. tabacum* was in pre-Columbian use, doubtless often in cultivation, in the West Indies, much of Mexico, Central America, Colombia, Venezuela, the Guianas and Brazil. Spinden . . . apparently would extend this range to Peru, Boliva, Chile and Argentina, since tubes 'for taking snuff, presumably of tobacco, occur far and wide' in those areas . . . . There is, however, considerable doubt that the material snuffed in the tubes so familiar in remains of certain ancient civilisations in the Americas was 'tobacco' obtained either from early races of *N. tabacum* or from progenitors of the species of *Nicotiana* which today are native in the regions concerned. In other words, there is little evidence that *N. Tabacum* was in pre-Columbian use in western North America or in lower South America."

Tobacco in snuffing—whether the source of the snuff be *Nicotiana Tabacum* or some other species of the genus—seems quite generally to have been used alone, although there are occasional reports that it is sometimes mixed with *Anadenanthera*. Amongst the tribes of the Guaporé River in Amazonian Brazil, tobacco snuff was mixed with "crushed angíco leaves [*angíco* refers to leguminous trees, especially to *Anadenanthera*] and ashes of a certain bark" (*12*). During my years of field work amongst the Indians of the northwestern Amazon, I witnessed the preparation of tobacco snuff on many occasions and actually employed the snuff myself instead of smoking. The species used was *Nicotiana Tabacum*, and with two exceptions, I never saw the admixture of any other plant to the snuff—that is, other than ashes. These two exceptions were with the Witotos of the Rìo Igaraparaná and the Yukunas of the Río Miritiparaná of Colombia, where powdered coca (*Erythroxylon Coca*) is added to the tobacco. It is my belief that the ashes (usually from bark of *Theobroma* or leaves of *Cecropia*) serve mainly or wholly a physical function to help keep the finely pulverised and sifted tobacco particle from absorbing humidity from the excessively wet atmosphere and lumping so that the material could not be used as a snuff.

South America boasts a wide variety of containers and implements for the administration and self-administration of snuffs. Since there is normally, I believe, no relationship between these paraphernalia and the botanical source of the snuffs, I need not here discuss this intricate topic which has already been thoroughly investigated by a more competent specialist (*27*).

A critical survey of tobacco snuffing in South America, incorporating all of the extensive literature interpreted against the background of intensive field observations, is overdue. I venture to predict that, as such a study unravels the enigmas, we shall see other narcotic snuffs assume greater roles and tobacco find a progresively less important role than it has been given in our ethnobotanical evaluation.

One of the most interesting and enigmatic snuffs of South America is yopo or niopo, prepared from the beans of the leguminous tree *Anadenanthera peregrina*. During its botanical history, this plant has been placed in the related genera *Acacia* and *Mimosa*. It is perhaps best known under the binomial *Piptadenia peregrina*, but recent studies have indicated that it is most appropriately accommodated within *Anadenanthera* (*1*).

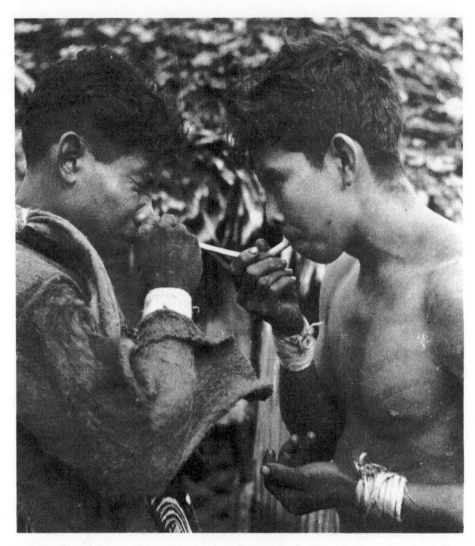

FIG. 1.—Use of the straight bird-bone snuffing-tube for administration of the tobbaco-coca snuff of the Yukuna Indians, Río Miritiparaná, Amazonas, Colombia. Photograph by R. E. Schultes.

Of possible significance is the curious fact that *Anadenanthera peregrina* is or has been employed not only in northern South America but probably in the Antilles as well. Tobacco snuffing was a well established custom in the West Indian islands long before the arrival of Europeans, and the snuffing in Hispaniola of a narcotic, vision-producing powder called *cohoba* was no cause for intellectual curiosity, since most early writers assumed that cohoba was merely another tobacco snuff. It was the American enthno-botanist Safford who first identified, quite correctly, I believe, the West Indian cohoba snuff with the yopo of the Orinoco basin of Venezuela and Colombia (*16*).

There were a number of reports in the literature ascribing the sources of Amazonian snuffs to various leguminous trees, and its was Bentham who "came to the conclusion that all South American trees . . . referred to as the source of narcotic snuff were probably one species and were identical with Linnaeus' *Mimosa peregrina*, which was first described in 1737 from a seedling growing in the celebrated Clifford Garden in Holland" (*16*). It seems that one of the most extraordinarily mistaken generalisations in ethnobotany—that all of the narcotic snuffs of the Amazon that were not obviously tobacco must have been prepared from *Anadenanthera peregrina*— has stemmed from Benthem's conclusions. This generalisation, of course, has not been without influence, judging from the state of confusion and lack of clarity encountered in many of the earliest reports of "smoking" and "snuffing." We have no clear distinction, in many early instances, as to whether tobacco or cohoba represented the plant the use of which was being described, since tobacco was snuffed in the Caribbean area at the time of the arrival of the Spaniards.

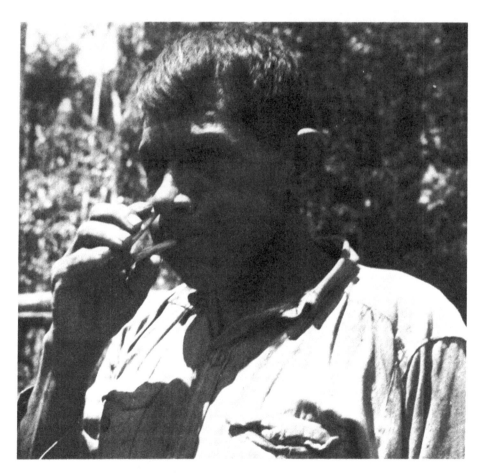

Fig. 2.—Tanimuka Indian administering tobacco-coca snuff with the V-shaped bird-bone snuffing tube employed for self-administration. Río Miritiparaná, Amazonas, Colombia. Photograph by R. E. Schultes.

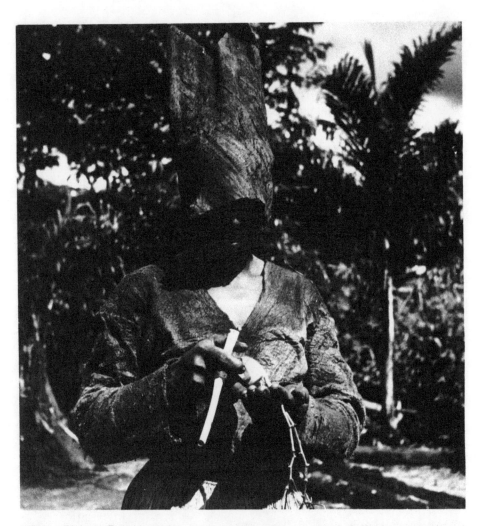

FIG. 3.—Yukuna Indian pouring out into the hand from a snail-shell case a quantity of tobacco-coca snuff for insertion into the bird-bone snuffing tube. Río Miritiparaná, Amazonas, Colombia. Photograph by R. E. Schultes.

A recently published map (*4*), showng the distribution of snuffs made from *Anadenanthera*, includes the entire Orinoco basin and adjacent areas of southern Venezuela to the east; westward across the northern Colombian Andes, much of the Magdalena Valley; down the Andes through Columbia, Ecuador, Peru and Bolivia; the coastal region of Peru, and scattered isolated areas in northern Argentina, and the central and western Amazon Valley. One must remember that this map refers not to one species but to a genus—and there have been suggestions that species other than *Anadenanthera peregrina* have entered the South American snuff making picture. Furthermore, one must recall that Cooper himself cautioned that "our tribal records on which the . . . distribution map . . . is based are probably very incomplete. On the other hand, some of the attributions may not be correct, since in some cases the lack of exact botanical identification makes

296

it doubtful whether we have to do with *Piptadenia* snuff, tobacco snuff or snuff from some other plant . . . ."

When I first went to the northwesternmost Amazon in Colombia—a region the flora of which I investigated in the field from 1941 to 1953—I fully expected to meet with the use of yopo snuff. One of my reasons for choosing this geographcal area for my studies was our knowledge that here the aborigines were reported to be using more kinds of narcotic preparations than in any comparable region of the world. Consultation with the sparse literature for this part of the Amazon basin led me to believe that yopo snuff from *Anadenanthera peregrina* was known and employed throughout the area. True, amongst the Witotos, Kubeos, Yukunas, Tanimukas, Tukanos, Makunas and other native groups, I met with the use, oftentimes excessive use, of tobacco snuff. I never met with anything called yopo or niopo, and what was more confusing to me as a botanist was my failure to encounter, wild or cultivated, a single tree of *Anadenanthera peregrina*. This species grows cultivated in the Llanos of Colombia—the Orinoco drainage area of Colombia, northerly adjacent to its Amazon area. Furthermore, from the writings of Spruce (*24*) and other earlier travellers, as well as from reports of missionaries of the present day, we know that this hallucinating snuff was and is employed extensively and in large amounts by the naitves of the Llanos. My later explorations and researches in the Colombian Amazon convinced me that generalisation from reports in the available literature had led to gross error; that, in effect, yopo snuff not only is *not* used but is actually unknown, and that the tree does not occur, at least in the northwesternmost Amazon. Furthermore, since I was resident for three years in country of the Tikuna Indians of the uppermost Amazon River at the point where Brazil, Colombia and Peru join, I was especially interested in the assumption that these natives formerly made snuff from *Anadenanthera* (*3*). Inasmuch as I met no tree of this species in the area nor did I see the Tikunas (who do make tobacco snuff) prepare snuff from leguminous seeds, I must conclude that this specific instance is also one of the numerous erroneous generalisations.

How can we assume, or justify an assumption, that natives over such a vast area as the Amazon make a snuff from a plant that they do not know, that does not grow in their region, wild or cultivated, the seeds of which they would have to import for many, in some cases, for several thousand miles?

Let us contemplate what is known of the distribution of *Anadenanthera peregrina*. Safford, who apparently concurred with the ideas that such widely scattered Amazonian peoples as the Omaguas of Amazonian Peru and the Murus of the Rio Negro of Brazil prepared snuff from this leguminous tree, truthfully wrote that *Anadenanthera peregrina* "has a most appropriate specific name, for it has a wide geographical range." He further pointed out that its range had "undoubtedly been increased by human agency." But, when Safford cites for *Anadenanthera peregrina* a range comprising Hispaniola and Puerto Rico, Venezuela, northeastern Peru, southern Peru, Argentina, Guiana and "many parts" of Brazil, he was including with *Anadenanthera peregrina* two other species of the genus which he presumed to be employed as the source of making snuff. He cites no herbarium voucher specimens,

262-016 O-67—21

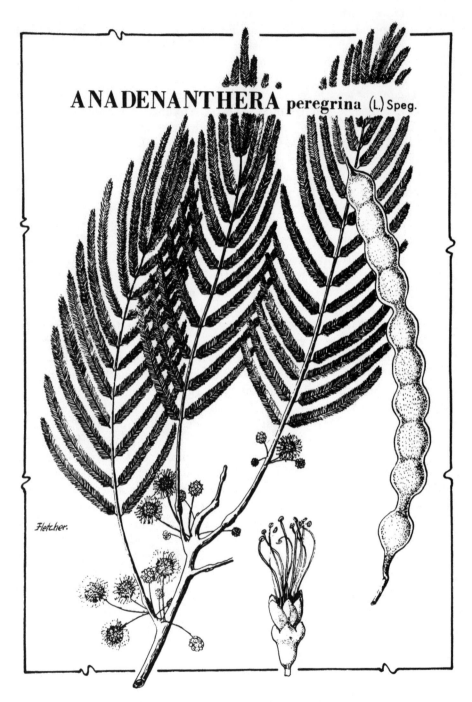

ANADENANTHERA peregrina (L.) Speg.

Fletcher.

FIG. 4.—Anadenanthera peregrina (Piptadenia peregrina).

instead giving references to the use of snuffs in the literature and assuming that they did refer actually to snuffs from *Anadenanthera*.

Fortunately, we have several botanical studies of monographic nature that shed light on the distribution of *Anadenanthera peregrina*. It is these data, not "interpreted" literature reports, that must guide any definitive generalisations. Ducke, renowned Brazilian botanist who spent more than half a century studying the Amazon flora in field and laboratory, specialised in the Leguminosae. In his "Leguminosas da Amazonia", he (*5*) cites all known collections of *Anadenanthera peregrina* (under *Piptadenia peregrina*). If the species had been much commoner in the Amazon, Ducke would have made more collections than those that he cited. More recently, Altschul, in her studies of the genus of the yopo snuff (*1, 25*), has treated *Anadenanthera* monographically, citing only collections, wild or cultivated, from South America. Thus, we know that, at least in the present century, *Anadenanthera peregrina* is far from common in the Amazon basin.

It is, therefore, somewhat exaggerated to expect us to conclude that many tribes are preparing an important hallucinogenic snuff, and a product often taken in excessive amounts, from a tree that is uncommon or even not found in their environment. Trees of this species are reported in Venezuela as "being forest dominants, belonging to secondary forests, inhibiting savannas, light forests and riversides," in British Guiana confined to "savannas and riverside forests," while in Brazil represented mostly in the *campos* or savannas (*1, 6*). The distribution of *Anadenanthera peregrina* in the Amazonas of Brazil is, significantly, confined to savanna-like areas, usually in or near the lower Rio Madeira and the Rio Branco basins—significantly, I say, because the Maué and other tribes of the Madeira area have, probably correctly, been reported as using snuff from *Anadenanthera*. I have seen excellent specimens of *Anadenanthera peregrina* recently collected by Mr. Georg Seitz along the Rio Negro, in the vicinity of the mouth of the Rio Branco, in Amazonian Brazil; these were undoubtedly cultivated from material brought in from the savannas of the Rio Branco.

Now, let us contemplate the problems that arise. If *Anadenanthera peregrina* is not the source of a snuff employed over wide areas in the Amazon, what are the sources of the numerous snuff preparations that we know are or have been prepared in isolated localities from the mountains of Venezuela and the Guianas south to the Argentine and from the eastern slopes of the Andes to the Atlantic Ocean? We cannot fully answer this query at the present time, but we can offer several tentative approaches towards a solution.

To begin with, it is very probable that several, if not many, different plants formed the basis for the snuffs employed similarly and for similar purposes over such a vast area. We know very definitely that this is true. We do not, to be sure, know all of the plants involved in this complicated enigma, but we know enough to arrive at an overall picture to guide future research.

It was apparently Safford (*16*) who first suggested that species of *Anadenanthera* other than *peregrina* may be the source of narcotic snuffs in South America. He identified the *vilca* or *huilca* of southern Peru and Bolivia, and the *cébil* of northern Argentina, with seeds of what he called *Piptadenia macrocarpa*, now correctly referred to as *Anadenanthera colubrina* var. *Cébil*. Although the evidence is, in my opinion, rather weak, several other species and varieties may have been employed in isolated localities in southern South America. Inasmuch, however, as a paper in the series is devoted precisely to the problem at hand, I shall refrain from considering it at greater length.

When I first went to the northwesternmost Amazon in Colombia, I heard numerous reports of a strongly hallucinogenic snuff made from the bark of forest trees. Known in the area as *yakee* or *paricá*, it was obviously not tobacco snuff nor was it prepared from seeds of *Anadenanthera*.

After eight years of search, I discovered that yakee was prepared from several species of *Virola*, *V. calophylla*, *V. calophylloidea* and, perhaps, *V. elongata* of the Myristicaceae (17, 18). The natives strip bark from the trunks before the sun has risen high enough to heat up the forest. A blood-red resin oozes from the inner surface of the bark. It is scraped off with a machete or knife and boiled in an earthen pot for hours, until a thick paste is left. This paste is allowed to dry and is then pulverized, sifted through a fine cloth, and finally added to an equal amount of ashes of the stems of a wild cacao species. The ashes give the snuff consistency to withstand the excessive dampness of the air which might otherwise quickly "melt" the powdered resin-paste to a solid lump.

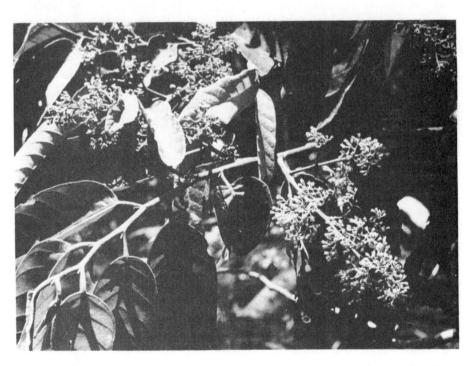

FIG. 5.—Leaves and flowers of *Virola calophylloidea*, one of the species of *Virola* from which a strongly hallucinogenic snuff is prepared. Mitú, Vaupés, Colombia. Photograph by R. E. Schultes.

300

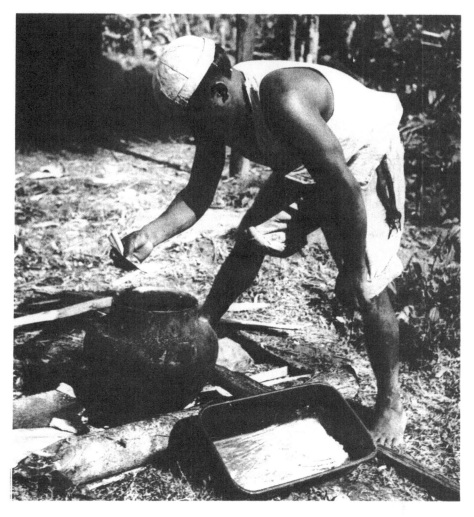

FIG. 6.—Puinave Indian preparing yakee-snuff from the red resinous exudate from the bark of *Virola*-trees. Río Apaporis, Vaupés, Colombia. Photograph by R. E. Schultes.

At the beginning of this century, the German ethnologist Koch-Grünberg mentioned (*11*) an intoxicating snuff prepared from the bark of an unidentified tree by the Yekwana Indians of the headwaters of the Orinoco in Venezuela. There seems to be every reason to believe that this snuff was made from a species of *Virola*. Seitz (*23*) has identified the *epená* snuff of the Waika Indians (who now live in the Rio Negro basin of Brazil, but who have migrated from the headwaters of the Orinoco) as representing *Virola calophylloidea*.

At one time, I presumed that the active principle in this myristicaceous snuff must be the same essential oil—myristicine—that is common throughout the family and that has been thought to make nutmeg a dangerous narcotic in appropriate amounts. Myristicine may have some effect, but Holmstedt has recently isolated tryptamine derivatives from *Virola*—snuff which itself could account for the hallucinogenic properties of the powder (*10*).

301

It may be interesting to append a few observations which I made personally after taking yakee (*17*). I took about one-third of a teaspoonful in two inhalations, using the characteristic V-shaped bird-bone snuffing tube. This represents about one-quarter the dose that a diagnosing medicine man will take to bring on an eventual state of unconsciousness.

The dose was snuffed at five o'clock one afternoon. Within fifteen minutes, a drawing sensation was felt over the eyes, followed very shortly by a strong tingling in fingers and toes. The drawing sensation in the forehead gave way to a strong and constant headache. Within a half hour, the feet and hands were numb and sensitivity of the fingertips had disappeared; walking was possible with difficulty, as with beri-beri. I felt nauseated until eight o'clock, and experienced lassitude and uneasiness. Shortly after eight, I lay down in my hammock, overcome with a drowsiness, which, however, seemed to be accompanied by a muscular excitation except in the hands and feet. At about nine-thirty, I fell into a fitful sleep which continued, with frequent awakenings, until morning. The strong headache lasted until noon. A profuse sweating and what was probably a slight fever persisted throughout the night. The pupils were strongly dilated during the first few hours of the intoxication.

Though performed under primitive conditions in the jungle by myself, this experiment does, I think, indicate the great strength of the snuff as a psychotropic agent. The witch doctors see visions in color, but I was able to experience neither visual hallucinations nor color sensations. The large dose used by the witch doctor is enough to put him into a deep but disturbed sleep, during which he sees visions and has dreams which, through the wild shouts emitted in his delirium, are interpreted by an assistant. That it is a dangerous practice is acknowledged by the witch doctors themselves. They report the death, about 15 years ago, of one of their number from the Puinave tribe during a yakee-intoxication.

Sources of Snuffs of Lesser Importance

We are aware from the literature of references to narcotic snuffs in South America the botanical identities of which are still uncertain or unknown.

A most mysterious snuff of which we still know almost nothing is said to be prepared from the fruits of the gigantic moraceous jungle tree *Olmedioperebea sclerophylla* (*19*). It is reputedly employed in the central part of Brazil, especially along the upper Xingú, but is known only by the general Portuguese term *rapé dos indios* ("Indian snuff"). So far as I have been able to ascertain, chemical examination of the fruits of this tree has not yielded substance with psychotomimetic effects.

It would be satisfying to know the plant source of the clear amber-coloured and aromatic resin that is procured from a large forest tree, and that forms part of the sacred accoutrements of every medicine man of the Tukanoan tribes in the Apaporis and Vaupés Rivers of Amazonian Colombia (*17, 22*).

In particularly difficult cases of diagnosis of disease, divination or other magic practice, minute amounts of this resin, powdered, are snuffed. Although it is said to induce dizziness, it is not reputed to have hallucinogenic properties. Nevertheless, botanical identification and chemical study of this resin-snuff should be made, if only because of the intriguing fact that it is quite generally referred to as *paricá*, the same name that is applied to the highly hallucinogenic snuff prepared from the blood-red resin of the inner bark of several species of the myristicaceous tree-genus *Virola*, by the same people in the same part of the Amazon.

A number of years ago, a missionary working in the headwaters of the Orinoco in Venezuela handed me a partially rotted, matted roll of plant material which he said was the source of one of the narcotic snuffs of the Waika Indians. The condition of the material was very poor, but it seemed to represent a species of *Justicia*. This identification was tentatively corroborated by Dr. E. C. Leonard, the American specialist on the Acanthaceae. I have never been able to visit this region to investigate the problem personally. With the unsatisfactory preservation of the material and the failure of other botanists who had visited the general region to report it (*31*), I more or less dismissed *Justicia* as a serious contender for inclusion in our list of hallucinogens. I am now, however, convinced that this problem must be investigated thoroughly in the field, for recently, the Brazilian botanist, Prof. João Murça Pires, informed me personally that the Waikas do indeed employ a species of *Justicia*, a species close apparently to *J. pectoralis*, in the preparation of a vision-producing snuff. We know that alkaloids have been reported from several species of *Justica*, and there has been some question of synonymy of *Justica* with *Adhatoda*, which is known to contain harman-type alkaloids. Several other genera of the Acanthaceae have been reported as alkaloidal, and this family might well bear an intensive phytochemical study. In this connexion, I might report here that one of the minor fish poisons that I found in use amongst the Taiwanos of the Río Kananarí of Colombian Vaupés is the root of an acanthaceous shrub, the genus of which is as yet phytochemically wholly unknown: *Mendoncia aspera* (*22*).

There is, apparently, a fertile field for the study of narcotic snuff preparations in the general area of the headwaters of the Orinoco. In fact, this part of South America would seem perhaps to represent the centre of complexity of this curious culture trait.

The Waikas of the upper Orinoco basin have been reported to prepare their yopo snuff from three plants (*27*). One source enumerates *hisioma*, *Anadenanthera peregrina*, as one ingredient; a second is called *masho-hara* or *yauardi-hena* and is said to be a piperaceous species; a third is a powder known as *bolek-hena*. It is a temptation to wonder whether or not this bolek-hena or "leaves of the spirit of death" might be a *Justicia*. Other sources (*2, 23, 27, 32*) assert that the snuff of the Waikas and of a related tribe, the Samatari, was prepared from the bast of a tree called *epéna-kési* (referrible probably to *Virola*); the ashes of the outer bark of *ama-asita*, which has been identified in the literature as an *Acacia;* and the powder of *mashi-hiri*, a plant of about one foot in height which might conceivably also represent

303

Justicia. The Surára and Pakidái make their snuff (*30*) from seeds of *Anadenanthera peregrina*, ashes of *hekurahihená*, the bark of a tree of uncertain identity but possibly representing also this same species, a piperaceous species, *maxarahá*. The Karimé, culturally related to and neighbours of the Waikas, elaborate a snuff powder (*30*) from leaves of "a small plant called *kokoime*." Again, are we warranted in suspecting that kokoime might be the *Justica?*

The Kashuena of the Rio Trombetas in Amazonian Brazil, are reported by one source to have several kinds of snuff in addition to that made "simply of tobacco" (*7*). One is prepared by "blending the dried and powdered bark of a tree and a quantity of paricá with other substances taken from kernels or seeds of a variety of wild fruits." A third comprises a mixture of these two kinds of snuff. We are left in the dark about the species of tree from which the bark is taken, although it may possibly be referrible to an *Anadenanthera*, and the "wild fruits" remain unidentified. Could one be the fruits of *Olmedioperebea sclerophylla?*

Final Query

The several attempts to synthesise and summarise our knowledge of the precise botanical identification of plants entering into the preparation of South American snuffs (*26, 28*) have met with the same difficulties that I find in trying to discuss this topic here. Because of similarities in the tools and methods of snuffing, and especially as a result of the lack of voucher botanical specimens, we are too often reduced to conjecture as to the plants involved. In view of the importance of snuffing in many cultures—past and present—and of the possibility that a number of plants hitherto unknown as ingredients of narcotic snuffs might be uncovered, further field investigation of snuffs in South America is clearly indicated.

In connexion with the possibility of finding new plants as sources of narcotic snuffs, there is one point that has disturbed me for a long time. Why should only several of the narcotic plants be administered as snuff? Snuffing is a widespread New World culture trait. It is a relatively easy method of self-intoxication. It lends itself easily to ritual or ceremonial use. Snuffs usually tend to keep over longer periods, especially in the humid tropics, than infusions or decoctions. Why then are not more narcotics taken in this form? One limiting factor, to be sure, would be the requirements that the activite principle must be absorbable through the membranes to enter directly into the blood stream and be active. Nicotine, of course, answers these reqirements. Obviously, the active principles of the snuffs from *Anadenanthera peregrina* and *Virola* also satisfy these requirements. But would not the active constituents of other narcotics likewise follow this pattern? Why, for example, have we never found the sundry species of *Datura* powdered and employed as snuffs?

Would snuffs prepared from the bark of *Banisteriopsis* provide the desired psychotropic effects? And what about the narcotic properties of *Ery-*

throxylon Coca—would they be lost if the powdered leaves were introduced into the nostrils as a snuff? The rich variety of toxic plants in the flora of South America—would not many of these species have psychotomimetic effects which would be more controllable or perhaps less dangerous as snuffs then decoctions or infusions of the same plants? All of this leads to two questions that I would leave with you: Was not the snuffing of narcotic powders much more widely practiced in South America than it is at present? Was and is not the number and variety of plants snuffed for their peculiar physiological properties greater than we at present believe? The answer to both questions, I suspect, is "Yes." But only more intensive and extensive search and interpretation of the literature, and more immediate and insistent ethnobotanical field studies can provide us with answers.

BIBLIOGRAPHY

(1) ALTSCHUL, SIRI VON REIS. "A taxonomic study of the genus Anadenanthera." Contrib. Gray Herb., Harvard Univ. 193 (1964), 1.

(2) BARKER, JAMES. "Memoria sobre la cultura de los guaika." Bol. Indig. Ven. 1 (1953), 433.

(3) BATES, HENRY W. "The naturalist on the River Amazons," (1863). John Murray, London.

(4) COOPER, JOHN M. "Stimulants and narcotics" in Handbook of South American Indians, Bull. No. 143, Vol. 5, Bur. Am. Ethnol. (1949), 525.

(5) DUCKE, ADOLPHO. "As leguminosas da Amazônia brasileira." Bol. Tecn. Inst. Agron. Norte 18 (1949).

(6) DUCKE, ADOLPHO and GEORGE A. BLACK. "Phytogeographical notes on the Brazilian Amazon." An. Acad. Bras. 25 (1953), 1.

(7) FRIEKEL, PROTÁSIO. "Mori — a festa do rape (indios kachiryana, rio Trombetas)." Bol. Mus. Para. Emilio Goeldi, n.s., Anthrop. 12 (1961), 1.

(8) GARCILASO DE LA VEGA, (El Inca) "Primera parte de los commentarios reales. . . ." Pt. 1, Book 2 (1723), Chapt. 25.

(9) GOODSPEED, THOMAS HARPER. "The genus Nicotiana" (1954), Chronica Botanica Co., Waltham, Mass.

(10) HOLMSTEDT, BO. "Tryptamine derivatives in epená, an intoxicating snuff used by some South American Indian tribes." Arch. Int. Pharmacodyn. Therap. 156 (1965), 285.

(11) KOCH-GRÜNBERG, THEODOR. "Zwei Jahre unter den Indianern." 1 (1909) 298. Ernst Wasmuth A.-G., Berlin.

(12) LEVI-STRAUSS, CLAUDE. "Tribes of the right bank of the Guaporé River" in Handbook of South American Indians, Bull. 143, Vol. 3, Bur. Am. Ethnol. (1948), 378.

(13) MASON, J. ALDEN. "Use of tobacco in Mexico and South America." Field Mus. Nat. Hist. Anthrop. Leafl. 16 (1924).

(14) NIMUENDAJÚ, CURT (Ed. R. H. Lowie). "The Tukuna" Univ. Cal. Publ. Am. Arch. Ethnol. 45 (1952).

(15) ROWE, JOHN HOWLAND. "Inca culture at the time of the Spanish Conquest" in Handbook of South American Indians, Bull. 143, Vol. 2, Bur. Am. Ethnol. (1946), 292.

(16) SAFFORD, WILLIAM EDWIN. "Identity of cohoba, the narcotic snuff of ancient Haiti." Journ. Wash. Acad. Sci. 6 (1916), 548.

(17) SCHULTES, RICHARD EVANS. "A new narcotic snuff from the northwest Amazon." Bot. Mus. Leafl., Harvard Univ. 16 (1954), 241.

(18) ———. "Un nouveau tabac à priser de l'Amazone du nord-ouest." Journ. Agric. Trop. Bot. Appl. 1 (1954), 298.

(*19*) SCHULTES, RICHARD EVANS. "Native narcotics of the New World." Texas Journ. Pharm. 2 (1961)', 141.

(*20*) ———. "Hallucinogenic plants of the New World." Harvard Rev. 1 (1963), 18.

(*21*) ———. "Ein halbes Jahrhundert Ethnobotanik amerikanischer Halluzinogene." Planta Medica 13 (1965), 124.

(*22*) ———. "The search for new natural hullucinogens." Lloydia 29 (1966), 293.

(*23*) SEITZ, GEORG. "Einige Bemerkungen zur Anwendung and Wirkungsweise des Epená—Schnupfpulvers der Waika—Indianer." Ethnolog. Studier No. 28 (1965), 117.

(*24*) SPRUCE, RICHARD (Ed. A. R. Wallace). "Notes of a botanist on the Amazon and Andes." 2 (1908), 426. Macmillan & Co., Ltd., London.

(*25*) VON REIS, SIRI S. P. "The genus Anadenanthera : a taxomomic and ethnobotanical study." Ph. D. Thesis (ined.) (1961), Radcliffe College, Cambridge, Mass.

(*26*) WASSEN, S. HENRY. "Some general viewpoints in the study of native drugs, especially from the West Indies and South America." Ethnos 29 (1964), 97.

(*27*) ———. "The use of some specific kinds of South American Indian snuff and related paraphernalia." Ethnolog. Stud. 28 (1965).

(*28*) ———. "Sydamerikanska snusdroger." Nytt och Nyttigt, No. 1 (1966), 1.

(*29*) ——— and Bo Holmstedt. "The use of paricá, an ethnological and pharmacological review." Ethnos 28 (1963), 5.

(*30*) WILBERT, JOHANNES. "Indios de la región Orinoco—Ventuari." Monografía No. 8, Fundación La Salle de Ciencias Naturales, Caracas (1963).

(*31*) WURDACK, JOHN. "Indian narcotics in southern Venezuela." Gard. Journ. 8 (1958), 116.

(*32*) ZERRIES, OTTO. "Das Lasha—Fest der Waika—Indianer." Di Umshau 21 (1955), 662. Frankfurt-am-Main.

Vilca and its Use

SIRI VON REIS ALTSCHUL
Botanical Museum of Harvard University, Cambridge, Mass.

It generally has been assumed that the Peruvian substance known as *Vilca* is, or was, a snuff made from a *Piptadenia* in the family *Leguminosae* (Safford, 1916; and later authors). However, there is evidence in the literature and in unpublished materials that *Vilca* may involve other plants as well, and that it may have been used in forms different from snuff. I would like to examine this evidence with a view to opening new areas in the search for psycho-active drugs.

The discussion which follows is based in part on research in the ethnobotany of the strictly New World genus *Anadenanthera*, which formerly was considered as section *Niopa* of the genus *Piptadenia* and is known commonly as the source of some hallucinogenic snuffs. The genus *Anadenanthera* contains two very similar species which have not been shown to differ significantly with respect to their psycho-activity, and which may have been used interchangeably. One species is *Anadenanthera colubrina*, found in southern Peru, Bolivia, northern Argentina, Paraguay and southern Brazil. The other species is *A. peregrina*, ranging from southeastern Brazil to the Greater Antilles. (von Reis, 1961; von Reis Altschul, 1964).

The discussion also will make use of information which recently has become available. This information has been selected from nearly 6,000 field notes from a search of almost 2,500,000 herbarium specimens at Harvard University (von Reis, 1962). Dr. Richard Evans Schultes and I have just completed this project and intend to publish our data as soon as it is feasible.[1]

Let us look first at the earliest references to *Vilca*, which are to be found not in the herbarium but in the post-conquest literature of Peru. Around 1571, Polo de Ondegardo reported that the witch doctors of the Incas [2] foretold the future by speaking with the devil in some dark place by means of various ceremonies, for which office they intoxicated themselves with an herb called *Villca*, pouring its juice into *chicha* or taking it another way. The reporter stated that, although only old women were reputed to practice this craft, in fact its use was widespread but concealed among men and boys, as well. In 1695, Santa Cruz Pachacuti spoke of a medicine called *villca* which was the seed of a tree. Two years later, González Holguín said that *Villca* referred to a tree with a purgative fruit. An early report by Falcón (1946 ed.; in Yacovleff & Herrera, 1935) indicated that the Indians took a purge called *Vilcas*

---

[1] This project was carried out through the sponsorship of The Botanical Museum of Harvard University. It was supported by Smith, Kline & French Laboratories; the National Institute of Mental Health; and the Lilly Research Laboratories. We are very grateful to the staffs of the Gray Herbarium and Arnold Arboretum of Harvard University, especially to Professors Reed C. Rollins and Richard A. Howard, respective directors, for generous permission to use their facilities and herbarium materials.

[2] Murdock's *Outline of South American Cultures* (1951) has been used for classifying all the Indian cultures dealt with in this paper.

(or *elilcas*) which was beneficial to those who worked too hard. In 1629, Vásquez de Espinosa said that the pods of the *vilca* tree had small, round seeds which were the common purge of the Indians for all sorts of humors. Some years later, in 1653, Bernabé Cobo stated that the Indians used a decoction of the roots of a *Polypodium* fern with two or three *Vilca* seeds to remove phlegm and choler without pain or nausea. He gave a fair, but not diagnostically adequate, description of the tree called *Vilca*, and maintained that the Indians cured a variety of illnesses with the purgative seeds taken in *chicha*. These seeds were said to be both laxative and emetic and to dispel melancholy. Cooked and drunk in honey, they cleared the chest, stimulated urination and made women fruitful.

Modern writers usually identify the name *Vilca* with the species here called *Anadenanthera colubrina* (Herrera, 1934; Lastres, 1951). In 1916, Safford stated that seeds labelled *Huillca* and secured from an Indian drug vender in southern Peru had been identified as belonging to *Anadenanthera*. Herrera reported in 1940 that the seeds of *Huillca* (*Herrera 3210*) are a narcotic-cathartic element in the indigenous pharmacopoeia. Yacovleff & Herrera (1935) have said that the seeds are sold as purgatives in the local markets. Recently, Vargas confirmed in a letter (1966) from Cuzco that herb doctors in that vicinity continue to use the seeds for this purpose. Cárdenas has stated from Bolivia that the same species, known as *Willca*, is used as a stimulant and aphrodisiac by the *callahuayos* (1943), or itinerant medicine men who travel today between Chile and Mexico (H. C. Cutler in conversation, 1966). The seeds also have been used in our time as charms or fetishes by the Quechua Indians of northwest Bolivia. At the market in La Paz one may buy, among other goods for similar purposes, seeds of *A. colubrina* and of other leguminous species in the genus *Ormosia*. These seeds and other items are buried, for magical purposes, under houses in the process of construction (Nordenskiöld, 1907; Pardal, 1937).

In the course of the herbarium search mentioned above, we found two specimens labelled *Vilca*. Both belonged to *Anadenanthera colubrina*. One was from southern Peru (Departamento de Huancavelica, *Weberbauer 6505*). The other was from east of La Paz, Bolivia (Cañamina, *White 254*). These data indicate that *A. colubrina* indeed is identifiable with *Vilca*, but they do not insure that *Vilca* is referable exclusively to this plant.

For one thing, it is especially difficult to establish botanical identifications in the early literature. Apparent inconsistencies or omissions in plant descriptions, and the lack of voucher specimens require that we habitually entertain the possibility of altogether new interpretations, particularly among groups like the legumes, where many similar species may be mistaken one for another. In fact, the widespread representation of the *Leguminosae* in native medicine suggests that a pharmacological screening of its New World genera for psycho-active compounds might be a worthwhile undertaking.

In conjunction with our herbarium search at Harvard, we found three species with common names similar to *Vilca* but from families other than the legumes. These were a Peruvian specimen of *Banisteria leiocarpa* (*Malpighiaceae, Vargas 2044*) labelled *Vilca bejuco*, or climbing *Vilca;* a Venezuelan specimen of *Virola sebifera* (*Myristicaceae, Steyermark 60758a*) labelled *wircaweijek*, whose inner bark is said to be dried and smoked by witch doctors to cure fevers; and a Peruvian specimen of *Baccharis floribunda* (*Compositae, West 3735*) labelled *Ullccochilca*, a species also reputedly curative (*Macbride & Featherstone 1631*).[3]

In addition to these interesting attributions, our herbarium search revealed information which does not relate directly to *Vilca* but which I will present here because it very much bears upon the search for psychoactive drugs. This information consists of common names of *Anadenanthera* species which have come to light in connection with new plants. The accompanying map (Fig. 1) shows the distribution of the common names of *Anadenanthera* species in South America, based upon labels of specimens examined. With these names and their locations in mind, I would suggest that the following species be examined chemically for possible pharmacological activity: in the *Asclepiadaceae, Asclepias curupi* (*Balansa 1361*) from Paraguay, labelled *Curupí*, the powdered leaves and a decoction of the plant said to be applied to snake bite; in the *Euphorbiaceae*, three species of *Sapium* from Uruguay, labelled *Curupí* (*S. gibertii, Lombardo 3048; S. haematospermum, Lombardo 3047; S. linearifolium, Lombardo 3344*); in the *Rubiaceae, Guettarda viburnoides* from Brazil, labelled *Angico* (*Mexia 5583*); and in the *Leguminosae* from Brazil an undetermined *Pithecellobium* (*Krukoff 1887*), *Piptadenia contorta* (*Mexia 4438*), both labelled *Angico Branco;* and *Mimosa malacocentra* (*Mexia 5624*) labelled *Angiquin*, whose leaves are used to make a tea for pain.

Further afield from *Anadenanthera* but pertinent to the objectives of the conference are a few surprising new combinations: in the *Convolvulaceae*: two species of *Ipomoea* (*I. denticulata, I. tiliacea, W. H. & B. T. Hodge 3323, 3318*, respectively) from the island of Dominica, West Indies, labelled *Caapi;* in the *Leguminosae, Calliandra calothyrsis* (*Standley 23846*) and *Leucaena guatemalensis* (*Standley 73562*), both from Guatemala and labelled *Yaje;* in the *Compositae, Trichocline incana* (*Meyer 3982*) from Argentina, labelled *Coro* and said to be smoked with tobacco. The word *Coro* has appeared now and then in the early chronicles and has been linked previously with *Anadenanthera* and (the root of) wild tobacco (Cobo, 1890–93 ed.; Uhle, 1898) but never, to my knowledge, with this plant: According to Cobo, *Coro* powder was drunk in water for detention of urine, or taken as snuff for headache and to clear the vision.

I would like to return now to *Vilca* and to review some of the botanical common names similar to it in the published literature. The species ascribed to these names perhaps should receive critical attention, too. *Vilcarán* has been associated with *Piptadenia rigida* (Burkart, 1949) in Argentina. *Vilcaparu* is a word for yellow maize (González Holguín, 1607) from Bolivia (A. Grobman in conversation, 1961). *Huillko* means species of *Ipomoea* and

---

[3] Any pharmacological research on these and other species cited in this paper should be preceded by a verification, by a competent botanist, of the correct identification of the specimens cited. The research should be based on the specimen cited, as designated by the collector's name and field number. All specimens are in the collections of the Arnold Arboretum and Gray Herbarium of Harvard University, Cambridge, Mass.

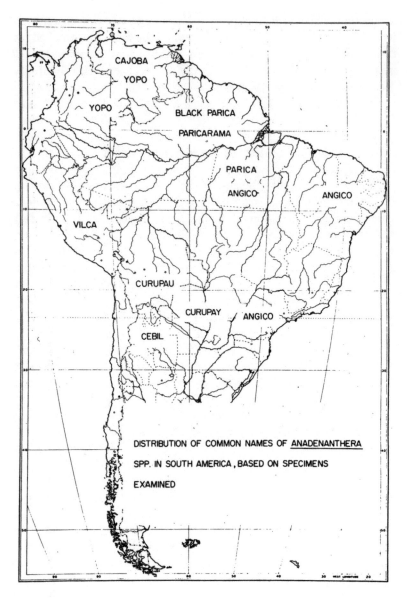

DISTRIBUTION OF COMMON NAMES OF ANADENANTHERA SPP. IN SOUTH AMERICA, BASED ON SPECIMENS EXAMINED

FIG. 1

the Nyctaginaceous genus *Mirabilis* (Herrera, 1934). *Tara Huillca* has been identified as *Anadenanthera colubrina* (Yacovleff & Herrera, 1935), but *Tara*, alone, refers to another legume, *Caesalpinia tinctoria* (Herrera, 1934). *Wilca Tarwi* has been assoicated with the leguminous genus *Lupinus* (Lastres, 1941). The chronicler Poma de Ayala (1936 ed.; Lastres, 1941) reported that the Indians purged themselves once a month with *bilca tauri*, made from some kind of seeds ground into a liquid, half of which was drunk and half of which was taken as an enema which was said to give the Incas strength, health and a 200 years life span. At the time of the conquest, the word *Vilcu* referred in Aymará to a plant with yellow, bird-like flowers (Cobo,

310

1890 ed., Vol. I). It also meant ivy (*Villcu*) González Holguín, 1607). Our herbarium search unearthed two specimens of the climbing *Compositae*, *Mikania cordifolia* (*Mexia 8042*) from Peru labelled *Huaco verde*, and *M. houstoniana* (*Caec. et Ed. Seler 5475* (*396*)) from the ruins of Palenque, Mexico. *Villca* or *Huacca* both meant idol (González Holguín, 1607) or something sacred to the Incas. Hence, the possibility that *Mikania* species might have been ritual plants deserves a thought.

One might sum up what generally has been known of the role of *Vilca* in Peru at the time of the conquest by saying that it seemed to be confined mostly to simple folk-medicine, its divinatory aspects divorced from formalized religion. Rowe has stated (in Steward, 1946) that narcotics were unimportant to the Inca culture and that none was taken expressly to obtain visions; the strongest substances reputedly used were *coca*, tobacco and *Vilca*. The main curatives were *Chicha*, *Vilca* and tobacco (Fornée, 1885 ed.), and Peruvian medicine consisted primarily in blood-letting, purging with *Vilca*, and in taking tobacco (*sayri*) snuff (Garcílaso de la Vega, 1688 ed.).

Besides its occurrence with reference to medical botany, the term *Vilca* appears so frequently and in such a variety of contexts in the historical narratives of Peru that one is led to suspect that it may have had a great antiquity and that plants passing under its name may have had greater ritual importance in earlier times than at the time of the conquest. Various forms of the word meant enema or clyster (*Vilca* or *Vilcas* in González Holguín, 1607; *Vilca Tarvi* or *Vilcatauri* in Lastres, 1941; *Vilcachima* in Lastres, 1951; *Vilcana* in González Holguín, 1607, Lavorería, 1902, Mossi, 1860); the giving of an enema (*Vilcani* in D'Harcourt, 1939, González Holguín, 1607, Mossi, 1860, Lavorería, 1902); a syringe (*Vilcana* in Mossi, 1860; *uilcachina* in Poma de Ayala, 1936 ed., Lastres, 1951); or a small stick commonly used to clean the rectum in the Cuzco area (*Vilcachina* in Lastres, 1951). The same root is found in the words for doctor or surgeon (*Vilca-Cama* in Velasco, 1840 ed.); priest or informant (*Villac* in Lastres, 1951); and ostrich-like chief (*Surivilca* in Lastres, 1941); and in designations of familial relationships (*Vilca* or *Vilcay* in González Holguín, 1607, in Mossi, 1857, 1860). In 1671, Ogilby stated that in the Chilean language *Vilca* meant mother-in-law; ˚*Hilca* meant one-eyed person. Among the Araucanians, a *pivillca* was a flute (Medina, 1882). In the area of the Diaguita culture, *Vilka* is today a surname of Quechua or Calchaquí origin (Ambrosetti, 1917).

Essentially, however, *Vilca* was one of the two names mentioned earlier by which the Peruvian Indians called their idols or gods. It was used to describe whatever was first, original or important (Lastres, 1941), and to refer to any sacred place or thing (Cobo, 1890–93 ed.; Garcílaso de la Vega, 1688 ed., 1941–44 ed.; González Holguín, 1607; Mossi, 1860). These include words for an idol (*Huacavilca* in Lastres, 1941), a temple (*Huarivilca* in Cieza de León, 1864 ed.), a town or village (*Vilca* or *Vilcas* in Cobo, 1890–93 ed.), bodies of water (*Vilca* or *Vilcas*, a river in Garcílaso de la Vega, 1688 ed.; *Vilca-Mayo*, a river in St. Cricq, 1873–74 ed. *Vilca-cocha*, a lake which flows into the *Vilca-Mayo* in St. Cricq, 1873-74 ed.), a valley called the Paradise of Peru (*Vilca-Mayo* in Cieza de León, 1864 ed.), a mountain peak (*Vilcanota* in Garcílaso de la Vega, 1688 ed., 1941–44 ed.; *Huanca Vilca* in Lastres, 1941; *Vilcaconga* in Cobo, 1890–93 ed.) or a sierra (*Vilca* or *Vilcas, Vilcanota* in Cobo 1890–93 ed.), a province (*Vilca Pampa* in Cobo, 1890–93 ed., Garcílaso de la Vega, 1688 ed., 1941–44 ed.; *Vilca* or *Vilcas* in Cobo, 1890–93 ed., Cieza de León, 1864 ed.) or a people (*Vilca* or *Vilcas* in Garcílaso de la Vega, 1688 ed., 1941–44 ed.; *Chumbivilcas* in Cobo, 1890–93 ed., Garcílaso de la Vega, 1688 ed., 1941–44 ed.; *Huancavilca* in Cieza de León, 1864 ed.).

Among the ritual paraphernalia which seem to relate to *Vilca* are the *vilca ronco* (González Holguín, 1607), small *coca*-filled baskets which were thrown into the fire at animal sacrifices in Cuzco. One might mention, also, the *vilques*, earthenware jugs with which the Indians toasted their dead, after which the *chicha* contained in them was poured over a round stone which they worshipped in the middle of a plaza (Cobo, 1890–93 ed.). The chronicler Acosta (1584, folio 104) relates that the Spanish conquerors ordered the Incas to stop worshipping the sun, moon and so on, ". . . ni tengays villcas, ni guacas, ni figura de hombre, . . ."

An Incaic version of the origin of the medicinal *Vilca* (Santa Cruz Pachacuti, 1927 ed.; Yacovleff & Herrera, 1935) states that an Inca captain named *Villcaquire*, being struck down in war by his nation's enemies, the Chanca, requested that he be buried in the trunk of a nearby tree which, he foretold, would produce *villca* seeds, to dispell all bad humors and choler from his people. The story takes place above a river on the Aporima road. Specimens of *Anadenanthera colubrina* (*West 3679, 3845*) have been identified from the Department of Apurimac. I would not be surprised to learn that the story was a relatively modern one which served the needs of the Incas to attribute to their own invention something which had its origins in much earlier times. It is tempting to wonder whether the medicinal *Vilca* had had an important role among the people named *Vilca*, who were numbered among the Chanca (Garcílaso de la Vega, 1688 ed.). Legend has associated the *Vilca* with edifices whose art and grandeur, built centuries before the Inca monarchy, was much admired and emulated by the Inca culture (Cobo, 1890–93 ed.).

Modern archaeology has cast doubt as to the veracity of some of the histories in the early narratives, and, geographically, it is not easy to locate many of the places referred to in the sixteenth and seventeenth century writings on Peru. However, a number of names incorporating the term *Vilca* can be found today on a map of southern Peru, correlating in general with the distribution of *Anadenanthera* in that country.

Archaeological data suggest that the use of enemas was more widespread in pre-conquest times than it was when the Spaniards arrived (Heizer, 1944; Nordenskiöld, 1930; Vélez-López, 1930). What was used in these enemas and in the tubes and tablets of the neighboring regions has not been determined, to my knowledge. *Anadenanthera* seeds have not been found at any Peruvian sites, as far as I know. The *Cebil* snuffs used at the time of contact among the Mataco and Vilela cultures of northern Argentina appear to have been *Anadenanthera*-derived. But the use of this genus further south beyond its natural distribution is less likely. Yet there, further south, the Comechingon Indians took something called *Sebil* through the nose (Sótelo Narvaez, 1915 ed.), and the Huarpe Indians chewed a substance called *Cibil* for endurance (Ovalle, 1703). Perhaps one even should ask whether the monumental weeping god with the tear-streaked cheeks at Tiahuanaco in Bolivia might be depicted in a state of intoxication from a powerful snuff or emetic.

This paper has posed many more questions than it has attempted to answer, but it has been instrumental in pointing out some unusual approaches to a better knowledge of *Vilca*, which could serve as a model for studies on other little known so-called narcotics. The facts gathered here suggest that a number of hitherto unsuspected species should be analyzed for psycho-activity, and that the drug plants used by man in the New World may prove to constitute a richer and more elaborate complex than we yet have been led to believe. The early writings deserve to be read again, and herbarium information should be sought more assiduously.

BIBLIOGRAPHY

ACOSTA, J. DE. Doctrina Christiana y Catecismo para instrucción de los Indios. Lima, 1584.

AMBROSETTI, J. B. Supersticiones y Leyendas. Buenos Aires, 1917.

BURKART, A. "Leguminosas Nuevas O Criticas, III." Darwiniana, 9: 63–96, 1949.

CÁRDENAS, M. Notas Preliminares sobre la materia medica Boliviana. Cochabamba, Imprenta Universitaria, 1943.

CIEZA DE LEÓN, P. DE. The Travels of Pedro de Cieza de León, A.D. 1532–1550. London, 1864 ed.

COBO, B. Historia del Nuevo Mundo. Sevilla, 1890–93 ed.

D'HARCOURT, R. La médicine dans l'ancien Pérou. Paris, 1939.

FALCÓN, F. "Daños que hacen a los indios." Pequeños Grandes Libros de Historia Americana Ser. I, 10: 141. Lima, 1946 ed.

FORNÉE, D. N. ED. "Descripción del Corregimiento de Abancay . . . In Jiménez de la Espada, M." Relaciones Geográficas de Indias, II: 218. Madrid, 1885 ed.

GARCÍLASO DE LA VEGA. The Royal Commentaries of Peru. London, 1688 ed.

GARCÍLASO DE LA VEGA. Los Comentarios Reales de los Incas. Lima, 1941–44 ed.

GONZÁLEZ HOLGUÍN, D. Vocabulario Qquichua, que es la lengua general de todo el Piru. Lima, 1607.

HEIZER, R. F. "The use of the enema among the aboriginal American Indians." Ciba Symposia 5: 1686–1693, 1944.

HERRERA, F. L. "Botánica Etnológica," Filológica Quechua III. Rev. Mus. Nac. Lima 3: 39–62, 1934.

HERRERA, F. L. "Plantas que curan y plantas que matan de la flora del Cuzco." Rev. Mus. Nac. Lima 9: 73–127, 1940.

LASTRES, J. B. "La medicina en la obra de Guamán Poma de Ayala." Rev. Mus. Nac. Lima 10: 113–164, 1941.

LASTRES, J. B. Historia de la Medicina Peruana, I. Lima, 1951.

LAVORERÍA, D. E. "El arte de curar entre los antiguos peruanos." An. Univ. Mayor San Marcos de Lima 29: 159–263, 1902.

MEDINA, J. T. Los aborígines de Chile. Santiago, 1882.

MOSSI, F. H. Ensayo sobre las Escelencias y Perfección del Idioma Llamado comunmente Quichua. Sucre, 1857.

Mossi, F. H. Diccionario Quichua-Castellano. Sucre, 1860.

Nordenskiöld, E. "Recettes magiques et médicales de Pérou et Bolivie." Jour. Soc. Am. Paris Nouv. Sér. 4 : 153–174, 1907.

Nordenskiöld, E. "The use of enema tubes and enema syringes among Indians." Compar. Ethnogr. Stud. 8 : 184–195, 1930.

Ogilby, J. America : Being the Latest and Most Accurate Description of the New World. London, 1671.

Ovalle, A. de. "An Historical Relation of the Kingdom of Chile." In Churchill, A. & J. Collection of Voyages and Travels. London, 1703.

Pardal, R. Medicina Aborigen Americana. Buenos Aires, 1937.

Polo de Ondegardo, J. Informaciones, acerca de la Religión y Gobierno de las Incas. In Urteaga, H. H. Collección de Libros y Documentos referentes a la Historia del Perú (Lima) 3 : 29–30, 1916 ed.

Poma de Ayala, F. G. "Nueva Coronica y Buen Gobierno." Trav. et Mém. l'Inst. d'Ethnol. Paris 23 : 71, 1936 ed.

Reis, S. von. The genus *Anadenanthera:* a taxonomic and ethnobotanical study, Part II. Unpublished Ph.D. thesis ms., Radcliffe College, 1961.

Reis, S. von. "Herbaria : sources of medicinal folklore." Economic Botany 16, 4 : 283–287, 1962.

Reis Altschul, S. von. "A taxonomic study of the genus *Anadenanthera*." Contr. Gray Herb., 193 : 3–65, 1964.

Safford, W. E. "Ethnobotany—Identity of Cohoba." Jour. Wash. Acad. Sci. 6 : 547–562, 1916.

Saint-Cricq, L. (Marcoy, P.) A Journey across South America. I–IV. London, 1873–34 ed.

Santa Cruz Pachacuti, J. de. "Historia de los Incas y Relación de su Gobierno." In Urteaga, H. H. Colección de Libros y Documentos referentes a la Historia del Perú (Lima) 2, 9 : 180, 1927 ed.

Sótelo Narvaez, P. "Relación de las Provincias Tucumán. In Freyre, J. El Tucumán Colonial 1 : 97–98. Buenos Aires, 1915 ed.

Steward, J. H., Editor. Handbook of South American Indians, I–II. U.S. Govt. Print. Off., 1946.

Uhle, M. "A snuffing-tube from Tiahuanaco." Bull. Free Mus. Sci. Art 1 : 158–177, 1898.

Vargas, C. Personal communication, Nov. 10, 1966.

Vásquez de Espinosa, A. "Compendium and Description of the West Indies." Smith. Misc. Coll. 102 : 1–862, 1942 ed.

Velasco, J. de. Histoire du Royaume de Quito I : 164. Paris, 1840 ed.

Vélez-López, L. "El clíster en el antiguo Perú." Proc. Intern. Congr. Am. 23 : 296–297, 1930.

Yacovleff, E. & Herrera, F. L. "El mundo vegetal de los antiguos peruanos." Rev. Mus. Nac. 4 : 31–102, 1935.

314

Epéna, the Intoxicating Snuff Powder of the Waika Indians and the Tucano Medicine Man, Agostino [1]

GEORGE J. SEITZ

Köln-Lindenthal, Dürenerstrasse 175, Germany

The WAIKA Indians belong to an isolated group of natives called YANO-AMA or YANONAMI. They live in the triangle formed by the Rio Branco in the southeast, the Uraricuera and Upper Orinoco Rivers in the north and the Rio Negro in the southwest. This territory lies on both sides of the boundary between Brazil and Venezuela.

During the last ten years, my wife and I made six expeditions to several WAIKA tribes in the region of the Upper Rio Negro, that is the southwestern part of that habitat, situated in the Brazilian Territory near the Venezuelan boundary. We found these tribes

(1) near the TUCANO IGARAPÉ, one of the headwaters of the Cauaborí River,

(2) on the Maturacá Channel, in the south of the Fall of HUÁ,

(3) on the Marauiá River, near the Igarapé IRAPIRAPÍ and

(4) on the Upper Maiá River, a branch of the Cauaborí River.

These Indians are nomads. We had a lot of difficulties in finding them and their primitive villages, called "SHABONO". They are always rather distant from the rivers, and we had to march hours and hours through the thick jungle to reach them.

Without the assistance and the experience of a Catholic priest—the only white man who had made contact with the WAIKA Indians before—our expeditions scarcely would have been successful.

The name WAIKA means KILLER—a nice, gentle sort of name. Undoubtedly, the group is one of the most primitive in South America. They have never found out how to make a boat or a raft. As nomads, these Indians make pots; they do not know anything about alcoholic drinks, or mandioc, the most important vegetable of the southern Hemisphere besides corn.

In a region where the rivers provide the most important traffic routes, they have never found out how to make a boat or a raft, As nomads, these Indians wander about the jungle. They live in primitive, wall-less, palm-thatched huts only as long as the food lasts in the neighborhood. When they eat up all the food around, they go to another village with huts just as primitive. They are a restless people that live off the land. And they live in a period that for us is prehistoric.

---

[1] The presentation of this paper was given in conjunction with the showing of an excellent, informative film. The photographs in this paper come from this film. (Editor)

They have never learned anything from their more advanced neighbors, the ARUAK group, represented by the TUCANO and BANIVA tribes.

The existence of these WAIKA Indians has been known for more than a hundred years. However, explorers of the region—Humboldt, and at the beginning of our century, Koch-Grünberg and Hamilton Rice—gave only brief reports about the WAIKAS. They had only occasional meetings with a few Indians from this group. These quick meetings did not give any basis for more than superficial notes.

In general, the explorers knew about the WAIKAS from the stories of other Indians, who described the Indians as terrible enemies, who used their poisoned arrows to keep out trespassers.

In the Brazilian territory, the WAIKAS made their first mark in modern history in 1929, when they attacked the settlements of rubber-tappers in the area between the Imeri Range and the Upper Rio Negro—along the Demití, Cauaborí, Marauiá and Padauirí Rivers. The Indians attacked suddenly, killed the men and carried off the women and children. The survivors fled to the Rio Negro. For 25 years, until 1954, everybody kept away from the area for fear of the Indians. In 1954, a Catholic priest of the Salesian mission in Tapuruquara, Rev. Antonio Goes, entered the territory, went up the Cauaborí River by boat and made the first peaceable contact with a tribe of the WAIKAS.

We met the priest in 1955 when we went through Tapuruquara on an expedition to the Colombian frontier. One year later, in 1956, we went with him to the WAIKA village situated near the headwaters of the Cauaborí River, a few miles from the Venezuelan boundary.

It was the priest's third visit to the tribe, where we found about 200 Indians in their original, primitive state. They never had any previous contact with civilized people other than the priest and then, ourselves.

In two later visits, we were able to observe and to film their daily village life, but we saw nothing of the snuff. We saw them dancing under the influence of the EPÉNA, but we were not able to see the snuff prepared. When we asked, they told us that the ingredients did not grow nearby.

Our relations improved with the repeated visits. On our fourth trip in 1960, we were received like old friends. We were shown the ingredients. We saw that they were neither seeds of PIPTADENIA PEREGRINA nor of any other tree. They turned out to be two kinds of bark and the leaves of a small plant. For the first time, we were able to get some of the snuff by exchanging gifts. It was the same powder that I sent to Professor Holmstedt, who analysed it. He found tryptamine derivatives to be the active components. In 1965, finally, we had a chance to film the snuff-making process.

The Preparation of the Epéna Snuff-Powder

We could observe and film the whole process of the EPÉNA preparation on the Upper Marauiá River in the village of the KARAUETARI tribe. First we looked, in the company of two Indians, for a tree of the species

316

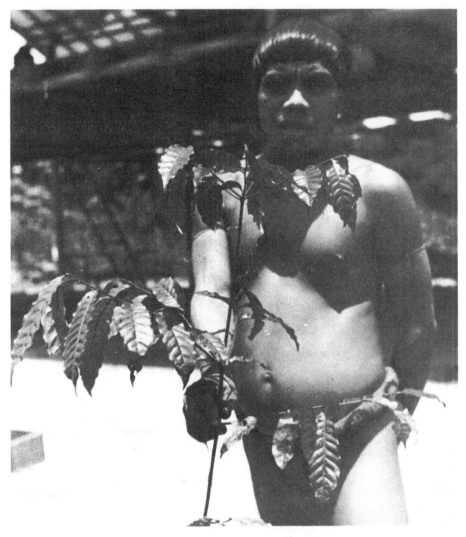

FIG. 1.—A sapling of "EPÉNA."

VIROLA CALLOPHYLLOIDEA, Markgraf, called by the Indians EPÉNA.

We had started in the early morning because the Indians said that the bark has to be stripped in the early hours of the day for the snuff powder to be good. The EPÉNA trees did not exist in any quantity. We marched three days through the jungle to find a group of them.

When the bark is stripped it appears white on its inner-side, but only a few seconds later a red brownish resin like liquid begins to exude in drops. The Indians told us that this "bleeding" is more intensive before the heat of the tropical sun begins to penetrate the forest.

The inner-side of the bark consists in a soft fibre-like layer that the Indians scrape off with a knife. These scrapings—moistened by the red brownish liquid—are collected on a palm-leaf and carried to the village for drying.

The drying process begins very slowly. The scrapings are fastened on a twisted disk which will be put approximately four feet above a slow fire, and there remain till the next morning. Then comes the second phase of the drying, more intensive, directly over the fire.

In this state the scrapings are stored till the second ingredient of the snuff-powder, called AMA ASITA, is ready. AMA ASITA is a tall tree that was not possible to classify as yet. But it seems to be a TRICHILIA species. Also, this tree seems to be scarce.

Before stripping the Indians looked for a specimen with smooth bark. They took only strips of bark whose outside was entirely perfect. This outside is important. It is the only part used. It was separated from the inner side of the bark immediately after the stripping and carried to the village. There these outside strips of the bark were cut in pieces and put in a fire. As soon as they began to glow, the Indians took them out of the fire and let them burn to ashes separately. They watched carefully, to see that no piece of any other wood or bark might be mixed with them.

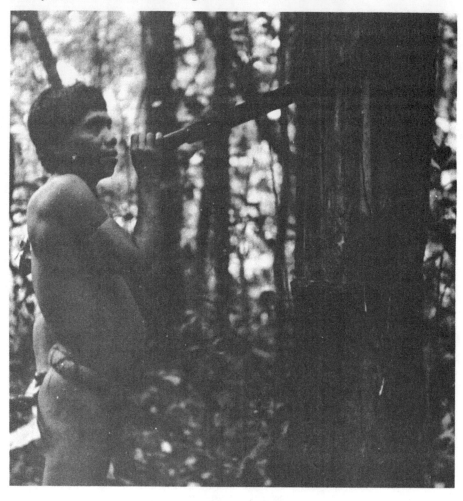

FIG. 2.—Stripping of the "EPÉNA" bark.

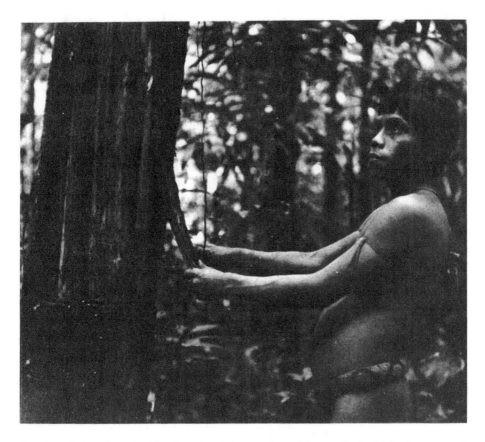

Fig. 3.—Only a few seconds after the stripping the red-brownish liquid begins to exude in drops and tinges the clearsighted wood of the trunk and the inner side of the bark.

These ashes of the AMA ASITA-bark are called by the WAIKA-Indians, "YUPU USHI".

While the bark was burning separately, our Indian began to rub down the dried EPÉNA scrapings with his hands. He did it sitting on the ground and pressing his knees against his hands.

After reducing the EPÉNA scrapings to a crumbled dust, the Indian roasted it for a short time over the fire. Then he mixed it with the ashes of AMA ASITA. The proportion of the mixture was 50:50. As it is measured by sight, the snuff-powders of the different manufacturers never have the same tone of colour.

The snuff was not yet sufficiently uniform and refined. It contained little spelts and crumbs that had to be eliminated. This was done in a little basket such as each WAIKA household owned. The Indian beat the basket gently, and the resulting dust was the final snuff-powder. It was kept in a bamboo-tube, the usual storage box of the WAIKAS. Four or five of these tubes are stuck between the palm-tree-leaves of each hut. The smaller tubes are usually used for snuff-powder, and the bigger ones for keeping feathers, arrow-heads and pigment for painting the body.

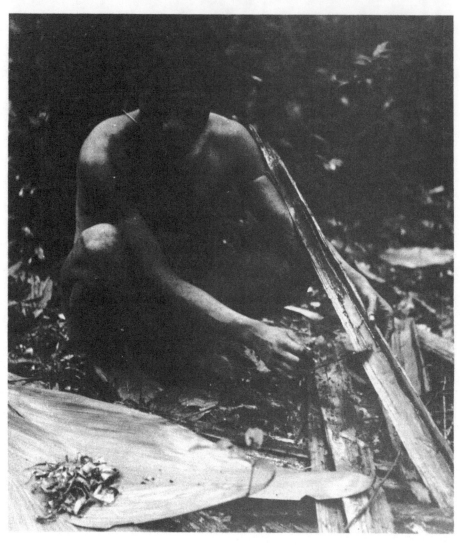

Fig. 4.—The inner side of the bark consists in a soft fibre-like layer that the Indians scrape off with a knife.

320

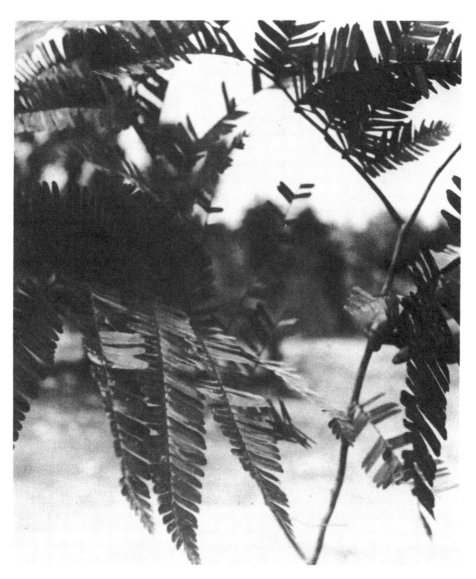

Fig. 5.—A branch of AMA ASITA.

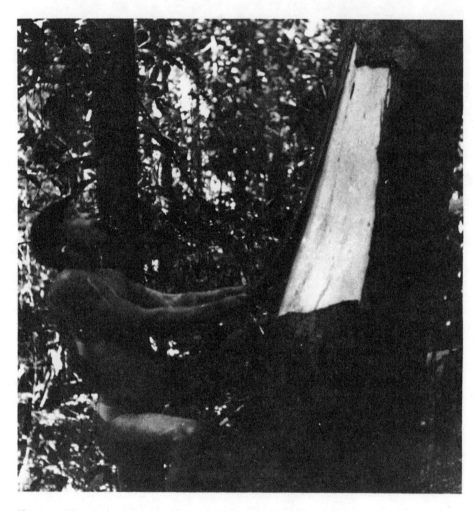

FIG. 6.—The AMA ASITA bark is stripped. Note that the wood of the trunk remains clear-sighted.

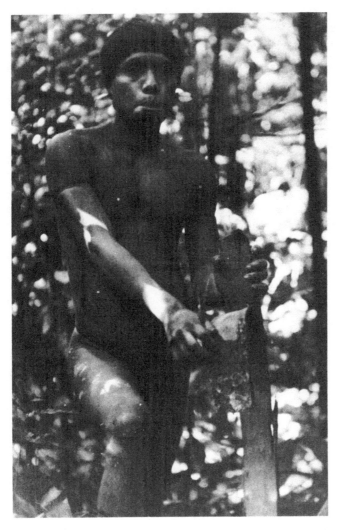

Fig. 7.—The outside of the bark is separated from its inner side.

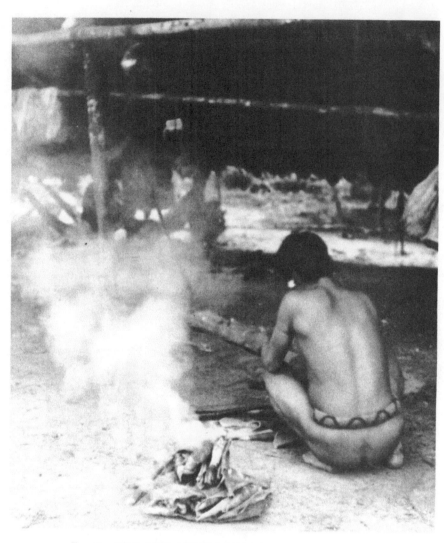

Fig. 8.—THE AMA ASITA bark burns to ashes separately.

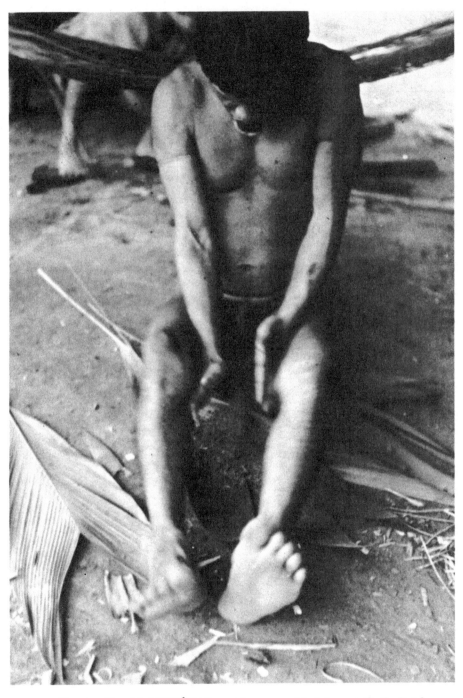

FIG. 9.—The dried "EPÉNA" scrapings are rubbed down with the hands.

In another WAIKA-village, near the Maturacá-channel, we saw that a third ingredient was added: the little leaves of a HERBACEUS-plant, called MASHI HIRI, like the EPÉNA-scrapings dried and powdered. These leaves, however, have no intoxicating effect. The Indians say they are merely aromatic. I don't know why the KARAUETARY didn't use the plant. Perhaps it was not available at the moment, or the Indians in the MA-RAUIÁ-River like another flavour.[1]

---

[1] There is also used another snuff powder which contains, besides the above mentioned three ingredients, the other vegetables:

    (1) The leaves of a plant called POSCHI-HAVE-MOSCHI-Hena ("hena" means "leaf")

    (2) The leaves of another vegetable called AI-AMO-Hena.

In the villages we visited, the Indians either could not or did not want to show us these two plants. They always said that they only grew in the higher region of the mountains, and not nearby. For this reason the powder compound of the five ingredients was not on hand.

In my opinion it is the same compound whose snuffing we saw in our first expedition, and whose effect was discribed as noxious for health. (People of the rain forest, page 167.) I cannot at the moment say more about this powder. Neither the missionary with whom I am corresponding and who lives in continued contact with several tribes, nor myself, saw in our other expeditions a similar effect again. And in no other visited tribe were we able to get this powder.

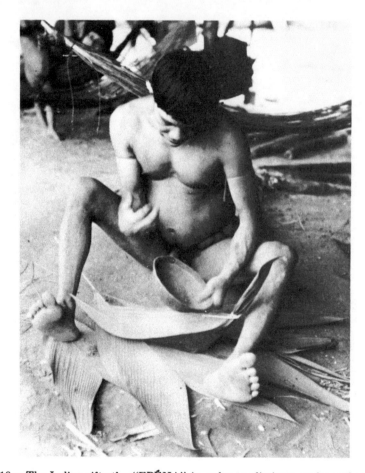

Fig. 10.—The Indian sifts the "EPÉNA" in order to eliminate spelts and crumbs.

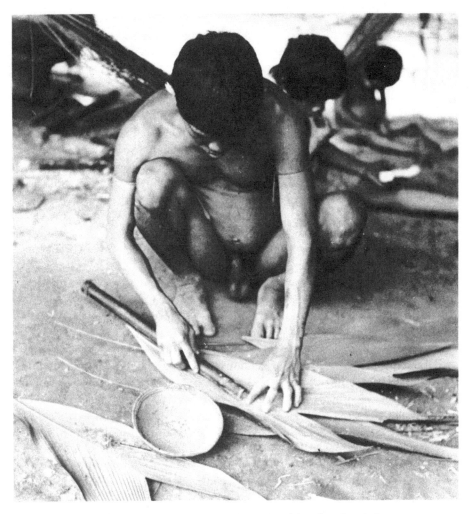

Fig. 11.—The final snuff powder is stored in a bamboo tube.

Some Remarks on the Use of Epéna

We watched the use of EPÉNA in four WAIKA-villages: (1) near the Upper Cauaborí River; (2) near the Upper Maiá River; (3) near the Upper Marauiá River, and (4) near the Maturacá Channel.

Firstly: The snuff was never inhaled in the morning. At this time, we saw some of the corresponding preparations, such as painting the face and the upper part of the body. Another Indian helped to paint the back and legs. The feather ornament is tied on the upper arm. All in all a certain festive preparation is part of the ceremony.

Secondly, The snuff-Inhaling ceremony generally began in the early afternoon; rarely in the evening.

Thirdly: Once, we saw two Indians blow snuff into each other's noses. Generally, only one person inhaled the EPÉNA.

327

Fourthly: Only adult men, but not women, took part in the ceremony.

Fifthly: The blowpipe, 23 to 28 inches in length, was used for inhalation with one exception. We did not see any other inhalation instrument.

Sixthly: Only once did we see an Indian inhale snuff without the aid of another man, and without instrument. (See also footnote Nr. 4). He poured the snuff from the bamboo tube into his open hand, lifted his hand to his nose and inhaled the powder simply and neatly.

Seventhly: When we became able to distinguish one Indian from another, we saw that there is no system for the snuff ceremony. For example: There were Indians who took EPÉNA powder every day at any time in the afternoon; there were others who practiced the ceremony only once in a fortnight. Seldom did we see any formal motive for taking the snuff, such as curing a sick person, invoking success in the hunt or thanksgiving for a successful hunt.

Only for the first motive, we saw snuff taking a few times. One or two men took snuff to bring about the curing of a sick child. So did the child's father, but not at the same time. I had the impression that in most cases, snuff was taken without any profound meaning—such as treating the ill, exorcism, contact with the HÄKULA spirits, cult. There seemed to be only a sort of swagger—an attempt to show "What a great guy I am!"

Otherwise how can we explain the fact that a great number of the Indians did not take any notice of the ceremony in the village square. Or that a dancer's girl friend sitting in her hammock, proudly watched the man stamping and yelling in front of the hut? Moreover, the interpreters occasionally burst out laughing at the dancer's movements and words. These words did not always seem to make sense.

The dose for inhaling in each nostril was a coffee-spoon full. The Indians usually take two doses. Only once, in the KARAUETARI-village near the Marauiá River, did we see an Indian take four doses, one after another.

Administration

The inhalation was practiced in general in the following manner: (with one exception observed in the KAUARETARI-village): At first the snuff power of one or two bamboo tubes was poured on a little board or plate, and the little crumbs—caused by the high humidity of the air—were carefully pinched between the fingers.

Then the two Indians, the carefully painted and adorned one as well as the "blower" cowered under the roof of a hut, one opposite the other. The "blower" filled a dose of powder with his fingers in the blowpipe, which the other Indian kept on his right nostril. With a forceful blow the powder entered the nose. The receiver immediately let fall the blow-pipe and held the back of his head with both hands.

Our interpreter, a portuguese speaking Indian, explained that he would feel in this moment a violent headache. Not seldom, the Indian curved himself, probably because of this headache. Saliva ran out his mouth and he vomited.

328

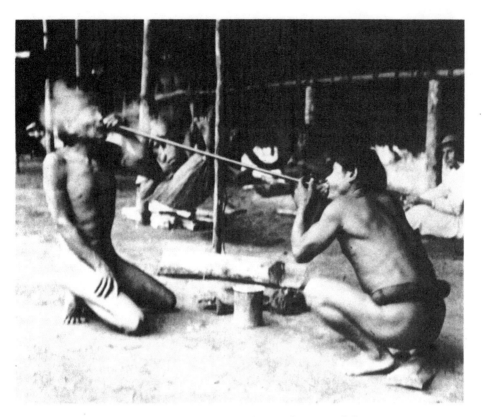

FIG. 12.—With a forceful blow the powder entered the nose.

After about 3 or 4 minutes it seemed that the first effect passed, and he took again the blow-pipe, which the other Indian, the "blower", had again filled up. The Indian now put the blow-pipe on the left nostril and got the second dose. The immediate consequences like headache, salivation and vomiting were repeated, however, not always so strongly.

Effect

After inhaling the two doses of EPÉNA, the usual quantity of snuff powder at the beginning of the ceremony, the Indian continued for about two or three minutes in his cowered position. Then he stood up and walked swaying like a drunkard. On his way his walk became faster and steadier. His stare became fixed and he experienced a violent perspiration. In a few minutes his face and body were completely wet.

Then his steps changed into a stamping that generally was adapted to a certain rhythm: three or four steps forward, one step on the same place. This "dance" the man accompanied with a recitative, monotonous singing, which was relieved about every five to eight minutes by a terrible yell. During

329

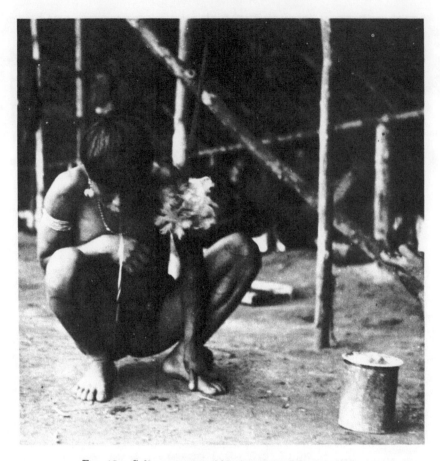

FIG. 13.—Saliva ran out of his mouth and he vomited.

this yelling the man generally stopped his "dance," and turned himself with high lifted or spread arms to the mountain-range that elevates itself, steep in the sky, a few miles to the north of the villages.[2,3]

After about half an hour of stamping and singing and yelling an interval took place in most of the observed cases. The Indian stood some minutes with straddled legs, the upper part of his body bowed forward, nearly the position which we took as children for playing leap frog. After this interval, either the singing and stamping continued or the Indian—still singing and

---

[2] In some of the cases observed by us, this yelling toward the mountain range certainly was a threat against another tribe, living in hostility against our Indians. Some weeks ago they had killed two members of that tribe and expected now the requital attack.

I see in these yellings against the mountains where the other tribe was living, no invitation to the HÄKULA spirits for help, but translate them more in this way:

"Come on over when you get up the courage!—We will make hash of you!" Conclusion: Nothing but boasting, in consequence of the macropsia provoked by the EPÉNA. Certainly, this makes the dancer think he is physically superior.

[3] In the cases when they had inhaled EPÉNA to cure a sick child, the dance was stopped in front of the child's hammock, and the Indian accompanied his yells with the vehement movements of his arms, or the softly passing of his hands over the child's body. So, he tried to take out the illness of the patient's body.

stamping—fetched from his hut some arrows, and continued dancing with these.[4]

The snuff powder EPÉNA provokes a strong intoxication but by no means an entire state of trance. Otherwise the man would not be able during his "dance" to find with sure hand the arrows in the hut or—as it had happened with me when I had gone with the camera in spite of warning—would have

[4] The Indian of the KARAUETARI tribe who inhaled the powder without the assistance of another man, snuffing the EPENA by himself from his open hand, was the only one whose "dances" differed from the general manner :

(1) The phases of his "dance" lasted not more than 15 minutes, (2) In the intervals of his "dance" he inhaled some further doses of EPÉNA. He was the only one we saw snuffing *during* the intoxicating state and not only *before* it.

It is possible that in his case the initial doses, inhaled without the powerful blow of another man, had not provoked the common intoxicating effect. So he was forced to snuff again.

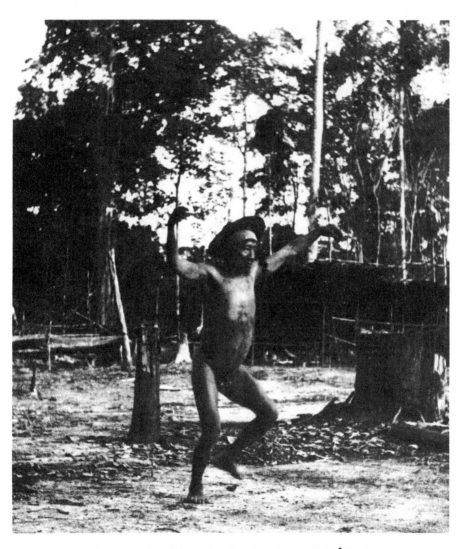

Fig. 14.—The "dance" under the effect of "EPÉNA."

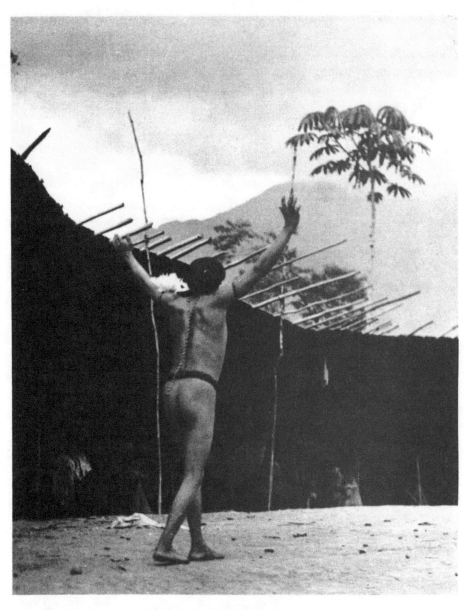

Fig. 15.— . . . turned himself with high lifted arms to the mountain-range.

been able to threaten to throw a poisoned arrow at me, if I had not disappeared. My interpreter, who had understood these words—in contrast to me—had hastened to fetch me back to the hut and translated the threat.

The "dances", the movements of the arms in the normal intoxication state—as such it could be said—were very different from those seen on our first expedition, in the few minutes when the two young men were dancing on the square under the effect of the other snuff powder, mentioned in footnote 1. These Indians doubtless had lost consciousness.

332

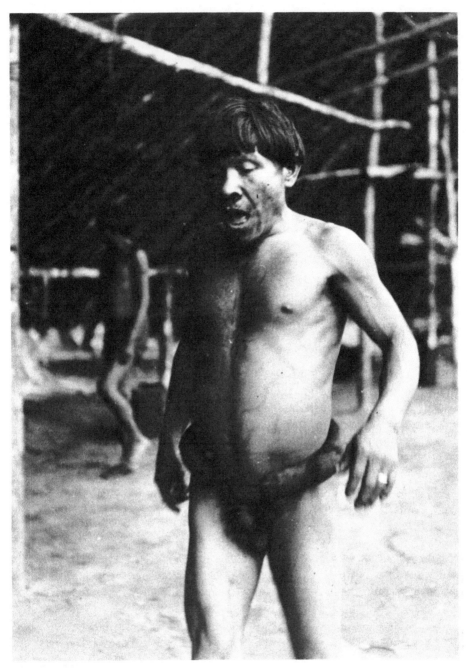

FIG. 16.—Typical face expression during the intoxication.

We talked with a young Indian of the KAUARETARI-tribe who had learned Portuguese in the mission-school in Tapuruquara. We gathered some explanations about the ceremony from this conversation:

We asked, "Do you snuff EPÉNA?" He answered, "No, I am not allowed to. I am not grown up yet!"

"When will you grow up?", we then asked.

"I don't know", he said, "but I think it will be soon."

Next question: "Who decides when you are grown up?"

"My father. He shows me how to make the EPÉNA powder, and tells me what happens when I sniff it."

Question: "What will happen then?"

Answer: "Then I will see the HÄKULA, who are big men living there above in big huts."—He pointed to the sky and continued: "The EPÉNA makes me so big that I can see them and talk with them!"

Another Indian named Daniel, who had lived in the Tapuruquara-mission for some years before returning to the tribe and marrying, told me that he had seen " A N G E L S " while under the effect of the EPÉNA. And that he had talked with them!

This one Indian tells us that he will see "big men". Another says that he saw "angels". This shows that the EPÉNA has two effects:

First: The real effect well-known from the experiments of Doctor Becher and Doctor Richard E. Schultes. The Indian feels that he is a giant; everything around him takes enormous and magnificent forms. In the midst of a super-dimensional world, he feels like a superman! Consequently his movements correspond to this state of excitation. These are braggart's gestures. These symptoms are accompanied by profuse salivation, a bad headache, a fixed stare and heavy perspiration. The symptoms reveal a state of strong intoxication.

The second effect is imagined. The Indian sees things he has been taught to see. One sees "big men" because his father has told him that he would. The other saw "angels" because he had been taught in the mission that they are more powerful than HÄKULA-spirits!

It can be assumed that these Indians think about the HÄKULA spirits and want to speak with them to cure a sickness or succeed in hunting. But my general impression is that many Indians take snuff only for kicks—to experience a bigger world.

After about an hour, the effects of the snuff diminish. The dancer slows, and goes to his hut to lie down in his hammock, where he apparently falls asleep. Several Indians who had taken snuff and danced early in the afternoon, were seen in the evening at about eight o'clock seated around the fire as if nothing had happened. The duration of the snuff effects is comparatively short. One of our interpreters said to me that they don't like to take snuff in the evening because they can't sleep afterward. We can conclude from this that perhaps the apparent sleep in the hammock after the dance is not really sleep but exhaustion, or the need to rest an aching head.

It is certain, however, that the violent headaches and nausea are caused by the way that the snuff is taken—blown into the nostrils—that the head-

334

ache is temporarily relieved by the drug. Otherwise, the Indian would not be able to behave so violently in the square. After about an hour, the exilarating, euphoric effect of the snuff backfires and turns into a hangover.

The "Paricá" of the Tucano-Medicine Man Agostino

Most of the Indians who live in the village of Tapuruquara on the Upper Rio Negro are TUCANOS, who abandoned their old tribe territory on the PAPURÍ River. Agostino is the "Pagé", the medicine man, in this village, and he still uses "PARICÁ", a snuff that he prepared in our presence. He uses the same raw-material as the WAIKA Indians—the inner layer of the bark from VIROLA CALOPHYLLOIDEA, Markgraf, but he prepared the powder in a very different manner.

With his knife he scraped off the inner layer of the bark moistened by the red-brown liquid. Then he threw these scrapings into a pot partly filled with water. In this water they were thoroughly kneaded, and squeezed so that the water turned muddy and took a reddish-brown colour. Then this muddy liquid was set to evaporate over a slow fire.

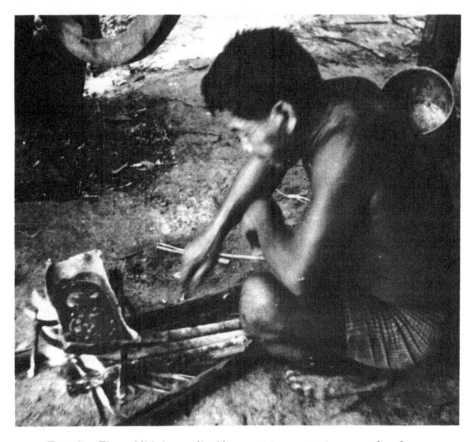

FIG. 17.—The reddish-brown liquid was set to evaporate over a slow fire.

"It should not boil very rapidly", explained Agostino. And, indeed, three hours passed before the quart of liquid had become a hard, dark crust on the bottom of the bowl. From time to time a dirty foam rose to the surface, and the "Pagé" Agostino removed it with a little branch. Also, other impurities like fibres of the bark rose up with the bubbling and were eliminated in the same way. Finally nothing remained except a thick, dark brown syrup with a strong smell. Now, Agostino lowered the fire still more. The final drying was done very slowly, probably to prevent burning.

The residue was a hard crust that was scraped off with a knife. It was the concentrate of that red-brown liquid that had begun to exude from the inner side of the bark, as well as from the trunk of VIROLA CALOPHYLLOI-DEA, Markgraf. The scraped residue was ground into a fine powder with a smooth stone.

With this process the "paricá" was ready as Agostino said. It was not mixed with ashes or other ingredients. He explained that he, the medicine man, is the only one allowed to inhale the snuff powder.

We didn't see the intoxicating effect, here, but it was confirmed by inhabitants of the village that it is very strong. Therefore Agostino can snuff his "PARICÁ" only twice a month at the most. He inhales the "PARICÁ", as he told us, before diagnosing the trouble with his patients. In the intoxicated state he stammers confused words which are interpreted by his brother. Later on he tries to cure the patient, using for the treatment the rattle "NASH SÃ" and the quartz crystal "MARIA PIRÍ".

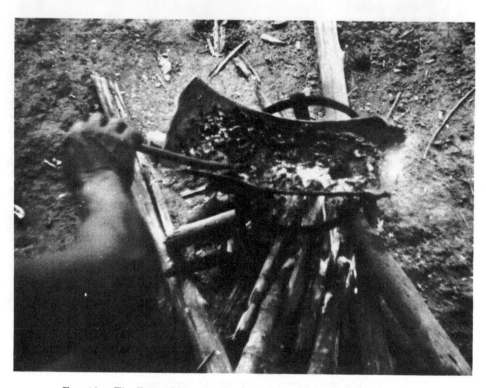

Fig. 18.—Finally nothing remained except a thick, dark-brown syrup.

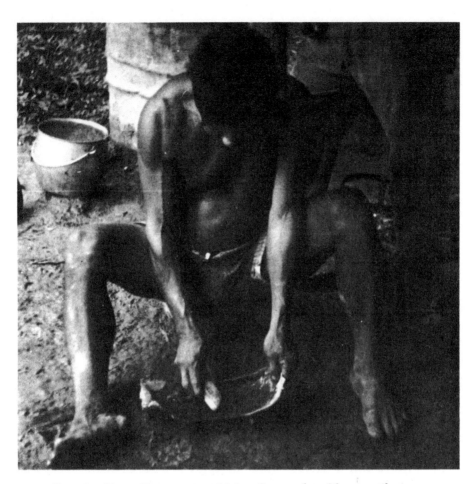

Fig. 19.—The residue was ground into a fine powder with a smooth stone.

BIBLIOGRAPHY

Bechler, H. "Die Surára and Pakidái, zwei Yanonámi-Stämme in Nordwestbrasilien." Hamburg, Cram, De Gruyter & Co. 1960, 133 pp.

Holmstedt, B. "Tryptamine Derivatives in Epena, An Intoxicating Snuff used by some South American Indian Tribes." Arch. int. Pharmacodyn. 156: 2, p. 285–305. 1965

Koch-Grünberg, Th. "Vom Roroima zum Orinoco, Erlebnisse einer Reise in Nordbrasilien und Venezuela 1911–1913," Stgt. Band III (1923) 386 pp.

Schultes, R. E. "A new narcotic snuff from the Northwest Amazon." Bot. Museum Leaflets, Harvard Univ. 16 (1954), 297–316.

Schultes, R. E. "Ethnobotanik amerikanischer Halluzinogene," Planta Medica, 13. Jahrgang, Heft 2, Mai 1965, Hippokrates, Stgt.

Seitz, G. J. People of the rain forest, Heinemann, London, 1962

Wassén, S. H. "The Use of Some Specific Kinds of South American Indian Snuff and Related Paraphernalia," Etnologiska Studier, vol. 28, Göteborg 1965

Wassén, S. H., and Holmstedt, B. "The use of paricá, an ethnological and pharmacological review," Ethnos 28, 5–45, 1963

Zerries, O. "Medizinmannwesen und Geisterglauben der Waika-Indianer des Oberen Orinoco," Ethnologica 2, Köln, E. I. Bill (1960), 487–507.

ZERRIES, O. "Waika, Die kulturgeschichtliche Stellung der Waika-Indianer der Oberen Orinoco in Rahmen der Völkerkunde Südamerikas." 1964. Klaus Renner Verlag, München (Ergebnisse der Frobenius-Expedition 1954/55 nach Südost-Venezuela. Band I. Waika.)

Chemical Constituents and Pharmacology of South American Snuffs[*]

BO HOLMSTEDT AND JAN-ERIK LINDGREN
Department of Toxicology, Swedish Medical Research Council
Karolinska Institutet, Stockholm, Sweden

About ten years ago E. C. Horning and co-workers isolated from seeds of *Piptadenia peregrina*, a leguminous plant, indole alkaloids which were identified by means of paper chromatography, colour reactions, fluorescence and infrared spectra (Stromberg 1954, Fish, Johnson and Horning 1955). They found the seeds to contain dimethyltryptamine-*N*-oxide (DMT-*N*-oxide) and Bufotenine (5-OH-DMT) and its corresponding N-oxide. The seeds of *Piptadenia peregrina* is the most commonly known botanical source of snuffs made by South American Indian tribes, and is inhaled to produce visions and hallucinations. The interest of Horning and co-workers arose from the properties of the crude drug. As a result of these analyses synthetic dimethyltryptamine (DMT) has come to be used experimentally by psychiatrists, in order to produce shortlasting states of illusions and hallucinations (Szara et al. 1957, 1961, Böszörményi and Grunecker 1957).

Ethnological and botanical evidence in recent years demonstrates clearly that *Piptadenia peregrina* by no means is the main constituent of all snuffs used by South American Indians. In view of this it was felt necessary to make a general investigation of whatever material of this kind that could be collected. The first results of these studies are reported here. Modern techniques of analysis such as gas chromatography and the combination of gas chromatography and mass spectrometry (Ryhage 1964) offer possibilities for an accurate analysis even of very small amounts of material, such as can usually be obtained from museum specimens.

Material and methods

List of abbreviations used

DMT   =*N*,*N*-Dimethyltryptamine
MMT   =*N*-Monomethyltryptamine
5-MeO-DMT=5-Methoxy-*N*,*N*-dimethyltryptamine
5-MeO-MMT=5-Methoxy-*N*-monomethyltryptamine
5-OH-DMT   =5-Hydroxy-*N*,*N*-dimethyltryptamine (bufotenine)
GLC   =Gas-liquid-chromatography
MS   =Mass spectrometry

Ethnological and botanical specimens

Epéna snuff collected in 1965 at Rio Marauiá. Epéna snuff collected in 1965 at Rio Maturacá. Snuff prepared by Pagé Agostino collected in 1965 in Tapuruquara. All were obtained from Mr. Georg J. Seitz, Caixa Postal 2605, Rio de Janeiro.

Paricá obtained from Dr. Stig Rydén at the Ethnographical Museum in Stockholm.

[*]This investigation was supported by Grant MH–12007 from the National Institute of Mental Health, U.S. Public Health Service, Chevy Chase, Md.

The specimen was collected in 1955 by the late Gustav Bolinder among the Piaroa Indians (Orinoco region, Venezuela). Sample No. 56–7–282 Statens Etnografiska Museum, Stockholm.

Yopo snuff, obtained from Mr. Donald Overton, School of Tropical and Preventive Medicine, College of Medical Evangelists, Dept. of Biotoxicology, Loma Linda, Calif., collected in Colombia 1956. Sample No. P56–70–11.

Epéna snuff, obtained from Dr. H. Becher, Niedersächsisches Landesmuseum, Abteilung für Völkerkunde, Hannover, collected among the Surára Indians in 1956.

Seeds from *Piptadenia peregrina*, obtained from the Abbott Laboratories, collected in 1948 in San Juan, Puerto Rico, Sample No. (N–2003–C).

Seeds from *Piptadenia peregrina*, obtained from Dr. W. Haberland, Museum für Völkerkunde, Hamburg, collected by Dr. Franz Caspar among the Tupari Indians (Caspar 1953).

Bark from *Piptadenia peregrina*, obtained from Mr. Donald Overton, collected in Colombia 1956. Sample No. P56–70–7.

Bark from *Virola calophylla*, obtained from Mr. William A. Rodrigues, Manaus, Brazil, 1964.

Material used in gas chromatography—mass spectrometry

Gas Chrom P 100–120 mesh, Applied Science Lab., State College, Pa., U.S.A. F–60 (a methyl *p*-dichlorophenylsiloxane polymer, Dow Corning, Midland, Mich., U.S.A.). EGSS–Z (= Z a copolymer from ethylene glycol, succinic acid and methyl phenyl siloxane monomers, Applied Science Lab.). SE–30 silicone, Applied Science Lab. PDEAS (phenyldiethanolamine succinate, Wilkins Instrument & Research, Walnut Creek, Cal., U.S.A.).

Dichlorodimethylsilane, Hopkins & Williams Ltd., Essex, England.

Reference compounds and reagents

5-Methoxy-N,N-dimethyltryptamine, 5-methoxy-N-monomethyltryptamine, N-mono-methyltryptamine bioxalate were kindly placed at our disposal by Dr. A. Hofmann, Sandoz A.G., Basle. Harmine and tetrahydroharmine hydrochloride were kindly placed at our disposal by Dr. K. Bernauer, F. Hoffmann-La Roche & Co., A.G. Basle. *N,N*-Di-methyltryptamine (Aldrich Chemical Co., Inc., Milwaukee, Wis., U.S.A.). Harmine (Fluka A.G. Buchs SG, Switzerland). Bufotenine was prepared from *Piptadenia peregrina* by E. C. Horning, Baylor University, College of Medicine, Texas Medical Center, Houston, Texas, U.S.A. All other reagents used were of "reagent grade" and from different manufacturers.

Isolation of organic bases

5–20 g of the powdered material was treated according to a procedure known to be satisfactory for phenolic amines in the indole series (Fish, Johnson and Horning 1955). The isolation procedure was followed in detail but the amounts of solvents were reduced with respect to the initial weight of the sample.

The steps of isolation procedure were followed by tests using Ehrlich's reagent. After drying with magnesium sulphate the final product was obtained upon removal of the solvent. The total alkaloids obtained were then dissolved either in methanol or in tetrahydrofurane.

Gas chromatography (GLC)

Gas chromatographic analysis was performed with an F & M Model 400 apparatus equipped with a hydrogen flame ionization detection system.

The column support, 100–120 mesh Gas Chrom P, was acid washed and silanized according to the method described by Horning et al. (1963). The coating was applied by the filtration technique (Horning, et al. 1959, 1963). The stationary phases used were (1) 6% F–60 and 2% EGSS–Z (2.25 m x 3.2 mm glass tube), (2) 5% SE–30 (4 m x 3.2 mm glass tube). The F–60–Z column was operated at 190° and the SE–30 column at 210°. The flash heater and detector cell were kept 30–40° above the column temperature. The flow rate of the carrier gas, nitrogen, was 60 ml/min. Samples were injected in methanol or tetrahydrofuran solution with a Hamilton syringe.

Gas chromatography-mass spectrometry (GLC-MS)

The principles of the technique have been described in detail by Ryhage (1964). The mass spectrometry work was carried out with LKB 9000 gas chromatograph-mass spectrometer including a fast scan system and the Ryhage "molecule separator." The ion source was 270°, the electron energy was 70 eV and the electron ionization current 60μA, respectively. The separations were made on systems consisting of 3% PDEAS at 190° or 5% SE–30 at 200°. The column consisted of a 2 m x 3.2 mm glass tube. Helium was used as the carrier gas. At the outlet of the column, the separated compounds were concentrated and continuously fed into the mass spectrometer. The mass spectrometer simultaneously serves as a gas chromatographic detector and for recording of mass spectra of the compound as they emerge from the column. The reference compounds were run through the column, and the mass spectra of the compounds recorded. The alkaloid fractions prepared as described above, were then run under identical conditions, and mass spectra were recorded from the gas chromatographic peaks having the same retention times as those of the reference compounds.

Results

The results of the authors' analysis of crude drugs such as paricá, epéna, etc. and corresponding botanical specimens are contained in Fig. 1–14. In table 1–2 our own results as well as those of previous investigators have been included. In every case the peaks in the gas chromatograms have been corroborated by mass spectra obtained with the combination instrument. This method assures complete identity with the reference compounds, and gives direct evidence for identity in contrast to indirect methods such as relative retention times.

Snuffs

In all six snuffs were examined (Table 1). In the crude drugs we have identified the various tryptamines. In three of them 5-MeO-DMT was the main component. DMT was identified in five but was nowhere found to be the main component. 5-OH-DMT was found in substantial amounts in two snuffs. One drug proved to have as much Bufotenine as DMT. This snuff has very little 5-MeO-DMT but in addition to simple indoles also contains harmine. Only one drug has 5-OH-DMT as its main constituent but contained in addition DMT and 5-MeO-DMT. Two compounds hitherto unidentified in South American snuffs were found to be present namely MMT and 5-MeO-MMT. Only one snuff contained exclusively β-carbolines.

Plants

As a comparison, plant material from *Piptadenia peregrina* and *Virola calophylla* were examined in identical ways. Piptadenia seeds from two various locations proved to contain in one case 5-OH-DMT and in another case 5-MeO-DMT as the main constituent. The bark from *Piptadenia* when examined contained the following substances: DMT, MMT, 5-MeO-DMT and 5-MeO-MMT where 5-MeO-DMT by far was present in the highest concentration. Finally, the bark from *Virola calophylla* proved to contain DMT, MMT and 5-MeO-DMT, the highest concentration in this case being DMT.

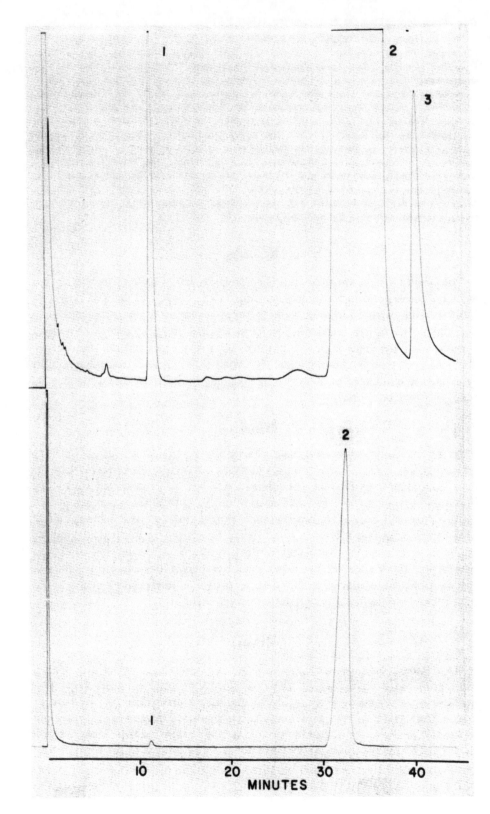

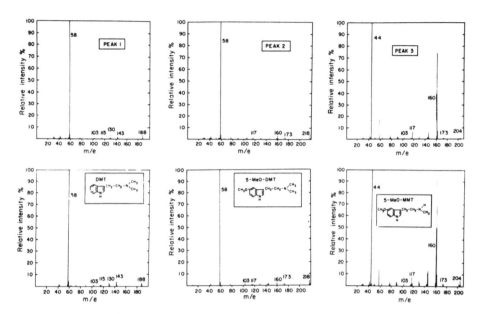

FIG. 2.—Mass spectrometric recording of compound in peak effluents from alkaloid fraction (Fig. 1) and reference compounds. Conditions: Column 2 m; i.d. 3.2 mm; 3% PDEAS; 100–120 mesh Gas Chrom P; temp. 190°.

FIG. 1.—Gas chromatogram of alkaloid fraction from South American snuff prepared by Pagé Agostino, obtained from Mr G. Seitz. Tucano Indians, Tapuruquara, 1965. GLC conditions: Column 2.25 mm; i.d. 3.2 mm; 6% F 60 and 2% EGSS—Z on 100–120 mesh Gas Chrom P; temp. 190°; flow 60 ml per min. Upper panel high magnification. Lower panel low magnification. Mass spectra recorded simultaneously from peak effluents of extract and model substances injected under similar conditions, see Fig. 2.

FIG. 3.—Gas chromatogram of alkaloid fraction of Epéna snuff obtained from Mr G· Seitz. Waica Indians, Rio Marauiá, 1965. GLC conditions: Same as for Fig. 1. Upper panel high magnification. Middle panel low magnification. Lower panel reference substance recorded simultaneously. Mass spectra from effluent from peak 2 and model substances injected under similar conditions, see Fig. 4. Mass spectrometric control of peak effluents: Peak 1 and DMT: Molecular ion at $m/_e$ 188; other peaks at $m/_e$ 58 (base peak), 103, 115, 130, 143. Peak 3 and 5-MeO-DMT: Molecular ion at $m/_e$ 218; other peaks at $m/_e$ 58 (base peak), 103, 117, 160, 173.

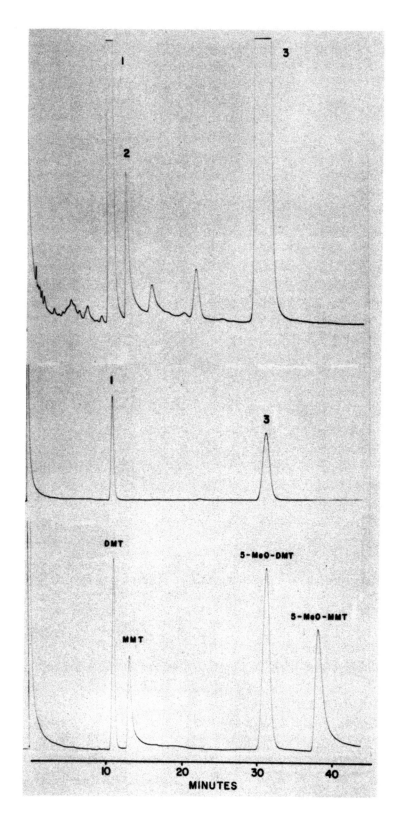

FIG. 4.—Mass spectrometric recording of compound in peak effluent from peak 2 from alkaloid fraction (Fig. 3) and reference compound. Conditions: Same as for Fig. 2.

346

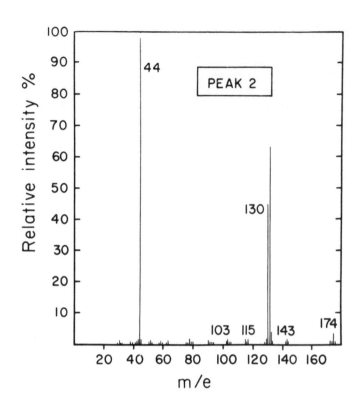

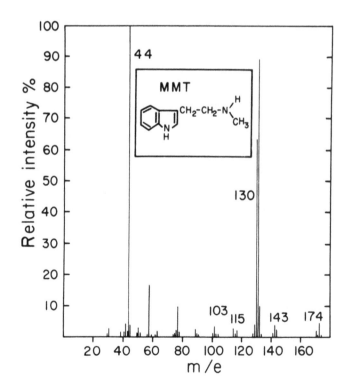

Fɪɢ. 5.—Gas chromatogram of alkaloid fraction of Epéna snuff obtained from Mr G. Seitz, Araraibo Indians, Rio Maturacá, 1965. GLC conditions: Same as for Fig. 1. Upper panel alkaloid fraction. Lower panel reference substances. Mass spectrometric control of peak effluents: Peak 1 and DMT: Molecular ion at $m/_e$ 188; other peaks at $m/_e$ 58 (base peak), 103, 115, 130, 143. Peak 2 and 5-MeO-DMT: Molecular ion at $m/_e$ 218; other peaks at $m/_e$ 58 (base peak), 103, 117, 160, 173.

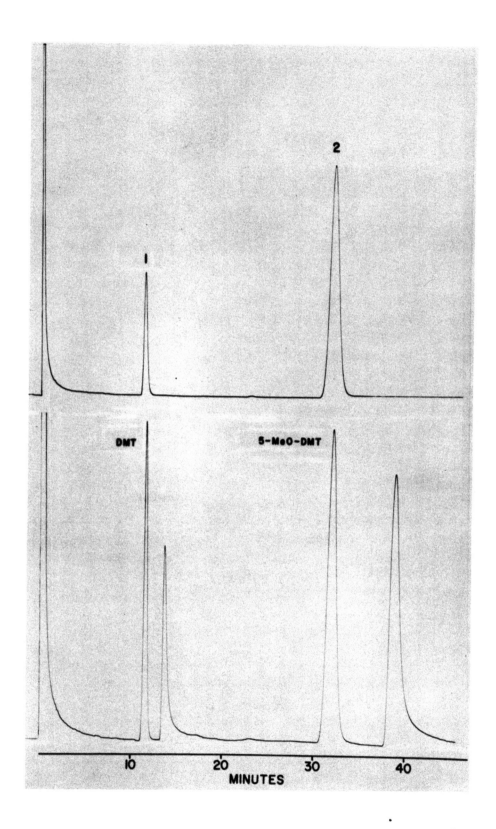

349

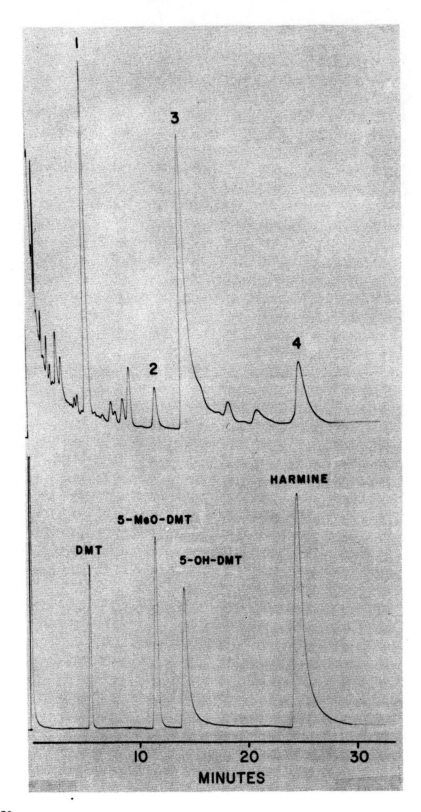

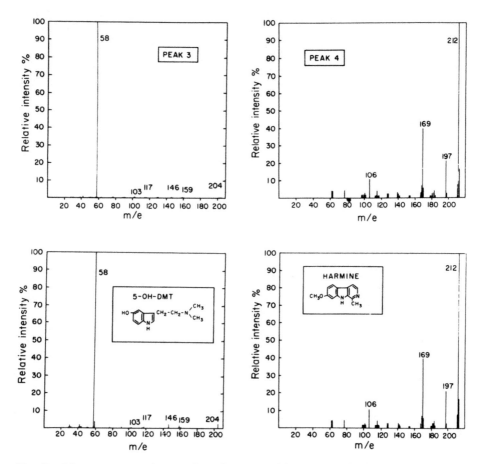

FIG. 7.—Mass spectrometric recording of compound in effluents from peak 3 and 4 from alkaloid fraction (Fig. 6) and reference compounds. Conditions: Column 2 m; i.d. 3.2 mm; 5% SE–30; 100–120 mesh Gas Chrom P; temp. 200°.

FIG. 6.—Gas chromatogram of alkaloid fraction from Paricá obtained from the Ethnographical Museum, Stockholm, collected by the late Prof. Bolinder. Piaroa Indians, Venezuela, 1955. Column 4m; i.d. 3.2 mm; 5% SE–30 on 100–120 mesh Gas Chrom P; temp. 210°; flow 60 ml per min. Upper panel alkaloid fraction. Lower panel reference substances. Mass spectrometric control of peak effluents: Peak 1 and DMT: Molecular ion at m/e 188; other peaks at m/e 58 (base peak), 103, 115, 130, 143. Peak 2 and 5-MeO-DMT: Molecular ion at m/e 218; other peaks at m/e 58 (base peak), 103, 117, 160, 173. Mass spectra from effluents from peak 3 and 4 and model substances, see Fig. 7.

351

FIG. 8.—Gas chromatogram of alkaloid fraction from Yopo, Colombia, 1956, obtained from Mr Donald Overton. Sample number P56–70–11. GLC conditions: Same as for Fig. 6. Upper panel alkaloid fraction. Lower panel reference substances. Mass spectrometric control of peak effluents: Peak 1 and DMT: Molecular ion at m/e 188; other peaks at m/e 58 (base peak), 103, 115, 130, 143. Peak 2 and 5-MeO-DMT: Molecular ion at m/e 58 (base peak), 103, 117, 160, 173. Peak 3 and 5-OH-DMT: Molecular ion at m/e 204; other peaks at m/e 58 (base peak), 103, 117, 146, 159.

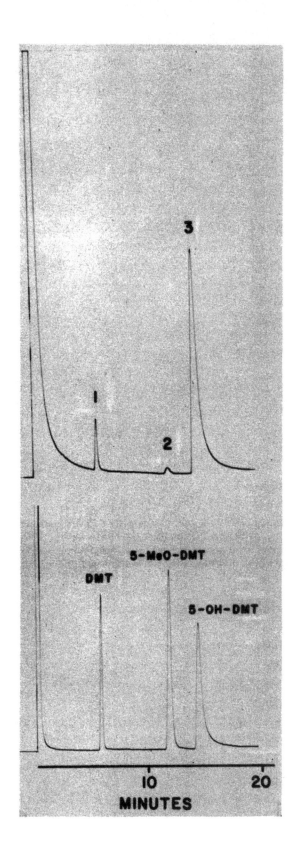

Fig. 9.—Gas chromatogram of alkaloid fraction from Epéna snuff obtained from Dr H Becher. Surára Indians 1956. GLC conditions: Same as for Fig. 6. Upper panel alkaloid fraction. Lower panel reference substances. Mass spectra recorded simultaneously from peak effluents of extract and model substances injected under similar conditions, see Fig. 10.

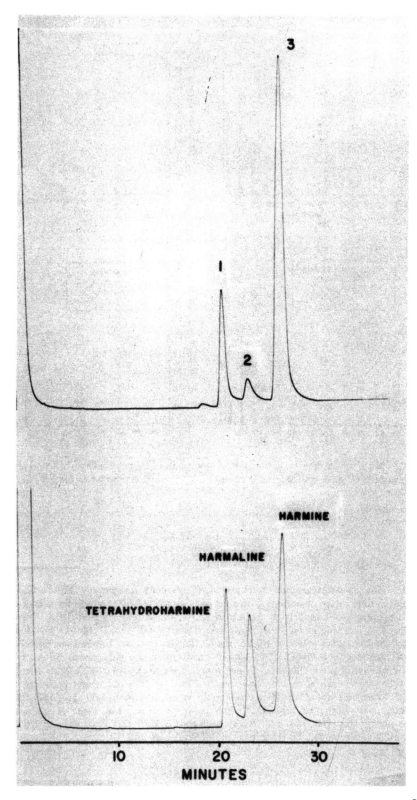

355

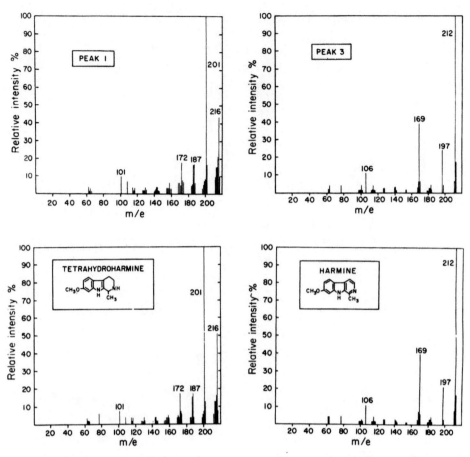

FIG. 10.—Mass spectrometric recording of compounds in peak effluents from alkaloid fraction (Fig. 9) and reference compounds. Conditions: Same as for Fig. 7.

FIG. 11.—Gas chromatographic comparison of alkaloid fraction in Piptadenia seeds obtained from various locations with reference substances. Upper panel seeds of Piptadenia peregrina obtained from Abbott No. N–2003–C, Puerto Rico 1948. Previously analysed by Horning et al. 1955. Main constituent 5-OH-DMT. Middle panel seed of Piptadenia peregrina collected by F. Caspar. Tupari Indians, Rio Branco, Brazil, 1953. Main constituent 5-MeO-DMT. Lower panel reference substances. Mass spectrometric control of peak effluents: *Upper panel*—Left peak and DMT: Molecular ion at $m/_e$ 188; other peaks at $m/_e$ 58 (base peak), 103, 115, 130, 143. Right peak and 5-OH-DMT: Molecular ion at $m/_e$ 204; other peaks at $m/_e$ 58 (base peak), 103, 117, 146, 159. *Middle panel*—Left peak and DMT: Molecular ion at $m/_e$ 188; other peaks at $m/_e$ 58 (base peak), 103, 115, 130, 143. Right peak and 5-MeO-DMT: Molecular ion at $m/_e$ 218; other peaks at $m/_e$ 58 (base peak), 103, 117, 160, 173.

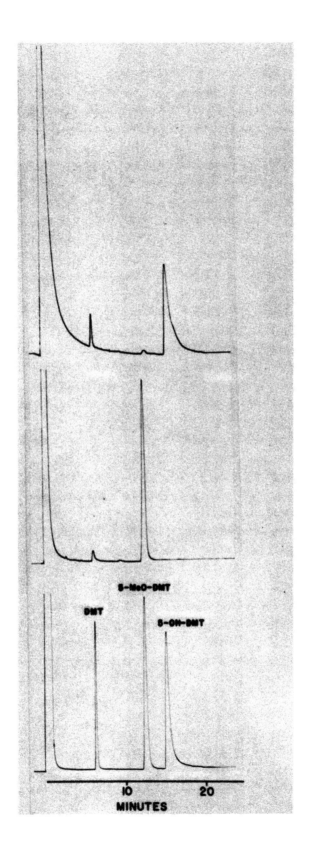

357

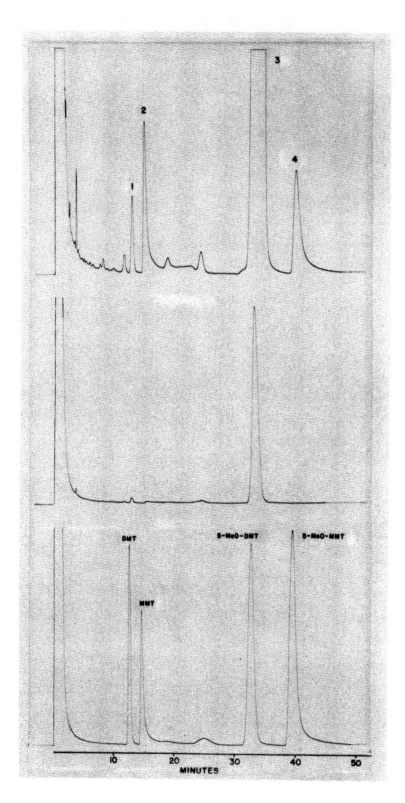

358

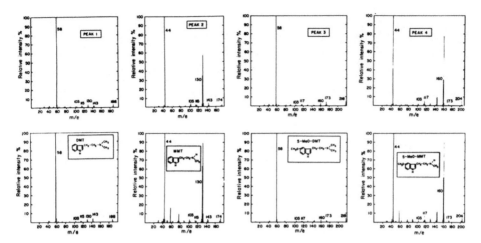

Fig. 13.—Mass spectrometric recording of compounds in peak effluents from alkaloid fraction in Fig. 12 and reference compounds. Conditions: Same as for Fig. 2.

Fig. 12.—Gas chromatogram of alkaloid fraction from bark of Piptadenia peregrina obtained from Mr. Donald Overton, collected in Colombia. 1956. Sample number P56-70-7. Column conditions: Same as for Fig. 1. Upper panel high magnification. Middle panel low magnification. Lower panel reference substances. Mass spectra recorded simultaneously from peak effluent of extract and model substances injected under similar conditions, see Fig. 13.

359

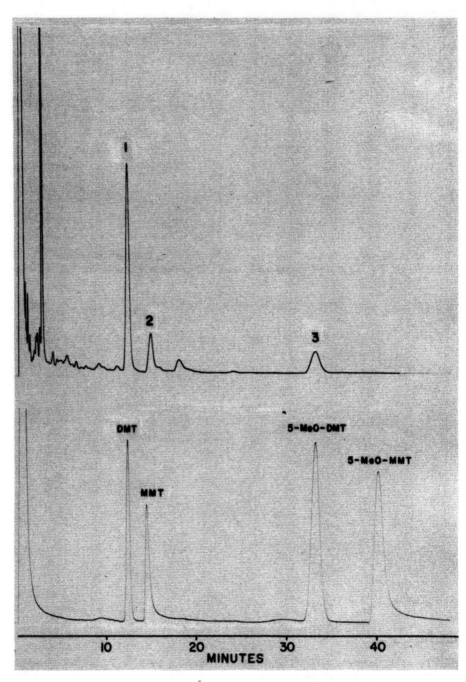

F ɪ ɢ. 14.—Gas chromatogram of alkaloid fraction from bark of Virola calophylla. Manaus 1964. GLC conditions: Same as for Fig. 1. Upper panel alkaloid fraction. Lower panel reference substances. Mass spectrometric control of peak effluents: Peak 1 and DMT: Molecular ion at $m/_e$ 188; other peaks at $m/_e$ 58 (base peak), 103, 115, 130, 143. Peak 2 and MMT: Molecular ion at $m/_e$ 174; other peaks at $m/_e$ 44 (base peak), 103, 115, 130, 131, 143. Peak 3 and 5-MeO-DMT: Molecular ion at $m/_e$ 218, other peaks at $m/_e$ 58 (base peak), 103, 117, 160, 173.

TABLE 1.—*Distribution of indole alkaloids in South American snuffs*

Name	Origin	Alkaloid	Reference
Paricà	Venezuela	5–OH–DMT	Fish and Horning 1956
Paricà	Colombia	5–OH–DMT	
Epéna	Waica Indians	DMT 5–OH–DMT 5–MeO–DMT	Holmstedt et al. 1964
Epéna	Yanonámi Indians	DMT DMT–N-oxide 5–OH–DMT 5–OH–DMT–N-oxide	Marini-Bettolo et al. 1964
Epéna	Surára Indians	Harmine Tetrahydroharmine	Bernauer 1964
Paricà	Tucano Indians	Harmine Harmaline Tetrahydroharmine	Biocca et al. 1964
Epéna	Tucano Indians	DMT 5–MeO–DMT 5–MeO–MMT	Present investigation
Epéna	Waica Indians	DMT MMT 5–MeO–DMT	
Epéna	Araraibo Indians	DMT 5–MeO–DMT	
Yopo	Colombia	DMT 5–OH–DMT 5–MeO–DMT	
Paricà	Piaroa Indians	DMT 5–OH–DMT 5–MeO–DMT Harmine	
Epéna	Surára Indians	Harmine Tetrahydroharmine	

361

TABLE 2.—*Distribution of indole alkaloids in South American plants used for snuff preparation*

Plant	Part	Origin	Alkaloid	Reference
Piptadenia peregrina Benth.	Seeds	Puerto Rico	5-OH-DMT	Stromberg 1954
Piptadenia peregrina Benth.	Pods Seeds	Puerto Rico and Brazil	DMT DMT-N-oxide 5-OH-DMT 5-OH-DMT-N-oxide	Fish, Johnson, and Horning 1955
Piptadenia peregrina Benth.	Seeds Seeds	Puerto Rico Rio Branco region, West Brazil	DMT 5-OH-DMT DMT 5-MeO-DMT	Present investigation
Piptadenia peregrina Benth.	Bark	Brazil	MMT 5-MeO-DMT 5-MeO-MMT	Legler and Tschesche 1963
Piptadenia peregrina Benth.	Bark	Colombia	DMT MMT 5-MeO-DMT 5-MeO-MMT	Present investigation
Piptadenia macrocarpa Benth.	Pods Seeds	Brazil	DMT DMT-N-oxide 5-OH-DMT 5-OH-DMT-N-oxide	Fish, Johnson, and Horning 1955
Piptadenia macrocarpa Benth.	Bark Pods Seeds	Argentine	5-MeO-MMT DMT 5-OH-DMT DMT 5-OH-DMT 5-OH-DMT-N-oxide	Iacobucci and Rúveda 1964
Piptadenia excelsa (Gris.) Lillo	Pods Seeds	Argentine	DMT 5-OH-DMT 5-OH-DMT-N-oxide	
Piptadenia colubrina Benth.	Seeds	Brazil	5-OH-DMT	Pachter, Zackarias, and Riberio 1959
Mimosa hostilis Benth.	Root	Brazil	DMT	
Virola calophylla	Bark	Manaus Brazil	DMT MMT 5-MeO-DMT	Present investigation

362

Discussion

Mass spectrometric fragmentation of tryptamines

In the past years the mass spectrometer has taken its place beside other methods in studies of natural products. The unique function of this instrument is to delineate the molecular size and composition of a compound; in many cases it can also provide information on the arrangement of atoms in the molecule. The classical application of mass spectrometry, one in which its precision is superior to that of any other method, is in determining the molecular weight of an unknown compound. More extensive deductions regarding structures of complex molecules may often be derived from careful examination of the entire mass spectrum of a compound.

The combination of mass spectrometry and gas chromatography as invented by Ryhage (1964) is even more advantageous, because it combines the means of identification described above with the best method so far described for the separation of a series of compounds.

In the instrument available (LKB 9000), a mass spectrometer is coupled to a gas liquid chromatography (GLC) column. As the compounds emerge from the column they are ionized in the ion source of the mass spectrometer and about 10% of the total ion current is used for continuous registration of the effluent. Two molecule separators are coupled in series between the column and the gas inlet line of the mass spectrometer. With this technique the sample-to-helium ratio is increased at least a hundred times. Less than one μg of material introduced into the column suffices for a good mass spectrum. GLC-MS has the great advantage not only to resolve various substituted and non-substituted tryptamines, but also to give accurate identification. It is conceivable that the nonspecificity of the most commonly used method spectrophotofluorometry has prevented the elucidation of other normally occurring compounds than serotonin and tryptamine, and that with the progress in GLC-MS additional biogenic amines of physiological and pharmacological importance may be found. No doubt, the combination of GLC and mass spectrometry will be one of the powerful tools used in biological research for years to come.

According to Budzikiewics, Djerassi and Williams (1964) simple indoles have a characteristic fragmentation pattern. By analogy with this the psychotomimetic substance 5-MeO-DMT discovered by us in South American snuff would have the following fragmentation pattern.

5-MeO-DMT   MW 218

Here the main cleavage occurs as follows:

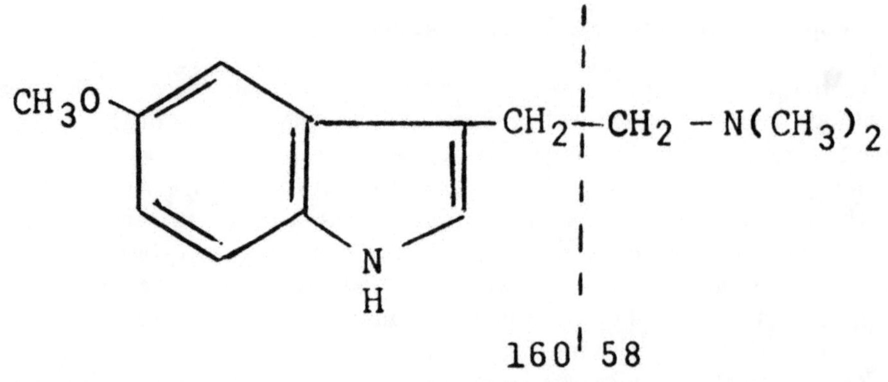

$$160 \mid 58$$

The ions $m/_e$ 160 and 58 are clearly seen in the mass spectrum. If one CH_3 on N is replaced by H such as occurs in 5-MeO-MMT the corresponding ions occur at $m/_e$ 160 and 44. The latter ion is found as the base peak of the spectrum. If one CH_3 on N are replaced by other groups such as acetyl in melatonine a corresponding ion is formed.

On the other hand $m/_e$ 160 will change according to different substitution in the indole nucleus such as occurs in bufotenine $(m/_e = 146)$.

$m/_e$ 173 may represent

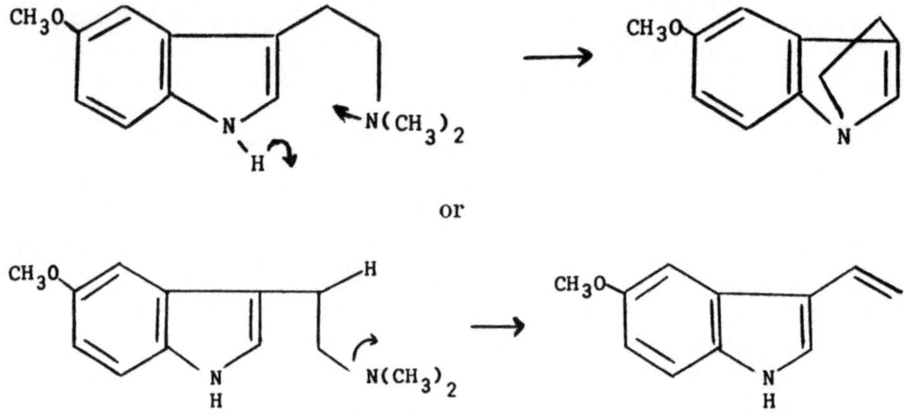

or

$m/_e$ 174 may represent

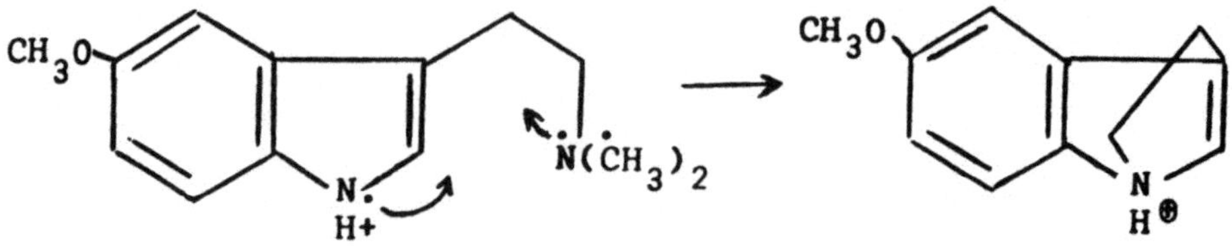

For $m/_e$ 115, 116, 117 in the spectrum the origin is not known, but the presence of these peaks seems to confirm previous belief that they are a good qualitative

364

indication of indoles. The mass spectra of 5-OH-DMT, 5-MeO-MMT and MMT when scrutinized confirm the fragmentation pattern proposed for 5-MeO-DMT.

Plants containing indoles

The first indoles in plants were isolated in the beginning of this century (Saxton 1965). Since then the number has been steadily increasing. Good accounts of their occurrence are available (Hochstein and Paradies 1957, Stowe 1958, Cerletti 1960, Downing 1962, Poisson 1965, Saxton 1965 and Morimoto et al., 1965, 1966). Unsubstituted and 5-substituted indoles command special interest with regard to pharmacological effects in two instances.

Firstly there are reports of cases of a disease called "staggers" in sheep pastured largely on a perennial grass, *Phalaris tuberosa L.* (Gallagher et al. 1964). Investigation of this and related species of Phalaris has led to the isolation of DMT, 5-MeO-DMT, 5-MeO-MMT and 5-OH-DMT (Wilkinson 1958, Culvenor et al. 1964).

Secondly, the same tryptamines as presented in table 1–2 of this review occur in the snuffs used in South America for intoxicating purposes. From the tables it is evident that tryptamines both unsubstituted and substituted in the ring (5-OH- and 5-MeO-) occur, and that both secondary and tertiary amines are present. In addition to this some snuffs contain β-carbolines, either in combination with the simple tryptamines or solely. In South American botany β-carbolines (harmine, harmaline and tetrahydroharmine) are usually associated with the species of *Banisteriopsis*, wherefore it is very likely that this is their origin in the snuffs. Very likely this is an admixture to the snuff, although definite botanical proof for it is lacking at the moment. To the knowledge of the authors, simple indoles and β-carbolines have not yet been isolated *from the same plant*.

The occurrence of both tryptamines and β-carbolines in the South American snuffs is pharmacologically interesting. The β-carbolines are monoamine-oxidase inhibitors (Udenfriend et al. 1958), and could potentiate the action of the simple indoles. The combination of β-carbolines and tryptamines would thus be advantageous. However, pharmacological actions of the β-carbolines unrelated to monoamineoxidase inhibition has also been proven to exist (Schievelbein et al. 1966). Further botanical and chemical studies are obviously needed to see if the two groups of compounds in the snuff are derived from one plant or a mixture of plants.

Deposition and absorption of snuffs

The equipment used for the administration of the powder in some cases consists of a straight tube equipped at one end with a palmkernel through which a hole has been bored. This end is fitted into the nostril of one person while another blows the powder forcefully through the opposite end of the tube. Another variation is a V-shaped tube, used for self-administration, where one end is put into the mouth and the other end into the nostril and the snuff is blown into the nasal cavity. Other equipment for the administration

365

exist among other tribes, the usual apparatus being the frequently described bifurcated tube (Safford 1916). This is used for administration by means of direct inhalation.

The two means of administration, forceful blowing or inhalation can be expected to differ in the effect produced. It is necessary to consider here the broad features of normal nasal physiology. The stream of inspired air does not pursue a straight course from anterior nares to choana, but passes in a wide curve beginning at the nostril, extending through the olfactory fissure, and ending in the choana (Proetz 1953). The negative pressure produced in the nose on inspiration, reaches a maximum figure of 55 mm. of mercury. The air fluctuations are rarely of sufficient force or magnitude to carry foreign particles into the sinuses. During normal sniffing (inspiration) air is projected against the nasal mucosa and the anterior portion of the nose, producing eddies. Harrison (1964) let volunteers sniff pinches of barium sulphate powder up one nostril. Inspection revealed that in every case the powder collected primarily in the middle meatus. By forceful blowing as with the straight and the V-shaped tube a more widespread deposition on the nasal mucosa may be expected, and some particles even reach the lungs (Chinachoti et al. 1957). However, we must assume that the main part of the administered material affects the brain from the nose. From a theoretical point of view several possibilities exist.

(a) The tryptamines reach the brain, via absorption from the richly vascularized nasal mucosa into the blood stream. It is well known that many other drugs have a very rapid action when applied in this way.

(b) The compounds act directly on the brain without having been transported through the general circulation.

Anatomical reasons have been proposed for the direct action on the CNS of certain drugs, such as cocaine, through the nasal mucosa (Lewin 1927). The following veins communicate directly with the cranial cavity, the concomitant veins of the *arteriae ethmoidales*, and a vein which accompanies a ramification of the anterior ethmoidal artery. The last one is an important connection between the nose and the cranial cavity. This vein accompanies the artery through the ethmoidale plate and makes connection within the cranial cavity, either with the network of veins of *Tractus olfactorius* or directly with a bigger vein in the orbital lobe. All the vessels mentioned are accompanied by lymph vessels, and it is conceivable that drugs can act directly on the brain without having to be transported through the general circulation. Experimental proofs for this are, however, lacking.

Several observers have described the passage of simple solutions from the nose into the cranial cavity. (For references see Yoffey and Drinker 1938). Clark (1929), for example, stated that a solution of potassium ferrocyanide and iron ammonium citrate, dropped into the nasal cavities of rabbits, reaches the surface of the brain *within one hour* (Sic!). He believed that there was a pathway along "the perineural sheaths of the olfactory nerves". The existence of a current running centripetally in these perineural sheath spaces of the olfactory nerves under normal conditions was postulated. Faber (1937), came to similar conclusions as a result of experiments on rabbits.

In the series of experiments by Yoffey and Drinker (1938), this was definitely not the case. The results were of especial interest since by cannulation of the cervical lymph duct it was possible to show that dye was present in the lymph in high concentration over many hours, and yet could never be detected in the interior of the cranium.

It seems evident that for anything but solutions of simple crystalloids, the cribriform plate offers an effective barrier to the passage of substance (non-living) from the nose to the interior of the skull. The rapidity of action of the tryptamines (minutes) also speaks against a direct transport from the nasal to the subarachnoidal cavity via the lymph vessels.

Symptomatology

The first written account of the action of the American intoxicating snuffs is that by Friar Ramon Pane on cohoba, published first in 1511 and quoted in detail by Wassén (this volume). Ramon Pane's observation of symptoms is revealing:

> . . . he takes a certain powder called cohoba, snuffing it up his nose, which intoxicated them so that they do not know what they do and in this condition they speak many things incoherently in which they say they are talking with the *cemis* and that by them they are informed how the sickness came upon him. Having snuffed cohoba into their nostrils (so they call the intoxicating plant by which the bovites also are thrown into a frenzy), they say that the house is turned upside down the roofs and floors being interchanged and that men walk with their feet upward. Such is the strength of the powder of cohoba that it takes away the senses of using it. When the stupefaction begins to go away, he hangs down his head and clasps his knees with his arms. He remains in this state of suspended animation for a little while; then he raises his head as one awakening from sleep and casting his eyes up at the sky at first he mutters a few rambling words to himself. The words which they say, none of our people understand. With this powder they lose consciousness and become like drunken men.

This undoubtedly constitutes the first written account of the psychotomimetic effects of the tryptamines, and is astonishing in its correctness when compared to later descriptions only some of which will be quoted here. Ramon Pane's description also corresponds very well to what one can see in the film about the use of the epéna among the Waicas made by Mr. Georg Seitz. Later explorers have, however, pointed out additional effects. Nimuendajú (1948), (quoted from Wassén 1965) says:

> . . . the powder caused a general state of excitement and exaltation with auditory hallucinations, and a condition of feverish activity which ended with prostration or unconsciousness. According to Martius, individuals who were overexcited by the narcotic and suffocated, died on the spot. On the morning following "a narcotic spree'" the bodies of persons were often found shot with arrows or stabbed with knives. These murders were not considered as crimes and were blamed on the paricà.

Cohoba, according to Columbus, Ramon Pane, Las Casas and others who observed and reported its use in Haiti, was employed by the medicine-men chiefly to induce a state of trance; more hedonistic uses have been described later (see Seitz this volume). The violent effect of this snuff indicated that its chief ingredient was a powerful substance. None of the early commentators on the custom says that the substance inhaled was derived from the tobacco plant, but before the close of the sixteenth century the snuff used in the cohoba ceremonies reported was assumed to be tobacco, and the association was continued up to our own time (Lovén 1935). Only a person entirely inexperienced in pharmacology and toxicology would, however, confuse the illusions and hallucinations described under the influence of cohoba, with a nicotine intoxication. The confusion of cohoba and tobacco was also largely dispelled by the paper by Safford (1916).

All modern evidence confirms the psychotomimetic action of the snuffs. Zerries (1964) and Seitz (this volume) describe how in the Waica tribe individuals quickly become intoxicated by repeated inhalation of the snuff. The somatic symptoms are headache, salivation, vomiting, profuse perspiration, unsteady gait and a typical facial expression. During the intoxication the Indians are able to establish contact with the Hekula, the spirits of rocks and waterfalls in order to induce them to bring mishap and sickness to the enemies of the village. The medicine man becomes possessed by spirits, excited and sometimes loses consciousness. The best description of the use of epéna is the one given by Becher (1960) relating details about the religious use of the compound, and how during the ritual the Indians become so obsessed with the spirits that they have to be exorcised. Under the influence of the drug, the Indians identify themselves with the gigantic spirits of animals and plants Hekura (Hekula), and also have the impression that they personify themselves the Hekura (Surára tribe). Becher, who became a member of this tribe, gives a rare description of his own experience when taking the snuff. His symptoms were the following (translation by the authors):

> A few minutes (after taking the snuff) I felt terrible with a headache and nausea just as the boy who comes into contact with the drug for the first time. Shortly afterwards, I had a very strange experience, I felt myself to be a giant among giants. Everybody around me, people as well as dogs and parrots, seemed suddenly to have become giants.

Interestingly enough this is a description of macroptic illusions.

Dysmegalopsia, synonymous with *dysmetropsia*, is a disturbance of the visual appreciation of the size of objects which occurs with certain drugs. It can be subdivided into *macropsia* and *micropsia*. These conditions may result from disturbances in the peripheral motor perception, *i.e.*, eye muscles, but they also occur in toxic psychoses. Macropsia has been described, particularly in alcoholic delirium. Its most famous manifestation is the well known "pink elephants." It also occurs in intoxications with *Amanita muscaria* (Kracheninnikov 1764). The macroptic phenomenon has been treated in detail by di Gaspero (1908). It is interesting to know that these experiences are described by people who are fully oriented in time and space, and that during experience living persons and animals *but not dead objects*, change size (compare Becher). The latter may be perceived in a different colour as to the giants. Macropsia seems to be more common than micropsia, but the latter has been described as a result of intoxication with ether, alcohol, cocaine, chloral hydrate and cannabis (de Clerambault 1909). Apparently it can occur also in intoxications with *Banisteriopsis* (Preuss 1921). Beringer (1934), who has devoted a study to optic illusions and hallucinations, describes a third phenomenon, a change in size in one direction or the other somewhat reminiscent of what can be achieved with a modern zoom lens of a camera.

Shortly after Horning et al. had isolated DMT and 5-OH-DMT from *Piptadenia peregrina*, Szara (1957), conducted experiments on himself with the injection of DMT. The symptoms he reported are in good agreement with what has been described by the explorers:

> In the third or fourth minute after the injection vegetative symptoms appeared, such as a tingling sensation, trembling, slight nausea, mydriasis, elevation of the blood pressure and increase of the pulse rate. At the same time eidetic phenomena, optical illusions, pseudohallucinations and later real hallucinations, appeared. The hallucinations consisted of moving, brilliantly coloured oriental motifs, and later I saw wonderful scenes, altering very rapidly. The faces of the people seemed to be masks. My emotional state was elevated sometimes up to euphoria. At the highest point, I had compulsive athetoid movement in my left hand. My consciousness was completely filled by hallucinations, and my attention was firmly bound to them; therefore I could not give an account of the events happening around me. After ¾–1 hour the symptoms disappeared, and I was able to describe what had happened.

Macropsia is also a frequent phenomenon in experimental DMT-intoxications (Isbell, personal communication).

The action of 5-OH-DMT (bufotenine) is more controversial. Fabing and Hawkins (1956), reported that intravenous injection, over a three minute period, of 8 to 16 mg of bufotenine in human volunteers resulted in primary visual disturbances, alteration of time and space perception, and paresthesias. It is difficult to judge by this account whether any illusions and hallucinations really occurred. It seems that the observed phenomena can as well be interpreted as general somatic symptoms of intoxication. Neither Isbell nor Turner and Merlis (1959) themselves in their carefully conducted studies, could substantiate the claim that bufotenine injections had any effect on the central nervous system, whereas DMT under the same experimental conditions had psychotomimetic effects.

Control experiments with various preparations of snuff have been carried out by two groups but have not proven the capability of the used preparations to produce the intoxication attributed to it by natives or explorers. In a letter, Dr. Harris Isbell describes his experiment with the same compounds in the following way:

> We studied several forms of the material: Untreated snuff, roasted snuff, limed and roasted snuff, fermented snuff, fermented and limed snuff, fermented, limed and roasted snuff. Our subjects inhaled the snuff through straws. We obtained no reports that there were any subjective effects after inhalation of this material in amounts ranging up to 1 gram, and we further were unable to obtain any evidence of objective effects on pupillary size, tendon reflexes, body temperature, respiration, blood pressure etc., after doses ranging up to 1 gram orally.
>
> Inhalation of pure bufotenine in aerosol suspension, or oral ingestion of bufotenine in doses running up to 100 mg (total dose) also were without effect.

The above quoted experiments were all performed with snuff made from the sample of *Piptadenia peregrina* in which Horning et al. had found

5-OH-DMT (bufotenine) to be the main component, and *this fully explains the negative results.*

One measure of the ability of compounds to penetrate the nervous system is the lipid solubility, as determined by the lipid solvent-water partition coefficients. Gessner and Page (1962), found a low value for the chloroform-water partition coefficient of 5-OH-DMT, indicating a low lipid solubility attributable to the hydrophilic phenolic hydroxy group. Hence, the low activity of 5-OH-DMT could be related to its relative inability to cross the blood-brain barrier. The 5-MeO-DMT shown by the present investigation to be the major component of most South American snuffs was, however, found to be a compound in which the right structure is present both for lipid solubility and central action.

The animal experiments by Gessner and Page (1962) have pointed to the strong action of synthetic 5-MeO-DMT on the central nervous system, and its important role in the elucidation of central nervous mechanisms. The effect of 5-MeO-DMT on the conditioned avoidance response of trained rats was compared quantitatively, using a shuttle-box, with that of several other substituted tryptamines and LSD-25. At a dose level of 19 μM/kg it had a pronounced effect on the conditioned avoidance response, much more pronounced than that due to DMT. A similar response was elicited by LSD-25 at a dose level of 6 μM/kg.

Benington et al. (1965), report that the effect of 5-MeO-DMT on cat behaviour is dramatic. An intense sham rage response was induced within a few minutes. Of all drugs examined that induce sham rage in the cat, 5-MeO-DMT is one of the most potent, and its potency was very close to that of LSD-25. From the rapid onset of the rage response induced by 5-MeO-DMT by any route of administration, it is evident that the drug reaches the sites of action rapidly. The nature of the response suggests a central effect of a relatively short duration.

It is outside the scope of the present investigation to go into the detailed effects of the various tryptamines with regard to their circulatory and other peripheral effects. (With regard to 5-MeO-MMT see Marczyński, 1959, 1960). It ought to be mentioned, however, that the effects of 5-MeO-DMT on the general circulation are negligible compared to those of 5-OH-DMT (bufotenine). Detailed pharmacological and metabolic studies of 5-MeO-DMT are still lacking. No doubt its resemblance to serotonine, its solubility properties, its relative lack of peripheral and marked central action of an obvious psychotomimetic nature will in the future make 5-MeO-DMT an important tool in psychopharmacological studies. Once again, one cannot but marvel at the ingenuity of the South American Indians who relentlessly seem to be able to find their way to the right herb containing the most active component.

Acknowledgement

We thank Dr. R. Ryhage (Department of Mass Spectrometry, Karolinska Institutet) for expert advice and laboratory facilities placed at our disposal in connection with the recording of mass spectra.

REFERENCES

BECHER, H. "Un viaje de investigación por los rios Demini y Aracá (Brasil) Trabajos y Conferencias." Seminarion de Estudios Americanistas, vol. II, 3 : 149–160, 1958.
"Die Surára und Pakidái, zwei Yanonámi-Stämme in Nordwest-Brasilien." Hamburg, Kommisionsverlag Cram, de Gruyter & Co., 1960.
"Dringende ethnologische Forschungsaufgaben in Nordwest-Brasilien." Sonderdruck aus Akten des 34. Intern. Amerikanistenkongresses Wien, 1960.

BENINGTON, F., R. D. MORIN and L. C. CLARK. "5-Methoxy-N, N-Dimethyltryptamine, A Possible Endogenous Psychotoxin." The Alabama Journal of Medical Sciences, 2 : 397–403, 1965.

BERINGER, K. "Optische Wahrnehmungsveränderungen und Sinnestäuschungen bei Rauschgiften." Augenärztliche Tagesfragen (Böhlein-Wegner), 77 : 2711, 1934.

BUDZIKIEWICS, H. C., C. DJERASSI and D. WILLIAMS. "Interpretation of Mass Spectra of Organic Compounds." San Francisco, Holden Day Inc., 1964.
"Structure Elucidation of Natural Products by Mass Spectrometry." San Francisco, Holden Day Inc., 1964.

BÖSZÖRMÉNYI, Z. and G. GRUNECKER. "Dimethyltryptamine (DMT) experiments with psychotics." Psychotropic drugs. Milano, ed. by S. Garattini and V. Ghetti, 580 pp., 1957.

CASPAR, F. "Ein Kulturareal im Hinterland der Flüsse Guaporé und Machado (Westbrasilien), dargestellt nach unveröffentlichten und anderen wenig bekannten Quellen, mit besonderer Berücksichtigung der Nahrungs- und Genussmittel." Hamburg. Dissertation, 1953.

CERLETTI, A. "Über Vorkommen und Bedeutung der Indolstruktur in der Medizin und Biologie." Progr. Drug, Res., 2 : 227–249, 1960.

CHINACHOTI, N. and P. TANGCHAI. "Case Report Section. Pulmonary Alveolar Microlithiasis Associated with the Inhalation of Snuff in Thailand." Diseases of the Chest, 32 : 687–689, 1957.

LE GROS CLARK, W. E. "Anatomical investigation into the routes by which infections may pass from the nasal cavities into the brain." Reports on Public Health and Medical Subjects No. 54. Ministry of Health. London. Published by his Majesty's Stationary Office 1929.

DE CLÉRAMBAULT, M. "Diskussionsbemerkung zu R. Leroy: Les Hallucinations liliputiennes." Ann. Med. Psychol., 286, 1909.

CULVENOR, C. C. J., R. DAL BON and L. W. SMITH. "The occurrence of indolealkylamine alkaloids in Pharalis Tuberosa L. and P. Arundinacea L." Australian J. Chem., 17 : 1301–1304, 1964.

DOWNING, D. F. "The chemistry of the psychotomimetic substances." Quart. Rev. of the Chem. Soc. of London, 16 : 133–162, 1962.

FABER, W. M. "The nasal mucosa and the subarachnoid space." Amer. J. Anat., 62 : 121–148, 1937.

FABING, H. D. and J. R. HAWKINS. "Intravenous Bufotenine Injection in the Human Being." Science, 123 : 886–887, 1956.

FISH, M. S., N. M. JOHNSON and E. C. HORNING. "Piptadenia Alkaloids Indole Bases of P. peregrina (L.) Benth. and Related Species." J. Am. Chem. Soc., 77 : 5892–5895, 1955.

GALLAGHER, C. H., J. H. KOCH, R. M. MOORE and J. D. STEEL. "Toxicity of Phalaris tuberosa for Sheep." Nature, 204 : 542–545, 1964.

DI GASPERO, H. "Über das Phänomen der Makropsie als Symptom bei akuter toxischer Halluzinose." J. Psychol. u. Neur., 11 : 115, 1908.

GESSNER, P. K. and I. H. PAGE. "Behavioral effects of 5-methoxy-N :N-dimethyltryptamine, other tryptamines and LSD." Am. J. Physiol., 203 : 167–172, 1962.

HARRISON, D. F. N. "Snuff—Its Use and Abuse." Brit. Med. J., 2 : 1649–1651, 1964.

HOCHSTEIN, F. A. and A. M. PARADIES. "Alkaloids of Banisteria caapi and Prestonia amazonicum." J. Am. Chem. Soc., 79 : 5735–5736, 1957.

HORNING, E. C., E. MOSCATELLI and C. C. SWEELEY. Chem. Indust., 751, 1959.

HORNING, E. C., W. J. A. VAN DEN HEUVEL and B. G. CREECH. "Methods of Biochemical Analysis." D. Glick, Ed., XI, Interscience, London 1963.

ISBELL, H. Letter to the author, October 25, 1957.

KRASHENINNIKOV, S. P. "Opisanie zemli Kamchatki (A Description of Kamchatka)." Akademia Nauk, 1755. New critical edition in 1949.

LEWIN, L. "Phantastica. Die betäubenden und erregenden Genussmittel." Für Ärtze und Nichtärtze. Zweite Auflage, Berlin, Verlag von Georg Stilke in Berlin, 1927.

LOVÉN, S. "Origins of the Tainan Culture, West Indies," Göteborg, 1935.

MARCZYNSKI, T. "Some pharmacological properties of a recently isolated alkaloid, 5-methoxy-N-methyltryptamine." Bull. Acad. Pol. Sci., 7 : 151–154, 1959.

MARCZYNSKI, T. and J. VETULANI. "Further investigations on the pharmacological properties of 5-methoxy-N-methyltryptamine." Dissertationes Pharmaceuticae, 12 : 67–84, 1960.

MORIMOTO, H. and H. OSHIO. "Über Lesbedamin, ein neues Alkaloid." Inhaltsstoffe von Lespedeza bicolor var. japonica, I. Liebigs Ann. Chem., 682, 212–218, 1965.

MORIMOTO, H. and N. MATSUMOTO. "Inhaltstoffe von Lespedeza bicolor var. japonica, II." Liebigs Ann. Chem., 692 : 194–199, 1966.

NIMUENDAJÚ, C. "The Mura and Piraha." HSAM, 3 : 245–254, 1948.

PANE, R. "Quoted from Pietro Martire d'Anghieras." Opera Babylonica Oceani decas Poemata Epigrammata Sevilla 1511.

POISSON, J. "Note sur 'Natem', boisson toxique péruvienne et ses alcaloides." Ann. Pharm. fr., 23 : 241–244, 1965.

PREUSS, K. T. "Religion und Mythologie der Uitoto." Vol. I. Göttingen 1921.

PROETZ, A. W. "Essays on the applied physiology of the nose." St. Louis, Annals Publishing Co., 2nd ed., 1953.

RYHAGE, R. "Use of Mass Spectrometer as a Detector and Analyzer for Effluents Emerging from High Temperature Gas Liquid Chromatography Column." Anal. Chem., 36 : 759–764, 1964

SAFFORD, W. E. "Identity of cohoba, the narcotic snuff of ancient Haiti." J. Wash. Acad. Sci., 6 : 547–562, 1916.

SAXTON, J. E. "The Alkaloids." Vol. VIII. New York, London, Academic Press, R. H. F. Manske (editor), 1965.

SCHIEVELBEIN, H., H. PETER, I. TRAUTSCHOLD and E. WERLE. "Freisetzung von 5-Hydroxytryptamin aus Thrombocyten durch Harmalin." Biochem. Pharmacol., 15 : 195–197, 1966.

STOWE, B. B. "Occurrence and metabolism of simple indoles in plants." Fortschritte der Chemie organischer Naturstoffe (Herausgegeben von L. Zechmeister), Springer Verlag, Wien, 16 : 248–297, 1958.

STROMBERG, V. L. "The isolation of Bufotenine from Piptadenia peregrina." J. Am. Chem. Soc., 76 : 1707, 1954.

SZARA, S. "The comparison of the psychotic effect of tryptamine derivatives with the effects of mescaline and LSD–25 in selfexperiments." Psychotropic drugs. Milano. Ed. by S. Garattini and V. Ghetti, 460–467, 1957.

"Hallucinogenic effects and metabolism of tryptamine derivatives in man." Fed. Proc., 20 : 885–888, 1961.

SZARA, S. and L. H. ROCKLAND. "Psychological effects and metabolism of N,N-diethyltryptamine, an hallucinogenic drug." Proceeding of the Third World Congress of Psychiatry, 1 : 670, 1961.

TURNER, W. J. and S. MERLIS. "Effect of some indolealkylamines on man." Arch. Neurol. Psychiatr., 81 : 121–129, 1959.

UDENFRIEND, S., B. WITKOP, B. G. REDFIELD, and H. WEISSBACH, Biochem. Pharmacol., 1 : 160, 1958.

WASSÉN, S. H. "The use of some specific kinds of South American Indian snuff and related paraphernalia." Etnologiska Studier 28, 1965.

WILKINSON, S. "5-Methoxy-N-methyltryptamine: A new indole alkaloid from Phalaris arundinacea L." J. Chem. Soc., 2079–2081, 1958.

YOFFEY, J. M. and C. K. DRINKER. "The lymphatic pathway from the nose and pharynx." J.. Exp. Med., 68 : 629–640, 1938.

ZERRIES, O. "Waika, Die kulturgeschichtliche Stellung der Waika-Indianer des oberen Orinoco in Rahmen der Völkerkunde Südamerikas." München, Klaus Renner Verlag, 1964. (Ergebnisse der Frobenius-Expedition 1954/55 nach Südost-Venezuela. Band 1. Waika).

Discussion on the Psychoactive Action of Various Tryptamine Derivatives

Chairman—Bo Holmstedt

Members of the Panel—John W. Daly
Efrén Carlos del Pozo
Evan C. Horning
Harris Isbell
Stephen I. Szara

CHAIRMAN DR. HOLMSTEDT: We have some questions from the audience, and I know that some of the participants are also prepared to elaborate upon what they have done themselves.

Perhaps we should start with Dr. Szara, who had the courage to use dimethyltryptamine as an experimental tool for the first time, and we would be glad if he would give us a description of the symptoms he observed.

DR. SZARA: I think the picture was very clear. We saw in Mr. Seitz's movie what the drugs can do, and how quickly; so I would rather like to give a little summary of what we have done in the past twelve years with dimethyltryptamine, and how we came to start using it. Actually it was when I first read an article by Fish, Johnson and Horning in the Journal of American Chemical Society 77, 5892 (1955). These authors have found N,N-dimethyltryptamine, together with bufotenine, in snuff powder prepared by Haitian natives from *Piptadenia peregrina* seeds which the natives used in their religious ceremonies. The psychotropic effect was blamed on bufotenine, but it was unknown whether dimethyltryptamine was hallucinogenic or not. So I decided to synthesize it, and then tried it out on myself and other volunteers and friends who were courageous enough to volunteer. It was not active orally. I started taking this compound in very small quantities up to 250 mgs, but it was inactive. Then we started giving it intramuscularly, doses of one mg/kg, which give a very fast and very strong reaction. This resembled very closely symptoms which were described by Dr. Freedman the day before yesterday about LSD, so I would rather just summarize those symptoms which are similar to those of LSD, and point out some striking differences.

The perceptual distortions are primarily visual in nature, and with closed eyes you can see illusions and color patterns, primarily geometrical patterns, moving very fast, having sometimes very deep emotional content and connotation.

There is an inability to keep attention focused on any outside task. It seems to be very difficult to maintain contact with reality, and this often leads to a panicky action. There is an enhanced dependence on the environment for structure and for symbolic meanings, and increased association and search for synthesis, as Dr. Freedman mentioned.

There are some dissimilarities, however, when you compare the effects of dimethyltryptamine with those from LSD. The main difference is the rapidity of the onset and the shortness of the duration of action. After being given an injection intramuscularly, the symptoms begin in two or three minutes, and they last for only about thirty to forty-five minutes, or a maximum of an hour, and then it is just hangover and nothing else. The effects of LSD and mescaline last for four, six, eight and sometimes twelve hours, depending on the dose and on the individual variations.

Some other minor differences exist. In dimethyltryptamine there are more primary visual hallucinations, light flashes, colors, abstract forms and figures with oriental designs. There is a consistently larger but short-lasting autonomic effect, consisting of increased blood pressure and dilated pupils. The rapid onset of the strange experience and the overwhelming loss of control can cause panic reaction much faster than other known longer lasting hallucinogens.

We have worked very extensively since this on the metabolism of dimethyltryptamine, and I don't know if now is the time to go into it. We have synthesized several compounds which are also hallucinogenic. They differ slightly in duration. They are slightly longer acting than dimethyltryptamine, and the autonomic reaction is slightly less.

We were interested in the metabolism of this compound, and we have suggested that 6-hydroxylation may be a way of producing a psychoactive metabolite. This has been questioned by Dr. Isbell and by some others, based on the work of 6-hydroxy-5-methoxydimethyltryptamine, which was supposedly metabolized and has been found inactive in the behavioral tests.

I have repeatedly stressed in the last couple of years that our data strongly supports the notion that the 6-hydroxy pathway is somehow involved, although not necessarily through the first, and the main metabolite, which has been found to be the 6-hydroxydialkyltryptamine. The data on which we rely for this judgent are primarily clinical, obtained first on normal volunteers, later on alcoholic patients, in double blind tests. These studies have shown strong correlation between the rate of 6-hydroxylation and the hallucinogenic action as measured by rating scales and psychological reports.

The other support for the role of 6-hydroxylation is the fact that if you prevent this pathway by substituting the 6-position by a fluorine, thus having a 6-fluorodiethyltryptamine, this compound has not been found to have hallucinogenic properties in patients. It does produce autonomic effects, pupillary changes, blood pressure changes; but it does not produce the drifting away into a dream world and other phenomena characteristic for the hallucinatory activity.

We have used these compounds mainly as tools in learning about the mechanism of action of this particular type of drug, in which there seems to be a very deep interest in psychiatry.

Perhaps I could mention some experiments with tritium-labeled dimethyltryptamine, which illustrate very nicely how quickly this compound penetrates the brain and reaches the area involved in the central nervous effects.

In one of the experiments we gave 10 mg/kg of DMT intraperitoneally to mice, the brain was taken out at various time intervals, and the small areas were analyzed by chromatography and scintillation spectrometry. In ten minutes you can get a maximum amount of unchanged DMT in the cortical areas, and slightly less in other areas which gradually subside, but some of the basic metabolites which contain the hydroxylated metabolite have a slightly different course, and reach different areas of the brain later in time, but not in the first couple of minutes.

This is just some of the data which we have not published yet, but we have done a lot of work combining these drugs with a precursor of serotonin, 5-hydroxytryptophan. In these experiments there seems to be a very delicate regional change in the serotonin metabolism, primarily the hypothalamus area, when we give hallucinogenic diethyltryptamine, but not when we gave the nonhallucinogenic, 6-fluoro analog.

We have published some of these data in the proceedings of a symposium on "Amines and Schizophrenia," (H. Himwich et. al., Editors: Amines and Schizophrenia, Pergamon Press, Oxford, New York, 1966).

I would like to stop now.

CHAIRMAN DR. HOLMSTEDT: Thank you.

The thing which I personally would like to know from the two psychiatrists on the panel is, what are the visual phenomena of these experimental patients? Do they have microptic and macroptic phenomena? Dr. Isbell.

DR. ISBELL: Do they have micropsia and macropsia? Yes, they do, and the same individual may have both, in rapid or alternating fashion, and this may involve not only extraneous objects and people, but also his own body image. He may feel that he is nine feet tall, and then he may shrink to a point where he begins to get worried that he is going to get so small that he will completely disappear. The same alterations in size will occur in the environment. The room gets very small or very big, and simultaneously there are distortions of shape, color; practically every kind of thing that you think of that would happen in the visual sphere does happen.

DR. KLINE: Are these alterations in part emotional, or do you think they are totally physiological?

DR. ISBELL: I can't answer you, Dr. Kline. Things will happen in the same man at almost one time, and you can sometimes get from the patients themselves very interesting explanations why these things happened.

DR. KLINE: Rinkle did some work with adrenolutin or adrenochrome in which the size of the person and the apparent distance from the observer was quite dependent, according to this report, on whether he liked the person or not. Some subjects even managed to see "through" certain people if they didn't like them. I have never heard any confirmation of this, and I was wondering whether it might not be an interesting subject for investigation.

DR. ISBELL: I have personally never been able to correlate any particular subjective experiences that a given individual has with anything, except if one has observed him under drug on a previous occasion, it is very likely that the same type of phenomena will be seen on the second occasion.

I think that I might speak a little bit about some of the tryptamines other than dimethyltryptamine. One of these is bufotenine. It has been said that bufotenine is not a psychotomimetic drug. I don't think we should say that.

The difficulty is that bufotenine is a drug that has extremely powerful and dangerous cardiovascular effects, and for that reason it is not possible to push the dose in man. Also, it would be difficult to differentiate whether psychotic reactions were due to central effects or to cardiovascular actions. Cardiovascular actions include hypertension and development of an arrhythmia which actually amounts to a ventricular standstill. The auricle does not beat, the beat drops out, and the ventricle takes over, and it is very frightening. Simultaneously with the hypertension and ventricular escapes, one sees spectacular cynanosis in the upper part of the body, similar to that which has been described in the carcinoid flush, which is presumably due to serotonin. So bufotenine is a difficult drug to work in man for this reason, and it would not be too surprising if it did not have some kind of a central action if it were possible to extract it out.

6-Hydroxydimethyltryptamine had no effect in a dose of 1 mg/kg in our subjects, in fact. In contrast, my subjects had spectacular reactions to dimethyltryptamine. My men spoke of taking trips long before this term came into general use. They used to say that with dimethyltryptamine, "You can go to the moon and get back in time for breakfast"—so, they went to the moon long before the rockets landed. I hope they left a flag up there, but the 6-hydroxy derivatives were without effect. The 5-methoxy congener, as Dr. Holmstedt said, has not been tested, and we are still awaiting animal pharmacology on it.

I think we are, perhaps, forgetting that the psilocybin and psilocyn found in the mushroom are derivatives of tryptamine and serotonin with the hydroxyl group in the 4-position. These drugs give us the same kind of effect as does DMT. They are somewhat longer acting, and slower to start.

One interesting thing is that the resemblance of the clinical phenomena one sees with dimethyltryptamine and LSD is very striking. If you get LSD daily you soon develop such a high grade of tolerance that one might as well be issuing water. Then, if you take people who are tolerant to LSD and test them with psilocybin and mescaline, you will find that they are markedly cross-tolerant. We were unable to show a high degree of cross-tolerance between dimethyltryptamine and LSD, so despite the similarity of chemical structure it may be that dimethyltryptamine and LSD may act by somewhat different mechanisms within the brain, although we cannot be sure of this. The only thing we can be sure of, is that there is no great degree cross-tolerance.

CHAIRMAN DR. HOLMSTEDT: I can mention that as far as the animal experiments undertaken with the 5-methoxy compound are concerned, they have shown it to have a very weak effect on the circulation. My statement that bufotenine was not a psychotomimetic agent was based on two things: First your own work, Dr. Isbell; secondly, that its solubility properties are such that it is not very likely to penetrate the blood-brain-barrier.

We have several questions. One is from Dr. Kline, and he wants to know whether all alkylated tryptamines are psychotomimetic. I don't think anybody can answer that fully. Dr. Szara did, however, try out a number of them.

DR. SZARA: N,N-dibutyl- and N-monohexyltryptamines, which are higher homologues, were inactive in a few patients. There is no systematic study.

CHAIRMAN DR. HOLMSTEDT: Another question: Can these states be terminated with phenothiazine derivatives, as is the case with LSD and mescaline?

DR. SZARA: We never had to terminate it, because it is so short acting, it is over before you realize it happens.

CHAIRMAN DR. HOLMSTEDT: Question: "What ingredients in the snuff do you think caused the untoward side effects, based on similar experiments with purified chemical constituents?"

The answer to that is that the tryptamines themselves may very well cause the side effects, as pointed out by Dr. Szara.

Somebody also wants to ask Dr. Schultes a question: Why does he use the words "narcotic snuffs" or "hallucinogenic snuffs", and what is the difference? Do you want to answer that question, Dr. Schultes?

DR. SCHULTES: There are any number of definitions of the word "narcotic". Having had a classical education, I use it as it was coined from the Greek, meaning any substance that benumbs the central nervous system, whether ever so slightly or producing a comatose state. There is no one good definition of the term.

In this country, a substance is not a narcotic unless the Senate has declared it so. It has to be so declared under the Harrison Narcotics Act. For this reason, marijuana is not legally a narcotic. Then you have the popular and newspaper definition, meaning only the addictive and dangerous ones. Faced with this plethora of "definitions", I have decided to stay with the Greeks.

CHAIRMAN DR. HOLMSTEDT: Thank you, Dr. Schultes.

May we return again to the phenomena of micropsia and macropsia. It has been said—this is mostly Mr. Gordon Wasson, who is of the opinion that these drugs have played a very great role in religion (not only the Christian religion but previous religions as well)—that such things as the ideas of giants and dwarfs may have come from these intoxications.

Can I ask Dr. Del Pozo, who is very familiar with the Mexican literature on this subject, if there are any indications of these distortions of perception in the Mexican literature. In other words, do the Gods have any definite size?

DR. DEL POZO: The Chroniclers describe the different hallucinatory visions that the Aztec priests used to have. They ate the mushrooms because they thought that those visions would provide them with some information about the future, or about the interpretation of different facts, but I don't know of any paritcular descriptions of macropsia. They usually mention devils, figures and colors.

I had an experience, I would say a collective experience: We were working with mushrooms, and a group of young collaborators who joined to celebrate the birthday of one of them suddenly decided to go to the laboratory in the evening and eat mushrooms.

They were so worried about the effects that they called me at about three o'clock in the morning. All of them were very amused because of the color visions, the forms and things that appeared to them. They were talking one to another and saying: "Look at this yellow color, look at this green color". I am sure they were simultaneous, but more or less the same type of visions. This makes me believe that it is a physiological action, in which there is little influence of the psychological background. There were no reports of macropsia or any other deformation in size.

Dr. Szara: I would like to emphasize something here which has not been overlooked, but it has not been emphasized enough, and that is the tremendous importance of the set and the setting in determining the kind of reaction which a person can get. If you suggest to the subject that you are a little mouse or you are an amoeba, you feel like it, or if you suggest that he is God, he is powerful, then he will have macropsia—so that setting is very, very important. I think here what Mr. Seitz has referred to, this initiation ceremony during the taking of the snuffs—the father tells the son what to expect, what to hallucinate and what to experience—is apparently very much imbedded into the ritual use of these drugs.

Dr. Schultes: You asked me to define "hallucinogenic", and I forgot to do so. I believe that the man who coined this very useful and definitive word is Mr. Wassén. I am happy to note that in this meeting the etymologically impossible word "psychedelic" has not frequently been used.

One of the "psychedelic giants" asked my advice when he planned to use the term *psychedelic* in the title of a journal. I pointed out that one does not, in coining an English word from Greek roots, make a combination with "e"; it is made with "o". The word then would have to be "psychodelic". He pointed out that *psycho* had acquired a very special meaning in English, and that it could not be used without intimating that specialized meaning. Still, with the many good terms available, this etymological error would seem superfluous.

Chairman Dr. Holmstedt: May I at this point ask Dr. Daly or Dr. Horning what one would expect from a chemical point of view, when the OH group in tryptamines sits in the 4, 5, 6 and 7 position? Would there be chemically important differences in these compounds?

Dr. Horning: We made an observation some years ago, which was never published, for the hydroxy compounds. I think it is very clear that the properties would be different both chemically and, I am sure, physiologically, with different positions of subtitution.

In the crystalline form, bufotenine has an ionic structure. However, by certain chromatographic techniques, it is possible to get a second form of bufotenine. I think that probably the second form has a phenolic amine (non-ionized) structure (Fig. 1) because of infrared spectroscopic evidence. It was obtained in the absence of polar solvents (a non-polar system was used).

I think it is fairly clear that in the ionized form, in a polar medium, the compound would not penetrate the blood-brain-barrier. This is one of the problems in talking about the 6-hydroxy compound, as Dr. Holmstedt said.

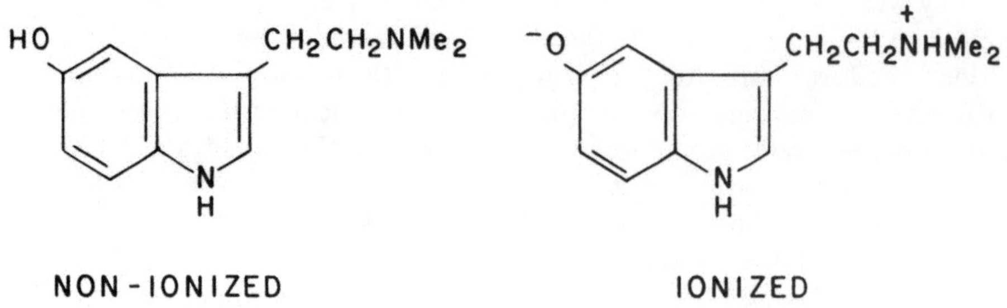

NON-IONIZED   IONIZED

Fig. 1.

CHAIRMAN DR. HOLMSTEDT: Why would it necessarily be in the 6-position?

DR. HORNING: This recalls the argument over specific and non-specific hydroxylation. I think that the other isomers are formed, too, but they are hard to find.

At any rate, the 6-position hydroxylation is a well-defined reaction. This would be the expected compound. On the other hand, I would expect no action for this metabolite.

DR. SZARA: How about psilocybin?

DR. HORNING: The question of active transport and mechanism of penetration into a cell runs through many areas of chemistry and pharmacology. If one has a phosphate, there may be an active transport mechanism. Also, polar compounds including glucose enter the brain. "Active transport" exists, although we know very little about the mechanism.

DR. SZARA: Psilocin is a free hydroxy. It has no phosphate.

DR. HORNING: I would ask what your own view of this is, since you have studied it so extensively.

DR. SZARA: What my feeling is about the hydroxy derivatives is that they don't have to penetrate the brain all the way, entirely. It might be enough to penetrate only some trigger points, where the blood-brain-barrier is more leaky, like the hypothalamus or other areas which have been shown to be able to let larger molecules through. It might be enough for a hydroxy derivative to penetrate those areas and produce some very fine regional changes, and this is, I think, really what happens with the hydroxylated derivatives.

DR. HORNING: You may not need to postulate transport as such.

DR. SZARA: This is hypothesis, really. I might mention here that the 6-flurodiethyltryptamine is equally lipid soluble, and it penetrates the brain but is not hallucinogenic.

DR. HORNING: You feel that the 6-position is indeed critical?

DR. SZARA: It might be.

DR. HORNING: I have one other thing to say: Dr. Holmstedt has been a pionere in many ways, and one of the ways is in the chemical techniques he is using to deal with these compounds. It is possible to study all of the materials in small quantities by gas chromotography, and this is due largely to a whole series of developments, not the least of which was the development in Stockholm by R. Ryhage of the "molecule separator". This permits the use of gas chromatography and mass spectrometry in a combined fashion.

This is at present the most powerful chemical way we have of investigating substances. I think this work will point the way for both pharmacologists and chemists, and investigations may go faster in the future.

I will ask if Dr. Daly agrees with any of these comments?

DR. DALY: It may be that in 4-hydroxytryptamines such as psilocybin, the nitrogen and the phenolic hydroxy group may interact intramolecularly in such a way as to increase the lipid solubility over that of other hydroxy-trytamines, and thus facilitate penetration into the brain. Again, while we assume that hydroxylation of tryptamines occurs only in the liver, we have no good proof that such hydroxylations do not take place in certain specific areas of the brain, in which case the hydroxytryptamine would be formed *in situ*, and would not have to penetrate the blood-brain-barrier.

In keeping with this idea, we thought to develop a sensitive assay for 6-hydroxylation based on the release of tritiated water from 6-tritiotryptamine on enzymatic hydroxylation. On studying this transformation with liver microsomes, we found that the tritium atom migrated to another position in the aromatic ring as a result of 6-hydroxylation. Similar migrations occur during the hydroxylation of other aromatic compounds, and cognizance of this unusual reaction should allow us to develop a sensitive and specific assay for the hydroxylation of tryptamines.

Regarding recent reports on hydroxylation of indoles in other than the 6-position, one finds that microsomal enzymes usually hydroxylate in positions of high electron density, so that for a 5-methoxyindole in which the electron density is higher in the 4- rather than the 6-position, one might expect preferential hydroxylation of the 4-position. We have done studies on microsomal hydroxylation of melatonin (5-methoxy-N-acetyltryptamine), and have isolated three products. The major product is 6-hydroxymelatonin, while one of the others has properties compatible with those expected of 4-hydroxymelatonin.

Our microsomal studies on hydroxylation of tryptamines support Dr. Szara's statement that the 6-fluorotryptamines do not undergo hydroxylation. Since 5-fluorotryptamines do undergo hydroxylation, to form what we believe is 5-fluoro-6-hydroxytryptamines, *in vivo* evaluation of the hallucinogenic properties of 5-fluoro-N,N-dimethyltryptamine would be of interest.

The 5-methoxy-N,N-dimethyltryptamine, found in plants and an active component of certain South American snuffs, also occurs in the skin of a certain toad. The presence of large amounts of this compound in these toads, and the occurrence in other toads of structurally related tricyclic indoles (dehydrobufotenine), led Dr. Witkop and myself to our present studies on O-methylnordehydrobufotenine, the cyclic analog of the 5-methoxy-N,N-dimethyltryptamine. This tricyclic indole prepared under the auspices of the Psychopharmacology Research Branch, NIMH, has CNS activity which is, however, markedly different from the open chain analog.

I would like to ask Dr. Holmstedt whether during his studies on the gas chromatographic and mass spectral analysis of snuffs, he also investigated the 4-methoxy, 6-methoxy and 7-methoxy-N,N-dimethyltryptamines, which would have virtually the same mass spectra as the 5-methoxy compound?

CHAIRMAN DR. HOLMSTEDT: That is right, but we have previously shown that the methoxy group was in the 5-position by using spectrofluorometric techniques and changing the pH of the solution; furthermore GLC resolves position isomers. This proves once more how advantageous the combination gas chromatrography-mass spectometry is.

DR. DALY: This might be worth looking at, whether other methoxy compounds occur which may not be separated in the snuffs and have hallucinogenic activity.

CHAIRMAN DR. HOLMSTEDT: Why has not anyone studied the 4-methoxy-N,N-dimethyltryptamine?

This session started out with anthropology, covered botany and pharmacology, and it now ends on a chemical note. I think it has been a good combination.

Thank you all.

SESSION V

AYAHUASCA, CAAPI, YAGÉ

Daniel H. Efron, *Chairman*

Psychotropic Properties of the Harmala Alkaloids

CLAUDIO NARANJO
Department of Anthropological Medicine
University of Chile, Santiago, Chile

The use of plant materials containing harmala alkaloids is probably very old. *Peganum harmala*, a zygophyllaceous plant, the seeds of which contain harmine (*1*), harmaline (*2*), and harmalol (*3*), is thought to be native to Russian Turkestan or Syria, and has been used throughout the Middle East both as a spice and as an intoxicant. Its medical and psychotropic properties are known in India, where it was probably taken by the Moslems, and where the seeds may now be purchased in bazaars (*4*). It is also believed that it was the Arabs who took the plant along the African Mediterranean and into Spain, where it may be found growing wild at present.

The species of *Banisteriopsis* that constitute a source of harmala alkaloids are used in an area lying between the rain forests of South America and the Andes. This is approximately the area designated as the "montaña" in the classification of South American cultures. It consists of a tropical elevated territory along the headwaters of the Amazon and Orinoco Rivers, where live some of the least known Indian groups.

Of much interest is the recent discovery of substances closely related to the harmala alkaloids in animals. One of these is adrenoglomerulotropine, a hormone of the pineal body, the chemical identity of which has been indicated as 2, 3, 4, 9-tetrahydro-6-methoxy-1-methyl-1H-pyrido(3, 4, 6)indole (*5*). This substance is identical to 6-methoxytetrahydroharman which has been shown to be formed *in vivo* from 5-methoxytryptamine and acetaldehyde (*6*). 6-Methoxytetrahydroharman is an isomer of tetrahydroharmine, one of the alkaloids in *Banisteriopsis* (*7*), and in the African *Leptactinia densiflora* (*8*). One more substance, 6-methoxyharmalan, has been shown to derive, at least *in vitro*, from melatonin (*9*), which in turn results from the methylation of acetylserotonin. The enzyme which makes this methylation possible, hydroxyindole-O-methyltransferase (HIOMT), has only been found in the pineal body. (See Fig. 1.)

6-Methoxyharmalan is an isomer of harmaline differing in the position of the methoxy group, which is attached to the same point of the ring as the phenolic group in serotonin or the methoxy group in ibogaine, a demonstrated hallucinogen (*10*). (See Fig. 2.)

As will be seen in the rest of the paper, I have found both synthetic 6-methoxyharmalan and 6-methoxytetrahydroharman to be hallucinogenic (*11*), a fact which invites speculation on the possible role of the metabolites on the psychoses. It is suggestive that the highest concentrations of serotonin have been found in the pineal glands of schizophrenics, and that 6-methoxyharmalan is a powerful serotonin antagonist.

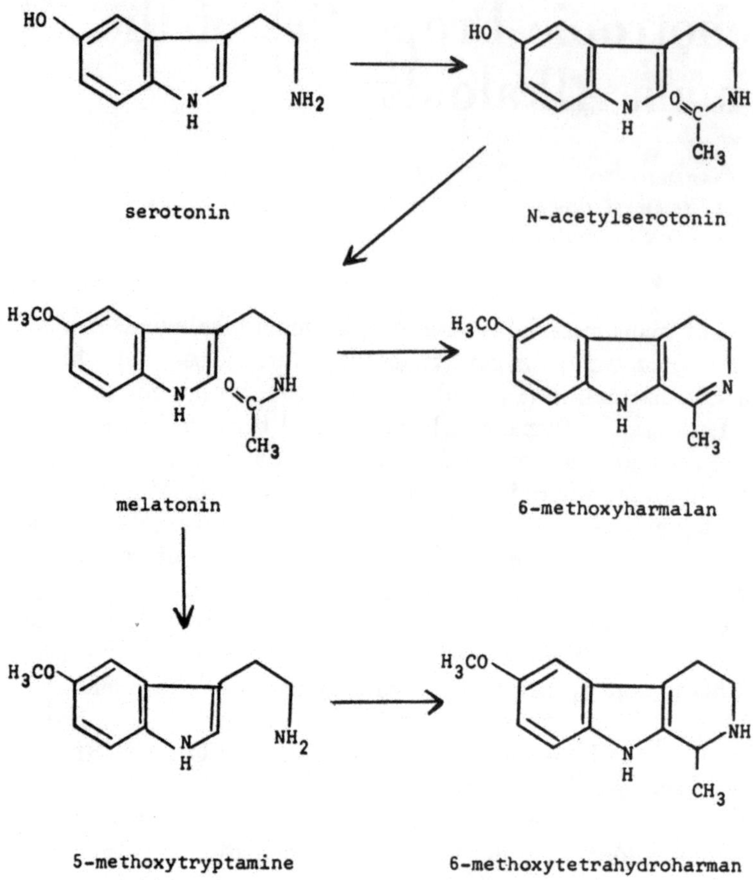
HO
NH2
N
H
HO
NH
N
H
O
C
CH3
serotonin
N-acetylserotonin
H3CO
NH
O
C
CH3
N
H
H3CO
N
N
H
CH3
melatonin
6-methoxyharmalan
H3CO
NH2
N
H
H3CO
NH
N
H
CH3
5-methoxytryptamine
6-methoxytetrahydroharman

FIG. 1.

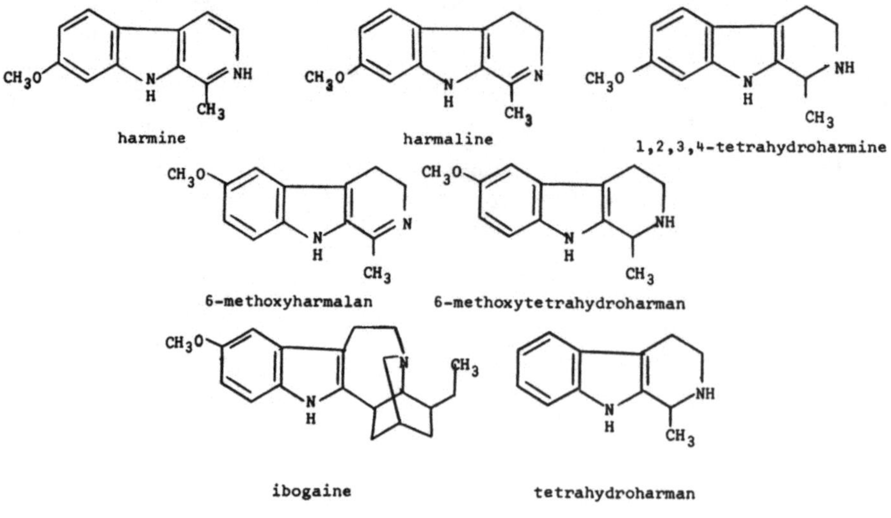
CH3O
NH
N
H
CH3
harmine
CH3O
N
N
H
CH3
harmaline
CH3O
NH
N
H
CH3
1,2,3,4-tetrahydroharmine
CH3O
N
N
H
CH3
6-methoxyharmalan
CH3O
NH
N
H
CH3
6-methoxytetrahydroharman
CH3O
N
CH3
N
H
ibogaine
NH
N
H
CH3
tetrahydroharman

FIG. 2.

It may be noted that the above reported finding constitutes the first demonstration of an endogenous hallucinogen, twenty years after the motion of a psychotoxic metabolite was proposed by Hoffer, Osmond and Smythies (*12*).

Lastly, one may wonder whether the pineal body—associated by Tibetan traditions with higher states of consciousness—may not actually play a part in the regulation of attention or the rhythm of sleep and wakefulness. An indirect indicated of this is the demonstration of increased pineal HIOMT activity in rats kept in constant darkness for six days (*13*).

Studies carried out some 30 years ago by Gunn et al., showed that some synthetic *beta*-carbolines had similar pharmacological properties, which in turn resembled those of quinine (*14*). Thus, both quinine and the harman derivatives were toxic to protozoa, inhibited the contraction of the excised muscle of the frog, caused relaxation of most smooth muscle, but contraction of uterine muscle, and caused convulsions followed by paralysis in mammals.

The only compound in this chemical group reported to have hallucinogenic properties, to my knowledge, is harmine (*15*), which may be regarded as identical to telepathine, yageine, and banisterine, and constitutes most of the alkaloid content in the *Banisteriopsis* extracts. Yet the question poses itself as to whether the qualitative similarity of harman derivatives, as evidenced by many pharmacological effects, would also apply to the psychological syndrome produced. For instance, Gunn finds that harmaline is twice as active as harmine, judging from the lethal doses of both compounds for the rabbit, and from their toxicity to protozoa. I have indeed found harmaline to be hallucinogenic at dosage levels above 1 mg./kg. i.v. or 4 mg./kg. by mouth, which is about one half the threshold level for harmine. It may be interesting to note at this point that the onset of effects of harmaline or other derivatives is about one hour after ingestion by mouth, but almost instantaneous after intravenous injection, if circulation time from elbow to brain is taken into account. In this, harmaline resembles the chemically related tryptamines and differs from the slow-acting phenylethylamines.

Tetrahydroharmine, the reduction product of harmaline, is another substance studied by Gunn and shown to be similar to its more saturated homologs, but three times less active than harmaline.

Racemic tetrahydroharmine, up to the amount of 300 mg. by mouth, was administered by us to one volunteer, who reported that at this dosage level there were subjective effects similar to those he experienced with 100 mg. of harmaline. More trials would be required to assess the mean effective dosage of tetrahydroharmine as a hallucinogen, but this single experiment suggests that racemic tetrahydroharmine is about one-third as active as harmaline, corresponding to Gunn's estimation on the basis of lethal dosage.

The effect of relocating the methoxy group of harmaline was not tested by Gunn but was of special interest here, in view of a possible function of the 6-methoxy homolog in the body. 6-Methoxyharmalan was indeed shown to be hallucinogenic, as was anticipated, subjective effects becoming apparent with approximate oral dosages of 1.5 mg./kg. The ratio between threshold doses of harmaline and its 6-methoxy analog is 3:2, 6-methoxyharmalan being the more active.

6-Methoxytetrahydroharman, probably identical with pineal adreno-glomerulotropine, was also shown to be psychoactive, eliciting mild effects at a dosage level of 1.5 mg./kg. The relative activities of the two 6-methoxyharmans are approximately 1:3, the harmalan being more active than its unsaturated homolog, which confirms once more Gunn's statement as to the relationship between double bonds and pharmacological effect.

It would seem premature to make any statement as to whether there is a qualitative difference in the subjective reaction to the different carbolines tested. Such appeared to be the case, in that experiences with the 6-methoxy compounds happened to be of a less hallucinogenic nature in the strict sense of the word, their effect being more akin to a state of inspiration and heightened introspection. Among the 7-methoxy compounds, harmaline seemed to cause more withdrawal and lethargy than harmine, but both substances showed a highly hallucinogenic quality in the visual domain. However, more systematic study would be needed to confirm differences such as these, in view of the variability which exists even between consecutive experiences of the same individual with the same chemical. This is well known for LSD–25, and was quite marked in four of the seven subjects to whom harmaline was administered more than once. Yet it seems clear that the various *beta*-carbolines are similar enough in their effect to be told apart from mescaline, as was shown by the comments of persons to whom mescaline, harmaline and some other harman derivative were administered on consecutive occasions. The third compound, the nature of which was not known to the experimental subjects, was invariably likened to harmaline rather than to mescaline. The same can be said of instances in which harmaline was administered on a second or third occasion without divulging the drug's identity. Regardless of the differences between consecutive harmaline experiences, these were classified together as distinct from that of mescaline.

It is quite possible that further research with a larger number of subjects may demonstrate qualitative differences of a subtle kind between the different carbolines, analogous to those shown for variously substituted phenylisopropylamines (*16, 17*). Nevertheless, it may be adequate for the time being to regard the effects of harmaline as an approximately valid indication of a syndrome shared, with minor variations, by compounds of similar structure.

This information that I am presenting here on the effects of harmaline is based on the reactions of 30 volunteers to whom the drug was administered as a hydrochloride, either by mouth or intravenously, under standard conditions. One aspect of these was the absence of all information regarding effects other than those primarily psychological in nature.

As part of the interest lay in knowing the difference between the harmaline syndrome and that of mescaline, both drugs were administered to each volunteer on different occasions.

In the case of every one of the 30 subjects it was evident to the observer that both the subjective and behavioral reactions of the person were quite different for the two drugs, and this was corroborated without exception by the subjects themselves. Yet the quality of the difference was not clearly the same in all instances, so that it is hard to find regularities to which no exception can be mentioned. Recurring differences between harmaline and mescaline can be observed however, and in what follows, the most salient of these are cited.

Physical sensations in general are more a part of the harmaline intoxication than of that produced by mescaline (or similar substances). Parasthesias of the hands, feet or face are almost always present with the onset of effects, and are usually followed by a sensation of numbness. These symptoms are most marked when the alkaloid is injected intravenously, in which case some subjects have likened them to those experienced under ether anesthesia. Distortions of the body image, which are quite frequent with mescaline or LSD–25, were very exceptional with harmaline. Instead, subjects indicated isolated physical symptoms such as pressure in the head, discomfort in the chest, or enhancement of certain sensations, as those of breathing or blinking.

Nausea was reported by 18 subjects and this sometimes led to intense vomiting. It was usually associated with dizziness or general malaise, which would in turn appear or disappear throughout a session in connection with certain thoughts or stimuli.

In the domain of perception, one of the most noticeable differences between the drugs is in the visual appearance of the environment. While distortions of forms, alterations in the sense of depth and changes in the expression of faces are of frequent occurrence under most hallucinogens, these phenomena were practically never seen with harmaline. The same was true in regard to color enhancement, or perception of apparent movement—flowers breathing, shapes dancing and so on—frequently seen with LSD–25. With harmaline, the environment is essentially unchanged, both in regard to its formal and its aesthetic qualities. Phenomena which most frequently occur with open eyes are the superposition of images on surfaces such as walls or ceilings, or the viewing of imaginary scenes simultaneously with an undistorted perception of surrounding objects. Such imagery is not usually taken for reality but there was an exception to this in the case of a man who saw a cat climbing a wall, then turning into a leopard, when in fact, not even the cat existed.

Other recurrent visual phenomena were a rapid lateral vibration in the field of vision and double or multiple contours in objects, especially when these were in motion or when the subject's eyes turned away from them. Some described lightning-like flashes.

With closed eyes, imagery was abundant and most often vivid and bright colored, with a predominance of red-green or blue-orange contrasts. Long dream-like sequences were much more frequent for harmaline than for mescaline. Certain themes, such as felines, negroes, eyes, and flying are frequent and have been reported elsewhere (18).

Perception of music was not altered or enhanced with harmaline as is the case with mescaline or LSD–25. Yet noises became very prominent and generally bothersome. Buzzing sounds in the head were reported by more than half of the subjects.

Synaesthesias were not reported, and the sense of time was unaltered.

Many of the differences between harmaline and mescaline may be related to the facts that the effect of the former on the emotions is much less than that of mescaline, and thinking is affected only in subtle ways, if at all. Concern with religious or philosophical problems is frequent, but there is not the aesthetic or emphathetic quality of the mescaline experience. Thus, the typical reaction to harmaline is a closed-eye contemplation of vivid imagery without much further effect than wonder and interest in its significance, which is in contrast to the ecstatic heavens or dreadful hells of other hallucinogens. Despite this lesser effect of harmaline on the intensity of feelings, qualitative changes do occur in the emotions, which may account for the pronounced amelioration of neurotic syptoms evidenced by 8 of our 30 subjects, as detailed in a separate report (19).

Desire to communicate is slight under the effect of harmaline, since other persons are felt to be a part of the external world, contact with which is usually avoided. Possibly related to this withdrawal is the extreme passivity which most subjects experienced in regard to physical movement. Most of them lay down for 4 to 8 hours and reported a state of relaxation in which they did not feel inclined to move a muscle, even to talk. In view of this observation, it is hard to understand how the Indians, according to some authors (20), engage in dancing or even whip one another under the effects of caapi.

Summing up, harmaline may be said to be more of a pure hallucinogen than other substances whose characteristic phenomena are an enhancement of feelings, aesthetic experiences, or psychotomimetic qualities such as paranoid delusions, depersonalization, or cognitive disturbances. Moreover, harmaline appears to be more hallucinogenic than mecaline (the most visually acting drug in its chemical group), both in terms of the number of images reported and their realistic quality. In fact some subjects felt that certain scenes which they saw has really happened, and that they had been as disembodied witnesses of them in a different time and place. This matches the experience of South American shamans who drink ayahuasca for purposes of divination.

The remarkable vividness of imagery viewed under the effect of harmaline, together with phenomena such as double contours and persistence of after images, had led us to suspect a peripheral, i.e. retinal, effect of the drug, and this was tested by the recording of electroretinograms in cats. The suspicion was confirmed, in that harmaline causes a definite increase in the alpha wave and a decrease in the beta wave of the electroretinogram, both of which become apparent before any change is observed in the brain cortex.

It would be beyond the scope of this paper to deal with electrophysiological studies, but I will briefly mention some recent results we have obtained in cat experiments at the University of Chile, which add to the general picture of the harmaline intoxication:

(1) Electrocorticograms recorded in chronically implanted cats showed either electrocortical desynchronization or synchronization in correspondence with the animal's behaviour, alternating between arousal and lethargy. In addition to this spindle bursts of high voltage and low frequency were observed in all instances and these did not seem to be related to the animal's behaviour.

(2) Experiments performed in cats with a chronically isolated forebrain showed even more clearly the above mentioned spindle bursts in the brain cortex, and regular wave bursts of high voltage in the pontine reticular formation, which we have not seen described under other pharmacological conditions. These cats were behaviourally overactive.

These facts may be interpreted as an indication that harmaline acts as a stimulant on the midbrain reticular formation. The direct action of harmaline on the brain cortex is hard to interpret and seems more that of a depressant, but this is counteracted in the intact animal by the arousing influence of the reticular formation. The neurophysiological picture matches well that of traditional yagé "dreaming", in that the state we have described involved lethargy, immobility, closed eyes and generalized withdrawal from the environment, but at the same time an alertness to mental processes, and an activation of fantasy.

REFERENCES

(1) GOEBEL, Annalen, 38, 363, 1841.
(2) FRITSCHE, Annalen, 64, 365, 1847.
(3) FISCHER, O., Chem. Soc. Abstr., 1901 (i), 405.
(4) MAXWELL, M. M. "Caapi, its source, use and possibilities." Unpubl. MS., 1937.
(5) FARREL, G. and W. M. McISAAC, "Adrenoglomerulotropin." Arch. Biochem. Biophys., 94: 443–544, 1961.
(6) McISAAC, W. M. "Formation of 1-methyl-6-methoxy-1,2,3-tetrahydro-2-carboline under physiological conditions." Biochem. Biophys. Acta 52: 607–609, 1961.
(7) HOCHSTEIN, F. A. and A. M. PARADIES. "Alkaloids of Banisteria Caapi and Prestonia Amazonicum." J. Am. Chem. Soc. 79, 5735, 1957
(8) PARIS, R. R., F. PERCHERON, J. MANLIL and GOUTAREL. Bull. Soc. Chim. France, 750, 1957.
(9) McISAAC, W. M., P. A. KHAIRALLAH and I. H. PAGE. "10-methoxyharmalan, a potent serotonin antagoinist which affects conditioned behaviour." Science 134, 674–675, 1961.
(10) NARANJO, C. Psychological effects of Ibogaine. In preparation.
(11) NARANJO, C. and A. SHULGIN. Hallucinogenic properties of a pineal metabolite: 6-methoxytetrahydroharman. Science. In press.
(12) HOFFER, A., H. OSMOND and J. SMYTHIES. "Schizophrenia: a new approach II." J. Ment. Sci., 100: 29–45, 1950.
(13) AXELROD, J., R. J. WURTMAN, and S. SNYDER. "Control of hydroxyindole-O-methyl-transferase activity in the rat pineal gland by environmental lighting." J. Biol. Chem. 240: 949–954, 1965.
(14) GUNN, Arc. Int. Pharmacodyn., 50, 793, 1935.
(15) PENNES, H. H., and P. H. HOCH, Am. J. Psychiat. 113, 885, 1957.
(16) SHULGIN, A., T. SARGENT and C. NARANJO. "Chemistry and psychopharmacology of nutmeg and related phenylisopropylamines." Paper presented at the Symposium "Ethnopharmacologic Search for Psychoactive Drugs." U. of Calif., S. F., 1967.
(17) NARANJO, C. MMDA in the facilitation of psychotherapy. Book in preparation.
(18) NARANJO, C. "Psychological aspects of the yagé experience in an experimental setting." Paper presented at the Annual Meeting of the American Anthropological Association, 1965.
(19) NARANJO, C., Ayahuasca, the Vine of the Dead. Book in preparation.
(20) TAYLOR, N., Flight from Reality. 1949.
(21) VILLIBLANCA, J., C. NARANJO, and F. RIOBÓ. Effects of harmaline in the intact cat and in chronic isolated forebrain and isolated hemisphere preparations. Psychopharmacologia. In press.

The Making of the Hallucinogenic Drink from Banisteriopsis Cuapi in Northern Peru

DERMOT TAYLOR
Department of Pharmacology, University of California
Los Angeles, California

A moving-picture film showing the ceremonies and procedures for the preparation of the drink was presented.

Chemical Compounds Isolated from Banisteriopsis and Related Species

VENANCIO DEULOFEU

Facultad de Ciencias Exactas y Naturales, Buenos Aires, Argentina

The Malpighiaceae, to which the genus *Banisteriopsis* belongs, is a family distributed in tropical and sub-tropical humid regions of Africa and America. The genus *Banisteriopsis* is represented by about 75 species, which grow in America from Mexico and Cuba to Argentina, most of them in South America (*1*).

Only a few species of *Banisteriopsis* have been investigated chemically, and the first stimulus for the chemical work was the finding in the middle of the last century by the British explorer Spruce that a woody vine, which he classified as *Banisteria caapi*, later known as *Banisteriopsis caapi*, was the main ingredient employed in the preparation of an intoxicating drink by certain tribes living in the Amazonian Brazil. It was later found that the preparation and use of a similar beverage extended to a larger region, to what is today known as the eastern parts of Colombia, Ecuador, Perú and Bolivia, where it was given different vernacular names: ayahuasca, caapi, yagé, yajé, natem, natema, etc., names which were also applied to the plants employed for their preparation. Other plants were added and mixed with the former.

The history of the botanical, chemical and pharmacological implications of the beverage has been told in several opportunities and from several angles (*2*, *3*). While at the beginning there were difficulties in the identification of the alkaloids isolated from the extracts of the plants, and which were made responsible for the activity of the intoxicating drink, it seems that today, with the improvement of the methods of identification and the use of new techniques, we know exactly which are the bases isolated. There seem to be more difficulties from the botanical side. The lack in many chemical studies of plant specimens, or of a rigorous identification of the botanical material worked by the chemists, makes it impossible to know exactly which were the species employed. It is with this qualification that some of the botanical names are quoted in this paper.

Early chemical investigation of the plant employed in Colombia by the natives indicated the presence of an alkaloid which was given the name of telepathine as early as 1905 by Zerda Barron (*4*). A base supposed to be responsible for the activity of the drink was isolated in 1923, no doubt in impure form, by Fischer Cardenas (*5*) who conserved the name of telepathine.

Another isolation was carried out two years later by Barriga Villalba (*6*), who seems to be the first who obtained a crystalline product, to which he gave the name of yajéine. From the assigned formula, $C_{14}H_8N_3O_3$ and from its m.p.206°, we have now to conclude that it was an impure substance, although the lack of rotation is in agreement with what can be expected for an aromatic β-carboline structure. Another base was present in the mother liquors and named yajénine, but no constants were mentioned in the paper. According to Barriga Villalba, he worked the stems of a vine which was known by the vernacular name of yajé, and which according to Reinburg was *Haemadictyon amazonicum* (*Prestonia amazonica Spruce*), which is an Apocynaceae. Rios, in his review on the ayahuasca, mentions that in a later paper, Barriga Villalba states (*7*) that the plant he worked was not *P. amazonica*, but *B. caapi*, which is in agreement with the investigations of Schultes and Raffauf (*8*) on the use of the former species as a narcotic.

From what can be considered an authentic specimen of *B. caapi*, Perrot and Raymond-Hamet (*2*) isolated for the first time in pure condition one of the bases present in the plant (m.p.258°), for which they conserved the name of telepathine. A year later Lewin (*9*) described the isolation of an alkaloid from the same source, which he called banisterine. In his paper, Lewin says that the chemists from E. Merck (Darmstadt, Germany), considered banisterine identical to the base harmine (*I*), an alkaloid isolated more than a century ago from *Peganum harmala* L. (Zygophyllaceae). Two papers on the identification were published the same year almost simultaneously; one by Elger (*10*) and the other by Wolf and Rumpf (*11*), the latter workers being members of the Merck laboratories.

Elger employed plant material supplied by Raymond-Hamet and which was identified as *B. caapi*, according to A. W. Hill, then Director of the Kew Botanical Gardens. Sir Robert Robinson compared the alkaloid isolated by Elger (m.p.263–264°), with the harmine (*I*) from *P. harmala*, and with a synthetic sample, and concluded that they were identical. He comments on the difficulties of purifying harmine, which can explain the low melting point of the base obtained by Barriga Vallalba. Chen and Chen (*12*), who worked also with an authentic botanical specimen, confirmed the identification, and could isolate harmine from stems, leaves and roots.

A plant identified as *B. caapi* Spruce was investigated many years later by Hochstein and Paradies (*13*). It was harvested near Iquitos, in Peru, where it was named ayahuasca. They confirmed the presence of harmine (I) and isolated also harmaline (II) and (+)-tetrahydroharmine (III). They state that the two latter alkaloids were found in a rather large amount. The same bases were also present in an aqueous extract of the plant "as used by the natives" but which appeared richer in harmaline and tetrahydroharmine than the extracts of the plant. They suggested that these two alkaloids may be the most active psychotomimetic components of the extracts.

All the bases isolated from *B. caapi* have a β-carboline skeleton, with different degrees of hydrogenation in the pyridine ring. Their structure was already known because of the interest of the chemists in similar alkaloids isolated from *P. harmala L.*, harmine (I) and harmaline (II), which culminated in the synthesis of harmaline (II) by Manske, Perkin and Robinson (*14*).

Although the racemic tetrahydroharmine had already been prepared in the laboratory, it was the first time that one of the enantiomers, (+)-tetra-

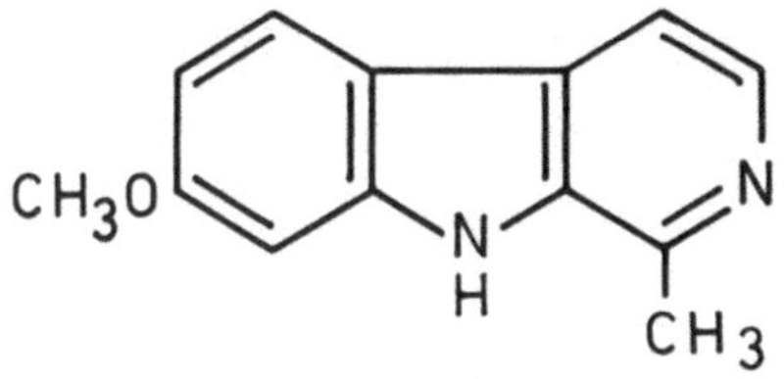

(I)

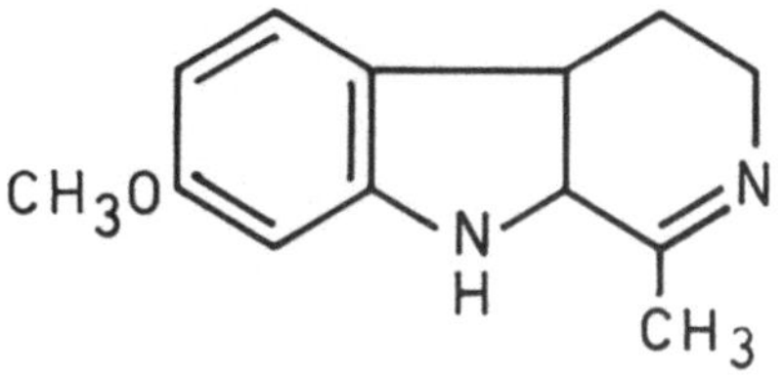

(II)

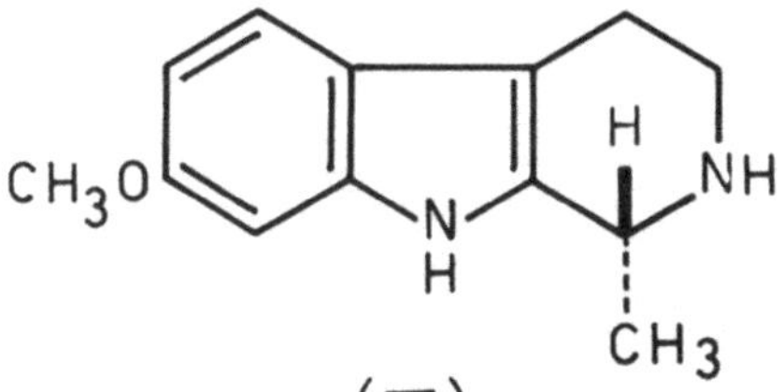

(III)

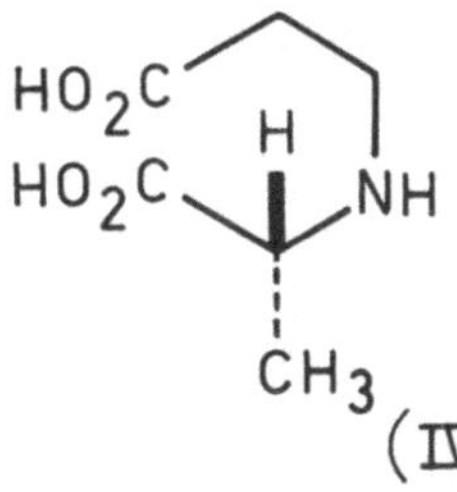

(IV)

hydroharmine (III), had been found in Nature. The dextro compound isolated by Hochstein and Paradies (*13*) was in fact a new natural base, and
because of its pharmacological activity it was of interest to determine its
absolute configuration. This was done recently by Koblicová and Trojánek
(*15*), who found that its asymmetric carbon atom has the same chirality as
the asymmetric carbon of D-alanine (IV), which is opposite to that of the
protein aminoacid L-alanine.

Another species investigated has been *B. inebrians* Morton. O'Connell and
Lynn (*16*) isolated harmine (I) from the stems of an authentic specimen
collected by Schultes, and found that the leaves probably contains the same
base. They could not detect harmaline nor harmalol. The same species was
worked again by Poisson (*17*) in 1965, the plant being collected in a place
named Nazareth, on the shores of the Marañon River, in Perú. He confirmed
the presence of harmine in the stems and pointed out that another base, with
the chromatographic properties of harmaline (II), was present in small
amount.

Poisson investigated also the leaves of another species, *B. rusbyana*
(Niedenzu) Morton, known to the natives as yajé, which were added to the
stems of *B. inebrians* when ayahuasca was prepared. Surprisingly, this
species did not contain alkaloids with a β-carboline structure, and the only
base which he could identify was dimethyl-tryptamine (V). The amount was
rather high (0.64%).

The species worked by Poisson were identified by Cuatrecasas. The finding
of dimethyltryptamine (V) in *B. rusbyana*, a species used together with
B. inebrians for the preparation of ayahuasca, is interesting for several
reasons. One is that the same base was isolated by Hochstein and Paradies
(*13*) from the extract of a plant which they considered to be *P. amazonica*,
which received the local name of yagé, and which was used by the natives

395

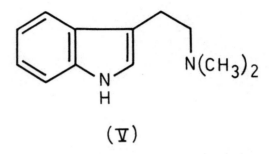

(V)

to prepare ayahuasca as an additional component to *B. caapi*. Hochstein and Paradies received only an extract of the plant, whose identification is doubtful (*8, 18*).

The second point of interest is that bases of the tryptamine type are typical components of other plants which have been used by the natives in many places of South America and in the Caribbean, for the preparation of intoxicating snuffs. They belong to the *Piptadenia* (Leguminosae) (*19*) and *Virola* (Myristicaceae) genus (*20*).

Other *Banisteriopsis* species have been mentioned as the main or additional ingredients employed in the preparation of ayahuasca. They are *B. quitensis* (Ndz) Morton (*21*), which according to Cuatrecasas (*1e*) is identical to *B. caapi* Spruce, *B. longialata* (*21*), and *B. metallicolor* Juss. (*B. lutea* Ruiz) (*3*).

I have not found in the literature any indication that authentic specimens of those plants have been submitted to chemical research, but because they are used in the preparation of intoxicating drinks, their investigation will be of much interest.

On the other hand, *B. crysophylla* Lam. a species which grows in Australia, is reported to contain alkaloids (*22*) and *B. nitrosiodora* Griseb, which is one of the species found in Argentina, is practically devoid of alkaloids (*23*). There remain a large number of species which have not even been submitted to a preliminary chemical investigation.

Harmine (I) has been isolated by Mors and Zaltzman (*24*) from the stems and leaves of another South American Malpighiaceae, *Cabi paraensis* Ducke, which is closely related to the *Banisteriopsis* genus. It grows in Brazil, in the upper Amazonian region and also in Perú (*3*). According to Duke (*25*), it is employed in popular medicine, although not for the preparation of intoxicating drinks.

It is worthwhile to note that only a few other species of Malpighiaceae have been investigated for alkaloids. One of them is *Lophantaera lactecens* (*L. longifolia*) which grows in the Amazonian, and is employed for the preparation of a kind of tea. Ribeiro and Machado (*26*) isolated from extracts of that plant a new base, lophanterine, which structure is unknown.

In his review on the Botanical Sources of the New World narcotics, Schultes (*21*) mentions in relation with the preparation of ayahuasca, two Malpighiaceae which, if botanical material became available, will deserve chemical attention. They are *Tetrapterys methystica*, from which an hallucinogenic drink is prepared in Colombia, on the limits of Brazil, and *Mascagnia psilophylla* var. *antifebrilis*, which was pointed out by Niedenzu as a source for the preparation of ayahuasca which in the opinion of Schultes is doubtful.

To my knowledge harmine (I), harmaline (II) and tetrahydroharmine (III), have never been isolated from other original American plants. They have been found to be present in intoxicating snuffs prepared by the natives from unknown botanical sources. We have two almost simultaneous reports. One is by Biocca, Galeffi, Montalvo and Marini-Bettolo (*27*), who from a snuff prepared by Tukano and Tariana Indians living in the valley of the Uaupes River, isolated harmine (I), harmaline (II) and tetrahydroharmine (III), exactly the same bases found in *B. caapi* by Hochstein and Paradies (*13*). According to the Italian authors, the snuff is named paricá and is prepared from a vine, which is also employed for the preparation of a drink. The species remained undetermined.

On the other hand, Bernhauer (*28*), has investigated a snuff employed by the Surara and Pakidai Indians, living near the River Demeni, a subsidiary of the Negro River, which he says is known as paricá, yopo, ebená or epená. He could isolate harmine (I) and (+)-tetrahydroharmine (III), while harmaline (II) was absent. The series of names given by Bernhauer to the drug that he investigated, shows how confused is its identification because samples of snuffs named epená, which were investigated not long ago by Holmstedt (*20*) and Marini Bettolo, Delle Monache and Biocca (*29*), contained only tryptamine bases. In my opinion this is a nice proof of the importance of the future interdisciplinary work, which is needed to clarify the botanical sources and the chemically active substances in the plants and in the drugs prepared by the natives.

Both types of bases isolated from *Banisteriopsis* species are related to tryptamine. Tryptamine or a precursor, is one of the intermediates in the biogenesis of a large number of indole alkaloids, most of them with a more elaborate structure than the simpler β-carboline bases.

The type and distribution of the simple tryptamine bases found in plants have been recently reviewed (*30*). Work done in several laboratories in recent years have shown that bases with a typical β-carboline structure are also, like the tryptamines, not restricted in botanical or geographical distribution (see Table I).

The earlier representatives were isolated from *Peganum harmala* L. (Zygophyllaceae) more than a hundred years ago: harmaline (II) (1841), and harmalol (XVIII) (1841). The simplest base, harman (XI), was isolated from a Rubiaceae growing in Brazil in 1861 (*Arariba rubra* Mart., *Sickinga rubra* K. Schumm), and a few years later (1878) from *Symplocos racemosa* (Symplocaceae), indigenous to India.

Research in the last few years has lead to the isolation of other β-carbolines from plants growing in America. Bächli *et al.* (*31*), were isolated from *Strychnos melinoniana* Baill. (Loganiaceae), the quaternary base which is known as melinonine-F (XIV), and Antonaccio and Budzikiewicz (*32*)

TABLE I. OTHER β-CARBOLINE BASES FOUND IN PLANTS[a]

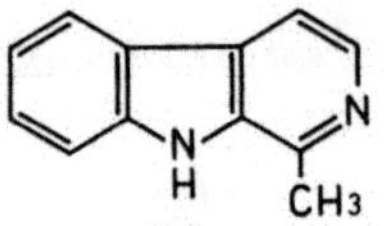

(XI)

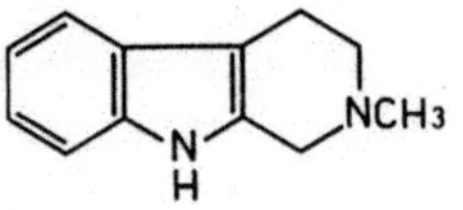

(XII)

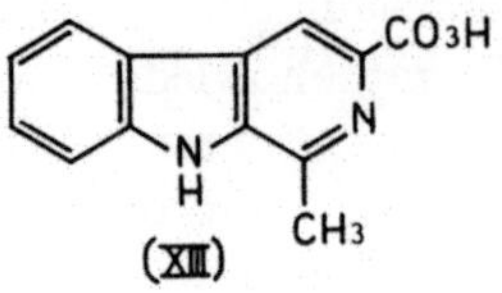

(XIII)

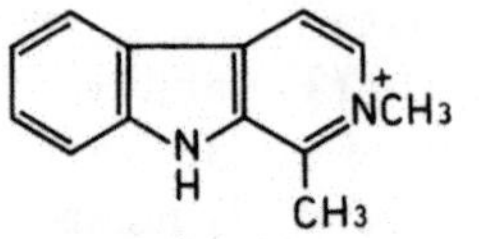

(XIV)

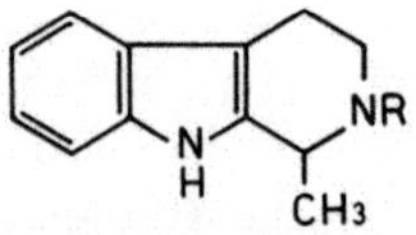

(XV) R = H ;(XVI) R = CH₃

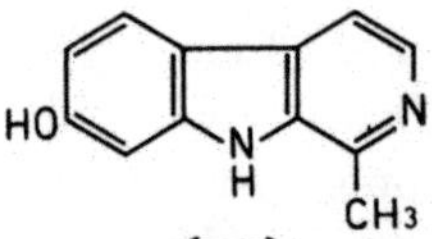

(XVII)

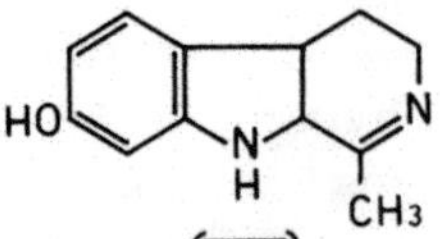

(XVIII)

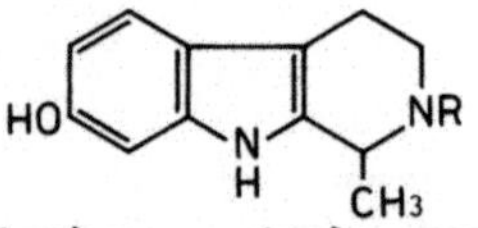

(XIX) R = H ; (XX) R = CH₃

(XI) Harman. *Peganum harmala* L. (Zygophyllaceae) ; *Passiflora* spp. (Passifloraceae) (*39*) ; *P. incarnata* L. (*40, 41*) ; *Calligonum minimum* Lipski (Polygonaceae) (*42*).

(XII) N-Methyl-tetrahydro-β-carboline. *Hammada leptoclada* M. Iljin (*Arthrophytum leptocladum* Popov) (Chenopodiaceae) (*43*).

(XIII) Harman-3-carboxylic acid. *Aspidosperma polyneuron* Müll. Arg. (Apocynaceae) (*32*).

(XIV) Melinonine F. *Strychnos melinoniana* Baillon (Loganiaceae) (*31*).

(XV) Tetrahydroharman, elaeagnine (R=H). *Petalostyles labicheoides* R. Br. (Leguminosae) (*44*) ; *Elaeagnus angustifolia* L. (Elaeagnaceae) (*45*) ; *Leptactina densiflora* Hook. f. (Rubiaceae) (*38*) ; *Hammada leptoclada* M. Iljin (*46*) ; *Calligonum minimum* Lipski (*42*).

(XVI) N-Methyl-tetrahydroharman, leptocladine (R=CH₃). *H. leptoclada* M. Iljin (*43*) ; *Acacia complanata* A. Cunn. (Leguminosae) (*47*).

(XVII) Harmol. *P. incarnata* L. (*40*) ; *Zygophyllum fabago* L. (Zygophyllaceae) (*48*).

(XVIII) Harmalol. *P. harmala* L.

(XIX) Tetrahydroharmol (R=H). *Elaeagnus angustifolia* L. (*49*).

(XX) N-Methyl-tetrahydroharmol (R=CH₃). *E. angustifolia* L. (*49*).

[a] This list of species is not exhaustive. They have been selected to show the distribution of bases in different families.

harman-3-carboxilic acid (XIII) from *Aspidosperma polyneuron* Müll. Arg. (Apocynaceae).

Recently, in our laboratory Sanchez and Comin (*33*), found β-carbolines in *Aeschrion crenata* Vell., a Simaroubaceae which grows is Southern Brazil, Paraguay and Argentina. Although it is used in popular medicine, there is no indication that its extracts have intoxicating properties. The bases crenatine (VI) and crenatidine (VII) were isolated, together with 1-carbomethoxy-β-carboline (VIII), which has been formerly found in *Pleiocarpa mutica* Benth. (Apocynaceae) (*34*).

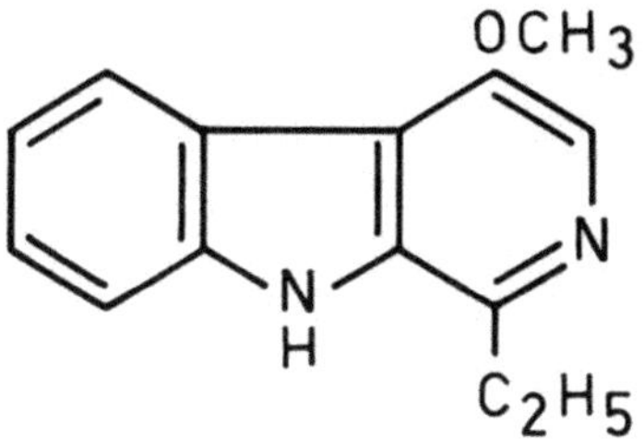

OCH$_3$

C$_2$H$_5$

(VI)

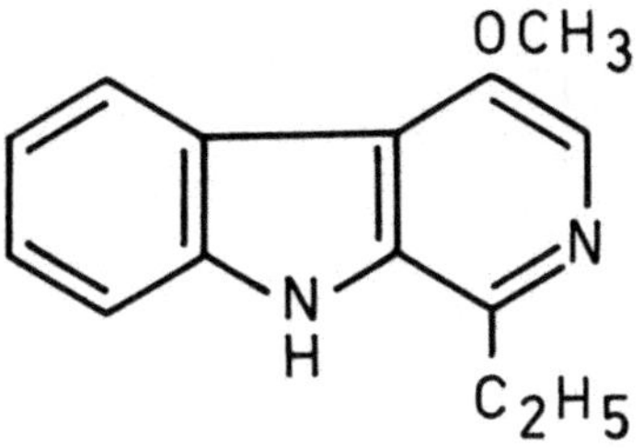

OCH$_3$

C$_2$H$_5$

(VII)

CO$_2$Me

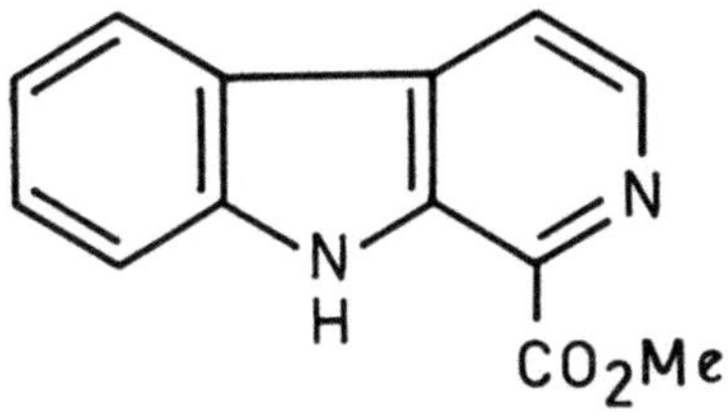

(VIII)

A β-carboline alkaloid with a more elaborated, novel type of structure, was isolated also in our laboratory by Brauchli et al (*35*), from *Pogonopus tubulosus* (DC) Schum. a Rubiaceae which grows in the Central and Northern part of Argentina, where in some places it is employed against fever. The base was named tubulosine (IX), and is structurally related to emetine (X) the tetrahydroisoquinoline moiety of the latter alkaloid being replaced by a β-carboline. Bases with this typical skeleton have been latter identified in *Alangium lamarckii* Thw. (Alangiaceae) (*36*) and in *Cassinopsis ilicifolia* Kuntze (Icacinaceae) (*37*).

It is of interest to note that besides *P. harmala*, the typical β-carbolines present in the *Banisteriopsis* species, have been isolated from a few species indigenous to other continents. In an African Rubiaceae, *Leptactine densiflora* Hook (±)-tetrahydroharmine (leptaflorine) (III) have been found (*38*). *Passiflora incarnata* L. and possible other *Passiflora* species (Passifloraceae) (*39*), contain harmine (I), which has also been found in *Zygophyllum fabago*, (*48*).

Other simple β-carbolines closely related in structure to the *Banisteriopsis* alkaloids have been isolated from other plants. They are listed in Table I with an indication of the source of isolation.

Many of the species containing β-carboline alkaloids have been used in popular medicine and several of the bases isolated have been submitted to pharmacological studies, and a few of them even employed in therapeutics. But outside America, so far as I know, plants containing those alkaloids have not been employed for their hallucinogenic properties.

(IX)

(X)

BIBLIOGRAPHY

(1) (a) NIEDENZU, F. in A. Engler and K. Prandl, *Die Naturlichen Pflanzenfamilien*, III, 4: 41–74. Leipzig, W. Engelmann, 1896. (b) NIEDENZU, F. in A. Engler, *Das Pflanzenreich*, IV, 141. Leipzig, W. Engelmann, 1928. (c) O'DONELL, C. A., and A. LOURTEIG. Malpighiaceae Argentinae. Lilloa, 9: 221–316, 1943. (d) PEREIRA, E., Contribuçao ao Conhecimento da familia Malpighiaceae. Arquiv. Servic. Forestal (Rio de Janeiro). 7: 11–70, 1953. (e) CUATRECASAS, J., Prima flora Colombiana. Webbia, 13: 343–664, 1957/1958.

(2) PERROT, E., and RAYMOND-HAMET. "Yagé, Ayahuasca, Caapi et leur alcaloïde: tele-pathine ou yagéine." Bull. Scienc. Pharmacol., 34: 337–347, 417–426, 500–514, 1927.

(3) RIOS, O. "Aspectos preliminares al estudio Farmaco-Psiquiátrico del Ayahuasca y su Principio Activo." Anales Fac. Med. Univ. Nacl. Mayor San Marcos, Lima. 45: 22–66 (1962). Chem. Abstr. 59: 3215, 1963.

(4) ZERDA BARRON, B. Quoted by E. Perrot and Raymond-Hamet in reference (2) and by O. Rios and reference (3).

(5) FISCHER CÁRDENAS G. "Estudio sobre el principio áctivo del Yagé." Thesis, Fac. Medic. Cienc. Natural. Bogotá, 1923. Quoted by E. Perrot and Raymond-Hamet in reference (2) and by O. Rios in reference (3).

(6) BARRIGA VILLALBA, A. M. "Yajéine. A new alkaloid." J. Soc. Chem. Ind. 44: 205–207, 1925.

(7) BARRIGA VILLALBA, A. M. El yagé. Bebida especial de los indios ribereños del Putu-mayo y el Amazonas." Bol. Lab. Semper-Martinez, N° espec. 9, 1927. Quoted by O. Rios in reference (3).

(8) SCHULTES, R. E., and R. F. RAFFAUF. *"Prestonia:* An Amazon narcotic or not." Bot. Museum Leafl. Harvard Univ., 19: 109–122, 1960.

(9) LEWIN, L. "Sur une substance enivrante, la banisterine, extraite de *Banisteria caapi.*" Compt. Rend., 186: 469–471, 1928.

(10) ELGER, F. "Ueber das Vorkommen von Harmin in einer südamerikanischen Liane (Yagé)." Helv. Chim. Acta, 11: 162–166, 1928.

(11) WOLFE, O., and K. RUMPF. "Ueber die gewinnung von Harmin aus einer südamerikanischen Liane." Arch. Pharm., 266 : 188–189, 1928.

(12) CHEN, A. L., and K. K. CHEN. "Harmine, The Alkaloid of *Caapi.*" Quart. J. Pharm.
Pharmacol., 12 : 30–38, 1939.

(13) HOCHSTEIN, F. A., and A. M. PARADIES. "Alkaloids from *Banisteria caapi* and *Prestonia amazonicum.*" J. Am. Chem. Soc., 79 : 5735–5736, 1957.

(14) MANSKE, R. H. F., W. H. PERKIN, and R. ROBINSON. "A synthesis of harmaline."
J. Chem. Soc., 1–14, 1927.

(15) KOBLICOVÁ, Z., and J. TROJÁNEK. "The Absolute Configuration of (+)-1,2,3,4-
Tetrahydroharmine." Chem. Ind. (London) 1342, 1966.

(16) O'CONNELL, F. D., and E. V. LYNN. "The Alkaloid of *Banisteriopsis inebrians* Morton." J. Am. Pharm. Assoc., 42 : 753–754, 1953.

(17) POISSON, J. "Note sur le 'Natem' boisson toxique péruvienne et ses alcaloïdes."
Ann. Pharm. Franc., 23 : 241–244, 1965.

(18) RAFFAUF, R. F., and M. B. FLAGLER. Alkaloids of the Apocynaceae. Econ. Botany,
14 : 37–55 (1960).

(19) DEULOFEU, V. "Chemical Aspects of American Medicinal Plants." Lecture, III
Internat. Pharmacol. Congress. Sao Paulo, Brazil, July 24–30, 1966.

(20) WASSÉN, S. H., and B. HOLMSTEDT. "The use of paricá, an ethnological and Pharmacological review." Ethnos, 5–45, 1963. Holmstedt, B., Tryptamine derivatives
in epená, an intoxicating snuff used by some South American indian tribes. Arch.
Intern. Pharmacodyn., 156 : 285–305, 1965.

(21) (*a*) SCHULTES, R. E. "The identity of the Malpighiaceous narcotics of South
America." Bot. Museum Leafl. Harvard Univ., 18 : 1–56, 1957. (*b*) SCHULTES, E. R.
"Botanical Sources of the New World Narcotics." Psychedelic Rev., 1 : 145–166,
1963. (*c*) SCHULTES, R. E. "Ein halbes Jahrhundert Ethnobotanik amerikanischer
Halluzinogene." Planta Medica, 13 : 125–157, 1965.

(22) WEBB, L. J. Australian Phytochemical Survey. Part I, Bulletin 241. Melbourne,
CSIRO, 1949. pag. 34.

(23) Unpublished results from our Laboratory.

(24) MORS, W. B., and P. ZALTZMAN. "Sobre o alcaloide da *Banisteria caapi* Spruce e
do *Cabi Paraensise* Ducke." Bol. inst. quim. agr. (Rio de Janeiro) Nº 34 : 17–27,
1954. Chem. Abstr., 49, 14906, 1955.

(25) Quoted by Mors and Zaltzman in reference 24.

(26) RIBEIRO, O., and A. MACHADO. Lophanterine, a new alkaloid. Anais assoc. quím.
Brasil, 5 : 39–42, 1946. Chem. Abstr., 41, 3109, 1947.

(27) BIOCCA, E. C. GALEFFI, E. G. MONTALVO, and G. B. MARINI-BETTOLO. "Sulle sostanze
allucinogene impiegate in Amazonia. Nota I. Osservazioni sul Paricá dei Tukâno
e Tariâna del bacino del Rio Uaupés." Ann. Chim. (Roma), 54 : 1175–1178, 1964.

(28) BERNHAUER, K. "Notiz ueber die Isolierung von Harmin und (+)-1,2,3,4-Tetrahy-
dro-harmin aus einer indianischen Schupfdroge." Helv. Chim. Acta., 47 ; 1075–
1077, 1964.

(29) MARINI-BETTOLO, G. B., F. DELLE MONACHE, and E. BIOCCA. "Sulle sostanze allucinogene impiegate in Amazonia. Nota II. Osservazioni sull'Epená degli Yanoáma
del bacino del Rio Negro e dall'Alto Orinoco." Ann. Chim. (Roma), 54 : 1179–
1186, 1964.

(30) STOWE, B. R. "Occurrence and Metabolism of Simple Indoles in Plants." Prog.
Chem. Org. Nat. Prod., 17 : 248–297, 1959. Saxton, J. E. The Simple Bases. In
R.H.F. Manske, The Alkaloids, Vol. 8 : 1–25. New York, Academic Press, 1965.

(31) BÄCHLI, E., C. VAMVACAS, H. SCHMID, and P. KARRER. "Uber die Alkaloide aus der
Rinde von *Strychnos melinoniana* Baillon." Helv. Chim. Acta, 40 : 1167–1187,
1957.

(32) ANTONACCIO, L. D., and H. BUDZIKIEWICZ. "Harman-3-carbonsäure ein neues Alkaloid aus *Aspidosperma polyneuron.*" Monatsh. Chem., 93 : 962–964, 1962.

(33) SANCHEZ E. and J. COMIN. Unpublished results.

401

(34) ACHENBACH, H., and K. BIEMANN. "Isotuboflavine and Norisotuboflavine. Two new Alkaloids Isolated from *Pleiocarpa mutica*." J. Am. Chem. Soc., 87: 4177–4181, 1965.

(35) BRAUCHLI, P., V. DEULOFEU, H. BUDZIKIEWICZ, and C. DJERASSI. "The Structure of Tubulosine, a Novel Alkaloid from *Pogonopus tubulosus* (DC.) Schumann." J. Am. Chem. Soc., 86: 1895–1896, 1964.

(36) PAKRASHI, S. C. "Indian Medicinal Plants XI. A new Alkaloid from the root bark of *Alangium lamarckii*." Indian J. Chem., 2: 468, 1964.

(37) MONTEIRO, H., H. BUDZIKIEWICZ, C. DJERASSI, R. R. ARDT, and W. H. BAARSCHERS. "Structure of Deoxytubulosine and interconversion with Tubulosine." Chem. Comm., 317–318, 1965.

(38) PARIS, R. R., F. PERCHERON, J. MAINIL, and R. GOUTAREL. "Alcaloïdes du *Leptactina densiflora* Hook." f. Bull. Soc. Chim. France, 780–782, 1957.

(39) NEU, R. "Inhaltssoffe der *Passiflora incarnata*. 3. Mitt." Arzneimittel-Forsch., 6: 94–99, 1956.

(40) LUTOMSKI, L. "Isolation of the major alkaloids from *Passiflora incarnata* L." Biul. Inst. Roślin Leczniczych. 6: 209–219, 1960. Chem. Abstr., 55: 21479, 1961.

(41) HULTIN, E. "Partition coefficients of ether extractable passionflower alkaloids." Acta Chem. Scand., 19: 1431–1434, 1965.

(42) ABDUSALAMOV, B., A. S. SADYKOV, and KH. A. ASLANOV. "Alkaloids and aminoacids of *Calligonum*." Nauchn. Tr. Tashkentsk. Gos. Univ., N° 263: 3–7, 1964. Chem. Abstr., 63: 3314, 1965.

(43) PLATONOVA, T. F., A. D. KUZOVKOV, and P. S. MASSAGETOV. "Alkaloids of Chenopodiaceae: *Anabasis jaxartica* and *Arthrophytum leptocladum*." Zhur. Obshchei Khim., 28: 3128–3131, 1958. Chem. Abstr., 53: 7506, 1959.

(44) BADGER, G. M., and A. F. BEECHAM. "Isolation of Tetrahydroharman from *Petalostyles labicheoides*." Nature (London), 168: 517, 1951.

(45) MENSHIKOV, G. P., E. L. GUREVICH, and G. A. SAMSONOVA. "Alkaloids of *Elaeagnus angustifolia*. Structure of eleagnine." Zhur. Obshchei Khim., 20: 1927–1928, 1950. Chem. Abstr., 45: 2490, 1951.

(46) ORAZKULIEV, I. K., O. S. OSTROSHENKO, and A. S. SADYKOV. "An adsorption method for the separation of alkaloids of *Hammada leptoclada*." Zhur. Prikl. Khim., 37: 1394–1395, 1964. Chem. Abstr., 61: 11014, 1964.

(47) JOHNS, S. R., J. A. LAMBERTON, and A. A. SIOUMIS. "Alkaloids of the Australian Leguminosae VII.N_b-Methyltetrahydroharman from *Acacia complanata*." Australian J. Chem., 19: 1539–1540, 1966.

(48) BORKOWSKI, B. "Chromatographic determination of alkaloids of *Zygophyllum fabago*." Biul. Inst. Roślin Leczniczych. 5: 158–168, 1959. Chem. Abstr., 54: 15844, 1960.

(49) PLATONOVA, T. F., A. D. KUZOVKOV, and P. S. MASSAGETOV. "Alkaloids of plants of the Elaeagnaceae family. Isolation of tetrahydroharmol and *N*-methyl-tetrahydroharmol." Zhur. Obshchei. Khim., 20: 3220–2323, 1956. Chem. Abstr., 51: 8765, 1957.

SESSION VI

AMANITA MUSCARIA (FLY AGARIC)

Daniel H. Efron, *Chairman*

Fly Agaric and Man

R. GORDON WASSON
Botanical Museum of Harvard University
Cambridge, Massachusetts

For the past three or four years I have devoted some of my time to the quest for information about the fly agaric, as this mushroom is called in England, *Amanita muscaria* Fr. as it is known to mycologists, and especially concerning its historic role in the Eurasian cultures, where its use as an inebriant has survived down to recent times. The results of my inquiries have led me to write a book on the subject, which is almost ready for the printer. Today it is my privilege to lay before you some of my findings and conclusions.

My theme has surprising ramifications, as I think you will agree when I have done. Indologists will review my evidence, but if I am right, it will be necessary for us all to make room in our own remote past for the part played by this mushroom, and the fly agaric will take its place by the side of alcohol, hashish, and tobacco as an outstanding inebriant utilized by *Homo sapiens* living in Eurasia.

The documented history of this inebriant goes back only to the 17th century and is confined to the northern reaches of Siberia. That its unwritten history begins earlier is certain, but how much earlier and how widespread its use was, are questions that remain to be answered. So far as I can learn, my inquiries mark the first fumbling effort to arrive at those answers.

The intellectual element in Europe learned for the first time of the fly agaric as an inebriant in 1730, when Philip John von Strahlenberg, a Swedish army officer, published in Stockholm a book written in German on the twelve years he had spent as a prisoner of the Russians in Siberia. This work, translated into English, came out in London in two printings, in 1736 and 1738, under a lengthy title beginning *An Historico-Geographical Description of the North and Eastern Parts of Europe and Asia* (1). Somewhat earlier, in 1658, a Polish prisoner in Siberia had observed the fly agaric being consumed for its inebriating effect by the Ostyak (or Khanty) in the valley of the Irtysh, a tributary of the Ob in western Siberia; but his diary was not published until 1874 (2). The first Russian to record the practice seems to have been Stepan Petrovich Krasheninnikov in 1755 (3), who, like von Strahlenberg, was writing about the Koryak, in the extreme Orient. Since their time more than a score of observers have given us accounts of this curious custom. They have included Russian anthropologists, linguists (many of these Hungarian or Finnish), and a varied assortment of travelers and adventurers, some of whom are remarkably superficial and supercilious. In my forthcoming book I am planning to publish *in extenso*, in English, what these men have had to say about the consumption of the fly agaric in Siberia. In addition to these primary sources, whether good or bad, there are a number of serious writers who have concerned themselves with the problem: the pharmacologists Ernst von Bibra (*4*), C. Hartwich (*5*), and Louis Lewin (*6*)—all German—and the Frenchman Philipe de Félice (*7*), the Swede Åke Ohlmarks (*8*), and the Hungarian J. Balázs (*9*). In addition, there have been innumerable literary allusions traceable to the marvelous properties of the fly agaric. One need only mention as examples, in English, Oliver Goldsmith in his *Letters from a Citizen of the World* (No. 32), an immensely popular book in the 18th century, and the celebrated mushroom in *Alice in Wonderland*.

The Distribution of the Practice

We possess reliable testimony permitting us to say that in recent centuries there have been two foci where the fly agaric has been used as an inebriant.

1. In the Ob Valley, in the extreme west of Siberia, and along the Ob's eastern tributaries until they interlock with the tributaries of the upper Yenisei, and along the upper Yenisei (Map 1). In this region tribes belonging to the Uralic family of languages have been historically dominant, and these are the ones that have been addicted to the fly agaric. Along the Ob and its tributaries dwell the Ostyak and the Vogul, called in the Soviet Union the Khanty and the Mansi, respectively. They are Ugrians, linguistically the nearest of kin to the Hungarians, who together with the Finnic peoples constitute the Finno-Ugrian linguistic group. The Ostyak and Vogul historically have been great consumers of the fly agaric. Their next of linguistic kin, the Hungarians, have no recollection of the practice, but *bolond gomba*, a familiar expression or cliché in the Hungarian language, means "mad mushroom," as when one says to a person behaving foolishly, "Have you eaten of the *bolond gomba?*", and this may well be a linguistic fossil dating from a time when the Magyar people still shared in the eating of the fly agaric. Among the Finnic peoples, as distinct from the Ugrian, none take the fly agaric today. However, it is of the highest interest that T. I. Itkonen, a reliable investigator, has reported that according to a tradition of the reindeer Lapps of Inari, their shamans formerly ate it, and that it had to have seven white spots. This places the practice well within Europe's borders, on the assumption that the Inari Lapps have not migrated to the West since they abandoned the practice. In the upper Yenisei the Selkup (a Samoyed people), called in the West the Ostyak-Samoyed, and in addition the southern-most of the Yurak-Samoyed, until recent times still used the fly agaric as an inebriant. (The peoples speaking Samoyed languages and those speaking Finno-Ugrian languages together constitute the Uralic family.) Their neighbors, the Ket, also have consumed it. The Ket, called in the West the Yenisei Ostyak, speak a language without known affiliation.

2. In the extreme northeast of Siberia there are three tribes—the Chukchi, the Koryak, and the Kamchadal—who have used the fly agaric (Map 2). They are neighbors and linguistically closely inter-related, but their language family, like the Ket, is unrelated to any outside linguistic family. The Yukagir, surviving in tiny communities in the extreme north and to the west of the Chukchi, recall that their forebears made use of the fly agaric. They

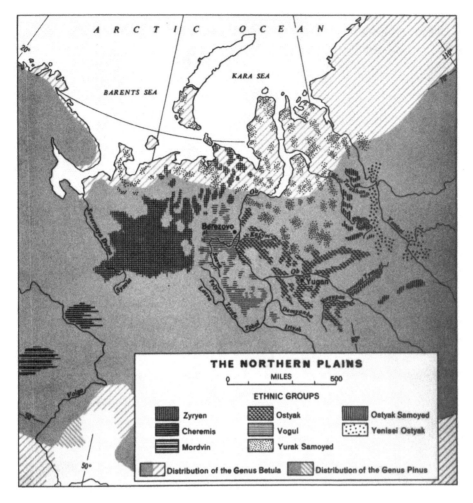

Map 1

also speak an isolated language. It is perhaps worth noting that the Gilyak, and the Ainu in Hokkaido, also peoples linguistically isolated, know nothing of the fly agaric as an inebriant.

The remoter communities of these peoples that I have been discussing did not know alcohol until the Russians or western whalers brought it to them. On a number of occasions the question has been put to individuals, when they have known both alcohol and the fly agaric, as to which they preferred. The answer, so far as it is recorded, was invariably the fly agaric.

What about the vast expanse of territory between the Uralic peoples on the West and the Chukchi group in the Far East (Map 3)? When the Russians arrived on the scene in the 17th century, this intermediate area was already occupied by the numerous Tungus tribes (including the Lamut), and by the Yakut, both of them belonging to the Altaic linguistic family identified with the Manchu, the Mongolian, and the Turkic-Tartar languages. Some western writers who have not visited these peoples have included them among the eaters of the fly agaric, but I can find no eye-witness authority for

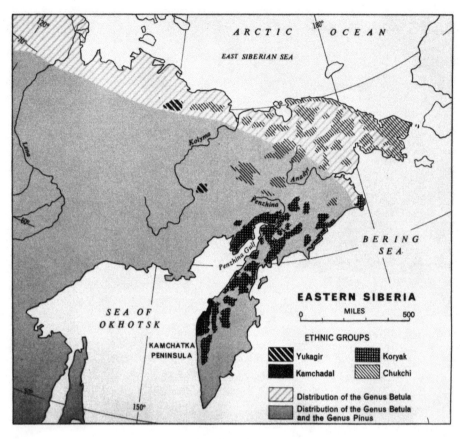

Map 2

this. S. M. Shirokogorov, the authority on the Tungus peoples, never mentions such usage, and Ivan A. Lopatin, also with extensive personal experience, has assured me in a personal communication that their shamans know nothing of the practice.

I think the answer to this question lies in history. The Tungus and Yakut erupted into northern Siberia in historic times. It was they who, forming a wedge, split apart the peoples using the fly agaric. Soviet historians say that the migration of the Tungus people took place at the end of the first millennium A.D., and the invaders came from the steppes far to the south, where the fly agaric does not grow. As they were the conquering people of somewhat superior culture, they were less likely to adopt the practices of those whom they conquered and dislodged.

The Linguistic Evidence

A strange linguistic pattern marks the name used for fly agaric among the Siberian tribes. This word pattern undoubtedly holds the key to cultural secrets, but the key proves difficult to use.

408

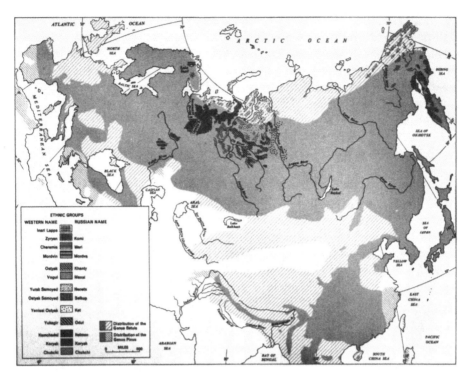

Map 3

The Obugrian peoples—the Ostyak and Vogul—and the Ket share the same work for "fly agaric". In Vogul that word takes the shape of *panx* or *peŋk*. In Ostyak the more northerly settlements say *poŋ;* the Irtysh folk, *pāŋ*. The Ket say *haŋgo*. The Selkup and the Yurak Samoyed use words of their own, except that from one village of the southern Yurak Samoyed *pōŋka* is reported.

Franz Boas (*10*) tells us that the Chukchi form for "mushroom" is *pómpo* (from a stem *poŋ*), to which *pósṇposṇ* corresponds in Koryak. But in these tribes on the Pacific Coast the words in every case is generic for all mushrooms, and the fly agaric is specifically named *wapaq*.

It seems that words derived from a single root circulate in the western and the eastern area of fly agaric addiction, and this lends support to my supposition that in former times (before the intrusion of the Tungus) the Western and Eastern groups were contiguous. We do not know what the Yukagir and the Inari Lapp words for the fly agaric are.

The story of this word cluster does not end here. Two Finnic peoples living in Eastern Europe, the Mordvinians and the Cheremis, known in the Soviet Union as the Mordva and the Mari, make use of this same word as a general term for all mushrooms. The Mordvinians say *paŋga* or *paŋgo*, and the Cheremis say *poŋgo*. But these two peoples do not know the fly agaric as an inebriant.

This word cluster has stimulated some discussion among philologists, chiefly Hungarian and Finnish. Is the root *poŋ* originally Finno-Ugric

409

(Vogul, Ostyak, Mordvinian, Cheremis, etc.) and is its resemblance to the Indo-European word represented by Greek (s)*póngos*, the English (s)*punk*, accidental? Or did the Finno-Ugrians (or some branches of them) borrow the word from Indo-European? If so, they did not borrow it from the Slavs because the wide spread of the word would indicate a much earlier contact between our Siberians and Indo-European, at a time when the Slavs (or Proto-Slavs) had had no contact with the Siberians-to-be.

In 1907 B. Munkácsi, the Hungarian philologist, suggested that the Iranian word *baṅha*, appearing already in the Avesta and meaning hemp, *Cannabis indica*, was the source, since in addition to its use for fibre, it serves as an inebriant, yielding hashish, otherwise known as marijuana or "pot". To me this suggestion seems in the highest degree unlikely. Here we have primitive Siberian communities living from of old in the birch and pine forests that they know intimately, their knowledge embracing of course the fly agaric growing in mycorrhizal relationship with these trees. In each of these languages they must have had a name or several names for this mushroom going back into the mists of time. We are asked to believe that suddenly, discovering the inebriating property of this mushroom, they go to Iran, a country where the birch and pine are not familiar trees, to borrow a name of an utterly different plant, *Cannabis indica*, to gve to the fly agaric.

When specialized mushroom vocabularies grow from within a cultural milieu, the rule is that the specific names precede the generic term. But this rule does not apply when words are borrowed from an outside source. In this case a general term may be borrowed and given a specific meaning, or a specific name may acquire a new application, and the same name may be clothed with different applications in different communities, and may change its application according to the evolving use of the various wild mushroom species in the given cultural milieu.

If the root *poη* was borrowed from an Indo-European people, the loan of the word must have marked a new and significant utilization of a species of mushroom, a use that must have swept across Siberia with the word, perhaps rather quickly. Let us suppose that an Indo-European people making use of the inebriating effect of the fly agaric in their religious life imparted this practice to the Siberian tribes; or perhaps in war-time to help their soldiers screw their courage to the sticking point. This application of a mushroom to a supernatural use or as a secret weapon would surely have been a sufficient reason for them to adopt the Indo-European name of that mushroom.

But in our preoccupation with the inebriating effect of the fly agaric we must not overlook an alternative possibility. The basic fungal sense of the word (s)*póngos*, identical with the Germanic *Schwamm* and the Slavic *gomba*, is "sponge". The generation of fire was of overwhelming importance in the lives of the northern tribes, indeed making life possible in the northern latitudes. Whether by percussion or by friction, the spark that was struck had to be received in inflammable tinder, and the best tinder for this purpose has long been considered *Fomes fomentarius*, a heavy shelf or bracket fungus

410

that grows on many species of trees, but that is generally identified with the birch. When it is dried it is light as a feather and quickly converts a spark into a flame. In archaeological diggings *Fomes fomentarius* has been found next to the stones of fire places in dwellings at Maglemose in Denmark and Star Carr in Yorkshire, these diggings going back almost to the last ice age, some nine or ten thousand years ago. If an Indo-European people introduced to the Siberian tribes the use of this *punk*, or *spunk* (sic), or touchwood (all of these meaning primary tinder), the Indo-European name for it would probably accompany the product wherever it went. That name meant "sponge", and it is striking that the original "sponge" was probably fungal and not marine, the marine sponge being a substitute given us by the Greeks after they had arrived in the Aegean. The preparation of this fungus for its purpose must have been one of the earliest industries of mankind in the northern latitudes—the making of the *amadou* of the French, the *esca* or *yesca* of the Italians and Spaniards, the *Zunderschwamm* of the Germans, the *trut* of the Russians.

Either this or the inebriating property of the fly amanita or a combination of both would have been of sufficient meaning in the lives of the ancestors of the Siberian tribesmen to explain the adoption of the root *(s)pon*, meaning "sponge" or "fungus", into the languages of Siberia. By a startling coincidence, the birch is the primary host for both *Fomes fomentarius* and the fly agaric, and the special place occupied by the tall Siberian birch in the imaginations of the Siberian peoples is certainly due not only to the ethereal beauty of the tree itself, but also to the fact that the fly amanita grows in mycorrhizal relationship with the roots of the birch, and that *Fomes fomentarius* grows from its trunk. It is true that the pine also is host to the fly agaric, but less often than the birch, and it is true that the beech and other trees are hosts to the *Fomes fomentarius*, but it is most commonly found on the birch. The birch is the Tree of Life for the man of the forest or taiga, supplying him with fire for his body and fire for his soul.

Surely I do not need to emphasize the speculative nature of these thoughts. To be dogmatic in terrain such as this is to court disaster. The etymology of words, the sequence of events, where there is so little to go on, is little more than guesswork. But I would have been derelict had I failed to call your attention to the linguistic problem presented by the wide diffusion of the root *pon* among the scattered Siberian tribesmen.

As those of you who are familiar with the writings of Mircea Eliade will perceive, I am forced to part company with him both on the etymology of the peculiar fungal word of the Siberian tribes and on the antiquity of the role of the fly agaric as an inebriant in Siberian shamanism (*11*). What Munkácsi advanced as a bold surmise he has converted into a statement of fact, elaborating on the etymology of *pon* with frightening self-assurance. His view that the use of narcotics to attain ecstasy is recent and only a "vulgar substitute for 'pure' trance" seems to run counter to such evidence as we have. For as far back as our records go, the area where the fly agaric was used by shamans has been shrinking, until its use is now virtually extinct. Consider primitive man groping his way forward, leading a precarious existence, and in his ever urgent quest for food experimenting with every plant and animal and insect and fish: his fund of knowledge and beliefs being derived exclusively from his own experience and from what he learned by word of mouth from his parents and neighbors. He must sooner or later have discovered the properties of the hallucinogenic plants, a discovery made almost certainly before he discovered how to control the processes of fermentation and to make beer or wine or mead. These hallucinogenic plants opened the doors for him to horizons beyond any he had known in his cruel daily existence. They translated him to utterly different planes of existence, where ecstasy reigned. The discovery of these plants must have had an explosive effect on his soul. He would resort to them in moments of soul-hunger. They would suggest to him possibilities sparking his imagination and inventive zeal. Surely this creature, limited in his range of knowledge and living by rules taught him by his own experience, his imagination peopling the world with invisible spirits benevolent and malevolent, would regard the hallucinogenic plants as miraculous gifts of the gods, and in moments of need he would resort to them without hesitation as a channel of communication with the Immortals. Only after having known them and in default of them would he devise ways through disciplined austerity and self-imposed mortification of the flesh to achieve the same result, and later, having attained sophistication in these matters, would he perceive what many regard as the moral superiority of this road to beatitude.

The Hallucinogenic Properties of the Fly Amanita

We do not know nearly enough about the fly agaric as an hallucinogen. But the evidence indicates certain traits to be defined thus:

a. It begins to act in fifteen or twenty minutes and the effects last for hours.

b. First it is a soporific. One goes to sleep for about two hours, and the sleep is not normal. One cannot be roused from it, but is sometimes aware of the sounds round about. In this half-sleep sometimes one has coloured visions that respond, at least to some extent, to one's desires.

c. Some subjects enjoy a feeling of elation that lasts for three or four hours after waking from the sleep. In this stage it is interesting to note that the superiority of this drug over alcohol is particularly emphasized: the fly agaric is not merely better, it belongs to a different and superior order of inebriant, according to those who have enjoyed the experience. During this state the subject is often capable of extraordinary feats of physical effort, and enjoys performing them.

d. A peculiar feature of the fly agaric is that its hallucinogenic properties pass into the urine, and another may drink this urine to enjoy the same effect. Indeed it is said that the urine of three or four successive drinkers may be thus consumed without noticeable loss of inebriating effect. This surprising trait of fly agaric inebriation is unique in the hallucinogenic world, so far as our present knowledge goes.

The soporific and kinetic effects of the fly amanita are utterly unlike anything produced by the mushrooms of the genus Psilocybe of Mexico.

The Indo-Aryans and Soma

An Indo-European people who called themselves Aryans conquered the valley of the Indus in the middle of the second millennium B.C. Their priests deified a plant that they called Soma, which has never been identified: scholars have almost despaired of finding it. The hymns that these priests composed have come down to us intact in the RgVeda, and many of them concern themselves with Soma. Lately there have been a number of fresh translations of the RgVeda, better than any of their predecessors.

This plant, Soma, was an hallucinogen. The juice was extracted from it in the course of the liturgy and forthwith drunk by the priests, who regarded it as a divine inebriant. It could not have been alcoholic, for various reasons; for one thing, fermentation is a slow process which the Vedic priests could not hurry.

I have studied these recent translations and it is apparent, I think, that Soma was the fly agaric. There are many touches in the lyric poems that fit the fly agaric as a glove, and I believe there are none that contradict it. To detail them here today would take too long, and I must ask you to wait for my book for the full dress presentation of my thesis.

If I am right that Soma is the fly agaric, we must revise our judgment about the role of fungi in the cultural history of Eurasia. The RgVeda is the earliest literary monument in the Hindu religion, and behold! it is a paean to the fly agaric! The RgVeda is one of the earliest texts that we possess from the Indo-European world, and behold! it is a paean to the fly agaric! If the Indo-Iranians really used the fly agaric, it means at an early date, before they left their homeland somewhere north of the Caucasus-Caspian-Oxus line, these tribes were consumers of the fly agaric. They or their congeners, fellow Indo-Europeans, may have given the fly amanita cult to the ancestors of the Obugrians of today, and the root $(s)po\eta$ to their languages. If I am right, the adoration of the fly agaric was at a high level of sophistication 3,500 years ago (and who can say how much further back?) among the Indo-Europeans, and we are witnessing in our own generation the final disappearance of a practice that has held the peoples of northern Eurasia enthralled for thousands of years.

REFERENCES

(1) PHILIP JOHN VON STRAHLENBERG: An Historico-Geographical Description of the North and Eastern Part of Europe and Asia, but More Particularly of Russia, Siberia and Great Tartary, Both in Their Ancient and Modern State, Together with an Entire New Polyglot-table of the Dialects of 32 Tartarian Nations, London, 1936. The citation is from p. 397 of the English edition.

(2) ADAM KAMIEŃSKI DLUZYK: "Dyarusz Wiezienia moskiewskego, miast i miejsc" (A diary of Muscovite Captivity, Towns and Settlement), published in Warta, a Collection of Articles, edited by the Rev. A. Maryański, Poznań, 1874, pp. 378–388.

(3) STEPAN PETROVICH KRASHENINNIKOV: "Opisanie zemli Kamchatki" (A Description of Kamchatka), Akademiía Nauk, 1755. New critical edition in 1949.

(4) ERNST VON BIBRA: "Die narkotischen Genussmittel und der Mensch" (Narcotic Substances and Mankind), Nüremberg, 1855, pp. 135–139.

(5) C. HARTWICH: "Die menschlichen Genussmittel: ihre Herkunft, Verbreitung, Geschichte, Anwendung, Bestandteile, und Wirkung" (Human Stimulants: their Origin, Distribution, History, Use, Components, and Effects), Leipzig, 1911, pp. 255–260.

(6) LOUIS LEWIN: This work, written in German and published in 1924, was translated into English and French, and the English edition, Phantastica: Narcotic and Stimulating Drugs, their Use and Abuse, was reprinted in 1964 by Routledge & Kegan Paul, London. The passage about the fly agaric is on pages 123–129 of this edition.

(7) PHILIPPE DE FÉLICE: "Poisons Sacrés Ivresses Divines: Essai sur quelques Formes Inférieures de la Mystique" (Sacred Poisons Divine Inebriations: Essay on Some Inferior Forms of Mysticism), Paris, 1936, pp. 110–113.

(8) ÅKE OHLMARKS: "Studien zum Problem des Schamanismus" (Studies on the Problem of Shamanism), Lund, 1939, pp. 100–125.

(9) J. BALÁZS: "Über die Ekstase des ungarischen Schamanen" (On the Ecstasy of the Hungarian Shamans), in Glaubenswelt und Folklore der Sibirischen Völker, edited by V. Diószegi, Budapest, 1963, pp. 57–83.

(10) FRANZ BOAS: "Handbook of American Indian Languages," Smithsonian Institution, Bureau of American Ethnology, Bulletin 40, Washington, 1922, p. 693.

(11) VIDE, e.g., MIRCEA ELIADE: Shamanism, Archaic Techniques of Ecstasy, Pantheon Books, New York, 1964; originally published in Paris by Librairie Payot in 1951 as Le Chamanisme et les techniques archaïques de l'extase. In the English edition, pp. 400–410; in the French edition, p. 360.

414

Ethnopharmacological Investigation of Some Psychoactive Drugs Used by Siberian and Far-Eastern Minor Nationalties of U.S.S.R.*

I. I. Brekhman and Y. A. Sam

Institute of Biologically Active Substances, Far Eastern Branch,
Siberian Department of the Academy of Sciences, U.S.S.R., Vladivostok, U.S.S.R.

The authors discuss the practice of eating the fly agaric in the extreme east of Siberia, among the Kamchadals, the Koryak, the Chukchi, and the Yukagir. They quote from the writings of Stepan Krasheninnikov, the Russian traveler who first reported in Russian the practice in the 18th century, from G. V. Steller, a junior colleague of Krasheninnikov's, and from the work on the Chukchi of V. G. Bogoras, a Russian anthropologist who wrote in English and whose work was later translated into Russian. According to Krekhman and Sam, the use of the fly agaric was unknown among the Tungus. The fly agaric was used in its natural state, gathered in the spring or summer or less often the fall, and swallowed whole in a slightly desiccated condition; or else by infusion, after soaking for five or six days in water. Sometimes the infusion was taken with *Epilobium angustiforlium* L., the latter being soaked in water and then boiled down into a sweet, thick liquor. Sometimes underproof vodka was added. The mushrooms are personified as little men, one dwarf to a mushroom, and when under its influence one used to speak of these dwarfs as all-powerful. Only men took the fly agaric; it was not used by women.

The Kamchadals made also a wine from a 'sweet herb'—*Heracleum dulce* Fisch., fam. Umbelliferae. It was eaten, like betel nut, in its fresh state, and the effects were similar to alcoholic intoxication. Various other plants were taken for their psychic effect by the Tungus tribes, among them *Ledum palustre* L. and *Ledum hypoleucum* Kam. The dried leaves were laid on a hearth or in a frying pan, and the fumes had a stupefying effect, this serving perhaps as an analgesic for the sick. All these drugs need further study.

---

*Paper submitted but not read at the meeting. We are presenting here only a summary of the paper.

Isolation, Structure and Syntheses of Central-Active Compounds from Amanita Muscaria (L. ex Fr.) Hooker

CONRAD H. EUGSTER

Department of Organic Chemistry, University of Zurich, Zurich, Switzerland

It has been desecribed that the carpophores of Amanita muscaria belong to the class of plant drugs affecting the central nervous system and possibly producing hallucinatory effects (*1*).

Since the classical work of Schmiedeberg and Koppe in 1869, the chemical investigation of these active substances has, until the present day, been almost exclusively concerned with muscarine, whose chemistry is now fully understood (*2*). The pharmacological investigations have shown in fact, that muscarine itself is not the prime cause of the previously mentioned central-activity of A. muscaria. The low plant content (2–3 mg per kg undried fungus), in conjunction with its relatively weak activity on oral consumption, leads to the conclusion that muscarine can only be considered as a minor active component of A. muscaria.

During the last few years it has been proposed that one or another of the bases *bufotenine, atropine, hyoscyamine* and *scopolamine* could be responsible for the main central-activity of A. muscaria (*3*). With regard to these suggestions the following comments can be made. The amounts of these compounds reported to have been isolated (0.1–0.2 mg atropine; 0.4–0.7 mg scopolamine per kg undried carpophores), although not rigorously confirmed, in relation to their known activity, exclude them as possible causes of A. muscaria poisoning. Moreover, other authors have demonstrated that Belladonna alkaloids (atropine, hyoscyamine, scopolamine) do not occur in A. muscaria (*4*). In addition in our hands, investigation of both Swiss and South German varieties of A. muscaria has led to the isolation of several indolic substances, the structures of which have not yet been elucidated. Bufotenine, however, was found not to be present.

Recently the, in contrast to the above-mentioned products, highly active muscimole and ibotenic acid have been isolated from A. muscaria (*5*).

The pharmacological tests (narcosis-potentiation), which were used as an aid in the isolation of these substances, lead us to the conclusion that they are in fact active on the central nervous system. Their structures have been elucidated and several syntheses published (*6*).

Muscimole, $C_4H_6N_2O_2$, mp. 155–156° (from water), 174–175° (from methanol-water), is a very polar and extremely water soluble substance. It is the enol-betaine of 5-aminomethyl-3-hydroxy-isoxazole (formula I), i.e., it is an unsaturated cyclic hydroxamic acid. Muscimol is easily formed by decarboxylation and loss of water from ibotenic acid, $C_5H_8N_2O_5$ mp. 145°

(dec.). The latter is the zwitterion of α-amino-α-[3-hydroxy-isoxazoylyl-(5)]-acetic acid monohydrate (formula II). It is to be considered a principal active constituent of A. muscaria, being present to the extent of 0.3–1 g per kg of undried carpophores.

The pharmacologically less active muscazone (7), $C_5H_6N_2O_4$, mp. 190° (dec.), co-occurs in varying proportions with muscimole and ibotenic acid in A. muscaria. It is also an amino-acid, namely α-amino-α [2(3H)-oxazolonyl-(5)]-acetic acid (formula III), and can be produced in the laboratory by UV-irradiation of ibotenic acid. It is probable that, in the plant also, ibotenic acid acts as a precursor for muscazone. We therefore assume that the widely known variation in toxicity of A. muscaria results from fluctuations in the ibotenic acid-muscazone ratio.

I   II   III

Our latest investigations have shown that A. muscaria produces still further physiologically active substances, the structures of which are not yet known.

REFERENCES

(1) GESSNER, O., Die Gift- und Arzneipflanzen von Mitteleuropa, Winter, Heidelberg 1953; RAMSBOTTOM, J., Mushrooms and Toadstools, Collins, London 1959; WASSON, V. P., and WASSON, R. G., Mushrooms, Russia and History, N.Y. 1957; HEIM, R., Les champignons toxiques et hallucinogènes, Paris, Boubée 1963.

(2) EUGSTER, C. H., "The chemistry of muscarine," in Advances in organic chemistry, Vol. II, Interscience, N.Y. 1960; WILKINSON, S., "The history and chemistry of muscarine," Quarterly reviews of the Chemical Society (London) 15: 153 (1961).

(3) FABING, H. D., and HAWKINS, J. R., Science 123: 886 (1956); TYLER, V. E., Amer. Jour. Pharmacy 130: 264 (1958); LEWIS, B., South African Medical Jour. 29: 262 (1955); MANIKOWSKI, W., and NIEZGODZKI, L., ref. Chem. Abstr. 58: 11703 (1963); TYLER, V. E., Lloydia 24: 71 (1961).

(4) SALEMINK, C. A., TENBROEKE, J. W., SCHULLER, P. L., and VEEN, E., Planta medica 11: 139 (1963); KWASNIEWSKI, V., Süddeutsche Apoth. Zeitung 94: 1177 (1954).

(5) (a) MÜLLER, G. F. R., and EUGSTER, C. H., Helv. Chim. Acta 48: 910 (1965); EUGSTER, C. H., MÜLLER, G. F. R., and GOOD, R., Tetrahedron Letters 1965: 1813; GOOD, R., MÜLLER, G. F. R., and EUGSTER, C. H., Helv. Chim. Acta 48: 927 (1965); MÜLLER, G. F. R., Beiträge zur Kenntnis der Inhaltsstoffe des Fliegenpilzes (Amanita muscaria), Dissertation, Universität Zürich 1961.

(b) TAKEMOTO, T., NAKAJIMA, T., and SAKUMA, R., Yakugaku Zasshi 84: 1233 (1964).

(c) BOWDEN, K., DRYSDALE, A. C., and MOGEY, G. A., Nature, 206, 1359 (1965); Tetrahedron Letters 1965, 727.

(d) EUGSTER, C. H., and TAKEMOTO, T. Zur Nomenklatur der neuen Verbindungen aus Amanita-Arten, Helv, Chim. Acta 50, 726 (1967).

(*6*) Review: Eugster, C. H., Über den Fliegenpilz, Neujahrsblatt Nr. 169 der Natur-
forschenden Gesellschaft in Zürich, Verlag Leemann AG. Zürich, 1967;
    Synthesis of muscimole: Patents to J. R. Geigy AG. Basle (Swiss Priority of
Dec. 6th, 1963, Belg. Pat. No. 656.759 of Dec. 7th, 1964; see Chem. Abstr. 63:
16356 (1965)); Gagneux, A. R., Häfliger, F., Good, R., and Eugster, C. H., Tetrahedron Letters 1965: 2077.
    Synthesis of ibotenic acid: Patents to J. R. Geigy AG. Basle (Swiss Priority
of July 22nd, 1964, Belg. Pat. No. 665.249 of Dec. 10th (1965) :, see Chem. Abstr.
65, 2266 (1966); Gagneux, A. R., Häfliger, F., Meier, R., and Eugster, C. H.,
Tetrahedron Letters 1965: 2081; Sirakawa, K., Aki, O, Tsushima, S., and Ko-
nishi, K., Chem. Pharm. Bull. (Japan) 14: 89 (1966); Kishida, Y., Hiraoka, T.,
Ide, J., Terada, A., and Nakamura, N., Chem. Pharm. Bull. (Japan) 14: 94 (1966).
(*7*) Isolation: see (*5*) (*a*); Structure: Fritz, H., Gagneux, A. R., Zbinden, R., and
Eugster, C. H., Tetrahedron Letters 1965: 2075; Reiner, R., and Eugster, C. H.,
Helv. Chim. Acta 50: 728 (1967); Reiner, R., Dissertation, Universität Zürich
1966; Synthesis: Göth, H., Gagneux, A. R., Eugster, C. H., and Schmid, H., Helv.
Chim. Acta 50: 137 (1967).

The Pharmacology of Amanita Muscaria

PETER G. WASER

Department of Pharmacology, University of Zurich, Zurich, Switzerland

Introduction

Rarely, to-day, are new natural products with an interesting pharmacological action found in Swiss plants. Most alkaloids have been discovered and extensively investigated in the past 50 years. For us remains the search for new active compounds (alkaloids, amines and aminoacids etc.), which are present only in small concentrations, or which show interesting biological properties not yet investigated.

The starting point most often is the centuries-old knowledge of remarkable and unusual actions of a plant or its crude drug form, on man after ingestion. Intoxication after an overdose is the overall response of the organism to the toxic principles in the plant. This reaction is a sum of very different pharmacological actions, and may be very complicated. As plants vary in metabolism and production of active principles corresponding to their environment, comparison of intoxication symptoms will show regional differences. Different varieties of the same species may produce quite different metabolites.

The pharmacologist first has the problem of carefully scrutinizing the symptoms of intoxication, or, if these are already known, the therapeutic use by primitive tribes. He then must try to classify these symptoms as pharmacological actions on different organ systems, following the large knowledge of typical drug-actions. Then he develops a method for screening the active principles to isolate and concentrate these from the extracts, with the help of specific tests. For this part, cooperation with an interested chemist is the most important mutual help. Both have to adjust their extraction and screening methods in order to isolate the active compounds. Very often the pharmacologist works with several independent tests, or a test battery which allows him to differentiate between several active principles. Finally, he has the rewarding task of investigating the actions of new and pure compounds of a plant, which so far were known only in primitive medicine.

The investigation of the pharmacology of amanita muscaria is a typical example of this procedure. It gave us the opportunity to investigate for the first time muscarine in its pure form. Now, the psychoactive principles are getting more of our interest. Already important facts are known and new active principles are discovered, but we feel that more must be found to explain the different astonishing effects of the fly agaric on man. My report therefore is not a final explanation and scientific description of active compounds, but more an account of our present knowledge and experiments under way. Finally, I want to describe our mode of detecting new hallucinogenic principles.

Muscarine

General

Because of its potent pharmacological actions muscarine, the best known alkaloid of amanita muscaria, has been studied by pharmacologists for over 100 years. It was the first drug with a selective action on organs innervated by the autonomic nervous system. The findings of these investigations, however, were uncertain and inaccurate until the isolation and crystallization of muscarine chloride from amanita muscaria (Eugster and Waser, 1954) (Table 1). The first preparations contained large amounts of choline, which is biologically less active, and unstable acetylcholine, which may be found in different mushrooms. These contaminations made standardization inaccurate.

All screening methods used for isolation of muscarine are based on its strong parasympathomimetic activity. Until to-day, muscarinic activity is the most used term for direct peripheral action on cholinergic receptors, situated in different smooth muscles, especially of the gastrointestinal tract and eye, exocrine glands and heart. Nicotinic action is reserved for cholinergic receptors in ganglionic synapses and endplates of skeletal muscle, where nicotine is stimulant and depressant, and where muscarine has only small or no action. Lately, even in the central nervous system these types of muscarinic (cortical neurons, Betz cells), nicotinic (Renshaw cells) and intermediate synapses (thalamic neurons, caudate nucleus), have been demonstrated (McLennan, 1965). Without doubt acetylcholine plays a major role as a chemical neuro-transmittor in the brain.

Screening methods for muscarine

As other investigators (Kögl, Duisberg and Erxleben, 1931) before us, we used the isolated frog heart of Straub, which is very sensitive, (0.003–0.01μg muscarine-chloride) for small amounts of cholinergic drugs, their action be-

TABLE 1.—*Compounds isolated from Amanita muscaria (1966)*

(structure)	Muscarine 0,0002 %
(structure)	Acetylcholine
(structure)	Choline
(structure)	Muscaridine ?
(structure)	Bufotenine ?
(structure)	Ibotenic acid 0,03 - 0,1 %
(structure)	Muscimol
(structure)	Muscazon

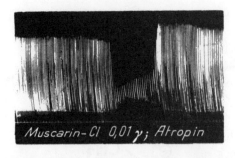

Fɪɢ. 1a.—Isolated frog heart (Straub). Muscarine diminishes amplitude of contraction and slows heart rate. Atropine (10^{-6} m) is an immediate antagonist.

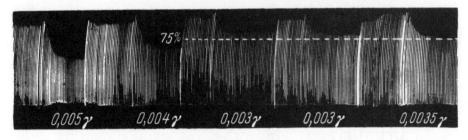

Fɪɢ. 1b.—Quantitative determination of muscarine with isolated frog heart. 25% paralysis is produced by 0.0035 μg muscarine-chloride.

ing immediately antagonised by atropine (Fig. 1). Concentration of muscarine from extracts by chromatography was followed until the final crystallization of pure muscarine-chloride. Biological methods are indispensable for the first isolation of the active principle, but later more specific coloration methods of the paper chromatograms were used.

Less suited for screening purposes are miosis and salivation of mice after intraperitoneal injection of 60–130 μg/kg, and chromodacryorrhoea produced in rats by subcutaneous or intraperitoneal injection of 20–35 μg/kg muscarine-chloride. The diameter of mouse-pupils is normally 0.3–0.4 mm wide, and must be measured with a magnifying device (low power microscope) (Pulewka, 1932). Mydriatic opening of the pupil is much easier to measure than miotic contraction. Furthermore, quantitative determination of salivation, lacrimation or chromodacryorrhoea is quite difficult. It may be accomplished by sucking these fluids from mouth or eye on filter paper and measuring the wet or coloured area (Malone and Robichaud et al., 1961).

Effects on the animal

In addition to the secretory and miotic action on larger animals (rabbit, cat, dog, monkey), a variety of other effects may be seen (Waser, 1961). The cardiovascular system is very sensitive to muscarine. Blood pressure is lowered rapidly by small intravenous doses, (cat: 0.002–1.0 μg/kg) and heart rate is slowed. Cardiac arrest may occur when the action of muscarine is not antagonized by atropine (Fig. 2). Vagotomy does not influence the only peripheral action of muscarine. Respiratory effects are noted with small doses: increase in volume and rate of respiration (0.02–1.0 μg/kg i.v.), probably due to stimulation of the chemoreceptors of the carotid body, is followed by bronchoconstriction and obstruction of the respiratory pathways by profuse secretion of mucus. Again all these effects are antagonized by atropine.

Transmission through ganglionic synapses (superior cervical ganglion) is not changed with high intravenous doses (500 μg/kg) of muscarine, and no neuromuscular block develops in atropinized cats. But with isolated and perfused ganglion preparations, higher concentrations of muscarine evoke postganglionic response, especially when the ganglion has been chronically denervated (Konzett and Waser, 1956).

Effects on isolated organs

The intense action of muscarine on the isolated frog heart has already been mentioned. Most investigations were done on smooth muscle organs for the purpose of comparing its potency with that of acetylcholine. The preparation best suited is the ileum of the guinea pig. Acetylcholine makes an immediate contraction during 15–30 minutes and later spontaneous relaxation

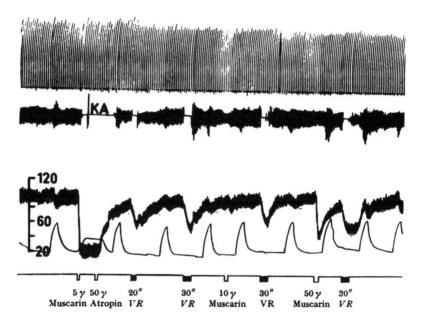

FIG. 2.—Cat in dial-nembutal narcosis. Registered are from top: twitches of m. gastrocnemius stimulated from n.ischiadicus tracheal respiration, blood-pressure in a.carotis, contractions of nictitating membrane stimulated from preganglionic sympathetic nerve. Signal: injected doses and denation of vagal stimulation (VR). Muscarine has no action on endplates in skeletal muscle, stops respiration by bronchoconstriction (KA=artificial respiration), lowers blood pressure and contracts nictitating membrane directly, atropine acts as antagonist.

423

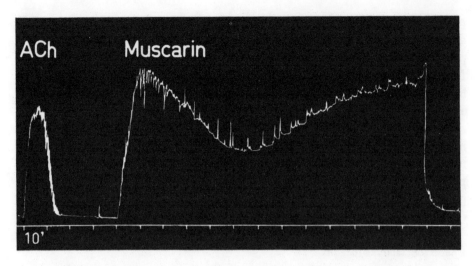

FIG. 3.—Guinea pig ileum. Contraction by acetylcholine (5×10^{-8} m Ach) and muscarine (3×10^{-8} m). Washing after 125 minutes. Slow and persistent contraction by muscarine with little twitches.

of the smooth muscle, by hydrolytic destruction of the molecule by tissue cholinesterases (Fig. 3). Muscarine shows a biphasic action. A rather quick but interrupted contraction is followed within 30 seconds by a slow phase of maximal contraction during 5–10 minutes. The relaxation after washing is at least two times slower than that after acetylcholine. Muscarine is not destroyed by cholinesterases; accordingly its action persists until the drug is removed by washing. Other contractions and twitches may follow.

Similar effects of muscarine on smooth muscle of other organs are found in many different species of animals. The average potency of contraction is much greater than with acetylcholine (Table 2). The isolated sphincter of the iris of pigs contracts with 10 times smaller concentrations of muscarine (10^{-7}m) than with acetylcholine (3.5×10^{-6}m). This explains well the miotic action on the intact animal (Fig. 4). Even high concentrations of muscarine (500 μg/ml) are not able to induce contraction of rectus muscle of the frog, and on nerve-muscle preparations no neuro-muscular block develops, as with curare.

TABLE 2.—*Spasmogenic activity of muscarine in isolated muscles. Average values from different animal species, activity ratio of muscarine to acetylcholine ($=1$)*

Tracheal chain	(guinea pig, rabbit)	150
Bladder wall (longitudinal and circular)	(guinea pig, rabbit, dog, rat, frog, horse, monkey)	46
Ureter	(horse)	29
Intestine (longitudinal and circular of duodenum, ileum, colon)	(frog, mouse, guinea pig, rabbit, dog, cat, horse, monkey)	8, 4
Uterus (longitudinal and circular)	(mouse, guinea pig, rat, horse, dog, rabbit)	4, 5

Central nervous effects of muscarine

Until to-day nobody has been able to show a direct psychotropic action of muscarine on animal or man. This is probably due to its difficulty as a quaternary amine in passing the blood-brain barrier. Passage may be possible in combination with an amino acid or lecithin. The low oral toxicity of d,1-muscarine on mice (200 mg/kg), compared to its intravenous action (0.8 mg/kg), shows that resorption through the intestinal wall probably by a transport system, as with other depolarizing agents, is slow (Lüthi and Waser, 1965 and 1967). An interesting experiment on the monkey showed muscarine to have little effect orally (Fraser, 1957). No effect followed oral administration of 2 mg, despite the fact that the amount given was many times that which causes poisoning by the ingestion of amanita muscaria in the human being.

Gyermek and Unna (1960) attempted to eliminate the peripheral actions of muscarine by blocking the cholinergic receptors with atropine-methyl-bromide 15–20 minutes before the administration of muscarine. By this procedure the intravenous minimal lethal dose of d,1-muscarine was elevated from 1 mg/kg to over 160 mg/kg, but no central effects were recorded.

The electrophoretical local administration of acetylcholine, d,1-muscarine and other cholinomimetics has shown quite different neurones of the central nervous system (pyramidal cells of the cortex, cerebellar and thalamic neurons and Renshaw cells) to possess excitable muscarinic and nicotinic receptors (Curtis et al., 1961, 1964, 1966) (Krnjevic and Phillis, 1963). Cortical cells are extremely sensitive to acetylcholine, muscarone, muscarine and acetyl-β-methylcholine. There may be many other neurons which behave in a similar way, and we have to conclude that muscarine entering the brain will have different central and psychotropic actions. Although *choline* is well absorbed through the intestinal wall, most of it is rapidly metabolised and esterified in the tissue. Generally the action of free choline is similar to

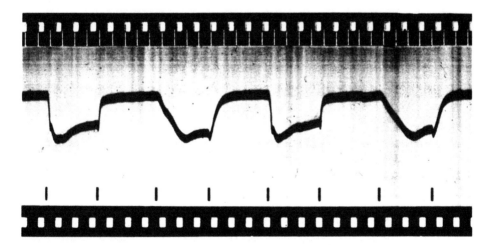

FIG. 4.—Contractions of m.sphincter iridis of pig by acetylcholine ($1:3,5 \times 10^{-6}$ m) and muscarine ($2:10^{-7}$ m). Time in minutes. Slow, gradual contraction by muscarine.

425

acetylcholine, but the dose needed in different experiments is 200–100,000 times higher (Bovet, 1948). Direct electrophoretical application of choline to different neurons in the brain has no effect.

Centrally Acting Compounds

Atropine and tryptophane derivatives

As we have seen, the oral ingestion of muscarine cannot be responsible for the colourful amanita-intoxication of asian people described by travellers touring Siberia. Different explanations were given and additional central active ingredients were proposed. The unknown active principle was unfortunately given the name *Pilzatropin* or *muscaridine* by Kobert in 1891. The search for an atropine-like alkaloid in amanita muscaria has continued since then. Lewis (1955), reported the isolation of hyoscyamine from amanita muscaria and amanita pantherina in South Africa. Later, Polish chemists made a similar statement concerning their local mushrooms. Regardless of the very small concentration found in the mushrooms (<0.0001%), the symptoms of the intoxication do not fit the central effect of 10–30 mg of orally ingested atropine or belladonna-alkaloids, as scopolamine. Profuse salivation and perspiration, nausea, vomiting, bradycardy, mydriasis, are found, together with central excitation and delirious intoxication. Even small doses of atropine with hallucinations would immediately block the peripheral actions of muscarine (salivation, perspiration etc.). It would be prejudicial to treat here the pharmacology of atropine and similar bases before the presence of these alkaloids in the mushroom is demonstrated with certainty by chemical methods. Until now this evidence has not been substantiated or repeated by other research groups.

Another dubious proposal as a psychotropic principle in amanita muscaria is *bufotenine* (Table 1). This amine was isolated in considerable quantities from Amanita mappa, and detected in small amounts by paper chromatography in Amanita muscaria and Amanita pantherina (Wieland et al., 1953). When injected intravenously, bufotenine may have some hallucinogenic activity in man. This is denied by other research groups using oral administration of 50 mg bufotenine and intravenous injections of 20 mg. Eugster and Müller (1961) were not able to find bufotenine in Amanita muscaria.

Finally another quaternary amine, "*muscaridine*", (Table 1) was found in Amanita muscaria (Kögl, Salemink and Schuller, 1960) but chemical data on it are scarce and no pharmacological investigations were made.

Ibotenic acid, muscimol and muscazon

Lately, Eugster and co-workers have isolated and identified different new active substances from amanita muscaria which may—at least partly—explain its psychotropic action. The pharmacological screening of the isolation process was developed by W. Theobald.[1] It is based on the potentiating effect of these compounds on the narcosis produced by a short acting hypnotic (2-methoxy-4-allyl-phenoxyaceticacid-diethylamide), (Müller and Eugster, 1965; Good, Müller and Eugster, 1965). The narcosis potentiating principle of the mushroom consists of three different compounds (table 1). Sedative action of *muscazon* was much less than with *ibotenic acid* and *muscimol*. These two have a very pronounced hypnotic effect, and it is very probable that they also are psycho-active, although nothing definite has been described.

In order to demonstrate this sedative/hypnotic effect, we have injected mice with different doses intraperitoneally, and put them together with controls in activity cages (Fig. 5, 6). Sedative action is evident with 4–8 mg/kg ibotenic acid and 1–2 mg/kg muscimol. Oral administration is approximately half as effective as intraperitoneal injection.

These new compounds are rather toxic for mice. Muscimol is roughly 5–10 times more potent than ibotenic acid. Rats seem to be less sensitive (Table 3).

TABLE 3

		i.p.	p.o.
Toxicity in mice (LD 50)	Ibotenic acid	25 mg/kg	50 mg/kg
	Muscimol	6 mg/kg	12 mg/kg

Typical signs of intoxication develop similarly from both substances: nervousness, excitation, wide open eyes and dilated pupils, convulsions, twitches, tonic cramps, typical signs of catalepsy, irregular often accelerated respiration, later sedation and sleep.

Screening Methods for Hallucinogenic Drugs

In order to search for new active principles, we have to use other screening methods, which should be especially useful for finding compounds with psychotonic activity. The symptoms of intoxication most often show pharmacological effects resulting from the stimulation of central sympathetic structures. We find three methods to be of value for a general screening of numerous fractions of extracts with mice.

The most simple may be to measure the diameter of the mouse pupil during the toxicological assay. We use groups of ten mice per dose. Most hallucinogens, as LSD, Psilocybin, produce a marked dilatation. When the starting diameter with a standardized light source is small, this effect may be measured with ease. Of the new compounds, muscimol is especially effective (Fig. 7). The best way of application is intraperitoneal injection, but for comparision with the intoxication symptoms with the mushroom, oral ingestion may be preferred (Fig 8). Direct application of muscimol (0.5%) on the eye has no dilatory effect.

---

[1] Dr. W. Theobald, J. R. Geigy, A. G. Basel.

Ibotenic acid i.p

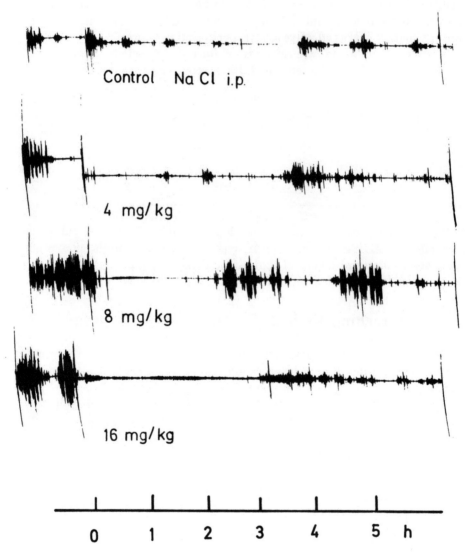

FIG. 5.—Mice in jiggle cage, intraperitoneal injection of ibotenic acid. 8 and 16 mg/kg produce sedation of 2 and 3 hours. In the first phase muscle twitching was recorded.

Muscimol i.p.

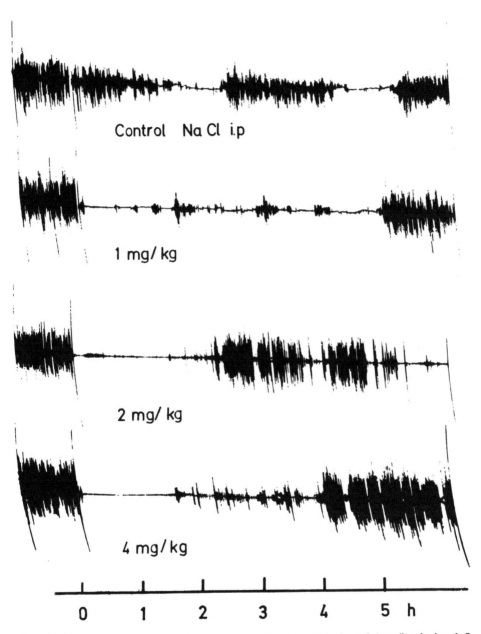

Control   Na Cl i.p

1 mg/ kg

2 mg/ kg

4 mg/kg

| 0 | 1 | 2 | 3 | 4 | 5 h |

FIG. 6.—Muscimol sedates mice in jiggle cage with doses of 1, 2, and 4 mg/kg during 1-2 hours. Myoclonic cramps were recorded.

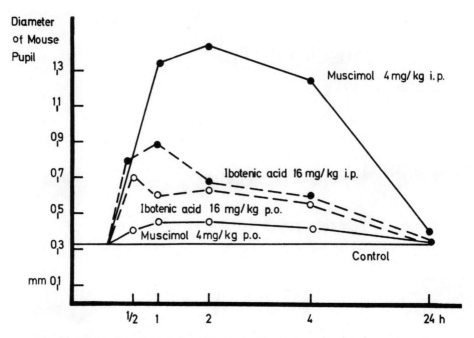

FIG. 7.—Dilatation of pupils by ibotenic acid and muscimol (groups of ten mice, statistical error not marked).

Another method we use is similar to the determination of antidepressant activity of neuro- and thymoleptics. It is based on the antagonism of reserpine-induced hypothermia. Liberation of catecholamines and serotonine in the brain makes mice sensitive to psychostimulating drugs (Askew, 1963). Mice are injected subcutaneously with 2 mg/kg reserpine and kept overnight at room temperature of 20° C. The rectal temperature is measured using a thermo-couple inserted to a depth of 2 cm. Groups of 8 mice are then injected intraperitoneally with the test drug or saline as control. CNS-stimulants (phenmetracine, amphetamine, methamphetamine, cocaine) and hallucinogenic drugs (LSD, Psilocybin), reverse the effect of reserpine and increase the rectal temperature within a few hours to normal values (Fig. 9, 10). The only exception is mescaline; it strongly depresses the temperature. Muscimol has an increasing effect on temperature like other hallucinogens, but only after 2–4 hours, whereas ibotenic acid keeps rectal temperature low (Fig. 11).

A third simple method to test psychotomimetic drugs is checking their effect on food intake. Hunger or appetite are the strongest drives in animal or man. They are easily influenced by central drug action. We have developed over the years different test methods to measure anorexogenic action (Spengler and Waser, 1957, 1959). Rats with a well controlled food intake are trained to a feeding period between 10 a.m. and 4 p.m. One hour before feeding time the test drug is injected intraperitoneally. At 12 a.m. and at the end of the feeding period (4 p.m.), the consumption of food is measured.

430

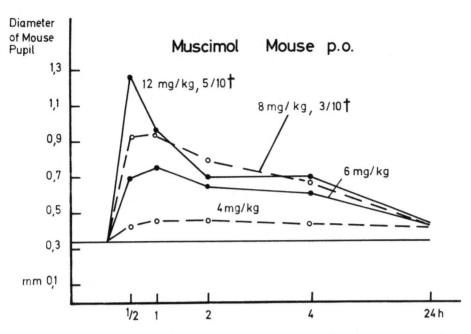

Fig. 8.—Action of muscimol per os on pupils of mice. Strong dilatations with toxic doses.

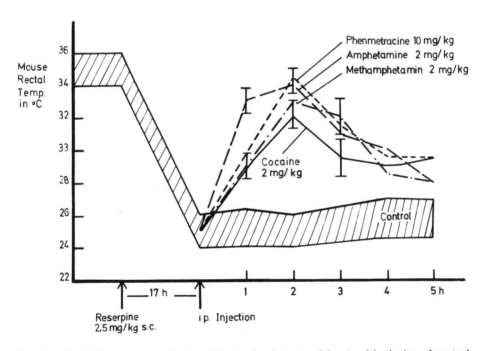

Fig. 9.—Rectal temperature of reserpinized mice (groups of 6 animals). Action of central stimulating drugs compared to control.

431

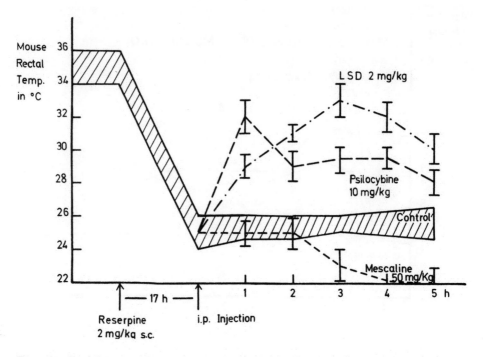

FIG. 10.—Rectal temperature of reserpinized mice under the influence of hallucinogenic drugs.

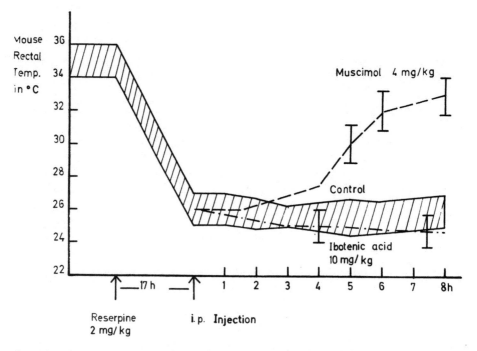

FIG. 11.—Rectal temperature of reserpinized mice under the influence of muscimol and ibotenic acid from Amanita muscaria.

Most sympathomimetics and hallucinogens have a pronounced anorexogenic effect during some hours, probably by stimulating the satiety center in the hypothalamus (Waser and Spengler, 1963) (table 4). Muscimol and ibotenic acid act in a similar way in doses which are not hypnotic. After the experiment the rats may recover during two days with standardized feeding period before the next injections.

TABLE 4.—*Anorexogenic activity of drugs in diminishing normal food intake of rats to one half (ED 50)*

	mg/kg i.p.	Excitation
d-Amphetamine	2, 5	+ +
Ephedrine	17	+
Phenmetrazine	15	+
Methylphenidate	17	+
Scopolamine	0, 8	
Atropine	2, 5	+
Carbachol	1, 0	
Parpanit	35	
Mescaline	90	(+)
LSD	1	(+)
Psilocybin	18	+
Cocaine	30	+
Caffeine	250	+
Ibotenic acid	5, 0	
Muscimol	4, 0	

We have adapted this method to mice for a screening of small amounts of Amanita extracts. Mice are not as clean and trainable as rats, and we have not finally decided on the best technique. Using a special food container from which the fine grain cereal cannot be scattered and which remains tolerably clean, we are able to determine small differences in food intake. On mice the effects of muscimol and ibontenic acid are even stronger than the actions of LSD and amphetamine (Fig. 12, 13). We therefore think this kind of approach to be very promising for the screening of psychotropic compounds.

Central Nervous Effects In Man

Besides the well known descriptions of amanita-intoxication, not much is known about experiments with pure substances on man. Ibotenic acid and muscimol are now under careful investigation by a psychiatrist.[2] The work of the pharmacologist ends at this stage.

Curiosity is one of the main qualities of a scientist, and this may be the reason why a pharmacologist watching the behaviour of his animals under

---

[2] Prof. H. Heimann, Clinique psychiatrique universitaire Lausanne.

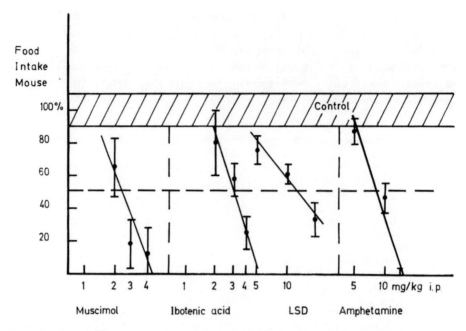

Fig. 12.—Diminished food intake of mice with different psychotropic drugs. Mice are much less sensitive to LSD and amphetamine than rats.

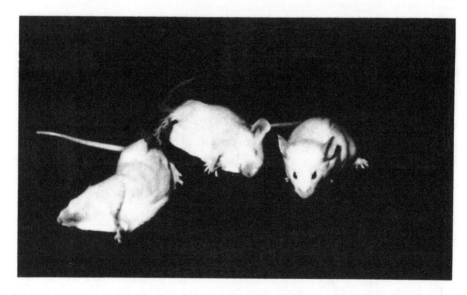

Fig. 13.—Mice two hours after i.p. injection of 5 mg/kg muscimol: different phases of sedation, catatonia, myoclonic cramps, with eyes open or closed.

434

certain drugs wants to know more about the emotions and changes in reaction they produce. Another reason is ethical. We have to foresee the accidents and dangerous actions new compounds of general interest may produce on man. My report on some experiments done on myself by ingesting ibotenic acid and muscimol under careful psychiatric control [3] may give you an unauthoritative view on this.

A 20 mg ibotenic acid dose ingested in water tastes like mushrooms, but produces little immediate action. Within half an hour a warm and slightly flushed face was noticed, without changes in blood pressure or heart rate with no psychic stimulation, but lassitude followed by sleep. One day later a migraine with classical one sided visual disturbance developed for the first time in my life. The occipitally localized headache continued in a milder form for two weeks.

Next I turned to muscimol. A dose of 5 mg in water orally ingested had little effect except a feeling of laziness. Ten mg produced a slight intoxication after 90 minutes with dizziness, ataxia and elevated mood, psychic stimulation (in psychological tests), no hallucinations but slight changes in taste and colour vision. Some myoclonic muscle twitching followed, then sleep with dreams. After two to three hours I felt normal, rested and able to undertake anything, even work. During the next night I slept well, deep and long. No other signs followed.

With 15 mg muscimol administered orally the intoxication started after 40 minutes and was more pronounced. Dizziness made walking with closed eyes impossible, but reflexes were not changed. Speech was sometimes inarticulate and dysarthric. Appetite and taste were diminished. After a phase of stimulation, concentration became more difficult. Vision was altered by endlessly repetitioned echo-pictures of situations a few minutes before. Hearing became noisy and sometimes was followed by echo. Most disturbing were repeated myoclonic cramps of different muscle groups. I felt sometimes as if I had lost my legs, but never had hallucinations as vivid and colourful as with LSD. The pupils remained always the same size. After 2 hours I fell asleep, but I cannot remember any dreams. Two hours later I awoke again and was glad that the muscle twitching was less frequent. I did not feel relaxed and fresh as after 10 mg. muscimol but rather dull and uncertain. Blood pressure was only a little elevated during the psychoactive phase. In preliminary experiments muscimol was detected in the urine by ion exchange separation and thin layer chromatography (C. H. Eugster).

Muscimol makes a toxic psychosis with confusions, dysarthria, disturbance of visual perception, illusions of colour vision, myoclonia, disorientation in situation and time, weariness, fatigue and sleep. Concentration tests show an improved performance with small doses (5 mg), but diminished performance and learning with an increased number of errors with higher doses (10–15 mg).

---

[3] PD Dr. J. Angst, Psychiatrische Universitätsklinik Zürich.

Discussion

Different biologically active principles have been isolated from amanita muscaria. Some, as muscarine, acetylcholine, choline, ibotenic acid, muscimol and muscazon, were found by different scientists, but others were not confirmed by later research.

The action of muscarine is well known today, and it is generally accepted that muscarine is one of the most active parasympathomimetic drugs. This is partly due to its stability, as it is not hydrolized by cholinesterases. On the other hand, muscarine does not inhibit acetyl-cholinesterase in concentrations up to 10^{-4} m. It acts on the same receptors as acetylcholine, but its action is restricted predominantly to peripheral effector organs innervated by the autonomous nervous system. All cholinomimetic effects are antagonized by atropine.

Muscarine affects ganglionic synapses only by much higher doses than acetylcholine. With electrophoretic application on cortical Betz cells, muscarine shows an action 1–4 times as powerful as acetylcholine (Crawford and Curtis, 1966). But as we have seen, muscarine passes only with great difficulty through the intestinal wall, and the oral toxicity is remarkably low. The same must be said for the passage through the blood-brain barrier. Therefore, with the very low concentration of muscarine in the orally ingested mushroom, it is impossible that this alkaloid produces the psychotomimetic symptoms observed in amanita intoxication.

Acetylcholine and choline which are found in small, but varying amounts in the mushroom can as well not be held responsible for this action. Acetylcholine is immediately hydrolyzed by ubiquitous cholinesterases, and choline is practically inactive, especially when applied directly on central neurons.

The central action of amanita muscaria must be caused by the new aminoacids and amines detected in considerably high concentration in the mushroom. The described screening methods show especially for muscimol an intense central action, which is linked with the sympathetic system of the brain stem, as shown by the typical hyperthermic effects of reserpinized mice, central pupillary dilation and anorexia. Furthermore, the pyramidal and extrapyramidal motor systems are probably involved in some of the classical reactions as ataxia, catalepsy, convulsions and muscle twitches. But only with a further analysis may these symptoms be linked to specific sites of action as central ganglionic nuclei or spinal interneurons. The amines are considerably more active than the aminoacids, which are different with other centrally active catecholamines or tryptamines.

The most important finding surely is the psychotic action of muscimol as demonstrated in man. Although intense hallucinations as with LSD were missing with doses of 10–15 mg, there resulted considerable disturbance of psychic functions, such as orientation in situation and time, visual perception, process of thinking, speech, and some new psychic phenomena of illusions and perseveration of optical perception (echo pictures). Here again muscimol was more active than ibotenic acid, which showed only some unpleasant effects on the local circulation.

When we compare now my personal psychotropic experiences with some descriptions of intoxications by amanita muscaria, we see in some respects an interesting parallelism. In the old literature (Donalies and Völz, 1960, Buck, 1963) and during this symposium (Brekhman and Sam, Wasson), the following symptoms were mentioned after ingestion of 1–4 mushrooms: dizziness, nausea, vertigo, somnolence, euphoria, sense of lightness, and coloured visions. Slight acoustic and optic hallucinations were noticed within the next few hours. A higher dose (5–10 mushrooms) produces severe effects of intoxication such as muscular twitching, leading to twitches of limbs; raving drunkenness with agitation and vivid hallucinations. Later, partial paralysis with sleep and dreams follow for many hours. Ingestion of more than 10 mushrooms is usually fatal. The hallucinogenic principle is excreted in the urine. It evokes the same symptoms when the urine is drunk again.

With 15 mg muscimol symptoms of the first group and muscular twitching were noticed. Hallucinations were not as vivid and colourful as expected. The picture would fit best for a dose of 5 mushrooms. As ibotenic acid produces only slight central action, probably muscimol is mainly responsible for these central effects. Further studies will show if muscimol is excreted unchanged and quantitatively in the urine. Other compounds in the mushroom may be responsible for its complex psychotic effect.

Summary

Because of its extraordinary pharmacological activity muscarine, the best known alkaloid of amanita muscaria, has been investigated for more than 100 years by chemists and pharmacologists. It was the first known drug with selective action on the autonomous nervous system. After its isolation in a pure and crystalline form (Eugster and Waser, 1954), its chemical structure and synthesis were established (Reviews by C. H. Eugster, S. Wilkinson). During the isolation process different screening methods were used. They are based on the strong parasympathomimetic activity of muscarine (Review by P. G. Waser, 1961). Until today nobody was able to show a direct psychotropic effect of muscarine on animal or man, probably due to its difficulty in passing the blood-brain barrier. In contrast, muscarine applied directly into the brain was shown to have an excitatory effect.

The active principles responsible for hallucinogenic or sedative symptoms described by different authors are only partly identified. Belladonna-like alkaloids, serotonin and bufotenin have not been extracted from the mushroom with certainty, but possibly there are other hydroxy-indoles present.

Lately Eugster, Theobald and colleagues (1965) discovered muscimol, ibotenic acid and muscazon in different varieties of amanita muscaria. These α-aminoacids and amine have pronounced sedative and hypnotic actions in mice, but little is known on their hallucinogenic activity. Their pharmacology on small animals was investigated with different methods. The temperature of reserpinized mice (2 mg/kg i.p.) is increased with orally 4 mg/kg muscimol as with LSD, psilocybin, amphetamine or cocaine, but not changed with 10 mg/kg ibotenic acid.

The diameter of mouse pupils is enlarged by intraperitoneal injection and oral ingestion of muscimol (4–8 mg/kg) and ibotenic acid (16 mg./kg). Both compounds showed a marked anorexogenic effect on mice (2–3 mg/kg oral) with sedation, hypnosis, muscle twitchings and catalepsy.

Most important is the psychotomimetic effect on man. Muscimol (10–15 mg oral dose) creates a toxic psychosis with confusions, dysarthria, disturbance of visional perception and hearing, illusions of colour vision, muscle twitching and myocloni, disorientation in situation and time, weariness, fatigue and sleep with dreams. Small doses (5 mg) improve performance in concentration tests, but large doses diminish psychic performances and learning. Ibotenic acid and muscazon have less central action. Muscimol is excreted in the urine.

Using different screening methods, we are now looking for other psychoactive principles in amanita muscaria.

REFERENCES

ANDERSEN, P., CURTIS, D. R., "The pharmacology of the synaptic and acetylcholine induced excitation of ventrobasal thalamic neurons." A. physiol, scand., 61: 100–120 (1964).

ASKEW, B. M. "A simple screening procedure for imipramine-like antidepressant agents." Life sciences, 10: 725–730 (1963).

BOVET, D., BOVET-NITTI, F. Médicaments du system nerveux végétatif. S. Karger, Basel, 1948.

BREKHMAN, I. I., SAM, Y. A. "Ethnopharmacological investigation of some psychoactive drugs of siberian and far-eastern minor nationalities of U.S.S.R." Ethnopharmacological Search for Psychoactive Drugs. Proceedings of a Meeting. Ed. Daniel H. Efron. Public Health Service Publication, U.S. Printing Office, 1967.

BUCK, R. W. "Toxicity of Amanita muscaria." J. Amer. Medical Assoc., 185; 663–664 (1963).

CRAWFORD, J. M., CURTIS, D. R. "Pharmacological studies on feline Betz cells." J. Physiol., 186: 121–138 (1966).

CRAWFORD, J. M., CURTIS, D. R., VOORHVEVE, P. E., WILSON, V. J. "Acetylcholine sensitivity of cerebellar neurons in the cat." J. Physiol., 186: 139–165 (1966).

CURTIS, D. R., PHILLIS, J. W., WATKINS, J. C. "Cholinergic and non-cholinergic transmission in the mammalian spinal cord." J. Physiol., 158: 296–323 (1961).

CURTIS, D. R., RYALL, R. W. "The excitation of Renshaw cells by cholinomimetics." Exp. Brain Res., 2: 49–65 (1966).

DONALIES, G., VÖLZ, G. "Ein Selbstmordversuch mit Fliegenpilz" Der Nervenarzt, 31. Jahrgang, Heft 182–185, 1960.

EUGSTER, C. H., WASER, P. G. "Zur Kenntnis des Muscarins." Experientia, 10: 298–300 (1954).

FRASER, P. J. "Pharmacological actions of pure muscarine chloride." Brit. J. Pharmacol., 12: 47–52 (1957).

GOOD, R., MÜLLER, G. F. R., EUGSTER, C. H. Prämuscimol und Muscazon aus Amanita muscaria." Helv. Chim. Acta., 48: 927–930 (1965).

GYERMEK, L., UNNA, U. R. "Spectrum of action of muscarone and its derivatives." J. Pharmacol. exp. Therap., 128: 30–36 (1960).

KOBERT, R. "Ueber Pilzvergiftungen." St. Petersburg med. Wochenschrift, No. 51: 463–466, No. 52: 471–474 (1891).

Kögl, F., Duisberg, H., Erxleben, H. "Untersuchungen über Pilzgifte I: Ueber das Muscarin I." Liebigs Ann., 489: 156–192 (1931).

Kögl, F., Salemink, C. A., Schuller, P. L. "Ueber Muscaridin." Rec. Trav. chim. Pays-Bas, 79: 278–281 (1960).

Konzett, H., Waser, P. G. "Zur ganglionären Wirkung von Muscarin." Helv. physiol. Acta, 14: 202–206 (1956).

Krnjevic, K., Phillis, J. W. "Acetylcholine sensitive cells in the cerebral cortex." J. Physiol., 166: 296–327 (1963).

Krnjevic, K., Phillis, J. W. "Pharmacological properties of acetylcholine sensitive cells in the cerebral cortex." J. Physiol., 166: 328–350 (1963).

Mc Lennan, H. "Synaptic transmission in the central nervous system." Page 399 in Physiological Pharmacology, volume II, Academic Press, New York, 1965.

Lewis, B. "Atropine in mushrooms—therapeutic implications." South African Medical Journal, 29: 262–263 (1955).

Lüthi, U., Waser, P. G. "Verteilung und Metabolismus von ^{14}C-Decamethonium in Katzen." Arch. int. Pharm., 156: 319–347 (1965).

Lüthi, U., Waser, P. G. "Verteilung und Metabolismus von ^{14}C-Carbachol bei atropinisierten Katzen." Arch. int. Pharm., 1967 (in press).

Malone, M. H., Robichaud, R. C. Tyler, V. E. Jr., Brady, L. R. "Bioassay for muscarine activity and its detection in certain inocybe." Lloydia, 24: 204–210 (1961).

Müller, G. F. R., Eugster, C. H. "Muscimol, ein pharmakodynamisch wirksamer Stoff." Helv. Chim. Acta, 48: 901–926 (1965).

Pulewka, P. "Das Auge der weissenMaus als pharmakologisches Testobjekt." Arch. exp. Path. Pharm., 186: 307–318 (1932).

Spengler, J., Waser, P. G. "Ein Apparat zur Messung des Futterverzehrs und zur Registrierung des Fressverhaltens von Ratten." Helv. Physiol. et Pharmacol. Acta, 15: 444–449 (1957).

Spengler, J., Waser, P. G. "Der Einfluss verschiedener Pharmaka auf den Futterkonsum von Albino-Ratten im akuten Versuch." Arch. exp. Path. Pharm., 237: 171–185 (1959).

Waser, P. G. "Chemistry and Pharmacology of muscarine, muscarone and some related compounds." Pharmacol. rev., 13: 465–515 (1961).

Waser, P. G., Spengler, J. "Die pharmakologische Beeinflussung von Hunger und Sättigung." Schweiz. med. W'schrift, 93: 90 (1963).

Wasson, R. G. "Fly agaric and man." Ethnopharmacological Search for Psychoactive Drugs. Proceedings of a Meeting. Ed. Daniel H. Efron. Public Health Service Publication, U.S. Printing Office, 1967.

Wieland, T., Motzel, W., Merz, H. "Ueber das Vorkommen von Bufotenin im gelben Kollenblätterpilz." Liebigs Ann., 581: 10–16 (1953).

439

Discussion [4]

Chairman—DANIEL H. EFRON
Members of the Panel—VENANCIO DEULOFEU
CONRAD H. EUGSTER
CLAUDIO NARANJO
DERMOT TAYLOR
PETER G. WASER
R. GORDON WASSON

DR. KLINE: I would like to start with a philological question for Dr. Wasson: Why is *Amanita muscaria* called Fly Agaric?

MR. WASSON: The origin of the name Aminita Muscaria is a folk word; it goes back in the Germanic world many generations. Mukhamor is the Slavic word, the fly killer, and in Japan one of the names used for this mushroom is Haitori, the fly killer, and that is quite independent of Europe.

This mushroom has weak insecticidal powers. If fresh fly agarics are cut up properly and laid out, flies will suck the juice and succumb in a stupor. They do not die as a rule, and will revive in a matter of hours or a couple of days. This is the current explanation. I think the name can be explained in another way: the association throughout the middle ages and earlier, of madness with the fly. People who were possessed were believed to be infested with flies. This was true throughout northern Eurasia. In Russia, Denmark, Germany, England, the fly spelled insanity. When you were treated, they waited for a fly to emerge from your nostril and you were cured. The mad mushroom, the Bolond gomba of the Hungarians, the Narren Schwamm of the Germans—these were the fly agaric.

DR. EUGSTER: I would like some comments. I agree with Mr. Wasson's view; these flies in Fly Agaric are in my opinion, symbols for the demonic power of Fly Agaric.

The insecticide properties of these compounds (e.g. muscimole and ibotenic acid) are very, very weak, and you have to use starved flies for these tests, so your explanation is the best one, in my opinion, too.

CHAIRMAN DR. EFRON: This question is to Dr. Waser: "How might one treat an intoxication by Amanita Muscaria?"

DR. WASER: The intoxication is not caused only by the small amount of muscarine, and, generally, atropine is of no big value. (Atropine is of big value only if you have an intoxication with *inocybe lateraria* where you have muscarine intoxication). Amanita muscaria creates intoxication of the central nervous system with hallucinogenic principles, and you should probably use chlorpomazine.

---

[4] This discussion covers papers of Sessions V and VI, as well as a general discussion of the entire meeting. In addition to the members of the panel, other members of the Faculty participated in the discussion.

441

CHAIRMAN DR. EFRON: The next question is the following—it is not addressed to anybody: "Is there a pharmacological explanation for the retained activity of Fly Agaric in the urine?" Who would like to answer this question?

DR. WASER: I can only say we do not know yet; we are investigating that Dr. Eugster found a compound in my urine which looks like muscimole, but this has to be confirmed.

CHAIRMAN DR. EFRON: I may speculate on this problem. There is a probability that the active principle of Fly Agaric—I don't want to say which one of the compounds it is—is not enzymatically metabolized. In the same way as we can find penicillin in urine after penicillin has done its job in the body, we may find also the active principle of Fly Agaric in the urine of the user. This is only pure speculation; I don't have any proof.

MR. WASSON: There is one factor: it is possible that some of the objectionable aspects of the raw mushroom, especially the emetic effect, is filtered out when you get it into the urine, and the urine seems to be popular as a beverage.

CHAIRMAN DR. EFRON: This question is for Mr. Wasson: "Would you speculate as to why the use of Fly Agaric has been decreasing during the last two hundred years?"

MR. WASSON: I don't think it is a matter of speculation. The superior and stronger culture of the Russians among Siberian tribes have brought lots of pressure to bear on these tribes to abandon their native ways. This is universal. I think we are just as guilty, if you wish to call it guilty, or we are just as noble, if you wish to call it noble, but the superior culture does not like native ways. In fact, we had a paper submitted to us for this session by Dr. Brekhman of Vladivostok, and he boasted at the end that this thing is being abolished by the beneficent influence of the great Soviet Union, and that is obvious; but before the Soviet Union, it was the Czars.

There is the commercial aspect that Vodka is sold to the natives, and if the natives prefer Fly Amanita, which they go out and gather in the field, they wouldn't drink vodka.

DR. HOLMSTEDT: Dr. Eugster and Dr. Waser, after this magnificent work that you presented, what is it that makes you think there are still other psychoactive principles in the Amanita?

DR. WASER: This is, I should say, only a feeling related to research work underway. Mr. Wasson has told, and we know of other statements, about the very vivid hallucinations; but I did not have this kind of hallucinations that we expected. Surely the dose and the psychoactive state of the volunteer are important—maybe I am a very sober Swiss man! But if you take at the same time maybe alcohol or other plant extracts, which we do not know, you might have a stronger reaction. Do you agree, Mr. Wasson?

MR. WASSON: Five of us took the mushrooms three days running in 1965. Three of us took the mushrooms three days running in 1966. We took it raw, we took it with the juice pressed out, and drank the pure juice. We mixed the juice with milk, we toasted the caps and then mixed the juice with *miso shiru*, the Japanese soup. Only one of us had the right reaction. We all threw up, we all slept then for two hours, but the feeling of elation was con-

442

spicuous in only one of us, and that man was a compulsive speaker for the next three or four hours. He was in a state of bliss beyond compare. He said, "This is nothing like alcohol, it is so superior, it belongs to a different class." He was one of the foremost mycologists of Japan.

DR. WASER: Maybe I should add about muscimole, that it gives me a very interesting feeling with small doses (5–10) mg). I felt just like walking on glass or on ice. The thinking was just like gliding on ice; if I started to think on something I would go like a curling stone without any friction. It was so easy to think about everything; but no distinct hallucinations were experienced.

CHAIRMAN DR. EFRON: Maybe Dr. Eugster would like to add something to this, because I saw his smile before.

DR. EUGSTER: There are some reports in the literature about Amanita Muscaria eating. You remember, Mr. Wasson, it also mentioned that the liquor made of *Epilobium angustifolium* L., an alcoholic drink, is taken simultaneously, and we don't know anything yet about the joint action of alcohol, for instance, and these compounds.

CHAIRMAN DR. EFRON: This question is to Mr. Wasson: "Have you ever seen a picture in Indian Art of a mushroom, or mention of mushroom itself in Indian literature to support your theory that Soma might be Fly Agaric?"

MR. WASSON: There is no mention in Indian literature and there is no picture in the hall of Indian art. Of course, that is perfectly easy to explain; it disappeared before there was any literature, except the RgVeda; it disappeared long before Christ; it disappeared about the time of Buddha, from which epoch we have no statuary, we have no art. Of course, there is mention of a mushroom in Indian history, a famous, famous mushroom. It is in connection with the death of Buddha; he is supposed to have died of mushrooms. The circumstances of Buddha's death are rather baffling, but I don't advance this theory of his death seriously. The oldest of the stupas in India, the ones that survive from the first to the third century before the Christian era, are topped with what the Indians call a 'parasol', a *chattra*. This *chattra* or parasol is the symbol of lay authority in Indian culture, of the rajput caste. Chattra means not only 'parasol' but mushroom, and I was much impressed by the triple-capped mushroom when I saw it surmounting the stupa at Ranchi.

DR. EUGSTER: Please explain ambrosia, your opinion about ambrosia.

MR. WASSON: Of course, it seems to me an insoluble problem. In Sanskrit the same word is *amrita*, and Sanskrit is just as old as Greek; you can say it is even older. Soma is called amrita, time and again in the RgVeda. My own view is that amrita is Soma, and that Soma is a mushroom.

CHAIRMAN DR. EFRON: This question says: "Have kinesthetic flying sensations been noted when taking Amanita Muscaria?"

MR. WASSON: I don't remember any in the literature, any flying sensation. We had no flying sensations, certainly.

The one man who had what would be called a perfect reaction—he wished to exert himself—he shouted at the top of his lungs to a man who was standing three feet from him; and the literature is full of that kind of thing. Of course, the thing behind this is, I suppose, witchcraft, the flying of the witches going to the Sabbat. But in the records of witchcraft, there is no mention of anything resembling mushrooms.

FROM THE FLOOR: Natives took mushrooms and they were flying off in the Yukagi, the Shaman. It is a well known thing in Asia, and you have the Shaman, they go up into the clouds.

MR. WASSON: With mushrooms?

FROM THE FLOOR: Yes.

MR. WASSON: Can you give me the citations?

FROM THE FLOOR: Shaman flying is not associated with mushrooms.

FROM THE FLOOR: They drink mushrooms, and they pass it on in the urine.

FROM THE FLOOR: The experience of your body leaving is very prominent in Muscaria intoxication; the body is separated or called the astro body.

DR. FREEDMAN: There is a recent article in the British Journal of Psychiatry on witchcraft.

DR. KLINE: Barnett has a recent article in which he tells us about the witches' sabbath, but I don't think he mentions mushrooms.

DR. NARANJO: I would like to comment that the experiences with harmaline have been similar, not only to tropical American Shamanism, but to Shamanism as described for Siberia. Siberian Shamans often describe an experience that involves flying and transformation into a vulture, or that of being taken by a big bird, or torn into pieces by a bird of prey, and the persons under the influence of the harmaline either felt transformed into birds of prey or had a very vivid imagery of the same type, which was blended with the motives of the big cats. Another way in which the idea of flying was expressed in harmaline visions is that many of them were scenes viewed from above, as if the person were soaring through space.

MR. WASSON: I find no difference between the flying episodes that have been pointed out and the flying episodes in people who have not taken any drugs, and I eliminated them for that reason.

It seems to be part of the cultural tradition that you fly, not as a part of the cultural tradition that after taking mushrooms you fly. The Tungus fly, too, or am I mistaken?

DR. WASER: I had a question: "You did not mention the use of Amanita Muscaria by the Norse Bersekers that you discussed in your article found in Psychopathology. Have there been any further findings on the use of the mushrooms by this prehistorical group?"

MR. WASSON: I don't remember having discussed it in any article for Psychopathology, but everybody in Scandinavia, almost everybody learned it in school, and it is in the encyclopedias, that Berseker-raging was provoked by Amanita Muscaria. A man named Odman in about 1760 propounded this thesis, after having read von Strahlenberg's book dealing with Siberia. That has led to a great debate pro and con, in Sweden, Norway and Denmark. There is no mention in the sagas of the mushrooms. I think there is no tradition in any remote valley in Norway or Sweden about mushrooms.

The symptoms of the Berseker-ragers do suggest exhilaration and the desire for physical activity that mushrooms would cause, but until we get

444

some positive evidence that the cause was mushrooms, it seems to be hazardous to assume that there were mushrooms.

CHAIRMAN DR. EFRON: Next question: "Is there any evidence of Fly Agaric among the Eskimo or northern Athabaskan peoples? Did it cross the Behring Strait from the Koriak, etc?"

MR. WASSON: I have looked through this literature with great care, and many of the people who are reading the literature have been asked to tip me off for any possible reference to it, and there is none.

CHAIRMAN DR. EFRON: Question: "Could Fly Agaric have been used in Tibetan magic—Bon Culture, 2000 B.C.?"

MR. WASSON: I don't think we have any report of Bon Culture that far back.

CHAIRMAN DR. EFRON: "Has anyone taken the urine and analyzed the chemicals present?"

MR. WASSON: I am ashamed that no one has analyzed the urine, no one has tasted it, except the natives of Siberia. Among the anthropologists there are some who feel they should participate in any native culture they are studying. I have never read of any anthropologist in Siberia who lived up to this idea!

CHAIRMAN DR. EFRON: Question: "Is the drinking of urine of people that used mushrooms considered a better source of the hallucinogen?"

MR. WASSON: There is no comment in the Siberian sources distinguishing the qualities of the urine from the mushroom. Naturally more take the urine, because there is more of it. I have a hunch that the urine would filter out some of the objectionable qualities of the mushroom, and that you might get a pure inebrient in the urine, but that is just a hunch.

CHAIRMAN DR. EFRON: Question: "Why a urine culture in association with "trips?" Does it happen in any other culture?"

MR. WASSON: I don't know, I have never heard of it with LSD.

CHAIRMAN DR. EFRON: I have the last two question for Dr. Naranjo: "Dr. Naranjo spoke of electrical changes in retina with harmaline. Are there similar changes with other hallucinogens,.or does this characterize harmaline only?"

DR. NARANJO: There has been a report of retinal changes of LSD in a cat, and this paper has been debated, and others have tried to reproduce the results, with no success.

What we have studied in Chile thus far is only harmaline, but we are planning to compare these results with those brought about with other substances.

CHAIRMAN DR. EFRON: The other question is: "Could banisteriopis have been used in Tibetan brews of this and later eras? For example, Millerepa, the mystic hermit, spoke of a root brew that was made from vines. It is found in Turkestan?"

DR. NARANJO: I am practically sure that banisteriopsis did not grow in this region. The climate is the absolute opposite. Peganum Harmala does grow in Asia, and probably in the frontiers of Tibet, and I feel attacted to the idea that Soma could be Peganum Harmala because I am impressed with the similarity of the effects of hamaline with presumable effects of Soma. What harmaline produces resembles states of Yogic trance, and involves withdrawal from the environment, instead of the LSD experience of communication and empathy.

MR. WASSON: "When has Peganon last been identified? Not the modern Peganon, but the Greek Peganon?"

That is what some people have talked about as being Soma, the Green Peganon. It is not the modern plant with the same name. There was a plant in antiquity, and if there is any connection with Soma it would have to be the plant called Peganon.

DR. NARANJO: My only information on this is what you told me yourself, which is that Angnetil Duperron, the translator of the Avesta, was the first to propose that Soma was Peganum.

CHAIRMAN DR. EFRON: The last question is for Dr. Wasson, and then we have to go to the general discussion. "Why did you say Fly Agaric mushrooms are better or stronger than *Psilocybe mexicana?*"

DR. WASSON: I did not say they are better, I did not say they are stronger; they are entirely different.

DR. KLINE: In the fifteen or twenty minutes remaining there are some general questions which may point to the direction in which we are going in the future.

One of the things which concerns me as a clinician is that there are certain entities which are untreatable at present. I have a half suspicion that either my colleagues in anthropology or my colleagues in the laboratory have on occasion looked at solutions to my problems but not recognized that they had them in hand, because they don't know what I'm looking for.

I suspect likewise that there are questions which the anthropologists and the laboratory scientists are asking, to which I have the answers. However, I, in turn, don't know that I have these answers.

For instance, in psychiatry, we have no fully satisfactory treatment of patients with obsessive, compulsive behavior. These are individuals who repeat things over and over either in terms of action, thinking or feeling. If those of you observing laboratory animals or peoples in other cultures happen to chance across anything that either produces or seems to rectify this condition, it would be a great boon to us in the clinical field.

I will add one or two other problems, and if anyone can provide a quick solution, we will ask Dr. Holmstedt to arrange for a Nobel Prize.

There are the problems of arteriosclerosis and the diseases of the senium, which constitute slightly more than twenty-five percent of admissions to mental hospitals in the United States. If there are either in laboratory animals or in other cultures some agent or technique which reverses the process or preferably retards or prevents it, we would very much like to know.

Further, in the treatment of certain kinds of mental deficiency, there is now at least some evidence that these may be due to such things as phenyl-pyruvic acid. This would suggest that there are specific proteins or other chemical substances, the presence or absence of which are necessary for the disease to occur. It may well be that there are other disorders of this kind.

CHAIRMAN DR. EFRON: During the three days of this meeting we have found—and we expected this—that there exist some substances for which there is evidence that they are active in the central nervous system, but that they are not used or checked for use in patients. During the meeting we described their activity; sometimes it was a very harsh description or a very broad description, without any particulars or details. We spoke very much about hallucinogens, or hallucinogenic activity. Why? Very simply, because the hallucinogenic activity is the easiest to observe, and even a man not trained in medicine or pharmacology can observe it. So, this was the easiest observation to make by different people going to remote parts of different countries to observe their native culture, customs and medicine. But in reality we are not specifically interested in hallucinogenic activity. This may be only an indication of central activity, and this is our main interest.

For the future we would like very much to gather more information about more compounds used in native medicine and culture, and to find out their mechanism of action. By doing the type of job Dr. Shulgin was doing—changing the molecules by replacing different chemical groups or adding or removing radicals—we could change the pharmacological activity of the compounds. Maybe by this type of chemical manipulation, we could lose also their undesired hallucinogen activity but keep their other central actions, and create new compounds that could be used in the clinic. They may enable us to treat some of the problems Dr. Kline has mentioned.

This would be the point where we would like now to start for the future. But we may think about these compounds not only as drugs, but also as pharmacological tools which will help us to elucidate information as to how the central nervous system is working. We may find also the locus of action of a compound. Some of this type of investigation has been done already by many researchers with other compounds. We now have new beautiful and powerful analytical chemical techniques. I will mention here only Drs. Holmstedt and Horning, who represent the most advanced techniques of the use of gas chromatography connected with mass spectrometry, which permits us to find very minute amounts of compounds either in plants or in brain or in other biological tissues, and chemically characterizes them. We have other pharmacological tracing techniques that can be used for the same purposes. This shows us that we are now equipped for doing the proper job with the compounds spoken about during the meeting.

The time is late. We are in the last moments where we can catch the information about the use of compounds and plants in native cultures. The intrusion of civilization and the changing ways of life destroy both the sources of information about them, as well as the uses of them.

DR. KLINE: Your reference brings up another acute clinical problem, namely that all the antidepressants, although they are a tremendous advance, still average two or three weeks before they act.

We would like to have an antidepressant that works effectively in twenty minutes—we would even wait forty minutes. Perhaps there may be some

447

modification of the drugs described which could do this. The absence of hallucinations would be an advantage, but perhaps their occurrence may be a lead.

Dr. Holmstedt has given a good deal of thought to the matter of why the conference was held, and what he hoped it might do in terms of future investigation; and I think he deserves the credit as the second Godfather in the field, and certainly the Godfather of the modern generation of ethnopharmacology, by reopening the whole area. Would you give us the advantage of your knowledge on this, Dr. Holmstedt?

DR. HOLMSTEDT: We have been working on this conference for four years, I guess, and filled many, many files with correspondence of various kinds. The idea was to bring together, as we have done, people in very many different fields in order to see what this would produce. I think it has been amply proven during this conference that there are problems that should be attacked.

Think of the discrepancies and the opinions of how Kava Kava acts. For example: Think of Dr. Deulofeu's brilliant report of harmaline alkaloids, of which there must be two dozens, of which only three or four have been worked on, and so the idea would be for the future to take advantage of what has been presented here in some way—just exactly how I don't know. That is up to Dr. Efron, I believe—to organize the future in such a way that people in these various fields know about the different advances or, for that matter, about the lack of knowledge that exists.

DR. KLINE: How would you educate anthropologists in terms of going out into the field? Would there be some way, perhaps, of even preparing a field guide for them? Perhaps it should be prepared by a botanist in terms of what should be looked for from the botanical point of view, and perhaps from a clinical point of view.

Professor Ford raised the question as to what to do with it after you get the specimen.

DR. HOLMSTEDT: That is a problem, and I can add to that the following: When we were working with the methoxytryptamines, we approached an eminent specialist in this country, Dr. Axelrod, who knows everything about the methylating enzymes, to find out if the collected plants had these enzymes. Dr. Schultes at this time was going down to one of the places he loves best in the world, a small town called Leticia in Southern Colombia, and Dr. Alexrod prepared a package for him with ampoules and instructions for everything that Dr. Schultes was supposed to do to collect the desired material for enzymological studies. That package, including the radioactive methionine, has disappeared into the interior of South America. It was disastrous, and I think something should be done to prevent such a recurrence in the future.

DR. KLINE: I would like to point out a problem that Dr. Efron raises; with current regulations of the Food and Drug Administration, even if Dr. Schultes had brought it back, he might not have been able to do anything with it in terms of human testing.

448

DR. HOLMSTEDT: That was not the point. Dr. Schultes was going to investigate whether there was a methylating enzyme, and he was going to incubate the radioactive ampoules on the spot.

DR. SCHULTES: These packages were apparently sent through the Embassy and I was not in contact with the Embassy at all.

DR. HOLMSTEDT: It completely disappeared.

CHAIRMAN DR. EFRON: I have already made three contacts about going farther in this field. I spoke with Dr. Ford, and he didn't have to be educated in the field; he knew about all procedures. He only didn't know how to avoid the bureaucracy, and we made arrangements for discussion on how to facilitate the sending of investigational material from abroad to this country.

I have invited Dr. Schultes and Dr. Altschul to Washington to give us more information, because their presentation was a real mine of new information on active compounds in plants.

MR. WEIL: May I suggest that an area of research which seems to have been largely neglected at this conference, and which may be helpful in attaining some of the larger goals, is anthropological research in this country.

For example, take a clue that can be gotten from tribes in San Francisco who use tryptamines. People here smoke DMT; they don't snuff it as we saw in the film. Significantly, they don't have many of the toxic effects we saw. This observation might suggest that the violent intoxication caused by the South American snuff is not primarily due to tryptamines.

If we paid attention to the ways in which many of these compounds are now being used close at hand, (and there is extensive self-experimentation by many persons looking for new effects) we might get important leads which we can follow up in the laboratory.

DR. HOLMSTEDT: You opened up this field. You gave an excellent account of this.

FROM THE FLOOR: There is an incredible amount of information among people who experimented with themselves. They could give their firsthand accounts to some of the scientists.

DR. KLINE: I am volunteering Mr. Weil, who has established his credentials as a reliable non-informer.

FROM THE FLOOR: I am not terribly worried about this question.

DR. KLINE: It would be very useful if those of you who had an interest, from both sides of the fence, were to set up an information bureau of this sort. If Mr. Weil would be agreeable, we will try to protect him so he might well become a center of information. He is interested in the problem and obviously sympatico in discussion of it. Could you have information of this sort directed to him? His address is in the program, or you can send it to any of us and we would forward it to him. Perhaps at the next congress of this sort, which we will start planning immediately—since they take four years on the average to create—he will be able to give much more detailed information than he presently has.

I think he in turn would know where to direct those inquiries which seem to him to have therapeutic or other relevancy. Are you agreeable to this?

MR. WEIL: Very much.

DR. KLINE: He is very much agreeable; we have it for the record.

FROM THE FLOOR: I want to volunteer to be on that thing.

DR. KLINE: He can appoint such assistants as he likes. He should be the responsible individual and be vested with privileged communication.

DR. TREANOR: I am a neurologist, and the neurologists seem to have been left out. I think that a great deal might be accomplished in brain physiology, as Dr. Efron has suggested, if a compilation of the important articles that have appeared be cataloged—those articles that have to do with brain localization and brain function after the use of these drugs—and be given some circulation among Neurologists who would be in a position to think about it and perhaps to give help.

DR. KLINE: I think that is an excellent suggestion. We did neglect the field, but I might point out, as my friend and colleague Dr. Henry Brill has pointed out, sometimes the site of highest concentration is not necessarily the site of action. He proved this once and for all by pointing out that the highest concentration of most ingested drugs is the bladder, and this is usually not the site of action. Thus there is a danger involved in work which assumes that concentration implies activity.

The same is true for digitalis, since the heart is not the site of greatest concentration.

DR. TREANOR: A neurologist would not be restricted to such a narrow concentration. Dr. Harvey Cushing, whose assistant I was at one time some fifty years ago, used to say that he was probably a neurologist and surgery became secondary, but brain function does not entirely depend on drug concentration. When you are concerned with a patient who has a physical-mental disturbance, it is important to know as much as you can about brain function, and we do not have the information that we could have, say, from Dr. Efron's department, which he could give us.

You might say a compilation of those articles that appeared among the two thousand that would lead the way to or indicate the localization within the nervous system.

DR. KLINE: In bureaucratic fashion, we will go back to the Institute of Neurological Diseases.

CHAIRMAN DR. EFRON: Everybody who is really interested in research can go through Index Medicus every month.

To do such a job as is requested would be very costly and time consuming, and we will end again with a big book.

DR. KLINE: The National Library of Medicine is excellent in compiling these articles from the Index Medicus.

DR. TREANOR: It is not only the comprehensive item but looking through this. . . .

DR. LEAKE: I suggest another important source of information. Historically, we have a huge amount of untapped information, especially in the herbals that became so prominent in the 16th century. There is a vast amount of manuscript material which needs the same kind of examination that you have given in the field.

450

CHAIRMAN DR. EFRON : Before closing this session, I think we should thank all the participants for their contribution, and especially the local organizers from the University of California; the Dean, Dr. Seymour Farber, Dr. Roger Wilson and their staff, Mrs. Florence Webster, Mrs. Pat Black and Miss Virginia Barrelier. Their help was invaluable, and contributed to a very large extent to the success of this meeting.

Thank you.

Index

453

Analgesics, 159, 191, 415
Andes, 45, 275, 292, 296, 299, 385
Anesthesia, 134, 137, 178, 180
Anger, 92
Angico, 309
Angiquin, 309
Anguish, 65
Anhalonium, 21, 22
Animals, XV, 82, 106, 134, 157, 160, 176, 177, 207, 228, 377, 385, 425, 430, 433, 437
Anorexia, 436
Anorexogenic, 430, 433, 438
Anterior Nares, 366
Anthropology, 15, 35, 55, 105, 175, 181, 186, 233, 292, 382, 445, 446, 448, 449
Antianxiety Drug, 159, 175
Anticholinergic Activity, 226
Anticonvulsant Activity, 137, 176
Antidepressants, 223, 225, 226, 430, 447
Antidiuretic, 44
Antiepileptic Activity, 106, 176
Antiinflammatory, 137
Antilles, 233, 242, 294, 307
Antimetrazol, 176
Antimissionary Movement, 119
Antiparkinsonian Agents, 226
Antipsychotic Effect, 157
Antipyretic Action, 137
Antireserpine, 226
Antirheumatic, 44
Antiserotonin Activity, 143, 147, 149, 176
Antistrychnine Effect, 155
Anxiety, 77, 84, 92, 141, 186, 198, 227
Aphrodisiac, 191, 308
Apocynaceous Species, 42, 48, 51, 53, 394
Appetite, XV, 108, 430, 435
Arabs, 6, 190, 191, 385
Arawak, 235
Archaeoethnobotany, 34
Archeology, 4, 233, 243, 274, 312
Argentina, 245, 246, 271, 293, 296, 297, 299, 300, 307, 309, 312, 393, 396, 398, 399
Aristotle, 7
Arm, 23, 121
Aroma, 188, 189
Aromatic Chemistry, 188, 191, 204–206, 208–210, 213, 381, 394
Arousal Response, 145, 177, 179, 390, 391
Arrhythmia, 377
Arrow Poisons, 3, 15, 27

Arteriosclerosis, 446
Aryans, 53, 413
Asarone, 228
Asclepias Curupi, 309
Ashes, 300, 304, 319, 336
Asia, 4, 51–53, 170, 193, 195, 444, 445
Aspidosperma Polyneuron, 398
Aspirin, 35, 159
Association, 374
Asthma, 191
Astro Body, 444
Astrology, 60
Astromythology, 27
Astronomical Data, 69
Astrophytum, 38
Asymmetric Carbon Atom, 395
Atacama Region, 246
Ataxia, 121, 122, 134, 145, 149, 174, 435, 436
Athabaskan Peoples, 445
Atropine, 13, 84, 137, 416, 422, 423, 426, 436, 441
Attention, 374
Auditory Hallucinations, 367
Auditory Sensation, 227
Auricle, 377
Australia, 396
Australs, 108
Authority, 92, 93
Automobile, 80
Autonomic Nervous System, 25, 229, 420, 436, 437
Autonomy, 92, 93, 95
Autoradiography, 84
Awareness, 85, 175
Axillae, 157
Ayahuasca, 26, 34, 47–49, 390, 393–396
Aztec Civilization, 43, 59, 62–66, 69, 71, 75, 378
Aztekium, 38

Baccharis Floribunda, 309
Bad Trips, 97
Balkans, 53
Banda Islands, 188, 190
Banisterine, 23, 26, 387, 394
Banisteriopsis, 39, 47, 51, 53, 304, 308, 365, 369, 385, 393, 395–397, 399, 445
Banisteriopsis Caapi, 23, 42, 48, 267, 393, 394, 396, 397
Banisteriopsis Extracts, 387
Banks Islands, 162
Barbiturate Sleep Time, 129
Barbiturates, 80, 135, 176, 177
Barium, 137
Bark, 316–318, 335, 340, 341
Beatniks, 193

Behavior XV, 82–86, 88, 92, 95, 99, 152, 226, 375, 433
Belladonna Alkaloids, 416, 426, 437
Belligerence, 26
Bemused Enlightenment, 97
Benzocaine, 137
Benzodiazepines, 176
Beri Beri, 302
Bering Strait, 445
Beringer, 23
Berlin, 13
Berseker Ragers, 444
Beta-Carbolines, 341, 365, 387, 388, 394, 395, 397, 399
Beta Wave, 390
Betel, 52, 162, 170, 179, 193, 415
Betz Cells, 420
Bibra, 9
Bilateral Vagotomy, 137
Bilca Tauri, 310
Biochemical Lesions, 8
Biogenic Amines, 363
Biological Regularity, 77
Birch, 411
Birth Control, 121
Blocking Moiety, 160
Blood-Brain Barrier, 228, 370, 377, 379, 380, 381, 425, 436, 437
Blood Pressure, 121, 137, 156, 227, 369, 375, 422, 435
Blood Stream, 304, 366
Bloodletting, 311
Body, XV, XX, 192
Bohuti, 238
Boletus, 53
Bolivia, 34, 39, 44, 293, 296, 299, 307–309, 313, 393
Bon Culture, 445
Bone, 64, 237, 267, 268, 270
Borrachera, 44
Botany, XIX, 19, 55, 63, 69, 71, 179, 186, 188, 291, 292, 299, 302, 303, 339, 365, 382, 393, 394, 397, 448
Bradycardia, 23, 137, 426
Bradykinin, 137, 148
Brain, 25, 28, 84, 86, 99, 144, 148, 160, 291, 366, 375, 377, 380, 381, 387, 420, 425, 426, 430, 437, 447
Brain Acetylcholine, 84
Brain Chemistry, XX, 82
Brain Cortex, 390, 391
Brain Function, 187, 450
Brain Homogenates, 219
Brain Localization, 450
Brain Mechanisms, 82
Brain Monoamines, 84
Brain Physiology, 450

Brain Serotonin, 84, 144
Brain Stem, 436
Brain Syndrome, 194
Brain Wave Activity, 179
Brazil, 34, 41, 44, 46, 48, 235, 271, 293, 297, 299, 301, 302, 304, 307, 309, 315, 393, 396–398
Bretonneau, 4
British Administrative People, 176
British Commerce, 191
British Guiana, 299
British Missionaries, 176
Bronchoconstriction, 423
Brunfelsia, 44, 45
Brunfelsia Hopeana, 44, 268
Brunfelsine, 44
Bufontenine, 339, 341, 364, 369, 374, 377, 379, 416, 426, 437
Bureaucracy, 449
Butadienyl, 129
Butylene, 129
Buzzing Sounds, 389

C6 Substitutions, 128, 133
Caapi, 26, 34, 42, 47–49, 51, 265, 309, 390, 393
Caapi Intoxication, 48
Caapi Pinima, 48
Cabi Paraensis, 396
Cactus, 21
Caesalpinia Tinctoria, 310
Caffeine Stimulant, 46
Calliandra Calothyrsis, 309
Calmecac, 68
Camphor, 206
Cannabis, 52, 83, 85, 195, 199, 200, 368
Cannabis Indica, 410
Cannabis Sativa, 52
Capsicum, 41, 107
Carbolines, 388
Carbonyl Group, 244
Carbuncles, 84
Carcinoid Flush, 377
Cardiac Arrest, 422
Cardiovascular System, 137, 192, 228, 377, 422
Cargo Cult, 119, 120, 175
Caribbean, 189, 203, 295, 396
Caroline Islands, 108, 162
Carotid Body, 423
Carpophores, 416, 417
Carrageenin, 137
Cassava, 266
Cassinopsis Ilicifolia, 399
Catalepsy, 427, 436, 438
Catechol Derivatives, 84
Catecholamines, 216, 430, 436

Scopolamine, 13, 26, 416, 426
Scopoletine, 44
Screening, 129, 131, 419, 420, 422, 426, 427, 433, 436–438
Sculpture, 69, 237, 275, 277
Search for Synthesis, 92, 374
Sebil, 269, 313
Sedation, 13, 87, 141, 156, 157, 177, 179, 191, 216, 427, 437, 438
Seeds, XIX, 42, 53, 188, 242, 265–268, 270, 304, 307, 308, 310, 312, 339–341, 374, 385
Self, 91, 92
Self-Awareness, XVI, XVII, 78, 93, 98
Self-Experiments, 13, 22, 26, 80, 304, 437, 449
Self Help Groups, XVII, 78, 93, 96
Senium, 446
Sensation, XV, 172, 178
Sensitivity, 199, 302, 427, 430
Sensory Function, 65, 86, 121
Septal Area, 142, 144, 149
Serotonin, XIX, 137, 143, 144, 147, 149, 153, 363, 370, 376, 377, 385, 430, 437
Set and Setting, 379
Sexual Behavior, 121
Shamanism, 59, 66, 265, 370, 390, 411, 444
Siberia, 54, 66, 405, 406, 408, 410, 411, 415, 426, 442, 444, 445
Side Effects, XVI, 15, 23, 98, 105, 160, 194, 195, 200, 226, 378
Singing, 329, 330
Situation, 435, 436, 438
Skeletal Muscles, 149, 177
Skin, 106, 107, 156–158, 160, 164, 177, 381
Sleep, 7, 13, 22, 105, 108, 122, 128, 131, 157, 177, 178, 302, 427, 435, 437, 438, 442
Smoking, 52, 225, 253, 292, 295, 309, 449
Smooth Muscle, 423, 424
Snake Bite, 44, 309
Sneezing, 291
Snuff, 193, 195, 235, 237, 242, 244, 245, 253, 262, 265–271, 275, 279, 283, 291–293, 295–297, 299–304, 307, 309, 311, 312, 315–319, 327, 328, 331, 334–336, 339–341, 363, 365, 367–369, 374, 378, 379, 382, 396, 397, 449
Snuffing Ceremonies, 235, 243, 262, 265, 266, 271, 273, 274, 291, 292, 294, 296, 304, 316

Snuffing Paraphernalia, 235–237, 246, 253, 255, 256, 261, 266, 267, 271, 275–277, 280, 282, 283, 304
Sociocultural Background, 59, 77, 78, 80, 105, 110, 170, 172
Solisia, 38
Solubility, 133, 160, 370, 377
Soma, 53, 54, 413, 443, 445, 446
Somatic Symptoms, 23, 186, 368, 369
Somnolence, 122, 437
Sophora Secundiflora, 42
Soporific, 177, 191, 412, 413
Sorcery, 64–66, 117
South Africa, 52, 426
South America, 9, 34, 51, 170, 233, 242–244, 256, 262, 265, 273, 291–293, 296, 299, 300, 302-305, 339, 341, 363, 365, 370, 381, 385, 390, 393, 396, 449
South Pacific, 105, 106, 126, 141, 170, 171
Spain, 292, 385
Spaniards, 62, 233, 295, 312
Specificity, 132, 177, 446
Specimens, 69, 71, 304, 448
Spectator Ego, 87, 90
Spectrophotofluorometry, 363, 382
Speech, 23, 435, 436
Spices, 185, 186, 188–191, 193, 195, 211, 385
Spinal Cord, 135, 177, 436
Spindle Bursts, 390, 391
"Sponge," 410, 411
Stability, 117, 436
Staggering, 199, 365
Sternutation, 291
Steroids, 82
Stimulants, 10, 21, 40, 41, 156, 185, 192, 216, 221, 291, 308, 389, 391, 420, 435
Strophanthine, 27
Structure, 84, 92, 127, 160, 363, 374, 416
Structure Activity Relationship, 131, 185, 225, 228
Strychnine, 27, 128, 129, 135, 155, 158, 160
Strychnos Melinoniana, 397
Students, 193, 195
Stupor, 191, 194, 215, 242, 415, 441
Subarachnoidal Cavity, 367
Subcortical Areas, 177
Subfractions, 143, 144, 147, 149, 215, 220, 221
Subjective Experience, 81, 156, 223, 388
Substitution Isomers, 126, 129, 211, 224, 228, 370

U.S. GOVERNMENT PRINTING OFFICE : 1967 O—262-016

also from SYNERGETIC PRESS

VINE OF THE SOUL:
MEDICINE MEN, THEIR PLANTS AND RITUALS
IN THE COLOMBIAN AMAZONIA
by Richard Evans Schultes and Robert F. Raffauf
Foreword by Sir Ghillean Prance
Preface by Wade Davis

CHANGING OUR MINDS:
PSYCHEDELIC SACRAMENTS AND THE NEW PSYCHOTHERAPY
by Don Lattin

AYAHUASCA READER:
ENCOUNTERS WITH THE AMAZON'S SACRED VINE
(New Expanded Edition) Edited by Luis Eduardo Luna and Steven F. White

ZIG ZAG ZEN: BUDDHISM AND PSYCHEDELICS
(New Expanded Edition)
by Allan Badiner and Alex Grey
Foreword by Stephen Batchelor, Preface by Huston Smith

MYSTIC CHEMIST:
THE LIFE OF ALBERT HOFMANN AND HIS DISCOVERY OF LSD
by Dieter Hagenbach and Lucius Werthmüller
Foreword by Stanislav Grof

BIRTH OF A PSYCHEDELIC CULTURE:
CONVERSATIONS ABOUT LEARY, THE HARVARD EXPERIMENTS,
MILLBROOK AND THE SIXTIES
by Ram Dass and Ralph Metzner with Gary Bravo
Foreword by John Perry Barlow

WHAT HAS NATURE EVER DONE FOR US?:
HOW MONEY REALLY DOES GROW ON TREES
by Tony Juniper
Foreword by HRH Prince Charles

Synergetic Press is pleased to print this book with Bang Printing, a green initiative company, which is FSC, SFI, and PEFC certified. Bang works with publishers, printers, paper manufacturers and others in the book industry to minimize social and environmental impacts, including on endangered forests, climate change, and communities where paper fiber is sourced. This book is printed on paper certified by the Sustainable Forestry Initiative.
www.sfiprogram.org

Find us at www.synergeticpress.com

Published in association with the HEFFTER RESEARCH INSTITUTE.
For more information on their ground-breaking medical research with psychedelics,
visit heffter.org.

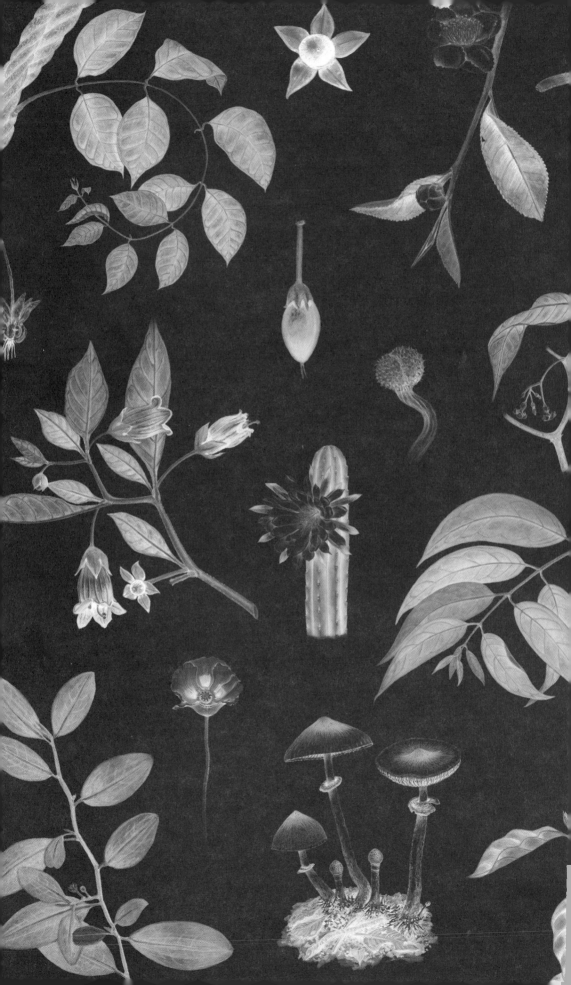

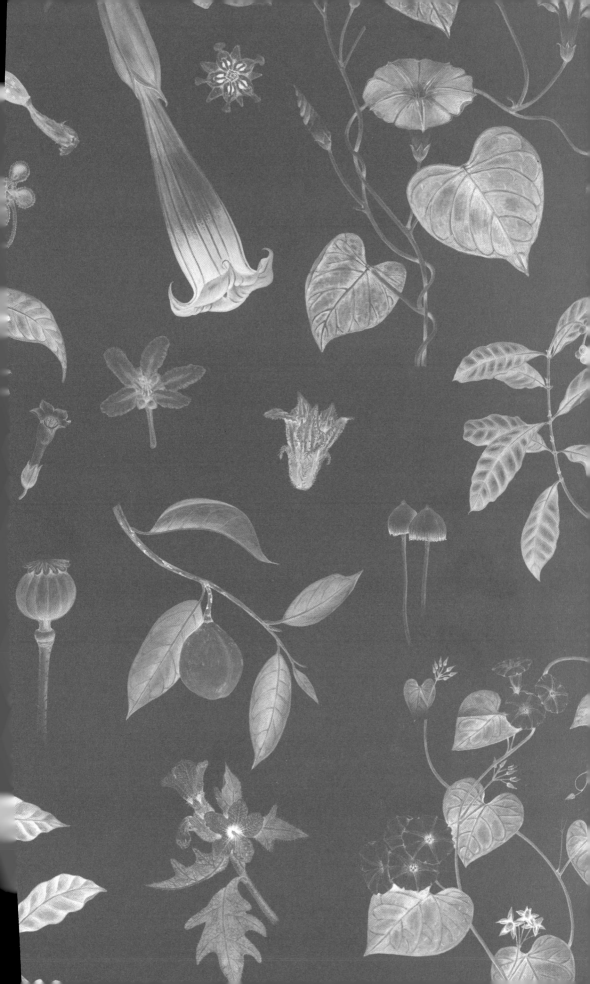

ETHNOPHARMACOLOGIC SEARCH
for PSYCHOACTIVE DRUGS · 2017

50th Anniversary Symposium › June 6 – 8, 2017
ESPD50.com

Vol. II

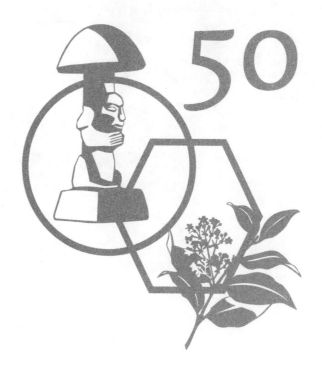

ETHNOPHARMACOLOGIC SEARCH
for PSYCHOACTIVE DRUGS · 2017

50th Anniversary Symposium › June 6 – 8, 2017
ESPD50.com

Vol. II

EDITOR IN CHIEF

Sir Ghillean Prance
[FRS, FLS, FRSB]
Director (ret.), Royal Botanic Gardens, Kew

MANAGING EDITOR

Dennis J. McKenna
[PhD, FLS]
Director of Ethnopharmacology
Heffter Research Institute

ASSOCIATE EDITORS

Benjamin De Loenen
[MA]
Founder & Executive Director
ICEERS (International Center for
Ethnobotanical Education, Research and Service)

Wade Davis,
[PhD, O.C.]
Professor of Anthropology and BC Leadership Chair
in Cultures and Ecosystems at Risk, University of British Columbia
Formerly Explorer in Residence, National Geographic Society

PUBLISHED BY
SYNERGETIC PRESS
Santa Fe | London

In association with the
HEFFTER RESEARCH INSTITUTE

Published by Synergetic Press, Ltd.
1 Bluebird Court, Santa Fe, NM 87508
24 Old Gloucester St. London, WC1N 3AL, England

Library of Congress Cataloging-in-Publication Data

Names: ESPD Symposium (2017 : Buckinghamshire, England), author. | Prance, Ghillean T., 1937- editor. | McKenna, Dennis J., 1950- editor. | Loenen, Benjamin de, editor. | Davis, Wade, editor. | Heffter Research Institute, issuing body.
Title: Ethnopharmacologic search for psychoactive drugs : 50th anniversary symposium, June 6- 8, 2017. Vol. II, 2017 / editor in chief, Sir Ghillean Prance; managing editor, Dennis J. McKenna ; associate editors, Benjamin De Loenen, E. Wade Davis (PhD, O.C.); book design and typesetting by Hugo Amadeu; Botanical illustrations on box set case and end sheets by Donna Torres.
Description: Santa Fe : Synergetic Press, in association with Heffter Research Institute, [2018] | Includes bibliographical references and index.
Identifiers: LCCN 2018003553 (print) | LCCN 2018002719 (ebook) | ISBN 9780907791720 (pbk. : alk. paper) | ISBN 9780907791683 (box set with reprint of vol. I : alk. paper) | ISBN 9780907791690 (ebook) | ISBN 9780907791690
Subjects: | MESH: Psychotropic Drugs | Ethnopharmacology | Congresses
Classification: LCC RM315 (ebook) | LCC RM315 (print) | NLM QV 77.2 | DDC 615.7/88--dc23

LC record available at https://lccn.loc.gov/2018003553

Book design and typesetting by Hugo Amadeu Santos
Botanical illustrations on box set case and end sheets © Donna Torres

Printed by Bang Printing, USA
This book was printed on SFI Certified #60 Offset
Typeface: Dolly Pro, Underware

DEDICATION

The 2017 ESPD 50th Anniversary Symposium and The Symposium Proceedings are respectfully dedicated to Dr. Stephen Szára, MD DSc.

For his many contributions to Psychopharmacology and to the early days of NIMH and NIDA. His pioneering and courageous investigations definitively established for the first time the psychedelic properties of DMT (N,N-dimethyl-tryptamine) in humans

We would also like to recognize and honor some other pioneers of Ethno-pharmacology, who presented at the 1967 ESPD conference, for their dedication to the science and the inspiration they provided for a younger generation.

Richard Evans Schultes (1915-2001) Harvard Botanical Museum	**S. Henry Wassén** (1908-1996) Gothenburg Ethnographic Museum
Bo Holmstedt (1918-2002) Karolinska Institute, Stockholm	**R. Gordon Wasson** (1898-1986) Harvard Botanical Museum
Siri von Reis Altschul (b. 1931) Harvard University	**Andrew T. Weil** (b. 1942) University of Arizona College of Medicine
John W. Daley (1933-2008) National Institutes of Health	**Daniel H. Efron** (1913-1972) National Institute of Mental Health
Daniel X. Freedman (1921-1993) University of Chicago	**Claudio Naranjo** (b. 1932) Escuela de Medicina Universidad de Chile
Nathan S. Kline (1916-1983) Rockland Research Institute	**Alexander T. Shulgin** (1925-2014) University of California
Evan C. Horning (1916-1993) Baylor University College of Medicine	**Harris Isbell** (1910-1994) University of Kentucky Medical Center

Proceedings of a commemorative Symposium held at Tyringham Hall, Buckinghamshire, UK, in the spirit of, and in honor of, the first ESPD Symposium which took place at the San Francisco Medical Center, University of California, on January 28-30, 1967.

The original 1967 Symposium was produced under the auspices of the program in Continuing Education in Medicine and Health Sciences of the San Francisco Medical Center, sponsored by:
Pharmacology Section, Psychopharmacology Research Branch
National Institute of Mental Health
Public Health Service Publication #1645
U. S. Department of Health, Education, and Welfare

This Anniversary Symposium and the 2017 Symposium Proceedings are an affirmation of our belief that many significant discoveries in this field took place in the five decades since the first ESPD symposium; and that the future holds great promise for many more to come.

ACKNOWLEDGEMENTS

The 2017 ESPD Symposium and the Symposium Proceedings could not have been done without the generous support of our sponsors and donors. Additionally, the Symposium and the Proceedings reflect the hard work and dedication of many volunteers and support staff.

INDIVIDUAL DONORS	INSTITUTIONAL SPONSORS
Anton Bilton	**Tyringham Initiative** tyringhaminitiative.com
Robert Barnhart	**Institute of Ecotechnics** ecotechnics.edu
Cody Swift	**RiverStyx Foundation** riverstyxfoundation.org
Betsy Gordon	**Heffter Research Institute** Heffter.org
Jerry & Linda Patchen	**MAPS** MAPS.org
Giancarlo Canavanesio	**Beckley Foundation** beckleyfoundation.org
Carey & Claudia Turnbull	**International Center for Ethnobotanical Education, Research & Service** ICEERS.org
David Petrou	**Erowid** www.erowid.org

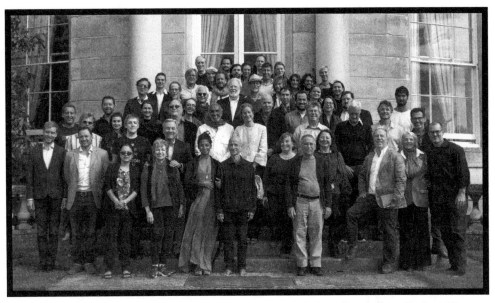

ABOVE: Conference Speakers, Organizers and Participants at Tyringham Hall, Buckinghamshire

ESPD50 Symposium and publication would not have been possible without our amazing team:

Rory Spowers
Tyringham Hall Logistics

Max Baring
Tyringham Video Production

Annette Badenhorst
Conference Coproducer, Communications and Coordination

Jeronimo Mazarrasa
Communication Support

**Mike Margolis
& Brian Normand**
[Psymposium.org] – ESPD Facebook page, webstream livecast

**Mitch Schultz
& Steve McDonald**
[AADII.org, DMT: The Spirit Molecule Facebook Page] – Video production, website support, ebook design and promotion

Deborah Parrish Snyder
Publisher, Synergetic Press; Director, Institute of Ecotechnics; Production Manager – ESPD50 Symposium Volume

Hugo Amadeus Santos
Layout Editor – ESPD50 layout and book design

**Caitlin McKenna
& Frank Cernik**
Scoria Press – developmental and copy editing

**Estaban Gonzalez
& Georges Chaulet**
ESPD50 logo design, ESPD50.com website

Linda Sperling
Editorial Support

Jasmine Virdi & Ivan Veller
Proofreading

Donna Torres
Botanical artwork on cover

OUR THANKS

To the chefs, housekeeping, and hospitality staff of Tyringham Hall – for keeping us well-fed, comfortably housed, and well-lubricated from beginning to end of the conference.

To the many people who placed pre-orders for the ESPD50 Symposium Volume, many thanks! Your faith in our vision has helped to make this publication possible.

To the 50,000 to 60,000 people who followed our conference on the Facebook Live Stream (at least occasionally), you have helped make "Ethnopharmacology" a household word.

To all members of the psychedelic community and beyond, who recognize the power of plant medicines, and believe in the importance of their scientific investigation, and in the preservation of traditional knowledge.

ESPD50 2017
SYMPOSIUM SPEAKERS

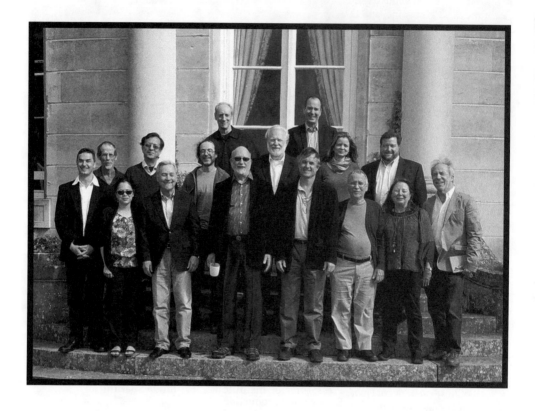

FRONT ROW, L TO R:
Jean-Francois Sobiecki; Dr. Jeanmaire Molina; Jerry D. Patchen;
Dr. Dennis McKenna; Dr. Glenn Shepard; Dr. Manuel Torres;
Dr. Stacey Schaefer; Dr. Mark Plotkin

SECOND ROW, L TO R:
Keeper Trout; Dr. Luis Eduardo Luna; Snu Voogelbriender; Dr. David Nichols;
Dr. Evgenia Fotiou; Dr. Christopher McCurdy

BACK ROW, L TO R:
Dr. Kenneth Alper; Dr. Nigel Gericke

NOT SHOWN:
Dr. Stephen Szára; Dale Millard; Dr. Michael Heinrich

Kenneth Alper, MD
Associate Professor of Psychiatry and Neurology at the New York University School of Medicine. He is internationally recognized as an authority on the chemistry and pharmacology of Iboga and Ibogaine, and the clinical use of Ibogaine in the treatment of substance use disorders.

Evgenia Fotiou, PhD
Assistant Professor of Anthropology, Kent State University. She is recognized for her work in cultural anthropology and Amazonian shamanism, in particular the *ayahuasca* tourism phenomenon.

Nigel Gericke, MD
South African medical doctor, botanist, ethnopharmacologist and entrepreneur has published many peer-reviewed scientific papers on ethnobotany and ethnopharmacology; he is co-author of books on S. African ethnobotany including *Medicinal Plants of South Africa* and *People's Plants: A Guide to Useful Plants of Southern Africa*. He is the world's foremost authority on Kanna, an indigenous psychoactive plant used by the San and Khoi peoples.

Michael Heinrich, PhD
Professor of Ethnopharmacology and Medicinal Plant Research (pharmacognosy) at the UCL School of Pharmacy, London, UK. He is Specialty Editor-in-Chief of *Frontiers in Pharmacology* (Ethnopharmacology section), and Review Editor of the *Journal of Ethnopharmacology*. He is co-editor with Anna Jaeger of a textbook, *Ethnopharmacology*.

Luis Eduardo Luna, PhD
Director, WasiWaska Research Center for the Study of Psychointegrator Plants, Visionary Art and Consciousness. (wasiwaska.org) Dr. Luna is internationally recognized as an authority on the ethnography of *ayahuasca*.

Christopher R. McCurdy, PhD, BS Ph, FAAPS
Professor of Medicinal Chemistry, College of Pharmacy, University of Florida, Gainesville, FL. Dr. McCurdy is Director of the UF Translational Drug Development Core and the 2017-2018 president of the American Association of Pharmaceutical Scientists. He is internationally recognized as an authority on Kratom, *Mitragyna speciosa*.

Dennis J. McKenna, PhD
Director of Ethnopharmacology, Heffter Research Institute; Assistant Professor, University of Minnesota. He has studied the botany, chemistry and pharmacology of *ayahuasca* and other South American shamanic plants over the last forty years.

Dale Millard
Ethnobotanist, naturalist and biodiversity explorer, with research interests ranging from herpetology to the study of plants used to treat tropical diseases and immune disorders. He has traveled and collected extensively in South Africa, Brazil, and Indonesia.

Jeanmaire Molina, PhD
Assistant Professor of Biology, Long Island University. She specializes in plant systematics, ethnobotany, and in the flora of the Philippines, including the giant-flowered Rafflesia, and uses phylogenetic and genomic tools in her research.

David E. Nichols, PhD
Distinguished Professor Emeritus of Medicinal Chemistry and Molecular Pharmacology, and former Robert C. and Charlotte P. Anderson Chair in Pharmacology, Purdue University. Founder and President of the Heffter Research Institute (heffter.org). He is recognized as a world authority on the chemistry and pharmacology of psychedelic medicines.

Jerry D. Patchen
Texas attorney and trial lawyer who has represented the Native American Church (NAC) to help secure access to their sacrament, peyote, and to preserve their rights to religious freedom. He was also on the legal team that secured the right of the *União do Vegetal* (UDV) to use *ayahuasca* in U.S. religious services.

Mark J. Plotkin, PhD, LHD
Ethnobotanist, educator, filmmaker co-founder and President of the Amazon Conservation Team (ACT.org). He is widely recognized for his advocacy for the protection of indigenous knowledge and Amazonian ecosystems. Plotkin was a protege of Richard Evans Schultes, and gave a unique and insightful look at his mentor as part of ESPD50.

Stacy B. Schaefer, PhD
Stacy B. Schaefer is Professor Emerita, Department of Anthropology, California State University at Chico. Her expertise from long-term ethnographic fieldwork with the Huichol people of Mexico includes their ritual use of peyote. She has also studied peyote and its importance in the Native American Church.

Glenn H. Shepard, PhD
Staff Researcher at Goeldi Museum, Belem, Brazil. His writing, research and photography on shamanism, traditional environmental knowledge and indigenous rights has appeared in *Nature, Science, National Geographic* and *The New York Review of Books*, among other prestigious publications. He has participated in several TV documentaries including an Emmy Award-winning Discovery Channel film.

Jean-Francois Sobiecki, B.Sc. Hons.
Ethnobotanist, Research Associate at the University of Johannesburg & founder of the Khanyisa Healing Gardens project, specializing in African psychoactive plants.

Stephen Szára, MD, DSc
Dr. Szára has had a long and distinguished career as a psychiatrist, medicinal chemist, and pharmacologist. He began his career as an Assistant Professor of Biochemistry at the Medical University in Budapest. After he emigrated to the U.S., he held several positions as scientist and section chief at NIMH and NIDA, as well as Associate Professor of Clinical Psychiatry at George Washington University. He has received numerous honors and awards. He is perhaps best known for his determination, through self-experiments, to ascertain whether DMT is a psychedelic in humans.

Constantino Manuel Torres, PhD
Professor Emeritus, Art and Art History Department, Florida International University. Dr. Torres specializes in the art and iconography of ancient cultures of the Central Andes. He is recognized for his excavations of shamanic burial sites in the Atacama Desert, and is a recognized expert on the use of Anadenthera snuffs in ancient South America.

Keeper Trout
Self-taught ethnobotanist, scholar and photographer. Author of *Trout's Notes* series of ethnobotanical references, formerly technical editor of *The Entheogen Review*. He is active in the Cactus Conservation Institute and the Shulgin Archives Project.

Snu Voogelbriender
Ethnobotanist, an authority on the Australian Acacias and author of *The Garden of Eden: Shamanic Use of Psychoactive Flora and Fauna and the Study of Consciousness*.

TABLE OF CONTENTS

FOREWORD

The contents of this book and the ESPD50 symposium from which these papers are derived shows that the investigation of psychoactive drugs is now a serious scientific endeavour. It is no longer the playground of a few adventurers. The indigenous peoples of the world have been fantastic explorers of the properties of the plants and fungi around them. They have discovered and used many psychoactive compounds, and often these plants are central to their cultural and religious life. But these discoveries have also been significant in a broader context, in that they have provided leads to the development of significant therapeutic medicines. The preservation of this knowledge under the stewardship of indigenous cultures has been an invaluable contribution to the advancement of science and medicine. This book clearly shows that this is a worldwide phenomenon, as it reports discoveries from the Amazon to Australia and from Mexico to South Africa. It also shows the broad range of organisms that contain psychoactive compounds, from Mexican fungi to tall Amazonian trees or desert Acacias of Australia. Many of us involved with this volume owe much to the encouragement or tutelage of Richard Evans Schultes, who was the pioneer who could justifiably be recognized as the founder of the interdisciplinary field of psycho-ethnopharmacology. Schultes' role as an explorer, an ethnobotanist extraordinaire, and a scientist who encouraged his colleagues to investigate the biodynamic compounds in the plants he discovered, opened a new frontier in the study of naturally-occurring psychoactive compounds. Without his encouragement to publish a paper about a visit to the Yanomami where I reported on their hallucinogenic snuff, I might never have followed this up in many other places and with several other tribes.

The rich ethnomedical heritage of indigenous peoples is now being scientifically studied and applied in many different ways, as is apparent from chapters of this volume. As someone who has spent much time with the tribal peoples of the Amazon and studied many different psychoactive compounds, it is my hope that those of us involved in research do all we can to maintain the cultures and the knowledge of these indigenous pioneers. Their discoveries would never have come to the attention of science had it not been for their role as guardians of this knowledge. In return for these inestimable gifts, it is our responsibility to be active in the preservation of the habitats in which tribal people live. But our responsibilities as members of the scientific community do not end there. We must also become strong advocates for the recognition and protection of the intellectual property rights of indigenous peoples. The sort of research reported here is leading to a much wider application of these indigenous discoveries, potentially yielding novel medicines worth billions of dollars to the global pharmaceutical industry. We must make sure that our indigenous friends also benefit for their role in making these discoveries and preserving this knowledge as part of their intellectual and cultural heritage. We must make sure that indigenous peoples and their knowledge are recognized and preserved. At the same time, we must encourage them to develop at their own pace and make their own choices when it comes to the decision to share (or not) their ethnomedical treasures.

Sir Ghillean Prance, FRS, FLS, FRSB
Director (Ret.), Royal Botanic Gardens, Kew
Currently: Scientific Director of the Eden Project

What a Long, Strange Trip it's Been: Reflections on the Ethnopharmacologic Search for Psychoactive Drugs (1967-2017)

Dennis McKenna, PhD

Director of Ethnopharmacology,
Heffter Research Institute

THE FIRST ETHNOPHARMACOLOGIC SEARCH FOR PSYCHOACTIVE DRUGS
— SAN FRANCISCO, 1967

In 1967, a landmark symposium in the history of psychedelics was held in San Francisco, California, under the sponsorship of the National Institute of Mental Health, which was part of the U.S. Department of Health, Education, and Welfare (HEW). This agency is now called the Department of Health and Human Services (HHS). The title of the invitational symposium was the Ethnopharmacologic Search for Psychoactive Drugs, and a volume of the proceedings was published under the same name and sold through the U.S. Government Printing Office. The symposium volume, now rare, has become a classic reference in the ethnobotanical literature.

This was the first time that an interdisciplinary group of specialists, ranging from ethnobotanists to neuroscientists, gathered in one place to share their findings on a topic of widespread interest at the time: the use of psychoactive plants in the context of indigenous and non-Western societies. In 1967, the word "psychedelic" had not yet become stigmatized. There were still expectations in the psychiatric and neuroscience communities that these little-known and curious agents, used for centuries in the ethnomedicine and rituals of more traditional cultures, might yield new healing materials that could be used therapeutically in our own troubled society, as well as being important tools in the exploration of the human mind.

The roster of those attending the original 1967 symposium reads like a who's who of ethnopharmacology: John Daly, Richard Schultes, Bo Holmstedt, Gordon Wasson, Alexander Shulgin, Andrew Weil, Stephen Szára, Nathan Kline, Daniel Efron, Daniel X. Freedman, and many others lesser known, and now all but forgotten. Only a few of the researchers who attended the original symposium are still alive, and of those, even fewer remain active in the field. Their work contributed to making the first ESPD symposium one of the most unusual and interdisciplinary scientific convocations ever organized.

Originally, follow-up symposia were planned to be held about every ten years; that time frame, it was thought, was sufficiently ample to accommodate the stately progress of scientific research, yet frequent enough to enable researchers in various specialties to come together in a collegial environment to share research results in a timely fashion.

Following the summer of 1967, the prevailing political winds shifted, and psychedelic substances soon after became demonized, feared, and banned. There was no further interest on the part of the federal government to sponsor any similar symposia. In fact, their sponsorship of the original symposium, as valuable as it was for the dissemination of research findings, became an embarrassment, and as a result, no follow-up symposia were ever held. The Symposium Proceedings, available for a time from the U.S. Government Printing Office (U.S. Public Health Service Publication #1645), eventually went out of print, closing that particular chapter in the history of psycho-ethnopharmacology.

In the fifty years that have passed since that first symposium, numerous federal administrations have come and gone. Our recent past and current administrations, along with most of their affiliated institutions, remain as far from developing a viable, realistic drug policy today as they were then. In the decades since, a new generation of researchers, many inspired by the giants represented at that first conference, has continued to investigate the outer limits of psycho-ethnopharmacology. Some outstanding discoveries have been made, and the work continues. At the same time, there has been a sea change in public and medical perception of psychedelics. There is now a renaissance in research around the world, and the therapeutic potential of some of these agents is being reinvestigated. While psychedelic substances have become less stigmatized than in the past, they remain controversial. Much work in this field remains unfinished, and the most significant discoveries may still lie in the future.

HOW ESPD CHANGED MY LIFE
— SUMMER 1968

When the first ESPD symposium was held in 1967, I was 16 years old, a bored teenager living in a small town in Western Colorado. More than anything, I longed to escape my dreary life and travel to San Francisco, the Mecca for the counterculture, the epicenter of the psychedelic revolution. My brother, Terence, a lifelong friend and mentor, had escaped our soft prison a few years earlier and was a student at Berkeley at the time. We were both just beginning to discover the wondrous world of psychedelics, and we agreed that they were the most fascinating things that we had encountered in our young lives. The fascination we felt then continued to guide our interests and even careers for the rest of our lives.

Terence passed on in 2000 after a long fight with brain cancer. I have continued the quest for understanding on my own, grateful to him for introducing me to psychedelics, and for the passionate curiosity we shared. I do the best I can, but every day I miss having his wisdom and humor in my life. He was, as he kindly said of me in his book *True Hallucinations*, "my brother and a colleague of long standing."

In 1967, while we were fascinated by psychedelics and wanted to immerse ourselves in the counterculture, neither of us had much of a clue about them. Terence was living in Berkeley, and I managed to get away from my small town and visit him during the height of the Summer of Love. Neither one of us was aware of the obscure private symposium that had taken place in San Francisco just a few months earlier.

Like most of our like-minded contemporaries, we had no context from which to understand the emergence of these ancient compounds into mass consciousness in the 1960s. Timothy Leary had transformed from a mild-mannered Harvard researcher to the Messiah of LSD, and although we resonated with much of his message, we were slow to plunge full tilt into the hippie movement. Part of the reason for this is because we identified as intellectuals, and were put off to some degree by the distinctly anti-intellectual trappings of hippie culture. We felt there had to be more to psychedelics than their superficial depictions in the mass media, but we had no idea where to find a more in-depth and balanced perspective.

Sometime in 1968, while we were busy trying to sort all this out, two books surfaced in our world; these works were able to provide for us a deep background context in which psychedelics made sense. One of these was *The Teachings of Don Juan*, Carlos Castaneda's first book of many, detailing his apprenticeship with a Yaqui shaman (Castaneda, 1968). Although subsequent events have shown that much of Castaneda's work is highly fictionalized, if not a complete fabrication, we did not know that at the time. For me at least, that first book was influential because it provided a cultural context for psychedelics, based on traditions older and richer than anything I had encountered in mass media sources. It made clear that there was nothing new about psychedelics; in fact, these sacred plants and fungi had been used in indigenous shamanic practices for hundreds, if not thousands, of years. While Castaneda's book was not scientific or even accurate, it gave me insights into shamanism, a set of practical technologies and beliefs involving the use of these materials for healing and the exploration of consciousness. Terence gave me a copy of the first edition of the *Teachings of Don Juan* for my 18th birthday in 1968; it was a very special gift. I still have it, and I still cherish it.

The proceedings of the first Ethnopharmacologic Search for Psychoactive Drugs were published some months after the symposium, in 1967. The volume was issued by the U.S. Government Printing Office as U.S. Public Health Service Publication #1645, published under the sponsorship of the Pharmacology Section, Psychopharmacology Research Branch of the National Institute of Mental Health (Efron et al., 1967).

I have no recollection of how this volume first came into my hands. All I remember is that somehow a rather well-used copy came into my possession sometime in the summer of 1968. I dropped whatever else I was reading and devoured the book from cover to cover! This book provided the perfect balance to the *Teachings of Don Juan*. While that work had made me aware of the cultural contexts related to the indigenous uses of psychedelics, the *Ethnopharmacologic Search for Psychoactive Drugs* was even more influential, because through it I became aware that this discipline – ethnopharmacology, or more accurately psycho-ethnopharmacology – was a real field of scientific investigation. Moreover, it was my first introduction to the people working in this field, people like R. E. Schultes, Bo Holmstedt, Alexander Shulgin, R. Gordon Wasson, and others, who became iconic figures in my personal pantheon, and in some cases, as with Schultes and Shulgin, mentors and friends.

The realization that real science was being pursued in this field was a revelation to me, not least because it opened up the possibility that one day I, too, might be able to achieve a place in this exclusive fellowship. And eventually I did, but when it first came into my hands, I thought at least I would be able to prove to my parents that I was serious about psychedelics, and not just a confused hippie in search of cheap thrills. They were not very reassured, but over the years they came to recognize the merits of my chosen career in science.

TWO DECADES LATER ...

The shabby volume of that first edition resides on my shelf to this day. While I don't remember exactly how it came into my hands, I remember very well how my second copy came to me, in 1986. I had completed my PhD at the University of British Columbia in 1984 under the supervision of Dr. Neil Towers, another one of my lifelong mentors and friends. My thesis was an ethnopharmacological investigation of the ethnobotany, chemistry, and pharmacology of *ayahuasca* and another hallucinogen, a relatively more obscure preparation known as *oo'ko-ey*, derived from *Virola* species. Though derived from entirely different botanical sources, both *ayahuasca* and *oo'koey* were orally active tryptamine hallucinogens, and my thesis was a comparative study of their active constituents and pharmacology.

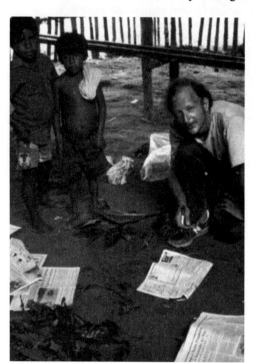

Dennis the aspiring ethnopharmacologist & helpers. Rio Ampiyacu, 1981

Following the completion of my thesis in early 1984, I moved to San Diego and began the first of three post-docs. About a year after I had moved, my thesis publications came out, and one attracted the attention of Dr. Juan Saavedra, a researcher at NIMH. When Dr. Saavedra requested a reprint of my publication on *ayahuasca* in the *Journal of Ethnopharmacology*, (McKenna et al., 1984), I was surprised. I recognized his name from an early paper he had published with Julius Axelrod on the endogenous synthesis of DMT in rabbit lung (Axelrod later won the Nobel Prize for his work on mechanisms of neurotransmission).

Figuring it was a long shot, I enclosed a letter with my signed reprint, timidly enquiring if there might be a chance I could come to NIMH and work with him on endogenous tryptamines. A few weeks passed (things moved slowly in those days), and one day I received a kind reply. He thanked me for my reprint, and mentioned that he had been in the Amazon in 1979 with Schultes and my mentor, Dr. Towers, along with a dozen other researchers on the R.V.[1] *Alpha-Helix*, operated by the Scripps Institute of Oceanography. He informed me that there was a fellowship program at NIMH, the Pharmacology Research Associate Traineeship (PRAT), that was targeted to young investigators wanting to expand their scientific training outside their field of specialization. He said it was a perfect fit for me, and encouraged me to apply. I did so, was accepted into the program, and began my second post-doc in the fall of 1986, in the hallowed environs of the Laboratory of Clinical Pharmacology at NIMH.

I had been in the lab for less than two weeks when Dr. Saavedra pointed to an upper shelf in a cabinet in the lab. He said there was a box up there containing some research chemicals that he and Axelrod had used in their research on endogenous tryptamines. He suggested I go through it and see if there was anything useful, and to send the rest to the hazardous waste disposal center on the NIH campus. I didn't waste any time; I stayed late one afternoon until most of my fellow workers had called it a day, then got up on the bench and retrieved the box. And something more: a mint-condition copy of the *Ethnopharmacologic Search for Psychoactive Drugs*! How many years it had languished on the shelf next to that box of chemicals I had no idea, but it had clearly never been opened.

Here I was, just beginning my post-doctoral studies in the heart of NIMH, the very institution where the original ESPD had originated, and suddenly the book that had so enthralled me as a curious teenager magically, reappeared. How cool was that? I took it as a very good omen. It quietly disappeared into my library, where it sits beside my first copy from 1968. Some of those research chemicals turned out to be interesting as well. Along with a couple of vials of DMT and 5-methoxy-DMT, there was an interesting assortment of other derivatives such as 5,7-dihydroxy-DMT, 6-methoxy-DMT, and so on. I kept those for many years, but never found the courage to bioassay them.

ESPD RETURNS: FIFTY YEARS LATER

So that is the story of my own personal history with this book. It has haunted most of my professional career. It opened my eyes to the science of ethnopharmacology, and later, I was fortunate to meet and befriend some of the people who presented at that 1967 symposium. Though its contents are dated now, that book influenced my life and career in profound ways, and I am sure that my career in ethnopharmacology, such as it has been, would never have happened had I not encountered that obscure tome in the summer of 1968.

I have wanted to organize a follow-up symposium for many years. In fact, I first drafted a proposal about it in 1995, hoping to stage it in 1997, the 30th anniversary of the San Francisco symposium. It never happened for various reasons, mostly due to lack of funds, time, and an appropriate venue. Now it is 2017, the 50th anniversary of the ESPD, and all of those necessary elements have come together almost miraculously.

I hope that this commemorative symposium and the publication of both symposium volumes, 1967 and 2017, will attract the attention of younger investigators working in the field of ethnopharmacology, and will inspire them to continue this valuable work. There is still more – much more – to be discovered. I hope that the quest represented in the book's title – *Ethnopharmacologic* **Search** *for Psychoactive Drugs* – will be carried on by a new generation, who one day will report their discoveries to the world at a future ESPD symposium. I also hope that it will not take another 50 years!

SIGNIFICANT DISCOVERIES OF
THE LAST FIFTY YEARS

Psycho-ethnopharmacology has not stood still over the last fifty years. Significant discoveries have been made, and are still being made. The ESPD50 anniversary conference in June 2017 included presentations on some of the most interesting discoveries made in those decades, but this volume must necessarily omit many others that are just as worthy. Though it's not my intention to discuss them in any detail, a few are worth mentioning in brief:

Ayahuasca Admixtures – The importance of the many admixtures to *ayahuasca* had not received much attention in 1967. Some of Schultes' students were reporting on the use of admixtures including the DMT-containing admixtures that give *ayahuasca* its psychedelic properties, but most of this work was not published until 1968 or later (Pinkley, 1969). Interestingly, the word "*Psychotria*,"

....

1. R. V. = Research Vessel

the genus that includes the most widely utilized admixture, *Psychotria viridis* R&P, occurs only once in the entire 1967 edition. In the 1980s, Eduardo Luna and I also published research on the many other species that are occasionally used as admixtures (McKenna, Luna, and Towers, 1986, 1995[2]). Many of these remain poorly investigated both as to their chemistry and their pharmacology. In a later publication (McKenna et al., 2011), I screened many of these species using neuroreceptor-binding assays as part of a broad sampling of purported CNS-active plants with potential anti-dementia and anti-schizophrenic activity. I have contributed a condensed version of that paper to this volume.

Salvia divinorum Epling & Játiva and Salvinorin A – Although ethnographic reports of the use of this member of the mint family (Lamiaceae) in Mazatec shamanism had been reported in the '30s (Johnson, 1939a, 1939b), it was not discussed in the '67 symposium. The primary active constituent, the diterpene Salvinorin A, was isolated and characterized in the '90s (Valdés, 1994), and its potent activity as a highly selective kappa-receptor agonist was described in 2002 (Roth et al., 2002). This initial discovery has led to a flurry of research on the chemistry and pharmacology of Salvinorin A and its analogs. Over 30 papers on Salvinorin A have been published since (for a review, cf. Cunningham et al., 2011). Dr. Michael Heinrich and his student, Ivan Casselman, contribute a retrospective on this interesting plant in this volume (Heinrich and Casselman, 2017).

Kava - Piper methysticum (G. Forst) – Kava, known under many names, is a mildly psychoactive beverage prepared from the roots of this member of the pepper family. It was reported on in the first ESPD symposium in 1967 (cf. Session II, ESPD 1967), but much additional work has been done on this plant in subsequent decades. It is now widely available as a dietary supplement; and its anxiolytic, muscle-relaxant, and sedative properties have made it a popular alternative to pharmaceuticals such as benzodiazepines (for review cf. LaPorte et al., 2011).

Mitragyna speciosa (Korth) Havil. – Known by its folk name of kratom, this Rubiaceous tree is the source of mitragynine and related alkaloids that are potent mu-receptor agonists. The plant can cause addiction like any opiate, but in traditional contexts it is often used as an alternative to opium, and as a way to gradually end dependence on opium and heroin. The *Mitragyna* alkaloids do not cause respiratory depression, unlike heroin and other opiates, and hence show promise as less toxic, and less addictive, analgesics. It is not illegal in the U.S. at the time of this writing, but has been identified as a "drug of concern" by the DEA, and may be scheduled in the near future. At the same time, some investigators, such as Dr. Christopher McCurdy, have urged that it not be prohibited as it may enable many opiate addicts to overcome their habits, as a kind of herbal methadone (Ward et al., 2011; Babu et al., 2008). Dr. McCurdy has reported on his research and the current "state of the art" with respect to Mitragyna in this volume.

Iboga – Tabernanthe iboga Baill. and Ibogaine – Iboga, sometimes spelled eboga, is used in traditional initiation rites among the Bwiti peoples of Gabon. In those rites, young men and women of the tribe, coming of age as adults, undergo an initiation in which they consume large – sometimes nearly lethal – amounts of iboga root. They experience a deep trance, sometimes lasting up to 36 hours, during which they are visited by their ancestors and are initiated and given the ancestral wisdom. Ibogaine, the major alkaloid, has received recognition and notoriety, as it is effective for the treatment of opiate and other addictions (Alper, 2001). Although a Schedule 1 controlled substance in the U.S., it is unregulated in many countries, and is used in treatment centers in various parts of the world, especially Mexico (Brown, 2013). Dr. Kenneth Alper, a leading authority on the chemistry and pharmacology of ibogaine, reports in this volume on The Ibogaine Project: Urban ethnomedicine for opioid use disorder.

Kougoed – Sceletium tortuosum (L.) N.E. Br. – Kougoed, also called canna or kanna, is a succulent in the family Azioaceae whose roots contain a spectrum of alkaloids with CNS activities. Some, such as mesembranone, mesembrine, and mesembranol, are potent 5HT-uptake inhibitors and phosphodiesterase 4 inhibitors. These are only 3 of more than 30 alkaloids that have been isolated; the pharmacological properties of most have not been thoroughly characterized (Gericke et al., 2008). In this volume, Dr. Nigel Gericke reports on his research with *Sceletium tortuosum* that has led to the commercial development of Zembrin™, a natural herbal anxiolytic and antidepressant sold as a dietary supplement (Gericke, 2017).

Jurema – Mimosa hostilis (C. Mart.) Benth.[3] and yuremamine – This species has long been known as the source of Vinho de Yurema, a psychoactive beverage that has DMT as its main active

---

2. This paper was originally published in Spanish in the journal, *America Indigena* in 1995; an English translation was published as a chapter in an anthology, *Ethnobotany: Evolution of a Discipline*. See bibliography for details.

3. Note: *Mimosa hostilis* (C. Mart.) Benth. is considered a synonym of the currently accepted name, *Mimosa tenuiflora* (Willd.) Poir. cf. http://www.theplantlist.org/tpl1.1/record/ild-20760

constituent. However, it has been an ethnopharmacological enigma because DMT is not orally active unless potentiated by a monoamine oxidase inhibitor. Yet there are no admixture plants with MAOI activity that have been reported to be added to the mixture. Recently, a novel compound, yuremamine, was isolated from the roots of *M. hostilis* at about the same concentration as DMT (Vepsäläinen et al., 2005). This compound has an interesting structure in that the structure of DMT is "caged" within the larger molecule, which may be a prodrug that is converted to DMT *in vivo*. The initially proposed structure has been challenged, and total synthesis has so far been elusive (Calvert and Sperry, 2015). It may also be an MAO inhibitor itself, and thus could potentiate the DMT. So far, there have been no human bioassays of this compound, so its pharmacological properties in a pure form are unknown.

Acacia spp. and tryptamines – The large genus *Acacia* (Fabaceae) has proven to be an unusually rich source of DMT and other psychoactive·tryptamines. At the time of the first ESPD conference in 1967, the tryptaminic *Acacias* were unknown to science. The earliest reference in Pubmed is Wahba and Elkhier (1975). Since that time, tryptamines have been detected in over 60 *Acacia* spp. worldwide, with about 40 species native to Australia, as documented in the review paper in this volume by Snu Voogelbreinder, *Australian Psychoactive Acacia Species and Their Alkaloids* (2017). Many more *Acacia* spp. contain unidentified alkaloids, and phenylethylamines, β-carbolines, tetrahydroisoquinolines, pyridines, and still other structural classes have been reported. Interestingly, much of what science knows about the chemistry of psychoactive *Acacia* spp. is due to investigations by amateur scientists who have conducted research outside conventional academic channels, and as a result, much of it does not appear in the peer-reviewed literature.

Frog and Toad medicines – Psychoactive and psychedelic amphibians – frogs and toads – have attracted attention recently as potentially being therapeutic. Among these are the so-called sapo medicines, more properly termed kambô, from *Phyllomedusa bicolor* (Giant Leaf Frog), a frog containing a variety of neuroactive peptides in their skin secretions. This species is used by the Matses tribe as hunting magic, and taking "sapo" is becoming a popular pastime among tourists in Peru. So far the peptides identified include phyllocaerulein (a hypertensive), phyllomedusin (tachykinin, potent vasodilator, and secretagogue), phyllokinin (a potent arterial smooth muscle dilator), and several delta-selective opiate peptides (the deltorphins), as well as mu-active peptides (the dermorphins). Many of these compounds may have therapeutic potential, and the neuroactive peptides are only a part of this rich peptide cocktail. For reviews and more information, see: Erspamer et al., 1993; Daly et al., 1992; den Brave et al., 2014.

In addition to the *Phyllomedusa* peptides, the venom of *Bufo* species contains psychedelic tryptamine derivatives, either bufotenine or 5-Methoxy-DMT, and its use has gained popularity in various neo-shamanic practices. Although the subjective effects of *Bufo* venom were first reported by Weil and Davis (1994), there is little evidence that these species were ever utilized as psychedelic medicines in any ethnomedical or shamanic tradition. A comprehensive review of the use of *Bufo* spp. as psychedelics, and an unpacking of some of the controversies surrounding this practice, can be found in Lyttle et al. (1996).

Old yet new: Harmine and related β-carbolines – Harmine is the major β-carboline in *Banisteriopsis caapi* (Spruce ex Griseb.) Morton, and is the primary MAO inhibitor in *ayahuasca*. Harmine is an "old" alkaloid. By that, I mean that it's been around for a while, having first been identified in the seeds of Syrian rue, *Peganum harmala* L., in 1847 by chemist J. Fritsch, over ten years before *ayahuasca* came to the attention of science as a result of Richard Spruce's discovery in 1858. However, recent investigations have shown that even old alkaloids can still harbor secrets; new research has shown that harmine and some of its derivatives can display a diverse array of biological activities. It has been shown to have antimicrobial, anti-diabetic, anti-depressant, anti-cancer, neuroprotective, and other effects. It interacts with a number of neuroreceptors including 5-HT2A, 5-HT2C, imidazoline, and DAT. Significantly, it has recently been shown to be a potent inhibitor of DYRK1A, a kinase involved in a variety of intracellular signaling functions related to cell proliferation and neurogenesis, and has been shown to potently stimulate proliferation of neural cell progenitors, an effect linked to its inhibition of DYRK1A (Dakic et al., 2016). For recent reviews on the pharmacology of harmine and other β-carbolines, see Cao et al., 2007; Patel et al., 2012; and the paper in this volume by Dale Millard (2017).

ACKNOWLEDGEMENTS

I want to express my profound thanks to those who have made contributions to this 50th Anniversary ESPD symposium volume, and the website and e-book, as well as to the many individuals who saw and shared my vision, and stepped up to help make it happen in so many ways.

The idea may have been mine; the time and effort that made it happen came from all of us.

- *Dennis McKenna*

REFERENCES

Alper, K., 2017. The ibogaine project: Urban ethnomedicine for opioid use disorder, in: Prance, G.T., McKenna, D.J., De Loenen, B., Davis, W. (Eds), *Ethnopharmacologic Search for Psychoactive Drugs: 50th Anniversary Symposium Volume* (2018). Synergetic Press, Santa Fe.

Alper, K.R., 2001. Ibogaine: A review. *The Alkaloids. Chemistry and Biology* 56, 1-38.

Babu, K.M., McCurdy C.R., Boyer E.W., 2008. Opioid receptors and legal highs: *Salvia divinorum* and kratom. *Clinical Toxicology* (Philadelphia) 46, 146-52.

Brown, T.K., 2013. Ibogaine in the treatment of substance dependence. *Current Drug Abuse Reviews* 6, 3-16.

Calvert, M.B., Sperry, J., 2015. Bioinspired total synthesis and structural revision of yuremamine, an alkaloid from the entheogenic plant *Mimosa tenuiflora*. *Chemical Communications* (Cambridge) 51, 6202-5.

Cao, R., Peng, W., Wang, Z., Xu, A., 2007. Beta-carboline alkaloids: Biochemical and pharmacological functions. *Current Medicinal Chemistry* 14, 479-500.

Castaneda, C., 1968. *The Teachings of Don Juan: a Yaqui Way of Knowledge.* University of California Press.

Cunningham, C.W., Rothman, R.B., Prisinzano, T.E., 2011. Neuropharmacology of the naturally occurring Kappa-opioid hallucinogen Salvinorin A. *Pharmacological Reviews* 63, 316-47.

Dakic, V., Maciel, R.M., Drummond, H., Nascimento, J.M., Trindade, P., Rehen, S.K., 2016. Harmine stimulates proliferation of human neural progenitors. *PeerJ.* 2016 Dec 6;4: e2727. eCollection. *PubMed.*

Daly, J.W., Caceres, J., Moni, R.W., Gusovsky, F., Moos, M. Jr., Seamon, K.B., Milton, K., Myers, C.W., 1992. Frog secretions and hunting magic in the upper Amazon: Identification of a peptide that interacts with an adenosine receptor. *Proceedings of the National Academy of Sciences USA* 89, 10960-10963.

den Brave, P.S., Bruins, E., Bronkhorst, M.W., 2014. Phyllomedusa bicolor skin secretion and the Kambô ritual. *Journal of Venomous Animals and Toxins Including Tropical Diseases* 20, 40.

Efron, D.H., Holmstedt, B., Kline, N.S. (eds.), 1967. *Ethnopharmacologic Search for Psychoactive Drugs – 1967.* Workshop Series of Pharmacology Section, NIMH No. 2. Sponsored by Pharmacology Section, Psychopharmacology Research Branch, National Institute of Mental Health. Public Health Service, U.S. Department of Health, Education, and Welfare. Public Health Service Publication No. 1645, U.S. Government Printing Office.

Erspamer, V., Erspamer, G.F., Severini, C., Potenza, R.L., Barra, D., Mignogna, G., Bianchi, A., 1993. Pharmacological studies of 'sapo' from the frog phyllomedusa bicolor skin: A drug used by the peruvian Matses Indians in shamanic hunting practices. *Toxicon.* 31, 1099-111

Gericke N., Viljoen, A.M., 2008. Sceletium: A review update. *Journal of Ethnopharmacology* 119, 653-63.

Gericke, N., 2017. Sceletium species and mesembrine alkaloids - The past, present and future of *Kanna*, in: Prance, G.T., McKenna, D.J., De Loenen, B., Davis, W. (Eds), *Ethnopharmacologic Search for Psychoactive Drugs: 50th Anniversary Symposium Volume* (2018). Synergetic Press, Santa Fe.

Heinrich, M., Casselman, I., 2017. Ethnopharmacology – from Mexican Hallucinogens to a Global Transdisciplinary Science, in: Prance, G.T., McKenna, D.J. De Loenen, B., Davis, W. (Eds), *Ethnopharmacologic Search for Psychoactive Drugs: 50th Anniversary Symposium Volume* (2018). Synergetic Press, Santa Fe.

Johnson, J.B., 1939a. Some notes on the Mazatec. *Revista Mexicana de Estudios Antropologicoa* 3, 142-156.

Johnson, J.B., 1939b. The elements of Mazatec witchcraft. *Etnologiska Studier* 9, 128-150.

LaPorte, E., Sarris, J., Stough, C., Scholey, A., 2011. Neurocognitive effects of Kava (*Piper methysticum*): A systematic review. *Human Psychopharmacology* 26, 102-11.

Lyttle, T., Goldstein, D., Gartz, J., 1996. Bufo toads and bufotenine: Fact and fiction surrounding an alleged psychedelic. *Journal of Psychoactive Drugs* 28, 267-90.

McCurdy, C.R., 2017. Kratom (*Mitragyna speciosa*): A summary of scientific knowledge leading to a potential therapy for opioid dependence, in: Prance, G.T., McKenna, D.J. De Loenen, B., Davis, W. (Eds), *Ethnopharmacologic Search for Psychoactive Drugs: 50th Anniversary Symposium Volume* (2018). Synergetic Press, Santa Fe.

McKenna, D.J., Luna, L.E., Towers, G.H.N., 1986. Ingredientes Biodinamicos en las Plantas que se Meszclan al Ayahuasca. Una farmacopea tradicional no investigada. *America Indigena* 46, 73-101 (Spanish with English abstract).

McKenna, D.J., Luna, L.E., Towers, G.H.N., 1995. Biodynamic constituents in *ayahuasca* admixture plants: An uninvestigated folk pharmacopoeia, in: von Reis, S., and Schultes, R. E. (Eds.), *Ethnobotany: Evolution of a Discipline.* Dioscorides Press, Portland.

McKenna, D.J., Ruiz, J.M., Hoye, T.R., Roth, B.R., Shoemaker, A.P., 2011. Receptor screening technologies in the evaluation of Amazonian ethnomedicines with potential applications to cognitive deficits. *Journal of Ethnopharmacology* 134, 475-492.

McKenna, D.J., Towers, G.H.N., Abbott, F.S., 1984. Monoamine oxidase inhibitors in South American hallucinogenic plants: Tryptamine and β-carboline constituents of *ayahuasca*. *Journal of Ethnopharmacology* 10, 195-223.

Millard, D., 2017. Broad spectrum roles of harmine in *ayahuasca*, in: Prance, G.T., McKenna, D.J. De Loenen, B., Davis, W. (Eds), *Ethnopharmacologic Search for Psychoactive Drugs: 50th Anniversary Symposium Volume* (2018). Synergetic Press, Santa Fe.

Patel, K., Gadewar, M., Tripathi, R., Prasad, S.K., Patel, D.K., 2012. A review on [the] medicinal importance, pharmacological activity and bioanalytical aspects of beta-carboline alkaloid "harmine." *Asian Pacific Journal of Tropical Biomedicine* 2, 660-4.

Pinkley, H.V., 1969. Plant admixtures to *ayahuasca*, the South American hallucinogenic drink. *Lloydia* 32, 305-14.

Roth, B.L., Baner, K., Westkaemper, R., Siebert, D., Rice, K.C., Steinberg, S., Ernsberger, P., Rothman, R.B., 2002. Salvinorin A: A potent naturally occurring non-nitrogenous Kappa opioid selective agonist. *Proceeding of the National Academy of Sciences USA* 18, 11934-9.

Valdés, L.J. 3rd., 1994. *Salvia divinorum* and the unique diterpene hallucinogen, Salvinorin (Divinorin) A. *Journal of Psychoactive Drugs* 26, 277-83.

Vepsäläinen, J.J., Auriola, S., Tukiainen, M., Ropponen, N., Callaway, J.C., 2005. Isolation and characterization of Yuremamine, a new phytoindole. *Planta Medica* 71, 1053-7.

Voogelbreinder, S., 2017. Australian psychoactive acacia species and their alkaloids, in: Prance, G.T., McKenna, D.J. De Loenen, B., Davis, W. (Eds), *Ethnopharmacologic Search for Psychoactive Drugs: 50th Anniversary Symposium Volume* (2018). Synergetic Press, Santa Fe.

Wahba, Khalil S.K., Elkheir, Y.M., 1975. Dimethyltryptamine from the leaves of certain acacia species of northern Sudan. *Lloydia* 38, 176-7.

Ward, J., Rosenbaum, C., Hernon, C., McCurdy, C.R., Boyer, E.W., 2011. Herbal medicines for the management of opioid addiction: Safe and effective alternatives to conventional pharmacotherapy? *CNS Drugs* 25, 999-1007.

Weil, A.T., Davis, W., 1994. *Bufo Alvarius*: A potent hallucinogen of animal origin. *Journal of Ethnopharmacology* 41, 1-8.

A Scientist Looks at the Hippies[I]

▬▬ *Stephen Szára*, MD, DSc [II, III]

I. Report to the Director, SMHRP, NIMH.

II. Chief, Section of Psychopharmacology, Laboratory of Clinical Psychopharmacology, SMHRP, NIMH, Saint Elizabeth's Hospital, Washington, D.C.

PRELIMINARIES

On the suggestion of the Director, SMHRP, NIMH, I agreed to take a visit to the San Francisco (SF), Los Angeles (LA) and New York City (NYC) hippie centers in order to obtain firsthand acquaintance with the "hippie" movement and with the role hallucinogenic drugs play in this psychedelic cult. I was to consult medical, psychological and sociological authorities well acquainted with this cult, as well as obtain personal impressions during the site visits. The main goals were:

1. To check on the validity of sensational newspaper and magazine stories on the "hippie" movement and drug usage associated with it.

2. To formalize scientific hypotheses on the possible biochemical, psychological or social mechanisms involved.

3. To suggest possible lines of approach for research relevant to handling the public health problems associated with this cult.

My credentials include over twenty years of experience in research, discovery of the hallucinogenic activity of a series of tryptamine derivatives (including DMT) and supervision as well as participation in over one hundred administrations of these drugs to volunteer subjects for research purposes.

At first my intention was to contact psychiatrist friends, and through them get acquainted with drug-taking youngsters who came to them for help. But I realized very soon that the psychedelic culture has widespread social and psychological manifestations and the drug usage is only a part, although probably a significant part, of it. To approach it from the psychiatric side would be similar to an attempt by a visiting foreigner to learn about the role of automobiles in American life today by interviewing victims of accidents in the hospitals.

The picture obtained this way would obviously be a lopsided one, ignoring positive aspects, which might perhaps be important. Because of limitations of time, (four days each in San Francisco, Los Angeles and New York City) I decided to meet only a few personal acquaintances in each city (psychiatrists, psychologists and sociologists) and see as many manifestations of the psychedelic

III. Editor's Note: This is a historic document, written in an era when certain norms of expression were accepted, for example the use of gender terms like "man" or "he" in referring to people of all genders. There are other instances of terms and expressions that would not be used in contemporary writing. These are not "errors" in fact, but reflect accepted idiomatic norms in use at the time of writing, and exemplify the "period" character of this work. Therefore, we have not "corrected" them.

culture in each location as possible. In addition, I kept a close watch on the Washington, DC psychedelic scene throughout the summer of 1967.

In the following report, I shall use primarily the observations made on these trips and my personal experience with the hallucinogenic drugs discussed, but I shall also use, whenever it is necessary, the information obtained from interviews with knowledgeable persons and from material published by the Underground Press Syndicate (U.P.S.) collected on my visits to the various "hippie" areas in San Francisco, Los Angeles, New York City and Washington, DC.

My observations and comments are organized around five basic questions about the hippies:

1. Who are they?

2. What are they doing which is of public concern?

3. Where and when are they active?

4. Why are they doing what they are doing?

5. What can or should be done about potential problems?

Finally, as a scientist I shall suggest certain areas of research to be explored if we are to cope with the problems arising from the activities of the hippies.

WHO ARE THE HIPPIES?

Time Magazine gives the etymology of the word "hippie" as deriving "from the pre-World War II jitterbug adjective 'hep': to be with it; hep became 'hip' (in noun form, 'hipster') during the bebop and beatnik era of the 1950's, then fell into disuse, to be revived with the onslaught of psychedelia" (Brown, Time, July 7, 1967).

I did not find a concise definition of a hippie, but a good approximation seems to be *a person who has the subjective feeling of being aware of reality and all that is taking place about him in nature, in life and society, and who is seeking a better world where an ethic of individual freedom, love and personal honesty prevails.*

The definition given above would exclude pseudo-hippies, such as hangers-on who move into a hip community, grow long hair, wear psychedelic garb and identify with the action, but do not have a serious commitment to the hippie ethic or to its social consequences and secretly receive sustenance from their parents, knowing that they can return to their security any time.

The real hippie is an idealist, continually and sincerely reaching for eternal matters of ultimate concern such as love, beauty and liberation, is deeply committed to an enlightened existence and has nothing to escape to. As the outside reflection of his conviction, he grows long hair and a beard, wears psychedelic clothing and joins a hippie community to participate in communal living aimed at the complete realization of these ideals. (A lucid discussion of this "hang-loose ethic" is by Simmons and Winograd, 1966).

The part-time, or "plastic" hippie, who may "drop out" for a night or two each week but would hold onto their job or go to school during the rest of the time might be covered by the given definition if they have the "awareness" and are sincere about the ethical ideas of the hippies, but for some reason they wouldn't join the hippie community full time.

It is my conviction that the use of hallucinogenic drugs like LSD, marijuana, DMT, mescaline and STP are instrumental in producing the subjective feeling of awareness of reality which, in turn, is probably playing an important part in changing the value system of the individual and inducing them to seek a better world by joining the hippie movement. The frequent use of hallucinogenic drugs also creates a number of legal, social and medical problems which will be touched upon later.

H. G. Shane, Professor of Education at Indiana University, calls attention to the variety of groups associated with the "hang-loose" movements (Shane, 1967):

1. Beatniks of the 1950's with a new label and minor changes in garb.

2. A strongly dedicated activist subgroup believing in and seeking social change.

3. A dedicated but more passive group seeking reforms.

4. Some misfits who feel less conspicuous amidst a cluster of people with unconventional beliefs.

5. The "synthetic" hippies who seem to think that psychedelic drugs are just another fad.

6. Racketeering types who, through the sale of drugs and other psychedelic items, prey upon the gullible or maladjusted.

This grouping seems to be related to my proposed categories in the following ways: Groups 1 and 4 are pseudo-hippies, according to my categorization. The second group, partially, and the third group, totally, cover the real hippies. The rebellious "new" leftists, the so-called "peaceniks," are essentially different from the followers of "flower power." The real hippies do seek social change through reform. Group 5 can be considered as a transitory stage between the "plastic" and "real" hippies.

I prefer to call "plastic" those hippies who have taken psychedelic drugs and are open to and aware of the psychedelic message, and who are ready to change their lifestyle if the situation permits. The "real" hippies use the term "plastic" in a derogatory sense to refer to those who lack the stamina and/or courage to give up the affluent life, but occasionally enjoy indulging in what the hippie way of life promises: love, compassion and the taste of the eternal "now," mainly by means of the drug experience. Shane's group 6 consists of an economic stratum composed of real, pseudo and plastic hippies.

The magazines and newspapers stress the almost exclusive white, middle-class origin of the hippie youngsters as opposed to the fairly mixed, integrated "beat" generation of the 1950's. As far as I can tell, the visible hippie population is an integrated community, reflecting the cross section of the area's ethnic population. In San Francisco, I saw quite a few Asian-American descendants among them, while in Los Angeles a proportional number of African-American, and in New York African-American and Puerto Rican hippies, were mingling freely with the white hippies.

WHAT ARE THEY DOING WHICH IS OF PUBLIC CONCERN?

The American sociologist W. I. Thomas set forth a theorem for his professional associates: "If men define situations as real, they are real in their consequences (Thomas and Thomas, 1929)." Time has proven the validity of this theorem and it is clearly applicable to the hippies. If they have the subjective feeling of being aware of certain "truths" about themselves or about the world around them, they will act according to this newly-found "reality" and the consequences of their actions should be regarded as real. Many of these actions do affect other people; therefore, they are of public concern. I shall review here only two types of activities which I have paid close attention to: the drug taking and the artistic activities.

A. DRUG TAKING

The drug taking, which seems to be a central activity by hippies, is clearly of the foremost public concern.

Practically all the drugs they are taking have been declared illegal to manufacture, sell or possess. Many of the problems have actually been created by this illegality, and the evidence is plentiful in the daily press. Besides this, many medical dangers (hepatitis, malnutrition, sexually transmitted infections, upper respiratory infections, possible chromosome damage, etc.), possible psychological dangers (temporary panic reactions known as "bad trips" or "freak-outs," longer-lasting psychotic breakdowns, vivid recurrences of the drug experience long after the acute drug effect has worn off ("flashbacks," permanent personality changes, etc.), and social problems (creation of an isolated subculture, the group activities in public places during "love-ins," association between hippies and "peaceniks," etc.) are related to the drug-taking activity, and many of them are of serious public concern.

Since talking about the drug experience is not illegal, much valuable information can be obtained through direct or indirect personal contacts with drug-taking individuals and from the pamphlets and "Underground" newspapers circulating in the hippie communities.

It is not my purpose to go into a detailed discussion of the drugs, since I reviewed them recently (Szára, 1967), but I would like to authenticate the evidence of widespread illegal drug-taking by the hippies in all the sites I visited.

In the rooms of the "Hippie Clinic" at Haight and Clayton in San Francisco, I saw some 30 to 40 hippies either waiting for medical attention or sleeping off a bad trip. The manager of the clinic explained that they see some 70 to 100 patients a day, but they have difficulties obtaining and retaining the services of the volunteer physicians and nurses. One of the attending pharmacologists,

Dr. Frederick Meyers[1], drops in frequently to supervise the legal drug supply (donated mostly by the pharmaceutical houses themselves) and to pick up samples of illegal drugs submitted by hippies for analysis and purity checks. He stressed the significance of the existence of the clinic as the only link in San Francisco between illicit drug users and the Establishment, in the sense that straight society can keep a finger on the pulse of illegal drug commerce.[2]

MARIJUANA: "POT"

In Berkeley, I met a graduate student who is working on his thesis about the commercial aspects of marijuana (pot, grass, weed) traffic. He has interviewed over 200 students and other marijuana users. The major conclusions of his survey were that marijuana traffic has the typical characteristics of individualized, part-time, small business merchandizing patterns, and in spite of this, the volume of the illegal marijuana trade is tremendous, estimated to be about 10 times as large as the amount seized by the narcotics authorities. In New York City alone, the Narcotics Bureau seized 1,680 pounds of marijuana in 1966. One pound yields as many as 1,000 joints, or cigarettes. The West Coast traffic is even heavier; in California and Arizona during the three summer months of July, August and September 1967, about 16,000 pounds of pot was seized by US Customs authorities (*Washington Post*, November 18, 1967). The price of marijuana depends on the quantity bought and upon the momentary market situation. One kilo (= 2.2 pounds) usually sells between $20-80, which is then retailed usually at $.25 to $1.00 per joint (cigarette).

The use of marijuana does not seem to be limited to 17-25 year olds, but has also spread to younger high school children (13-15 years of age). It is difficult to measure the significance of this. College students can go back to school after a week, month or year of "dropping out," if they have had enough "expansion" of their minds or for some other sobering reasons. But younger high school kids don't go back to school once they drop out; they are lost to society. Dr. William Soskin of the University of California at Berkeley has a group-therapy project exploring the problems these high school children have and in which he tries to lead them back to normal life. He had only four or five boys and girls coming in regularly at the time I visited him, but he would not have had a problem recruiting 100-200 similar young hippies from the San Francisco and Berkeley area.

LSD-25: "ACID"

Lysergic acid diethylamide (LSD-25, or acid) is the second major drug on the hippie scene. While marijuana is widely and frequently used for short-lasting mood manipulation and for its mild hallucinogenic effect, LSD is taken much less frequently (usually more than a week apart if taken regularly) and produces 10 to 16-hour "trips" consisting of profound perceptual and emotional experiences. In the setting it is taken, the major psychological effect seems to be a temporary suspension of the primacy of one's habitual perceptions of the self, environment, beliefs, values and a subjective feeling of freedom, awareness and insight. The bodily changes are the usual pupillary dilation, paresthesia, feeling of floating, etc.

All black-market LSD is produced illegally (the original Sandoz LSD-25 is not available anymore), and there is a wide variation in the quality of "acid" circulating in Hippiedom. "Owsley's Acid" is considered the best-quality material, but after police raids it tends to disappear and be replaced by poorer-quality LSD, often mixed with methedrine or even heroin, as Dr. Meyers of San Francisco explained.[3]

Dr. Sidney Cohen at the V.A. in Los Angeles has no problem recruiting subjects who are regular users of LSD. His project involves testing the subjects for organic brain damage; and they are glad to cooperate in order to find out whether or not any harmful effect has occurred.

Washington Post staff writer Nicholas von Hoffman, who spent three months with the hippies in San Francisco and described his experiences about the "Acid Affair" very vividly in the columns of his newspaper (October 15 through 31, 1967), conservatively estimates the monthly acid market in the Haight area to be 200,000 doses, selling at not less than 50 cents (usually $2.00 to $2.50) apiece.

....

1. Note: Dr. Frederick Meyers was a Bay Area physician and pharmacologist who played a key role in the founding of the Haight Ashbury Free Clinic. (SF Gate, 1998)

2. The clinic has been temporarily closed for about a month due to financial difficulties, but it is open again.

3. Augustus Stanley Owsley III, with four alleged associates, was arrested and an amount of psychedelic drugs (LSD and STP) potentially worth $11 million was seized by federal agents on December 21, 1967 (*New York Times*).

13

METHAMPHETAMINE: "SPEED"

The third major drug in the hippie scene seems to be methamphetamine (methedrine, "meth," "speed"). It is a stimulant which is usually taken intravenously, hence its significance in the incidence of hepatitis. Since it is also an anorectic agent, the lack of food and nourishment leads to avitaminosis, general debility and wasting. The subjective feeling produced by "meth" is distinctly different from that produced by the hallucinogens. The elevation of mood and feeling of well-being comes on very fast (therefore the name "speed"); the feeling induced of tremendous energy has been compared to trying to drive a Ferrari with the gas pedal stuck to the floor all the time. There is no feeling of awareness or insight, just a "coming of power ... this churning cloud of light with sparks shooting off" and "a continuous orgasm without a lover" until the drug effect wears off. A recent *Time* article estimates the "meth" users in San Francisco to be about 4,000 in number (October 27, 1967).

DANGERS OF MAJOR DRUGS QUOTED

All three drugs have been characterized by the WHO Expert Committee on Addiction-Producing Drugs (1966) as:

Moderate or variable psychic dependence.
Absence of physical dependence.
Development of tolerance is practically none in the case of marijuana, slow and considerable in the case of amphetamines, and greatly manifested with LSD, in which it develops rapidly and disappears rapidly.

The dangers of the hallucinogenic drugs LSD and marijuana are described by the same committee as follows:

1. The impairment of judgment can possibly lead to dangerous decisions or an accident.

2. The subjective feeling of increased capability with corresponding failure might lead to psychotic episodes or to development of depression and even suicide.

3. Society is harmed by the economic consequences of the impairment of the individual's social functions.

The dangers of the use of drugs of the amphetamine type are:

1. Facilitates the transition to the physically addicting "hard" narcotics, such as heroin and morphine.

2. Increases the incidence of hepatitis.

3. May lead to malnutrition, avitaminosis and wasting.

4. May precipitate paranoid psychosis (often indistinguishable from schizophrenia).

5. May lead to aggressive and dangerous antisocial behavior.

THE MINOR DRUGS

The other hallucinogenic drugs seem to play a minor role in the whole movement. N, N-dimethyltryptamine (DMT) is available, but is more expensive than LSD. DMT, also called the "businessman's lunchtime psychedelic" because of its short duration of action, is usually smoked in the form of dried parsley leaves soaked with the drug.

It seemed to me to be significant that the grocery store in the small rural community of Topanga Canyon, outside of Los Angeles, had a brisk business in dried parsley leaves at the time I visited.

DMT seems to be accessible in New York also. I received several calls from doctors at Bellevue Hospital requesting information about DMT on occasions of admission of patients with a history of having taken DMT.

In the middle of last summer, about 10,000 doses of a drug called STP were distributed among the West Coast hippies, which created some unusual problems. The drug (identified by the FDA as

4 methyl – 2,5 dimethoxy amphetamine) produced an unusually long effect lasting for 3-4 days, and attempts to "bring down" the subjects with thorazine seemed to aggravate the anxiety rather than to diminish it. The *East Village* Other, the U.P.S. paper for New York hippies, suggested "Tranquinol" as "the new come-down for STP freakouts" (Vol. 2/17, p. 7, August 1-15, 1967).[4]

B. PSYCHEDELIC ART

Another important aspect of the hippie subculture is the close relationship between the drug-produced psychological state and so-called psychedelic art.

This relationship is mutual, in the sense that on the one hand, the drug state seems to inspire many individuals to express their experience in various artistic forms – paintings, drawings, poetry, music, etc.—but on the other hand, many of the products of this "psychedelic" art are used to recreate or facilitate the production of a psychological state similar to the drug-induced state, but without taking drugs.

The importance of this positively reinforcing feedback effect on the social level is nowhere more visible than in the history of the development of the hippie subculture itself, and in the role the popular media, newspapers, magazines, TV, radio and especially rock music groups have played in spreading the psychedelic message and in reinforcing the subjective beliefs of the hippies.

I shall touch upon the history of the hippie subculture a little later, but now I would like to describe my experience in the so-called psychedelic theaters or dance halls.

My first experience of this type was in the Avalon Ballroom in San Francisco on a Sunday evening. The setting seems to be typical for most of the other so-called Total-Environment entertainment places I have visited subsequently, so I am going to describe it in detail.

The ballroom is dimly lit, and has projection screens on three walls around the room. Onto these about a dozen slide projectors project various abstract color patterns inspired by hallucinations experienced under LSD, or faces, or pictures of statues or paintings (usually of a religious character).

Superimposed on these occasionally changing patterns are constantly dancing patterns from six overhead liquid projectors. These project the image from large watch glasses filled with an oil-water mixture, dyed with a non-mixing single color and moved by hand, or squeezed by another watch glass on the surface of the liquid, creating single or multiple amoeba-like images moving and dancing to the rhythm of the music.

In some corners of the screen, still superimposed on the slide-projected images, there is a continuous, repeated projection of a short sequence from an old movie, a Mickey Mouse cartoon or some other, usually sexually suggestive, sequence of animated or real scenes.

As an additional visual stimulus, a flickering strobe light is turned on occasionally, under which the dancing people appear mechanized, their movements as jerky as in old-time movies.

The type of music called "acid rock" is played continuously by two or sometimes three orchestras, alternating with each other. It is called "acid" not only because many of the song lyrics allude to "acid" (LSD) and to "pot," but also because it employs a monotonous, harshly amplified drone-like sound which can act as a psychedelic stimulus. In the midst of a routine rock-and-roll number for instance, the players may focus on a particular pattern which is repeated again and again, louder and louder until the limit of the human eardrum is reached, upon which it suddenly stops.

Only part of the audience is actually dancing on the floors. A large portion of youngsters (mostly teenage girls) are lying in front of the screens and orchestras, practically "stoned" under the barrage of visual and auditory bombardments.

I saw similar arrangements and "happenings" in the "Magic Mushrooms" and "Genesis IX" of Los Angeles, in the "Electric Circus" in New York and in the "Ambassador Theater" in Washington, DC.

More sophisticated and artistic shows suggested by and suggestive of the psychedelic experience are being put together by young artists. I saw one of them at Cinema Discothèque in New York,

---

4. Snyder, Faillace, and Hollister (1967) recently reported that STP is not as active as the hippies reported it to be (the effect of up to 10 mg of STP on volunteers lasted for about 12 hours), and chlorpromazine did not seem to aggravate the psychological effects.

A variety of STP seemed to create other problems in the East Village at the end of August 1967. Posters in hippie shop windows warned:

> "Don't Do Blue STP
> It's Belladonna
> And makes you sick
> Like s..t."

On one of these posters, a P.S. in pencil added, "It's fatal, too."

entitled "After the IIIrd World Raspberry," by Al Rubin. The reference to "pot" by the projected pictures was unmistakable and the audio-visual manipulation was clearly aimed at the reproduction of the perceptual aspects of the psychedelic experience. When it was over (it lasted a little more than one hour), the audience seemed to be stunned. I was the first one to stand up and start walking out. Behind my seat there were two hippie girls sitting in a trance-like state, seemingly unaware that the show was over. It was not unusual to see about half of the audience in a similar reverie for minutes after the show had ended.

I have described these experiences in detail not only because the acid rock music seemed to be an essential part of the hippie scene, but also because it is likely to be the main carrier of the psychedelic message into the future, even if the hippie subculture as we know it today passes. The Beatles turning to Asian mystical meditation and changing their style, adapting Hindu raga music to acid rock, is clearly a sign of searching for new ways of expressing the same message and carrying it into the future. And the audience at these shows are not the typical hippies (they could not afford the whopping [in 1967] $3.50-$4.50 admission fee), but the college and high school kids who can afford it. The significance of this is that they, due to their higher educational development, might be more successful in formulating a convincing social philosophy and integrating the psychedelic experience with ongoing life.

WHERE AND WHEN ARE THE HIPPIES ACTIVE?

It seems to be most convenient to follow the ecological approach in answering these questions together about hippie communities. Human ecology is concerned with the influences of the environment on the structural pattern of a community, and with the forces behind its constant change. It helps to describe the development in space and time of a social movement in terms of five major processes, i.e., concentration, centralization, segregation, invasion and succession.

A. The pleasant climate, permissive atmosphere and local situations were probably important factors in inducing youngsters to concentrate in the Haight-Ashbury area of San Francisco in order to follow Timothy Leary's advice to "tune in, turn on and drop out" and form their own community to pursue these goals. In other cities, it is also possible to point to an already existing artistic or bohemian district to serve as points of concentration. Hollywood in the LA area, Greenwich Village in New York and the Georgetown area in Washington, DC clearly provide this type of permissive social climate.

B. The second process is centralization, i.e., the tendency to form a "Main Street" or perhaps several central areas, and this is clearly visible in all the places I visited.

- Haight Street in San Francisco, California
- Telegraph Avenue in Berkeley, California
- Sunset Strip in Hollywood, California
- N. Fairfax Avenue in Los Angeles, California
- St. Mark's Plaza in East Village, New York
- McDougal Street in West Village, New York
- "M" Street in Georgetown, Washington, DC
- DuPont Circle in Washington, DC

These are the focal points where the "action" takes place in psychedelic shops, coffee houses, print and button shops, psychedelic theaters and "meditation rooms." The action consists of meeting other hippies, buying or selling marijuana and other drugs, finding a pad where drugs can be taken undisturbed and, in general, participating in the activities of the hippies' subculture.

C. Segregation is the third process and it is not along racial lines, but is rather determined by the hippie's age, educational background and type of drug preferred.

- The Haight-Ashbury hippies clearly segregate themselves from the high school-age teeny-boppers from Berkeley.
- The N. Fairfax Avenue hippies in LA do not mix with the lower educational-level, hard narcotic user, homosexual hippies (pseudo-hippies) from the Sunset Strip area.

- The St. Mark's Plaza-area hippies in New York seemed to be the more committed, genuine types, while the West Village hippies were mostly the pseudo- or plastic-type, engaged more in exploiting the busy tourist business than pursuing an enlightened hippie existence.

D. The fourth process, invasion, is the tendency of a socio-economic group, usually of lower status, to move into the territory occupied by another. The attempts of gangster-type elements to move in and disrupt the hippie community could probably be considered such an invasion. The signs of this were the flooding of the black market with LSD and methedrine mixed with heroin in an obvious attempt to "hook" hippies on hard narcotics (Dr. Meyers), and the murders of a hippie called "Superspade" in San Francisco in the summer, and Linda Rea Fitzpatrick and James (Groovy) Hutchinson in New York's East Village hippieland in the fall of 1967.

E. An obvious and visible result of this invasion is the process of succession, as the original inhabitants of the areas are completely displaced by another type of group.

This process seemed to be in the making as news came about the symbolic "Funeral of the Hippie" in San Francisco's Golden Gate Park on October 6, 1967. A gray casket labeled "Summer of Love" and filled with beads, charms, peacock feathers, bread, flags, crucifixes and a marijuana-flavored cookie was set on fire as a shout went up: "Hippies are dead; now the Free Man will come through" (*Time*, October 13, 1967).

The hippie population, at least as of this writing (November, 1967), seems to be gradually disappearing from the center scenes. The pseudo-hippies went back to their parents and to school, and the plastic hippies went back to work or to study, but the real hippies, especially the artistic types, have begun to move out since the middle of the summer to the countryside to establish hippie communities in Marin, Sonoma and Mendocino Counties to the north and Big Sur to the south in California, and to the Santa Fe area in New Mexico, as well as to other areas of the country.

Other hippies, the "searchers," have started to establish their own psychedelic churches, partly as a means of keeping the movement alive, but mainly to avoid legal problems by declaring the psychedelic drugs to be sacraments. As of this writing, there are at least seven such groups: The League for Spiritual Discovery, Kerists, The Water Brothers, The Neo-American Church, The Church of the Awakening and the oldest of all in America, the Native American Church. The seventh was established by hippies who have moved to Kathmandu, Nepal (newspaper and magazine sources).

WHY ARE THEY DOING WHAT THEY ARE DOING?

It seems that there are as many answers to this question as there are subgroups or even individuals in the hippie movement. I would like to offer only some random psychological and philosophical notes on the origin of the hippie.

The hippie's crucial claim of greater "awareness of reality and all that is taking place about him in nature, in life and society" after a "transcendental" experience with LSD or the other psychedelic drugs brings up the validity of their awareness in relation to the generally-accepted concepts of "reality."

The definition and meaning of objective reality has been a major epistemological controversy for many philosophical schools from Descartes through Kant, Bergson, Berkeley, James and others to Whitehead, Carnap and today's existentialists.

For science, however, the most general definition of reality is that "it is the universe of discourse of a conceptual system that serves to correlate and predict, deterministically or statistically, the data of experience" (Lenzen, 1956).

The development of this scientific concept of objective reality is a long way from the "blooming, buzzing confusion" of the sense perception of a newborn by means of a long learning process to separate it from the subjective realities of dreams, visions, play and aesthetic realities which are mingled with objective realities in childhood and in primitive cultures (James, 1950; Piaget, 1959; Werner, 1961).

It has been borne out from several studies that LSD and similar drugs produce a regression of mental functioning to a primitive, childlike level, and I would like to examine some notions about the role of this naive thinking in the hippie movement.

Primitive thinking has been characterized as subjective, concrete and diffuse (Werner, 1961). I would like to elaborate on the concrete as opposed to the abstract of this type of thinking, because I feel it is very crucial in the immediate and perhaps lasting action of psychedelic drugs used so widely by the hippies.

Concrete reality is the three-dimensional outside world with which we are in contact through our five senses. We, as human beings, have learned to cope with this concrete reality by forming concepts and communicating with each other by a written or spoken system of symbols which constitute a language.

Thus, man created a conceptual world, which helped him to conquer nature, to fight his enemies, to search for happiness, and to discover the laws of nature, the nature of his fellow beings and of himself. Language, thereby, has become his second and foremost reality (Cassirer, 1955; Langer, 1948).

At the same time, language acts as a socially conditioned filter, meaning that experience can enter into awareness only if it can penetrate the filter of language, logic and the socially conditioned content of experience (Fromm, 1960).

It is interesting to speculate on how this development from concrete to abstract has occurred, and how much of a role the ubiquitous physiological process of habituation plays in decreasing our awareness of three-dimensional concrete reality to the point where we perceive it only to the extent it fits into our abstract world of concepts and socially accepted norms.

Habituation is a very general phenomenon in the biological world and refers to the decreased responsiveness of the organism to monotonously repeated stimuli if they are not rewarded (Jasper, 1966).

Since this perception of the concrete world is rewarded (reinforced) primarily through our thinking process, which is entirely in the conceptual sphere of reality, the first will be habituated (suppressed until we become unresponsive to it) and the abstract conceptual world becomes our main reality.

Science and philosophy have evolved during our struggle for survival into our foremost abstract reality, comprising the organized set of laws, values and formal solutions to recurrent problems which probably has a very practical purpose: It shows us the way to act in order to decrease our anxiety. Art, religion and love have remained in our lives as the main links to concrete, three-dimensional reality, giving us delight, spiritual lift and happiness.

There seems to be ample evidence that psychedelic drugs block the process of habituation, making even repeated stimuli appear to have special significance and meaning to the user.

At the animal level, Key and Bradley have shown this with LSD rather conclusively (1960). At the human level, we can quote a series of observers, professional and otherwise:

> During the drug state, awareness becomes intensely vivid while self-control over input is remarkably diminished; customary boundaries become fluid and the familiar becomes novel and portentous. Events take on a trajectory of their own; qualities become intense and gain a life of their own; redness is more interesting than what is specifically meant; connotations balloon into cosmic allusiveness; the limits of sobriety are lost. The very definition of the importance of the external world shifts when most mental activity is absorbed either in monitoring the novelty of experience or in maintaining the integrity of the self. (Freedman, 1967)

> The effect of LSD ... was ... to remove certain habitual and normal inhibitions of the mind and senses, enabling us to see things as they would appear to us if we were not so chronically repressed. Little is known of the exact neurological effects of LSD, but what is known suggests that latter possibility." (Watts, 1967)

The same author, talking about "cosmic consciousness," notes:

> All that I have been describing is a subjective feeling. It gives no specific direction as to what is or is not a proper use of intelligence in varying the course of nature which must always be a matter of opinion and of trial and error. What it does give is what I feel to be a correct apprehension of the continuum, of the context, in which we are working, and this seems to me to be prior to, basic to, the problem of what exactly is to be done. Much as we discuss the latter question, is it really sensible to do so until we are more aware of the context in which action is to be taken? That context is our relationship to the whole so-called objective world of nature—and relationship as something concrete, as more than an abstract and theoretical positioning of billiard balls, is practically screened out of consciousness by our present use of intelligence." (Watts, ibid)

An hour and a half after taking mescaline, Aldous Huxley (1954) found himself looking intently at a small glass vase:

> The vase contained only three flowers – a full-blown Belle of Portugal rose, shell pink with a tint at every petal's base of a hotter, flamier hue; a large magenta and cream-colored carnation; and, pale purple at the end of its broken stalk, the bold heraldic blossom of an iris. Fortuitous and provisional, the little nosegay broke all the rules of traditional good taste. At breakfast that morning I had been struck by the lively dissonance of its colors. But that was no longer the point. I was not looking now at an unusual flower arrangement, I was seeing what Adam had seen on the morning of his creation – the miracle, moment by moment, of naked existence ... My eyes travelled from the rose to the carnation, and from that feathery incandescence to the smooth scrolls of sentient amethyst which were the iris. The Beatific Vision, Sat Chit Ananda, Being-Awareness-Bliss – for the first time I understood, not on the verbal level, not by inchoate hints or at a distance, but precisely and completely what those prodigious syllables referred to." (Huxley, ibid)

When college kids read and hear reports like the ones quoted above, no wonder they sincerely feel they should confront an experience advertised to be so important. Some of them see the drug as an emotional fitness test, somewhat analogous to physical fitness. A "need to feel" – to gain access to themselves and others – and a pervasive sense of being constricted seems to characterize some of the college takers of LSD whom Dr. D. X. Freedman studied.

Anyone who has experienced this intense episode must come to deal with it, to integrate it somehow into the normal fabric of living. Some will borrow stability from ready-made explanations. Others will isolate the experience or set it aside in an attempt to master it, but they may end up with various pathological symptoms of a traumatic neurosis, delayed panic, depression or anxiety and be finally forced to seek professional help.

However, quite a few do not isolate the experience, but do search for synthesis either in various self-help groups, which appear to be peer groups, or in various religion-oriented groups which use the psychedelic drugs as sacraments.

In the hippie movement, there are quite a few self-help groups and religious groups which seem to fill the need for synthesis with more or less success. It is illuminating to read Dr. William McGlothlin's comments on the role psychedelic drugs and certain social forces played in the development of the hippie movement:

> The reason why the hippie movement has had such a sudden spurt in the last few months is that it has reached the point (particularly in California) where the subculture provides effective reinforcement of the drug-induced alterations of beliefs and values. The LSD trip provides a common ground on the experiential level which serves as the unifying principle for hippie communities, and for thousands of otherwise strangers at hippie gatherings. In turn, the subculture both suggests and sustains the new beliefs, and acts as a buffer against the faith-eroding forces of the dominant culture. The advent of large-scale communities and gatherings has turned the phenomenon of isolated drug use into a full-fledged, self-reinforcing movement." (McGlothlin, 1967)

WHAT CAN OR SHOULD BE DONE ABOUT POTENTIAL PROBLEMS?

Several possibilities seem to be open:

A. Ignore them. Every century and every land has had its hippies, but by different names. There have always been way-out non-conformists, whirling dervishes, bohemians and beatniks living on the fringes of society, and they constitute but a very small fraction of the population.

But we cannot easily ignore today's hippies for at least four reasons:

1. There is a segment of the hippie society which is clearly visible because of their unorthodox clothing and behavior, and because they often manage to stir up headlines

(c.f. the recent Dame Margot – Nureyev – affair in San Francisco)[5]. Although they are peaceful, they are very much in evidence in most of our great cities.

2. The visible segment – like that of an iceberg – is only a small portion of the large-city college and even high-school students (the estimates vary between 10% and 35%) who have experimented with psychedelic drugs. Only a few of them have joined the ranks of the openly defiant hippies. The parents seem to have a certain feeling of guilt and continue supporting them.

3. The drug usage leads very often to medical and psychiatric emergencies which cannot be ignored by society.

   Major emergencies are:
   - Spread of venereal diseases.
   - Frequent "freakouts," or bad trips.

   Minor in number but still serious emergencies are:
   - Hepatitis from the use of unclean needles for injecting amphetamine-type drugs.
   - Turning to "hard" narcotics (heroin).
   - Occasionally longer-lasting psychotic reactions requiring hospitalization.

4. The usage of drugs might contribute to criminal negligence, e.g., driving an automobile under this influence. The gross distortion of perception may lead to accidents which would add to the already high rate of traffic fatalities.

B. There are several possibilities at the legal level which could be pursued to face the problems drug abuse by hippies creates, but it is not my duty to comment on these here.

C. More research is needed along the following lines if society is to meet the challenge of the hippies:

1. The uncontrolled use of drugs creates medical problems. More research is needed in toxicology and into the mechanisms of psychotropic drug action at the basic biochemical, physiological and psychological levels. Particularly promising would be the exploration of the biochemical and physiological mechanisms for the process of habituation, which may be specifically affected by the drugs used and could be the basis for the observed behavioral and psychological phenomena.

2. Research into the mechanisms of non-drug means by which people are being turned on. The induction of a trance-like state akin to hypnosis, apparently by "driving" subcortical structures with rhythmic sensory stimuli, may be a reflection of an effect upon the abovementioned habituation mechanism. There are potential medical dangers to which people should be alerted, for instance, deafness (due to the high volume of music) and psychological damage via distorted perception, etc.

3. Research in social psychology on the significance of changes in personality, changes in value systems and their role in making adjustments to the existing social order.

OUTLOOK

Since hippies are a minority of the younger generation and are peaceful non-militants who do not want to overthrow the government but want to change its value system, they represent no immediate threat to society. They are mostly young, defiant members of the mainstream middle class society; and where there is serious concern, it is at the individual level.

Drug taking is a basic part of the hippie movement; consequently, there should be serious concern about the medical, psychiatric and possible genetic dangers which may result from careless

---

5. Editor's Note: This refers to an incident that took place in San Francisco in 1967 in which the famous ballet dancers, Rudolf Nureyev and Dame Margot Fonteyn, got 'caught up' in a hippie party-cum-riot outside the War Memorial Opera House following a performance of Romeo and Juliet. The incident was humorously recounted in the *San Francisco Chronicle* in April, 2016: The Great Haight Ballet Bust of 1967, authored by Bill Van Niekerken, library director of the *San Francisco Chronicle*. http://www.sfchronicle.com/thetake/article/The-great-Haight-ballet-bust-of-1967-7230386.php#photo-9749248

drug usage. The obvious medical dangers will only slowly penetrate this subculture because of its deliberate isolation from the dominant culture and the essentially irrational mode of their thinking. It will take some time until the biological and economic necessities of life will force them to integrate into the mainstream of society. Nevertheless, a subtle, almost imperceptible change does seem to result from even occasional drug taking, which may have some significance.

One of the results of drugs like LSD is that a tremendous array of possibilities present themselves, which first overwhelm the subject and give a powerful subjective feeling of freedom in terms of choices available. Since most of these possibilities have been suppressed by the traditions of culture, it is understandable that an impatience with traditional ways and values arises and a revolutionary, rebellious attitude emerges. However, a sober re-evaluation of the potential damage versus the potential gain after the drug wears off could convince many of the subjects about the time-proven wisdom of tradition and convince them to return to the fold of society.

A long way lies ahead in creating and disseminating information through research and education before intelligent decisions can be assured at the individual level. In the meantime, the widespread illegal and mostly uncontrolled use of psychedelic drugs creates some non-medical problems as well. A subtle rearrangement of the subjective value system of these young people might remain, and might play a part in future decision-making affecting both the individuals and the society.

It is within this changing system of values where the impact of the drug movement can best be seen, and it is very hard to predict the effects this change may have on the final outcome of the hippie movement itself and on the future of our established society.

ACKNOWLEDGEMENTS

The help of Christopher and Jeanne Szára in editing and formatting this manuscript is gratefully acknowledged.

REFERENCES

Brown, J. D. (Ed.), 1967. *The Hippies*. Time, Inc.

Cassirer, E., 1955. *The Philosophy of Symbolic Forms*, Vol. 2. Yale University Press, New Haven.

Freedman, D. X., 1967. Perspectives on the use and abuse of psychedelic drugs, in: *Ethnopharmacologic Search for Psychoactive Drugs*, Efron, D. H. (Ed.), PHS Publication, 77.

Fromm, E., 1960. *Psychoanalysis and Zen Buddhism*. Harper, New York.

Huxley, A., 1954. *The Doors of Perception*. Harper and Brothers, New York.

James, W., 1950. *The Principles of Psychology*. Dover Publications, New York.

Jasper, H. H., 1966. Pathophysiological studies of brain mechanisms in different states of consciousness, in: *Brain and Conscious Experience*, Eccles, J. C. (Ed.), Springer, New York, 256-282.

Key, B. J., Bradley, P. B., 1960. The effect of drugs on conditioning and habituation to arousal stimuli in animals. *Psychopharmacologia* 1, 450-462.

Langer, S., 1948. *Philosophy in a New Key*. Mentor Paperback, New York.

Lenzen, V. F., 1956. Philosophy of science, in: *Living Schools of Philosophy*, Runes, D. D. (Ed.), Littlefield, Adams Co., Ames, Iowa, 94.

McGlothlin, W. H., 1967. *Hippies and Early Christianity*. Unpublished manuscript.

Piaget, J., 1959. *The Language and Thought of the Child*. Humanities Press, New York.

San Francisco Chronicle, April 6 2016. The Great Haight Ballet Bust of 1967. http://www.sfchronicle.com/thetake/article/The-great-Haight-ballet-bust-of-1967-7230386.php#photo-9749248 (accessed 09/06/2017)

SF Gate, November 17 1998. Obituary for Frederick Meyers. http://www.sfgate.com/news/article/Frederick-Meyers-2978524.php. Accessed 09/06/2017

Shane, H. G., November 1967. Letter to the Editor. *NEA Journal* 56, 6.

Simmons, J. L., Winograd, B., 1966. *It's Happening*. McNally and Loftin, Santa Barbara.

Snyder, S.L, et al. 1967. 2,5-dimethoxy-4-methyl-amphetamine (STP): A new hallucinogenic drug. *Science* 158, 669-670.

Szára, S., 1967. Hallucinogenic drugs – curse or blessing? *Am. J. Psychiatry* 123, 1513.

Thomas, W. I., Thomas, D., 1929. *The Child in America*, 2nd ed. Alfred Knopf, 572.

WHO expert committee on addiction-producing drugs, 1966. *Psychopharmacology Bulletin* 3 (3).

Watts, A. W., 1967. *This is It*. Collier Books Edition, MacMillan Company, New York.

Werner, H., 1961. *Comparative Psychology of Mental Development*. Science Editions, New York.

AYAHUASCA & THE AMAZON

Ayahuasca: A Powerful Epistemological Wildcard In a Complex, Fascinating and Dangerous World

■ *Luis Eduardo Luna,* PhD ■

Wasiwaska Research
Center for the Study
of Psychointegrator
Plants, Visionary Art and
Consciousness
Florianópolis, Brazil

INTRODUCTION

Yagé and *ayahuasca* are the best-known preparations made of *Banisteriopsis caapi* Spruce ex. Griseb (Morton), a giant Malpighiaceous vine, which in the wild can climb through the forest up to 40 meters or more. It flowers in the canopy among other climbers and epiphytes. The terms *yagé* and *ayahuasca* are used to refer both to the preparations and to the *Banisteriopsis* vine itself. *Yagé* is made by adding the leaves of another Malpighiaceous vine, *Diplopterys cabrerana* (Cuatrecasas) B. Gates. This combination is used in the Colombian and Ecuadorian Amazon. *Ayahuasca* is prepared by adding the leaves of *Psychotria viridis* Ruiz & Pav., of the coffee family (Rubiaceae), to *B. caapi*, and is used in the Peruvian, Brazilian, Bolivian and Ecuadorian Amazon, where it coexists with *yagé*. In fact, indigenous and *mestizo* practitioners consider *P. viridis* the principal ingredient, with the other plants such as tobacco being possible additions. Some indigenous groups use the vine by itself. Anthropologists working in various areas of the Amazon have reported myths of origin of this plant, but not of the admixture plants (cf. Luna & White, 2016), probably indicating that the use of *Banisteriopsis caapi* alone is the most ancient one. In some areas, the vine is used as a tool to learn the properties of other plants, or 'to get to know their spirits' (Bristol, 1965; Luna, 1984). Indigenous and *mestizo* practitioners also recognize several "kinds" of the main vine, using taxonomic distinctions not yet studied by Western ethnobotanists.

This chapter is mainly focused on *ayahuasca*, although the preparation has to be understood within a much larger historical context of South American visionary plant knowledge and experimentation. Constantino Manuel Torres presents convincing evidence for this in his chapter in this book. It is also important to take into account that the pre-Columbian Amazon had larger populations than was previously thought, organized in great part through societal networks of diverse complexity, with extraordinary plant and soil knowledge (Heckenberger & Góes Neves 2009; Erikson 2014). Amazonians were the creators of *terra preta*, the extremely rich, charcoal-based, anthropogenic soils found in many areas. Contrary to other civilizations, Amazonians actually improved their environment, probably contributing to its biological diversity (cf. Tindall, Apffel-Marglin & Shearer, 2017).

During the last three to four decades, *ayahuasca* has moved from being almost hidden among indigenous and *mestizo* healing rituals to becoming the central player in a burgeoning number of religious, spiritual and therapeutic centers with worldwide distribution (cf. Labate & Jungaberle 2011). Few who take it remain indifferent to it, provided that the setting is safe, that the brew is well prepared and that enough of it is ingested. This explains the attention *ayahuasca* is getting in the media, the many popular and scientific publications and the conferences and symposia in full or part dedicated to this preparation. *Ayahuasca* is also embedded within a larger contemporary resurgence of interest in plants, fungi and substances that possess remarkable effects on human cognition. Depending on one's own cosmology, *ayahuasca* may be conceived as an intelligent entity, a gift of nature conveying messages from the biosphere, a portal to spiritual dimensions, or an agent of cognitive shamanic transformation. It is at least a complex alkaloid cocktail with extraordinary physiological, perceptual, emotional and cognitive properties, an astonishing tool for the study of the human mind-body connection. The phenomenology of the *ayahuasca* experience, similar to other psychedelic agents, challenges our ideas of identity, consciousness and reality itself. For some, it amounts to revelations of dormant unsuspected visionary worlds. For others, it may elicit significant insights, bring vivid memories, enhance perception or improve performance. Some may find resolution to mental or physical ailments, yet others may plunge into confusion – particularly if it is taken under poor guidance – or succumb to narcissistic behavior. The experiences may reinforce one's beliefs or shatter them. They may intensify the feeling of awe at the mystery of temporality, or may be rendered nearly ineffective due to repetition and dogma. *Ayahuasca* experiences may also increase fully-sensed body-and-mind awareness of the current perils of environmental destruction, nuclear disaster and social turmoil.

GLOBALIZATION OF AYAHUASCA: POINTS OF DISPERSION

There have been two main areas of dispersion of *ayahuasca*: the Peruvian Amazon, especially around the cities of Iquitos, Pucallpa, Tarapoto and Lamas, in the so-called vegetalista tradition (Chevalier, 1982; Luna, 1984ab, 1986, 2011; Beyer, 2009; Barbira-Freedman, 2014); and the Amazonian states of Acre and Rondônia in Brazil, where highly syncretic religious organizations, created by leaders originally from the Brazilian Northeast, adopted *ayahuasca* as a sacrament. A third, less well-known point of dispersion has been the Putumayo area in southern Colombia. Indigenous practitioners of various ethnic groups (Kamentsá, Inganos, Siona, Kofán, Coreguaje) at some point started to travel and work as healers among the *mestizo* and white population via the Sibundoy Valley and the city of Pasto.

My own discovery of *yagé* is linked to this tradition. Apolinar Yacanamijoy, an Ingano originally from the Putumayo, moved to Yurayaco, about sixty kilometers from Florencia, the capital of the Department of Caquetá in the Colombian Amazon, where I was born. As he used to go to the city from time to time, I had seen him since my childhood. In 1971, when on holiday in Colombia after an absence of seven years in Spain and Norway, I met Terence McKenna and his partner at that time, Erica Nietfeld, both Americans. Through Hans Herbert Mosler, a German citizen who had a restaurant in town, we met Kálmán Zsabó, whom we all called "Carlos," a Hungarian living in the Colombian Amazon. He was in contact with Don Apolinar, who gave him some *yagé*. The four of us took it in my family's humble country house (cf. Luna, 2016).[1] This meeting was one of the early stages of the globalization of *yagé/ayahuasca*.

Peruvian psychologists and psychiatrists had written about *ayahuasqueros* operating in the Amazon region of their country, but their work was not translated into English and thus had little international impact (Del Castillo, 1982; Chiappe & Costa, 1979; Lemlij & Millones Santa Gadea, 1985). American anthropologist Marlene Dobkin de Rios wrote about *mestizo* practitioners living in Iquitos (1970ab, 1971ab, 1972, 1973), but her early work remained mostly confined to anthropological circles. Something similar happened with my own early work (Luna 1984, 1986) until 1991, when *Ayahuasca Visions: The Religious Iconography of a Peruvian Shaman*, which I co-authored with Peruvian painter and former *vegetalista* Pablo Amaringo, was published. Some researchers claim that this book is largely responsible for the initial international surge in interest in *ayahuasca* (Beyer, 2012; McKenna, 2013), and the subsequent flow of foreigners to the Peruvian Amazon.[2] Amaringo's paintings were presented in the book within a cultural context that included the basic Amazonian ideas of diet and isolation in order to "learn from the plants," which became part of the subsequent assimilation of *ayahuasca* by Westerners.

....

1. I wish to express here my gratitude to Mr. Mosler, still living in Caquetá, who provided me with Carlos' full name. He also mentioned Frans Wolloch, another Hungarian interested in *yagé* at that time. According to Mr. Mosler, he had been with the Hungarian Olympic team in Berlin in 1936, escaping as a refugee when the games were over. Both Hungarians are now deceased.

2. I am referring here only to the anthropological literature concerning *mestizo vegetalismo*. There were, of course, publications of anthropologists working with indigenous groups using *yagé* or *ayahuasca*, such as the Tukano (Reichel-Dolmatoff, 1970, 1972, 1975,1978), the Yagua (Chaumeil, 1983), the Siona (Langdon, 1979ab), the Kofán (Robinson, 1976), the Matsigenka (Baer, 1984), the Aguaruna (Brown, 1978), etc.

The second most important point of dispersion of *ayahuasca* is located in the Brazilian Amazon. Three religious leaders who arrived in this area from the Brazilian Northeast created syncretic Brazilian religious organizations in which *ayahuasca* was incorporated as a sacrament. Raimundo Irineu Serra (1892–1971) in the thirties, and Daniel Pereira de Matos (1904– 1958) in the forties, created in Rio Branco, the capital of the State of Acre, organizations that called the brew *Santo Daime*. José Gabriel da Costa (1922–1971) created in the sixties, in Porto Velho, capital of the State of Rondônia, the UDV (*União do Vegetal*). He called *ayahuasca Vegetal*, a term that shows its link to the Peruvian *vegetalista* tradition.

These religions present an amalgam of elements from various traditions. Afro-Brazilian components are particularly evident in the religions created by the first two leaders, especially in the case of Daniel Pereira de Matos, who created a *Barquinha* (the small boat), a new religious organization mostly restricted to the State of Acre. He was heavily influenced by *candoblé* and *umbanda*, Afro-Brazilian religions with mediums that incorporate entities: *pretos velhos* (spirits of black slaves), *caboclos* (Indians), *erés* (children), and *encantados* (princes and princesses incarnated in plants and animals). Popular Catholicism is also a very important element, with the profusion of images of Jesus, Mary and various saints, and the recitation of hymns and prayers. In the case of José Gabriel da Costa, who created the UDV (*União do Vegetal*), Afro-Brazilian elements as well as those from popular Catholicism have been eliminated. All of these religions have been influenced by *kardecism*, a religion based on the books of French spiritualist Alan Kardec (born Léon Denizarth Hippolyte Rivail) (1804–1869), and also by various organizations linked to European esoteric traditions cultivating meditation and telepathy. All of these religions believe in reincarnation. Amazonian elements, apart from the use of *ayahuasca*, are minimal. The standing of Amerindians in the church's understanding of its history is either practically ignored or, in the case of the UDV, relegated to an inferior position in its mythology. Dancing is a prominent element in some of the rituals of the organizations that use *Santo Daime*. This is not so at all in the UDV, in which "the power of the word," the oral discourse of the religious leader under the effects of *Vegetal*, has predominance. In terms of organization, regarding those using *Santo Daime*, political power is based on the charisma of their leaders, with the succession going to their kin, while in the UDV, leadership is elected. The UDV is organized across a four-tier hierarchical structure, the upper level not accessible to women.

Disagreement about secession arose after the death of Irineu Serra, resulting in a split and the formation of a new congregation led by Sebastião Mota de Melo (1920–1990). This is the branch of *Santo Daime* that has expanded most, with communities in Europe, North and South America and Japan. The UDV is also present in many countries worldwide. According to Alex Polari, one of the main leaders of the branch that follows the doctrine of Sebastião Mota, there are now around 10,000 members drinking *Santo Daime*, not including transient participants that take the brew here and there (personal communication). Without having access to clear data, he believes that the members of the UDV should be around twice this number.

The third most important point of dispersion of the *Banisteriopsis* complex is linked to the healing activities of various indigenous practitioners, or *taitas*[3], of the Putumayo-Caquetá in the Colombian Amazon. They worked first among the lower classes of the Putumayo and other areas, and from the nineties also among educated middle-high-class people, especially university students of the city of Pasto (capital of the Department of Nariño) and other Colombian cities. White and *mestizo* practitioners initiated by indigenous shamans, such as Pacho Francisco Piaguaje (Siona) and Martín Agreda (Kamentsá), created *malocas* near Pasto in which a growing number of Colombians as well as foreigners participate in rituals, some heavily influenced by Catholicism, but stressing always their indigenous roots (cf. Pinzón & Suárez, 1991; Taussig, 1987; Weiskopf, 2004; Caicedo Fernández, 2014).

Engineer and prominent politician Antonio José Navarro Wolf, Governor of Nariño during 2008-2011 and currently a senator, took *yagé* with *taita* Querubín Queta Alvarado (Kofán). One of the results of his experience was the motivation to organize in 2009 the First International Encounter of Andean Cultures, with the active participation of numerous representatives of various ethnic groups. This was dedicated in great part to Amerindian traditional medicine, including the use of *yagé*. Well-publicized subsequent meetings took place in 2010, 2011 and 2014, all with the presence of *taitas* and shamans from various countries, as well as high-ranking official representatives. The program included not only academic presentations and exhibitions, but also ceremonies with *yagé*, *yopo* (*Anadenanthera peregrina* (L.) Speg.), *peyote* and sweat lodges, or *temazcals*, from North American indigenous traditions.

----

3. A Spanish colloquial term meaning 'Dad' or 'uncle'. A term of respect and endearment.

AMAZONIAN ANIMISM AND EVOLUTIONARY COGNITION: AN APPROACH TO CLOSING AN EPISTEMOLOGICAL GAP?

In Amerindian cosmology from Alaska to Tierra del Fuego, and especially in Amazonian cultures, humans are not the only persons on this planet. They share personhood with certain animals, plants and non-living objects and processes (winds, whirlpools, etc.) endowed with intention, volition and therefore subjectivity. Humans are not unique or special: They have to establish complex social relationships with other subjects, such as the master of animals, the master of fish, the master of the plants in a garden, or the "soul" of any particular species. There is therefore no clear distinction between nature ("out there") and culture, the world of the human and their institutions and symbols. Moreover, these subjectivities see themselves as human, appearing to us – or to other species – in their animal (or *vegetal*) clothes. At the same time, they see us as animals (predators or prey). Eduardo Viveiro de Castro (2005) calls this "perspectivism," which includes the idea that non-humans see their world as humans see their own world. Instead of multiculturalism, Amerindians would think in terms of multinaturalism.

A shaman has a special relationship with non-human entities: he/she is able to perceive them as they perceive themselves, as anthropomorphic. He/she is even able to transform into one of them, for instance a jaguar, an idea found not only in the Amazon, but also in the whole of Central and South America (Reichel-Dolmatoff, 1975; Stone, 2011). In mythic time, all animals were humans. The process of speciation was a process away from humanity, although the humanity of plants and animals is still perceptible through certain epistemological techniques – that is, through trance, dreams or illness. If, from the point of view of evolutionary biology, humans share with animals their animality, in Amerindian thought animals share with us their *humanity* (Viveiro de Castro, 2005). This is a radically different way of dealing with other species: Amazonian hunters, for example, often refer to their prey as "brother" or being other kin, and their relationship with the animals they hunt is one of respect (Descola, 2005). The disruption of the life-energy flow for no reason is a transgression: Killing an animal and not eating it, or cutting a tree and not using it, may result in illness (cf. Reichel-Dolmatoff, 1971, 1976).

Form seems to be fluid in Amazonian thought. A certain animal may appear as another one; it may take "different clothing" to deceive humans or other animals. A forest spirit may take the shape of a hunter's relative to attract him and trick him into getting lost. As Evgenia Fotiou points out in her chapter in this book, plants are taken to imbue the body with certain properties, to "construct" the body. Plants are taken to strengthen and refine perception, and to transfer to the body certain qualities from non-human persons. Shepard (2011), for example, reports that the Matsigenka take a certain mushroom-infected *Cyperus* to transfer to the hunter the predatory abilities of a harpy eagle (chemicals in the fungi may have physiological effects, such as giving the hunter sharper vision, or other properties). Fotiou gives other relevant examples in her chapter in this book. Don Emilio Andrade Gómez, my *mestizo ayahuasquero* teacher, said that *ayahuasca* is among the plants one should take in order to become strong, *para ser fuertes y mantener la mente despejada* ("to be strong and keep the mind clear"). Another expression often used by *ayahuasqueros* is to *limpiar y cerrar el cuerpo* ("cleanse and protect the body"), so that no illness gets through. Interestingly, a physical and visual motif many people report is that of being "scanned" with invisible hands, and of spirits, small serpents or other animals going through the body, stopping at specific parts and taking away illnesses. In the Amazon, dieting with plants, often in isolation, is equivalent to getting allies, to maintain a strong body and mind and to be able to learn from them through songs that need to be sung perfectly in order to later use them in healing ceremonies. For practitioners this is especially important, given that illness is believed to always be caused by an agent – be it human or spiritual. Healing requires either a confrontation with this agent or an arduous inner journey to restore the soul(s) of his/her patient.

In some cases, the invocation of plants and animals would suffice for this transferral. A shaman may summon an armadillo to transfer the strength of its legs to a child having difficulties with starting to walk; slippery animals or plants may be called to transfer this quality to a woman giving birth (Luna, 1992). Claude Lévi-Strauss, in his analysis of an indigenous ritual, attributes the efficacy of healing to a *psychological manipulation* of the symbols, an *inductive property* by which "formally homologous structures, built out of different materials at different levels of life – organic processes, unconscious mind, rational thought – are related to one another. Poetic metaphor provides a familiar example of this inductive process, but as a rule it does not transcend the unconscious level. Thus, we note the significance of Rimbaud's intuition that metaphor can change the world" (Lévi-Strauss, 1949:225).

Western science tries to totally disengage the subject from the object he is studying, even when that object is his own brain. The Amerindian way is to approach the subjectivity of the object, even identifying or transforming (cognitively) into it (the basis of shamanism). The idea that *ayahuasca*, other plants (especially large trees like the giant *Ceiba*) and animals are sentient is found in the three main areas of diffusion of *ayahuasca*. In the Peruvian Amazon, where I conducted fieldwork in the early eighties, animistic ideas are very much present (Luna, 1982, 1984, 1986). Don José Coral, another one of my teachers, pointed one day at the bubbles boiling on the surface of the *ayahuasca* being cooked. He said to me: "These are people." One may hear practitioners asserting: "The plants are our university." I found similar ideas in the Sibundoy Valley, where a young *mestizo* refers to the medicinal garden of his Kamentsá teacher Miguel Sibundoy as *el jardín de la ciencia* (the garden of science). In the *Santo Daime* tradition created in the State of Acre in the Brazilian Amazon, the sacrament is called *o professor dos professores* (the teachers' teacher). Former *vegetalista* and painter Pablo Amaringo excelled in making extraordinary depictions of all these motifs in his astonishing creation of inner realms.

One may wonder if any of these cosmological ideas are absorbed by Westerners – informed as they are by their individual cultural and personal histories and with no common coherent worldview – when they go to the Amazon to take *ayahuasca*, or when they take it in various settings all over the world. Surprisingly, the idea that *ayahuasca* is a sort of "mother," "grandmother," or "grandfather" is quite common, as one can see in reports of various kinds in the media. Often one hears statements such as "*ayahuasca* told me." I personally have gathered hundreds of statements after ceremonies from people from many countries and professions. I am amazed how many of them spontaneously and without apparent indoctrination refer to *ayahuasca* and other plants as volitional subjects, as teachers. Of course, people trained with indigenous or *mestizo* practitioners often accept at least some of the views of their teachers. But even therapists working with this medicine openly refer to *ayahuasca* as kin, or as a spiritual entity (cf. Harris, 2017).

There is no doubt the states of consciousness elicited by this preparation predisposes one to animistic ideas. This may of course have practical consequences. From a purely cognitive point of view, it is perhaps difficult to fully accept the rights of plants and forests as sentient beings. But emotionally-charged experiences with psychedelic plants or substances can do the trick. Given our current state of the world, with impending ecological disasters nearly everywhere, and with little comfort in the idea that we are alone as a conscious species, it is not surprising that some may have the urge to seek company, as our ancestors did, and invoke Gaia, Pachamama, Mother Earth, etc. as an entity that protects us and that also needs respect and protection. It is existentially uplifting to "feel" the world as one teeming with intelligence.

This is what prominent biologists in the field of evolutionary cognition are saying. The study of nonhuman intelligence is gradually coming to the fore, thanks to the work of scientists like Frans De Waal, who titled his latest book *Are We Smart Enough to Know How Smart Animals Are?* (2016). Only people who have never had pets or any close contact with animals may have difficulty assigning "personality" to them. The same is true not only of animals, but also of plants, as plant-behavioral biologists and ecologists are discovering: Plants are able to learn; exhibit memory; take decisions; react to the environment, nutrients and predators; show neighbor avoidance and plant competition; communicate with other plants through mycorrhizal networks; interact with the soil; and even take care of their offspring or transfer nutrients to plants of different species. This has been proved through experiments, for example giving radioactively labeled carbon to a tree and detecting it in independently growing saplings around them. (cf. Simard, 2009; Mancuso & Viola, 2013; Wohlleben, 2015; Gagliano, 2015; Vieira et al., 2017). It is, of course, difficult to recognize behavior in plants in our everyday experience, because plants operate at a different time scale than we do: We are not wired to recognize minute or extremely slow movement, and anyway much of it takes place out of our sight, whether under the ground or in the canopies. Plants move slowly and communicate through chemistry or even acoustically, processes mostly undetected by us (Gagliano 2012, 2013). Might it be true that not only animals but also plants have some sort of internal horizon? Could shifts in consciousness affect our perception in such a way as to make us sensitive to such signaling? This is what some indigenous societies say happens under appropriate conditions (cf. Callicott, 2013).

Philosophers, scientists of various disciplines, artists and religious leaders are increasingly discussing animism, posthumanism, panpsychism, the priority of consciousness and related ideas.

Animism may have been the original cosmology of most cultures, and still is in some parts of the world. World religions have been fighting it fiercely. Going back to animistic thinking is perhaps a necessity, as most of humanity has been severed from direct contact with these other *persons* with whom we share this precious and limited planet. In any case, animistic ideas are pragmatically much better than the current radical separation of nature and culture, with nature being simply instrumental to our own needs and composed of objects to be exploited commercially. In this critical situation, we need to look without arrogance into the philosophical repository of ideas of the past and of other cultures and to try and find solutions.

AYAHUASCA, A MIND-BODY PUZZLE

The extraordinary visionary and cognitive effects of *ayahuasca* have taken precedence in the general public over its physiological ones. However, recent research is concentrating on the physiological effects not only of the brew as a whole, but also on the alkaloids present in it: DMT (Frecska et al., 2013), and various beta-carbolines (cf. Riba et al., 2002, 2003, 2004, 2006). Dale Millard in this book makes a detailed review of the extraordinary multifunctional effects of harmine, the main alkaloid in *Banisteriopsis caapi*. It is intriguing that the same molecules that have such an important role in the immune system are also responsible for such powerful cognitive effects, an indication of the deep body-mind relationship.

Shanon (2000: 18), working mostly with non-indigenous people (and with himself), was the first to point out that *ayahuasca* seems to "improve performance": technical agility, accuracy, motor coordination and aesthetic delicacy, something I have also heard from practitioners and regular users of the brew in various settings. If *ayahuasca* improves your talents, whatever they are, then there must be a common underlying neurophysiological or psychological mechanism that needs to be investigated.

One area in which clear improvement is often felt is musicality. Many claim to have developed their musical capacities, or at least to have increased their musical sensitivity. A great number of current practitioners of *ayahuasca* sessions sing and play instruments. This is interesting, taking into account that learning *icaros*, magical songs or melodies to communicate with nonhumans and to exercise healing or malevolent power, is one of the essential elements in the process of becoming a shaman among indigenous and *mestizo* practitioners (Luna, 1986, 1992b, 1995; Beyer, 2012; Callicott, 2013; Bustos, 2016), who strive to establish performative ontological relationships with nonhuman persons (Brabec de Mori, 2011, 2015). Also of great importance are the *hinos* and *chamadas*, the songs "received" by members of the Brazilian organizations that have *ayahuasca* as a sacrament, in which doctrinal aspects and teachings are embedded (Labate & Pacheco, 2009).

Enhanced perception and observation may also play a role in the diagnosis of illnesses by practitioners, perhaps in the form of a greater capacity to receive factual information – as good doctors and therapists do – from small visual and psychological clues. *Ayahuasca* facilitates mental associations and the creation of symbols and metaphors during the exchange with the patients, a language "by means of which unexpressed, and otherwise inexpressible, psychic states can be immediately expressed," as Lévi-Strauss (1958: 198) wrote, referring to shamanic healing in general.

Perhaps one of the roles of contemporary Western *ayahuasca* facilitators is to help participants generate and interpret their own mythology and to identify with the appropriate archetypes, in order to regain strength and restore order and meaning to their lives. The cause-effect mode of healing, perceived as external, is in many cases less effective than the emotionally-charged mythopoeic process that affects the body and the mind simultaneously.

An area of great potential is to use *ayahuasca* as a tool for problem solving, whatever the problem's nature. The "afterglow" of the *ayahuasca* experience – around 3-4 hours after ingestion – is particularly interesting. It is a time in which the spirit is calm and the mind receptive to active imagination and creativity, a time propitious to cement the insights one has received during the session. Most people report a remarkable feeling of well-being after the ceremonies, which may last for some time. A recent study shows that *ayahuasca* reduces anxiety and promotes mindfulness even two weeks after a session (Sampedro et al., 2017).

It is almost unthinkable today, given the view of most people about these matters, to use these particular states of consciousness to discuss matters of great political and international importance. Yet I envision groups of people working on specific problems, symposia taking place, in the afterglow of *ayahuasca* experiences. Political leaders, religious and medical authorities, powerful business people, artists and philosophers could use their transcendent experiences to try to solve the impending problems humanity is facing in our times. It is perhaps unrealistic to imagine that this will happen soon, or naïve to expect that automatic consensus would be reached simply by taking the brew (a proof that this is not so is manifested in the various competing Brazilian religious institutions that share *ayahuasca* as a sacrament). But if attention is shifted from the strictly "visionary" aspects of *ayahuasca*, of which many are afraid, to the medicinal and psychological ones, a better understanding of the possibilities of this extraordinary preparation will gradually emerge. More and more influential people, although it seems so far only in the Western countries, are having extraordinary experiences and insights with *ayahuasca* and other such preparations and substances. Some of them are trying hard to show its many positive aspects and making a difference.

NATURE

Many people claim to rediscover their connection with nature during *ayahuasca* sessions, the deep realization of our commonality with the rest of life. This is especially so with urban dwellers, who may have forgotten the magic of the night and the miracle of the breaking of dawn. Adopting environmental practices, raising ethical questions related to animal food consumption, getting involved in sustainable projects and the feeling of bonding with other people or with life in general (biophilia) are some of the results for those who are deeply touched by their experiences with the brew, often described in mystical or spiritual terms. In many cases, people say they feel as if they had gone "home," as if these astonishing unsuspected inner realms were somehow totally natural, something forgotten, something that we may have experienced when we were children.

While humankind is making extraordinary advances in understanding the nature of the physical world and the depth of time, we are under the imminent threat of total annihilation of higher complex life due to environmental degradation and the permanent risk of nuclear cataclysm. Like the frog being heated slowly and not realizing that she is being cooked alive, we witness the gradual destruction of our environment as if it were a totally natural process. More than ever, we need creative thinking and imagination to determine ways we might come out of the terrible mess that our proud "civilization" has put us in.

Experiencing unity with other human beings, with the Earth or even with the cosmos may give a higher perspective on the mystery of existence, enhance solidarity and help to overcome the limitations of cultural identifications. When describing their experiences with *ayahuasca*, many use the word "love" to express them, extending to other human beings and the whole of nature. Within religious communities, the concept of "brotherhood" or "sisterhood" is often uttered. This may also happen in nonreligious therapeutic or exploratory circles. Bonding is perhaps one of the most striking consequences of taking *ayahuasca* within a group, something often more effective than with isolated experiences.

INNER WORLDS AND CREATIVITY

In our mostly urban and technical contemporary world, exploration of the natural environment is generally limited. However, the positive exploration of inner worlds is open to nearly anyone if the circumstances are right (appropriate set, setting and integration), and may be a source of awe and inspiration. *Ayahuasca* is one of the instruments that may open the gates of the "imaginal," that cognitive aspect of consciousness beyond simple cognition and "imagination." Jeffrey Kripal, not referring specifically to psychedelic experiences, conceives "the possibility that, in very special moments, the human imagination somehow becomes temporarily empowered or 'zapped' and functions not as simply a spinner of fantasies (the imaginary) but as a very special organ of cognition *and* translation (the symbolic) as a kind of supersense that is perceiving some entirely different, probably inhuman or superhuman order of reality but shaping that encounter into a virtual reality display in tune with the local culture" (Streiber & Kripal 2016).

Ayahuasca experiences are to a great extent the product of co-creation (Shanon, 2002; Luna, 2016). Our personal experiences and memories (at times extremely vivid), our aspirations and desires, interplay with something in us of which we are mostly unaware, and which may emerge effortlessly from a hidden dimension in a swift, elegant way, independent of our own volition. During the *ayahuasca* experience, the person is navigating between insights and projections, mind-wandering and mindfulness. Information stored in the mind seems to be at times readily available for reappraisal and integration, and rich narratives unfold while we try to make sense of them by trying to recognize and interpret their various components. Even if the process is interrupted by putting the attention onto the external world or by letting the mind wander into normal thinking, when the attention goes back to the inner world, a new narrative may unfold.

Ayahuasca may provide states of consciousness in which things lose their boundaries. The person may enter a fluidity in which the borders between the individual and the social, the inside and the outside, between wakefulness and dreaming, are eroded. Elements from normal reality may be embedded in the vision, or our fears of war and ecological disasters may play out. Indigenous people may see cities, pharmacies, doctors and so on; and Westerners may see Indian villages, jaguars and serpents. Idiosyncratic worlds may be constructed with repetitive experiences, or when the sessions are embedded within particular worldviews (Luna, 2016:261). On the other hand, it may happen that during the *ayahuasca* experience, perceptions may go undetected by the "central" ego-mind, so that at the end only dim memories of the experience may remain.

Humor, "a gentle form of transcendence" (Jeffrey Kripal, personal communication), seems to be embedded in some of the *ayahuasca* experiences. I can attest to it. On one occasion during a session, I was seeing the usual extraordinary visions. I was wondering, "What is behind it all?" My point of view then shifted. I was taken gently behind a huge screen on which "my visions" were projected, held up with great effort by small, strange creatures. On another occasion, I was in one of those extraordinary worlds. I lifted my gaze and I could see small windows up high from where I was being watched, like a guinea pig, by what looked like scientists. In yet another session, after another fantastic display of visions, credits played like in a film, moving from bottom to top, although too faint to be able to read the names. These are the kinds of jokes my mind is playing with me.

DANGERS AND PITFALLS

So far, I have presented a rather rosy picture of *ayahuasca*. But like everything that is of value, there are also problems involved. First of all, the growing demand for *ayahuasca* may lead to overharvesting of the plants. Michael Coe, working on his doctoral dissertation for the University of Hawaii, now in the field in the Peruvian Amazon, sent me the following provisional report:

> There is anecdotal evidence to suggest that there has been increasing scarcity of both *Banisteriopsis* and *Psychotria*, notably around the city of Iquitos, where prices are increasing for both plants due to demand linked to an estimated 200 retreat centers in the area and to its export out of the Amazon. In addition, it has been suggested that within a 130-mile radius of both Iquitos and Pucallpa, it has become more difficult to find wild populations of Banisteriopsis and *Psychotria*, indicating that harvest regimes are likely focused in areas further into the jungle. There is the concern by communities who have adopted a management plan that unauthorized harvest is occurring due to settlers in the area and to increased economic interests associated with *ayahuasca*. There is also potential for collateral damage with respect to *Banisteriopsis* harvests, as the companion plants (often large trees) have sometimes been cut down in order to gain access to the vine. It can take anywhere from 5 to 10 years before the vine is mature enough to harvest for preparation of *ayahuasca*, depending on soil, water and light conditions. Potential for sustainability is, on the other hand, likely to occur if mindful management practices are employed by *ayahuasca* retreats/centers, planting enough *Banisteriopsis* and *Psychotria* to meet the demands of harvest pressure and consumption. In addition, relationships built on reciprocity (i.e., living wages) with respect to working with communities who actively manage, grow, and harvest these plants are essential to long-term sustainability, especially when these cultural communities may provide *Banisteriopsis* or *Psychotria* for practitioners that live in areas where the plants may not grow due to biotic and abiotic factors.

Banisteriopsis is on the other hand an ideal high-value agro-forestry species, although not suited to be a monoculture. It is best planted in association with fast-growing pioneer species of trees. It has enormous potential to produce large amounts of biomass for recuperation of poor soils through falling leaves and twigs. The large root system is composed of fine roots that bind the soil and prevent erosion. It is capable of growing in many different soil types and therefore could grow in deforested and eroded areas damaged by cattle (Dale Millard, personal communication).

A second problematic area regarding *ayahuasca* is, of course, how it is used. Among indigenous and *mestizo* communities, a long and arduous apprenticeship is required to deal with this preparation. But as Peluso (2014, 231) points out, the globalization of *ayahuasca* is bringing together individuals with very divergent epistemologies and experiences, with the possibility of contradictions and misunderstanding. There are now probably hundreds of practitioners – Amazonian and non-Amazonian and with very different backgrounds – leading ceremonies of some kind, often without having undergone proper training or having acquired sufficient personal experience. For some, the experiences are such that they feel the urge to tell others about it, take practitioners to their countries or even take the great responsibility of dispensing the medicine themselves. It is easy to yield to the temptation to "initiate" other people without enough personal experience and basic pharmacological and psychological know-how. I know examples of young people who, after having spent a relatively short time in the Amazon, call themselves "shamans." They may have followers eager to experience and learn from them, but they are unaware of how delicate it is to deal with the peculiar states of consciousness elicited by the brew. Facilitators need continuous training and a broad education to be able to more effectively help others in their explorations. One is dealing with the innermost depths and heights of other people, and with the mysteries of the human mind. That is sacred. Hopefully, there will be a gradual integration of psychotherapy and pharmacology (Sessa, 2012; Lattin, 2017; Richards, 2015), but no academic or religious qualification guarantees that *ayahuasca* will not be misused by some. Integrity and a humble attitude are needed, as well as sufficient personal experience ("flight hours," in the language of pilots).

There are, unfortunately, also cases of people who need urgent therapy after participating in *ayahuasca* ceremonies that have minimal reintegration procedures. Regardless of setting – religious, therapeutic or "shamanic" – ego inflation is always one of the greatest dangers when dealing with this preparation (Luna, 2016:275-7).

There are external dangers as well: misunderstandings, prejudices, ignorance and persecution, as *ayahuasca* is still illegal in some countries due to its DMT content. An exemplary negative case is that of France, in which all the components of *ayahuasca* and *yagé* have been made illegal, both the plants and the alkaloids. On the other hand, because *ayahuasca* is such a powerful substance, there is the danger of a rush towards trying to control it, either in the name of religion or through strict medicalization. What is most needed is interdisciplinary education so that we can all learn from many sources, from indigenous practitioners as well as from therapists, scientists, artists and philosophers. This is already happening, as proved by the many meetings either totally dedicated to *ayahuasca* and other psychotropic plants or substances, or at conferences where *ayahuasca* has also found a niche.

FINAL REMARKS

Ayahuasca experiences are, for many, epistemologically challenging, obliging one to accommodate within one's worldview the evidence that reality seems to be much more intricate than had previously been deemed possible. Such fundamental concepts as time and space are perceived in a different way. Experiences of multidimensionality are common. There are many anecdotal reports of such phenomena as precognition and apparently telepathic episodes by seemingly "down-to-Earth" people that are impossible to comfortably ignore. One of the main indigenous uses of *ayahuasca* is for divination: locating game, seeing faraway places, finding the cause of illnesses, etc. In the past, it was even used to learn about the plans of the enemy in times of war. This amounts to obtaining information from the outside via the inside (Frecska & Luna, 2007). It is necessary to go beyond traditional scientific (and religious) paradigms. We need a radical empiricism that has no qualms about dealing with alternate states of consciousness, regardless of how awkward it is to write or talk about such things. We are really navigating in unknown – perhaps unknowable – waters, but we have to make an effort to know, with the best of our scientific tools as well as with introspective and meditative techniques developed by other cultures. We need to have the courage to investigate first-hand, with our own consciousness as part of a variety of methods, the vast inner universe of which we are most of the time unaware.

I remember well the stir and enthusiasm caused, especially among young people, by the film *The Matrix* (1999), an indication that this film seemed to have touched something deeply, felt by many. There is a suspicion that there must be something beyond the fascinating, but ultimately not totally satisfying world presented to us by academic science (which is, to a certain extent, a new religion). There seems to be something not quite right in the way we conceive and perceive reality. We experience small hints here and there, dreams and synchronicities, that seem to point towards something other, but to which we commonly pay little attention or dismiss as mere curiosities or coincidence. These kinds of phenomena seem to happen (or perhaps are perceived) more often around psychedelic experiences. This is puzzling and disconcerting and cannot be ignored. One of the most important consequences of psychedelic experiences is the suspicion that reality seems to be much more complex than we had imagined, that the mind is intrinsically intermingled with the material world. *Ayahuasca* expands our ideas of what is possible. It enhances the senses, heightens emotions, produces visions and elicits particular ways of cognition that point towards something other than phenomenological reality. It is a tool for which we must be profoundly thankful to the Amerindian cultures that discovered it and preserve its use. In the crucial moment in history in which we are immersed, anything that expands our creativity and our imagination, anything that connects us with all that exists, is a sacred instrument which we need to cherish and deeply respect.

REFERENCES

Baer, G., 1984. *Die Religion der Matsigenka Ost-Peru*. Wepf & Co. AG Verlag, Basel.

Barbira-Freedman, F., 2014. Shamans' networks in Western Amazonia, in: Labate, B., Cavnar, C. (Eds.), *Ayahuasca Shamanism in the Amazon and Beyond*. Oxford University Press.

Beyer, S. V., 2009. *Singing to the Plants. A Guide to Mestizo Shamanism in the Upper Amazon*. University of New Mexico Press, Albuquerque.

Beyer, S. V., 2012. Special *ayahuasca* issue introduction: toward a multidisciplinary approach to *ayahuasca*. *Anthropology of Consciousness* 23 (1), 1-5.

Brabec de Mori, B., 2011. *Die Lieder der Richtigen Menschen. Musikalische Kulturanthropologie der indigenen Bevölkerung im Ucayali-Tal, Westamazonien*. Doctoral dissertation. Vienna University.

Brabec de Mori, B., et al. (Eds.), 2015. *Sudamérica y sus mundos audibles. Cosmologías y prácticas sonoras de los pueblos indígenas*. Gebr. Mann Verlag, Berlin.

Bristol, M. L., 1965. *Sibundoy Ethnobotany*. Doctoral Dissertation. Harvard University, Cambridge, Massachusetts.

Brown, M. F., 1978. From the hero's bones: three aguaruna hallucinogens and their uses, in: Ford, R.I. (Ed.), *The Nature and Status of Ethnobotany*. Museum of Anthropology, University of Michigan. *Anthropological Papers* 67, 118-136.

Bustos, S., 2016. Healing *icaros* in Peruvian vegetalismo, in: Luna, L.E., White, S.F. (Eds.), *Ayahuasca Reader: Encounters with the Amazon's Sacred Vine*, 2nd edition. Synergetic Press, Santa Fe.

Caicedo-Fernández, A., 2014. Yagé-related neo-shamanism in Colombian urban contexts, in: Labate, B., Cavnar, C., (Eds.), *Ayahuasca Shamanism in the Amazon and Beyond*. Oxford University Press.

Callicott, C., 2013. Interspecies communication in the Western Amazon: music as a form of conversation between plants and people. *European Journal of Ecopsychology* 4, 32-43.

Chaumeil J. P., 1983. *Voir, Savoir, Pouvoir. Le Chamanisme chez les Yagua du Nord-Est Peruvien*. Editions de l'École des Hautes Études en Sciences Sociales, Paris.

Chevalier, J. M., 1982. *Civilization and the Stolen Gift: Capital, Kin, and Cult in Eastern Peru*. University of Toronto Press.

Chiappe Costa, M., 1979. Nosografía curanderil, in: Seguín, C.A. (Ed.), *Psiquiatría Folklórica. Shamanes y Curanderos*. Ediciones Ermar, Lima.

De Waal, F., 2016. *Are We Smart Enough to Know How Smart Animals Are?* W.W. Norton & Company, New York.

Del Castillo, G., 1963. La *ayahuasca* planta mágica de la Amazonía; el ayahuasquismo. *Perú Indígena*, Vol. X, nos. 24 & 25, Lima 88-98.

Descola, P., 2005. Ecology as cosmological analysis, in: Surrallés, A., García-Hierro, P. (Eds.), *The Land Within. Indigenous Territory and the Perception of the Environment*. IWGIA (International Work Group for Indigenous Affairs), Copenhagen.

Dobkin de Rios, M., 1970a. *Banisteriopsis* used in witchcraft and folk healing in Iquitos, Peru. *Economic Botany* 24 (35), 296-300.

Dobkin de Rios, M., 1970b. A Note on the use of *ayahuasca* among *Mestizo* populations in the Peruvian Amazon. *American Anthropologist* 72(6), 1419-1422.

Dobkin de Rios, M., 1971a. *Ayahuasca*, the healing vine. *International Journal of Social Psychiatry* 17 (4), 256-269.

Dobkin de Rios, M., 1971b. Curanderismo con la Soga alucinógena (*ayahuasca*) en la selva Peruana. *América Indígena* 31(3), 575-592.

Dobkin de Rios, M., 1972. *Visionary Vine. Hallucinogenic Healing in the Peruvian Amazon*. Chandler, San Francisco.

Dobkin de Rios, M., 1973. Curing with *ayahuasca* in an urban slum, in: Harner, M. (Ed.), *Hallucinogens and Shamanism*. Oxford University Press.

Frecska, E., Luna, L.E., 2007. The shamanic healer: master of nonlocal information? *Shaman* 15 (1-2).

Frecska, E., Szabo, A., Winkelman, M.J., Luna, L.E., McKenna, D.J., 2013. A possibly sigma-1 receptor mediated ole of dimethyltryptamine in tissue protection, regeneration, and immunity, *J Neural Transm* 120 (1), 295–303.

Gagliano, M., 2015. In a green frame of mind: perspectives on the behavioural ecology and cognitive nature of plants. *AoB PLANTS* 7, plu075.

Gagliano, M., 2013. The flowering of plant bioacoustics: How and why. *Behav Ecol* 24 (4), 800-801.

Gagliano, M., 2012. Green symphonies: a call for studies on acoustic communication in plants. *Behav Ecol*. 24, 789–796.

Harris, R., 2017. *Listening to Ayahuasca. New Hope for Depression, Addiction, PTSD, and Anxiety*. New World Library, Novato, California.

Heckenberger, M., Neves, G. 2009. Amazonian archeology. *Annual Review of Anthropology* Vol. 38: 251-266.

Labate, B.C., Jungaberle, H. (Eds.), 2011. *The Internationalization of Ayahuasca.* LIT Verlag, Vienna & Berlin.

Labate, B.C., Pacheco, G. 2009. *Música Brasileira de Ayahuasca.* Mercado de Letras, Campinas.

Langdon, J. E. 1979a. Yagé among the Siona: Cultural patterns in visions, in: Browman, D., Schwartz, R.A. (Eds.), *Spirits, Shamans and Stars.* Mouton Publishers, The Hague, Paris, New York.

Langdon, J. E., 1979b. The Siona hallucinogenic ritual: Its meaning and power, in: Morgan, J.H. (Ed.), *Understanding Religion and Culture: Anthropological and Theological Perspectives.* University Press of America, Washington, 58–86.

Lattin, D., 2017. *Changing Our Minds. Psychedelic Sacraments and the New Psychotherapy.* Synergetic Press, Santa Fe.

Lemlij, M., Millones Santa Gadea, L., 1985. *Alucinógenos y shamanismo en el Perú contemporáneo.* El Virrey, Lima.

Lévi-Strauss, C., 1963. *Structural Anthropology.* Basic Books, New York. Translated from French, originally published in 1958.

Lévi-Strauss, C., 1949. Needham, Rodney, ed., *Les Structures élémentaires de la parenté* [The Elementary Structures of Kinship] (in French), J. H. Bell, J. R. von Sturmer, and Rodney Needham, Translators (1969 ed.), Traviston

Luna, L.E., 2016. Some observations on the phenomenology of the *ayahuasca* experience, in: Luna, L.E., White, Steven F. (Eds.), *Ayahuasca Reader: Encounters with the Amazon's Sacred Vine,* 2nd edition. Synergetic Press, Santa Fe.

Luna, L.E., 2011. Indigenous and *Mestizo* use of *ayahuasca:* An overview, In: Santos, R.G. (Ed.), *The Ethnopharmacology of Ayahuasca.* Research Signpost, Trivandrum.

Luna, L.E., 1995. A barquinha. Una nueva religión en Río Branco, Amazonía Brasileña. *Acta Americana* 3 (2), 137-151. Stockholm.

Luna, L.E., 1992a. Therapeutic imagery in Amazonian shamanism: Some observations. *Scripta Ethnologica* Vol. XIV: 19-25. Centro Argentino de Etnología Americana, Buenos Aires.

Luna, L.E., 1992b. Function of the magic melodies or *icaros* of some *Mestizo* shaman of Iquitos, in the Peruvian Amazonas, in: Jean Matteson Langdon, J.M., Baer, G. (Eds.), *Portals of Power: Shamanism in South America.* University of New Mexico Press.

Luna, L.E., 1986. *Vegetalismo: Shamanism Among the Mestizo Population of the Peruvian Amazon.* Almqvist & Wiksell International, Stockholm.

Luna, L.E., 1984a. The concept of plants as teacher among four *Mestizo* shamans of Iquitos, Northeast Peru. *Journal of Ethnopharmacology* 11, 135-156.

Luna, L.E., 1984b. The healing practices of a Peruvian shaman. *Journal of Ethnopharmacology* 11, 123-133.

Luna, L.E., 1982. *Don Emilio y Sus Doctorcitos (Don Emilio and His Little Doctors).* 16mm, 27 m. film. Helsinki: Yleisradio (www.youtube.com/watch?v=2NJBnCKSjmM).

Luna, L.E., Amaringo, P., 1991. *Ayahuasca Visions: The Religious Iconography of A Peruvian Shaman.* North Atlantic Books, Berkeley.

Luna, L.E., White, S. F., 2016. *Ayahuasca Reader: Encounters with the Amazon's Sacred Brew,* 2nd ed. Synergetic Press, Santa Fe.

Mancuso, S., Viola, A., 2013. *Brilliant Green. The Surprising History and Science of Plant Intelligence.* Island Press, Washington, Covelo, London.

McKenna, D., 2013. *Ayahuasca* yesterday, today and tomorrow. Perspectives on the past and future of *ayahuasca.* Horizon Conference, October 11-13, 2013. https://vimeo.com/79992380

Peluso, D., 2014. *Ayahuasca's* attractions and distraction. Examining sexual seduction in shaman-participant interactions, in: Labate, B., Cavnar, C. (Eds.), *Ayahuasca Shamanism in the Amazon and Beyond.* Oxford University Press.

Pinzón, C., Suárez, R. (Eds.), 1991. Los cuerpos y los poderes de las historias. Apuntes para una historia de las redes de chamanes y *curanderos* en Colombia, in: Pinzón, C., Suárez, R. (Eds.), *Otra América en Construcción.* Colcultura. Instituto Colombiano de Antropología, Bogotá.

Reichel-Dolmatoff, G., 1970. Notes on the cultural extent of the use of yagé (*Banisteriopsis caapi*) among the Indians of Vaupes, Colombia. *Economic Botany* 24(1), 32-34.

Reichel-Dolmatoff, G., 1971. *Amazonian Cosmos: The Sexual and Religious Symbolism of the Tukano Indians.* University of Chicago Press.

Reichel-Dolmatoff, G., 1972. The cultural context of an aboriginal hallucinogen: *Banisteriopsis caapi,* in: Furst, P. (Ed.), *Flesh of the Gods. The Ritual Use of Hallucinogens.* New York, Washington, Praeger Publishers, 84-113.

Reichel-Dolmatoff, G., 1975. *The Shaman and The Jaguar. A Study of Narcotic Drugs Among the Indians of Colombia.* Temple University Press, Philadelphia.

Reichel-Dolmatoff, G., 1976. Cosmology as ecological analysis: A view from the rainforest. *Man New Series* 11 (3), 307-318.

Reichel-Dolmatoff, G., 1978. *Beyond the Milky Way.* UCLA Latin American Center, Los Angeles.

Riba J., S. Romero, E. Grasa, E. Mena, I. Carrió, M.J. Barbanoj, 2006. Increased frontal and paralimbic activation following *ayahuasca,* the Pan-Amazonian inebriant. *Psychopharmacology* 186, 93–98.

Riba J., Anderer, P., Jané, F., Saletu, B., Barbanoj, M.J., 2004. Effects of the South American psychoactive beverage *ayahuasca* on regional brain electrical activity in humans: a functional neuroimaging study using low-resolution electromagnetic tomography (LORETA). *Neuropsychobiology* 50, 89–101.

Riba J., Valle, M., Urbano, G., Yritia, M., Morte, A., Barbanoj, M.J., 2003. Human pharmacology of *ayahuasca:* subjective and cardiovascular effects, monoamine metabolite excretion and pharmacokinetics. *Journal of Pharmacology and Experimental Therapeutics* 306, 73–83.

Riba J., Anderer, P., Morte, A., Urbano, G., Jané, F., Saletu, B., Barbanoj, M.J., 2002. Topographic pharmaco-EEG mapping of the effects of the South American psychoactive beverage *ayahuasca* in healthy volunteers. *British Journal of Clinical Pharmacology* 53, 613–628.

Richards, W. A., 2015. *Sacred Knowledge. Psychedelics and Religious Experiences.* Columbia University Press, New York.

Robinson, S., 1976. *Towards an Understanding of Kofan Shamanism.* Doctoral thesis. Department of Anthropology. Cornell University.

Sessa, B., 2012. *The Psychedelic Renaissance: Reassessing the Role of Psychedelic Drugs in 21st Century Psychiatry and Society.* Muswell Hill Press

Sampedro F., de la Fuente Revenga M., et al., 2017. Assessing the psychedelic "after-glow" in *ayahuasca* users: post-acute neurometabolic and functional connectivity changes are associated with enhanced mindfulness capacities. *Int. Journal of Neuropsychopharmacology* 2017 May 19. doi: 10.1093/ijnp/pyx036. [Epub ahead of print] PubMed PMID: 28525587.

Shanon, B., 2002. *The Antipodes of the Mind: Charting the Phenomenology of the Ayahuasca Experience*. Oxford University Press.

Shanon, B., 2000. *Ayahuasca* and creativity. *Maps Bulletin* Vol. X, number 3.

Shepard, G., 2011. *The Hunter in the Rye: Ergot, Sedges and Hunting Magic in the Peruvian Amazon*. http://ethnoground.blogspot.com.br/2011/10/.

Simard, S., 2009. The foundational role of mycorrhizal networks in self-organization of interior Douglas Fir forests. *Forest Ecology and Management* 258, 95-107.

Stone, R. E., 2011. *The Jaguar Within: Shamanic Trance in Ancient Central and South American Art*. University of Texas Press.

Strieber, W., Kripal, Jeffrey J. 2016. *The Super Natural. A New Vision of the Unexplained*. Jeremy P. Tarcher, New York.

Taussig, M., 1987. *Shamanism, Colonialism, and the Wild Man. A Study in Terror and Healing*. The University of Chicago Press, Chicago.

Tindall, R., Apffel-Marglin, F., Shearer, D., 2017. *Sacred Soil: Biochar and the Regeneration of the Earth*. North Atlantic Books, Berkeley.

Vieira, P., Cagliano, M., Ryan, L. (Eds.), 2015. *The Green Thread: Dialogue with the Vegetal World*. Lexington Books.

Viveiro de Castro, E., 2005. Perspectivism and multiculturalism, in: Surrallés, A., García Hierro, P. (Eds.) *The Land Within. Indigenous Territory and the Perception of the Environment*. IWGIA (International Work Group for Indigenous Affairs), Copenhagen.

Weiskopf, J., 2004. *Yagé, the New Purgatory. Encounters with Ayahuasca*. Villega Editores, Bogotá.

Wohlleben, P., 2015. *The Hidden Life of Trees. What They Feel, How They Communicate*. Greystone Books, Vancouver.

From Beer to Tobacco: A Probable Prehistory of *Ayahuasca* and *Yagé*.

Constantino Manuel Torres, PhD

Professor Emeritus, Art and Art History Department, Florida International University

Origin, although an entirely historical category, has, nevertheless, nothing to do with genesis. The term origin is not intended to describe the process by which the existent came into being, but rather to describe that which emerges from the process of becoming and disappearance. Origin is an eddy in the stream of becoming, and in its current it swallows the material involved in the process of genesis.

The Origin of German Tragic Drama, p. 45,
Walter Benjamin. Verso, 2009.

INTRODUCTION

The iconography related to ancient South American snuff powders obtained from the seeds of trees of the genus *Anadenanthera* has been the primary focus of my research. These seeds, rich in bufotenine (5-OH-DMT) and related tryptamines, were reported by early Spanish chroniclers as an additive to fermented drinks. In the course of my studies on *Anadenanthera*, I began to inquire whether these drinks could be analogous to *ayahuasca* and *yagé*, and whether these could be linked to the origins of these complex beverages. The recipes for these potions presently available include plant combinations that provoke synergy between diverse alkaloids present in the component plants. It should be stressed that these are not fixed or standardized recipes, but rather are distinct beverages that adapt to regional demands, including plant availability and culturally determined methods of administration (e.g., smoking, snuffing, drinking, enemas and/or unguents). Consequently, instead of a fixed recipe, a construct related to plant synergy and modulation becomes apparent.

Ayahuasca and *yagé* share a basic potion composed of *Banisteriopsis caapi* (Spruce ex. Griseb.) Morton stems to which different plants are added (Beyer, 2009; Labate and Cavnar, 2014; América Indigena, 1986; Ott, 1994; Schultes, 1957). The *Banisteriopsis* (Figure 1) vine contains several β-carboline alkaloids – harmine, harmaline, and tetrahydroharmine – which are potent inhibitors of the enzyme monoamine oxidase (MAO). Frequently, *ayahuasca* and *yagé* are combined with the leaves of *Psychotria viridis* Ruiz & Pav. (Figure 2) or *Diplopterys cabrerana* (Cuatrec) B. Gates (Figure 3), respectively. The leaves of these two species contain N,N-dimethyltryptamine (DMT), which is not orally active. However, its combination with the MAO-inhibiting harmala alkaloids allow for its activity. Solanaceous additives are also common, and include *Nicotiana*, *Brugmansia*, and *Brunfelsia* species (Figure 4). Approximately 100 species from 40 plant families are reported as *ayahuasca/yagé* admixtures, many of them also psychoactive plants (Ott, 1994). Several other beverages, distributed throughout South America, employ similar notions of plant interaction. Among these, *vinho de jurema* (Samorini, 2016), *yaraque* (Reichel-Dolmatoff, 1944), *vino de cebil* (Califano, 1976), and *chicha* with an admixture of *Anadenanthera* seeds (Ondegardo, 1916), are of importance and are indicative of indigenous knowledge of plant synergy (Map 1, Table 1).

DMT is deaminated by the enzyme monoamine oxidase (MAO); the ingestion of β-carbolines may protect the DMT from deamination by MAO, and allow for oral activity. Unlike DMT, bufoten-

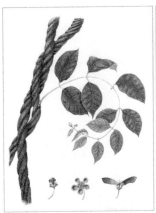
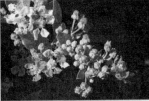
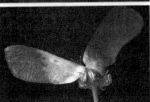

Fig. 1 *Banisteriopsis caapi* (Spruce ex Griseb) Morton (Malpighiaceae). Watercolor drawing courtesy of Donna Torres.

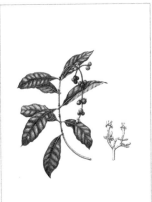
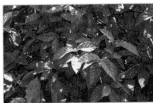
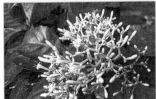

Fig. 2 *Psychotria viridis* Ruiz & Pav. Watercolor drawing courtesy of Donna Torres.

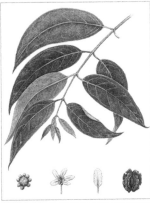

Fig. 3 *Diplopterys cabrerana* (Cuatrecasas) Gates. Watercolor drawing courtesy of Donna Torres. Photo courtesy of Kathleen Harrison.

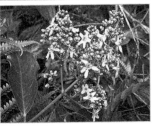
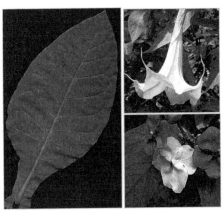

Fig. 4 Solanaceous admixtures to *ayahuasca* and *yagé* include a. Nicotiana, b. *Brugmansia*, and c. Brunfelsia species. Photos by C. M. Torres.

Table 1. Selected *ayahuasca*-like potions.

AYAHUASCA	*Banisteriopsis caapi* *Psychotria viridis*	Amazon Basin of Peru and Brazil
YAGÉ	*Banisteriopsis caapi* *Diplopterys cabrerana*	SE Colombia
JUREMA, AJUCA	*Mimosa hostilis*	NE Brazil
VINO DE CEBIL	*Anadenanthera colubrina* seeds added to aloja (fermented algarrobo pods)	Wichi, Gran Chaco
CHICHA CON VILCA	*Anadenanthera colubrina* seeds added to germinated corn chihca	Quechua, Central Andes
YARAQUE	*Anadenanthera peregrina* seeds added to fermented cassava	Guahibo, Colombia
TETRAPTERYS METHYSTICA	No admixture plants	Makú, Vaupés, Colombia
GÜEYO	Unknown admixture plants	Taino, Greater Antilles

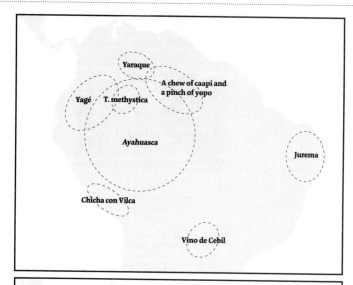

Map 1. Map of South America indicating approximate area of potions mentioned in the text.

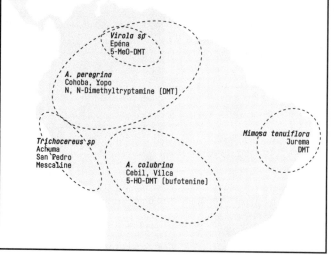

Map 2: Map of South America with approximate distribution of tryptamine use.

ine (5-OH-DMT) and 5-MeO-DMT maintain some oral activity, but oral ingestion notably diminishes the effect (Ott, 2001, 103-104, 110). Fifty years ago, in the first *Ethnopharmacologic Search for Psychoactive Drugs* conference, Holmsted and Lindgren (1967, 365) proposed the notion of synergy between β-carbolines and tryptamines when they detected the presence of harmine and harmaline in Piaroa and Surará *Anadenanthera* snuffs of the Orinoco Basin. These researchers stated:

> ... some snuffs contain β-carbolines, either in combination with the simple tryptamines or solely. In South American botany, β-carbolines (harmine, harmaline, and tetrahydroharmine) are usually associated with the species of *Banisteriopsis*, wherefore it is very likely that this is their origin in the snuffs. Very likely this is an admixture to the snuff ...

> The occurrence of both tryptamines and β-carbolines in the South American snuffs is pharmacologically interesting. The β-carbolines are monoamine oxidase inhibitors, and could potentiate the action of the simple indoles. The combination of β-carbolines and tryptamines would thus be advantageous.

My inquiry initially focused on the origins of *ayahuasca* and *yagé*. However, it soon became apparent that questions of origin were not restricted to sets of specific recipes, prescriptions, and localities. Instead, a construct related to plant interaction and modulation began to emerge. To investigate *ayahuasca* as a separate and distinct phenomenon is not an advantageous strategy. It should be considered in terms of the specific needs and circumstances that gave rise to these formulations and from the contemporary, perhaps privileged, point of view that makes it possible for us to contemplate a large sample of psychoactive preparations in South America. *Ayahuasca* and *yagé* should be seen within the wider South American visionary plant complex (smoking, snuffing, enemas and unguents), and not as isolated classes of psychoactive drinks (Map 2).

An investigation into the origins of *ayahuasca* reveals numerous beverages distributed throughout South America, each being distinct and varying according to plant availability, cultural predilections for ingestion and ritual requirements. It should be stressed that there are no fixed recipes, but instead, there is constant variation even within the practice of an individual practitioner—it is a methodology marked by continuous change. Instead of pursuing the origins of a specific recipe, this inquiry attempts a search for the origins of a concept that understands issues of synergy between plant components, such that an effect can be modulated, enhanced and prolonged.

ORIGIN STORIES OF AYAHUASCA AND YAGÉ

Tukano stories tell of a *yagé*-woman who gave birth to a luminous child born in a blinding flash of light:

> The first men had gathered in the House of the Waters ... They were trying to find a beverage ... that would take them beyond the narrow confines of everyday experience, and so they were concocting different kinds of fermented beer ... There was a woman among them, the first woman in Creation ... When the Sun Father had created her ... he had impregnated her body through the eye; ... and now she was about to give birth and so she left the house and walked into the darkness of the forest. While the men continued to sing she gave birth to a male child, a child that was going to be yagé ... born in a blinding flash of light ... Slowly, the *Yagé* Woman walked toward the house and entered it ... The men were watching her and they almost fainted; the brilliant light and the sight of the blood-red child were causing them to lose their senses. They felt as though they were drowning in swirling waters ... The woman looked around and asked, "Who is the father of this child?"... Then all the men rose and cried: "We are all fathers of this child!" And they took hold of the infant's body and tore it to bits. Each man tore off a part and kept it for himself. And ever since, each tribe ... had its own vine (Reichel-Dolmatoff, 1978, 3-4).

Archaeological evidence about the use of *ayahuasca* and *yagé* is lacking. Harmine has been detected in the hair of two mummies from archaeological sites (ca. AD 500-1000) in the Azapa Valley, northern Chile, although the results of the analyses are arguable (Ogalde et al., 2009, 471; see also Trout, 2008). Species of *Banisteriopsis, P. viridis,* and *D. cabrerana* have not been detected in archaeological sites. This is to be expected, since the habitat of these plants is not conducive to the preservation of organic remains. In addition, the great distance and climatic difference between the Atacama Desert and the Amazon makes the presence of *Banisteriopsis* in the Azapa Valley unlikely. DMT was not detected in the hair of these mummies (Ogalde et al., 2009, 471). The presence of β-carbolines in the hair of these mummies could be explained by the practice of smoking, and also of blowing tobacco smoke on patient's hair, frequent in South American healing practices (plus decades in museum storage rooms). Tobacco smoke contains harman and norharman, known MAO inhibitors (Herraiz and Chaparro, 2005).

The earliest printed reports of *ayahuasca* (Table 2) are those of Pablo Maroni (1737) and José Chantre y Herrera (1901). Chantre y Herrera compiled a history of Jesuit activity in the Marañon River area from 1637 to 1767. His compilation includes a detailed description of an *ayahuasca* ritual and a clear reference to the mixing of a liana with other plants. He did not provide a specific date for the following observation within the range of his history (1637 to 1767):

> ... an entire night is dedicated to divination. In order to achieve this, the most appropriate house in the community is chosen because many people will be attending the ceremony. Benches are placed on one side for the men and the rest of the space is left clear for the women. The diviner hangs his hammock in the middle and makes his raised platform or small stage and, beside it, places an infernal beverage that they call ayahuasca, which is singularly efficient in depriving one of one's senses. They make this concoction of lianas or bitter herbs, which, after a great deal of boiling, becomes very thick. Since it is so strong as to derange a person even in small quantities, the dose is minimal, and fits in two small receptacles. The sorcerer, each time he drinks, consumes very small amounts, and knows very well how many times he can drink the potion without losing his sanity in order to carry out the ceremony with due solemnity and direct the chorus, since everyone responds to his invocation of the devil (Chantre y Herrera, 1901, 80).

Pablo Maroni (1737, 172), another Jesuit missionary to the Marañon River area ca. 1738-1740, attributed healing and divinatory qualities to *ayahuasca*:

> For divination they drink the juice, some of white floripondio (*Brugmansia* spp.), that because of its shape they also call Campana, others use a liana that is called *ayahuasca* vulgarly, both very effective to deprive one of the senses, and even of life, in over-loading the hand. This they also sometimes use to cure themselves of habitual diseases, mainly of headaches. Drink, then, because he who wishes to divine conducts certain ceremonies, and being deprived of his senses lays face down, to avoid being suffocated by the power of the herb, he is thus many hours and sometimes even two and three days, until the inebriation takes its course. After this, he reflects on what the imagination represented, who alone and at times must remain in a delirious state, and this he takes as a fact and prophesies as an oracle.

The first botanist to identify the liana that forms the basis of *ayahuasca* and *yagé* as belonging to the genus *Banisteriopsis* was Richard Spruce (1873, 184). Spruce encountered the use of *Banisteriopsis* several times during his travels, ca. 1852-1853. He states:

> In the accounts given by travelers of the festivities of the South American Indians, and of the incantations of their medicine-men, frequent mention is made of powerful drugs used to produce intoxication, or even temporary delirium. Some of these narcotics are absorbed in the form of smoke, others as snuff, and others as drink; ... Having had the good fortune to see the two most famous narcotics in use, and to obtain specimens of the plants that afford them sufficiently perfect to be determined botanically, I propose to record my observations on them, made on the spot. The first of these narcotics is afforded by a climbing plant called *Caapi*. It belongs to the family of Mal-

Table 2. Earliest mention of *ayahuasca* potions.

Pablo Maroni - Noticias auténticas del famoso rio Marañón y ... en los dilatados bosques de dicho rio	Description of the use of *ayahuasca* and floripondio blanco (*Brugmansia spp.*)	Written ca. 1737
José Chantre y Herrera - Historia de las misiones de la Compañia de Jesús en el Marañón español.	Detailed description - no specific date given for this statement.	Information compiled from Jesuit documents covering the period 1637 - 1767
Juan Magnin - Breve descripción de la Provincia de Quito,... y de sus misiones... a las orillas del gran Rio Marañon.	Brief mention, no details given.	ca. 1734 - 1740
Manuel Villavicencio - Geografia de la República del Ecuador.	One of the first descriptions of self-experimentation.	Written ca. 1850 - 1858
Alfred Wallace - Narrative of travels on the Amazon and Rio Negro.	One among a series of researchers almost simultaneously reporting the use of *ayahuasca*: Wallace, Villavicencio, Simson, Spruce.	Written 1851
Richard Spruce - On Some Remarkable Narcotics of the Amazon Valley and Orinoco	First botanical description (*B. caapi*), mentions admixtures to the potion.	Observations conducted 1852 - 1853

Table 3. Documentation of admixtures to *ayahuasca* potions.

Richard Spruce - On Some Remarkable Narcotics of the Amazon Valley and Orinoco	."..with the addition of a small portion of slender roots of the *Caapi-pinima.*"	1852
Alfred Simson - Travels in the wilds of Ecuador, and the exploration of the Putumayo River.	Earliest mention of specific plants as admixtures. Differentiates between *ayahuasca* and *yagé*.	1874 - 1875
Theodor Koch-Grünberg - Zwei Jahre unter den Indianem. Reisen in nordwest-Brasilien (1903 - 1905)	Distinguishes two species of *caapi*.	1903 - 1905
Joaquín Rocha - Memorándum de viaje.	Probable identification of *Diplopterys cabrerana* as an admixture to *yagé* ("yerba que llaman chiripanga")	1905
P. Reinburg - Contribution à l'étude des boisson toxiques des indiens du Nord-ouest de l'Amazone, l'*ayahuasca*, le yagé, le huanto.	Leaves of *yagé* (*Diplopterys cabrearana*) as admixture to a *Banisteripsis* potion.	1921
William Burroughs - The *yagé* letters redux.	First mention of a Rubiacea as an admixture plant.	1954 - 1956
Homer V. Pinkley - Plant admixtures to *ayahuasca*, the South American hallucinogenic drink.	First botanical identification of *Psychotria viridis* as an admixture to *ayahuasca*.	1965 - 1967

pighiaceae, and I drew up the following brief description of it from living specimens in November 1853 – BANISTERIA CAAPI, Spruce ... The lower part of the stem is the part used. A quantity of this is beaten in a mortar, with water, and sometimes with the addition of a small portion of the slender roots of the *Caapi-pinima* [*Tetrapterys methystica?*]. When sufficiently triturated, it is passed through a sieve, which separates the woody fibre, and to the residue enough water is added to render it drinkable. Thus prepared, its colour is brownish-green, and its taste bitter and disagreeable.

The history of admixtures to a basic *Banisteriopsis* potion is unclear (Table 3). Chantre y Herrera (1901) and Spruce (1873, 184) mention plant additives but are not specific about their purpose or identity. *Psychotria viridis* Ruiz & Pavon (Rubiaceae) was identified as an admixture plant in 1967. Pinkley collected specimens identified as *Psychotria viridis* among the Kofán. The Kofáns add leaves and fruits of this plant for the same reason that they add leaves of *Diplopterys cabrerana*, in order to ."..increase their visions and to make them of longer duration" (Pinkley, 1969, 309).

William Burroughs, novelist and author of *The Yagé Letters* and *Naked Lunch*, during his search for *yagé* between 1952-1956, witnessed the addition of leaves to a *Banisteriopsis* potion while on a visit to Pucallpa (Burroughs et al., 2006, 95-97). He collected samples of the leaves and, with the help of an unnamed Peruvian botanist, identified the leaves as belonging to a species of *Rubiaceae*.

Ayahuasca and *yagé* could have points of origin in Northwest Amazonia, not earlier than the initial period of contact with Europeans (late 1500s?). The paucity of archaeological data and the lack of information about *ayahuasca* in early colonial documents, as well as imprecise descriptions of its use prior to AD 1850, suggest this approximate date. In contrast, snuffing and smoking are present in the archaeological record since at least 4,000 years ago (Table 4; Fernández Distel, 1980; Oyuela-Caycedo and Kawa, 2015, 32) and were documented by Spanish chroniclers from the earliest moments of the encounter (e.g., Aguado, 1956; Pané, 1999).

The question that results from this investigation is, If *ayahuasca* is indeed of recent invention, how and when did the knowledge of complex mechanisms of plant interaction develop? Essential to the answer are notions of: a) sequential use – chewing a *Banisteriopsis* stem previous to snuff inhalation, ingesting a simple *Banisteriopsis* tea in preparation for snuffing sessions, and simultaneous use of coca and tobacco; b) addition of *Anadenanthera* seeds to fermented drinks; and c) location, time period, and plant availability.

A CHEW OF CAAPI AND A PINCH OF YOPO
(*Anadenanthera peregrina* (L.) SPEG.)

Questions of origin should consider other methods of consumption that benefit from knowledge of plant interaction. Throughout the Orinoco River and its tributaries, there is ample documentation of chewing *caapi* stems in preparation for snuffing sessions in order to modify and prolong the effect of the DMT present in the snuffing powders (Gragson, 1997, 380; Reichel-Dolmatoff, 1944, 480; Rodd, 2002, 2008; Spruce 1970, 428). Sequential chewing of *Banisteriopsis* stems and nasal inhalation of *Anadenanthera* seeds were witnessed by Spruce (1970, 2, 428) in 1852. He described the chewing of *Banisteriopsis caapi* bark in conjunction with snuffing *yopo* (A. peregrina). This practice is also documented among the Guahibo, Pumé, and Piaroa.

Investigations among the Piaroa of southern Venezuela have shed light on the relationship between *Anadenanthera peregrina* (*yopo*) and *Banisteriopsis caapi*. Piaroa shamans consume B. *caapi* prior to snuffing and include *caapi* cuttings in the preparation of the snuff powder (Rodd, 2002, 2008).

The ethnographic evidence and pharmacologic research on the MAO-inhibiting effects of the harmala alkaloids clearly suggest that sustained chewing of *caapi* stems and/or drinking a *Banisteriopsis* tea could enhance the effects of the tryptamine-containing snuffs. This sequential consumption utilizes the human body to process the synergy between the harmala alkaloids present in *caapi* and the tryptamines in *yopo*.

ANADENANTHERA POTIONS

Previous to the accounts of Maroni and Chantre y Herrera there is no mention of *ayahuasca* by the early chroniclers, and the archaeological record is silent about the subject. It should be stressed that the important issue is to acknowledge that native peoples had an understanding of plant interaction, and that plant exploration was guided by this knowledge. In South America, no plant

Table 4. Antiquity of selected psychoactive plants in South America.

Anadenanthera	Inca Cueva, Argentina (Fernadéz Distel, 1980).	ca. 2100 BC (smoking) ca. 1200 BC (snuffing)
Banisteriopsis	Chantre y Herrera Pablo Maroni	ca. 1637 - 1787 AD ca. 1737 AD
Brugmansia	*Brugmansia* representations, Chavin sculpture (Torres, 2008).	ca. 900 -700 BC ca. 1400 AD
Nicotiena	Chiripa, Bolivia (Oyuela-Caicedo & Kawa, 2015) Niño Korin, Bolivia (Wassén, 1972).	ca. 1200 BC ca. 300 - 500 AD
Erythroxylum (coca)	Culebras, Ancash Perú (Engel 1957). Asia, Cañete, Perú (Engel, 1963).	ca. 2000 BC ca. 1800 BC
Trichocereus	Las Aldas, Perú (Polia Meconi, 1996). Garagay, Perú (Burger, 1995).	ca. 2000 BC ca. 1200 BC

is used as the sole ingredient of visionary preparations. Multiple ingredients are mixed in snuffs, fumatories, enemas and potions, or are of concurrent use, such as in the case of tobacco and coca.

Oral ingestion of *Anadenanthera* seeds has been recorded among diverse Amazonian cultures. The Guahibo prepare a drink called *yaraque*, which includes *yopo* powder. The Wichi of the Gran Chaco ingest *vino de cebil*, a fermented drink made from algarrobo (*Prosopis* spp.) and *Anadenanthera colubrina* (Vell.) Brenan seeds.

The addition of *vilca* (*A. colubrina*) to fermented drinks has been documented in the Central Andes during the early Colonial period (Cobo, 1964, 158, 272; Ondegardo, 1916, 29-30). Polo de Ondegardo (1916, Vol. 3, 29-30) made the first-known reference to *vilca* (*A. colubrina*) as a *chicha* additive in 1571:

> ... Those who wish to know an event of things past or of things that are to come ... invoke the demon and inebriate themselves and for this practice in particular make use of an herb called *vilca*, pouring its juice in *chicha* or drinking it by another way. Note that even though it is said that only old women practice the craft of divination and of telling what happens in remote places and to reveal loss and thievery, it is also used today by Indians not only by the old but also by the young.

Bernabé Cobo (1964, 272), writing ca. 1653, reported that *vilca* seeds were added to *chicha*. Garcilaso de La Vega (1970, 499; published 1609) documented a particularly strong *chicha*, known as *uiñapu*, made from sprouted corn: ."..some Indians, more passionate about inebriation than the rest of the community, steep the corn (*sara*) until it begins to sprout. They then grind it and boil it in the same water as other things. Once this is strained, it is kept until it ferments. A very strong drink, which intoxicates immediately, is thus produced ..." It should be noted that de la Vega references other ingredients to the brew but does not identify them.

THE ARCHAEOLOGICAL EVIDENCE

Direct archaeological evidence for psychoactive potions is difficult to identify. I am unaware of published chemical analysis of archaeological *chicha* residues. Unlike smoking and snuffing, which require distinctive paraphernalia specific to their respective tasks, the sole presence of elaborate drinking vessels should not be seen as evidence of visionary potions (Figure 5). Supporting evidence for the antiquity of *ayahuasca* relies on an elaborately carved ceramic vessel attributed to the Milagros-Quevedo culture (500 BC - 500 AD), and other ceramic vessels of native cultures of Ecuador dating as early as 2400 BC (Naranjo, 1986, 121-122). There is no evidence to support the proposal that these receptacles were ever used to drink *ayahuasca* or *yagé*.

Previous to the descriptions provided by Maroni (1737) and Chantre y Herrera (1637-1767), evidence for *ayahuasca* or *yagé* is totally lacking. Documentation of the addition of *Anadenanthera* seeds to fermented drinks by Cobo, Ondegardo, and others raises the possibility of the existence of drinks

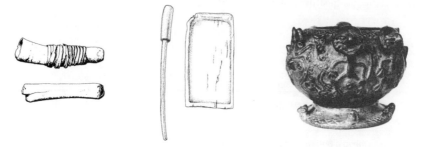

Fig. 5 Comparison of instruments for smoking and snuffing with a cup with elaborate designs. **Left:** puma (Felis concolor) bone pipes, ca. 2100 BC, 13 cm (top), 11.2 cm (bottom), Inca Cueva, Puna de Jujuy, Argentina, Museo Etnográfico Juan B. Ambrosetti, Buenos Aires, Argentina. **Center:** whale bone snuff tray (11.7 cm), and bird and fox bone tube (17.5 cm). ca. 1200 BC. American Museum of Natural History, NY. **Right:** carved ceramic vessel, Milagros-Quevedo culture, 500 BC - 500 AD. Museo Arqueológico del Banco Central, Quito,Ecuador.

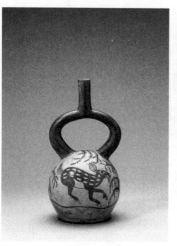

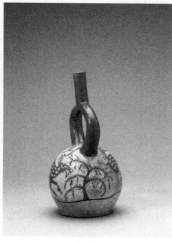

Fig. 6 Moche Stirrup Vessel painted with male and female deer and *Anadenanthera* trees, 26 cm h., Fowler Museum at UCLA, collection number X73.237. Photograph by Don Cole.

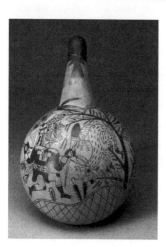

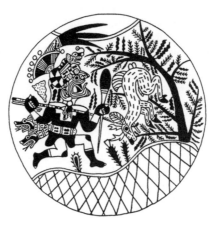

Fig. 7 Deer hunting scene, ladle (29.9 cm h), Moche, North Coast, Peru. **Left:** Art Institute of Chicago, Kate S. Buckingham Endowment, 1955.2277. **Right:** drawing by Donna McClelland, PH.PC.001-0166, Christopher B. Donnan and Donna McClelland Moche Archive, 1963-2011, Image Collections and Fieldwork Archives, Dumbarton Oaks, Trustees for Harvard University, Washington, D.C.

analogous to *ayahuasca* in the Central Andes prior to Spanish contact. Since direct archaeological evidence is absent, the iconography of two ancient Andean cultures, the Moche and the Wari, could divulge the existence of visionary potions and brews.

The Moche territory encompassed the arid north coast of present-day Peru, near the city of Trujillo, between ca. AD 100 and 900. They were not a unified entity, but independent polities that shared an iconographic system. For the purposes of this study, Moche fine-line painting on ceramic vessels (Donnan and McClelland, 1999) offers a large iconographic sample that allows a glimpse into the probability of an *Anadenanthera*-based potion consumed in pre-Columbian times. Depiction of *Anadenanthera* trees in Moche ceramics was first proposed by Peter Furst (1974, 84), based on the design on a pottery dipper painted with a deer-hunting scene. Bipinnate leaves, pods contracted between seeds, a bifurcated trunk, and slightly arched branches are characteristic of *Anadenanthera* (Figure 6).

Representations of deer in association with *Anadenanthera* trees are restricted to painted stirrup-spout vessels and ladles from Phase IV (ca. AD 500-650) of the Moche cultural sequence (Koons and Alex, 2014, 1050-1051). Male and female animals are depicted, although male representations are twice as common as female (Donnan, 1982, 238). *Anadenanthera* trees generally form part of deer-hunting scenes (Figure 7). Elaborately dressed individuals with supernatural attributes conduct the hunt. The ritualistic character of the event is further supported by the lack of evidence for eating deer meat in the Moche archaeological record (Donnan, 1982, 246). There is no evidence for smoking or snuffing.

Deer-hunting scenes painted on four stirrup-spout vessels suggest the possibility that *Anadenanthera* preparations might have been administered orally (Figs. 8-11). The first I will discuss here represents a scene that takes place within a clearly delimited space (Figure 8). Above the painted scene, an elaborately dressed individual armed with a spear thrower sits next to a deer. Below, in the painted scene, a personage seats on a litter, and two elaborately dressed individuals hunt deer assisted by dogs in contorted poses. Spruce (1970, 2: 429) observed a Catauixí hunter administering *Anadenanthera* seed enemas to himself and his hunting dog "...to clear their vision and render them more alert!" The Piro of the upper Ucayali River also gave *Anadenanthera* to their dogs prior to hunting. To the right, next to a wall with stepped designs, two women walk carrying jars with domed lids and attached branches that correspond in shape to those trees identified as *Anadenanthera* on vessels with deer-hunting representations.

In the second vessel (Figure 9), the two female figures are associated with seven jars with domed lids and attached *Anadenanthera* branches. The domed lids of two of the vessels are replaced by deer heads; the deer's nose attachment is similar to the one seen on the individual seated on the litter in the previous case. The deer heads substituting for the neck and lid of the jars suggest *Anadenanthera* as an ingredient of the liquid contained in these vessels. In the register above, an important personage and attendants are armed with spear throwers. A third vessel (Figure 10) represents a deer-headed human being holding a cup. Three vessels with attached *Anadenanthera* branches, one with the lid removed, are located just below the deer-headed individual. This vessel demonstrates, once again, a connection between deer and *Anadenanthera* trees. Deer are also associated with visionary plants in other cultures. The *Wixárika* (Huichol) identify deer with peyote (Furst, 1976, 113); and in Siberia, reindeer are equated with *Amanita muscaria* (Wasson, 1972, 161).

A fourth stirrup-spout vessel (Figure 11) depicts, in modeled clay, a mutilated human being bound to a tree stump. The mutilated individual stands over a painted scene with similar elements to those on the second described vessel (Figure 9). On the lower register of the painted scene, a woman sits tending jars with *Anadenanthera* branches, while above her an individual standing on a platform and surrounded by armed attendants is offered a drinking cup.

Moche iconography related to the deer hunt provides rare evidence for the use of visionary potions by pre-Columbian inhabitants of South America. The constant association and identification of the deer with fruiting *Anadenanthera* trees, and the tree's association with these ceramic vessels and dippers, underscores the possibility of oral administration among the Moche. This is further supported by the scene where the drink contained in the jars is offered to an important personage (Figure 11).

Further evidence for visionary brews is seen in the iconography of the Wari (ca. AD 300-900). Wari territory encompassed the south central Andes and the adjacent coast. Patricia Knobloch (2000), in her study of Wari ceramics found at the site of Conchopata, near Ayacucho, Peru, presents suggestive evidence for potions containing *Anadenanthera* seeds (Figure 12). She has identified an icon as a probable representation of *Anadenanthera* flowers, leaves, and seedpods. Her identification is based on an image painted on a large ceramic vessel related to *chicha*-drinking ceremonies (Kno-

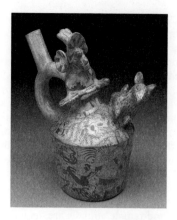

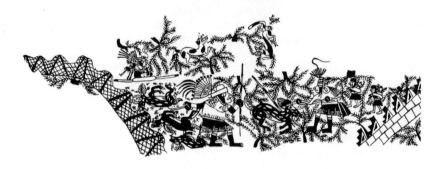

Fig. 8 Top, Moche stirrup-spout vessel depicting a deer hunt (23 cm h.). Dallas Museum of Art, The Eugene and Margaret McDermott Art Fund, Inc., 1969.2.McD. **Bottom,** Drawing by Donna McClelland, PH.PC.001-0111, Christopher B. Donnan and Donna McClelland Moche Archive, 1963-2011, Image Collections and Fieldwork Archives, Dumbarton Oaks, Trustees for Harvard University, Washington, D.C.

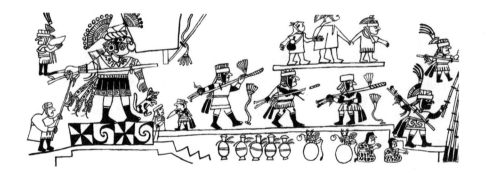

Fig. 9 Moche stirrup-spout vessel painted with warriors armed with spear throwers and with jars and deer heads. Drawing by Donna McClelland, PH.PC.001-0074, Christopher B. Donnan and Donna McClelland Moche Archive, 1963-2011, Image Collections and Fieldwork Archives, Dumbarton Oaks, Trustees for Harvard University, Washington, D.C.

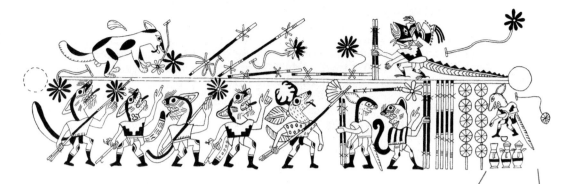

Fig. 10 Moche ceramic vessel painted with deer-headed warriors armed with spear throwers. Drawing by Donna McClelland (after Donnan and McClelland, 1999: Figure 4.91).

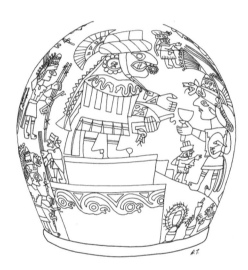

Fig. 11 Moche ceramic vessel depicting an important personage on a platform holding a cup. Drawing courtesy of Donna Torres.

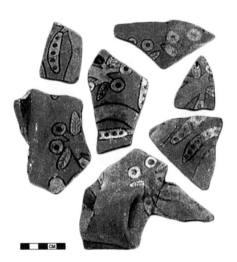

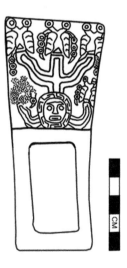

Fig. 12 Two representations of *Anadenanthera* icon. Left, ceramic fragments from the Wari archaeological site of Conchopata, Peru. Photo courtesy of Patricia Knobloch. Right, snuff tray, wood, 12.8 cm, Tiwanaku, Bolivia. Peabody Museum of Archaeology and Ethnology, Harvard University, Alexander E. Agassiz collection number 75-20-30/8649.

bloch, 2000, 398). In addition to Wari ceramics, this icon is seen in monumental stone sculpture at Tiwanaku, Bolivia; additionally, the *Anadenanthera* icon is frequent in snuff trays from San Pedro de Atacama, Chile (Torres, 1987). A snuff tray from Tiwanaku is inscribed with an *Anadenanthera* tree emerging from a disembodied head (Figure 12). Given the absence of snuffing paraphernalia in the Wari area, Knobloch (2000, 397-398) suggests that *Anadenanthera colubrina* could have been ingested as a drink. Citing Polo de Ondegardo (1916, Vol. 3, 29-30), she proposes that *A. colubrina* was added to *chicha* and was likely the beverage held by the large urns and jars found at Conchopata.

Several authors (Goldstein, 2005, 208-210; Janusek, 2004, 224; Moseley et al., 2005, 17267, Figures 5-6) have reported clear evidence of extensive *chicha* production at the archaeological sites of Tiwanaku and Lukurmata in Bolivia, and Cerro Baúl in Peru. Apparently, these archaic *chichas*, as reported in early colonial documents, might have contained vegetable admixtures to the fermented corn *molle* (*Schinus molle* L.) or *Prosopis* base, the most frequent bases for fermented drinks in the Central Andes.

CONCLUSIONS

Origin and invention are totally different categories of experience. Origin, as Walter Benjamin eloquently states, is the manner through which things or ideas come into life. Discovery and invention, however, are related to actual processes of creation. Selection of specific plants is guided by an intimate knowledge of environment and cultural needs of the community, and speaks directly about creativity and discovery. Any healer, any shaman, is keenly aware of all details of the landscape and of his/her life-space – not only plants, but also minerals, soil, weather patterns, etc. The exchange of knowledge with neighboring communities would most likely not be restricted to material goods. It would surely include transmission of ideas, pharmacological information, stories, and mytho/historical information, constructing a network that contributes to the creation of symbolic systems and complex approaches to the use of plants to modify states of consciousness.

The origin of *ayahuasca* and *yagé* must be seen within the large scale of interaction and ideological exchange that characterized native communities in the Amazon and the Andes. The evidence suggests multiple origin locations for *ayahuasca*, *yagé*, and analogous potions, and not a center from which a fixed recipe diffused. This incessant interaction is what gives origin to the potions and brews under consideration in this study. The origins of *ayahuasca* must be considered from two complementary points of view. The first should consider events that took place after European contact, and the second should take into account developments that occurred in the Andes during pre-Columbian times, including consideration of fermented drinks.

Bufotenine retains about one third of its activity when orally ingested (Ott, 2001, 103-104, 110). Its potency as a smoke or snuff was well known, a factor that could suggest to a user to seek ways to enhance its oral activity. Issues of plant availability could also motivate a search for more efficient ways to prepare and consume psychoactive plants. The absence of *A. colubrina* in the western slopes of the Andes could have motivated a search for more effective ways of consumption and of enhancing and prolonging the oral activity of bufotenine.

The problem to be resolved in proposing *chicha* with an admixture of *Anadenanthera* seeds, as well as other plants, as one of the the the precedents for modern *ayahuasca* and *yagé*, is whether there are β-carboline alkaloids present in the brew that could potentiate the psychoactive tryptamines. The alcohol present in *chicha* is metabolized into β-carbolines. Alcohol hydrogenase converts some of the alcohol into acetaldehyde; this compound reacts with tryptamines to produce β-carbolines. Drinking *chicha* could thus potentiate the bufotenine present in *Anadenanthera* seeds added during the fermentation process. *Chicha* is most frequently made of sprouted corn, but in northern Chile, southern Bolivia, and northwest Argentina, seeds and pods of Prosopis species are the source of the beer known as *aloja*. Tryptamine and β-carbolines have been detected in fresh leaves of *Prosopis nigra* Hieron, a tree present in northwest Argentina (Moro et al., 1975, 827). Also, *P. chilensis* (Molina) Stuntz and *P. alba* Griseb. contain tryptamine (Astudillo et al., 2000, 569, 571) that could easily convert into β-carbolines in the presence of acetaldehyde. This information suggests that these pre-Columbian beers could be predecessors of *ayahuasca* and *yagé*, and imply knowledge of plant interaction. The widespread use of tobacco in healing and shamanic rituals should also be considered. Origins of knowledge of synergy between tryptamines and β-carbolines emphasize the importance of tobacco, a constant presence in healing rituals (Bondeson, 1972; Oyuela-Caycedo and Kawa, 2015; Wassén, 1972). Tobacco smoke contains two β-carbolines, harman and norharman, which are well-known MAO inhibitors.

The key to understanding this origin phenomenon lies in the interaction and flow of ideas surrounding moments of population displacement. Cultural interaction patterns suggest that *ayahuasca* and *yagé* could have originated in the northwest Amazon, not earlier than the initial period of contact with Europeans ca. 1550-1650. I propose that *ayahuasca* and *yagé* resulted from the interaction of several visionary traditions coinciding in the northwest Amazon in the sixteenth century, stimulated by extensive population movements. Causes of population displacements during the early colonial period (1538-1767) include events that caused great disturbances in their respective areas. Among these, several are relevant to this discussion. The collapse of the Inca empire was motivated by many factors, including the execution of Atahualpa in 1533 and the capture of Cuzco by Francisco Pizarro (1533-1535). Subsequently, Spanish slave trading stimulated eastward movement of large percentages of populations from areas along the base of the Andes adjacent to centers of Spanish colonization. Portuguese slave trading along the lower Amazon provoked migration west upriver. Slavery produced a crisis in the area of the mouth of the Napo, which Spain and Portugal claimed. Indigenous people were forced to migrate upriver and seek refuge in Jesuit missions. After 1767, Jesuit missions disbanded, causing further population movement. This was followed a century later by the Rubber Boom (1880-1920). Healing and shamanic lore spread with these journeys. Population displacements carried knowledge of visionary preparations and familiarity with plants, environmental conditions, and historical information.

To the east of the proposed area of origin of *ayahuasca*, there is intensive use of sequential or simultaneous dosing, and of fermented drinks with an admixture of *Anadenanthera peregrina* seeds (Gragson, 1997, 380; Reichel-Dolmatoff, 1944, 480; Reis Altschul,1972, 31). In the mid and upper tributaries of the Orinoco, the simultaneous consumption of *caapi* and *yopo* could be seen as *ayahuasca* analogues. The Piaroa chew *caapi* stems for 2 to 3 hours prior to snuff inhalation to enhance and prolong the visionary state. When the Piaroa desire a particularly strong snuff experience, a potion with *Banisteriopsis* as the sole ingredient is ingested prior to the use of DMT- and bufotenine-containing snuff (Rodd, 2002, 2008). For the people of the tropical grasslands (llanos) of the Orinoco Basin in Colombia and Venezuela, the chewing and drinking of *caapi* prior to inhalation of powdered *Anadenanthera* seeds was a frequent modality for enhancement of the bufotenine present in the seeds. Sequential use, as seen among the Piaroa and the Guahibo, could likely be a precursor to the invention of complex potions such as *ayahuasca* or *yagé*, and clearly indicates a knowledge of issues of plant synergy.

From northwestern Amazonia, the use of *ayahuasca* may have spread following routes of colonial/missionary expansion (Map 3; Shepard, 2014, 16). Brabec de Mori (2011) proposes, first, an expansion from the Tukano or their predecessors to Kichwa speakers related to Jesuit missions in Ecuador and Peru; and second, to the Quechua de Lamas (Lamas prov.) and Shawi people (Loreto prov.), and third, up the Ucayali and to the Brazilian state of Acre, probably associated with the movements of rubber workers (Brabec de Mori, 2011, 42). In its movement to the southwest, *ayahuasca* reached the Shipibo about two centuries ago (Brabec de Mori, 2014, 207). Gow, (2015, 57) demonstrates how the Piro of the Urubamba River in Peru may have known of the existence of *ayahuasca* ca. 1880, although they did not begin to use it until much later, probably ca. 1930. He proposes that *ayahuasca* is a recent introduction to the healing practices of indigenous populations of the southwest Amazon (Gow, 2015, 45). The recent distribution of *ayahuasca* in western Amazonia supports a date for the creation of *ayahuasca* sometime ca. 1550-1650.

Connections between the northern and northwestern Amazon and the Andes are evident in shared iconographic themes; this region has been a crossroad for exchange between the highlands and the tropical forest since early pre-Columbian times (Map 4). For example, connections between the highland Chavín culture (ca. BC 300-900) and the northwest Amazon are clear (Lathrap, 1971). The Tello Obelisk (Figure 13), a stone sculpture from Chavín de Huántar, depicts a caiman with supernatural attributes. The habitat of the caiman does not include the high Andes; instead, they thrive in the tropical forest. Sculpture in the Chavín style has been found in the upper drainage of the Marañon River, indicating accessibility and ideological exchange with the lowlands to the east of Chavín (Burger, 2008, 163; Morales Chocano, 2008, 148). Another example of Andean contact with the Amazon area is apparent in the culture of San Agustín, ca. BC 100-AD 500, located on the eastern slopes of the Colombian Andes. San Agustín is characterized by the presence of hundreds of stone carvings. There are details in the sculpture that clearly connect San Agustín with Amazonian cultures. Several sculptures depict an iconographic theme known as the "double" or "alter-ego," commonly associated with shamanism in the Andes and in the Amazon (Figure 14). Stone sculptures in the San Agustín style have been found in the Upper Caquetá River (Friede, 1946, 196; Silva Celis, 1963, 397). The Caquetá and tributaries provide direct routes to the Amazon River.

49

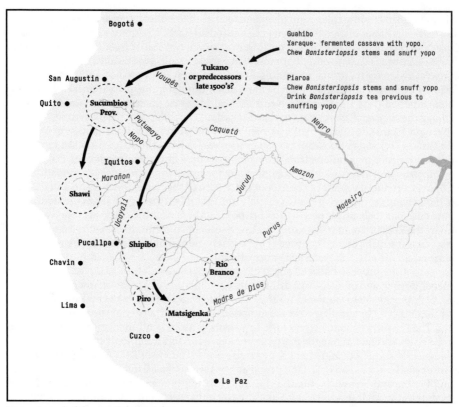

Map 3 Spread of the use of *ayahuasca* in western Amazonia.

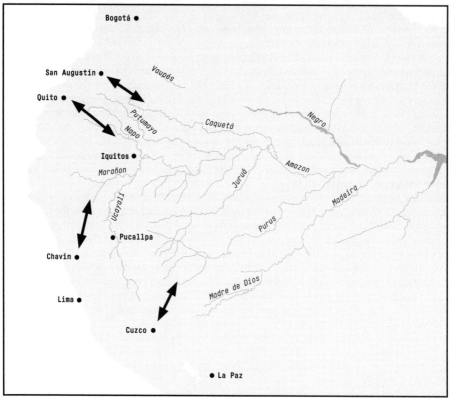

Map 4 Map showing zones of interaction between the Amazon and the Andes previous to contact with Europeans.

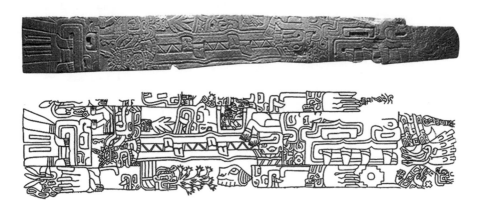

Fig. 13 The Tello Obelisk, 2.52 m high, granite. Chavín de Huántar. Museo Nacional de Arqueología, Antropología e Historia, Lima (after Burger 1995: Fig. 141).

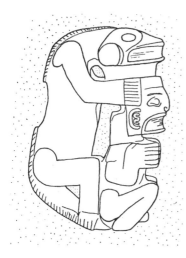
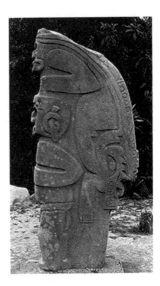

Fig. 14 Alter-ego or double representations. Left, snuff powder container, stone, 17.5 cm, Trombetas River, Brazil. Museum of World Cultures, Gothenburg, Sweden, collection number 25.12.1. Right, stone sculpture, 3 meters, Alto de las Piedras, San Agustín, Colombia.

Information obtained from early colonial documents, and iconographic information from pre-Columbian cultures such as the Moche and the Wari, prove that potions and brews analogous to *ayahuasca* were in use in the Central Andes and adjacent coast since at least 500 AD. Sequential or simultaneous practices, such as those of the Piaroa and the Guahibo, including the chewing and drinking of *caapi* to potentiate snuffing sessions, combined with knowledge of fermented drinks (with the addition of *vilca* seeds, as well as other unknown plant ingredients) could have motivated a search of the local flora to create numerous potions and plant combinations. The numerous variations and lack of fixed recipes found in Andean and Amazonian visionary preparations attest to a dynamic pharmacopoeia, constantly inventing and reinventing itself in search of access to alternate states of consciousness. The importance of beer and tobacco should be stressed, as these two are shared by all of South American shamanism and provide a clear link through time and space.

The most important factor gleaned by this investigation is knowledge of an understanding of the combined effect produced by varied admixture plants, and that plant selection is guided by an exacting familiarity with the immediate living space, and not by simple trial and error. This concept enabled and created multiple visionary preparations not limited by locality, or by the spread of a fixed recipe and related issues of plant availability. Multiple origin locations interacted with each other to create numerous plant combinations and delivery methods, such as drinking, smoking, snuffing, enemas, and unguents, each being appropriate to location, time period, and specific communities, and not to a center from which a fixed recipe diffused.

ACKNOWLEDGEMENTS

I am indebted to Carlo Brescia, Jace Callaway, Javier Echeverría, Kathleen Harrison, Luis Eduardo Luna, Dennis McKenna, Jonathan Ott, Giorgio Samorini, Donna Torres, Keeper Trout, and Steven White for generously sharing their knowledge of *ayahuasca* botany, pharmacology, and history.

REFERENCES

Aguado, P. de, 1956. *Recopilación Historial*, 4 vols. Biblioteca de la Presidencia de Colombia, Bogotá.

América Indígena, 1986. Chamanismo y uso de plantas del género *Banisteriopsis* en la hoya amazónica. Proceedings of a symposium organized by Luis Eduardo Luna, XLV Congreso Internacional de Americanistas, Bogotá, 7-11 de Julio, 1985. América Indígena, vol. XLVI, no. 1. México DF, Instituto Indigenista Interamericano.

Astudillo. L., G. Schmeda-Hirschmann, J. P. Herrera, M. Cortés, 2000. Proximate composition and biological activity of Chilean prosopis species. *Journal of the Science of Food and Agriculture* 80, 567-573.

Beyer, S. V., 2009. *Singing to the Plants. A Guide to Mestizo Shamanism in the Upper Amazon*. Albuquerque, University of New Mexico Press.

Bondeson, W. E., 1972. Tobacco from a Tiahuanacoid culture period, in: *A Medicine-man's Implements and Plants in a Tiahuanacoid Tomb in Highland Bolivia*. Etnologiska Studier 32, 177-184, Göteborgs Etnografiska Museum, Sweden.

Brabec de Mori, B., 2011. Tracing hallucinations: Contributing to a critical ethnohistory of *ayahuasca* usage in the Peruvian Amazon, in: Labate, B. C., Jungaberle, H. (Eds.), *The Internationalization of Ayahuasca. Performances: Intercultural Studies on Ritual, Play and Theatre - Performanzen: Interkulturelle Studien zu Ritual, Spiel und Theater Series*, Book 16., LIT Verlag, Berlin, 23-47.

Brabec de Mori, B., 2014. From the natives' point of view. How Shipibo-Kanibo experience and interpret *ayahuasca* drinking with "Gringos," in: Labate, B.C.,Cavnar, C. (Eds.), *Ayahuasca Shamanism in the Amazon and Beyond*. Oxford University Press, Oxford, 206-230.

Burger, R. L., 1995. *Chavín and the Origins of Andean Civilization*. Thames and Hudson, New York.

Burger, R. L., 2008. The original context of the Yauya Stela, in: Conklin, W., Quilter, J., (Eds.), *Chavín Art, Architecture and Culture*. Los Angeles, Cotsen Institute of Archaeology, University of California, 163-179.

Burroughs, W., Ginsberg, A., and Harris, O., 2006. *The Yagé Letters Redux*. San Francisco, City Lights Books.

Califano, M., 1976. El Chamanismo Mataco. *Scripta Ethnologica* 3, Part 2, 7-60. Centro de Estudios de Etnología Americana, Buenos Aires, 16-18.

Chantre y Herrera, J., 1901. *Historia de las Misiones de la Compañía de Jesús en el Marañón Español*. Imprenta de A. Avrial, Madrid.

Cobo, B., 1964. *Historia del Nuevo Mundo*. Biblioteca de Autores Españoles, vols. 91, 92. Ediciones Atlas, Madrid.

Donnan, C. B., 1982. *La Caza del Venado en el Arte Mochica*. Revista del Museo Nacional 46, Lima, 235-251.

Donnan, C. B., McClelland, D., 1999. *Moche Fineline Painting. Its Evolution and its Artists*. Fowler Museum of Cultural History, University of California, Los Angeles.

Engel, Frédéric, 1957. "Early Sites on the Peruvian Coast." *Southwestern Journal of Anthropology* 13: 54-68, University of New Mexico, Albuquerque.

Engel, Frédéric, 1963. "A preceramic settlement in the central coast of Peru: Asia, Unit 1." *Transactions of the American Philosophical Society* 53 (3), Philadelphia.

Fernández Distel, A., 1980. Hallazgo de pipas en complejos precerámicos del borde de la Puna Jujeña (Republica Argentina) y empleo de alucinógenos por parte de las mismas culturas. *Estudios Arqueológicos* 5, Universidad de Chile, Antofagasta, 55-75.

Friede, J., 1946. Migraciones indígenas en el Valle del Alto Magdalena, in: *Compilación de Apuntes Arqueológicos, Etnológicos, Geográficos y Estadísticos del Municipio de San Agustín*, edited by Tiberio López. Coopgráficas, Colombia.

Furst, P. T., 1974. Hallucinogens in Precolumbian art, in: King, M.E., Traylor, I.R. (Eds.), *Art and Environment in Native America*. Museum of Texas Technological University, Lubbock, 50-101.

Furst, P. T., 1976. Hallucinogens and culture. Chandler and Sharp Publishers, San Francisco.

Goldstein, P. S., 2005. *Andean Diaspora: The Tiwanaku Colonies and the Origins of South American Empire*. University Press of Florida, Gainesville, Florida.

Gow, P., 2015. Methods of tobacco use among two Arawakan-speaking peoples in Southeastern Amazonia: A case study of structural diffusion, in: Russell, Andrew, Rahman, Elizabeth (Eds.), *The Master Plant: Tobacco in Lowland South America*. Bloomsbury Academic, London, 45-61.

Gragson, T. L., 1997. The use of underground plant organs and its relation to habitat selection among the Pumé Indians of Venezuela. *Economic Botany* 51 (4), 377-384.

Herraiz T, Chaparro C., 2005. Human monoamine oxidase is inhibited by tobacco smoke: Beta-carboline alkaloids act as potent and reversible inhibitors. *Biochemical and Biophysical Research Communications.* Jan 14;326(2):378-86.

Holmstedt, B., Lindgren, J. E., 1967. Chemical constituents and pharmacology of South American snuffs, in: Efron, D.H, Holmstedt, B., Kline, N.S. (Eds.), *Ethnopharmacologic Search for Psychoactive Drugs.* Public Health Service Publication 1645, U.S. Department of Health, Education, and Welfare, Washington, D.C., 339-373.

Janusek, J. W., 2004. *Identity and Power in the Ancient Andes: Tiwanaku Cities through Time.* Routledge, New York.

Knobloch, P. J., 2000. *Wari Ritual Power at Conchopata: An Interpretation of Anadenanthera Colubrina Iconography.* Latin American Antiquity 11 (4), 387-402.

Koch-Grünberg, T., 1909-1910. *Zwei Jahre unter den Indianern. Reisen in Nordwest-Brasilien 1903/1905.* 2 Vols. Ernst Wasmuth, Berlin.

Koons, Michele L., Alex, Bridget A., 2014. Revised moche chronology based on Bayesian models of reliable radiocarbon dates. *Radiocarbon* 56 (3), 1039-1055, University of Arizona, Tucson.

Labate, Beatriz Caiuby, Cavnar, Clancy (Eds.), 2014. *Ayahuasca Shamanism in the Amazon and Beyond.* Oxford Ritual Studies, Oxford University Press.

Lathrap, D. W., 1971. The tropical forest and the cultural context of Chavín, in: Benson, E. (Ed.), *Dumbarton Oaks Conference on Chavín.* Dumbarton Oaks Research Library and Collection, Washington, D. C., 73-100.

Luna, L. E., 1986. Vegetalismo - Shamanism Among the *Mestizo* Population of the Peruvian Amazon. *Stockholm Studies in Comparative Religion* 27. Almqvist & Wiksell International, Stockholm.

Magnin, J. 1988. Breve descripción de la Provincia de Quito, en la América meridional, y de sus Missiones de succumbíos de Religiosos de S. Franc.o, y de Maynas de PP. de la Comp.a de Jhs. a las orillas del gran Río Marañón, hecha para el Mapa que se hizo el año 1740. In *Noticias auténticas del famoso río Marañón y misión apostólica de la Compañía de Jesús de la Provincia de Quito,* ed. J. P. Chaumeil, pp. 463-492. Iquitos: Monumenta Amazonica, Instituto de Investigaciones Científicas de la Amazonía Peruana.

Maroni, P., 1737. Noticias auténticas del famoso Río Marañón y Misión Apostólica de la Compañía de Jesús de la Provincia de Quito en los dilatados bosques de dicho río, escribialas por los años de 1738 un misionero de la Misma Compañía, in: Chaumeil, J. P. (Ed.),. 1988. *Monumenta Amazonica,* Volume 4, Instituto de Investigaciones Científicas de la Amazonía Peruana. Iquitos.

Morales Chocano, D., 2008. The importance of Pacopampa architecture and iconography in the Central Andean formative, in: Conklin, W., Quilter, J. (Eds.), *Chavín Art, Architecture and Culture.* Cotsen Institute of Archaeology, University of California, Los Angeles, 143-160.

Moro, G. A., Graziano, M. N., and Cousio, J. D.,1975. Alkaloids of Prosopis nigra. *Phytochemistry* 14, 827. Pergamon Press.

Moseley, M. E., Nash, D. J.,Williams, P. R., deFrance, S. D., Miranda, A., and Ruales, M., 2005. Burning down the brewery: Establishing and evacuating an ancient imperial colony at Cerro Baúl, Peru. *Proceedings of the National Academy of Sciences of the United States* 102 (48), 17264–17271.

Naranjo, P., 1986. El *ayahuasca* en la arqueología ecuatoriana. América indígena. Chamanismo y uso de plantas del género *Banisteriopsis* en la Hoya Amazónica. Proceedings of a symposium organized by Luis Eduardo Luna, XLV Congreso Internacional de Americanistas, Bogotá, 7-11 de Julio, 1985. *América Indígena,* vol. XLVI, no. 1, 117-127. México DF: Instituto Indigenista Interamericano.

Ogalde, J. P., Arriaza, Bernardo T., Soto, E. C., 2009. Identification of psychoactive alkaloids in ancient Andean human hair by gas chromatography/mass spectrometry. *Journal of Archaeological Science* 36, 467-472. Elsevier Science, London.

Ondegardo, P. de, 1916. *Informaciones Acerca de la Religión y Gobierno de los Incas, in Colección de Libros y Documentos Referentes a la Historia del Perú,* edited by H. H. Urteaga. Lima.

Ott, J., 1994. *Ayahuasca Analogues: Pangæan Entheogens.* Natural Products Company, Kennewick.

Ott, J., 2001. Pharmañopo–psychonautics: Human intranasal, sublingual, intrarectal, pulmonary and oral pharmacology of bufotenine. *Journal of Psychoactive Drugs* 33(3), 273-281.

Oyuela-Caycedo, A., Kawa, N. C., 2015. A Deep History of Tobacco in Lowland South America, in: Russell, Andrew, Rahman, Elizabeth (Eds.), *The Master Plant: Tobacco in Lowland South America.* Bloomsbury Academic, London, 27-44.

Pané, Fr. R., 1999. *An Account of the Antiquities of the Indians.* Duke University Press, Durham. (Spanish version, *Relación Acerca de las Antigüedades de los Indios.* Siglo Veintiuno Editores, México.).

Pinkley, H. V., 1969. Plant admixtures to *ayahuasca,* the South American hallucinogenic drink. *Lloydia* 32, 305-314.

Polia Meconi, Mario, 1996. "Despierta, remedio, cuenta...": Adivinos y medicos del Ande, 2 vols. Fondo Editorial, Pontificia Universidad Católica del Perú, Lima.

Reichel-Dolmatoff, G., 1944. *La Cultura Material de los Indios Guahibo.* Revista del Instituto Etnológico Nacional 1 (2), 437-506.

Reichel-Dolmatoff, G. 1978. *Beyond the Milky Way. Hallucinatory Imagery of the Tukano Indians.* Latin American Center Publications, University of California, Los Angeles.

Reinburg, P., 1921. Contribution à l'étude des boissons toxiques des Indiens du Nord-Ouest de l'Amazone: L'ayahuásca, le yagé, le Huánto. Étude comparative toxico-physiologique d'une expérience personnelle (suite). *Journal de la Société des Américanistes* 13 (2), 197-216.

Reis Altschul, S. V., 1972. *The Genus Anadenanthera in Amerindian Cultures.* Botanical Museum, Harvard University, Cambridge.

Rocha, J., 1905. *Memorandum de Viaje (Regiones Amazónicas).* Casa Editorial de El Mercurio, Bogotá.

Rodd, R., 2002. Snuff synergy: Preparation, use and pharmacology of *yopo* and *Banisteriopsis caapi* among the Piaroa of Southern Venezuela. *Journal of Psychoactive Drugs* 34 (3), 273-9.

Rodd, R., 2008. Reassessing the cultural and psychopharmacological significance of *Banisteriopsis caapi:* Preparation, classification and use among the Piaroa of southern Venezuela. *Journal of Psychoactive Drugs* 40 (3), 301-307.

Samorini, G., 2016. Jurema, la planta visonaria. *Dal Brasile alla Psiconautica di Frontera.* ShaKe Edizioni, Milan.

Schultes, R.E., 1957. *The Identity of the Malpighiaceous Narcotics of South America*. Botanical Museum Leaflets 18 (1), 1-56.

Shepard Jr., G. H., 2014. Will the real shaman please stand up? The recent adoption of *ayahuasca* among indigenous groups of the Peruvian Amazon, in: Labate, B.C., Cavnar, C. (Eds.), *Ayahuasca Shamanism in the Amazon and Beyond*. Oxford University Press, Oxford,16-39.

Silva Célis, E., 1963. Movimiento de la civilización Agustiniana por el alto Amazonas. *Revista Colombiana de Antropología* 13, 389-400. Instituto Colombiano de Antropología e Historia, Bogotá.

Simson, A., 1886. *Travels in the Wilds of Ecuador and the Exploration of the Putumayo River*. Sampson Low, Marston, Searle, and Rivington, London.

Spruce, R., 1873. On some remarkable narcotics of the Amazon Valley and Orinoco. *The Geographical Review*, New Series 1, 184-193. Also published in *Spruce, R.*, 1970, 414-425. Ocean Highways, London.

Spruce, R., 1970. *Notes of a Botanist in the Amazon and the Andes*. Johnson reprint, New York (orig. ed. 1908, MacMillan, London).

Torres, C. M., 1987. The Iconography of Prehispanic Snuff Trays from San Pedro de Atacama, Northern Chile. *Andean Past* 1, 191-245. Latin American Studies Program, Cornell University, Ithaca, NY.

Torres, C. M., 2008. Chavín's psychoactive pharmacopoeia: The iconographic evidence. In: *Chavín: Art, Architecture and Culture*, eds. W. J. Conklin and J. Quilter, Cotsen Institute of Archaeology, University of California, Los Angeles.

Trout, K., 2008. Old hair and tryptamines. *The Entheogen Review* 16 (4), 146-149.

Vega, G. d. L., 1970. *Royal Commentaries of the Incas, and General History of Peru: Part One*. University of Texas Press, Austin (orig ed. Lisbon, 1609).

Villavicencio, Manuel, 1858. *Geografía de la República del Ecuador*. Imprenta Robert Craighead, New York.

Wassén, S. H., 1972. A medicine-man's implements and plants in a Tiahuanacoid tomb in highland Bolivia. *Etnologiska Studier* 32, 7-114. Göteborgs Etnografiska Museum, Gothenburg, Sweden.

Wasson, R. G., 1972. Soma: Divine mushroom of immortality. *Ethno-Mycological Studies* 1. Harcourt Brace Jovanovich.

Plant Use and Shamanic *Dietas* in Contemporary *Ayahuasca* Shamanism in Peru

■■■ *Evgenia Fotiou*, PhD ■■■

| Assistant Professor of Anthropology, Kent State University

ABSTRACT

Ayahuasca is a psychoactive plant mixture used in a ceremonial context throughout Western Amazonia, and its use has expanded globally in recent decades. As part of this expansion, *ayahuasca* has become popular among Westerners who travel to the Peruvian Amazon in increasing numbers to experience its reportedly healing and transformative effects. In and around Iquitos, Peru, shamanism is reinvented as local shamanic practices converge with Western ideas of spirituality and healing and create a hybrid and highly dynamic practice, which I call *shamanic tourism*. I use this term because the experience often involves the participation in a shamanic *dieta*, which involves fasting and the ingestion of non-psychoactive plants. In addition, it is a common practice in this context to use a variety of plants for bodily and energetic cleansing in the form of purges and ritual baths. Drawing from ethnographic fieldwork in and around the area of Iquitos, the epicenter of *shamanic tourism*, this paper will focus on some of the plants that *curanderos* and *ayahuasqueros* use in the area alongside *ayahuasca* and the ways these are perceived by healers and participants. I will show that the use of plants in this manner is intricately connected with Amazonian conceptions of the body.

INTRODUCTION

Ayahuasca is a psychedelic plant mixture consumed in the form of a brew, which is prepared from the stems of the jungle liana, *Banisteriopsis caapi* (Spruce ex Griseb.) Morton most often combined with the leaves of *Psychotria viridis* Ruiz & Pav. or *Diplopterys cabrerana* (Cuatrec.) B. Gates to produce visionary and purgative effects. The *Banisteriopsis caapi* vine is indigenous to the western and northwestern Amazon, but its use has expanded globally. For decades, *ayahuasca* was the stuff of legend, associated with scientists and literary writers, from the pioneer field ethnobotanist Richard Evans Schultes to the poet Allen Ginsberg and the writer William Burroughs. Today its use has expanded to a global level and has had an enormous impact on religious and neo-shamanic currents in the West. It has also attracted the attention of scientists internationally, who conduct research with *ayahuasca* in order to determine possible therapeutic uses.

In indigenous Amazonian shamanism, *ayahuasca* had a variety of uses. Depending on the ethnic group, it was used in communal rituals of men, singing and dancing, for locating game animals, divination, in warfare and conflict, to see faraway places, and for healing by communicating with spirits. It was also important in native art, cosmology, and ethnoastronomy, and in the Jaguar complex (Reichel-Dolmatoff, 1975). Among indigenous Amazonians, *ayahuasca* is very important in maintaining social order and in interpreting daily life events. Shamans, being mediators between the spirit and the human worlds, used *ayahuasca* to move freely between the two and negotiate and restore relations between them. Shamans also contact the "master spirits of the animals in order that the hunters may find game and influence the spirits of the seasons so that harvests will be abundant" (Langdon, 1979, 64). *Ayahuasca* is so fundamental for some groups like the Shuar (Jívaro) of the Ecuadorian Amazon that, as Michael Harner (1973) points out, the *ayahuasca* induced experience is seen as the true reality whereas normal waking life is considered simply an illusion. For the Shuar, the true forces behind daily life are in the supernatural realm and can only be accessed through the psychedelic experience. In addition, in many tribal cultures, *ayahuasca*, along with other mind-altering plants, is viewed as an intelligent being possessing a spirit (*ayahuasca* mama) who is able to communicate and transmit knowledge to humans through the visionary state (Whitten, 1976).

This paper is based on research that started with my dissertation fieldwork on *shamanic tourism* in Iquitos, Peru (Fotiou, 2010) and has evolved into an ongoing project focusing mainly on interculturality. The central anthropological issue I wanted to explore was how *ayahuasca* shamanism is constructed in different settings and contexts. More specifically, the question I set out to answer was: "Why do westerners pursue shamanic experiences and how are these experiences constructed in the context of shamanic tourism?" I argued that I do not see *shamanic tourism* as an anomaly but as consistent with the nature of shamanic knowledge, which has always been exchanged across and between cultures. Traditionally, in South American shamanism power and symbolism has been sought outside a particular cultural milieu. Moreover, in the West, esoteric knowledge has often been sought in faraway places (Helms, 1988); thus, this intercultural exchange is also consistent with Western tradition. I do not see tourism as an external force that imposes meaning on local shamanism; rather I showed that there is a two-way exchange and westerners adopt shamanic discourse as well, especially one that involves relationships with non-human persons. In addition, I argue that this phenomenon should be looked at in the context of a new paradigm, or rather, a shift in the discourse about plant hallucinogens, a discourse that tackles them as sacraments, medicines or teacher plants. Ritual, in this context, is instrumental and fosters self-transformation while at the same time challenging the participants' very cultural constructs and basic assumptions about the world.

Recent scholarship (Winkelman, 2005) has shown that the western interest in *ayahuasca* is much more than a pretext for drug use but rather has a spiritual component and seeks to address an urgent need for self-transformation. In the Iquitos milieu, shamanism is reinvented as local shamanic practices converge with western ideas of spirituality and healing and create a hybrid and highly dynamic practice, which I call *shamanic tourism*. *Ayahuasca* is viewed by westerners as a healing force for bodily and mental disorders that stem from what is perceived as Western culture's spiritual impoverishment. For participants in *ayahuasca* ceremonies, this healing is also part of a larger project for healing and transforming humanity.

I chose to use the term *shamanic tourism* as opposed to the more often used term *drug tourism* to refer to this phenomenon because I see a substantial difference between the two. The latter tends to be used when speaking of travel for the recreational consumption of drugs or, on rare occasions, travel to exotic places (popular destinations are Amsterdam, Southeast Asia, and South America) with the intention to smuggle illegal drugs. This is not the case with *ayahuasca* shamanism as others have pointed out (Winkelman, 2005). Even though there is a number of tourists that will try the experience out of curiosity – because it is so widely talked about in Iquitos – most people will begin their quest with a specific motive in mind. The physical and physiological unpleasantness of the experience alone disputes any claims for the recreational use of *ayahuasca*, as well. Finally, the experience often includes the participation in a shamanic *dieta*, which involves fasting and the ingestion of other "teacher plants."

Shamanic tourism is a relatively new phenomenon that has escalated in the last decade. However, the western fascination with shamanism – including psychoactive plants and substances and the changes in consciousness that they produce – is deeply rooted in western intellectual tradition and the relationship of the West with the exotic and spiritual "other," a history that has gone hand in hand with colonialism and exploitative relationships. The recent interest in *ayahuasca* is a continuation of this long history and belongs to its latest chapter that has been called the "psychedelic renaissance" (Joy, 1992; Cloud, 2007; Kotler, 2010; Sessa, 2012) – a renaissance dominated by the themes of healing, self-transformation, and the sacramental use of hallucinogens.

In this paper, I want to draw attention to our use of the word "drugs" in the context of the indigenous use of psychoactives and stimulants. These are usually used in specific contexts alien to the context where the discourse of drugs arose and carries certain political weight. These substances are often used alongside a multitude of other plants and substances that we often overlook because they have no apparent psychoactive effect. I argue that these dichotomies might be limiting the scope of our research efforts. I propose that we focus on these other plants, the contexts in which they are used and the ideologies surrounding that use. In Amazonia, where plants are not used to change the user's consciousness but to imbue the body with certain properties, we need to work with local categories and not impose our own.

The idea for this paper came from my discussions with contemporary *ayahuasca* practitioners and my last couple of visits in the Peruvian Amazon. There is a large body of literature focusing on *ayahuasca* and its healing effects, but the large array of plants used around it are understudied. In this paper, I want to draw attention to these other plants and encourage future researchers to focus on them. I will first address Amazonian conceptions of the body that inform contemporary *ayahuasca* shamanism and will help illustrate how plants are used in this context. Then, I will discuss several examples of plants that are used in conjunction with *ayahuasca*, either before or after ceremonies. I will follow with a discussion of *dietas* as tools for transformation and knowledge acquisition including a recent ethnographic example.

BODIES AND SUBSTANCES IN AMAZONIA

A review of the ethnographic literature on indigenous Amazonia reveals elaborate theories of the body and its creation through substances. There is an emphasis on fabricating the body relating to perspectivism, according to which all living beings have a soul, while bodies are markers of difference (Viveiros de Castro, 1998). Since the soul is the constant among living beings while bodies are unstable, there is a need for the management and fabrication of bodies through different substances and techniques. For groups such as the Muinane (Londoño Sulkin, 2012), social life is centered on the production of human bodies on the basis of substances. Substances have their own agency and are of divine origin. They were given to each Muinane lineage by divinities or mythical heroes and their misappropriation could turn them into poison (Londoño Sulkin, 2012). For the Cashinahua, the body is not a taken-for-granted biological fact nor does it "grow naturally"; rather, bodies are unstable and constantly constituted (McCallum, 2014) and "made" often with the ingestion of certain substances. According to Santos-Granero, persons "are not born as such, but must be intentionally manufactured or shaped through the input of a variety of substances and effects provided by parents and kin" (Santos-Granero, 2009, 7).

A variety of substances of plant and non-plant origin are used to infuse the body with their properties at different stages of a person's life. Cashinahua boys are initiated into hunting via a prolonged diet that begins with using the frog skin to induce vomiting and then killing a boa to eat its tongue (McCallum, 2001). The idea is that the abilities of the boa are transmitted to the hunter and help them to kill large game animals. Among the Napo Runa, the location of the body's power is the flesh (Uzendoski, 2005); and one's body must change form and become strengthened, over the course of one's life. The Ashéninka use leaf baths to strengthen the body (Lenaerts, 2006). Among the Urarina, bodies are leaky and permeable; and there is a continuous process of sealing/ hardening/ ensouling the body through a variety of techniques involving objects and songs to develop and solidify the heart-soul (Walker, 2013). In addition, eating well is important for mental and emotional well-being (Walker, 2013). Similarly, the Barasana theory of the body "places extreme value on the regulation of exits and entrances" (Hugh-Jones, 1979, 119).

The role of altered states of consciousness and their relationship to acquiring knowledge should not be overlooked. For the Napo Runa, to be drunk is to open one's body to the spirit world so that one's "essence" is manifested; drunken states are seen positively, as a means of attaining knowledge (Uzendoski, 2005). For the Urarina, most knowledge has its source outside of human society and learning comes through ingesting herbal medicines or remedies, while keeping a strict regimen of fasting and other prohibitions (Walker, 2013). While acquiring a new skill there is an imprinting phase centered on disciplined practice (Walker, 2013). For example, to obtain spearfishing ability, one must tie strips of the inner bark of the bijiurara tree around the forearm, which leaves lasting scars (Walker, 2013); likewise, during the imprinting phase, the novice must throw the spear repeatedly, which incorporates the ability into the body. For the Cubeo, the brain and heart are connected, with the mind storing a replica of its knowledge within the heart; in addition, painting and ornamentation are meant to set the body in "a straight direction;" lastly, leaving the body in a disorganized state has the risk of illness or death (Goldman, 2004). McCallum has also stressed the relationship between knowledge and health, showing on the one hand that among the Cashinahua the same substances and experiences that can be transformed into knowledge may also become ill-ness-causing agents; and on the other hand, that "illness can be understood as a disturbance in the body's capacity to know" (McCallum, 1996, 363).

Healing involves active manipulation of these principles and there is a variety of remedies for purposes beyond healing. For the Matsigenka, for whom illness is caused by harmful spirits that en-ter the body, toxic plants are used to "expel such intruders" (Shepard, 1998, 323). Illness is often con-sidered to be the result of breaking food (Hugh-Jones, 1988) or behavioral taboos (Lenaerts, 2006), of which there are many. Among the Iquito, dieting is central during healing (Jernigan, 2011). Chevalier notes that healing prescriptions center around the same theme; for example, the patient must re-frain from cultural exchanges with other persons (sexual, social and spatial isolation is required) (Chevalier, 1982); they must also not ingest cultural foods; basically, "anything that is cooked or highly valued by men but is quite superfluous to other living species" (Chevalier, 1982, 347). An Ura-rina remedy for strength involves drinking a decoction of the chuchuhuasi tree, crushed tapir bone and piri-piri (Walker, 2013). During the fast, all food must be cold and salt, gruel, sugar, manioc beer and banana drink are prohibited; in addition, the person must bathe continuously. If the fast is followed correctly, the novice will become brave but if not, they will emerge weak (Walker, 2013).

While these processes are utilized throughout a person's life, they are instrumental in the sha-manic apprenticeship during which knowledge and power are embedded in the shaman's body. For the Achuar, shamanic apprenticeship involves "a change in the ecology of his physical system" (De-scola, 1997, 338). This is achieved through "ascetic discipline" involving purging and a strict diet (De-scola, 1997). At the end of the Desana "shaman's" training, there is a closing ceremony which leaves the knowledge acquired dormant in the initiate's body; therapeutic spells are put in his brain, while evil ones in his belly (Buchillet, 2004). For the Siona, a substance called *dau*, the root of the shaman's power, forms and grows in the shaman's body as he continues to ingest *yagé* (Langdon, 1992). Part of this power might leave the shaman's body in the form of a dart or other object directed at some-one else (Langdon, 1992). This accumulation of knowledge in his body makes a shaman vulnerable and in need for constant protection to avoid potential damage to his *dau* (Langdon, 1992). A similar process is present with the shamanic phlegm and *virotes* (darts) found among the Shuar as well as *mestizo* shamans in the area around Iquitos today, who still practice fasting and sexual abstinence during their apprenticeship.

PLANTS USED IN CONJUNCTION WITH AYAHUASCA IN CONTEMPORARY AYAHUASCA RETREATS

During my fieldwork, I found that a multitude of plants are often used alongside with *ayahuasca*, often with similar objectives, as discussed above. First, there are a number of admixtures that *cu-randeros* add to the brew itself in order to influence its effects, depending on what a patient is trying to heal or what qualities they are trying to incorporate in the brew. Some have a list of admixture plants and barks that they always include in their *ayahuasca* brew. By adding these extra plants, they incorporate the spirits and the properties of these plants into the brew. These plants (and any plants used in this type of shamanism) are used for their energy and their spirit as much as they are for their pharmacological qualities. In fact, the difference between the two is not always clear. Plants are treated as living beings and their external characteristics reveal their spirit and qualities. Many tree barks that are used in the brew are used precisely for their strength and endurance, which is revealed by their vertical shape. This has a symbolic meaning as well; just like the physical trees support the *ayahuasca* vine, in the same way the bark from the trees in the brew supports the vine spiritually.

What follows is a list of plants and trees that might be included in the brew, and the properties they are meant to add to it: *Mapacho* – strength and protection; Toé – strength; Ayahuma – protec-tion and healing susto; Capirona – cleansing and protection; Chullachaquicaspi – physical cleans-ing and healing; Lupuna Blanca – protection; Punga Amarilla – protection and drawing out of nega-tive spirits and energies; Remocaspi – moving dense or dark energies; Huayracaspi – create purging, help with gastro-intestinal ailments, bring mental calmness and tranquility; Uchu Sanango – pro-tection, power and strength; Shiwawaku – healing and protection. It is obvious that protection from malevolent spirits and attacks from malevolent shamans is paramount, and several of the additive plants aim to this.

Some shamans have strong feelings about using additives in their brew and they are proud to report that they only use *ayahuasca* and *chacruna* or chacropanga. Most will add small amounts of *mapacho* and other plants such as toé (*Brugmansia suaveolens*) (Humb & Bompl. ex. Willd.; Bercht. & J. Presl.). Toé is a very controversial plant because it is considered to be used by *brujos* (sorcerers). Everybody agreed that it is a very powerful spirit; but I was told that it is a very defensive spirit as well. Some shamans will use a small amount of it, small enough to not cause any visionary effect, precisely for this protective quality. This is what one shaman had to say on the subject of additives:

> We use a number of plants that a lot of other shamans consider to be plants that you don't use. And then they often use plants that we won't use. For instance, we use cata-hua, a lot of shamans say they won't use. They say it's venomous, they say it's a poison, they say it's dark, they say it turns you into the dark side and all these things. We don't believe it to be that way. We see it as a completely different spirit. Although they'll use piñon rojo, and the spirit of piñon rojo for us by the nature of it being a red plant is basically based in red magic, or red arts, which are all negative and have to do with black magic, or becoming basically a witch doctor to do witchcraft on people. (Anonymous, 2005; interview with shaman by author, n.d.)

Purification and cleansing are thought to be instrumental in *ayahuasca* healing; and not only is it a part of the *ayahuasca* experience itself, but it often precedes it by means of diet and purgatives. Certain dietary restrictions are meant to keep the body pure before the ceremony; these require refraining from spices, sugar, salt, oils, meat (especially pork, which is to be avoided for 30 days after the last ceremony), stimulants, and sex. Pork, especially its fat, is to be avoided because of its "dirty energy." Diet is very important in other shamanic traditions as well; Siikala mentions that Siberian shamans fast, meditate and go into seclusion before ceremonies (1992).

The diet includes abstinence from sex for a few days before the *ayahuasca* ritual and for eight days afterwards. The idea behind this is that the plants remain in one's body for days after the ceremony and will continue to work and heal or teach the person, provided that they stay pure. Even though I could not get a consensus from my consultants on the reasons behind some of the rules, most shamans agreed on the prohibitions themselves. The only disagreement was on the topic of fruit. While some shamans would allow fruit to be consumed, other would not allow them because they contain sugar. On the day of the ceremony, one is not supposed to eat anything after noon; and it is advised to eat a light meal or just fruit and herbal teas throughout the day. On the day following the ceremony, one is not supposed to eat before noon nor use soap or toothpaste. Some shamans prefer to "break" the diet on the following day using salt and lemon taken directly under the tongue.

Regarding the sexual abstinence rule, shamans would have different theories as to why sex is prohibited—as well as different observational approaches. One shaman of European descent said that from what he had been taught, the spirit of *ayahuasca* is very jealous and does not want people to have sex when it resides in their body. In his opinion and from a western point of view, the rationale behind the prohibition is because sex is a very strong, very open, energetic exchange. The energies of the persons interfere with each other and it can "defocus" someone who is dieting and doing spiritual work. He added that it could also be because of taboos that were imposed by the Catholic Church, although there is no evidence to support that.

As mentioned, participants are encouraged to keep the diet for some time after the ceremony as the medicine continues to be in the body and bodily purity is desired for it to continue working. But if the diet is broken, the healing or spiritual work stops and there is the possibility of dire consequences; for example, Peruvian consultants have told me that they got skin rashes from breaking the diet early. Shamans and patients alike are known to be "punished" by the spirits for not following the dietary restrictions. In one ceremony in which I was present, a young man who had eaten a full meal in the afternoon of the day of the ritual insisted on drinking with the rest of the group despite the warning of the shaman not to do so. After much persistence, he was allowed to drink and during the ceremony, he had a really hard time, vomiting and generally feeling sick, as well as having unpleasant and scary visions. The shaman pointed out to him several times during the ceremony that *ayahuasca* was punishing him for not having fasted.

On occasion, I have witnessed purgative plants being used to purify the body before an *ayahuasca* ceremony. This is usually done in the morning of the day of the ceremony. These plants will induce vomiting or diarrhea (or both). On one occasion, the latex of the *ojé* plant (*Ficus insipida* Willd.) was used. *Ojé* is quite toxic and a large quantity of water needs to be drunk to avoid poisoning, which induces powerful purging. On another occasion, the shaman gave *piñones blancos* (probably the nut of the *Jatropha curcas* L.), to a large group of tourists at an *ayahuasca* retreat. Most people retired in their individual rooms but throughout the day one could hear the purging sounds all over the camp. One of the guests said jokingly that the shaman was a "naughty witch" who had created a "vomit camp." The shaman told me that she did this so that people would have less to purge during the ceremony and would suffer less. A similar practice is reported by Langdon among the Siona who use emetics to make the body lighter before *yagé* ceremonies (Langdon, 1992, 56).

TOBACCO

I will finish this section with a discussion of the plant that accompanies *ayahuasca* most often and is considered most powerful by many groups in Western Amazonia. Tobacco, a plant vilified in Western cultures, is probably the most important plant in South American shamanism and one that contributes to its ambivalence. Fausto notes the absence of tobacco in "neoshamanic sites and rites" (Fausto, 2004, 158), while others have emphasized the importance of tobacco as food for the spirits in indigenous shamanism (Shepard, 1998; Freedman, 2015). The best-known study that focuses on indigenous use of tobacco and its importance is the one by Johannes Wilbert (1972, 1975, 1987). In the cultures he discusses, tobacco was not used recreationally but always consumed in the context of a shamanic ceremony. In fact, nicotine, in appropriate dosages, is particularly well suited to produce in the shaman the chemical changes that activate the attack behavior of his jaguar-self (Wilbert, 1987). Today, tobacco is an important agent of the Jaguar shaman transformation complex of Amazonian shamanism, but nicotine is often considered of lesser significance than hallucinogenic compounds. For some ethnic groups, however, such as the Campa, it is the most important hallucinogen in high doses (Weiss, 1973). The Campa word for shaman is *sheripiári*, which contains the root *sheri*, which means tobacco. The Matsigenga word for shaman is *seripi´gari*, which can be translated as "the one intoxicated by tobacco" (Baer, 1987, 73).

Tobacco is used in shamanic initiations in order to experience symbolic death; it is believed that nicotine is exceptionally well suited to manifest the continuum of dying. Mentally, it is experienced as a journey of the soul outside the body; along the celestial road, the soul of the person in trance repeatedly encounters and escapes death (Wilbert, 1987). Among the Ayoreo of the north Chaco (Paraguay and Bolivia), it is said that the apprentice will drink nearly a liter of pulverized green tobacco and will fall into a coma; if he survives, he becomes a shaman (Califano, et al. 1987). Shipibo apprentices will also ingest great quantities of tobacco water in order to acquire their powers, but also use a variety of ingestion techniques such as chewing, drinking, smoking, snuffing and enema (Wilbert, 1987). Wilbert mentions six indigenous groups that use four or more ingestion techniques: Campa, Jívaro, Piro, Matsigenka, Shipibo, and Tucuna; these groups also consume *Ayahuasca* in a ceremonial context.

Additionally, tobacco is used to induce visions. The mention of visions following tobacco use is very frequent in the scholarly literature. As to the nature of the things seen, authors make occasional reference to the spirits, ancestors, demons, lightning, flashes, and a giant sun. Auditory hallucinations occurring simultaneously with visions include chanting and verbal messages. Unquestionably, however, tobacco ingestion is capable of provoking intense visionary experiences and of providing eschatological scenarios on a grand scale. Tobacco is also experienced as a sight-and-vision-altering drug that permits the tobacco shaman to view the spiritual world (Wilbert, 1987).

Tobacco is not only used as a hallucinogen. Karsten (1964) reports that the Shuar ingest tobacco for three major reasons: as a universal remedy for all sorts of illnesses, as a prophylactic to strengthen the body; and as a narcotic to induce dreams. Tobacco is an important substance for the Muinane (Londoño Sulkin, 2012). Despite their initial fragility, men, using tobacco become capable of dealing effectively with anything that could cause them harm (Londoño Sulkin 2012); tobacco also provides people with "moral sociable discernment and predatory capabilities" (Londoño Sulkin, 2012, 100).

Tobacco, from the species *Nicotiana rustica* L. – called *mapacho* – was ever present in the ceremonies I observed; its spirit was considered extremely powerful, even though some healers might consider its spirit "heavy" and will not "diet" it. It is used throughout the region during the preparation of the *ayahuasca* brew when the smoke is blown on the pot where the *ayahuasca* is cooking. *Mapacho* is also blown on the plants that are going to be used before they are harvested and before they are placed in the pot. At the beginning of the ceremony, a shaman blows smoke in the four directions, both for protection and to establish the ceremonial space. Tobacco smoke is also blown on the ritual objects, including the *ayahuasca* bottle and each individual cup serving of the brew, as well as on the participants to cleanse and protect them. In every ceremony, there were large bundles of *mapacho* cigarettes close to the shaman. One of my consultants who was an apprentice, told me that if someone wants to be a shaman, they have to be willing to smoke several *mapacho* cigarettes during the ceremony, even if they do not normally smoke. The cigarettes can be purchased rolled at the Iquitos market. In the Iquitos area, there are ritual specialists called *tabaqueros* who specialize in tobacco use and consider tobacco a much more powerful spirit than *ayahuasca*.

SHAMANIC DIETAS AS A TOOL FOR TRANSFORMATION AND KNOWLEDGE ACQUISITION

Shamanic initiation radically transforms the person who becomes initiated, but this transformation is not easy and is the result of years of training and isolation. In this context, the word apprenticeship is more appropriate than initiation, as there is a long training period before someone becomes a master shaman and it is a gradual process to get there. In the context of *mestizo* shamanism, shamanic knowledge is a combination of internal proclivity and apprenticeship and acquired knowledge. In this manner, a good shaman should have both the gift and a good teacher and they are expected to add their own creative touch to the teachings they receive. Some of the shamans I worked with started their apprenticeship after a life-threatening disease that was healed by a shaman – a theme very common in the literature from other regions, as well. In all cases, there was a radical transformation of those individuals who changed their life course and helped develop their confidence as healers.

Around the world, one is considered a shaman after they have received two kinds of teaching: ecstatic (in dreams and trances) and traditional, such as shamanic techniques (Eliade, 1959). The first one is given by the spirits and the second one by the master shaman. In Amazonia, often the training of the shaman requires fasting, vomiting, and sexual abstinence (Hugh-Jones, 1988); and the novice must obtain several spiritual weapons and tools of office. The novice also consumes strong hallucinogens and must master the trance state (Reichel-Dolmatoff, 1971) – all this while in isolation from the community and spending long periods of time in the jungle. During this time, the apprentice disconnects from society and comes closer to nature and the spirits from which he or she learns. Around Iquitos, the apprenticeship is a vital part of a shaman's credentials and the lineage of healers they belong to is very important, as there are significant differences between lineages. What is transmitted through the lineage is esoteric knowledge, ceremonial practices as well as other "property" or powers. *Icaros* (songs sang in *ayahuasca* ceremonies) and some of the shaman's powers are passed on by the teacher to the student, an example being the *yachay* (knowledge phlegm), which resides in the shaman's body and needs to be fed with tobacco (Freedman, 2015). A relationship with certain plant spirits is also expected; a respected shaman is someone who has received powers from his master shaman as well as the spirits of the plants directly.

A central theme in the stories of the shamans I interviewed is that physical, psychological and spiritual cleansing preceded the beginning of the apprenticeship. The future shamans had to purge all dark and negative elements before they could become healers and accept the spirits of the plants and their teachings in their bodies. Not only is this an element of purification, but it is an important step for self-transformation as well. In addition, the future shaman has to suffer and sometimes even experience death and rebirth as is found in many cultures around the world (Dobkin de Rios 1984). Another important part of the process is sacrifice in the form of strict dietary and sexual prohibitions. According to my consultants, traditionally shamans would undergo extensive periods of fasting called *dietas*[1] (diets). The practice of *dietas* by individuals who do not have the intention of becoming *curanderos* is a more recent phenomenon. Today, this is something that is available to westerners and some people will choose to undergo a *dieta* while participating in *ayahuasca* retreats; more recently, I was told that because of the increasing association of *ayahuasca* with sorcery, groups of people will go to the jungle to diet other plants only and refrain from taking *ayahuasca* while in Peru. One of my consultants said:

> In the jungle, I truly experienced the effects of witchcraft first hand and the power of those who use it. After talking with many healers in the area, I found out that all somehow experienced sorcery. Although Westerners may think it is something unreal, it is not. I know people from other parts of the world who also experienced it and decided not to drink *ayahuasca* in the jungle anymore. They only come here to diet and get more medicine, and go back to their countries as soon as they can, which I totally understand. (Anonymous, 2014, interview with shaman by author, June 18)

1. Note that *dieta* is not the same as the *ayahuasca* diet that has to be observed by everyone who intends to drink *ayahuasca*.

Plant *dietas* can be done for a variety of reasons, such as to be healed or to "learn medicine." *Brujos* or sorcerers will diet certain plants to learn sorcery. According to some lineages, it is good for healers to diet the same plants in order to learn how to protect themselves from sorcery. One of the shamans told me that:

> There are many types of *dietas*. There are *dietas* for more protection, more guardians; *dietas* that serve to heal bones, muscles, organs; others that enhance you spiritually; others to strengthen you physically; others to strengthen you mentally. Each plant has its way. Ultimately, if we focus and welcome each plant letting it take us to what the medicine gives us, I believe that the same plant can give a person one thing from another. That's why I do not focus so much on what the plant is for. Because I have seen that the same plant, which is being ingested by the same people, doing the same things, eating the same food, doing the same *ayahuasca* ceremonies, to some it brings certain things, and to others something different. The purpose of diets is to heal. (Anonymous, 2014, interview with shaman by author, June 18)

The principle behind *dietas* is simple: the shaman, patient or anyone who wants to acquire knowledge from the plants ingests one or more plants followed by a strict dietary regimen for a period of time ranging from a few days to a few months. The *dieta* starts off rather strict and gradually decreases in strictness allowing the person to eat or drink more things; it is generally advised to ease back into a regular diet. Plant *dietas* are rather tedious and physically challenging since most of the plants ingested have noticeable effects on the body, especially when one is fasting, meaning eating most likely only rice and plantains or manioc. Ideally, during the *dieta*, the person is not to have vigorous physical activity and they are expected to spend most of their time lying in their hammock or bed–in other words, they are supposed to behave like a sick person. Some consultants have said that any kind of activity, even reading and writing, as well as contact with other people should be avoided. This is especially important for apprentices, but today is often not adhered to, given the practical challenges.

There are a number of principles, restrictions, and plants that are followed by most of the shamans in the area but different lineages of shamans will have their own rules or plants that they diet. This is because each shaman works with different spirits, which may ask them to do things a certain way. Even within a lineage, there may be differences if the spirits impose different requirements on different shamans. Most diets last 8, 15 or 30 days, even though one often hears that a few decades ago shamans would diet for 6 months to a year at a time. One of my consultants said that his first diet was 30 days. Today this is rare and for most visitors, it is common to diet for an eight-day period; even if one diets for a longer period, they only drink the plants on the first four to five nights and some maestros will only give the plants on the first day. After that point, the *dieta* continues by following the dietary restrictions.

Things that are not allowed are sugar, alcohol, sex, pork, salt, spicy food, and drugs. Some consultants have said that the exclusion of these elements from the body allows the human spirit, body, and mind to be more open to the forest and the plants' teachings. Other things not allowed during the *dieta* are soap or toothpaste, and direct physical contact with others – except the shaman or other dieteros. After the *dieta*, no sexual contact – including masturbation – is allowed for 30 days, and pork is not allowed for at least six months. During the *dieta*, one should avoid the sun as well as any strenuous activity and should remain isolated as much as possible. For this reason, dieters will usually stay in a small hut in the jungle called a *tambo* for most of the duration of the *dieta*. In addition to rice, plantains, and *fariña* (manioc flour), some species of birds and fish are allowed. I was told that any fish with teeth are not allowed because they eat "basura" (garbage). Another shaman said that the reason they do not eat fish that have teeth is that they are aggressive. Fish with vivid colors or shapes on them are also not allowed to avoid the dieter's skin taking on these colors. The idea is that when one diets, they are ingesting not only the meat of the animal but also its spirit and properties. On the other hand, if one wants to be a brujo (sorcerer) they might want to eat fish with teeth to take on their aggressiveness. According to one of my consultants "to become a healing shaman, you will follow a very strict diet that will direct you into a place of pure medicine. In that place of medicine, you'll learn how to defend yourself, what they call *defensivas*. But that comes from medicine, it doesn't come from dark spirits" (Anonymous, 2005, interview with shaman by author, n.d.).

During the period of the *dieta*, the spirits of the trees or plants will enter the dieter's body, where they will start the teaching literally from the inside out. They will also come to the person during their dream time and teach them. The person is not supposed to do any activity unless the plant they diet requires them to bathe a certain number of times in a day. In that case they are allowed to go to the river and bathe and then continue to lie down. If the diet is broken, the teaching will stop and sometimes consequences will ensue. Usually, the person faces the consequences the next time they drink *ayahuasca*, during their visions–meaning that they will suffer and they will in a sense be "punished" by the spirits.

Different plants are considered to teach different things and certain plants are more suitable for certain people. Some of the common plants that people will diet are ajo sacha, ayahuma, huayra-caspi, lupuna blanca, capirona, huaca purana, huacapú, bobinsana, chullachaqui caspi, cumaceba, tamamuri, chuchuhuasi and remocaspi[2]. Each plant has certain properties and distinct teachings to offer. For example, ajo sacha is a plant that is said to treat problems of discomfort and general pain, generates heat in the body and reinforces overall physical strength, while chullachaqui caspi helps one to communicate with the spirit world. There is no standard way for choosing which plant to diet. If a person is dieting for healing, they diet the plant that the spirits will indicate to the shaman. Usually, at the beginning of the diet, an *ayahuasca* ceremony is done and the shaman determines which plant or plants the patient should diet. More experienced users might receive that information from *ayahuasca* themselves and they share that with the shaman.

Most people will participate in *ayahuasca* ceremonies during a *dieta*. This is considered danger-ous by some because it puts the dieter in a very vulnerable position as *ayahuasca* opens the person up to the spiritual world – whereas the *dieta* in itself does not. I was told that if there is a rival sha-man or negative energy in the area, they will not be able to "see" the dieter – he or she will not come into their awareness. But when one participates in *ayahuasca* ceremonies rival shamans can hear the *icaros*; they can hear the ceremony vibrating and see the mesa (ceremonial altar) shining; therefore, it is safer not to drink *ayahuasca* during the time of the *dieta*. However, if one is working with mas-ter shamans, it is considered reasonably safe to drink *ayahuasca* during the *dieta*, because they are watching over the dieter and are able to protect them. I was told that during the *dieta*, one feels closer to the jungle and the plants and animals and it can be difficult to return to normal life, especially to an urban environment. After a *dieta*, a person is very open to anything and the negative energy of a city can affect them much more than it would have before they dieted.

There is a disagreement over the number of plants that is ideal to diet at any given time. Most shamans will diet one plant at a time and learn from its spirit. I have worked with one shaman that diets as many as 25 plants at a time, a fact that is frowned upon by other shamans and experienced users. They argued that it would be impossible to learn anything if you had so many teachers trying to teach you at the same time. For them, it is optimal to diet one plant at a time and concentrate on the energy and teaching of the particular plant.

According to some, to be a traditional *ayahuasquero*, *dietas* are not necessary. An *ayahuasca* sha-man can only learn from *ayahuasca* and work with *ayahuasca*. *Ayahuasqueros* are considered by other specialists in the area, such as *paleros* or *tabaqueros*, to be weak and very easy to dominate. However, for *ayahuasqueros paleros*, experts in both *ayahuasca* and tree barks, *dietas* of trees barks are the most fundamental aspect of their practice. By ingesting them, they allow the spirits of the trees to enter their bodies and teach them directly. The greatest learning takes place within the period of the *dieta*, while during the ceremonies they learn how to utilize that medicine.

The frequency in which *dietas* are done varies. According to a European shaman I have come to know well over the years, it is good to diet at least once a year in order to cleanse and center oneself. He also saw dieting as an exercise in his own power. He believes that *dietas* are a good way for anyone to reflect on their lives, their patterns, and ways to change them. He said:

> These plants have their genios (spirits), their fairies, their goblins, whatever we want to call them. Their elementals. When you are dieting these eight days without salt, without sugar, as we are now, and you have taken the plant, and the plant is in you, you are allowing that plant to develop in you, but to your elemental as well. That month that you do not do certain things, let's say it's the valorization that you're going to give to that plant. If you are dieting well, then the spirit of that plant will be with you. If it is to cure a disease, it will help you cure the disease (if it is in your hands and in God's hands to heal it). If it is to learn, every time you need that plant in an icaro or something to heal someone, you will have the strength and power of that medicine in you. (Ano-nymous, 2014, interview with shaman by author, June 18)

---

2. For the botanical names of these plants, see Appendix.

Since 2013, I have been working on a collaborative book on sorcery together with a shaman, who I will call Juan, who is originally from Spain. According to Juan, sorcery has played an instrumental role in his life, often changing its course. Since we decided to work on the book together, he often experienced sorcery attacks during ceremonies and he was not able to complete any of his projects. During the attacks, he would often comment that "they don't want us to write the book." In 2014, I got severe diarrhea almost immediately after arriving in Iquitos and subsequently, probably due to dehydration, got a bladder infection, which went undetected until my body started shutting down. I had no desire to eat or energy to do anything at which point he took me to the hospital where I was diagnosed and took antibiotics.

Because of these events and because we were close and I had started perceiving certain things during ceremonies, Juan suggested that we both diet the ayahuma tree to fortify ourselves. His teacher had taught him that the spirit of ayahuma was very powerful and a very good guardian. It could teach one sorcery but at the same time how to protect oneself from it. Juan had an apprentice at the time who had just finished a long diet with ayahuma and felt extremely strong. The *dieta* consisted of drinking an infusion of the ayahuma bark on the first day and bathing with the pulp of its fruit on consequent days. In his lineage, the *dieta* also involved immersing oneself in water every morning, eating very little bland food, not talking or coming into contact with people and avoiding the sun.

Juan also had me diet camalonga, which I took on the second day of the *dieta* in order to heal. During one of our conversations, he said that it would help me accept the sickness and its larger significance. He said:

> The gift (of the illness) is to contemplate the negative parts that it brings you. Meditate, feel, think about it. Why are you here? What is the gift that you are bringing me? Whether it is physical, mental or what the disease is. What does it create in you when you think about the disease? What patterns of behavior? [...] Because the root, if it is a gift sent to you from above, the root is not here. It is not in the physical. Even if it looks to me as if it's here. But the root ... you see the tree, but the root you do not see. (Anonymous, 2014, interview with shaman by author, June 18)

In 2015, I was once again in Iquitos, ready to head to the jungle to begin a series of *ayahuasca* ceremonies, when my purse containing my passport was stolen on the night before we were scheduled to leave for the jungle. Putting this in the context of the attacks Juan was experiencing as well as my illness in the previous year, he determined that shamanic intervention was needed. He was concerned that our work on the book was not welcome by local shamans and that they were trying to stop it. He decided that a powerful purging, followed by a protective bath was necessary to cleanse and fortify my body against future attacks. The protective bath contained tobacco, toé leaves and patiquina (Elephant's ear), which is generally known in the area to be a protective plant. Other friends in Iquitos have commented on its protective qualities and often people plant it near a house door for protection. This course of action had worked for him in the preceding year when he was experiencing a lot of attacks. I was told:

> I learned about plants that sorcerers dieted, but could be used as protection as well. Dieting these plants for long periods of time could become a means to do evil. It is ideal to diet them for short periods of time so they become protectors. After my diet with tobacco and the baths with patiquina, tobacco and toé, I started feeling better and the ceremonies became more lucid. I felt much stronger, safer and protected. The attacks did not end, but I dealt with them better." (Anonymous, 2015, interview with shaman by author, June 7)

To induce the purge, he procured ojé, a plant mentioned in the literature as a powerful plant teacher (Luna, 1992). The plant is often ingested to get rid of parasites, but I have seen it used to cleanse the body before taking *ayahuasca*. A local shaman that was also present, told me repeatedly that after this cleanse I would feel stronger and that I would glow. I ingested the resin of the tree and spent the rest of the day by the riverside drinking gallons of water. This induced vomiting and diarrhea. By late afternoon I was exhausted and hungry, after which I rested and had a light meal. In the following days, we had several *ayahuasca* ceremonies. This last ethnographic example is not atypical of how people use plants alongside *ayahuasca* in contemporary *ayahuasca* retreats.

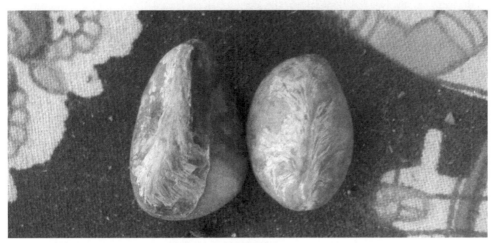

Fig. 1 A pair of camalonga seeds, thought to be male and female.

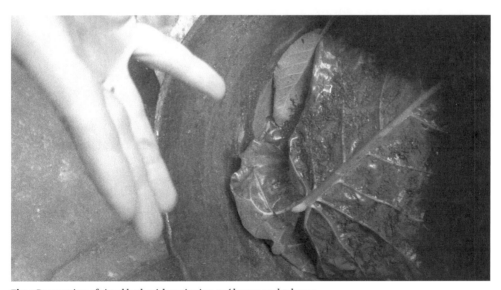

Fig. 2 Preparation of ritual bath with patiquina, toé leaves, and tobacco.

CONCLUSION

I have shown that *ayahuasca* shamanism both from the perspective of the practitioners as well as the patients, involves much more than the ingestion of *ayahuasca*. In addition, as I was recently told, because of the increasing discussions of sorcery involved in *ayahuasca* shamanism, many travelers will travel to the jungle to diet other plants and will not partake of *ayahuasca* itself. Not only do shamans in Peru include a variety of other interventions, baths and cleanses among others, utilizing plants, but there is a great degree of specialized knowledge as evidenced in the different types of specialists in the area such as paleros and *tabaqueros*. There is a vast body of knowledge that needs to be more at the center of our research efforts and understanding local conceptions of the body will help elucidate the ways that these modalities work. According to Hugh-Jones "an anthropology of "peculiar substances" might usefully begin by thinking more about the consumption of stimulants or psychoactive substances in relation to the consumption of more ordinary fare" (Hugh-Jones, 1995, 48). He suggests focusing on ethnographic evidence of behavior and social interaction and a "more cultural approach focusing on categorization" (Hugh-Jones, 1995, 49). I would also urge us to reconsider terms such as "drugs" as foreign to the majority of the contexts that we are discussing here. In this case, even though many of the plants I have discussed are not psychoactive, the study of their use within the context of *ayahuasca* shamanism can only enhance our understanding.

Finally, considering several *ayahuasca* related deaths, some of which seem to be related to tobacco ingestion (Macdonald, 2017), more research is needed from a variety of academic disciplines to determine and minimize risks. The discourse has predominantly been that *ayahuasca* is safe unless someone suffers from certain conditions, but most of the recent deaths have been of young and healthy people, which should be cause for concern. Although researchers have pointed out that many of the deaths are probably due to incompatible drug use or prior pathology (dos Santos, 2013) further research on admixture plants and other purgatives used in conjunction with *ayahuasca* can only enhance our understanding and prevent future fatalities. While research and exploration of the pharmacological properties of psychoactive plants is important, I argue that ethnography as well as ethnopharmacology are equally important when researching the plants used in conjunction with them. Venues such as this symposium and volume are important in forging these interdisciplinary collaborations and dialogue.

APPENDIX

LIST OF PLANTS

(As cited in McKenna, Luna, and Towers, 1995; Castner, Timme, and Duke, 1998; Duke and Vasquez, 1994; Duke, et al., 2009; Schultes and Raffauf, 1992; López Vinatea, 2000)

Vernacular name	Scientific name
Ajo Sacha	*Cordia alliodora* (Ruiz & Pav.) Oken
Ayahuma	*Couroupita* guianensis Aubl.
Ayahuasca	*Banisteriopsis caapi* (Spruce ex Griseb.) Morton
Bobinsana	*Calliandra angustifolia* Benth.
Camalonga	*Strychnos* spp.
Capirona	*Calycophyllum spruceanum* (Benth.) Hook.f. ex K.Schum. or *Capirona decorticans* Spruce (López Vinatea 2000)
Catahua	*Hura crepitans* L.

Chacruna	*Psychotria viridis* Ruiz & Pav.
Chagropanga, Chaliponga	*Diplopterys cabrerana* (Cuatrec.) B.Gates
Chiricaspi	*Brunfelsia chiricaspi* Plowman
Chiricsanango, Chuchuhuasha	*Brunfelsia grandiflora* D.Don
Chuchuhuasi	*Maytenus boaria* Molina or *Maytenus ebenifolia* Reiss. (Lopez Vinatea 2000)
Chullachaquicaspi	*Remijia peruviana* Standl. or *Tovomita* sp.
Cumaceba	*Swartzia polyphylla* DC.
Huacapú	*Minquartia guianensis* Aubl. or *Vouacapoua americana* Aubl. (Lopez Vinatea 2000)
Huacapurana	*Campsiandra comosa* Benth.
Huayracaspi	*Sterculia apetala* (Jacq.) H. Karst.
Lupuna, Lupuna blanca	*Ceiba pentandra* (L.) Gaertn.
Mapacho *	*Nicotiana tabacum* L. or *Nicotiana rustica* L.
Ojé	*Ficus insipida* Willd.
Piñon blanco	*Jatropha curcas* L.
Piñon rojo, piñon negro, piñon colorado	*Jatropha gossypiifolia* L.
Patiquina	*Dieffenbachia* spp.
Punga amarilla	*Pseudobombax munguba* (Mart. & Zucc.) Dugand
Remocaspi	*Pithecellobium laetum* (Poepp.) Benth.
Shiwawaku	*Dipteryx odorata* (Aubl.) Willd.
Tamamuri	*Brosimum acutifolium* Huber
Toé, floripondio	*Brugmansia suaveolens* (Humb. & Bonpl. ex Willd.) Bercht. & J.Presl
Uchu sanango	*Tabernaemontana sananho* Ruiz & Pavon.

* Editor's Note: Mapacho is often claimed to be *Nicotiana rustica* L. in popular literature, however, there is no evidence to support this. The term "mapacho" is listed under the entry for *N. tabacum* L. in the *Amazonian Ethnobotanical Dictionary* (1994) and *N. rustica* is not listed in that publication. My colleague at UNAP, Curator of the Herbarium Amazonensis, Juan Ruiz, also confirms that "mapacho" is in fact *N. tabacum* L.

REFERENCES

Baer, G., 1987. Peruanische *ayahuasca*-sitzungen - schamanen und heilbehandlungen, in: Dittrich, A., Scharfetter, C. (Eds.), *Ethnopsychotherapie: Psychotherapie Mittels Aussergewöhnlicher Bewusstseinszustände in Westlichen Und Indigenen Kulturen*. Ferdinand Enke Verlag, Stuttgart, pp. 70–80.

Buchillet, D., 2004. Sorcery beliefs, transmission of shamanic Knowledge, and therapeutic practice among the Desana of the Upper Rio Negro Region, Brazil, in: Whitehead, N.L., Wright, R. (Eds.), *In Darkness and Secrecy: The Anthropology of Assault Sorcery and Witchcraft in Amazonia*. Duke University Press, Durham, pp. 109–131.

Califano, M., Idoyaga Molina, A., Perez Diez, A.A., 1987. Schamanismus und andere rituelle heilungen bei indianischen voelkern Suedamerikas, in: Dittrich, A., Scharfetter, C. (Eds.), *Ethnopsychotherapie: Psychotherapie Mittels Aussergewöhnlicher Bewusstseinszustände in Westlichen Und Indigenen Kulturen, Forum Der Psychiatrie*. Ferdinand Enke Verlag, Stuttgart, pp. 114–134.

Castner, J.L., Timme, S.L., Duke, J.A., 1998. *A Field Guide to Medicinal and Useful Plants of the Upper Amazon*. Feline Press, Gainesville, FL.

Chevalier, J.M., 1982. *Civilization and the Stolen Gift: Capital, Kin and Cult in Eastern Peru*. University of Toronto Press, Toronto.

Cloud, J., 2007. Was Timothy Leary right? *Time* 169, 64.

Descola, P., 1997. *The Spears of Twilight: Life and Death in the Amazon Jungle*. New Press, New York.

Dobkin de Rios, M., 1984. *Hallucinogens, Cross-cultural Perspectives*. University of New Mexico Press, Albuquerque.

dos Santos, R.G., 2013. A critical evaluation of reports associating *ayahuasca* with life-threatening adverse reactions. *J Psychoactive Drugs* 45, 179–188.

Duke, J.A., Bogenschutz-Godwin, M.J., Ottesen, A.R., 2009. *Duke's Handbook of Medicinal Plants of Latin America*. Taylor & Francis, Boca Raton.

Duke, J.A., Vásquez, R., 1994. *Amazonian Ethnobotanical Dictionary*. CRC Press, Boca Raton, Fla.

Eliade, M., 1959. *The Sacred and the Profane: The Nature of Religion*. Harcourt, Brace, New York.

Fausto, C., 2004. A blend of blood and tobacco: Shamans and jaguars among the Parakana of eastern Amazonia, in: Whitehead, N.L., Wright, R. (Eds.), *In Darkness and Secrecy: The Anthropology of Assault Sorcery and Witchcraft in Amazonia*. Duke University Press, Durham, NC, pp. 157–178.

Fotiou, E., 2010. From medicine men to day trippers: *Shamanic Tourism* in Iquitos, Peru (PhD Dissertation). University of Wisconsin - Madison.

Freedman, F.B., 2015. Tobacco and shamanic agency in the Upper Amazon: Historical and contemporary perspectives, in: Russell, A., Rahman, E. (Eds.), *The Master Plant: Tobacco in Lowland South America*. Bloomsbury Publishing, London; New York, pp. 63–87.

Goldman, I., 2004. *Cubeo Hehénewa Religious Thought: Metaphysics of a Northwestern Amazonian People*. Columbia University Press.

Harner, M., 1973. The sound of rushing water, in: Harner, M. (Ed.), *Hallucinogens and Shamanism*. Oxford University Press, New York, pp. 15–27.

Helms, M., 1988. *Ulysses' Sail: an Ethnographic Odyssey of Power, Knowledge, and Geographical Distance*. Princeton University Press, Princeton, N.J.

Hugh-Jones, C., 1979. *From the Milk River*. Cambridge University Press, Cambridge.

Hugh-Jones, S., 1995. Coca, beer, cigars and *ayahuasca*: Meals and anti-meals in an Amerindian community, in: Goodman, J., Andrew Sherratt, Paul E.Lovejoy (Eds.), *Consuming Habits: Drugs in History and Anthropology*. Routledge, London; New York, pp. 47–66.

Hugh-Jones, S., 1988. *The Palm and the Pleiades: Initiation and Cosmology in Northwest Amazonia*. Cambridge University Press.

Jernigan, K.A., 2011. Dietary restrictions in healing among speakers of Iquito, an endangered language of the Peruvian Amazon. *Journal of Ethnobiology and Ethnomedicine* 7, 20.

Joy, D., 1992. Psychedelic renaissance, in: Stafford, P.G. (Ed.), *Psychedelics Encyclopedia*. Ronin Publishing, Oakland, pp. 21–60.

Karsten, R., 1964. *Studies in the Religion of the South-American Indians East of the Andes*. Societas Scientiarum Fennica, Helsinki.

Kotler, S., 2010. The new psychedelic renaissance. *Playboy* 51–52, 114, 119.

Langdon, E.J.M., 1992. *Dau*: Shamanic power in Siona religion and medicine, in: Langdon, E.J.M., Baer, G. (Eds.), *Portals of Power: Shamanism in South America*. University of New Mexico Press, Albuquerque, pp. 41–61.

Langdon, E.J.M., 1979. The Siona hallucinogenic ritual: Its meaning and power, in: Morgan, J.H. (Ed.), *Understanding Religion and Culture: Anthropological and Theological Perspectives*. University Press of America, Washington, pp. 58–86.

Lenaerts, M., 2006. Substances, relationships and the omnipresence of the body: An overview of Ashéninka ethnomedicine (Western Amazonia). *Journal of Ethnobiology and Ethnomedicine* 2, 49.

Londoño Sulkin, C.D., 2012. *People of Substance: An Ethnography of Morality in the Colombian Amazon*. University of Toronto Press, Toronto.

López Vinatea, L.A., 2000. *Plantas Usadas por Shamanes Amazonicos en el Brebaje Ayahuasca*. Universidad Nacional de la Amazonía Peruana, Iquitos.

Luna, L.E., 1992. *Icaros*: Magic melodies among the *Mestizo* shamans of the Peruvian Amazon, in: Langdon, E.J.M., Baer, G. (Eds.), *Portals of Power: Shamanism in South America*. University of New Mexico Press, Albuquerque, pp. 231–253.

Macdonald, B.H., 2017. *How an Ayahuasca Retreat Claimed the Life of a 24yo Kiwi Tourist in the Amazon*. URL http://www.abc.net.au/triplej/programs/hack/how-ayahuasca-retreat-claimed-the-life-of-a-24yo-kiwi-tourist/8350338 (accessed 8.25.17).

McCallum, C., 2014. Cashinahua perspectives on functional anatomy: Ontology, ontogenesis, and biomedical education in Amazonia. *AMET American Ethnologist* 41, 504–517.

McCallum, C., 2001. *Gender and Sociality in Amazonia: How Real People are Made*. Berg, Oxford; New York.

McCallum, C., 1996. The body that knows: From Cashinahua epistemology to a medical anthropology of lowland South America. *Med.Anthropol.Q.* 10, 347–372.

McKenna, D.J., Luna, L.E., Towers, G.H., 1995. Biodynamic constituents in *ayahuasca* admixture plants: An un-investigated folk pharmacopoeia, in: *Ethnobotany: Evolution of a Discipline*. Dioscorides Press, Portland Or., pp. 349–361.

Reichel-Dolmatoff, G., 1975. *The Shaman and the Jaguar: a Study of Narcotic Drugs among the Indians of Colombia*. Temple University Press, Philadelphia.

Reichel-Dolmatoff, G., 1971. *Amazonian Cosmos the Sexual and Religious Symbolism of the Tukano Indians*. University of Chicago Press, Chicago.

Santos-Granero, F., 2009. Introduction: Amerindian constructional views of the world, in: *The Occult Life of Things: Native Amazonian Theories of Materiality and Personhood*. University of Arizona Press, Tucson, pp. 1–29.

Schultes, R.E., Raffauf, R.F., 1992. *The Healing Forest: Medicinal and Toxic Plants of the Northwest Amazonia, Historical, Ethno- & Economic Botany Series*. Dioscorides Press, Portland, Or.

Sessa, B., 2012. *The Psychedelic Renaissance: Reassessing the Role of Psychedelic Drugs in 21st Century Psychiatry and Society*. Muswell Hill, London.

Shepard, G.H., 1998. Psychoactive plants and ethnopsychiatric medicines of the Matsigenka. *Journal of Psychoactive Drugs* 30, 321–332.

Siikala, A.-L., 1992. The Siberian shaman's technique of ecstasy, in: Hoppál, M., Siikala, A.-L. (Eds.), *Studies on Shamanism, Ethnologica Uralica*, 2. Finish Anthropological Society; Akadémiai Kiadó, Helsinki; Budapest, pp. 26–40.

Uzendoski, M., 2005. *The Napo Runa of Amazonian Ecuador*. University of Illinois Press, Urbana.

Viveiros de Castro, E., 1998. Cosmological deixis and Amerindian perspectivism. *Journal of the Royal Anthropological Institute* 4, 469–488.

Walker, H., 2013. *Under a Watchful Eye: Self, Power, and Intimacy in Amazonia*. University of California Press, Berkeley, Calif.

Weiss, G., 1973. Shamanism and priesthood in Light of the Campa *ayahuasca* ceremony, in: Harner, M. (Ed.), *Hallucinogens and Shamanism*. Oxford University Press, New York, pp. 40–47.

Whitten, N.E., 1976. *Sacha Runa: Ethnicity and Adaptation of Ecuadorian Jungle Quichua*. University of Illinois Press, Urbana.

Wilbert, J., 1987. *Tobacco and Shamanism in South America, Psychoactive plants of the world*. Yale University Press, New Haven.

Wilbert, J., 1975. Magico-religious use of tobacco among South American Indians, in: *Cannabis and Culture*. The Hague, pp. 439–461.

Wilbert, J., 1972. Tobacco and shamanistic ecstasy among the Warao Indians of Venezuela, in: *Flesh of the Gods: The Ritual Use of Hallucinogens*. New York, pp. 55–83.

Winkelman, M., 2005. Drug tourism or spiritual healing? Ayahuasca seekers in Amazonia. *J. Psychoactive Drugs* 37, 209–218.

Wright, R.M., 1998. Cosmos, self, and history in Baniwa religion: *For Those Unborn*. University of Texas Press.

69

Spirit Bodies, Plant Teachers and Messenger Molecules in Amazonian Shamanism

Glenn H. Shepard, PhD

Museu Paraense Emílio
Goeldi, Belém, Brazil

ABSTRACT

Western scientists and entheogen enthusiasts have used terms such as "psychoactive," "hallucinogenic," "psychedelic," or more recently, "entheogenic," to refer to shamanic plants and substances. Yet in all their permutations, such terms reinforce the foundational Cartesian dichotomy between body and mind, substance and spirit, the finite and the infinite. Indigenous peoples of the Amazon, by contrast, do not distinguish the mental or spiritual effects of shamanic plants and substances from their physiological or sensory properties. Among the Matsigenka people of Peru, for example, the term *kepigari* (which could be translated as "toxic," or "intoxicating") encompasses the physiological, sensory and cognitive dimensions of shamanic experience under a single, unified concept. The Matsigenka and other Amazonian peoples make no distinction between a shamanic plant's active pharmacological ingredients and what we might refer to as the anthropomorphized "soul" that animates and infuses it with agency. Indeed, for the Matsigenka and other Amazonian peoples, the body can sometimes be used as a synonym for what we would refer to as the soul, and vice versa. And yet just as ethnobotanists might overlook the philosophical ramifications of indigenous ways of knowing, anthropologists in Amazonia, increasingly concerned with ontological questions, often overlook the material and phenomenological basis of indigenous knowledge. Indigenous concepts surrounding the sensory properties, body/mind manifestations and spiritual properties of shamanic plants transcend Cartesian dualism. Specific plants and plant-based substances are sometimes personified by Amazonian shamans as "plant teachers." Scientific findings about the role of messenger molecules in plant communication and an emerging appreciation of "plant intelligence" provide new windows of understanding into the deep truth behind shamanic concepts.

STARS HAVE BODIES

Sitting out on a tropical night under a clear, shimmering sky, still reeling from the latest round of strong tobacco snuff, I ask Machipango why stars are alive. For over twenty years, Machipango has patiently endured these question-and-answer sessions about the most obvious things in the universe. Tonight, I am back on a subject that has intrigued me since my very first lesson in Matsigenka grammar: the animate/inanimate distinction. The Matsigenka language treats "animate" subjects and objects as grammatically masculine, taking the prefix i- at the head of possessed nouns and verbs and the suffix–ri for the direct or indirect object of verbs, while "inanimate" objects are grammatically feminine, taking the prefix o- at the head of possessed nouns and verbs and the suffix

–*ro* for direct and indirect objects. Most animals for the Matsigenka are animate (masculine), with some exceptions like frogs and deer (because they are mythological female seducers), while water, soil and rocks are inanimate (feminine). Curiously, most plants are *not* treated as animate things by the Matsigenka: they "grow," (*oshivokake*), but cannot move of their own volition (*tenga anutake*). On the other hand, money is animate, as are rubber, stars and other celestial objects such as the sun and moon. The basic distinction seems to be between things that exhibit locomotion or apparently volitional movement (doesn't money flee from the hands as inexorably as a bouncy rubber ball?), and those that mostly stand still.

I know all this, yet nonetheless, I ask probably for the twentieth time, "What about plants? What about stars?"

And Merino answers, predictably, "Plants don't move, they just stand there. The stars move across the sky." But then he says something I wasn't expecting:

"Stars have bodies."

But I'm translating. What he really says is, *Aiño ivatsa*.

Now *ivatsa* is a curious word, because it may be used to refer to the body in a very physical sense, as in meat, flesh, the whole body or physical presence, but can also be used in reference to the invisible human essence or "spirit body" of certain personified beings. So on the one hand, animal meat is *ivatsa*, as is raw flesh exposed in a wound. The human body is also *ivatsa* (*novatsa*, "my body"). One can use the same phrase as a question to ask whether so-and-so is actually home: *aiño ivatsa?* "Is his body there?" i.e., "Is he physically present? Is he home?" (compare with English, "Is any-*body* home?"). Of course, we, too, refer to stars and planets as "celestial bodies," but what we mean by this is something very different, indeed almost the opposite of what Machipango was saying. To refer to a star as a 'celestial body' is to emphasize its corporeal physicality while denying it any form of consciousness, animate nature or 'soul'. But when Machipango says 'stars have bodies', what he means is that they have *human* bodies, which necessarily implies that they, like humans, have spirits or souls.

The soul for the Matsigenka is not an invisible force relegated to the pineal gland, as it were. Rather, the soul is what activates all bodily functions and gives it appetite, manifesting itself as the muscle and fat on a healthy body. Without 'life essence' (*yani*), the body is merely skin and bones. 'Skin' (*itaki*, also 'tree bark') and 'bones' (*itonki*), rather than flesh, are considered to be the inert aspects of the body. Flesh, muscle, blood and fat are all signs of the life force (*yani*) present in a healthy body. The life essence of animals is passed on to those who consume their flesh. Without meat (*ivatsa*) in their diets, people grow hungry (*itasegaka*), skinny (*imatsataka*), and ill (*imantsigataka*). A sick person or an old person who is thin and frail is as good as dead: The soul has already left the body, the flesh has been eaten away, and all that remains are the inanimate skin and bones. A person stricken by sadness likewise loses their appetite, wastes away, and eventually dies due to the flight of their soul.

According to Matsigenka myths and origin stories, in ancient times all species of animals, as well as the sun, moon, stars, and other beings, were human, which is to say, they had human bodies, lived in human societies and possessed the trappings of human culture. Through a series of episodes related in Matsigenka myths and tales, these different beings were transformed into their current form, assuming the diverse bodies and habits of different animal species, celestial beings, spirits, certain plants, and so on. Primordial beings, the *Tasorintsi* or "blowing spirits" first used the transformative powers of tobacco and other psychoactive plants to breathe diversity into the animal and plant kingdoms. Thus, a transformative, shamanistic act is thought to underlie the observable taxonomic disjunctions between related species of organisms.[1] And yet, despite these transformations in their outward form and appearance in the current world of day-to-day existence, such spirit-beings still possess a human form that is invisible under ordinary circumstances, but which becomes visible in dreams and special states of consciousness. This underlying "body human" possessed by diverse cosmological beings is something we Cartesian Westerners wouldn't call a body at all; if we were to call it anything, we'd likely call it a "spirit" or "soul."

To distinguish between the mundane, visible form of such cosmological beings and their manifest, transcendent human body, I have heard a number of expressions that seem to defy our Cartesian, Western instincts. For example, the screaming piha (*Lipaugus vociferans*) or *vuimpuio* in

---

1. In this sense, the process we call evolution is driven, for the Matsigenka, by past and present shamans. The transformative cognitive effects of psychoactive plants are invoked by the Matsigenka to explain the same conundrum of evolution that Linnaeus once pondered: How did the world came to be filled with such a great diversity of plants and animals, all different and yet apparently more or less related to one another? For Linnaeus, the answer was the Mind of God. For the Matsigenka, the answer is God's Mind on Drugs (Shepard 1999).

Matsisgenka, is a drab forest bird with an unmistakable song that begins like a low cat-call and then builds as a rising, whistled crescendo and finally bursts out in a ringing, explosive finale: *vui-vui-vui... VUIM-PUI-OH!*, hence the Matsigenka name for the animal. The *vuimpuio* bird is considered to be a helper to the Matsigenka shaman. The true *vuimpuio*, the one that appears to the shaman in trance – what we might call its "spirit" – is called *ivatsa*, "his body," which is to say, *human* body. Its mundane form, visible to anyone walking in the forest, is merely *ivanki*, "his wings." By the same token, the snake we see in the forest is merely *ichakore*, "his arrow," the poison dart the snake uses to kill its human prey, just as humans use arrows to hunt wild boar. The true snake is an invisible human hunter, called *ivatsa*, "his body," possessing a human body and form, but who looks upon human beings as wild boar or tapirs to be hunted, killed and eaten (Shepard, 2002a). Jaguars and other predators likewise look upon human beings as game animals. By the same token, game animals like peccaries and tapir see themselves as human, while human hunters appear to them as jaguar-like predators.

Such concepts are widespread among Amazonian indigenous peoples, who conceive of the relationships among different beings of the cosmos in ecological terms (Reichel-Dolmatoff, 1976; Århem 1996). The notion of predation is especially important in Amazonian cosmologies (Fausto, 2007); and the status of different species, beings and bodies within the cosmic food chain depends upon their point of view. Hence, this theoretical paradigm has been dubbed "perspectivism" (Lima, 1996; Viveiros de Castro, 1996). What unites the various beings of the cosmos is not, as Western science would have it, their universal biological nature, but rather their universal *human nature* (Viveiros de Castro, 2002). Amazonian ethnography is replete with examples of perspectival relations with the animal world, and yet curiously, given the prominence of plants in the tropical rainforest ecosystem, contemporary anthropologists have showed far less interest in indigenous peoples' conceptions of and relationships with plants (but see Daly 2015; Oliveira 2016).

PLANTS HAVE SOULS

Continuing our conversation on the grammatical status of different "animate" vs. "inanimate" beings, I pressed Machipango on the subject of plants. Generally, the Matsigenka do not consider plants to be "animate" in the sense of possessing locomotion and volition: Plants "grow," and hence do possess a "life force" (*ainyo ani*). However, they don't "walk," and for that reason, they are generally not treated as animate (for grammatical as well as philosophical purposes). There are exceptions, however. For example, the rubber tree, and certain other plants containing latex, are treated as grammatically animate ("masculine"), due to the flowing latex and elastic nature of the dried resin. Most psychoactive plants are also considered to be animate beings with spirit "masters," (*itinkami*), owners (*shintarorira*) or "mothers" (*iriniro*) who can appear in human form during dreams or altered states of consciousness to pass along healing powers and other forms of knowledge to those who use them properly.

The Matsigenka word for soul or spirit, *suretsi*, can also be used to refer to the heartwood of a tree or the pith of an herbaceous plant. When the core of a tree dies and its leaves stop growing, the term to express this is *okamasuretaka*, "its core – its soul – has died." Moreover, *suretsi* also refers to the pharmacological principles of medicinal, toxic or psychoactive plants. The activity of medicinal plants is described as *okitsitingake osure novatsaku*, "its soul infuses my body" (Shepard, 1999a, 2004): Note the use of the inanimate, "feminine" prefix *o-* on both the verb *okitsitingake* ("it infuses") and the noun *osure* ("its soul"). When one cooks a medicinal plant, its "soul" infuses the herbal brew, often made visible by a change in the coloration of the liquid. Then, when one drinks the tea, the "soul" of the plant, manifest in its taste or odor as well as coloration of the liquid, then "infuses" the blood, nerves and muscles, spreading its medicinal, toxic, or other effects throughout the body. Thus, again contradicting our Cartesian instincts, not only can "inanimate" things have a soul, but also the "soul" can have observable, physical manifestations that are passed from one being to another.

MATSIGENKA: 'THE PEOPLE'

The Matsigenka are people of the MONTAÑA, the rugged rainforests of the upper Amazon fringing the eastern slope of the Andes. They currently number about twelve thousand people inhabiting the Urubamba, upper Madre de Dios, and Manu River basins in southeast Peru. The Matsigenka language belongs to the pre-Andine group of Arawakan languages, most closely related to Nanti, Ashaninka (Campa), Nomatsiguenka and Caquinte. The term *matsigenka* means simply, 'people;' and when referring to the human status of animals, certain plants and other beings, either in the mythical past or in the shamanic present, the noun is turned into a verb; *i-matsigenkatake* or *o-mat-sigenkatake*, "he/she takes on human form."

The Matsigenka have traditionally practiced long-fallow swidden agriculture, growing manioc, plantains and bananas, maize, sweet potatoes, cotton, annato, beans, peanuts, chili peppers and a variety of other crops in small gardens cleared out of the forest (Johnson, 1983). Fish, game, fruits and other wild foods gathered from the forests and rivers of their environment are also essential in their diet. The Matsigenka traditionally lived in small settlements of extended families clustered according to a matrilocal (or uxorilocal) pattern of residence: a man marries out of his home village and goes to live with his wife's family (Johnson, 2003). In the past, such matrilocal settlements were widely dispersed and highly autonomous. As the Catholic Church, Evangelical missionaries and the Peruvian state have increasingly penetrated into the hinterlands, Matsigenka families have settled near mission outposts or government school houses, forming more densely populated, formally recognized "Native Communities" that can total hundreds of families. Since the 1980s, oil and gas prospecting activities have increasingly affected Matsigenka communities in the lower Urubamba region (Izquierdo & Shepard, 2003). The recent construction of the Camisea gas pipeline has caused lasting social, economic and political transformations in the communities of that region (Shepard, 2012). Though I have worked in many communities throughout the broader Matsigenka territory, most of my work has been among communities within Manu National Park somewhat buffered from the rapid rate of cultural changes going on currently outside this protected zone (Shepard et al., 2010).

KEPIGARI: THE CONCEPT OF MEDICINES AS POISONS

Toxic, caustic, purgative, hallucinogenic, and other noxious plants figure prominently in the medical system of the Matsigenka. Like many indigenous peoples of the tropical rainforest, the Matsigenka are connoisseurs in manipulating plant compounds through domestication, preparation, and dosage to enhance desired effects while avoiding fatal toxicity. In describing toxic plants and their physiological activity, the Matsigenka use the term *kepigari*. The term invokes a chain of inter-related meanings: bitterness, toxicity, lethal poison, purgative and emetic properties, nausea and dizziness, psychoactivity, and shamanistic ecstasy. The relationship between plant toxicity and curative power is fundamental to the Matsigenka's understanding of illness and healing: Medicines are also poisons, used to purge the body and soul of illness and illness-causing spirits (Shepard, 2005).

The term *kepigari* is derived from the root *-piga-*, 'to turn around, spin around, feel dizzy,' and hence by extension 'nausea, intoxication.' *Kepigari* refers to all toxic, poisonous, narcotic and psychoactive substances: alcohol, tobacco and other psychoactive plants; purgatives, emetics and poisonous plants; venomous snakes, frogs, insects and toxic mushrooms; any substance – from vanilla orchids to gasoline – with an overpowering "intoxicating" odor; and menstrual blood, known as *ogepigariaate*, "the poison that flows" (Rosengren, 1987). Many plants and other substances that are *kepigari* are also *kepishiri* ("bitter") or else have an "intoxicating odor," *kepigarienga*. Bitter, pungent and other noxious plants are sought out by Matsigenka healers because their toxic properties are said to hurt, kill and expel intrusive illness-causing agents, whether spiritual or material in form (Shepard, 2004).

Kepigari refers to the physiological state of intoxication, including bouts of dizziness, fainting, nausea and vomiting, as well as drunkenness, shamanic ecstasy and even insanity. In chants that accompany shamanistic ceremonies, singers evoke the physical and cognitive sensations of these experiences, and *kepigari* is intoned frequently to denote the whirling, giddy sensation of ecstasy. Plants used to induce altered states of consciousness like tobacco, *ayahuasca* and *Brugmansia* (fundamental to the Matsigenka shaman's transformative powers) are all *kepigari*. I hesitate to use Western terms like "psychoactive," "narcotic," "hallucinogenic" or "psychedelic" to refer to these shamanic substances, since such terms reinforce the foundational distinction René Descartes drew between *res extensa* ("extended [i.e. in space] things"), or material substance, versus *res cogitans* ("thinking things"), or mental substance. Cartesian dualism between mind and body remains a fundamental problem in Western science and philosophy; in working with peoples who have different notions about the world and its various substances and beings, we find ourselves tripping over it all the time. For example, when we say a plant is "psychoactive" or "psychedelic," we focus on mental, emotional and psychic states, as if these were somehow separate from physiological effects in the body. By calling such substances "hallucinogens" we further denigrate them by assuming that the visions they produce are mere hallucinations, fantasies, fallacies.

The term *entheogen*, "revealing God (or the divine) within" (Ruck et al., 1979), was coined to overcome the bias and derogatory nature implicit in terms like "hallucinogen." And yet, the Greek term *theos* at the root of the expression ironically reinforces the tenets of Cartesian philosophy by emphasizing the third substance posited by Descartes, namely God, *res infinita*, a special kind of "thinking substance" that, unlike mortal human thought, is infinite in scope. Indeed, many entheogen users focus their enthusiasm on the spiritual and religious aspects of their experiences, while minimizing, or even consciously attempting to eliminate, unpleasant physiological side-effects like nausea. For the Matsigenka, there is no such thing as "side effects," since the physical, mental and spiritual dimensions of shamanic plants are all integrated with their overt chemosensory properties (bitter taste, toxicity) into the single concept of *kepigari*, "intoxicating." Transcendental effects in consciousness go hand-in-hand with unpleasant effects in the body such as nausea, vomiting, sweating, shaking and dizziness, which are in turn signaled, encapsulated, and transmitted through specific empirical, sensory properties (bitter, astringent, caustic) associated with toxicity. The more intense the toxic effects endured by the body, the more profound are the visions experienced by the soul: The stronger the poison, the better the medicine.

SUBSTANCE, SOUL, AND SENSATION: A SENSORY ECOLOGY OF MEDICINAL AND SHAMANIC PLANTS

Sensory properties like taste, odor, color, texture and so on serve for more than just identifying plants and transmitting this knowledge to others. Rather, sensory cues and perceptions are crucial to understanding how medicines interact with illness agents in the body, how illness enters and affects people, and how people relate to one another and to other beings in the cosmos. This approach, which I have called "sensory ecology" (Shepard, 2004), builds on the work of other anthropologists who have explored cultural variations in sensory experience (Stoller, 1989; Classen, 1990; Howes, 1991). Sensory ecology seeks to appreciate and analyze indigenous understandings of sensory experience, attending to the interwoven biological, cultural, experiential and cosmological dimensions of sensory experience. Here, I apply the approach of sensory ecology to a number of important toxic, medicinal, and psychoactive plants in the Matsigenka pharmacopoeia.

Tobacco and shamanism are synonymous for the Matsigenka: The shaman is *seripigari*, "the one intoxicated by tobacco" (Baer, 1992). Tobacco (*Nicotiana tabacum* L.) is consumed by the Matsigenka in many forms: smoked (*nopenatakero*) in pipes, drunk in liquid form (*oani*), chewed in a concentrated, bitter quid (*opatsa*) and blasted up the nostrils as powdered green snuff (*opane*). Tobacco is judged by how painful (*katsi*) it is to the taste or in the nostrils. The intensity of the tobacco's pain (*katsi*) is proportional to its intoxicating strength (*kepigari*), which is also a measure of the shamanic strength of the person who prepared it. The more painful the tobacco, the more powerful the shaman. Tobacco is like food for shamans and their spirit allies: As their powers grow, shamans come to relish the pungent nourishment of tobacco over ordinary food. By sharing tobacco snuff or quid in daily life, and especially during an *ayahuasca* session, Matsigenka men reinforce social bonds while performing a mystical exchange of powers through the physical medium of the tobacco substance (Shepard, 2015a). Tobacco snuff is prepared by drying and grinding fresh, green tobacco leaves to a fine powder, mixed with the ash of specific kinds of tree bark. In addition to its social and shamanic functions, tobacco can also be used to fight off the nasal congestion caused by colds, or to dispel bad dreams by physically "hurting" (*okatsitakeri*) the illness vector or harmful spirits causing discomfort. Likewise, tobacco quid tossed near the watery lair of an anaconda acts to 'burn' (*otegakeri*) the snake and frighten it away.

Tobacco quid or paste, *opatsa seri*, is prepared by boiling cured tobacco leaves with pounded *Banisteriopsis* liana until it is reduced to a thick, dark, bitter paste which is absorbed using native cotton (*ampei*) to form a quid that is stored in bamboo tubes. *Opatsa seri* is taken during *ayahuasca* sessions to augment the visionary experience, or can be taken alone to induce dreams. The master shaman swallows *opatsa seri* and then regurgitates it, giving it to his apprentice mouth-to-mouth in a mystical kiss, thereby passing on his shaman's soul and his supernatural powers.

One Matsigenka shaman explained *opatsa seri* in this way (Shepard, 1998: 325):

> *Opatsa seri* is a seed. When you swallow it, it is like planting a seed in your heart. Your tobacco (*pisere*) is your soul (*pisure*). Each time you take *opatsa seri*, your soul grows like a tree. Not the ordinary soul, but the shaman's soul, the soul of the *Saankariite*. Your brother. Not everyone has a tobacco soul, only the *seripigari*. My teacher long ago gave me his tobacco (*isere*), thus giving me his soul (*isure*). Just like I have now given you my tobacco (*nosere*), which is my soul (*nosure*).

He emphasized the similarity in the sound of the words *nosere*, "my tobacco," and *nosure*, "my soul," suggesting they were virtually synonymous: a clear example of how shamanic powers can be gained and transmitted through the transfer of specific, usually toxic, substances.

Like many other Amazonian peoples, the Matsigenka currently prepare the *ayahuasca* brew by boiling the liana *Banisteriopsis caapi* (Spruce ex Griseb.) C.V.Morton with leaves from one or more species of the *Psychotria* shrub. The Matsigenka name for *Banisteriopsis* is *kamarampi*, literally, "vomiting medicine," emphasizing the plant's purgative properties. Though *ayahuasca* is mostly known in Amazonia for its religious and medical uses, a main goal of *ayahuasca* use among the Matsigenka of the Manu River is to help men improve their hunting skills. Consumption of *kamarampi* is thought to cleanse a man's body of contamination from improperly cooked meat, menstrual blood and other sexual and dietary impurities (Shepard, 2002b; see below). While the emetic properties of *kamarampi* cleanse the hunter's body, the psychoactive properties allow the hunter's soul to visit the *Saankariite* ("invisible ones," benevolent forest beings) and convince them "not to be stingy" (*gani itsaneakaro*) with their pets, the game animals of the forest. Matsigenka men of the Manu take *Banisteriopsis* frequently throughout the rainy season, when many forest fruits are ripe and the game animals, especially large primates like woolly and spider monkeys, are fat. When you ask Matsigenka men why they take *ayahuasca*, they typically answer, "I take *ayahuasca*, the next day I go out and kill two monkeys." The Matsigenka avoid taking *ayahuasca* during the dry season, because they say the spirit world is full of dangerous fires caused by the *Saankariite* who, like the Matsigenka, burn their gardens during that time of year.

Prior to the 1960s, the Matsigenka of the Manu region did not use DMT-containing *Psychotria* species as an admixture to *Banisteriopsis*. Instead, they prepared *Banisteriopsis* by boiling it for long periods of time until it was reduced to a honey-like consistency, sometimes mixing it with tobacco in the preparation known as *opatsa seri*, noted above. Various other plants were used as admixtures, and their use appears at least partly related to the presence of brightly colored venation or markings on some species' leaves, said to produce colorful patterns during trance (see Shepard, 1998). The Matsigenka of the Manu region learned to use the *Psychotria* admixture from Matsigenka fellows from the neighboring Urubamba river who had come to the region, ironically enough, in the company of Protestant missionaries (Shepard, 2015b). The plant was already present in their environment, but since the knowledge came from the Urubamba region, they refer to it now as "Urubamba-leaf," *orovampashi*. Although *Psychotria viridis* Ruiz & Pav. is the most frequently mentioned *ayahuasca* admixture in the literature, the Matsigenka consider this to be a dangerous plant, used by sorcerers of rival tribes such as the Shipibo and Piro. The Matsigenka name for *P. viridis* is *irorovampashi pijiri* ("*Psychotria* of the bat") or *yakomamashi* ("anaconda leaf") since it is said to be "owned" by these animal spirits, who bring on terrifying visions of bats or snakes. The Matsigenka consistently use another as yet unidentified *Psychotria* species which they refer to as *orovampashi-sano* ("true *Psychotria*").This plant, they say, causes no unpleasant visions of bats or snakes, but only "good" visions of birds and happy, dancing *Saankariite* spirits (Shepard, 1998). Their observations appear to hint at different concentrations of different DMT-related compounds in closely related species. These examples also attest to the wide variety of traditional uses and preparations which preceded the more homogenous current *ayahuasca* tradition that apparently spread in the aftermath of the rubber boom (Shepard, 2015b).

The cultivated *Datura* relative, *Brugmansia suaveolens* (Willd.) Bercht. & C.Presl, is known to the Matsigenka as *jayapa*, *saaro*, or simply, *kepigari* ("intoxicant, poison"). Containing potent tropane alkaloids such as atropine and scopolamine, it is considered to be the most intoxicating (*kepigari*) and strongest of all medicines. Frequent use is considered to be dangerous, and I have documented several cases of deaths owing to overdose or excessive use (Shepard, in press). Great care is taken in the preparation and dosage of *Brugmansia* due to its high potency and toxicity. The fresh leaf can be heated and applied as an external plaster for broken bones, stomach aches, arthritic pains, swelling and other conditions, consistent with biomedical uses of atropine. A small dose may be given orally to a woman suffering from difficult childbirth, a practice that recalls the use of scopolamine to induce "twilight sleep" during childbirth in American hospitals in recent times. A larger, vision-inducing dose of *Brugmansia* infusion may be given orally as a last resort to treat people suffering from severe trauma, chronic illnesses, or suspected sorcery. During these sessions, the patient can spend days, even weeks in a trance where spirit beings, white-robed doctors or the spirit "mother" of the plant herself appear to them to reveal the true source of their suffering, remove any intrusive sorcery objects and repair the physical or spiritual damage. Apprentice shamans may take a large dose to open a channel of communication with the *Saankariite* forest spirits. During the intense, dream-like state of *Brugmansia* trance, shamans may also receive new agricultural varieties from the *Saankariite*, especially manioc cuttings and medicinal sedges (Shepard, 1998; Shepard, 1999b). *Brugmansia* plants that have gone to seed in old gardens or along river courses are referred to as "*Brugmansia* of the caiman" (*iayapate saniri*), and considered to be extremely dangerous when ingested, leading to soul loss or death.

Amazonian ethnobotanists in the tradition of Richard Evans Schultes have shown a special interest in psychoactive plants. Yet among the Matsigenka, the concept of *kepigari* is not restricted to vision-inducing shamanic plants, but embraces a wide range of other toxic, caustic, emetic and purgative plants used for a variety of purposes. For treating recently cut umbilical cords and the tropical skin disease leishmaniasis, the Matsigenka use a number of toxic plants including curare species[2] (*Curarea*) and the highly toxic cultigen *Solanum mammosum* L. The bitterness (*kepishiri*) and painful causticity (*katsi*) of these plants is said to "embitter" (*okepishitakeri*), "hurt" (*okatsitakeri*), and "kill" (*ogamagakeri*) the illness-causing vectors.

The Matsigenka attribute many gastrointestinal and skin conditions as well as ear, eye, and tooth infections to the activity of tiny worms (*tsomiri*) that enter the body and gnaw at the affected part. Although they are aware of parasitic intestinal helminths, the conception of *tsomiri* is broader, embracing microscopic illness-causing agents much like our own folk concept of "germs" or "microbes." Many illnesses are treated by ingesting or applying plants with strong, noxious sensory properties – bitter, astringent, pungent, caustic, sour (Shepard, 2004). Such properties are manifestations of the plant's soul (*osure*), a holistic healing force that infuses (*okitsitingakero*) the herbal decoction and the body of the patient. Pathogenic agents react to noxious properties much like humans, suffering pain and discomfort, retreating, and at high enough doses, perishing. In other cases, the Matsigenka take specific steps to detoxify overly poisonous plants to render their usage safe, especially for children. One species of *Anthurium* known as *matsontsorishi*, "jaguar leaf," is known to cause severe skin irritation when handled raw. However, when boiled long enough in water, the noxious properties are attenuated and the concoction is used to bathe newborns in order to protect them from illness.

EAGLE EYES: THE ETHNOPHARMACOLOGY OF HUNTING MEDICINES

A significant portion of the Matsigenka pharmacopeia is dedicated to what is often referred to in the literature as "hunting magic" (Daly et al., 1992). According to my observations, there seems to be more pharmacology than magic at work. Some 25% of the Matsigenka pharmacopoeia belong to a category that should be more properly called "hunting *medicines*," referred to in Matsigenka as *kovintsari*, "to have or achieve good aim." Being a good hunter is not only about having keen eyesight, good aim and a strong, sturdy grip on the bow. The hunter must, in the first place, be able to *see* the animals in the forest. A hunter who has "lost his aim" is not only unable to fire his arrow straight, he is, in a deeper sense, unable to locate and visualize game animals. This happens because he has violated behavioral, dietary and sexual taboos that offend the "masters" (*itinkami*) or "owners" (*shintarorira*) of game animal species (see also Fausto, 2008). (Note that the same terms are used to refer to the owners or spirit-masters of psychoactive and other powerful plants). Purity, both spiritual and bodily, are fundamental to a hunter's tracking skills, physical stamina and "aim."

---

2. I have collected and identified most of the plant species mentioned in this and other published works. However, in order to protect Matsigenka intellectual property rights, I refrain from publishing full species information for all but the most commonly known, widespread species.

A man can lose his aim by eating spoiled or improperly cooked meat. For example, if his wife allows a pot of meat to boil over and spill into the flames, the sizzling broth vaporizes and its odor wafts into the forest, where the "owner" of that particular species smells the telltale sign of improperly prepared meat and becomes angry, saying, "Who is wasting my pets?" The spirit owners of game animal species raise wild animals much like humans raise chickens or dogs, and they can reveal or hide their "pets" to specific hunters as they see fit. If possible, a man should avoid carrying the animal he has killed, lest his body become infused with the odor of the animal's blood, thereby warding off the animals and their master the next time he goes to the forest. A companion, typically a brother-in-law or teenage boy, carries it for him. A man should never eat the head of the animal he has killed. To eat the head is to take on, quite literally, the point of view of the dead animal, breaking down the balance in the predator-prey relationship. Sexual intercourse the night before a hunt, or any contact with menstrual blood or menstruating women, said to smell like carrion or raw meat (*janigarienka*), also takes away a man's aim: the strong odors of sexual fluids and menstrual blood likewise offend and frighten game animals and their spirit-masters.

When a man violates these norms, he thus loses not only his aim, but his ability to encounter animals in the first place. Such a man's body is said to reek with the carrion smell of spoiled meat or raw blood, and his soul becomes possessed with the spirit of the vulture. A number of species of purgative and emetic plants are taken by hunters to clean themselves of sexual, dietary, and ritual impurities. Fathers prepare their adolescent sons for manhood and hunting through a rigorous regimen of purgative, emetic or psychoactive hunting medicines belonging to a wide range of botanical families. Frequent use of *ayahuasca* during the rainy season is part of this broader practice associated with hunting medicine. Many hunting medicines are bitter or induce fits of vomiting or diarrhea of various degrees of severity. The more bitter and the more extreme the purgative effect, the better the medicine. The idea behind purgative remedies is to clean out the body of the spoiled meat and carrion-eating vulture spirit and replace it with the harpy eagle's hunting spirit. *Pakitsa*, the harpy eagle, is the epitome of hunting prowess for the Matsigenka.

Matsigenka men also apply the leaf-juice of numerous plant species (mostly Rubiaceae) to their eyes in order to clarify vision and instill the hunter with the soul of the harpy eagle, *Pakitsa* (Shepard, 2002b). The acidic or mildly caustic eye-drops cause the eyes to sting and water intensely for a few minutes, like getting lemon juice or chili peppers in the eyes. The stinging sensation is the sensory cue indicating that the "soul" (*osure*) of the plant is "infusing" (*okitsitingakeri*) the man's body, starting with the eyes, spreading through the head and descending into the torso, arms and hands through the muscles and veins. When hunting, the plant's soul also infuses the bow and the arrow with its power.

Cultivated sedges (*Cyperus* spp.), referred to as *ivenkiki*, are an especially important part of Matsigenka hunting lore, and of medicinal practices more generally. Individual Matsigenka men and women can cultivate dozens of sedge varieties in a single garden. There are sedge varieties for treating fevers and headaches, for dispelling nightmares, for healing arrow wounds and snake bites. Women cultivate sedge varieties for protecting babies from animal spirits, facilitating childbirth, for reducing or increasing fertility, for improving their skill in spinning and weaving cotton and resolving domestic disputes. Men cultivate a plethora of sedge varieties as hunting medicines, each sedge variety corresponding to a specific game animal. Many of the sedge varieties appear to be botanically identical, and only their owners are able to distinguish them. Given the tremendous diversity of uses for what appear to be nearly identical plants, ethnobotanists had long overlooked sedges in the Amazon, until it was discovered that cultivated sedge varieties in the Amazon harbor a systemic, mutualistic infection of the fungus *Balansia cyperi* (Plowman, et al., 1990), which belongs to the Clavicepitaceae, the same family as rye ergot (*Claviceps purpurea*) from which medically important ergot alkaloids, including psychoactive lysergic acid derivatives closely related to LSD, are extracted. Like rye ergot, the *Balansia* fungus (and not the sedge plant itself) produces a number of ergot-like compounds. Ergot alkaloids are known to constrict blood vessels, alter uterine contractions, and at high enough doses cause convulsions and hallucinations. The Matsigenka's use of different sedge varieties to treat wounds and snakebites, to staunch birth-related hemorrhaging and to alter fertility are consistent with the physiological properties of ergot alkaloids. Hunters carry specific sedges along on the hunt and consume them just before shooting an arrow. The hunter chews the root bulb, which has a bitter, aromatic taste, and then spits the masticated bulb onto his hands, on the bow, on the arrow, and towards the game animal. The sedge is said to infuse the hunter's body and weapon with its power, while mesmerizing the animal. The vasoconstrictive and psychoactive properties of ergot alkaloids may contribute to the hunter's heightened state of awareness, calm and perception.

Brunfelsia spp., belonging, like *Brugmansia* to the Solanaceae, are used widely throughout the Amazon for treating a variety of conditions, especially arthritic pains (Plowman 1981). The Matsigenka recognize several folk species: *sankenke* ("purifying shrub"), *oshetopari* ("spider monkey root"), *shimakoa* ("fish plant") and *pakitsapari* ("eagle root"). *Pakitsa*, the harpy eagle, is the epitome of hunting prowess for the Matsigenka. In ancient times, *Pakitsa* walked the earth in human form and taught these and other hunting medicines to the Matsigenka (Shepard 1998). *Kaviniri*, apparently a distinctive species of *Brunfelsia*, is said to instill such formidable hunting powers that the user turns into a jaguar and becomes a threat to his own family (Shepard 2014). *Brunfelsia* is prepared as a tea or cold infusion, and produces dizziness, nausea and a unique, needle-like prickling sensation in the hands and feet for several hours to several days. Depending on the dosage, *Brunfelsia* consumption can produce visions, convulsions or even coma. The Matsigenka describe the tingling, prickling sensation with the phrase, *tseki-tseki-tseki-tsek!*, the sensation of needles pricking the skin. This sensation is the physiological manifestation of the infusion of the plant's soul (*osure*) into the hunter's body, giving him the same clear eyesight and ferocious hunting ability as the plant's owner, the harpy eagle.

DISCUSSION: PLANT TEACHERS, PLANT INTELLIGENCE AND MESSENGER MOLECULES

The Matsigenka ingest a wide range of bioactive plants, following careful modes of preparation and administration, in order to infuse their bodies with chemical compounds that are selected and recognized according to specific sensory manifestations. The physical absorption of plant substances is understood to establish an intimate relationship with the personified "owners" or "masters" that infuse these plants with spiritual power: in short, transubstantiation. The concept of direct apprenticeship from plants is widespread among indigenous as well as non-indigenous peoples of the Amazon. As Luis Eduardo Luna (1984: 140, 142) writes in his study of *mestizo ayahuasca* healers or *curanderos* in Amazonian Peru,

> Crucial to shamanic practices is the belief that many plants, if not all plants, each have their own "mother" or spirit. It is with the help of the spirits of some of these plants, which I have called "plant teachers", that the shaman is able to acquire his powers... Informants insist that the spirits of the plants taught them what they know.

According to Eduardo Viveiros de Castro (2004: 468), such ways of knowing stand in direct opposition to the Western philosophical tradition, where knowledge is achieved through objectification, which is to say, de-subjectification:

> Amerindian shamanism is guided by the opposite ideal. To know is to personify, to take on the point of view of that which must be known. Shamanic knowledge aims at something that is a someone – another subject. The form of the other is *the person*.

For Viveiros de Castro (ibid.), Amerindian peoples view social relationships, as defined by cosmological perspective, to form the primary substrate of the universe, while physical substances are secondary:

> Our traditional problem in the West is how to connect and universalize: individual substances are given, while relations have to be made. The Amerindian problem is how to separate and particularize: relations are given, while substances must be defined.

Viveiros de Castro implies not only divergence between Western and Amerindian ways of knowing, but a nearly perfect, dichotomous inversion. Presenting indigenous ways of knowing as a mirror-image of our own risks simplifying the internal complexity of indigenous knowledge while at the same time reproducing the problematic Cartesian dichotomy (nature/culture, mind/body, matter/spirit) from the other side of the looking glass. In this review of Matsigenka pharmacology and pharmacognosy, I have sought to show how their understandings of illness agents, spirit beings, and shamanic powers are revealed through the direct experience of specific plant substances. In this sense, the Cartesian divide simply falls away. Plant-based chemical compounds are not so much material vehicles that open neural networks or pathways of communication with spirit beings, they *are* those spirit beings in and of themselves, manifested through specific sensory cues and transubstantiated in the physical process of infusion and absorption into the holistic spirit-body.

Ingold (2000) resists the anthropological tendency to dichotomize indigenous and scientific ways of knowing, emphasizing the holistic quality of environmental perception whether among indigenous peoples, field biologists or ethnobotanists. His description of how environmental knowledge is learned and transmitted captures the texture of my long apprenticeship with Matsigenka shamans, hunters and herbalists: "When the novice is brought into the presence of some component of the environment and called upon to attend to it in a certain way, his task, then, is not to decode, but rather to discover for himself the meaning that lies within it" (ibid: 20). Ingold draws a distinction between the symbolic *cipher*, that must be decoded, and the holistic *clue* that is revelatory in itself, that "opens up the world to perception of greater depth and clarity" (ibid). Odor, taste and other chemosensory properties used by the Matsigenka to ascertain and understand the powers of medicinal and shamanic plants are "clues" in this holistic sense.

In the case of psychoactive plants, their revelatory nature emerges directly from the material properties of specific chemical substances. In this sense, and contrary to Viveiros de Castro's (ibid) formulation, substance and relation are not only both equally "given," but indeed intimately entwined. Psychoactive compounds mimic the structure of specific brain hormones known as neurotransmitters, responsible for chemical communication across the junctions (synapses) between neurons. Due to their specific three-dimensional chemical structure, neurotransmitters bond with specialized receptor sites on the surface of the post-synaptic neuron, causing it to relay electrical impulses along its own axon. Due to their similar, but not identical, chemical structures, psychoactive compounds bond with specific neurotransmitter receptor sites, magnifying, suppressing, or otherwise altering their activity. For example, psilocin, found in hallucinogenic "magic mushrooms," is a tryptamine derivative that mimics the structure of 5-hydroxytryptamine (5-HT), the chemical name for the neurotransmitter serotonin. Psilocin, ibogaine, dimethyltryptamine (DMT – found in the *ayahuasca* brew), LSD, and other compounds found in traditionally used psychoactive plants and fungi belong to a class of compounds known as indole alkaloids, all derived from the same basic tryptamine structure.

Though a fair amount is now known about *how* psychoactive plants and compounds produce their peculiar effects on the human mind, it is still largely a mystery as to *why* certain plants produce such compounds. Alkaloids and other physiologically active compounds do not appear to be directly involved in the primary metabolic activities of plants. For this reason, they have been referred to as "secondary" plant compounds. And yet alkaloids contain nitrogen, a limiting element in plant growth, which means they are produced at a significant metabolic cost. Some have theorized that toxic compounds in plants evolved as chemical defenses to deter animals from eating their leaves, stems, roots, fruits, or seeds during particular life cycle phases.

Gottlieb and Borin (2005: 34) have pointed out that the most important secondary compounds driving animal-plant interactions, namely alkaloids and polyphenols, may not, in their evolutionary origins, have anything to do with attracting or deterring predators. Instead, these compounds likely evolved to communicate information across cell membranes:

> The primordial function of micromolecules in organisms, and probably the reason for their original appearance, does not concern attraction, defense or any other ecological function, but membrane construction… Considering the principal properties of micromolecules, e.g. small molecular mass, polarity, chirality, chemical reactivity (structural variation), different and variable half-lives, sporadic occurrence and antioxidant potential; it is possible to suggest that these molecules are messengers of information.

Up to 100,000 different compounds belonging to at least twenty different classes of molecules with communicatory roles have been identified for plants, and insights are now emerging as to their specific functions in transmitting information within cells, between cells of the same plant, among individuals of the same or different plant species, and with other organisms, notably animals and fungi. The analysis of such communication within, between and beyond different organisms is known as biosemiotics (Witzany 2008). Biosemiotics includes the analysis of combinations (syntax), context (pragmatics) and content-specific meanings (semantics) of chemical and other forms of signaling between organisms.

Traditional students of plant physiology have concluded that the growth patterns and developmental adaptations of plants in response to various stimuli such as light, water, nutrients, gravity and herbivory to be rote, genetically programmed adaptive responses. Trewavas (2003) reviews a wide range of research findings that suggest that plants show a capability for learning and problem-solving that goes beyond mere passive vegetative response, constituting a form of "plant intelligence." Trewavas (2003: 2) further points out that "the suite of molecules used in signal transduction are entirely similar between [animal] nerve cells ... and plant cells."

Such scientific findings give new levels of meaning to indigenous understandings of "plants as teachers." Compounds that may have originally emerged to facilitate communication of information within and between plant cells, now continue to serve as messenger molecules, transmitting information across multiple levels: the intra and inter-cellular, the inter-organismal and biospheric, as well as among multiple beings across different layers of the cosmos. By bringing indigenous understandings into dialog with biochemical insights, native and scientific concepts can illuminate one another, without privileging one perspective over the other. The empirical, sensory properties of plants can be seen, both by scientists and shamans, as concrete chemical signs that emerge within a complex web of information, transmission, communication and ultimately, relation between diverse beings, each with its own syntax, semantics, pragmatics and goals. The concept of plants as teachers is more than metaphor: it is a profound and accurate description of shamanic biosemiotics.

REFERENCES

Århem, K., 1996. The cosmic food web: Human-nature elatedness in the Northwest Amazon, in: Descola, P., Pálsson, G. (Eds.), *Nature and Society: Anthropological Perspectives*. Routledge, London and New York, pp. 185–204.

Baer, G., 1992. The one intoxicated by tobacco: Matsigenka shamanism, in: Matteson-Langdon, J., Baer, G. (Eds.), *Portals of Power: Shamanism in South America*. University of New Mexico Press, Albuquerque, pp. 79–100.

Classen, C., 1990. Sweet colors, fragrant songs: Sensory models of the Andes and the Amazon. *Am. Ethnol.* 17, 722–735.

Daly, J.W., Caceres, J., Moni, R.W., Gusovsky, F., Moos, M., Seamon, K.B., Milton, K., Meyers, C.W., 1992. Frog secretions and hunting magic in the Upper Amazon: Identification of a peptide that interacts with an adenose receptor. *Proc. Natl. Acad. Sci.* 89, 10960–10963.

Daly, L., 2015. The symbiosis of people and plants: Ecological engagements among the Makuxi Amerindians of Amazonian Guyana. PhD thesis, Dept. Anthropology, University of Oxford.

Fausto, C., 2007. Feasting on people: Eating animals and humans in Amazonia. *Curr. Anthropol.* 48, 497–530.

Fausto, C., 2008. Donos demais: Maestria e domínio na Amazônia. *Mana* 14, 329–366.

Gottlieb, O.R., Borin, M.R. de M.B., 2005. Insights into evolutionary systems via chemobiological data, in: Elisabetsky, E., Etkin, N.L. (Eds.), *Ethnopharmacology*. Encyclopedia of Life Support Systems, Theme 6.79. UNESCO/Eolss Publishers. http://www.eolss.net, Oxford, pp. 25–70.

Howes, D., 1991. *The Varieties of Sensory Experience: A Sourcebook in the Anthropology of the Senses*. University of Toronto Press, Toronto.

Ingold, T., 2000. *The Perception of the Environment: Essays in Livelihood, Dwelling and Skill*. Routledge, New York.

Izquierdo, C., Shepard Jr., G.H., 2003. Matsigenka, in: Ember, C.R., Ember, M. (Eds.), *Encyclopedia of Medical Anthropology: Health and Illness in the World's Cultures*. Kluwer Academic/Plenum Publishers, New York, pp. 823–837.

Johnson, A., 1983. Machiguenga gardens, in: Hames, R., Vickers, W. (Eds.), *Adaptive Responses of Native Amazonians*. Academic Press, New York, pp. 29–63.

Johnson, A.W., 2003. *Families of the Forest The Matsigenka Indians of the Peruvian Amazon*. University of California Press, Berkeley & Los Angeles.

Lima, T.S., 1996. O Dois e seu múltiplo: Reflexões sobre o perspectivismo em uma cosmologia Tupi. *Mana* 2, 21–47.

Luna, L.E., 1984. The concept of plants as teachers among four *Mestizo* shamans of Iquitos, northeastern Peru. *Journal of Ethnopharmacology*, Vol. 11, Issue 2, 135–156.

Oliveira, J.C. de, 2016. Mundos de roças e florestas. *Bol. do Mus. Para. Emílio Goedi, Ciências Humanas* 11, 115–131.

Plowman, T.C., Leuchtmann, A., Blaney, C., Clay, K., 1990. Significance of the fungus *Balansia cyperi* infecting medicinal species of *Cyperus* (Cyperaceae) from Amazonia. *Econ. Bot.* 44, 452–462.

Plowman, T.C., 1981. *Five New Species of Brunfelsia from South America (Solanaceae), Fieldiana*. Field Museum of Natural History. Chicago.

Reichel-Dolmatoff, G., 1976. Cosmology as ecological analysis: A view from the rain forest. *Man* 11, 307–318.

Rosengren, D., 1987. *In the Eyes of the Beholder: Leadership and the Social Construction of Power and Dominance Among the Matsigenka of the Peruvian Amazon*. Göteborgs Etnografiska Museum, Göteborg.

Ruck, C.A.P., Bigwood, J., Staples, D., Ott, J., Wasson, R.G., 1979. Entheogens. *J. Psychedelic Drugs* 11, 145–146.

Shepard Jr., G.H., 1998. Psychoactive plants and ethnopsychiatric medicines of the Matsigenka. *J. Psychoactive Drugs* 30, 321–332.

Shepard Jr., G.H., 1999a. Pharmacognosy and the senses in two Amazonian societies. PhD thesis, Dept. Anthropology, University of California at Berkeley.

Shepard Jr., G.H., 1999b. Shamanism and diversity: A Matsigenka perspective, in: Posey, D.A. (Ed.), *Cultural and Spiritual Values of Biodiversity*. United Nations Environmental Programme and Intermediate Technology Publications, London, pp. 93–95.

Shepard Jr., G.H., 2002a. Three days for weeping: Dreams, emotions and death in the Peruvian Amazon. *Med. Anthropol. Q.* 16, 200–229.

Shepard Jr., G.H., 2002b. Primates in Matsigenka subsistence and worldview, in: Fuentes, A., Wolfe, L. (Eds.), *Primates Face to Face: The Conservation Implications of Human and Nonhuman Primate Interconnections*. Cambridge University Press, Cambridge, U.K., pp. 101–136.

Shepard Jr., G.H., 2004. A sensory ecology of medicinal plant therapy in two Amazonian societies. *Am. Anthropol.* 106, 252–266.

Shepard Jr., G.H., 2005. Psychoactive botanicals in ritual, religion and shamanism, in: Elisabetsky, E., Etkin, N.L. (Eds.), *Ethnopharmacology*, Vol. 2, Encyclopedia of Life Support Systems. UNESCO/Eolss Publishers. http://www.eolss.net, Oxford, pp. 128-182.

Shepard Jr., G.H., 2005. Venenos divinos: Plantas psicoativas dos Machiguenga do Peru, in: Labate, B.C., Goulart, S. (Eds.), *O Uso Ritual Das Plantas de Poder*. Editora Mercado de Letras, Campinas, pp. 187–217.

Shepard Jr., G.H., Rummenhoeller, K., Ohl, J., Yu, D.W., 2010. Trouble in paradise: Indigenous populations, anthropological policies, and biodiversity conservation in Manu National Park, Peru. *J. Sustain. For.* 29, 252–301.

Shepard Jr., G.H., 2012. Shipwrecked: The sorry state of development in the lower Urubamba, in: Castro de la Mata, G., Majluf, P., Shepard, G.H. Jr. & R.C. Smith, *Independent Advisory Panel on Development Issues in South-Central Peru – 2011-2012 Report*. Centro de Sustentabilidade Ambiental, Universidad Peruano Cayetano Heredia, Lima, 21-34.

Shepard Jr., G.H., 2014. *Old and in the Way: Jaguar Transformation in Matsigenka*. Paper presented at the International Congress of Ethnobiology, Bhutan, June 2014 and the Conference of the Society for the Anthropology of Lowland South America (SALSA), Göteborg, Sweden, June 2014. https://www.academia.edu/15538299/Old_and_in_the_way_Jaguar_transformation_in_Matsigenka

Shepard Jr., G.H., 2015a. Agony and ecstasy in the Amazon: Tobacco, pain and the hummingbird shamans of Peru. *Broad Street* 2, 5–20. https://medium.com/@susanncokal/from-our-pages-agony-and-ecstasy-in-the-amazon-by-glenn-h-shepard-jr-8of00d6f085b

Shepard Jr., G.H., 2015b. Will the real shaman please stand up?: The recent adoption of *ayahuasca* among indigenous groups of the Peruvian Amazon, in: Labate B., Cavnar C. (Eds). *Ayahuasca Shamanism in the Amazon and Beyond*. Oxford University Press, New York, 16-39.

Shepard Jr., G.H., in press. Toé (*Brugmansia suaveolens*): O caminho do dia e da noite, in: Labate, B.C., Goulart, S.L. (Eds.), *O Uso de Plantas Psicoativas Nas Américas*. Compania das Letras, São Paulo.

Stoller, P., 1989. *The Taste of Ethnographic Things: The Senses in Anthropology*, Contemporary Ethnography Series. University of Pennsylvania Press, Philadelphia.

Trewavas, A., 2003. Aspects of plant intelligence. *Ann. Bot.* 92, 1–20.

Viveiros de Castro, E.B., 1996. Os pronomes cosmológicos e o perspectivismo Ameríndio. *Mana* 2, 115–144.

Viveiros de Castro, E.B., 2002. Perspectivismo e multinaturalismo na America Indigena, in: Viveiros de Castro, E.B. (Ed.), *A Inconstancia da Alma Selvagem e Outros Ensaios de Antropologia*. São Paulo, pp. 347–399.

Viveiros de Castro, E.B., 2004. The transformation of objects into subjects in Amerindian Ontologies. *Common Knowl.* 10.

Witzany, G., 2008. The Biosemiotics of Plant Communication. *Am. J. Semiot.* 24, 39–56.

Broad Spectrum Roles of Harmine in *Ayahuasca*

■■■ *Dale Millard* ■■■

Wasiwaska, Research
Center for the Study
of Psychointegrator
Plants, Visionary Art and
Consciousness, Florianópolis,
Brazil

ABSTRACT

Ayahuasca is an Amazonian psychoactive plant beverage used ceremonially, normally containing *Banisteriopsis caapi* (Spruce ex Griseb.) Morton as a base ingredient and an admixture plant, either *Psychotria viridis* (Ruiz & Pav.) Schult. in Brazil and Peru, or *Diplopterys cabrerana* (Cuatrec.) B. Gates in Colombia and Ecuador. In the latter case it is normally referred to as *yagé*. In the Amazon, *ayahuasca* is commonly prescribed to combat psychospiritual as well as physical ailments (Dobkin de Rios, 1972).

This paper seeks to provide an overview from both past and current literature on harmine, demonstrating its wide variety of therapeutic activity inducing antimicrobial, anti-diabetic, anticancer, antidepressant, antiparasitic, DNA-binding, osteogenic, chondrogenic, neuroprotective and other effects. Harmine is by far the most abundant constituent of the medicine *ayahuasca*. Its presence in pharmacologically active amounts may therefore provide a rationale for its contribution in *ayahuasca*'s wide application in traditional medicine and its general reputation for treating a broad range of diseases and ailments.

Some of the psychoactive and physiological roles of harmine have been known since Lewin published his paper on banisterine in 1928. Harmine has now received the attention of the international scientific community, looking at a broad range of activities that allude to the possible applications of harmine in several different areas of medicine. In more recent years studies have begun looking at both the endogenous and physiological roles of dimethyltryptamine. Similarly, β-carbolines are found in various body tissues and fluids.

A major role of harmine in the synergistic effect of *ayahuasca* chemistry is to function as a monoamine oxidase inhibitor (MAOI) that allows dimethyltryptamine to become orally active, though as a molecule on its own, harmine also shows some potent and broad-spectrum activities. The findings discussed in this paper may suggest future opportunities in areas where conventional medicine is facing challenges.

AIMS AND OBJECTIVES

This article explores the β-carboline constituents of *ayahuasca*, with special attention paid to the dominant alkaloid harmine, its potential role in primary healthcare and as a natural-product medicine. However, not all of the physiological properties of harmine have been discussed. Focus has been placed on those areas deemed of most value, as well as some of the interesting lesser-known effects. As *ayahuasca* is a complex brew of chemicals, it is not the author's intention to undermine the roles that any of the other chemical constituents may play in producing healing effects. Some of

82

this chemistry is likely to be synergistic in its effect, as is already known to be the case with harmala alkaloids and tryptamines.

It is hoped that this review may help readers, researchers, policy makers and consumers of *ayahuasca* explore some of the hidden potentials of harmine and raise general awareness as to its possible therapeutic role in this medicine.

METHODOLOGY

The material cited in this paper was derived from a variety of sources. In-depth online searches using the search engines Google, Science Direct and PubMed were conducted. Private libraries as well as the author's personal archives were consulted. Personal comments and ideas shared in general conversation have also been included. In the introduction, aims and objectives and conclusion sections, the personal beliefs and viewpoints of the author have been included.

INTRODUCTION

Ayahuasca is a Quechua term used to describe the sacred Amazonian medicine used ceremonially and for a host of other purposes. Aya + huasca, translated as death/spirit + vine, traditionally refers to the vine *Banisteriopsis caapi*. Other plants such as *chacruna* (*Psychotria viridis*) in Brazil and Peru, and *yagé* (*Diplopterys cabrerana*) in Colombia and Equador) (Shultes, 1957) are considered admixture plants incorporated for a desired effect. In several Amazonian tribes such as the Tukano (Shultes, 1976), *Banisteriopsis* preparations are consumed without the addition of admixture plants.

Ayahuasca has become a well-documented global phenomenon (Tupper, 2006) and in this global community *ayahuasca* generally refers to a preparation of *Banisteriopsis caapi* in combination with a dimethyltryptamine source plant.

Since the 1970's when anthropologists first started focusing on the uses of *ayahuasca*, much has been documented in terms of cultural use for many different purposes such as hunting, war, healing of psychosomatic illness, magical or ritual purposes, etc. (Dobkin de Rios 1972). Sadly, there are no systematic studies, and no major attention seems to have been paid to the use of *ayahuasca* in the treatment of various physiological diseases found in the Amazon. The author found only scant references (Rodrigues et al., 1982; Karsten, 1964; Karsten, 1935; Spruce, 1908) mentioning its use amongst *mestizos* for treating physical ailments. This was perhaps due to the astonishing visionary psychoactive effects of the medicine, which captivated the attention of early explorers and researchers. It can be supposed that since then, much of this type of medicinal knowledge may have disappeared, though this area should still remain open as an important avenue of research.

Ayahuasca certainly contains bioactive chemicals with a broad range of physiological properties, many of which can be exploited as medicine. More recently there has been much interest shown in the physiological properties of compounds contained in *ayahuasca*. The endogenous compound dimethyltryptamine (DMT) is believed to have important physiological properties. A sigma-1 ligand, DMT is known to play a pivotal role in many pathologies (Fontanilla et al, 2009; Frecska et al, 2013).

POSSIBLE ROLES OF HARMINE AND
β-CARBOLINES IN NATURE

β-carbolines are widely and commonly distributed in nature. These compounds have been detected as component substances in many different tissues of living organisms and continue to be discovered across many plants from different families, as well as fungi, mammals, reptiles, birds, and in humans. Although the exact evolutionary role these substances play in organisms and natural systems is at present poorly understood, some preliminary studies discussed here may disclose possible functional roles.

As β-carbolines are increasingly being discovered in nature and as endogenous substances in humans, the discovery of their many functions is important, regarding both the role they play in our intrinsic health/biological systems and when introduced through medicine or diet.

When *ayahuasca* vines are harvested with machetes in tropical conditions, they tend to recover rapidly. Many other plants would not tolerate such harvesting practices in such microbe-rich environments. This tendency to strongly resist rot and disease may point to the possible antifungal and antibacterial role of β-carbolines in plants such as *Banisteriopsis caapi* which contain high levels of these substances.

One study claimed that root hairs of the Peruvian root vegetable *oca* (*Oxalis tuberosa* Molina), propagated in sterile media, were found to produce β-carbolines/harmine only when challenged by the introduction of microbes. This article was subsequently retracted on the basis that the authors failed to prove that the fluorescent exudates from the roots were in fact harmine (Bais et al., 2002). A study screening for antimicrobial properties of harmine postulates that the results suggest that harmala alkaloids have a defense role in plants (Reza and Abbas, 2007).

β-carboline, also known as norharmane, is the prototype substance in the class of compounds known as β-carbolines. It is one of two known ultraviolet-fluorescing substances found in the cuticles of scorpions (Wankhede, 2004). The other is a methylated coumarin-type compound. Reasons why scorpions display this fluorescence remain unclear. As nocturnal creatures, they likely see in this spectrum of light, and this attribute would help them naturally select partners for reproduction. All species of scorpions display unique mating "dances." This suggests β-carbolines may be involved in signalling.

| Tetrahydroharmine | Harmine | Harmaline |

At least three β-carboline derivatives are endogenous chemicals found in the corneas (eye lenses) of human beings. Corneas are subject to continual oxidative and photic stresses. A study suggests these derivatives play a role in protecting tissues from oxidative stress (Pari et al., 2000). It is intriguing to find these compounds present in the lens, the area where photons enter the body and reach the brain. As β-carbolines are known to become activated or charged under ultraviolet light, it suggests a possible relationship to the photodynamic properties of these substances. Further research may well uncover the dynamics of such a relationship.

Harmine increases spatial learning in mice (Dandan et al., 2015). Spatial learning is an aspect that is important to the growth and survival of plants, especially jungle lianas like *Banisteriopsis* that hope to eventually reach the canopy, finding their place amongst fellow plant species. Although concepts such as plant intelligence, memory and learning have long been held to be the realm of quasi-science, new experiments are showing that in fact plants do possess such behaviors (Gagliano et al., 2014).

It seems that β-carbolines are polyfunctional in nature. In the human body they are certainly capable of performing several different functions, and this flexibility of function makes them good candidates for medicines targeting broad-spectrum activity.

NOTES ON THE CHEMISTRY AND PHARMACOLOGY OF BANISTERIOPSIS

To date, there has been much published on this subject. Refer to (Mckenna et al, 1984; Rivier and Lindgren, 1972) for comparisons of chemical profiles of *ayahuasca* brews. In summary, *ayahuasca* essentially consists of *Banisteriopsis* plus a DMT-admixture plant (usually *Psychotria viridis* or, in the case of *yagé*, *Diplopterys cabrerana*). *Banisteriopsis* is the main source of the three β-carbolines that typically occur in the brew—harmine, tetrahydroharmine and harmaline. Although much variation exists, a general estimate of the proportions in a "typical" *ayahuasca* brew could be in the order of harmine constituting around 45%, tetrahydroharmine 25% and harmaline 5%, with dimethyltryptamine making up the remaining 25% of the total alkaloid volume.

Although the scope of this article focuses mainly on harmine, both harmaline and tetrahydroharmine (THH) also play important roles in MAOI inhibition amongst other things. Tetrahydroharmine has shown to bind to serotonin transporters in blood platelets (Callaway et al., 1994), and given *in vitro*, it induces neurogenesis in the brain (Riba et al, 2017). THH also has approximately double the half-life (around 660 minutes) of harmine and harmaline, and has been anecdotally suggested to be partly responsible for the "afterglow" effect reported by many *ayahuasca* drinkers.

Harmine has some of the same properties as harmaline, though in some areas great differences are seen. For example, harmine has been shown to bind over 100 times more efficiently to DNA. Harmaline on the other hand is used in animal models to induce tremors and amnesia (Louis and Zheng, 2010). Although this is probably a dose-related phenomenon, it does raise some concern with respect to ingesting this compound in large doses, as essential tremor (ET) is a serious condition. Although this is unlikely to be a problem with *Banisteriopsis* species, the practice of preparation of "*ayahuasca* analogues" using Syrian rue (*Peganum harmala* L.), which has much higher levels of harmaline, should in the author's opinion be exercised with caution.

It is known that variation exists in the levels of these chemicals between individual plants and between different brews analyzed. The *Banisteriopsis caapi* varietal *tucunacá* appears to be the most common variety used in the preparation of *ayahuasca* these days. Compared to another variety of this species, *caupuri*, which is possibly what Spruce collected in 1853 (Luna, pers, comm.), and described as "Swollen at the joints", there is a vast difference in their chemical profiles. Considering the emerging evidence for β-carbolines' therapeutic role in so many pathologies, varieties like *caupuri* are in need of further study for their potential application in medicine. Varieties with higher levels of β-carbolines may find special application in conditions such as depression and neurodegenerative diseases.

Variety	Harmine	Harmaline	Tetrahydroharmine
Caupuri	8.68 mg/g	0.69mg/g	5.06mg/g
Tucunacá	5.50mgl/g	0.11mg/g	0.19mg/g

Source: Rosana Lucas Serpico, 2006. *Ayahuasca*: Revisao Teorica e Consideracoes Botanica sobre as species *Banisteriopsis caapi* e *Psychotria viridis*. Universidade Garulhos.

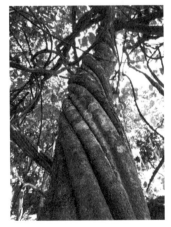

Banisteriopsis caapi var. tucunacá

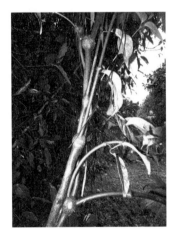

Banisteriopsis caapi var. caupuri

Some results reported by (Callaway, 2005a) found more equal, proportional amounts of harmine and tetrahydroharmine in brew samples. It was speculated that due to fermentation the beverage had become acidic with time, and that in an acidic substrate both harmine and harmaline degrade into tetrahydroharmine (Callaway, 2005b). It is significant to point out that the dominant alkaloid in all fresh *ayahuasca* brews analyzed thus far is always harmine and that the importance of this compound in producing the broad-spectrum effects of *ayahuasca* should not be underestimated.

NEUROLOGICAL EFFECTS

β-carbolines display broad psychopharmacological effects through binding to benzodiazepine, imidalozine, serotonin and opiate receptors and through inhibiting monoamine oxidase (MAO) and DYRK1.

Perhaps, due to the early discovery of the psychoactive properties of harmine in medicines such as *ayahuasca*, its effects on the nervous system have generated much research interest to date. Much of this research has been published elsewhere, but for the scope of this article only the highlights of this research are discussed. Some of these results have proven to be astonishing, and several studies suggest that both *Banisteriopsis* and harmine hold strong promise for the treatment of several neurodegenerative diseases, including Alzheimer's, Parkinson's, and Huntington's (Muhammad et al., 2010). It has been shown in animals and humans that harmine produces a marked degree of neurogenesis, which holds the possibility of reversing some of the neural damage caused in neurodegenerative conditions. In 2016, a Brazilian team showed that harmine stimulates proliferation of human neural progenitors (Dakic et al., 2016). In addition, harmine has shown an ability to stimulate the release of dopamine, validating its usefulness in certain diseases related to dopamine deficits.

Preliminary harmine studies with both harmine on its own and also in the *ayahuasca* brew are beginning to show great promise with regards to depression. Current global estimates report that around 350 million people have a major depressive disorder. The antidepressant effects of *ayahuasca* have shown to be immediate and long lasting. In 2015, a collaboration between a group of Brazilian and Spanish scientists reported on the rapid, acute antidepressant and anxiolytic effects observed after only a single dose of *ayahuasca* when compared to slower-acting traditional antidepressants (Sanches et al., 2016). At the time of writing, there are no further studies strongly supporting these findings.

Ayahuasca has been reported in several studies to be of great value in treating addictions. It is difficult to know for certain whether it is the experience itself or the pharmacological effects that are responsible for this efficacy. It is probable that both aspects are of value in treating addiction. *Ayahuasca* and specifically harmine have been the subjects of several studies focusing on substance dependence. In an increasing number of trials, harmine and β-carbolines have shown to be useful in treating cocaine, amphetamine, opiate and alcohol dependence (Owaisat et al., 2012). Harmine activity at a receptor level correlates with several receptors known to be important in treating addiction.

CANCER

Traditionally, *ayahuasca* has been used in the Amazon region for treating cancer. There is anecdotal evidence, especially from the Brazilian syncretic churches and the global *ayahuasca* community, of cases where *ayahuasca* has cured or been beneficial in cancer treatment (Schenberg, 2013). It is difficult to separate whether or not these reports are attributed to the *ayahuasca* experience itself or to the actual chemistry contained in the brew. It is true that both harmine and DMT have reported properties that can fight cancer, with harmine especially showing promise in the treatment of certain cancers.

The 2017 annual report for The American Cancer Society estimates that nearly 1,700,000 new cancer cases will be diagnosed in the United States alone per year, of which nearly 600,000 are expected to result in death. Out of the total data spectrum of cancers affecting all sites, 13% are considered to be rare cancers. Thus we can expect the emergence of new and rare types of cancer.

Modern society and lifestyles often dictate that individuals are exposed to abnormal levels of stress, whether psychological, dietary or environmental, as is often the case with industrial toxins and agrochemicals found in our food. The epidemic and emergence of viral disease, as well as smoking and other substance-related behaviours, are all capable of affecting us at a genetic level and causing mutations at a cellular level that potentially could develop into cancerous tumors. In addition, these unnatural stresses can lead to immune disorders, which further inhibit resistance to cancers.

Current conventional therapies in the treatment of cancer include surgery, radiotherapy, chemotherapy and molecular-targeted therapy. Existing chemotherapy drugs are not ideal and have numerous side effects, including myelosuppression, hepatotoxicity and immunosuppression (Leite et al, 2012). Therefore, there is an urgent and growing need to seek out safer alternative therapies and chemotherapy compounds. Harmine displays interesting, multiple anticancer properties in its ability to induce programmed cell death (apoptosis) in tumors, prevent proliferation and metastasis as discussed in the research results below.

The ability of harmine to effectively bind to DNA—100x more effectively than harmaline (Nafisi et al., 2010)—lends to interesting possibilities with regard to cancer therapies. Harmine is a small molecule, and biological responses caused by mutagenic, carcinogenic and anti-tumor agents are often associated with the binding of small molecules to DNA. Harmine interacts with DNA via intercalative modes and causes major DNA structural changes (Nafisi et al., 2010).

In several studies, harmine has demonstrated genotoxic abilities to damage the DNA of malignant cells, thus preventing proliferation and growth of tumors (Nafisi et al., 2010; Cao et al., 2005). In the reviewed literature, the terms 'genotoxic' (Boeira et al., 2002) and 'antigenotoxic' are used to describe properties of harmine. It should be understood that whilst genotoxicity is often confused with mutagenicity, all mutagens are genotoxic, whereas not all genotoxic substances are mutagenic. Based on evidence thus far, harmine falls into the latter category.

Harmine is named after the medicinal plant *Peganum harmala*. It has a long-standing reputation in the Middle East for treating cancers of the stomach. Recent research from China has shown that harmine induces pro-death autophagy and apoptosis in human gastric cancer cells (Zhang et al., 2013). The enzyme cyclooxygenase has been shown to be important in the development of cancers, specifically gastric cancers. The Chinese investigators showed that harmine was able to induce apoptosis and inhibited tumor cell proliferation, migration and invasion through downregulation of cyclooxygenase-2 expression in gastric cancer (Zhang, et al.,2013).

Harmine interferes and restricts blood supply to tumors (anti-angiogenesis). In mice infected with B16F-10 melanoma cells, , harmine significantly decreased tumor-directed capillary formation, at a dose of 10mg/kg, whilst it increased immune anti-tumor factors such as interleukin-2 (Hamsa and Kuttan, 2010).

A recent study proved *in vitro* that a harmine derivative called CM16 inhibited the growth of oligodendroglioma and melanoma cancer cell lines through targeting protein synthesis (Carvalho et al, 2017).

Melanomas are notorious for metastasis and for chemo resistance. As some forms do not respond well to current chemo or radiotherapy, often the only option is resection. Therefore, it is desirable to look for phytochemicals that show efficacy in melanomas. In a 2011 study in India, it was shown that harmine caused cell death in melanomas and regulated some transcription factors and proinflammatory cytokines (Hamsa and Kuttan, 2011).

An *in vitro* study demonstrated in several different types of cancer lines that harmine displayed a dose-dependent inhibitory effect on cell proliferation against all human carcinoma cells tested, and that harmine was identified as a useful inhibitor of tumor development (Jimenez et al, 2008).

Other β-carbolines and harmine derivatives are being investigated as potential anticancer drugs. A newly synthesized β-carboline called DH332 exerts effective anti-tumor activity *in vitro* and *in vivo*, and has the potential as a promising drug candidate for lymphoma therapy (Gao et al., 2014).

The harmine-containing medicinal plant *Peganum harmala* has also shown to have anti- growth properties in a cell line of breast cancer (Shabani et al., 2015).

CIRCADIAN RHYTHMS

A curious genetic effect of harmine has been observed in a study whereby harmine was shown to modulate circadian period. All living creatures are subject to biological rhythms. The master clock that generates these circadian rhythms in mammals is found in the suprachiasmatic nucleus of the hypothalamus. These rhythms control many processes in the body such as sleeping and waking, blood pressure, heartbeat and hormone secretion. Even cells have their own clock, known as the "cell autonomous clock." Genes are also controlled by these rhythms, which determine timely processes such as the order of protein folding. Harmine has been shown to affect these core clock gene networks and has been suggested as a new candidate to control period length in mammals. The results of this study suggest harmine affects clock genes in peripheral tissues such as the liver, and not at the master clock level in the hypothalamus (Onishi et al., 2012). What makes this important is that it is known that disruption of circadian period is linked to several different pathologies such as insomnia, cancer, depression and metabolic syndrome (Bechtold et al., 2010).

PARASITES

Ayahuasca has a strong reputation in the Amazon for its ability to treat parasitic infections. Parasitic infections are diverse and vary geographically, as well as the sites in the human body that they infect and colonize. In the developing world, as well as in rural areas of the developed world, parasitic infections often go unnoticed and are not diagnosed in time, resulting in potentially dangerous infections that are difficult to treat and often require the use of potentially toxic drugs. Treatments for parasitic infections through conventional medicines often have limitations, mostly due to toxicity issues and the development of drug resistance in parasites.

Several constituents of the *ayahuasca* brew are likely responsible for certain antiparasitic effects. For example, in gut-borne parasites, the various tannins in *ayahuasca* brews would likely bind with the proteins of foreign organisms as well as to gastric mucosa, thus inhibiting these organisms' ability to infect the body systemically and rendering them ineffectual. It could thus be expected that *ayahuasca* would be of some value in potentially treating common gastric infections such as giardia, flagellates and possibly even amoebic infections.

Harmine, being a small molecule, has the ability to cross membranes in the body. Of special interest is harmine's ability to enter cells and effectively kill blood-borne parasites for which many of the conventional medicines are not ideal and in some instances show serious side effects and toxicity. Harmine has been investigated in the treatment of some of these parasites.

Toxoplasmosis is a peculiar disease that has been around since humans started domesticating cats. It can be active for a lifetime in all mammals, though the tachyzoite parasite *Toxoplasma gondii* Nicolle & Manceaux needs to return to a feline to complete its reproductive cycle. Although this parasite may not cause obvious symptoms in humans, in certain instances, for example immunocompromised individuals such as HIV patients, infections can become acute and even potentially fatal. Up to half the world's population is believed to be infected with latent toxoplasmosis (Flegr et al, 2014). This disease has been listed as one of the "neglected parasitic infections" by the World Health Organization.

A number of studies have shown that this often asymptomatic infection may lead to other pathologies (Alomar et al., 2013). Of particular interest is this parasite's ability to affect the nervous system and cause changes in behavior. Experimentally infected rodents lose all fear of feline scents and urine, thus insuring the host will be captured by a feline and thus the parasite will complete its life cycle. Neurological pathologies including schizophrenia have been observed in humans, with the artwork of Louis Wain being partly responsible for bringing this disease to public attention. It has even been linked to the cause of a unique syndrome known as "crazy cat lady syndrome" popularized by the media (Flegr et al., 2014). Serological estimates suggest that between 30 and 50% of the global population is infected, while in some regions it is estimated that up to 95% of the population is infected (Flegr et al., 2014). *Toxoplasma gondii* is capable of invading many different tissues and forming cysts, and if acquired during pregnancy, it has been linked to a condition known as congenital toxoplasmosis. In newborn babies it is associated with chorioretinitis (which can cause blindness), hydrocephaly, microcephaly and abortion (Tamomh et al., 2016).

An *in vitro* study showed that low doses of less than 40 μM of harmine were shown to have a strong inhibitory effect on *Toxoplasma* parasite invasion and replication, and showed no toxicity to the host cells. The study recommended that harmine be explored in potential drug development as a treatment for this disease (Alomar et al., 2013).

MALARIA

Malaria remains a very serious disease with high incidence of both morbidity and mortality. The disease is associated with infection caused by parasites in the genus *Plasmodium*, of which about 200 species are known. Globally, five species are known to infect humans. Transmission takes place through female mosquitoes of the genus *Anopheles*. In 2015, the World Health Organization reported 212 million cases and an estimated 429,000 malaria deaths worldwide, with 90% of these occurring in Africa. In the last decade, substantial progress was made in its treatment and prevention. This was largely due to various global efforts to control the disease, and the development of artemesinin-type drugs based on the medicinal plant *Artemesia annua* L. At present, treatment globally consists largely of artemesinin-based drugs, together with a partner drug to limit development of resistance. Of great concern is the emergence of artemesinin-resistant strains from Southeast Asia and elsewhere.

Harmine has been identified as a potential drug in the treatment of malaria. Of relevant interest is the widespread traditional use of known β-carboline-containing plants such as *Guiera senegalensis* J.F.Gmel.in West Africa, and *Eurycoma longifolia* Jack in Southeast Asia for the treatment of malaria. Both species are highly regarded for efficacy in many ailments in the regions they come from. In 2012, a Canadian study showed that harmine is a potent antimalarial, and proved its mechanism in combating malaria by targeting heat shock protein 90 (Hsp90) (Shahinas et al., 2012). This is a very interesting target for drug development as heat shock proteins are among the most highly expressed cellular proteins across all species and are a known target in various forms of cancer (Csermely et al., 1998). This target has been identified as having potential application in many diseases. In *Malaria Journal*, exciting new research was published showing both *in vitro* and *in vivo* anti-malarial activity of novel harmine-analogue heat shock protein-inhibitors. The article recommends harmine analogues as a possible partner for artemesinin in the fight against malaria. In addition, this study showed that harmine analogues inhibited *Plasmodium falciparum* Welch, the most common and dangerous form of malaria, and reduced parasitaemia in micromolar concentrations, as well as having an additive synergistic effect when combined with dihydroartemesinin (Bayih et al., 2016).

LEISHMANIA

Leishmaniasis is a vector-borne parasitic disease spread by the bite of certain types of sandflies. These insects harbor parasites of the genus *Leishmania*, of which at least 20 species are known to infect humans. The World Health Organization estimates that between 4 to 12 million people are currently infected, with 2 million new cases and between 20,000 to 50,000 deaths occurring annually in some 88 countries, and has classified leishmaniasis as a neglected tropical disease. Leishmaniasis has a mortality rate that approaches 90% for untreated patients (Herwalt, 1999). A 2014 French study showed harmine had weak anti-leishmanial activity, while on the contrary harmaline, also a component of the *ayahuasca* brew, showed strong activity (Di Giorgio et al, 2004). Antimony-type compounds have been the first line of defense, though these need to be given intravenously or intramuscularly, and are not entirely satisfactory (Murray, 2000). Therefore, it is recommended that a search for new anti-leishmanial compounds be undertaken.

CHAGAS DISEASE

Chagas disease is one of the most serious protozoan diseases in Latin America and is categorized as a neglected tropical disease by the Centre for Disease Control and Prevention. It is caused by a parasitic infection normally involving *Trypanosoma cruzi* Chagas. The vector for this disease are the Triatomid bugs, also known as "kissing bugs." Harmine has been shown to inhibit the protozoan *Trypanosoma cruzi*. When this disease reaches a chronic stage, current medicines only slow the progression, but do not effectively cure the disease. The World Health Organization estimates 6.6 million people were infected in 2015, with mortality estimated at around 8000. An *in vitro* study showed harmine induced programmed cell death in cells infected with *Trypanosoma brucei* Plimmer & Bradford at a concentration of less than 100 μM (Rosenkranz and Wink, 2008).

ANTI-DIABETIC

Diabetes type 1 and 2 are serious disease burdens affecting an estimated 380 million people globally. Diabetes is caused by an insufficiency of the pancreatic β cells in producing insulin, which metabolizes sugar in the body. The growth of these cells declines dramatically after birth. A potential cure or treatment would be to facilitate the growth of more insulin-producing pancreatic β cells. An urgent need has been established to discover a compound capable of doing this.

At present, diabetes type 1 is normally controlled through insulin injections. This is not ideal, as often insulin resistance is encountered, necessitating an increase in insulin dosage. There is also the inconvenience of regularly having to test blood glucose levels to ascertain how much insulin is needed, as too much or too little can dangerously alter blood sugar levels.

In 2015, one group screened over 100,000 compounds, with only harmine showing ability to cause pancreatic β cell division in rats, demonstrating the uniqueness of this molecule. The proposed mechanism is due to the nuclear factors of activated T-cells (NFAT) family of transcription factors as likely mediators of human β cell proliferation as well as β cell differentiation (Wang et al, 2015) Harmine also induced an increased sensitivity to insulin. The partial regrowth of these cells is truly encouraging, as this is the first time it has been demonstrated. This approach also holds hope for a host of other sugar-metabolic conditions.

ANTI-INFLAMMATORY

Inflammation is currently understood as a major underlying factor associated with many chronic pathologies. An exciting new 2017 study showed evidence that harmine is an inflammatory inhibitor through the suppression of NF-κB signalling. In addition, it uncovered a new potential of harmine for treating infectious disease: "Our data suggest that harmine may be responsible for the anti-inflammatory effect of *P. harmala* and *ayahuasca*, and may have a potential role for inflammatory and infective diseases." (Liu, 2017)

BONES AND JOINTS

Diseases of bone and joint tissue are numerous. They include common pathologies such as osteoarthritis and immune-related rheumatoid arthritis, osteoporosis, fracture and less frequently, genetic disorders and cancers. In these diseases, bone or cartilage tissue damage is normally observed. Treatment at this stage is often symptomatic and requires the use of steroidal drugs such as cortisone. Though these steroidal drugs may provide symptomatic relief, they work by blocking certain immune processes and do not offer any real hope of curing the diseases. Furthermore, anabolic drugs that aggressively promote osteoblastogenesis and bone formation are insufficient for effective treatment of these diseases (Yonezawa et al., 2011a). The "Holy Grail" for preventing and treating these diseases would be to discover compounds that prevented degeneration of these tissues or could stimulate their outgrowth once the pathology has expressed. Harmine has shown some very interesting and encouraging results in this regard in several ongoing studies that were conducted in China and Japan recently. A study by Hu and Xie (2016) reports that harmine can exert regenerative and protective effects on bone and cartilage tissues by regulating the proliferation, differentiation and metabolism of osteoclasts, osteoblasts and chondrocytes. A Japanese study (Yonezawa et al., 2011a) report that harmine inhibits osteoclast differentiation and bone resorption *in vitro* and *in vivo*. In the same year, the same group proposed the mechanism, releasing a paper under the title "Harmine promotes osteoblast differentiation through bone morphogenetic protein signalling" Yonezawa et al., 2011b). Their findings suggest that harmine has bone anabolic effects and may be useful for the treatment of bone-decreasing diseases and bone regeneration. Bone morphogenetic proteins (BMPs) deserve some further explanation, as they are considered important in many processes in the body. They are multifunctional growth factors that interact with specific receptors on a cell surface. In the embryonic stage, they are considered important for the development of the heart, central nervous system and cartilage, as well as postnatal growth and skeletal development and formation. More recent research is showing importance in practically all tissues of the body, including the brain (Bragdon et al, 2010). In one author's eloquent phrasing, "BMPs are now considered to constitute a group of pivotal morphogenetic signals, orchestrating tissue architecture throughout the body" Milano et al, 2007). Over 20 BMPs have been discovered so far in the human body and the delicate balance of their signalling mechanisms is considered fundamental in many pathologies. Cancers are often associated with misregulation of BMP signalling systems. For example, the absence of BMP signalling is an important factor in the progression of colon cancer (Kodach et al, 2008), and conversely, overactivation of BMP signalling is believed to be important in development of adenocarcinoma of the gastrointestinal tract (Milano et al, 2007). The role harmine can play in modulating BMPs is an area of important research.

ANTIMICROBIAL PROPERTIES

There have only been a few studies reporting on the antimicrobial properties of harmine. Antimicrobial activity has been ascribed to both harmine and harmaline. The author has heard of Amazonians applying *ayahuasca* externally to treat skin infections, and β-carbolines may well be involved in killing microorganisms. Antifungal activity was also shown in one study (Ahmad et al., 1992) where harmine was effective against all eight dermatophytes (skin fungi) tested. In another study, antibacterial activity was shown against *Staphylococcus aureus* Rosenbach, *Escherichia coli* (ex. Migula) Castellani & Chalmers and *Proteus vulgaris* Hauser. Antifungal activity was also shown against *Candida albicans* (C.P. Robin) Berkhout (Nenaah, 2010). Harmine has also demonstrated activity against both gram-negative and gram-positive bacteria (Ahmed et al., 1991).

A fascinating effect first looked at in 1981 is the discovery that certain β-carbolines, including harmine, can be charged with ultraviolet light to display even greater antibacterial properties (McKenna and Towers, 1981). These are referred to as the "photodynamic" properties of a compound and is an area worthy of further research for its potential in drug development and therapeutic strategizing.

ANTIVIRAL PROPERTIES

Viral diseases are a great threat to many populations of the world. The risk of emergence of new viral disease and resistance is always present. Transmission in a population may be rapid, as is seen in the Ebola virus. Furthermore, climate change is expected to play a large role in the spread of these diseases. The numerous viral diseases that exist are beyond the scope of this paper, though it includes several epidemic diseases, for some of which there is currently no known cure—for example, Human Immunodeficiency Virus (HIV). Due to rapid resistance, monodrug therapies have limitations and it is always advisable to seek out new and safer antiviral compounds to keep up with emerging resistance. In line with this, β-carboline compounds structurally lend themselves to new drug design, and a number of these harmine derivatives have been investigated for antiviral properties.

Some of these compounds have shown important and intriguing antiviral effects. β-carbolines have received research in Dengue virus serotype 2, Herpes simplex virus (HSV 1 and HSV 2)(Deyan et al, 2015) and even Human Immunodeficiency Virus (HIV). Harmine, being such a small molecule, can cross nuclear membranes and potentially confer activity where viral particles encode within the DNA. As harmine is capable of affecting multiple targets challenged by viruses, it is likely that further research will reveal new antiviral properties.

The research in β-carbolines in Dengue virus is worth mentioning, as Dengue fever is the most prevalent and fastest-spreading viral disease worldwide. In an Argentinean study (Quintana et al, 2016), research was conducted not on harmine itself, but on two close derivatives: a natural β-carboline harmol, and a synthetic 9N-methylharmine. Interestingly, these two compounds showed inhibitory effects against all Dengue serotypes tested, with greatest inhibition for DENV2. In this study, it was discovered that the effects were due not to direct antiviral activity but rather to these β-carbolines impairing the maturation and release of viral particles out of the cell, thus impeding cell-to-cell transmissions. The authors of this paper recommend that "further investigation of β-carbolines by performing a structure-activity analysis of new derivatives obtained from the active compounds and additional study of their mechanism of action would represent a promising approach for the development of novel antiviral agents to deal with DENV infections" (Quintana et al, 2016).

A particular challenge is treating viral diseases where the virus is able to go into latency, as is the case with retroviruses. Herpes simplex viruses (HSV1 and HSV2) are retroviruses that are highly prevalent in many populations, and sadly, therapeutic options to treat them are limited. HSV1 infection may result in corneal blindness and encephalitis, and HSV2 infection leads to *herpes genitalis* (Deyan et al, 2015). Current treatment revolves around antiviral medications like acyclovir, to which resistance has already emerged. Harmine was found to potently inhibit HSV2 infection through several different mechanisms and has been suggested as a valuable candidate for further study as a potential agent for blocking the HSV infection (Chen et al, 2015).

With regards to HIV infection, a recent study (Brahmbhatt et al, 2010) screened a number of β-carboline derivatives as potential inhibitors of HIV, and identified 1-formyl-β-carboline-3-carboxylic acid methyl ester derivative as an active agent against HIV. Further investigation and modification of this lead compound is in progress.

CONCLUSION

It seems, at least to the author, that there has indeed been a bias in the Western understanding of *ayahuasca* towards visionary aspects and experiential phenomena. Although these are considered paramount to the experience and research into the potential for *ayahuasca* in treating psychiatric and psychological problems is gaining momentum. Little is known to date about the application of this medicine in treating diseases of the body. It is only through anecdotal information that we know that Amazonian practitioners use *ayahuasca* for a wide variety of physiological diseases and complaints.

Harmine already demonstrated a remarkably broad spectrum of activity, which supports the hypothesis that, if taken at regular intervals in nontoxic dosages, as is the case in the vast majority of *ayahuasca* drinkers, it may well have wide-reaching and positive health-enhancing properties. The evidence presented thus far, in particular concerning diseases for which conventional medicine is currently challenged, demonstrates the usefulness of this compound, and specifically of *ayahuasca*, as a potential medicine not only in the treatment of psychiatric and psychosomatic problems but in a wide variety of human physiological pathologies. The seemingly remarkable ability of harmine to interfere with crucial metabolic processes in such a wide range of pathological organisms and cancerous cells, but still promote the healthy outgrowth of neural networks, bone and joint tissues and pancreatic β cells, is of great interest and importance, especially as these tissues normally degenerate in all of us with age.

The role of harmine and *ayahuasca* in the treatment of depression is of considerable value and importance, considering the rising incidence of this disorder in global populations and the controversial, limited success of modern antidepressant medications.

The newly demonstrated effects that harmine is showing in many notoriously stubborn parasitic infections is an exciting area of research and can potentially help a great deal in preventing and treating these types of infections.

Finally, the ability of harmine to bind so strongly with DNA, resulting in predominantly positive effects and so far no demonstrated real toxic effects in a global population of *ayahuasca* consumers, is intriguing.

This leads to interesting speculation in a world where, in the last 200 years since the industrial revolution, we have undeniably reached a situation whereby we regularly place undue chemical stresses on our environment and our bodies, evidenced by mutations at a genetic level potentially causing modern-day cancers. It can be speculated that harmine and similar compounds common in nature may even provide organisms with an evolutionary advantage at a genomic level through this intercalation with DNA.

As both the β-carbolines and dimethyltryptamine are endogenous compounds and constitute the main areas of pharmacological activity in *ayahuasca*, perhaps these discovered effects point to possible functions that these compounds serve in the body. In addition, discovery of the function(s) these molecules serve in nature may help us in our targeting and development of new medicines.

Harmine and β-carbolines, being natural compounds that are available in a wide range of botanical sources and with such broad-spectrum activity, certainly have a potential role to play both in primary healthcare in the undeveloped world and in the discovery of new medicinal properties. The recent international research interest in harmine has evoked its exciting therapeutic potential. It is hoped that further research will help uncover and explain more of these mysteries.

ACKNOWLEDGMENTS

The author would like to thank Dr. Luis Eduardo Luna for his continued support and encouragement over the years, as well as Dr. Dennis McKenna for the invitation to be part of the ESPD50 symposium.

REFERENCES

Ahmad, A., Khan ,K.A., Sultana, S., Siddiqui, B.S., Begum, S., Faizi, S., Siddiqui, S., 1992. Study of the *in vitro* antimicrobial activity of harmine, harmaline and their derivatives. *J Ethnopharmacol.* 35, 289-94

Alomar, M., Rasse-Suriani, F., Ganuza, A., Cóceres, V., Cabrerizo, F., Sergio A., 2013. *In vitro* evaluation of β-carboline alkaloids as potential anti-Toxoplasma agents. *BMC Research Notes* 6, 193.

Bais, H.P., Park, S.W., Stermit, F.R., Halligan, K.M., Vivanco, I.M., 2002. Exudation of fluorescent β-carbolines from Oxalis tuberosa L Roots. *Phytochemistry* 61, 539-43.

Bayih, A.G., Folefoc, A., Mohon, A.N., Eagon, S., Anderson, M., Pillai, D.R. 2016. *In vitro* and *in vivo* anti-malarial activity of novel harmine-analog heat shock protein 90 inhibitors: a possible partner for artemisinin. *Malaria Journal* 15, 579.

Bleuming, S.A., He, X.C., Kodach, L.L., Hardwick, J.C., Koopman, F.A., Ten Kate, F.J., van Deventer, S.J., Hommes, D.W., Peppelenbosch, M.P., Offerhaus, G.J., Li, L., van den Brink, G.R, 2007. Bone morphogenetic protein signaling suppresses tumorigenesis at gastric epithelial transition zones in mice. *Cancer Research* 67 (17), 8149-55.

Boeira, J., Viana, A., Picada, J., Henriques, J., 2002. Genotoxic and recombinogenic activities of the two β-carboline alkaloids harman and harmine in *Saccharomyces cerevisiae*. Mutation Research/Fundamental and Molecular Mechanisms of Mutagenesis 500 (1&2), 39-48.

Bragdon, B., Oleksandra, M., Saldanha, S., King, D., Joanne, J., Nohe, A., 2011. Bone Morphogenetic Proteins: A critical review. *Cellular Signalling* 23, 609-620.

Brahmbhatt, K., Nafees, A., Sudeep, S., Debashis, M., Singh, I., Bhutani, K., 2010. Synthesis and evaluation of β-carboline derivatives as inhibitors of human immunodeficiency virus. *Bioorganic & Medicinal Chemistry Letters* 20, 4416–4419.

Callaway, J.C., Airaksinen, M.M., McKenna, D.J., Brito, G,S,, Grob, C.S. 1994. Platelet serotonin uptake sites increased in drinkers of *ayahuasca*. *Psychopharmacology* (Berl). 116, 385-7.

Callaway, J.C., Brito, G.S., Neves, E.S., 2005a. Phytochemical analyses of *Banisteriopsis caapi* and *Psychotria viridis*. *Journal of Psychoactive Drugs* 37, 145-50.

Callaway, J.C., 2005b. Various alkaloid profiles of vegetal Caapi. *Journal of Psychoactive Drugs* 37, 151-155..

Cao, R., Peng, W., Chen, H., Ma, Y., Liu, X., Hou, X., Guan, H., Xu, A., 2005. DNA binding properties of 9-substituted harmine derivatives. *Biochemical and Biophysical Research Communications*, 338, 1557-63.

Carvalho, A., Chu, J., Meinguet, C., Kiss, R., Vandenbussche, G., Masereel, B., Wouters, J., Kornienko, A., Pelletier, J., Mathieu, V., 2017. Data in support of a harmine-derived β-carboline *in vitro* effects in cancer cells through protein synthesis. *Data Brief* 12, 546–551.

Csermely, P., Schnaider, T., Soti, C., Prohászka, Z., Nardai, G., 1998. The 90-kDa molecular chaperone family: structure, function, and clinical applications. A comprehensive review. *Pharmacology and Therapeutics* 79 (2), 129 -168.

Dakic, V., Maciel, R., Drummond, H., Nascimento, J.M., Trindade, P., Rehen, S.K., 2016. Harmine stimulates proliferation of human neural progenitors. *PeerJ* 4, e2727.

Dandan, H., Wu, H., Wei, Y., Lui, W., Huang, F., Shi, H., Zhang, B., Wu, X., Wang, C., 2015. Effects of harmine, an acetylcholinesterase inhibitor, on spatial learning and memory of APP/PS1 transgenic mice and scopolamine-induced memory impairment mice. *European Journal of Pharmacology* 768, 96-107.

Deyan, C., Su, A., Fu, Y., Wang, X., Lv, X., Xua, W., Xu, S., Wang, H., Wu, Z., 2015. Harmine blocks herpes simplex virus infection through downregulating cellular NF-jB and MAPK pathways induced by oxidative stress. *Antiviral Research* 123, 27–38.

Di Giorgio, C., Delmas, F., Ollivier, E., Elias, R., Balansard, G., Timon-Davida, P., 2004. *In vitro* activity of the β-carboline alkaloids harmane, harmine, and harmaline toward parasites of the species *Leishmania infantum*. *Experimental Parasitology* 106, 67–74.

Dobkin de Rios, M., 1972. *Visionary Vine: Psychedelic Healing in the Peruvian Amazon*. Chandler Press.

Flegr, J., Prandota, J., Sovičková, M., Israili, Z., 2014. Toxoplasmosis – A global threat. Correlation of latent toxoplasmosis with specific disease burden in a set of 88 countries. *PloS One* 9, e90203; doi: 10.1371.

Fontanilla, D., Johannessen, M., Hajipour, A., Cozzi, N., Jackson, M. R., 2009. The hallucinogen N,N-dimethyltryptamine (DMT) is an endogenous sigma-1 receptor regulator. *Science* 323 (5916), 934-937.

Frecska, E., Szabo, A., Winkelman, M., Luna, L.E., McKenna, D.J., 2013. A possibly sigma-1 receptor-mediated role of dimethyltryptamine in tissue protection, regeneration, and immunity. *Journal of Neural Transmission* 120, 1295-1303.

Gagliano, M., Renton, M., Depczynski, M., Mancuso, S., 2014. Experience teaches plants to learn faster and forget slower in environments where it matters. *Oecologia* 175, 63-7.

Gao, P., Tao, N., Ma, Q., Fan, W.X., Ni, C., Wang, H., Qin, Z.H., 2014. DH332, a synthetic β-carboline alkaloid, inhibits b-cell lymphoma growth by activation of the caspase family. *Asian Pacific Journal of Cancer Prevention* 15, 3901-3906.

Hamsa, T.P., and Kuttan, G., 2011. Harmine activates intrinsic and extrinsic pathways of apoptosis in B16F-10 melanoma. *Chinese Medicine*. 6, 11

Hamsa, T.P., Kuttan, G., 2010. Harmine inhibits tumour-specific neo-vessel formation by regulating VEGF, MMP, TIMP and pro-inflammatory mediators both *in vivo* and *in vitro*. *European Journal of Pharmacology*. 64, 64-73

Herwalt, B.L., 1999. Leishmaniasis. *Lancet* 354, 1191–1199.

Hu, Y., Xie, H., 2016. Progress in study on effect of harmine on bone and cartilage metabolism. *Zhong Nan Da Xue Xue Bao Yi Xue Ban*. 41, 328-32 [Chinese]

Jiménez, J., Riverón-Negrete, L., Abdullaev, F., Espinosa-Aguirre, J., Rodríguez-Arnaiz, R., 2008. Cytotoxicity of the beta-carboline alkaloids harmine and harmaline in human cell assays *in vitro*. *Exp Toxicol Pathol*. 60, 381-389.

Karsten, R., 1935. The Head Hunters of Western Amazonas – The Life and Culture of the Jibaro Headhunters of Eastern Ecuador and Peru. Societas Scientarium Fennica. *Commentationes humanarum litterarum VII*. Helsinki.

Karsten, R., 1964. Studies in the religions of the South American Indians, East of the Andes. In: A. Rungerg and Michael Webster (eds.). Indians of South America. Scientarium Fennica. *Commentationes humanarum litterarum VII*. T 29 no. 1 Helsinki.

Kodach, L., Wiercinska, E., de Miranda, N.F., Bleuming, S.A., Musler, A.R., Peppelenbosch, M.P., Dekker, E., van den Brink, G.R., van Noesel, C.J., Morreau, H., Hommes, D.W., Ten Dijke, P., Offerhaus, G.J., Hardwick, J.C., 2008. The bone morphogenetic protein pathway is inactivated in the majority of sporadic colorectal cancers. *Gastroenterology* 134, 1332–41.

Leite de Oliveira, R., Deschoemaeker, S., Henze, A., Debackere, K., Finisguerra, V., Takeda, Y., Roncal, C., Dettori, D., Tack, E., Jönsson, Y., Veschini, L., Peeters, A., Anisimov, A., Hofmann, M., Alitalo, K., Baes, M., D'hooge, J., Carmeliet, P., Mazzone, M., 2012. Gene-targeting of Phd2 improves tumour response to chemotherapy and prevents side-toxicity. *Cancer Cell* 22, 263–277.

Lewin L. 1928. Ser un substance enivirante, la banisterine, extraite de Banisteria caapi. Compt. Rend. 186, 469-471.

Liu, X., Li, M., Tan, S., Wang, C., Fan, S., Huang, C. 2017. Harmine is an inflammatory inhibitor through the suppression of NF-κB signaling. *Biochem Biophys Res Commun*. 489,3 32-338

Louis, E., Zheng, W., 2010. β-carboline Alkaloids and Essential Tremor: Exploring the Environmental Determinants of One of the Most Prevalent Neurological Diseases. *The Scientific World Journal* 10, 1783–1794.

Luna, L.E., 2011.The Ethnopharmacology of *Ayahuasca* Indigenous and mestiso use of *ayahuasca*. An overview. Chapter 1, pp. 1-23 in: Dos Santos R. G., Pandalai S. G.(Eds.) The Ethnopharmacology of *Ayahuasca*. *Transworld Research Network*, Kerala, India

McKenna, D.J., Towers, G.H. 1981. Ultraviolet mediated cytotoxic activity of β-carboline alkaloids. *Phytochemistry* 20, 1001-1004.

McKenna, D.J., Towers, G.H., Abbott, F., 1984. Monoamine oxidase inhibitors in South American hallucinogenic plants: tryptamine and β-carboline constituents of *ayahuasca*. *J Ethnopharmacol*. 10, 195-223.

Milano, F., van Baal, J.W., Buttar, N.S., Rygiel, A.M., de Kort, F., DeMars, C.J., Rosmolen, W.D., Bergman, J.J., Van Marle, J., Wang, K.K., Peppelenbosch, M.P., Krishnadath, K.K., 2007. Bone morphogenetic protein 4 expressed in esophagitis induces a columnar phenotype in esophageal squamous cells. *Gastroenterology* 132, 2412-21.

Muhammad, L., Samoylenko, V., Rahman, M., Tekwani, B.L., Tripath, L.M., Wanga, Y., Khana, S.I., Khana, I.A., Millerd, L.S., Joshi, V.C., 2010. *Banisteriopsis caapi*, a unique combination of MAO-inhibitory and antioxidative constituents for the activities relevant to neurodegenerative disorders and Parkinson's disease. *Journal of Ethnopharmacology* 127, 357-367.

Murray, H.W., 2000. Treatment of visceral leishmaniasis (kala-azar): a decade of progress and future approaches. *Int. J. Infect. Dis.* 4, 158–177.

Nafisi, S., Bonsaii, M., Maali, P., Khalilzadeh, M.A., Manouchehri, F., 2010. Beta-carboline alkaloids bind DNA. *J Photochem Photobiol B.* 100, 84-91.

Nenaah, G., 2010. Antibacterial and antifungal activities of (beta)-carboline alkaloids of *Peganum harmala* (L) seeds and their combination effects. *Fitoterapia* 8, 779-82.

Onishi, Y., Oishi, K., Kawano, Y., Yamazaki, Y. 2012. The harmala alkaloid harmine is a modulator of circadian Bmal1 transcription. *Bioscience Reports* 32, 45–52.

Owaisat, S., Raffa, R.B., Rawls, S.M., 2012. *In vivo* comparison of harmine efficacy against psychostimulants: preferential inhibition of the cocaine response through a glutamatergic mechanism. *Neurosci Letters* 525, 12-16.

Pari, K., Sundari, C.S., Chandani, S., Balasubramanian, D., 2000. β-carbolines that accumulate in human tissues may serve a protective role against oxidative stress. *J Biol Chem.* 275, 2455-62.

Quintana, V.M., Piccini, L.E., Panozzo Zénere, J.D., Damonte, E.B., Ponce, M.A., Castilla, V., 2016. Antiviral activity of natural and synthetic β-carbolines against dengue virus. *Antiviral Res.* 2016 134, 26-33.

Reza, V., Abbas, H., 2007. Cytotoxicity and Antimicrobial Activity of Harman alkaloids. *Journal of Pharmacology and Toxicology* 2, 677-680.

Riba J., Perez-Castillo, A., Morales-García, A., de la Fuente Revenga, J.M., Alonso-Gil, S., Rodríguez-Franco, M.I., Feilding, A., 2017. The alkaloids of *Banisteriopsis caapi*, the plant source of the Amazonian hallucinogen Ayahuasca, stimulate adult neurogenesis *in vitro*. *Scientific Reports* 7, 5309.

Rivier, J., Lindgren, E., 1972. "*Ayahuasca*," the South American hallucinogenic drink: An ethnobotanical and chemical investigation. *Economic Botany* 26, 101–129.

Rodriguez, E., Cavin, J., West, J., 1982. The possible role of Amazonian psychoactive plants in the chemotherapy of parasitic worms: A Hypothesis. *Journal of Ethnopharmacology* 6, 303-309.

Rosenkranz, V., Wink, M., 2008. Alkaloids induce programmed cell death in bloodstream forms of trypanosomes (*Trypanosoma b.* brucei). (Special Issue: Spiro compounds). *Molecules* 13, 2462-2473.

Sanches, R.F., de Lima Osório, F., Dos Santos, R.G., Macedo, L.R., Maia-de-Oliveira, J.P., Wichert-Ana, L., de Araujo, D.B., Riba, J., Crippa, J.A., Hallak, J.E., 2016. Antidepressant Effects of a Single Dose of Ayahuasca in Patients With Recurrent Depression: A SPECT Study. *J Clin Psychopharmacol.* 36, 77-81.

Schenburg, E., 2013. *Ayahuasca* and cancer treatment. SAGE Open Med. 1:2050312113508389 [online]

Schultes, R.E., 1957. The identity of the malpighiaceous narcotics of South America. *Botanical Museum Leaflets*, Harvard University 18, 1-56.

Schultes, R.E., 1976. *Hallucinogenic Plants, A Golden Guide*. Golden Press.

Serpico, R.L., 2006. *Ayahuasca*: Revisao Teorica e Consideracoes Botanica sobre as species *Banisteriopsis caapi* e *Psychotria viridis*. Universidade Garulhos.

Shabani, S., Tehrani, S., Rabiei, Z., Enferadi, S., Vanozzi, G., 2015. *Peganum harmala* L.'s anti-growth effect on a breast cancer cell line. *Biotechnology Reports* 8, 138–143.

Shahinas, D., MacMullin, G., Benedict, C., Crandall, I., Pillai, D., 2012. Harmine is a potent antimalarial targeting Hsp90 and synergizes with chloroquine and artemisinin. Antimicrob. *Agents Chemother.* 56, 4207-13.

Spruce, R., 1908. *Notes of a Botanist of the Amazon and the Andes*. Macmillan and Co Limited, London.

Tamomh, A., Mohamed, H., Magboul, A., Hassan, I., Ibrahim, R., Ahmed, H., Dafaallah, M., Dafaallah, T., 2016. Prevalence of toxoplasmosis among pregnant gynecological women in Tendalty Hospital, Tendalty Town, White Nile State, Sudan. *World Journal of Biology and Medical Sciences* 3, 76-83.

Tupper, K., 2006. The globalization of *ayahuasca*: Harm reduction or benefit maximization? *International Journal of Drug Policy* 19, 297–303.

Wang, P., Alvarez-Perez, J., Felsenfeld, D., Liu, H., Sivendran, S., Bender, A., Kumar, A., Sanchez, R.S., Garcia-Ocaña, A., Stewart, A., 2015. Induction of human pancreatic β-cell replication by inhibitors of dual specificity tyrosine regulated kinase. *Nat Med.* 21, 383–388.

Wankhede, R. A. (2004). *Extraction, Isolation, Identification and Distribution of Soluble Fluorescent Compounds from the Cuticle of Scorpion* (Hadrurus Arkizonensis) (Doctoral dissertation, Marshall University Libraries).

Yonezawa, T., Hasegawa, S., Asai, M., Ninomiya, T., Sasaki, T., Cha, B.Y., Teruya, T., Ozawa, H., Yagasaki, K., Nagai, K., Woo, J.T., 2011a. Harmine, a β-carboline alkaloid, inhibits osteoclast differentiation and bone resorption *in vitro* and *in vivo*. *Eur J Pharmacol.* 650, 511-518.

Yonezawa, T., Ji-Won, L., Ayaka, H., Midori, A., Hironori, H., Byung-Yoon, C., Toshiaki, T., Kazuo, N., Ung-Il, C., Kazumi, Y., Je-Tae, W., 2011b. Harmine promotes osteoblast differentiation through bone morphogenetic protein signalling. *Biochemical and Biophysical Research Communications* 409, 260–265.

Zhang, H., Sun, K., Ding, J., Xu, H., Zhu, L., Zhang, K., Li, X., Sun, W., 2014. Harmine induces apoptosis and inhibits tumor cell proliferation, migration and invasion through down-regulation of cyclooxygenase-2 expression in gastric cancer. *Phytomedicine*. Feb 15;21, 348-55.

Viva Schultes - A Retrospective

[Keynote]

■■ *Mark J. Plotkin,* PhD,[I] *Brian Hettler* [II]
& Wade Davis, PhD [III]

I. President, Co-founder;
II. GIS & New Technologies
Manager: Amazon
Conservation Team
Arlington, Virginia
III. Dept. of Anthropology,
Univ. of British Columbia

*This paper is a companion piece to the Amazon Conservation
Team interactive map journal plotting thirteen years of work in
the Amazon by legendary ethnobotanist, Richard Evans Schultes.
This online resource follows Schultes' explorations through geo-
referenced herbarium specimens, photographs and field notebooks,
accompanied by historical digital maps. Wade Davis' biography of
Schultes, One River, was an invaluable source of information in
reconstructing his life and travels. The Schultes Map is available at
amazonteam.org/maps/schultes.*

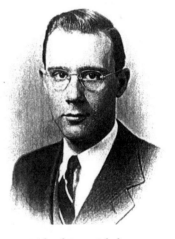

*Richard Evans Schultes,
a freshman at Harvard, 1933*

INTRODUCTION

Richard Evans Schultes was often called the Father of Ethnobotany.
He was quick to point out, however, that ethnobotany began when
Pharaoh Hatshepsut sent an expedition to the Land of Punt 3500
years earlier, and that he was not quite that old. Such self-deprecat-
ing humor was one of his hallmarks and played a large role in the
trust and friendship that friends, students, and his many informant
colleagues, from Oklahoma to the Amazon, placed in him.

Schultes – ethnobotanist, taxonomist, writer and photographer
– is widely regarded as one of the most important plant explorers
of the 20th century. In December 1941, he entered the Amazon rainforest on a mission to study and document how indigenous peoples
employed local plants for medicinal, ritual and practical purposes. He would follow in the tradition
of great Victorian era explorers, spending over a decade immersed in near-continuous fieldwork. In
total, Schultes would collect more than 24,000 species of plants, including some 300 species new
to science.

Schultes' geographic area of focus was the northwest Amazon, an area that had remained largely
unknown to the outside world, isolated by the Andes to the west and dense jungles and impassable
rapids on all other sides. Schultes lived amongst little-studied groups, mapped uncharted rivers,
and was the first scientist to explore some areas that have been little researched since. His notes and
photographs are some of the only existing documentation of indigenous cultures in a region of the
Amazon on the cusp of change.

Throughout his travels, Schultes' love of plants and respect for indigenous knowledge of the
forest helped him earn the trust of the communities he encountered. He found that the shamans he
met were often willing, if not eager, to discuss their plants and their practices with outsiders who
had a common appreciation for plants.

Schultes was not only an accomplished scientist: his teachings at Harvard University had a
profound impact on countless students. His vivid descriptions of Amazonian peoples and creative
classroom demonstrations, such as the use of a blowgun, inspired hundreds of students into careers

in biology, anthropology, medicine and conservation, and his many writings on the importance of shamanic wisdom and the therapeutic potential of psychotropic plants remain as important today as the day they were first published.

The special significance of Schultes' research derives in part from ideal timing: he arrived in the Amazon at a time of massive change for the peoples he encountered and ultimately for the great forest itself. In our map journal that accompanies this paper, available at www.amazonteam.org/maps/schultes, we retrace Schultes' journeys, exemplify his vast botanical collection – a great legacy to science – and explore the natural and cultural context of the environments he traversed, then and now, impressing upon us the immense importance of their conservation.

EARLY LIFE AND EXPLORATION
BEGINNINGS

Born in Boston, Massachusetts on January 12, 1915, Richard Evans Schultes was the grandson of immigrants; German on his father's side and English on his mother's. He was raised in East Boston in a house that still stands at 276 Lexington Street. At the time, East Boston was predominantly Irish – in fact, according to biographer Wade Davis, Schultes' mother attended school with Joseph Kennedy, Sr., father of JFK. That Schultes grew up in an Irish-American enclave as descendant of both Germans and English must have set him apart from most of the people of his age in his neighborhood. This ability to survive and thrive as an outsider in a challenging setting was to prove excellent training for life as an ethnobotanist.

At the age of eight, Schultes contracted a severe stomach ailment which kept him home and bedridden for many weeks. Looking for a book to read to the child, his father Otto visited the public library and checked out Notes of a Botanist on the Amazon and the Andes by 19th-century English botanist Richard Spruce, who had spent 15 years exploring the Amazon in the mid-19th century, meaning that Schultes heard about *ayahuasca* before he turned ten. Richard E. Spruce – who had the same initials as Richard Evans Schultes – became the personal hero of the young American who was to follow in Spruce's footsteps many years later.

As a young man, Schultes excelled in school and received a full scholarship to Harvard, in which he enrolled in the fall of 1933 to study pre-medicine. There, he took a job filing papers at Harvard's Botanical Museum on Oxford Street just north of Harvard Yard, earning thirty-five cents an hour. The museum's vast collections of plants and accounts of the people who used them intrigued young Schultes, and inspired him to enroll in a class entitled "Plants and Human Affairs," taught by Oakes Ames, a renowned orchidologist and Director of the Harvard Botanical Museum.

One day in class, Ames announced that each student would be expected to submit a term paper at the end of the semester, and they had to choose a subject based on one of the books at the back of the classroom. Determined to choose the shortest book possible, at the end of the class Schultes hurried to the bookshelf and selected Mescal: The Divine Plant and Its Psychological Effects, a 1928 publication by German psychiatrist Heinrich Klüver, one of the early studies of peyote. The author described the small, blue-green cactus native to the Texas – Mexico border that was said to induce powerful visions. Intrigued by what he had read, Schultes asked Ames if he could write his undergraduate thesis on the magical cactus. Ames agreed, but with one proviso - Schultes must study peyote in situ among the Kiowa of Oklahoma.

SCHULTES AMONG THE KIOWA

In 1936, Richard Evans Schultes headed west from Boston to Kiowa lands in Oklahoma on what undoubtedly represented the greatest adventure of his young life; he had never previously been west of the Hudson River. Schultes and anthropology graduate student Weston La Barre shared driving duties, making their way west in a broken-down 1928 Studebaker that La Barre had received in exchange for his train ticket. The pair arrived in Anadarko on June 24, 1936.

Their main local contacts were Charlie Apekaum (aka Charlie Charcoal), a local Kiowa leader, and his aunt Mary Buffalo, a Kiowa elder with extensive knowledge of plants. Mary Buffalo appreciated Schultes' and La Barre's willingness to listen and learn, and gave them deep insights into the Kiowa use of medicinal and ritual plants. Mary demonstrated how soaps were made from yucca roots and dyes from fruits, how willow bark was chewed to relieve toothaches, and how smoked sumac was employed for spiritual and physical purification before peyote ceremonies. She even revealed the contents of the "Ten Medicine Bundles", a sacred item that had been in her family for generations and was adorned with twelve scalps. Many evenings, Mary would build a sweat lodge out of hides and saplings over a hole in the earth filled with red-hot stones, where Schultes and La Barre would endure the heat for hours while listening to the Kiowa elders pray.

Over the course of the summer, they visited numerous villages, taking peyote two to three times a week. The ceremonies were led by a Roadman - the local term for traditional healer – which usually began with the participants smoking tobacco around a fire in contemplative silence. The Roadman would then pass around a leather bag full of peyote buttons and throw juniper on the fire, filling the tipi with aromatic smoke. He would chant songs accompanied by the fast-paced beating of a buckskin drum, which continued intermittently throughout the night as the participants fell into a world of rhythmic, colorful visions. Schultes typically took ten to twelve buttons of peyote, while some of the Kiowa men would consume as many as forty.

Schultes formed three lifelong bonds on that Oklahoma adventure. The first was with the plants themselves. Emerging from the Kiowa tipi, he reported that the cacti had brought him experiences beyond the description of contemporary science. The second inextricable link was with the nations and bands themselves: his mind-altering experiences under the guidance of the Kiowa Roadmen had opened his eyes to different ways of knowing and healing.

The third firm bond formed was that with his colleague, anthropologist Weston La Barre. Two years after their trip west, La Barre published The Peyote Cult as his first book. It was immediately considered a landmark psychological anthropology text. Schultes, in turn, observed how well-trained anthropologists could acquire a penetrating ability to perceive many otherwise invisible aspects of culture. Though today Schultes is widely regarded as the father of ethnobotany, some of his greatest work was done in collaboration with experts from other disciplines, such as the chemist Robert Raffauf or the mycologist Gordon Wasson – not to mention the shamans themselves.

Schultes recalled that Oklahoma experience fondly to the end of his life, and stated after that trip that he considered everything west of the Hudson River to be "Indian Country."

TEONANACATL: FLESH OF THE GODS

While researching peyote, Schultes encountered numerous references to intoxicating mushrooms employed by the Aztecs for divinatory purposes, known as teonanácatl or "flesh of the gods" in Nahuatl, the Aztec language. Accounts of teonanácatl being served at the crowning of the Aztec emperors Ahuitzotl in 1486 and Montezuma in 1502 intrigued Schultes.

Surviving pre-Columbian documents offer ample evidence of the cultural importance of teonanácatl. The 14th century Mixtec document Codex Vindobonensis Mexicanus includes repeated references to mysterious mushrooms: on the top left of the 14th page, seven gods each grip pairs of mushrooms. A prince holding two mushrooms is seated in front of Quetzalcoatl, who chants while beating a drum made from a human skull. Quetzalcoatl is also shown in a bird mask, carrying a woman on his back who is wearing a mask adorned with four mushrooms. The scene is believed to show the first encounter between the gods and teonanácatl.

The Spanish associated these rituals with devil worship and tried to identify the psychoactive mushroom so that they could eliminate these pagan ceremonies. Despite their best efforts, they never determined the source of the teonanácatl.

Despite the historical evidence of psychoactive mushrooms being used in Mexico, William Safford – a leading botanist with the U.S. Department of Agriculture - insisted that teonanácatl referred to peyote. He claimed that the Indians were trying to mislead the Catholic Church so they could consume their sacramental peyote in secret. Safford also cast doubt on the botanical knowledge of both the Aztecs and the early Spanish chroniclers.

Schultes was skeptical of Safford's theory. There was little resemblance between the peyote cactus and the fungi; furthermore, the Harvard ethnobotanist knew that peyote was a plant of the northern deserts rather than the tropical regions of southern Mexico. In an adroit bit of ethnobotanical detective work, Schultes located a letter addressed to the herbarium director J.N. Rose from an Austrian national in Mexico named Blas Pablo Reko.[1] Writing from Guadalajara, Reko stated that Safford was mistaken and that teonanácatl was a magic mushroom celebrated and consumed by the Mazatec in the state of Oaxaca. In 1936, Schultes headed to Oaxaca to investigate.

If the plains of Oklahoma and the Kiowas and their magic cacti seemed like a different country to the young scientist from East Boston, Oaxaca and the Mazatec must have appeared a different continent. Oaxaca in southernmost Mexico is somewhat remote even today, but in the 1930s it was

---

1. Reko, BP (1923) Letter to J.N. Rose, Herbarium Sheet No. 1745713. U.S. National Herbarium, Washington, D.C.

all but off the map. Home to 16 different indigenous nations, often separated by soaring mountain ranges that can reach 12,000 feet, Oaxaca remains the most ethnically diverse state in all of Mexico, home to the Mazatec, Zapotec, Mazateco, and Mixe cultures, among others.

Schultes met Blas Pablo Reko in Mexico City and traveled by rail to Huautla, the capital of Mazatec country, in search of a local shopkeeper who was said to have firsthand knowledge of the mushroom cults. They explored around Huautla and the nearby city of San Antonio Eloxochitlán with little success. There were rumors of mushroom cults, but Schultes and Reko were unable to find definitive proof.

One day, as Schultes was drying plants in town, he was approached by a middle-aged Mazatec man with a dozen fresh mushrooms. A local merchant identified these as 'los niños santos' (the "sacred children"). Schultes received an assortment of mushrooms, and within the handful Schultes identified a species of *Panaeolus* (later named *Panaeolus campanulatus* var. *sphinctrinus*) and *Psilocybe cubensis*. This was the first identifiable botanical collection of teonanácatl.

A later analysis by Schultes' colleague chemist Albert Hofmann of Sandoz Labs – who later became famous as the creator of LSD - eventually extracted compounds from these mushrooms that helped lead to the creation of some of the first beta blocker cardiac drugs.

OLOLIUQUI: VINE OF THE SERPENT
– THE MAGIC MORNING GLORY

Schultes had also heard of another plant sacred to the Aztec: coaxihuitl, "the vine of the serpent", more commonly known as ololiuqui. The seed was said to be taken orally and employed for divination. A native person's 1632 'confession,' recorded by a Spanish priest, confirms the cultural importance of the plant: "I have believed in dreams, in magic herbs, in peyote, and in ololiuqui, in the owl...."

The Spanish Chronicles described ololiuqui as having a twining habit, with heart-shaped leaves, long white flowers, and seeds similar to lentils. Based on this description, 19th century botanists suggested that ololiuqui was a plant in the morning glory family, the Convolvulaceae. In 1897, a Mexican botanist, Manuel Urbina, defined the plant as *Ipomoea sidaefolia*, and it is now known as *Turbina corymbosa*.

The ethnobotanically-challenged Safford once again disagreed, saying that no member of the morning glory family had shown narcotic or toxic properties and that ololiuqui could therefore not possibly be *Ipomoea sidaefolia*. Safford believed that the Native nations were again trying to hide the true identity of ololiuqui, which he believed was *Datura meteloides*, a well-known and highly toxic hallucinogen from the Solanaceae family.[2]

Schultes returned to Oaxaca in April of 1939, planning to investigate further. He began in the town of Chiltepec, on the eastern side of the Sierra Madre de Oaxaca, where he bought provisions and hired a young Chinantec named Guadalupe Martínez-Calderón to serve as a field assistant and guide. Over a series of expeditions from May to July 1939, they crisscrossed the Chinantla rainforest, climbing Cerro Zempoaltepetl, Cerro Cuasimulco, Cerro Zacate, and crossing the difficult Cerro de los Frailes. They passed through the territories of many different ethnic groups, visiting and collecting plants with Maztec and Zapotec colleagues.

One night in San Juan Lalana – the same town where Schultes was bitten by vampire bats several weeks before – he and Guadalupe struck paydirt when they found the house of an elderly *curandero* (traditional healer) covered by a giant morning glory vine, full of fruit. The *curandero*'s only source of revenue was selling the seeds from this massive climber. Guadalupe called the vine a-muk-ia, medicine for divination. Schultes knew that it must be ololiuqui. He identified the plant as *Rivea corymbosa*, finally determining the mysterious botanical identity of the Aztec's "vine of the serpent."

SCHULTES AND THE PSYCHEDELIC ERA

In 1952, the English poet (and author of I, Claudius) Robert Graves sent Schultes' paper on teonanácatl to Gordon Wasson, an American banker and Vice President of J.P. Morgan & Co. in New York, who had a deep and abiding interest in the role of mushrooms in European and Asian cultures. Intrigued by the paper, Wasson and his wife, a Russian physician, launched a series of expeditions in search of teonanácatl, ultimately locating and consuming the sacred mushrooms in 1955.

2. Safford W.E.,1915. An Aztec narcotic. *Journal of Heredity* 6:291-311 July
Safford W.E.,1923. Peyotl. Journal of the American Medical Association 77:1278-1279

Two years later, Wasson published Seeking the Magic Mushroom, a photo essay about his experiences with the fungi, in the May 13th, 1957 issue of *Life* magazine. The essay would become a cult hit, leading many spiritual seekers to Mexico in the 1960s. John Lennon, Bob Dylan, Mick Jagger and Keith Richards are said to have followed in Schultes' footsteps in search of "los niños santos." Schultes' research would eventually influence many other popular counterculture figures, like William S. Burroughs, Allen Ginsberg, Aldous Huxley, Carlos Castaneda, and Terence McKenna.

Ever sober-minded, Schultes had little patience for those who raved about their experiences with mind-altering plants. After William Burroughs described a *yagé* (*ayahuasca*) trip as a mind-opening metaphysical experience, Schultes' response was, "That's funny, Bill, all I saw was colors!"

Schultes' mission was to document sacred plants and investigate their potential to create new medicines. His trailblazing research into the hemisphere's most powerful mind-altering plants – peyote, magic mushrooms, *ayahuasca*, and *Datura* – unintentionally helped to spark the psychedelic era.

SCHULTES IN THE AMAZON
THROUGH THE EMERALD DOOR

"My own acquaintance with the promise of ethnobotanical conservation began in 1941, when I first went to the Amazon Basin. I had just earned my PhD at Harvard, and I had been offered two jobs. One was as a biology master at a private school in New England; the other was a ten-month grant from the National Research Council to go to the Amazon region to identify the plants employed in the many kinds of curare the Indians use for hunting. I decided on the Amazon – which is fortunate, because otherwise I would probably still be a biology [teacher]!"

In September 1941, twenty-six-year-old Richard Evans Schultes arrived in Colombia for the first time. The adventure commenced on his very first day when – on a lark – he took the Bogotá trolley to the southern end of the line. There, he followed a stone staircase up to foot of the lush, green mountains that bordered the eastern part of the city, where he noticed a small orchid nestled among some ferns at the base of a small tree. Gently, he plucked the specimen out of a soft bed of moss. Lacking plant-collecting equipment, he pressed the little specimen inside his passport for safekeeping. The orchid would prove to be new to science, later named *Pachyphyllum schultesii* in his honor, one of more than 120 species that would eventually bear his name.

THE SIBUNDOY VALLEY

In late 1941, Schultes headed south to the headwaters of the Putumayo River with the main goal of researching arrow poisons, which were then showing promise as muscle relaxants used alongside anesthetics, especially with abdominal surgeries. The young ethnobotanist also hoped to determine the botanical identity of yoco, a strong stimulant employed by local tribes that was mentioned in several historical accounts.

Schultes' entry point to the Putumayo was the Sibundoy Valley, a bowl-shaped depression at 2,200 meters above sea level on the edge of the southern Colombian Andes. The flat, roughly circular valley is surrounded on all sides by steep mountains, and is usually engulfed by clouds and inundated by heavy rains that are funneled into the valley, forming the headwaters of the Putumayo River.

Schultes had been in the field for hardly a week when he learned of the Japanese attack on Pearl Harbor. Disappointed to have to cut his trip short, he made plans to return to Bogotá to report to the American Embassy. On February 12, 1942, as travel preparations were being made, Schultes wandered up the mountains northeast of Sibundoy into the páramo of Tambillo where he found a new species of *Espeletia*, the bizarre genus of treelike daisies that give the páramo an otherworldly appearance. The species would later bear his name: *Espeletia schultesiana*.

Espeletia, commonly known as frailejón, is a genus in the sunflower family that lives in the páramo, a wet and windswept grassland ecosystem found above the tree line in the high Andes, typically around 3,000 meters. Páramo ecosystems have distinct levels based on elevation: higher areas are typically open fields of tussock grasses with scattered frailejónes and other low shrubs, while lower elevations contain fragmented forests with a high diversity of orchids, ferns and epiphytic bromeliads. Páramos are considered to be "evolutionary hot spots" for plant diversity.

Páramo vegetation is uniquely adapted to the cold temperatures, excessive moisture, overcast skies and strong winds found at high elevations. *Espeletia* has a thick trunk with a spiraling pattern of dense, hair-covered leaves that hang down after dying, acting as insulation. The succulent, hair-covered leaves help capture water vapor from the near-constant cloud cover, transferring it through their roots into the soil. The highly organic soils of the páramo support water retention, creating a layer of thick, waterlogged soil similar to peatlands.

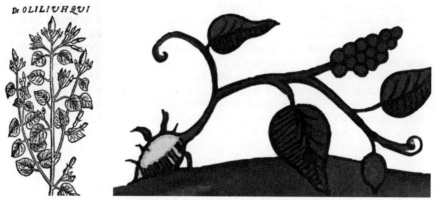

Fig. 1 Drawing of ololiuqui in the chronicles of Franciscan friar, Bernardino de Sahagún, 1905.

These highland wetlands are important water regulators in the health of the river systems, providing clean, naturally filtered water. Today, the páramos in Colombia cover just 1.7 percent of the national territory yet produce 85 percent of its drinking water.

After a brief stay in Bogota awaiting orders from the American Embassy, Schultes was told he had a few months before the Embassy required him for an undisclosed mission. He returned to Sibundoy in February 1942, stopping along the road from Pasto to collect plants on the páramo of San Antonio.

THE INGA AND KAMENTSÁ PEOPLE

The Sibundoy Valley is home to two indigenous ethnic groups: the Inga and the Kamentsá. The two groups speak distinct languages and have different mythologies and origin stories, but are nearly identical in their social organization, lifestyle, modes of subsistence, and worldview.

The Kamentsá say their ancestors are the original inhabitants of Sibundoy. They speak a language isolate, believed to be the sole surviving dialect of a lost language spoken by pre-historical and early historical Quillasingas, a political federation centered in the Pasto region of modern day Colombia (Sañudo, 1938). Kamentsá shamans are masters of both lowland and highland plants, including those of the páramo.

The Inga are more recent arrivals to the valley and speak a dialect of Quechua, the official language of the Inca Empire that is still widely spoken throughout the Andean regions of Peru, Ecuador and Bolivia. There are several theories as to how the Inga arrived in Sibundoy: some claim the Inga are the descendants of Inca nobility, or of a group of Peruvians relocated by the Inca. Other scholars argue the Inga could have arrived as yanaconas, an indigenous bureaucratic order brought by the Spanish from Quito to serve as interpreters and intermediaries. The Inga are also thought to have arrived in several waves, with the first group settling in Santiago some centuries ago, and a second group settling in San Andres in the 18th century, arriving from the Amazonian lowlands in the south (Levinsohn, 1976).

Led by the charismatic cacique (chieftain) Carlos Tamoabioy, the Inga and Kamentsá in the late 17th century created a political unification that endures to this day (Bonilla, 1972). Under this unification, the Inga-Kamentsá territory was defined by the high peaks around the valley: Patascoy, Bordoncillo, Aponte, Juanoy and Portochuelo. In March 1700, Tamoabioy fell ill. Already in his seventies and knowing he was dying, the great cacique decided to dictate his will with two Spanish noblemen as witnesses. In the will, Tamoabioy listed the locations of the major land holdings that constituted the roughly 12,000-hectare indigenous resguardo (reserve). Three copies of the will were made and entrusted to the cabildos (administrative councils) of Sibundoy Grande, Santiago and Aponte for safekeeping.

SCHULTES ENCOUNTERS AYAHUASCA

Schultes' main teacher in Sibundoy was Salvador Chindoy, a renowned Kamentsá shaman who could often be seen in public markets in Bogotá and Quito, talking about his medicinal plants and selling herbs. Chindoy believed that the plants themselves had taught him how to use them for medicinal purposes. He would consume *yagé* or borrachero, another hallucinogenic plant concoction, and have a young apprentice record his vision-induced insights throughout the night so that he could read them in the morning. One of Chindoy's most gifted students was his nephew, Pedro Juajibioy, who also became one of Schultes' closest friends, colleagues and guides.

Schultes often told journalists (including William Burroughs) that *ayahuasca* had little effect on him and that he only saw a few flashes of color. However, Pedro Juajibioy was there the first night Schultes took the potion, and many years later vividly recalled that Schultes sang and told stories the entire time. When asked what Schultes had said, Juajibioy shrugged his shoulders and replied: "We don't know – it was all in English!"

Schultes also wrote about taking another species of *ayahuasca* (*Tetrapterys methystica*) with the Bara Maku peoples of the Rio Tikie in Brazil and noting how powerful the effects were. In retrospect, Schultes was a very private man in some ways, and presumably chose not to share his personal visions with the many people who continually badgered him for details.

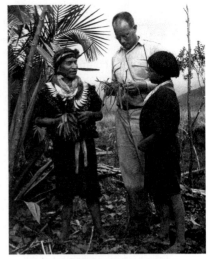

Schultes with shaman Salvador Chindoy, Sibundoy Valley, 1985.

BORRACHERO: THE TREE OF THE EVIL EAGLE

Schultes was particularly fascinated by the great diversity of *borrachero*, also referred to by South American cultures as "the tree of the evil eagle." Most *borrachero* medicines were derived from variations of the genus *Brugmansia*, rich in tropane alkaloids and highly psychoactive. These plants were grown and used by indigenous cultures from Colombia south to Chile, but no place holds more species diversity than Sibundoy.

No fewer than eleven variants of *borrachero* were employed in Sibundoy. The rarest versions were typically found in gardens near the houses of the most powerful and accomplished medicine men. Some of the species were dramatically different, highly atrophied forms with thin or deformed leaves, likely the result of centuries of cultivation by the shamans of the Sibundoy.

One of the strongest of the atrophied *Brugmansias* induced strong visions for hours, with effects lasting for several days. This was a stunted plant with deformed leaves that looked as though they had been eaten by caterpillars, and was fittingly called munchiro borrachero ("drunken caterpillar"). Varieties also were named after water (buyé), the hummingbird, the deer, and the boa constrictor.

The strongest of the local medicines and the most favored hallucinogen of Kamentsa payés (shamans) for prayer and divination was *Borrachero culebra* ("drunken snake"). According to local shamans, the effects were so deeply transformative that a dose could put a person to sleep for four days. The plant had a variety of other uses as well: the leaves were used to make an infusion, and, when heated in water, the leaves and flowers were used to relieve tumor, swollen joints, and persistent chills and fevers. *Borrachero culebra* was extremely rare, found only in the gardens of Salvador Chindoy and a handful of other shamans. Schultes planted it in the garden of the church and around the seminary, in keeping with of his droll sense of humor.

The plant appeared so dramatically different from other *Brugmansia* or *Datura* varieties that Schultes described it as a new genus: *Methysticodendron amesianum*, named in honor of his botanical mentor Oakes Ames. This classification has been debated, with some suggesting that the atrophied appearance was the result of a viral infection or the mutation of a single gene. Today the plant is most commonly referred to as *Brugmansia aurea* (*Hybrid*) *culebra*, a classification that Schultes agreed with later in life as genetic research helped elucidate the relationships between different varieties and species of plants.

INTO THE LAND OF THE KOFÁN

Schultes traveled down the road to Puerto Asís, stopping to collect plants with Inga communities along the Uchupayaco River and in Puerto Limon. He remained at Puerto Asís for two weeks before heading downriver to Puerto Ospina, a military base at the mouth of the Sucumbíos River. There, he met Colonel Gómez-Pereira, a Colombian officer who offered to mount an expedition up the Sucumbios when he heard of Schultes' desire to explore the headwaters. Along the way, the Colonel would also help teach him the basics of the notoriously difficult Kofán language.

The Sucumbíos, or San Miguel as it is more often called in Colombia, forms part of the international border between Colombia and Ecuador. Colonel Gómez-Pereira and his gunboat, the *Mercedes*, had been assigned to patrol the country's borders to prevent entry by the Brazilians, Ecuadoreans and Peruvians into a region that was still disputed in the early 20th century. On March 27, 1942, the *Mercedes* set off up the Sucumbíos.

The Sucumbíos drained the territory of the Kofán, a nation that had remained largely isolated from the outside world in the 1940s with the exception of a few missionaries and rubber traders. At the time of the Spanish Conquest, the Kofán were numerous and had successfully resisted Huayna Capac and the Inca Empire. By the 17th century, disease and enslavement had reduced their population to some twenty thousand individuals. Several waves of epidemics that the missionaries introduced in the 20th century further reduced Kofán numbers to fewer than a thousand at the time of Schultes' visit.

Their isolation from the outside world was reinforced by their warlike reputation and the variety and toxicity of their arrow poisons, but what repelled others often attracted Schultes. "I do not believe in hostile Indians," he remarked on many occasions. Schultes believed that "native people, if properly approached and treated, are friendly and sometimes willing to share their knowledge with the interested scientist."

The *Mercedes* arrived at the Kofán village of El Conejo on March 29, 1942. Schultes and Gómez-Pereira were greeted by an elder Kofán shaman, dressed in a blue cotton cusma (a type of long shirt), with layers of necklaces made from peccary tusks, seeds, and shells; his face was adorned with intricately painted red lines from achiote berries and a macaw feather jauntily inserted in his pierced nasal septum.

Schultes found that the Kofán had more shamans relative to population size than any other band or nation in the northwest Amazonia. He described them as "deeply knowledgeable men with unusual intelligence and imposing personality." By reputation, they were experts in manipulating spiritual forces to prescribe cures for illnesses and even solve socio-political problems. Some Kofán shamans believed that, when in a plant-induced trance, they could turn themselves into jaguars and roam the rainforest at night.

Other Amazonians considered the Kofán shamans exceptionally powerful. These medicine men regarded the ritual hallucinogenic brew *yagé* as their sacrament and consumed the beverage at least once a week. Entire villages would sometimes participate in the ceremonies.

At the time of Schultes' visit, ten Kofán villages were recorded: four on both the Aguarico and Sucumbíos rivers, and two more on the Guamués River to the north in Colombia. Schultes stayed at El Conejo for several days, collecting plants, observing the routines of daily life, taking photographs and spending the evenings learning from the shamans. With Conejo as a base, he paddled up the Sucumbíos to Santa Rosa, followed a traditional Kofán path south to the Aguarico River in Ecuador, and poled up the Quebrada Hormiga, crossing over the Guamués River.

CURARE: FLYING DEATH

Schultes had come to Kofán territory to document their renowned mastery of arrow poisons. Curare – a blanket term for all arrow poisons prepared from tropical plants, particularly those that cause respiratory paralysis – is one of the few words in the English language derived from Amazonian dialects. The use of curare was first brought to the attention of western science by the eccentric British explorer Charles Waterton in the early 19th century. Schultes began his fieldwork in the northwest Amazon just as curare medicines were becoming important muscle relaxants in abdominal surgery. He and others believed that the study of curare varieties and their admixtures could lead to both new medicines and a better understanding of the human nervous system.

The Kofán had an intricate cultural system built around the preparation of curare. Certain shamans specialized in curare production. They had to know the correct times to collect bark, what part of the liana to use, and how the plants should be prepared. ("Liana" are any slow-growing, woody vines.) This knowledge was passed from one generation of payés (shamans) to the next, following a long and difficult training period and starting with an apprenticeship at an early age.

Stipulated practices had to be followed for the creation of curare for special purposes, and the shaman had to observe strict fasting from certain foods when preparing curare. The intricate mixing of plants was accompanied by chanting, believed to maximize the toxicity of the plants; poison intended for use on large animals or humans required the chanting of two shamans.

Schultes would eventually identify and document more than 70 species of plants employed to make curare in the Amazon. The most common varieties consisted of highly poisonous plants, such as those of the *Chondrodendron* or *Strychnos* genera, combined with admixtures, typically non-toxic plants that the locals believed served as amplifiers. He also observed the Kofán employing the sap of the *Virola* tree, a hallucinogen, when producing certain curare poisons. Many years later, his student Homer Pinkley documented the Kofán along the Colombia-Ecuador border making curare from a relative of the cinnamon family.

FISH POISON: BARBASCO

The most commonly-employed Amazonian fish poison is derived from lianas of the genus *Lonchocarpus*, often readily identifiable by both a cucumber-like odor and a relatively bright yellow wood. The fish poison is generally known as barbasco in Spanish-speaking America, timbo in the Brazilian Amazon and neku in the Guianas. The phrase "fish poison" is a bit of a misnomer, because the active compound, rotenone, stuns the fish rather than killing them. The chemical enters the fishes' gills and interferes with their ability to intake oxygen, causing them to rise to the surface where hunters wait with bows and arrows drawn. (Today, in the western world, rotenone is employed as a biodegradable pesticide.) Such fishing expeditions are often followed by major celebrations and feasting.

Schultes remained on the Sucumbíos for several weeks before heading east to Puerto Ospina, where he briefly paused before traveling upstream on the *Mercedes* to explore the lower Guamués. When he returned to Puerto Ospina in early May 1942, he caught a military flight to Tres Esquinas on the Caquetá River, eager to find another flight to Bogotá so that he could deposit his Kofán plant collections at the city's herbarium and then return to his beloved rainforest. He spent several days waiting for his plane in a Koreguaje village on the Caquetá, where he observed their preparation and use of coca.

DOWN THE MIGHTY PUTUMAYO

In mid-May, Schultes flew to Puerto Leguízamo, a military base on the Putumayo River south of Puerto Ospina. There, Schultes met up with Nazzareno Postarino, a young Italian from Mocoa whom he hired as an expedition assistant. Schultes spent several days collecting on the Rio Caucaya before heading down the Putumayo on May 19, 1942 aboard the *Ciudad de Neiva*, a three-story, wood-burning paddle wheeler.

Schultes' plan was to explore two of the major tributaries of the Putumayo. First, he would ascend the Cara Paraná, meaning "river with canoes," and then cut overland to the Igara Paraná, the "river without canoes," a reference to its many rapids. From there, he hoped to purchase a dugout canoe from the natives and continue downriver all the way to Tarapacá near the Brazilian border.

Schultes and Postarino were entering the territory of the Witoto and related Bora, Andoke, and Ocaína peoples. The Witoto were exceptionally numerous: whereas most Amazonian bands numbered in the hundreds or low thousands, the Witoto population was estimated to be about 50,000 at the beginning of the 20th century, inhabiting a lowland territory ranging from modern day Colombia to Peru. Early Witotos were described as a peaceful people known for large ceremonies of singing and dancing.

AMBIL, THE TOBACCO PASTE

While he was on the Putumayo, Schultes observed Witotos preparing a tobacco paste known as ambil in Colombia and chimu in neighboring Venezuela. The Witoto would mix tobacco leaves and salt-like minerals extracted from other plants, cooking them down into a thick black paste periodically placed between the cheek and gums as a stimulant. Ambil was an important part of many ceremonies, and almost always taken when chewing mambe, a dried and powdered form of the sacred coca leaf.

Ambil is an unusual form of tobacco preparation most commonly found among the peoples of the northwest Amazon, although similar concoctions have been found in northern Colombia and in the Guianas. Ambil is also consumed in *ayahuasca* ceremonies by some bands, and often partaken as a stimulant and appetite suppressant on long boat rides or hikes though the forest.

Few people in the industrialized world realize that tobacco has long been considered a sacred plant in Native American cultures. Archeological sites associated with tobacco cultivation in use have been dated to well over a thousand years. Tobacco was and is a stimulant, digestive, emetic, fumitory, and trade item. Even today, it is commonly found in gardens throughout the Amazon.

MANGUARÉS: THE JUNGLE GRAPEVINE

At dawn in Witoto territory, Schultes often heard the sounds of manguarés, large drums fashioned from tree trunks that had been hollowed out with burning stones. Each drum had a narrow opening running lengthwise, with larger openings at the top and bottom. The drums were struck with drumsticks tipped with wild rubber; blows to either side of the opening produced distinct tones. Manguarés were suspended from the rafters of malocas (longhouses) and used as musical instruments for ceremonial occasions and for communicating over long distances to announce festivals or summon council meetings. Manguarés have been reported to have an audible range of six to ten miles, depending on the size of the drum and the surrounding topography. Amazonian historian John Hemming described manguarés in his book *Tree of Rivers*: "A code is arranged, based upon the difference of tones and the length and number of blows struck, so that all kinds of messages can be exchanged." As Schultes would later say: there really was a jungle grapevine.

In the 1970s, Schultes returned to the Amazon aboard the Alpha Helix research vessel, accompanied by several other eminent scientists. Schultes and his colleagues walked into a Witoto village, where they were met by two local women. The women welcomed the visitors in Spanish and asked them what they wanted. Schultes replied that what he really wanted was some coca powder – in fluent Witoto. Taken aback, the women squealed and laughed – and then brought the coca!

THE SEARCH FOR YOCO

Schultes arrived in Puerto Ospina in early July 1942. Thin and exhausted after nearly six months of nearly continuous fieldwork, he was eager to rest and recover. Schultes was relieved to receive a comfortable cabin on a Colombian military gunboat, thanks to his friend Colonel Gómez-Pereira.

One morning, Schultes was surprised to hear a knock on the door to his cabin. The visitor was a Colombian marine who told him that someone wished to speak with him. Schultes looked over the railing of the gunship to see a Kofán he had met on the Sucumbíos River. The Kofán was holding a section of the *yoco* liana, the plant Schultes had been fruitlessly searching for throughout his journey down the Putumayo. The Kofán told him the plant was in full bloom not far from Puerto Ospina.

Yoco had been in use for hundreds if not thousands of years, and was mentioned repeatedly in early Spanish chronicles. Schultes had first read about the plant in the book *Northwest Amazons*, written by the British Captain Thomas Whiffen, who spent a year in the lower Putumayo in 1908. Florent Claes, a Belgian botanist who traveled with the Capuchin priest Gaspar de Pinell in 1925, identified yoco as a forest liana in the genus *Paullinia* (related to the well-known guarana – *Paullinia guarana*), but was able neither to find a specimen in fruit or flower nor to determine it to species. The Spanish botanist José Cuatrecasas later found *yoco* growing on the forested banks of the Putumayo River at Puerto Piñuña Negra, but once more the plant lacked fruits and flowers and could neither be adequately described nor identified. The precise botanical identity of the plant remained a mystery that Schultes was eager to solve.

Locals said that *yoco* was almost impossible to cultivate, and was therefore collected in the rainforest. Indigenous communities consumed *yoco* in a beverage made by scraping off the bark and pressing the milky sap into cold water. Ingestion alleviates hunger and fatigue, often allowing one to go for up to two days without food while also providing a sense of focus and overall well-being. (A chemical analysis reveals that, in addition to other active ingredients, *yoco* bark yields about 3% caffeine, stronger than coffee.) Several Kofán communities insist that *yoco* consumption also helps prevent malaria.

The plant was a dietary staple of the bands living in western Caquetá and Putumayo in Colombia and adjacent parts of Ecuador and Peru. Most indigenous households of these areas kept a supply of yoco stems, and preferred never to leave for the forest without carrying the plant. Yoco was so important to them that they would simply pick up and move their village to another location when local supplies had been depleted. It also was an integral part of many of these cultures' morning rituals: they would rise at dawn, rinse their mouths in the river, and drink a gourdful of *yoco* before eating any food. The first gourd was followed by another about a half an hour later, with even more ingested for hunting or fishing trips. Regional bands were able to distinguish fifteen varieties of yoco, including *yoco blanco* and *yoco colorado*, all of which fell within a well-defined indigenous system of classification.

Schultes had seen *yoco* in use throughout his explorations of the Putumayo watershed. The first was with the German rancher Jorge Fuerbringer and some local natives, who had led him to *yoco* outside of Mocoa in 1941, but the plant was not in fruit or flower. He found other sterile specimens in an Inga community in the headwaters of the Uchupayaco River in February 1942, between the Putumayo River and Teteyé River in March 1942, and at the Kofán community of El Conejo on the Sucumbíos in April 1942.

On July 6, 1942, after twenty hours of travel, Schultes and the Kofán came to a spot in the forest about 15 km along the trail from Puerto Ospina to Puerto Asís where the ground was covered in small flowers. After the group felled a few small trees, a large woody vine came crashing to the ground. Schultes had identified another species new to science, and named it in honor of the indigenous appellation: *Paullinia yoco*.

> Many a liana had I cut down, only to find it flowerless and, in this condition, without value for taxonomic study. All the Indians of the upper Putumayo River knew of my quest. In June, when the rivers rose, flooding all the forests, I decided to end my trip and return to Bogotá. My legs were covered with ulcers from walking through the swamps and … when I arrived at the Colombian naval base on that river, the clean bunk which the commander of one of the river gunboats offered me pending the arrival of an aeroplane felt regal. Three days before the arrival of the plane, an Indian came paddling down with the news that he had located a flowering yoco. He assured me it was only four hours' walk through the forest. I hesitate. The pains in my legs, I confess, nearly won out. By, finally, I agreed to go, half expecting to find just one more flowerless liana. It was a terrible pilgrimage of six or seven hours on foot, most of the time knee-deep in water and mud. On arrival, I saw an enormous liana, the tiny flowers of which were strewn far and wide on the forest floor. We had to fell seven trees before the treasure would fall into our laps…that collection not only enabled us to identify an interesting drug but provided me with a species new to science. (From Schultes' Field Notes, 1946)

THE APAPORIS: WORKSHOP OF THE GODS

WORLD WAR II & SCHULTES' RUBBER MISSION

As Schultes made his way down the Putumayo River in 1942, Nazi Germany was consolidating control of continental Europe after conquering Poland in 1939 and France in 1940. German U-boats were devastating British shipping in the Atlantic while the German army turned its hungry gaze east towards the eastern European countries and the Soviet Union.

In early 1942, Schultes left the rainforest and presented himself at the American Embassy in Bogotá in order to enlist in the Allied cause. He expected to be sent back to the States to undergo basic training and then be shipped to the European battlefield. Much to his surprise, he was told he could do far more to help his country by returning to the Amazon on a special mission to find high-yielding and disease-resistant strains of rubber trees.

A steady supply of rubber was vital to the war effort. Each Sherman tank required a half ton of rubber; a heavy bomber required a full ton. Some warships contained 20,000 rubber parts. Rubber was not only a component on every single wheel of every single vehicle, it coated every wire. At the outbreak of World War II, 90% of the global supply of rubber was being produced in plantations in the European colonies of Southeast Asia, mostly the Dutch East Indies and British Malaya.

The day after the attack on Pearl Habor, the Japanese invaded British and Dutch colonies in Southeast Asia to secure access to rubber, a vital resource that had been cut off from Japan by economic sanctions. The Japanese nearly-simultaneously invaded the Philippines, British Borneo, Hong Kong and, later, British-controlled Singapore and Java and Sumatra in the Dutch East Indies. By May 1942, Japan had conquered a wide arc of territory, from Burma in the west to New Guinea to the south and north to Iwo Jima, thereby controlling a substantial portion of the world's rubber supply.

HEVEA: THE ODYSSEY OF THE TREE THAT CHANGED THE WORLD

Schultes later referred to rubber as "the tree that changed the world in one century." In fact, it was a remarkable set of circumstances that led to the global dependence on Asia for a product originally derived from an Amazonian tree.

Rubber was initially collected exclusively in the wild, often by corrupt enterprises led by ruthless rubber barons who enslaved local peoples through both insurmountable debt and extreme cruelty. All attempts to establish rubber plantations in South America ended in disaster, due to incessant depredations by leaf blight and Dothidella fungi. Attempts to transport rubber seeds out of South America also failed, as the oily seeds quickly spoiled and perished.

Henry Wickham, a British adventurer, spent many years living in the Amazon and Orinoco in the mid-19th century, and published a book on his travels. Wickham had a keen interest in economically useful plants. He collected the cinchona seeds in Peru and Ecuador that later became the source of quinine plantations in India and Ceylon, producing valuable anti-malarial drugs for the British Empire.

In 1876, Wickham was in Santarem when a steamship of recent vintage – appropriately named the S.S. Amazonas – forged up the Amazon River on an inaugural voyage from Liverpool to Manaus. While the ship was making its way downriver, Wickham learned that a corrupt businessman had left the S.S. Amazonas without cargo for the return trip. Seizing this opportunity, Wickham instructed his indigenous associates to collect rubber seeds that happened to be ripening at that moment. Previous seed shipments had been sent by sailing ships, and the few days saved by the faster steamboat helped ensure that some seeds survived the voyage to England. More than 70,000 seeds were collected and transported to the Royal Botanic Gardens at Kew outside London, of which 2,800 survived. The resulting seedlings were packaged in glass-domed cases and shipped through the Suez Canal to Ceylon, Singapore and other tropical European colonies.

After initial difficulties cultivating and efficiently harvesting the latex in Asia, rubber plantations grew in popularity as methods improved. In 1907, there were over 10 million rubber trees in Ceylon and Malaya. Just two years later, Malaya had planted more than 40 million specimens. New techniques for tapping trees were developed: by making only a light incision in the bark, the rubber trees could be harvested more frequently and at a younger age without impeding growth or killing the tree. Selective breeding of genetic lines doubled production within a generation. As the Asian plantations expanded and grew more productive, the Amazon rubber industry collapsed, and Southeast Asia became the dominant provider.

With the Japanese threatening the European colonies in Southeast Asia, the United States government realized that its reliance on rubber from these regions was a vulnerability. In response, the U.S. established the Rubber Reserve Company to determine how best to establish flourishing rubber plantations in the Americas.

Early accounts indicated that blight-resistant species of *Hevea* might exist in other less-explored regions of Amazonia, especially the northwest Amazon, which reports – including those by Richard Spruce in the mid-1800s – suggested might be the origin of the genus. Schultes' mission was to explore these remote areas and estimate how many such species, and members thereof, existed in a given region. His first assignment was to investigate three sites in the upper Caquetá watershed said to be rich in wild rubber.

> I joined this organization and immediately plunged into the rubber forests of Colombia as an explorer, searching out the densest [stands] and best type of rubber, mapping rivers, and reporting on their navigability and other tasks preparatory to the rebirth of the wild rubber industry. I became intensely interested in the rubber plant, the more so since I saw, from studies in the field, that botanically there was so much to do before we lay claim to even a preliminary understanding of the numerous wild species of the commercial rubber: *Hevea*. (Schultes' field notebook, 1952)

On December 26, 1942, Schultes left Bogotá by train, bound for Neiva to the southwest, from where he continued south to Pitalito to meet the expedition team. Over the next two weeks, the team made their way slowly across the mountainous terrain, crossing from the headwaters of the Magdalena River to the upper Villalobos River. As the expedition moved slowly over the rugged terrain, Schultes found several varieties of caucho blanco ("white rubber"), a high-quality rubber, and discovered a new species of *Hevea* known as *Hevea Colorado* or "red rubber." He and his colleagues also found many scarred trunks and disfigured stumps that indicated this area had been overharvested and ravaged by caucheros (rubber tappers) in earlier decades, leaving few healthy and productive mature rubber trees.

Schultes had hoped to reach the Inga community of Yunguillo in the headwaters of the Caquetá, but the terrain proved too difficult and the expedition had to turn back. The difficult conditions and low density of remaining rubber trees meant the area was of little use for their purposes.

CHIRIBIQUETE: THE LOST WORLD

Schultes' next mission was to investigate the remote rainforests of the Apaporis River, which, though one of the least-known rivers in Colombia, was yet believed to contain a huge supply of rubber. This assignment brought him to one of the most inaccessible and spectacular landscapes in the Amazon, inhabited by a mysterious people reputed to be fierce cannibals.

On March 3, 1943, Schultes arrived in Miraflores, a newly created rubber station on the upper Vaupés River in southeast Colombia. The expedition began with an ominous start: many supplies failed to arrive or were severely delayed. Schultes was also unable to find anyone familiar with the upper Apaporis to help guide the expedition, though a local chief in Puerto Nare did warn of its treacherous rapids.

Schultes assembled a small scouting team and ascended the Vaupés River to the confluence of the Unilla and Itilla rivers, a location known as Puerto Trinidad to local caucheros. From Puerto Trinidad, the team spent fourteen hours hacking their way through dense forests overland before finally reaching the Macaya River at a series of rapids.

That same evening, a young member of the expedition team attempted to swim across the river, but was caught in the current and pulled into and under the twisting rapids. His body was never recovered. The next day, Schultes returned to Miraflores to report the death. To commemorate this tragedy, the rapids were named "Cachivera del Diablo" – the "Devil's Cataract."

After a quick trip to Bogotá in early April, Schultes returned to Miraflores on April 18, 1943. There, he and Everett Vinton, a fellow explorer also working for the RRC, assembled an expedition team of 28 men and set to work establishing a twenty-mile supply trail from Miraflores to Puerto Trinidad and then on to the Macaya. After slowly accumulating the necessary supplies, they cleared a high piece of land and built a camp at the confluence of the Macaya and Ajajú rivers. The rustic camp included a kitchen, dining hall, store rooms, sleeping quarters for thirty men, and a rough landing strip on the opposite bank of the Macaya. They named the camp "Puerto *Hevea*" because of the high concentration of rubber trees in the area. This locale can still be seen as a clearing in satellite imagery.

On May 14, while the expedition crew was clearing the forest and setting up camp, Schultes set off across the Macaya to explore the immense sandstone mountain that had loomed in the distance for many weeks. As he climbed, the dense forests gave way to a rocky savannah. Arriving at the broad summit, a magical landscape was revealed: thousand-foot-high granitic domes and tabletop sandstone mountains emerged from the pristine rainforests all around him. Waterfalls roared over the edges of cliffs, through giant caverns, and into unspoiled rivers.

The sober-minded Schultes – never a man given to poetic flights of fancy – was deeply impacted by this enchanted landscape. He would later say that these eerie rock formations seemed like giant sculptures left over from God's workshop: "It was from these first tentative experiments," Schultes mused, "that He had gone out and built a world."

Schultes climbed to the summit of Cerro Chiribiquete, part of the larger Chiribiquete mountain range that runs for more than 240km from north to south. The Chiribiquete range can be divided into five distinct parts: the Chiribiquete, Cuñaré, Yarí and Araracuara ranges, and the Mesa de Iguaje. Chiribiquete is bordered to the east by the Apaporis River, whose two major tributaries, the Ajajú and Macaya, originate in the Yarí River to the west. To the south, the Yarí – also originating in the savannas – crosses through the southern portion of Chiribiquete, where it joins with its major tributary, the Mesay, originating in the least-explored central region of the range. The Caquetá River cuts through the Araracuara highlands, forming the spectacular thousand-foot-high canyons of Araracuara, memorably captured in one of Schultes' most famous photographs.

THE GUIANA SHIELD

Chiribiquete forms the westernmost extent of the Guiana Shield, an ancient geological formation stretching along the northern edge of South America from central Colombia to the northern Atlantic coast. It contains some of the oldest rocks on earth, dating back to the Precambrian era almost two billion years ago, long before the Andes were formed. This ancient mountain range has been grotesquely eroded over time, leaving unusual granitic rock formations and flat, table-topped sandstone mountains with sheer cliffs known as tepuis.

The Guiana Highlands harbor some of the world's most spectacular waterfalls, like Angel Falls in Venezuela and Kaieteur Falls in Guyana. Pico da Neblina, at over 9,800 feet, is the highest point in lowland Amazonia. Due primarily to its remoteness, the Guiana Shield contains some of the most

107

pristine rainforests in the world, features high levels of biodiversity, and is home to many endemic species, particularly in and on the isolated massifs.

On these mountaintops, Schultes gathered the first-ever botanical collections from this awe-inspiring region. In his book *One River* (1996), Wade Davis describes Schultes' experience on Cerro Chiribiquete:

> What Schultes found on the summit was a grassland interspersed with dense brush of low gnarled shrubs, an island of savannah perched a thousand feet above a tropical rain forest. Adapted to the dry conditions, the plants were reduced in size, and many bore glossy leathery leaves, often coated with heavy waxes or dense pubescence. Their bark was either thick and corky, or thin and coated with wax. Epiphytes had exaggerated pseudobulbs for water storage, and many plants grew low to the ground and had dense rosettes of leaves. The roots were especially well developed, penetrating the cracks and fissures in the rock, reaching like veins across the face of cliffs. The growth forms were exceedingly strange, the overall aspect of the flora elfin and bizarre. (*One River*, p.319)

Schultes found several new species that day, including *Vellozia phantasmagoria*, a ghostly herb from the small genus of monocots found in northern South America and adjacent Panama. As he cut through the forest, his clothes became covered with a sticky latex, leading to the discovery of two new rubber plants: *Senefelderopsis chiribiquetensis*, a relative of balata, and *Hevea nitidia* var. *toxicondendroides*.

The expedition completed construction of their first canoe in early June of 1943. Unfortunately, a motor that had been promised never arrived, so Schultes and a small crew paddled their way up the sweeping curves of the Ajajú River, surrounded on both banks by majestic and mysterious tabletop mountains. After several days on the water, the expedition passed a set of rapids near the mouth of the Macuje River, and continued upstream to the Yaya-Ayaya River. The ecosystem began to transition as they paddled west up the Ajajú: The rocky, sandy terrain gave way to flooded forests less likely to harbor rubber trees. Finding the Yaya-Ayaya ridden with rapids, the expedition turned back and descended the Ajajú.

THE BELL MOUNTAIN – CERRO CAMPANA

On June 6, Schultes and his crew turned north up the Caño Negro, a small tributary of the Ajajú on the northernmost side of the Chiribiquete highlands. In front of them loomed an imposing series of steeply sloped domes with soaring peaks, one of which was known as the Cerro Campana – the "Bell Mountain." Schultes described Cerro Campana in his book *Where the Gods Reign*:

> ...the isolated quartzitic mountains of [Chiribiquete] are sentinels of a mysterious past. The Cerro de la Campana is one of the westernmost vestiges of these hills and is so strikingly awesome that it is wrapped in legend in the Indian mind. All Indians believe that fierce thunderstorms and torrents can be caused by beating upon a thinly eroded slab near the summit. When struck with another stone, it sends forth a bell-like tone."

In his ascent of the isolated massifs, Schultes noted that those who once lived there had created strange and wonderful cave paintings on the walls and in rock shelters. These ancient designs, painted with dark red dyes, depict chaotic mosaics of people, animals, shamans, hunters, and dancers.

Jaguars with intricate spot patterns leap through the air. Shamans hold long staffs and palm fronds above their heads while hunters stand alert with barbed spears, ready to be launched. Abstract spiral designs emerge from the torso of animal-human hybrids as the creature undergoes a mysterious spiritual transformation. The paintings portray fish, frogs, birds, and unrecognizable animals. Hundreds of red handprints are the only remaining signature of a mysterious people that created this ancient artwork before disappearing into the jungle.

Schultes was one of the first explorers to observe these paintings, in what would turn out to be one of the largest concentrations of pre-Columbian cave paintings in all of Amazonia. Later research found as many as 8,000 paintings on a single wall. To this day, the region remains largely unexplored, with experts having little idea of the total number of cave paintings, their date of creation, or their precise origin.

CARIJONAS OF CHIRIBIQUETE

As he explored the Chiribiquete highlands, Schultes' guide was Barrera, a young Carijona he had met along the Vaupés River. Barrera accompanied Schultes along the visits to the Macaya and Ajajú Rivers, and had taught the ethnobotanist about the mythological importance of Cerro Campana as well as the local uses of various plants.

Near the Apaporis River, they found *Markea coccinea*, an epiphytic vine with red flowers valued by the Carijona for mystical ceremonies and to expel intestinal parasites. Carijona medicine men would treat dementia by traveling to the top of Cerro Chiribiquete to gather the leaves and stems of a species that was eventually named by Western science in Schultes' honor: *Piper schultesii*. They would soak these plants parts in water or a ferment them before giving them to elderly patients "who sit without talking all day." Schultes noted that these plants could be kept dry for several months without losing their strong pungency and were also used in a tea to relieve coughs and chest infections. The Carijona also knew and used herbal remedies for fevers, fungal skin infections, and ringworm, and to relieve the symptoms of malaria.

The Carijona had dominated the Chiribiquete region for more than four hundred years, at one point totaling more than 25,000 people. Within a hundred years of contact with the outside world, the Carijona were reduced to less than a thousand members. As Schultes journeyed through Chiribiquete, the former heart of Carijona territory, he knew he was recording important ethnobotanical information from a dying people who would soon cease to exist as an intact cultural entity. He was in a race against time as he traveled, recorded and collected plants with some its last members.

DOWN THE LITTLE-KNOWN APAPORIS RIVER

The expedition's next goal was to descend the 1,350-mile Apaporis, one of the most isolated and least-known of rivers in the Amazon basin. Schultes knew this task would not be easy: on a previous overflight, he had counted more than a dozen daunting rapids, including an enormous waterfall followed by a mile-long canyon that nearly obscured the river running through it.

Setting off down the Apaporis, they passed the first set of rapids, the Cachivera de Chiribiquete, some twenty miles from Puerto Hevea. After proceeding smoothly through 20 miles of open river, they encountered a set of fierce rapids that nearly capsized the canoe. Barely reaching the shore, they were forced to haul the boat ashore and hike back to Puerto Hevea overland through the trackless rainforest, all the while carrying an injured man. They needed additional workers to portage the upcoming rapids.

Nearly a week later, they once again continued down the Apaporis. Although slowed by a rainstorm that damaged many of their supplies, they were eventually able to advance nearly fifty miles through many treacherous rapids. Deciding they would not safely reach the mouth of the river, they once again decided to return to Puerto Hevea by land, leaving the canoe behind.

In his book *One River* (1996), Wade Davis describes Schultes' revelation on the trek back to Puerto Hevea:

> As he moved along the shore he realized that the counts he had been making from the water had been consistently low. When he factored this error into his survey results, he discovered that the upper Apaporis...supported more than a quarter million rubber trees. Properly exploited, they would yield almost a million pounds of rubber a year. (*One River*, page 321)

After a brief stint in Villavicencio and Bogotá to recover from a blood infection that nearly killed him (the "doctor" turned out to be a veterinarian), the undaunted Schultes returned to Miraflores on August 25, 1943. His next expedition would cross overland on a trail from Puerto Nare to the Apaporis, below the rapids that halted their progress down the river two months before.

It was a difficult journey, and the team struggled to carry an extraordinarily heavy, sixteen-meter boat overland across the thirty-six mile trail they had hacked through the forest. It was thankless, backbreaking work: the journey took fourteen days and left them exhausted and demoralized.

Beginning below the final rapids of Chiribiquete, Schultes was finally able to continue his descent of the Apaporis, which from that point remained unbroken by rapids for nearly three hundred miles. The work proceeded smoothly, and Schultes counted many mature and harvestable *Hevea guianensis* trees along the bank of the river. This was ideal rubber territory.

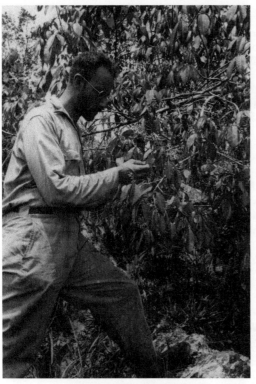

Schultes along the Rio Apaporis

As they proceeded, Schultes also mapped the course of the Apaporis using a tedious but surprisingly accurate technique: As they progressed, Schultes would actually pace a kilometer on the shore of the river, marking each end with a white flag. This also allowed him to measure the speed of the river as the boat drifted from one marker to the next. As they drifted down the Apaporis, Schultes used his compass to keep track of the boat's orientation. Together with his kilometer pacings, this permitted him to plot river's course and produce the first map of the Apaporis; it was an ingenious, low-tech approach more akin to those employed by early Victorian explorers like Alfred Russel Wallace (who had been trained as a surveyor) than the cartographers of today.

At one point, Schultes and his team observed a ridge rising in the distance, and the mouth of a blackwater river emptying into the Apaporis, known as the Kananarí. There they encountered a Taiwano, busy fishing for his dinner. So remote was the territory they had crossed that this fellow was the first person they had encountered for six months.

Later, with the Taiwano guiding them up the Kananarí, a massive sandstone plateau known as Cerro Isikburi rose abruptly out of the forest to their right, adorned with numerous ribbon-like waterfalls cascading from the summit.

As they ascended the Kananarí, they passed giant boulders engraved with highly stylized figures of unknown ancient origins. They spent the night in a Kubuyarí maloca on the Caño Paco with similar designs painted on the walls in yellow, red and black. Their hosts explained that the designs represented *yagé* visions.

ETHNOGRAPHIC NOTE: ETHNIC GROUPS OF
THE LOWER APAPORIS & VAUPÉS REGION

The lower Apaporis and Vaupés region represent one of the most complex linguistic areas in the Amazon, if not the world. It harbors some fifteen Tucano languages and a few other less commonly spoken and unrelated dialects, such as Makú. Tucano-speaking bands of the region include the Makuna, Barasana, Tanimuka, Cubeo, Taiwano, and Letuama.

Interestingly, many cultural groups in this region have a socially obligatory multilingualism wherein indigenous community members are expected to marry someone of a different language group and learn their language; to marry someone belonging to the same language group is considered akin to incest. Due to these social norms, the indigenous peoples of the region are able to speak a remarkable number of languages and maintain a diverse array of cultures and cultural traditions.

This linguistically and culturally diverse territory made for an exceedingly interesting research area for Schultes, as each ethnic group had different oral histories and different medicinal uses for local plants. However, the complex linguistic traditions often made it difficult for him to communicate, especially with elders who spoke little or no Spanish. Never easily discouraged, Schultes responded by learning the basics of some the local languages.

THE PALM OF THE SPIDER WEB

At dawn, Schultes emerged from the maloca and went to bathe in the river. Through the early morning mists, he noticed the graceful silhouette of a stand of palm trees growing on the nearby rapids. Known locally as caranaí, the palm would be a species new to science: *Mauritiella cataractarum*, found only on rocky riverbanks near rapids.

The Makuna call this tree bö-pö-ma – the tree of the spider web – due to the resemblance of the crown to gigantic spider webs as one looks upwards through the canopy from a canoe. They say the palm was planted before man came to earth from the Milky Way. In this primordial era, the "Spirit of the Sun" threw fishing nets (the spider web) from the sky onto the lands below, indicating where the Makuna should settle and build their malocas. Schultes would later observe that most Makuna settlements are found near rapids, giving their location a dually cosmological and ethnobotanical origin.

As they descended the Kananarí, the Kubuyarí chief warned Schultes of the perilous rapids that lay ahead. He claimed these were dangerous places inhabited by the spirits of the dead whose presence was manifested by strange spirit faces on the cliff walls.

Schultes had been ordered not to pass the falls of Jirijirimo, but now, with a barely functioning outboard motor, dwindling supplies, and little chance of successful hunting, this would be virtually impossible. He would have to face the rapids.

Schultes was an aficionado of the classics, often travelling with *The Illiad* or *The Odyssey*, which he would translate from the ancient Greek when he spent endless days in longhouses waiting for the rains to cease during the wet season. After such a risky and hazardous journey down the Apaporis, he likely recalled the famous lines from Virgil's *Aeneid*: "The descent to Hell is easy; the return, impossible!"

At the beginning of October 1943, Schultes and his small crew set off at dawn. As the river narrowed and increased in speed, Schultes heard a distant rumble and saw a plume of mist in the distance. Huge sandstone slabs emerged from the churning river. The crew navigated over to the right bank against the river's strengthening force. Tired as they were from the long journey, they slowly carried the boat along an overland trail.

ANCIENT RAMPARTS: JIRIJIRIMO & YAYACOPI

Schultes had arrived at one of the great natural wonders of Colombia: the falls at Jirijirimo. For much of its lower course, the Apaporis is broad and meandering, measuring 1,500 meters across before arriving at an ancient mass of hard, metamorphosed rock that forces the powerful river through a chasm just 40 meters wide.

Preceded by nearly a kilometer of rapids, the fall itself begins with several giant rock steps before the water tumbles over a vertical drop some 30 meters high. During the rainy season, the high water almost completely covers the rocks with churning whitewater; in the dry season, the water is barely visible as it falls between the rocks. Schultes mused that – when viewed from a plane during the dry season – it appeared that the falls could be forded by jumping from one rock to the next, "but such is not the case" (Field Notebook).

As his crew rested, Schultes carefully picked his way along the side of the gorge against the perpetual mists and deafening roar of the falls. There, Schultes noticed a strange plant with alga-like leaves clinging to the rocks. Unfortunately, he was travelling without his plant collecting equipment for the first time of his career, due to the journey's difficulty and many overland portages. He vowed to return to study this plant, which he did eight years later, in 1951.

He would learn that local Makuna called the plant moo-á, and they used it as a form of table salt by reducing its leaves to ashes. Sodium chloride, the basis of salt common to most of the world, does not exist in the Amazon, and for centuries indigenous communities throughout the Amazon have used the potassium-rich ashes of river herbs to flavor their food.

A species of *Rhyncholacis*, the plant is a member of the Podostemaceae family of aquatic plants. These herbs have developed remarkable adaptations to the difficult riverine habitat: "The podostemonaceous plants have tough, alga-like leaves that come out at the height of the rainy season and clothe the rocks where the flood will reach its fullest. The tiny white flowers have blossomed in time to set ripe fruit for the fullest sweep of the waters" (*Where the Gods Reign*, 98).

After hauling the canoe overland around the falls, they resumed their journey down the Apaporis, shortly thereafter to find a mysterious chasm.

> The mighty Apaporis, after it tumbles over the Falls of Jirijirimo, enters a long and narrow chasm walled in by high vertical cliffs. At one point the whole river disappears into a tunnel, flowing tranquilly and deep through the curious fault. This is a place of awful mystery to the Indians of the area who, except for the medicine-men, never travel through the chasm, and the tunnel is known to them only through hearsay. (*Where the Gods Reign*, 56)

111

After emerging from the Jirijirimo canyon, the Apaporis resumed its tranquil path for another 5 miles, until arriving at a massive, horseshoe-shaped falls known as Yayacopi. Schultes later wrote "the thundering falls of Yayacopi strike awe into the hearts of the Indians of the region, accustomed as they are to the titanic forces of angry waters everywhere in the Apaporis basin" (*Where the Gods Reign*, 62).

The rapids of the Apaporis – of which Yayacopi and Jirijirimo are the largest – have strong spiritual significance to the Makunas and other nations of the lower Apaporis. It is said that in ancient times a fierce group inhabited the headwaters of the Apaporis River. This warlike band would attack the Makunas, at one point nearly annihilating them. A primordial shaman determined to protect his people took *yagé* for seven days, allowing him to commune with friendly spirits. Together, they raised a series of mountains across the Apaporis, forming impassable rapids imbued with magical spells that have protected the people of the lower Apaporis ever since.

Schultes noted that Makuna shaman would make pilgrimages to perform elaborate incantations at the foot of Yayacopi. The Makuna would also paddle for several days to fish in the richly stocked whirlpools at the base of the falls. However, they never willingly traveled above the rapids, leaving the upper Apaporis uninhabited for many decades.

> In view of the natural beauty and complexity of this waterfall there can be little wonder why the Indians ascribe a supernatural origin to it. (*Where the Gods Reign*, 86)

At night, in the malocas of the indigenous groups living below the waterfalls, Schultes would sit with the shamans and other elders, imbibing coca powder and tobacco syrup. There, he listened to mythical stories about the ancient past and about the thunderous waterfalls of Jirijirimo and Yayacopi. The Tucano language family spans Colombia, Ecuador, Brazil and Peru. Members of an eastern group – the Coreguaje, Siona, and Secoya – are completely isolated from the western group. It is believed that the Carijona invasion of the 1500s led to the division of the Tucano-speaking groups, lending credence to the oral history that the great waterfalls were protection against fierce cannibal invaders.

THE ROCK OF NYI

Although low on supplies, Schultes turned north off the Apaporis to paddle up the Pira Piraná River, arriving at one of the most elaborate rock carvings in the entire northwest Amazon: the Rock of Nyi. Located on the banks of the Pira Paraná almost exactly on the equator, the Rock of Nyi is a remarkable feat of artistry: five and a half feet tall, the stylized anthropomorphic design is carved into an extremely hard granite boulder, at times cut half an inch deep.

The Rock of Nyi is revered by local indigenous groups. For them, this petroglyph honors four mythical cultural heroes who used the sacred trumpets of the Yurupari to create the rivers, mountains, ritual artifacts and cosmos, while confronting evil spirits and turning them into stone.

Schultes noted that the Pira Paraná featured more rock carvings then neighboring rivers. Most were located in inaccessible locations near swiftly flowing narrows in the river or at rapids or waterfalls. Sacred petroglyphs such as Nyi account for just a few of the many holy sites known to the peoples of the lower Apaporis and Vaupés, nearly all of which are connected to their view of the mythological origins of the world.

The Tucano-speaking nations of the lower Apaporis believe that humanity originates in the Amazon, known to them as the "River of Milk", and in the Pira Paraná, which they call the "River of Water of the Yurupari." The mouth of the Amazon is said to be the original maloca of the Yurupari and the "Door of the Waters" from which life emanated. It is here that ancestral anacondas lived, receiving great knowledge from the jaguar spirits of the Yurupari.

Per this mythology, in primordial times, a great noise sent the anacondas fleeing the maloca, and scattering out into the ocean. Supernatural "creators" gathered them, giving each a name such as the Celestial Anaconda, the Anaconda of Remedy, the Fish Anaconda, and the Water Anaconda. From the Door of the Waters, the Ancestral Anacondas emerged to migrate up the Amazon River, dividing into separate paths. As they ascended, the anacondas designated the territories of the lower Apaporis.

As the ancestral anaconda swam up the Amazon, they periodically halted to provide their gifts of knowledge and sacred plants, in the process creating a variety sacred sites imbued with spirits. The indigenous peoples of the lower Apaporis and Vaupés believe that these sacred sites are interconnected, spanning not only their territory but the entire Amazon basin as well.

These sites are divided into categories with distinct rules for how they must be maintained. Mountains and stones are believed to be sacred places of ancestral importance, and held in high reverence. Savannas, especially in swampy headwaters, are areas that cannot be utilized for any purpose. Rivers and lakes can be used, but with restrictions. Sometimes it is necessary to be accompanied by a shaman, or to first receive permission from them to visit sacred sites.

The sites are said to be inhabited by ancient spirits who local people believe are the true owners of the world. It is these spirits that ensure the health and prosperity of the surrounding peoples and forests, making sacred locales important areas of pilgrimage and concentration to help mankind maintain a connection to and equilibrium with nature.

The Tucano-speaking groups of the Apaporis and Vaupés region practice elaborate ceremonies in accordance with annual harvest calendars, which they believe maintain spiritual balance and prosperity within their territories. These ceremonies are led by traditional healers known as the "Jaguar Shamans of the Yuruparí," who, after ingesting *yagé*, coca, and chicha (a fermented beverage), undertake vast spiritual journeys between sacred sites, cleansing their territory as they travel, thereby preventing sickness and hunger while promoting spiritual well-being within their communities.

These ceremonies are accompanied by chanting, and punctuated by haunting music played on bamboo pan pipes, thumping sticks and leg rattles, all of which are made from locally available plants and designed to bring on a trance state as the shamans and their people connect with the Cosmos.

OVERLAND TO THE MIRITÍ PARANÁ

Immediately after arriving in Jinogojé in February 1952, Schultes made plans to travel overland south to the remote Mirití Paraná River, home to the little-known Yukuna, Tanimuka and Matapi. Born in the lightly forested lowlands between the Apaporis and Caquetá, the blackwater Mirití Paraná flows for more than three hundred miles over seven major rapids before emptying into the whitewater Caquetá River.

In early March of that year, Schultes and Jacome Cabrera descended the Apaporis from the mouth of the Pira Paraná and turned to paddle up the Popeyacá River for two days, passing several malocas along the way. Cabrera was the perfect guide: the son of a Colombian father and a Tukano mother, he had spent most of his life in the region and fluently spoke several of the local languages.

Approaching the narrow headwaters of the Popeyaca, they abandoned their canoe and proceeded on foot, undertaking the difficult overland hike through the forest to the headwaters of the Guacayá – the largest tributary of the Mirití Paraná.

After a day of walking, they came upon an isolated massif emerging from the forest. It seemed as if a titanic boulder had split in half, creating two small mountains. The Tanimuka know this odd peak as the "Mountain of the Little People" and believe that tiny people emerge in swarms from caves and crevices to attack intruders with powerful magic. Thunder and sickness are said to originate in these mountains when the chief of the little people is preparing magic and poisons.

Schultes and Cabrera continued on to the Guacayá, spending a week there with the Tanimuka, Yukunas and the Matapies, whose language had been lost a generation before. Cabrera knew that these communities would soon be hosting a great festival, one of five throughout the year corresponding to annual harvest cycles. The upcoming festival would be the spectacular *Kai-ya-ree* - the Dance of the Spirits - in celebration of the pupunha, or peach palm harvest.

BACTRIS GASIPAES: THE PEACH PALM

Known as chontaduro and peijibaye in Spanish, pupunha in Portuguese, and peach palm in English, *Bactris gasipaes* was domesticated in the western Amazon in Pre-Columbian times and spread as far north as Central America. The large, orange or reddish peach palm fruits are typically boiled or roasted. Some are instead used for dry meal, suitable for storage throughout the year, an important quality in the rainforest environment where food items usually spoil quickly. Peach palm fruits are also used to prepare a *chicha*, a delicious and mildly alcoholic drink prepared by kneading the flesh of the fruit in water to create a kind of mash, which is then tightly packed into baskets and buried for several weeks, allowing it to ferment into a nutritious beer. It is an essential component of multi-day indigenous ceremonies: entire canoes are filled with the beverage, and the festivities continue until the *chicha* is no more.

Kai-ya-ree — THE DANCE OF THE SPIRITS

Schultes returned to the Guacayá at the end of April 1952, as the final preparations for the festival were underway. Schultes referred to the ceremony as the *Kai-ya-ree*, but it is also known as the Baile de Muñeco - the Dance of the Dolls - a name believed to have been ascribed by outsiders in the 20th century but commonly used by indigenous inhabitants of the Mirití-Paraná river even today. The celebrants had begun to gather from as far as five days away, congregating about a day's walk away from the maloca where the ceremony would be held.

When ready for the festival to begin, the maloquero – the so-called "owner" of the maloca, typically a chief or a shaman – sends a signal using the enormous manguare drums made from hollowed tree trunks that are audible up to a six-hour walk away from the maloca, even further when the sound travels along the river rather than through the rainforest. As each participant arrives, the chief of the dance performs an unusual chant, recounting the events of the previous year. The Yukuna chief opens the ceremony by circling around the maloca three times while carrying a six-foot rattling wand.

The ceremony begins at midnight, and participants wear elaborate costumes of brown barkcloth shirts and long, free-flowing grass skirts, dyed pitch black along the bottom edge. Intricate, sometimes grotesque masks of black and yellow are worn to represent devils, spirits and many forest animals, including tapirs, bees, squirrels, monkeys, and jaguars. The ceremony consists of a long series of individual dances, each dedicated to a different animal or spirit and each with its own intricate step and chant. The dances dedicated the animal spirits mimic their movements and sometimes their vocalizations.

As far as we know, Schultes was the first western scientist to participate in this unique ritual, and described the various dances in his seminal paper "Palms and Religion":

> The young boys, those from eight to twelve years of age, dressed in the typical shirt but with the head covered with a hammered bark hood upon which the facial features of a monkey have been delineated, begin with the Monkey Dance. It is a quick, lithe dance mimicking the nervous jumping of monkeys from branch to branch; and the boys carry leafy branches which they wave rhythmically while chanting in high-pitched voices, very suggestive of the chattering of monkeys in the tree tops.

> The Jaguar Dance, with characteristics stealthy half steps interrupted on occasion with pounces and a whining, snarling catlike chant, is performed by only the nimblest and most experienced of dancers. The mask is a superb creation: a replica in black pitch of a jaguar head, replete with eyes flashing with tiny pieces of mirror. Whiskers, and snarling mouth set with wooden teeth.

> The Tapir Dance, slow and lumbering, has a fanciful tapir-head mask, and the Anteater Dance mask stands out among all the others because of its realistic, long, curved snout. In the Deer Dance, the movements are graceful and rapid in the extreme, consisting mostly of intricately interweaving in a running, darting step performed with and unbelievable mimicry of the deer's nervous and frightened manner. A low, sustained buzzing chant accompanies the Wild Bee Dance, and a similar song honors another insect in the Wasp Dance; the masks for both are most ingeniously fashioned with the tufts of tree cotton or kapok to simulate the hairiness of the insect. The most unexpected beauty attends the Dance of the Bats, the masks for which are strikingly representative of the bat and the chants for which are squeaky and shrill to mimic the bat's voice. (Schultes, 1972)

The ceremony continues for 56 hours, the dancers stopping only to fortify themselves with enormous quids of mambe (coca powder), peach palm beer, smoked game, and titanic snorts of tobacco snuff.

So important was this ritual to Schultes' thinking and worldview that he prominently displayed the photos of the Yukunas taking snuff and Yukunas wrestling in his office in the Harvard Botanical Museum.

> Tobacco is not smoked during the *Kai-ya-ree*, but great gourdfuls of snuff are made. The older men dry and pulverize finely the tenderest leaves of tobacco (*Nicotiana tabacum*) and mix with the powder equal amounts of the leaf ashes of the yam (*Dioscorea* spp.); the

resulting snuff is a greyish-white powder which is administered in teaspoonful doses through hollow bird-bone snuffing tubes. The Yukunas are excessive snuffers, just as they are extraordinary consumers of coca. ... It is an honor to be offered a snuffing by a friend who fills the tube with snuff, inserts one end in his mouth, the other end in the recipient's nostril, and gives a strong but quick puff. (Schultes, 1972)

In addition to celebrating the harvest of the peach palm, the ceremony is meant to commemorate the evolution of the nation and its place within the universe. The Dance is said to have originally been taught to the neighboring Letuama by a mythic ancestor so that the reverent could express their gratitude to the surrounding spirits, plants (particularly the peijibaye), and animals (particularly fish) for support and sustenance. Through this celebration, the animals are said to be both placated and domesticated, replacing the wildness of nature.

COSTUME PREPARATION

Schultes was intrigued by the ingenious use of plants to create the elaborate costumes used during the festival. The coarse brown shirts are created by hammering the inner back of the llanchama (*Olmedia aspera*), a common 20-meter tree of the fig family. The ankle-length skirt is made from the peeled bark of a large tree of the Brazil nut family. The lower section of these skirts are submerged in a dark grey water-clay mixture, causing a chemical reaction between the clay and the bark that permanently dyes the skirt a striking shade of glossy black. The dancers wore rattling anklets to help punctuate the rhythmic steps of the dance. They were made from the cultivated fruits of a vine of the cucumber family, the Cucurbitaceae. Schultes immediately recognized that this was a species previously unknown to science, and named it *Cayaponia kathematophora* when he returned to Harvard.

The intricate masks were made by spreading the pitch from the brea tree (*Symphonia* spp. and *Moronobea* spp. – tall, yellow-sap-bearing trees of the Clusiaceae family) across a bark cloth hood prepared from the same llanchama tree. The black dyes of the mask are created by extracting a yellow pitch from the tree and boiling it for several hours to darken the color, remove sticky properties, and cause it to harden faster. The end result is a shiny pitch black, adding an element of the macabre to some of the demon masks.

YUKUNA MALOCA DESIGN

The Yukuna malocas where these dances are performed represent the largest works of art in the Amazon rainforest, serving as a remarkably efficient architectural design with deep symbolic meaning. These longhouses can stand over three stories tall and over 15 meters in diameter.

They feature a unique and instantly recognizable shape: a round base topped by a semiconical roof with two gabled openings oriented to the east and west that permit air and sunlight to enter and cooking smoke to escape. The windows, sometimes called "ears" in local languages, are effectively designed and constructed to keep the maloca inhabitants dry despite the pervasive tropical downpours.

In the past, a Yukuna longhouse could serve as a home to 200 people and would last for about fifteen years. The Yukuna still build these magnificent structures entirely from wild plants: the great roofs were usually woven from "puy" (*Lepidocaryum tenue*) or "carana" (*Mauritia carana*) palm leaves, the latter when the malocas are built on or near white-sand savannas. The palisade walls are constructed of the wood of the *Aspidosperma excelsum* – a tall and strong forest tree, often used to make canoe paddles elsewhere in Amazonia – and the great structural support beams seem to be trunks of "acapu" trees (*Vouacapoua americana*). Most astonishing of all is that even today, these structures are built without nails: all materials are woven together or tied with rainforest vines and lianas.

According to Dr. Martin von Hildebrand, the leading authority on the people of this region, the Yukuna maloca serves as a place of residence, a ceremonial center, a cemetery, a sundial and a model of the cosmos. The central region between the four central posts is a sacred space that serves as the ceremonial center of maloca life. The surrounding area between the four inner posts and the second ring of posts is a public space. The periphery of the maloca near the outer palisade is where the families eat, sleep, rest and bury their dead.

The malocas are also divided along north-south and east-west axes, with certain sections reserved for traditionally male activities such as preparing and chewing coca, and others for traditionally female activities such as preparation of cassava. The triangular windows in the peak serve as an astronomical instrument, used by the Yukuna to track the equinox based on the movement of the sun across the floor. In sum, in the globe's hottest and wettest ecosystem, the maloca keeps her inhabitants cool and dry as well as spiritually nourished.

BETRAYAL BY THE USDA

In December 1943, after descending 600 miles down the Apaporis River, Schultes and his crew arrived at La Pedrera with less than a gallon of gas, as the outboard motor sputtered and died. Schultes had been declared missing months earlier after an overflight ordered by the Rubber Reserve Company failed to reveal the missing expedition crew. When he strolled into the herbarium in Bogotá several months later with a load of plant specimens under his arm, several colleagues were said to have nearly fainted.

Schultes felt a special connection to the Apaporis. From his groundbreaking explorations of its headwaters in Chiribiquete, to his long, perilous descent of the river, he knew it like no other foreigner.

On his initial descent of the Apaporis, he had meticulously charted the course of the river and made detailed counts of *Hevea* on its banks, finding and identifying unique and potentially valuable varieties. His mission would soon change from mere inventory to coordinating the collection of *Hevea* specimens, including seeds that might enable the creation of disease-resistant plantations in the Americas.

In the course of this work, Schultes often returned to the Apaporis, establishing rubber stations at Soratama and Jinogoje and coordinating rubber latex collection efforts in those regions. He and his indigenous colleagues had scoured some of the least-known and most inaccessible rainforests in the world to bring back a trove of rubber specimens of all shapes and sizes, some high-yielding, others pest-resistant.

The U.S. government decided that the only means to prevent future scenarios in which the U.S. might be deprived a supply of natural rubber was to create plantations in the New World. Schultes' new mission was to collect seeds from a variety of rubber species to establish a repository of *Hevea* genetic diversity for future research. With this germplasm bank, experts would be able to experiment with interbreeding to increase productivity and resistance to pests and diseases.

As denizens of equatorial regions, these trees could not be grown in North America, so another secure and ecologically suitable site was sought. The people in charge settled on a famous botanical station in Turrialba, Costa Rica due to its favorable microclimate and distance from areas already affected by the rubber blight. It was believed that Schultes' botanical treasures could be safely planted and nurtured by fellow scientists in the most stable of the Central American republics.

However, due to the end of the war and advances in synthetic rubber manufacture, the need to create a sustainable supply of natural rubber became less urgent. Even though many products still required natural rubber – automobile tires, surgical instruments, etc. – the World War was long over, eliminating the most pressing threat. In an act of great shortsightedness, the U.S. government eliminated the rubber program on October 12, 1953.

Schultes wanted to compile all of his rubber notes and knowledge into a comprehensive report, but his request for support was denied. Needing a source of income upon his return to the United States, Schultes took the only position available as curator at the Harvard Orchid Herbarium. This job had formal legal stipulations that demanded complete focus on orchids, making it impossible for Schultes to continue his rubber work for several years. He would never finish his comprehensive rubber report, an enormous loss to science.

THE AMAZON: THEN AND NOW
SCHULTES AS A CONSERVATIONIST

Once he began his work in South America in 1941, Schultes became a strong conservation advocate, championing partnerships with indigenous communities to protect the Amazon rainforest.

Schultes knew well that the rainforests of South America contained an extraordinary wealth of chemical compounds that could benefit humanity if properly researched and utilized. Felling the forest not only diminished biodiversity (and fueled climate change, as we now know), it also destroyed the hidden chemical wealth of plants that might provide the basis for lifesaving medicines or economically valuable products.

Throughout twelve years of immersive fieldwork, Schultes was continually impressed by the botanical and medical knowledge of his indigenous colleagues. He saw that in the rainforest, many indigenous people were able to distinguish plants far beyond even what a Harvard-trained botanist would be able to recognize. He observed indigenous people as they combined unrelated plants to create novel and powerful effects, and remarked that such understanding could be of great benefit to the world at large.

However, as Schultes often said: "The Indians' botanical knowledge is disappearing even faster than the plants themselves."

Schultes advocated for working with indigenous communities to record and transmit traditional knowledge. He believed this strategy would benefit the well-being of the communities and yield immense conservation benefits that could in turn, benefit humanity.

Seventy-five years after Schultes first explored the Amazon, reflecting on what has changed in these regions provides a valuable lesson on what has been lost, and what is left to protect.

SIBUNDOY VALLEY

In the early 1940s, Schultes was enchanted by Colombia's picturesque Sibundoy valley and its fascinating inhabitants. He explored the otherworldly highland páramo ecosystem, discovering many plant species new to science. He learned about these plants from Inga and Kamentsá, who possessed an extensive botanical knowledge and utilized the greatest diversity of the psychoactive plant remedies that Schultes encountered during his travels.

Today, there are some 13,000 Inga and Kamentsá people in the Sibundoy Valley, about one-third of the valley's total population. There are still many Inga and Kamentsá taitas (shamans) and elders working to protect their knowledge of medicinal plants, including members of the Union of Indigenous *Yagé* Healers of the Colombian Amazon (UMIYAC) and the Union of Women Healers (ASOMI). Many Kamentsá people still speak their unusual and unique language.

The Sibundoy Valley changed rapidly during the second half of the twentieth century. Improved road access led to rapid colonization and the displacement of Inga and Kamentsá communities from much of their ancestral lands. In recent years, the region has been embroiled in controversy due to extensive mining activity and the construction of a new highway leading from Pasto to Mocoa. Indigenous communities have led the protests against mining activity and the road, which they see as a threat to their way of life.

Since 2015, the Colombian government, local indigenous associations, and the Amazon Conservation Team have partnered to carry out the formal expansion of more than 80,000 hectares of indigenous reserves in the upper Putumayo River region. These expanded reserves provide Inga and Kamentsá communities with improved legal land rights over their ancestral territories, while also establishing a protective ring around the Sibundoy Valley, helping to protect water-rich páramo ecosystems in the headwaters of the mighty Putumayo River, the most important waterway in the Colombian Amazon.

KOFÁN TERRITORY

When Schultes visited in 1940s, the Kofáns were renowned for their powerful shamans, who possessed perhaps the most extensive plant pharmacopoeias of all the Colombian Amazon. They were masters of the plant-based poisons whose chemical compounds revolutionized surgical anesthetics. Schultes noted they knew numerous unstudied herbal remedies, including a potential anticoagulant that he felt had important commercial potential.

In the 1940s, Kofán territory reached from the Guamuéz River in southern Colombia to the Aguarico river in northern Ecuador. Schultes noted that this equatorial region had perhaps the highest amount of plant diversity he encountered throughout his travels.

Oil was discovered in Kofán territory in the 1950s, leading to extensive extraction and contamination from ruptured wells and pipelines. Oil extraction and the related development of roads and infrastructure sparked a flood of colonization, displacing the Kofán from their ancestral territories. Since the 1980s, the Kofán suffered terribly during Colombia's internal conflict.

The Kofán now live on several indigenous reserves on both sides of the Ecuador / Colombia border. Several protected areas have been established for the protection of Kofán lands. In 2008, Kofán communities partnered with the Colombian National Parks Service and the Amazon Conservation Team to establish the 10,204-hectare Orito-Ingi Ande Sanctuary for Medicinal Plants and Flora, marking the creation of a unique new land designation recognizing the botanical knowledge of indigenous communities and the cultural value of medicinal plants.

WITOTO

In 1942, Schultes traveled through the lower Putumayo river basin, finding Witoto communities still recovering from the terrors and abuses of the rubber boom less than a generation before. Even though their culture had been severely abused by rubber barons and later missionaries, the Witotos still maintained their language and much of their culture, employed many medicinal plants, and still danced to the sound of their *manguare* drums made from hollowed trees. Seventy years after Schultes began his work in their territory, the Witoto communities maintain many aspects of their culture.

To protect tribal lands, the Predio Putumayo Indigenous Reserve was created in 1988, encompassing a huge tract of land between the Caquetá and Putumayo rivers, a territory home to Witoto, Bora, Miraña, Andoque, Ocaina, Muinane, and Nonuya nations. The reserve now measures 5,819,505 hectares, making it one of the largest legally demarcated indigenous territories in the entire Amazon, nearly equal in size to the state of West Virginia. The Puerto Zábalo Los Monos and Monochoa Witoto reserves were also created in 1988, covering a combined 474,573 hectares north of the Caquetá River, later expanded by a combined 567,890 ha.

The creation of these vast indigenous reserves was part of a larger effort in the late 1980's to secure land rights for all indigenous peoples of the Colombian Amazon. During the Presidency of Virgilio Barco Vargas and following the leadership of Martín von Hildebrand as Head of Indigenous Affairs, the Colombian state legally demarcated an area of more than 100,000 square miles of communal indigenous lands through the creation of 162 Resguardos Indígenas, later encoded into law in the 1991 Colombian Constitution.

CHIRIBIQUETE

After his 1943 expedition to Chiribiquete, Schultes was deeply impressed with its spectacular lost world mountains, keeping a photo of the Cerro Campana prominently displayed on the wall of his Harvard office for over five decades. He was one of the first to report the prehistoric cave paintings in Chiribiquete, and was a constant advocate for the creation of a natural park to protect the cultural and botanical treasures of Chiribiquete.

Largely due to his initiative and his urging, in 1989, the 1,300,000-hectare Chiribiquete National Park was created by the Colombian government, thus protecting one of the most unique and pristine ecosystems and cultural sites in the entire Amazon.

In 2013, the Chiribiquete National Park was nearly doubled to more than 2,750,000 hectares, making it the largest national park in Colombia and the second largest national park in Amazonia. The park was expanded in part to protect as many as three uncontacted or isolated indigenous communities living in the region. The Chiribiquete park expansion represents just a part of Colombia's cutting-edge strategy to safeguard vulnerable isolated indigenous communities, through an innovative collaboration between local indigenous communities, the Colombian government, and the Amazon Conservation Team.

YAIGOJÉ-APAPORIS

Schultes spent years based in the lower Apaporis River region in the 1950s, learning about the complex culture and ethnomedical knowledge of the many Tucano-speaking groups in the region. These groups were remarkably multilingual and possessed perhaps the most complex and sophisticated worldview in the Amazon.

The lower Apaporis River region has seen persistent threat from mining activity seeking to exploit the minerals of the rivers, hills and forests sacred to the Tukano peoples. There are several existing mining titles with many more applications pending. The 2013 announcement of a "Strategic Mining Reserve" covering much of the Vaupés region was widely denounced and is on hold for now, thanks to efforts the local communities and the Gaia Amazonas Foundation.

These nations received legal title to their lands with the creation of the approximately 3,500,000-hectare Gran Vaupés Indigenous Reserve and the approximately 1,000,000-hectare Yaigojé Apaporis Indigenous Reserve. The Yaigojé Apaporis National Park was created in 2012 to provide increased protection and protect subsoil resources from potential mining activity. In 2011, UNESCO recognized the Jaguar Shamans of the Yuruparí as part of the intangible heritage of humanity in need of protection, marking the first time an entire culture complex has received this designation.

MIRITÍ-PARANÁ

In 1952, Schultes participated in the three-day-long *Kai-ya-ree* ritual dance with the Yukuna and Tanimuka of the Mirití-Paraná. This was just one of the Yukuna and Tanimuka's five annual dances, which had maintained the practice of many of their traditional ceremonies. Schultes adored the Yukuna, always saying that they ranked among the strongest, kindest, friendliest and most reliable peoples that he knew.

Today, the proud Yukuna and Tanimuka communities of the Mirití-Paraná still maintain their traditional dances and ceremonies, including the *Kai-ya-ree*, long ago danced by Schultes as he truly entered the rainforest realm. Thanks to the Colombian government, local colleagues and the Yukuna and Tanimuka themselves, the Mirití-Paraná Indigenous Reserve, encompassing the entire Mirití River watershed, was created in 1981 and now has an area of more than 1,500,000 hectares, larger than the state of Connecticut.

SCHULTES AND THE ETHNOPHARMACOLOGIC SEARCH FOR PSYCHOACTIVE DRUGS IN RETROSPECT

Schultes never failed to point out that he did not "discover" new hallucinogens – the indigenous peoples had been using them all along. From his first encounter with peyote in the Kiowas' Oklahoma tipis to his field research on teonanácatl / magic mushrooms, ololiuqui, *ayahuasca* and Virola snuff, he never wavered in his belief that these species and the wisdom of the shamans who employed them offered great potential for western patients and medicine. Schultes strongly believed that these shamanic approaches to treatment offered novel approaches to understanding, diagnosing and treating the human mind in ways beyond the reach of western physicians. Moreover, he believed that these plants harbored novel chemicals which could serve as the bases for new medicines. Given that the compounds extracted from the Mexican mushrooms played a role in the development of the first beta blockers and that western doctors are seeing promising results in the treatment of intractable ailments like PTSD and depression using compounds like mescaline and *ayahuasca* alkaloids, Schultes' wisdom and field results maintain their relevance and their promise – both today and in the foreseeable future.

REFERENCES

Davis, W. (1997). *One River*. New York: Simon and Schuster.
Davis, W. (2004). *The Lost Amazon: The Photographic Journey of Richard Evans Schultes*. San Francisco: Chronicle Books.
Schultes, R.E. (1988). *Where the Gods Reign: Plants and Peoples of the Colombian Amazon*. London: Synergetic Press.
Schultes, R.E. (1992). *Vine of the Soul: Medicine Men, Their Plants and Rituals*. Santa Fe: Synergetic Press.

Photos courtesy of the Richard Evans Schultes Estate and Synergetic Press.

AFRICA, AUSTRALIA & SE ASIA

Kabbo's !Kwaiń: The Past, Present and Possible Future of *Kanna*

■■ *Nigel Gericke,* MD ■■

Founding Director of HG&H
Pharmaceuticals (Pty), Ltd.,
Bryanston, South Africa

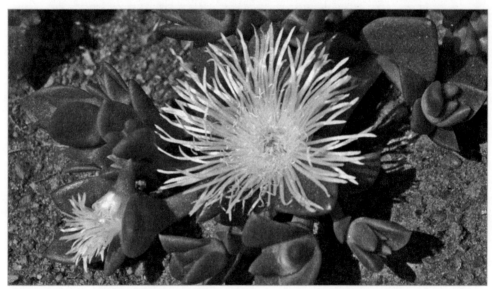

Flower of a low-mesembrine Sceletium cultivar.

ABSTRACT

PART I

The history of the use of *kanna*, the traditionally used plant material derived from a number of Sceletium species, is given from 1610-1971. This overview includes fragments of history documenting European ships docking in the Cape to search for *kanna* roots as a "ginseng" to trade in the Far East, and an ethnographic record from the 1700s transcribed directly from ||Kabbo, a /Xam San "Bushman" from the Breakwater Convict Station in Cape Town, who gave us the name *!k"waï* for *kaauwgoed*, the Dutch name for *kanna*, and his own account of the uses of the plant.

PART II

The recent ethnobotany, ethnopharmacology and pre-clinical research on a commercialized standardized extract of Sceletium (trademarked Zembrin®) is given for the period 1995 to 2017. *In vitro* studies have demonstrated that the major alkaloids of *kanna*, including mesembrine, mesembrenone and mesembrenol, are responsible for the psychoactivity of Sceletium, and have dual serotonin reuptake inhibitory (SRI) activity and phosphodiesterase-4 (PDE4) inhibitory activity. The effect of the extract of *Sceletium tortuosum*, Zembrin®, on brain electrical activity has been studied *in vivo*, demonstrating by discriminant analyses that the quantitative EEG electropharmacogram of the extract plots in close proximity to the plots for *Ginkgo biloba*, *Rhodiola rosea*, and also to the first-generation pharmaceutical PDE4 inhibitor Rolipram, indicating the potential of this extract for managing anxiety and depression and enhancing cognitive function.

PART III

Clinical experience with Sceletium is summarized and the results of pilot randomized, double-blind, placebo-controlled clinical studies on the extract of *Sceletium tortuosum*, Zembrin®, are presented, including:

- A safety and tolerability study.
- A pharmaco-Magnetic Resonance Imaging study.
- A study on cognitive function domains using CNS Vital Signs, a computerized neurocognitive test battery.
- A study looking at changes in brain electrical activity in response to cognitive and emotional challenges; changes in psychometric tests; and changes in the Hamilton Anxiety Scale (HAM-A).

PART IV

Scenarios on the future of *kanna* and alkaloids derived from *kanna* are considered.

Folk names for traditionally used Sceletium species

kanna	Nama-speaking Khoikhoi people. Sometimes also written *canna* and *channa*.
kougoed	Afrikaans-speaking people of European or mixed descent, derived from the earlier Dutch *kaauwgoed* or *kauwgoed*, meaning "chewing stuff."
!k"waï	Also *!k"wai:n*. /Xam-speaking San people. This language is now extinct.

BOTANY

The genus Sceletium of the Family Aizoaceae, Mesembryanthemoideae, is characterized by the distinctly skeletonized leaf venation visible in dried older leaves. Sceletium is a genus with a climbing, or decumbent, habit and succulent leaves that sometimes have prominent idioblasts, or bladder-like cells. The flowers range from white or yellow to pale pink. The fruit capsules contain numerous very small kidney-shaped seeds, brown to black in color.

The genus is distributed in the arid southwestern parts of South Africa, including parts of three provinces: Northern Cape Province, Western Cape Province, and Eastern Cape Province. The plant populations and individual plants are typically widely scattered, but in the *Kougoedvlakte* (literally translated as "Chewing Stuff Plains") of Namaqualand in the Northern Cape Province, and in the *Kannaland* district (literally, "The Land of Kanna") in the Western Cape Province, the plants were once locally abundant and traded widely.

Klak et al. (2007) proposed a single genus, Mesembryanthemum, that includes members of the genus Sceletium. However, for the purpose of this paper, the use of the genus Sceletium is retained, and the genus Mesembryanthemum (sometimes spelled Mesembrianthemum in former times) is used when quoting historical texts.

The taxonomy of Sceletium is complex, and will hopefully become clearer when species based on standard plant morphological features can be interpreted in the light of DNA-bar coding and plant chemistry. Eight Sceletium species are recognized in the revision by Gerbaulet (1996):

Sceletium tortuosum (L.) N.E. Br.
Sceletium crassicaule (Haw.) L. Bolus
Sceletium emarcidum (Thunb.) L. Bolus ex H.J. Jacobson
Sceletium exalatum Gerbaulet
Sceletium expansum (L.) L. Bolus
Sceletium rigidum, L. Bolus
Sceletium strictum L. Bolus
Sceletium varians (Haw.) Gerbaulet.

To illustrate the taxonomic complexity at the species level, the following synonyms have been used for *Sceletium tortuosum* (L.) N.E.: (Nortje, 2011).

Mesembryanthemum aridum Moench
Mesembryanthemum concavum Haw.
Mesembryanthemum tortuosum L.
Pentacoilanthus tortuosus (L.) Rappa and Camorrone
Phyllobolus tortuosus (L.)Bittrich
Sceletium boreale L. Bolus
Sceletium compactum L. Bolus
Sceletium concavum (Haw.) Schwantes
Sceletium framesii L. Bolus
Sceletium gracile L. Bolus
Sceletium joubertii L. Bolus
Sceletium namaquense L. Bolus var. *namaquense*
Sceletium namaquense L. Bolus var. *subglobosum* L. Bolus
Sceletium ovatum L. Bolus
Sceletium tugwelliae L. Bolus

PART I

HISTORICAL REPORTS, 1610 - 1971

Early visitors to the Cape of Good Hope in the 17th century frequently emphasized the value attached to *kanna*. The captains of trading ships en route to the East Indies thought of the roots of *kanna* as a Cape ginseng, and also called it *ningin* root or *ningimm* root, a corruption of vernacular names used for the ginseng root they had seen in Japan and China. Ships of the East India Company, stopping off at the Cape en route to Japan to stock up on fresh water, fruit and vegetables, were instructed to search for the roots as a valued item for trade.

1610

The English East Indiaman *The Globe*, under the command of Captain Hippon, stopped to replenish water supplies at the Cape of Good Hope en route to the East Indies. Captain Hippon's lieutenant, Peter Floris, reported:

> Being by Gods grace here arrived, wee presently fell to the ordering of the shippe, and hooping of our caske to fill freshe water, for much refreshing was not here to bee had att this tyme of the yeare, by the greate quantitie of rayne, being now in the chiefeste of winter so that the mountains laye covered with snowe : during which tyme wee used great diligence in seeking of the roote Ningimm according to our instruction, the aforesaid 2 Holland shipps being expressly come thether for the same purpose, being one of Japan that first discovered the secret; butt, being winter tyme, there was for this tyme no more to bee done but to go away as wyse as wee came, for the olde roote

being decayed and rotten, the new leaf began onely to come foorth, so that had it not bene by reason of some information that was gotten of one who here shalbee nameles for dyvers considerations sake, wee shoulde have bene fayne to have departed without notice thereof, the right time of gathering the same being in December, January, and February, being called by the inhabitants Canna. (Moreland, 1934)

1615

Purchas 1625: Saldanha Bay, approximately 130 kilometers north of the Cape of Good Hope: "The Countrey people brought vs downe of the Root Ningin, whereof wee bought one handful for a piece of Copper an inch and halfe broad, and two inches and halfe in length. Our men got [some], but not [so] full, nor ripe, this being not the [season], which in the full perfection is as tender and [sweet] as [anise seeds]. On the twentieth wee [set sail]." "Ningin, a medicinable root much prized in Japan" .

1660

"It was the control over fields of canna that made the Inqua king Hijkon "chief lord of all kings and potentates", for he was one of the patrons whose power flowed from the precious canna that grew in the desert" (Gordon, 1996, quoting from Jan van Riebeeck's journal, 21-22 Sep. 1660, from the Archives of the Nederlandsche Oost-Indische Compagnie).

1662

In 1652, the Vereenigde Oost-Indische Compagnie or VOC (the Dutch East India Company), founded a refreshment and recuperation station at the Cape of Good Hope for the benefit of the crews of its fleets trading between Europe and Asia. The station was to supply fresh fruit and vegetables, meat and clean water to the VOC ships whose crews were decimated by scurvy during the long ocean voyages. In 1662, the first commander of this station, Jan van Riebeeck, received *kanna* and sheep from the indigenous people in exchange for gifts, and pronounced that *kanna* is similar to Chinese ginseng (Smith, 1966).

1685

DUTCH EXPEDITION TO NAMAQUALAND (GERICKE, 2014)

In 1657, the first commander of the VOC's refreshment station at the Cape, Jan van Riebeeck, heard from an indigenous interpreter that the copper in indigenous tribal earrings and beads came from the Namaqua, a tribe of pastoralists who lived to the north of the Cape. Between 1659 and 1663, seven expeditions were dispatched north to the land of the Namaquas to look for copper and any other riches, but they all failed, unable to penetrate through the mountainous and difficult terrain. In 1679, Simon van der Stel was appointed commander of the settlement at the Cape of Good Hope by the VOC, and concerned himself with the development of agriculture and viticulture and the improvement of the company's botanical and herbal garden. In April 1682, some Namaqua people visited the VOC fort at Table Bay with pieces of good quality copper ore. Expeditions sent north to find the source of the copper ore failed, unable to cross the mountainous terrain.

In 1685, Hendrik van Rheede tot Drakenstein, a VOC commissioner, arrived at the Cape and gave Commander van der Stel permission to personally lead an expedition to find the Copper Mountains. In addition to the search for copper, the expedition was charged with cultivating friendly relations with the Namaquas, describing the country, and documenting useful plants. The expedition, which left the Cape of Good Hope on 25 August 1685, was a major undertaking. The party included van der Stel as commander, his three slaves, fifty-six people of mainly European extraction, a prince from Makassar (now within Indonesia), forty-six local people of mixed ancestry as drivers and leaders for the wagon train and accompanying stock animals, and a number of Khoikhoi translators. The expedition included a carriage, seven wagons, eight carts, a boat for river crossings, and two small cannon. Technical specialists accompanying the expedition included a navigator, a mineralogist, and the apothecary and artist Heinrich Claudius, who also served as the expedition's cartographer. Claudius had been sent to the Cape from Batavia in the East Indies to collect botanical specimens for a private collector, and was then retained at the Cape by the VOC on account of his exceptional abilities as naturalist and artist.

It is not known what became of the original journal of the 1685 expedition, or of Claudius' original drawings, but copies of excerpts from the expedition journal and accompanying drawings were made shortly after the expedition. One of the copies of the journal is in the collection of Trinity

College Library, Trinity College MS. 984 (TCMS), and is thought to have been removed from the Archives of the Dutch East India Company in 1691 or 1692. TCMS includes seventy-one pages of coloured drawings believed to be the work of Heinrich Claudius, with descriptive text on alternate folios. The drawings include two landscapes within the Copper Mountains, a Namaqua man and woman, forty-three plants, eleven birds, nine reptiles, one fish and eight insects. Watercolor copies of Claudius' drawings are in the collection of the Iziko South African Museum in Cape Town, known as the Codex Witsenii (CW). These copies were made in 1692 for Nicolaas Witsen, a prominent citizen of Amsterdam and a director of the Amsterdam Chamber of the VOC. A third manuscript on the expedition, written by Jan Commelin (JCMS) about 1687, is held by the Staatsbibliothek Kuturbesitz, Berlin, as ms. germ. qu. 238.

The journal entry in TCMS, which accompanies a fine painting easily recognized as Sceletium and including the flower and skeletonized lower leaves, states:

> This plant is found with the Namaquaas and then only on some of their mountains. It is gathered in October and is called Canna. It is held by them and the surrounding tribes in as great esteem as the betel or areca with the Indians. They chew the stem as well as the roots, mostly all day, and become intoxicated by it, so that on account of this effect and its fragrance and hearty taste one can expect some profit from its cultivation. Found on the 20th October. (Waterhouse et al., 1979)

The journal entry in Codex Witsenii, accompanying a copy of the painting of Sceletium, states:

> This is from the Namaquas and also other nations the famous *kanna*, which they carry in the mouth daily and chew, as the Indians do with Areca, and who do it often can easily get drunk from it, it is held in great esteem by them, like all things that corrupt the mind, and make drunk. And that there is something particular in these plants is seen not only from the activity, but also the pleasant and cordial taste, are found nowhere but on certain mountains in the country of the Namaqua and collected in October; found 20 October 1685.

1686

Guy Tachard (1651–1712), also known as Père Tachard, was a French Jesuit missionary and mathematician of the 17th century who was sent on two occasions to the Kingdom of Siam by Louis XIV, and en route spent time at the Cape of Good Hope. Translated from the original French,

> This captain, pleased with his gifts, sent us in gratitude two fat tail sheep, each tail weighing more than twenty pounds, with a large vessel full of milk, and a certain herb which they call Kanna, it is apparently this famous plant that the Chinese call Ginseng; for Monsieur Claudius, who has seen it in China, asserts that he had found two plants at the Cape, and shows us the whole figure which he had painted in nature." (Tachard, 1686)

1726

François Valentijn was a Dutch minister, naturalist and author. In his Beschryvinge van de Kaap der Goede (Descriptions of the Cape of Good Hope), he noted that the "Canna of the Hottentots closely resembles the Chinese root Nisi or Ginseng" (Serton, 1971).

1731

Peter Kolben was sent to the Cape of Good Hope with letters of introduction from the mayor of Amsterdam, with a mandate to compile a comprehensive description of South Africa for geographical research and surveying. He wrote detailed accounts of the geography, climate, flora and fauna, followed by a study of the indigenous Khoi people (called Hottentots at that time), covering their language, religion, lifestyle and customs:

> There is a Root, gather'd in the *Hottentot* Countries, called Kanna; which is in [such Esteem] among the *Hottentots* for its great vertues that they almost adore it. What greatly enflames the Value of this Root, is its Scarcity; for 'tis very rarely found. They look upon

it as the [greatest] Chearer of the Spirits, and the [noblest] Restorative in the world. They will give [almost] any Thing in Exchange for it; and will, any of 'em, run Twenty Miles upon an Errand, or perform a hard Day's Work, for a very small Bit of it. With a piece of Kanna you may manage 'em [almost] in any Manner you [please]. You win their hearts Forever by [presenting] them with the smallest Chip of it; and they will run, fetch and carry for you like your Slaves, under [so] charming an Obligation...I have often [seen] the Effects of *Kanna* upon *Hottentots*. They chew and retain it a [considerable] Time in their Mouths. But taking generally too much of it at a Time, it drowns 'em in Intoxications. They chew it not long, before their Spirits [visibly] [rise], their Eyes brighten, their Faces take a jovial Air, and they [Sport] and wanton under a [thousand] Gaieties of Imagination. But in the End it [Strips] 'em of their [Senses], and throws 'em into the [wildest] *Deliria* (Kolben, 1731).

1763

De la Caille (1763): "The Canna of the Hottentots is entirely different from [Ginseng]. I have seen both, they are entirely different. They harvest the root in the months of November and December, add water and put some honey in it, and leave it in the rocks to ferment. They drink it while it lasts, abruptly unable to do anything. When the supply is exhausted, they are long sick; eating orca restores them."

1772-1775

Carl Peter Thunberg was a Swedish botanist and physician who had been a student of Linnaeus. He made two journeys to the Eastern Cape region of South Africa between 1772 and 1774, and reported that valuable narcotic plants were found in the vicinity of the present-day town of Oudtshoorn in the Little Karoo, in an area formerly occupied by the Attaqua Khoikhoi. This area of South Africa is still known as Kannaland. According to Thunberg (Forbes, 1986),

Kon, was a name given by the Hottentots to a shrub that grew here (*Mesembryanthemum emarcidum*) and was famous all over the country. The Hottentots came far and near to fetch this shrub with the root, stalk and leaves which they stamp together, and afterwards twist them up like pig-tail tobacco; after which they let the mass ferment, and keep it by them for chewing, especially when they are thirsty. If it be chewed immediately after fermentation, it intoxicates. The word kon is said to signify a quid; the colonists call it canna root. It is found in the driest fields only, and is gathered chiefly by the Hottentots, who live near this spot. These afterwards hawk it about, frequently to a great distance, and exchange it for cattle and other commodities."

1851

The Great London Exhibition of 1851 may have been a pivotal moment in the history of Sceletium, where the plant was exposed to international visitors that would have included physicians, chemists and pharmacists. A collection of the most important Cape botanical medicines was sent to the exhibition from Cape Town by Messrs S.H. Scheuble & Co. (Gunn and Codd, 1981). Karl Wilhelm Ludwig Pappe, a German-born physician and botanist who moved to Cape Town to practice as a physician, wrote a small book as a commentary to accompany the exhibited medicinal plants. In the entry for *Sceletium tortuosum* (as *Mesembryanthemum tortuosum*. Lin.), Pappe wrote, "This species, a native of the Karroo, appears to possess narcotic properties. The Hottentots, who know it by the name *Kauw-goed*, are in the habit of chewing it, and become intoxicated, while the farmers use it in the form of decoction or tincture, as a good sedative" (Pappe, 1868).

1856

Confusion between *kanna* and ginseng seems to have persisted well into the 19th century, with a French-English Dictionary of the time describing *kanna* as a species of ginseng (Collot, 1856).

1858

The distinction between processed and unprocessed plant material, and differences in the activity of different Sceletium species, is made by Tully: "*Mesembryanthemum emarcidum*, like *Nicotiana tobacum*, is not narcotic until it has undergone a certain change in consequence of it being treated in a peculiar manner. *Mesembryanthemum tortuosum* is considered narcotic without any such change" (Tully, 1858).

1873

The Bleek and Lloyd Archive of the University of Cape Town is a remarkable collection of /Xam San oral literature, language and ethnography documented in Cape Town by W. H. I. Bleek and Lucy C. Lloyd between 1870 and the early 1880s. They became aware of a group of /Xam San prisoners at the Breakwater Convict Station in Cape Town and received permission for //Kabbo to stay in their Mowbray home as a research participant. Later, other San prisoners were also allowed to stay in the house, including ≠Kasiŋ. //Kabbo, meaning "Dream", stayed with Bleek and Lloyd between February 1871 and October 1873. He was sent from the Breakwater Convict Station, where he had been imprisoned for two years for stock theft or sharing in the spoils of theft, as prisoner Number 4628. ≠Kasiŋ arrived at Bleek and Lloyd for the first time from November 1873 until March 1874, after //Kabbo had left. He had been imprisoned at the Breakwater Convict Station for culpable homicide and served four years of a five-year sentence as prisoner Number 4435 (Digital Bleek & Lloyd, 2017).

//Kabbo and ≠Kasiŋ were shown a number of "Bushman medicines" that had been found in the hut of a "Bushman sorcerer", and their comments on these medicinal plants were transcribed into English by Wilhelm Bleek and Lucy Lloyd (MSS BC151 006; Prader-Samper, 2007). I was surprised to find that none of the botanical names of these plant medicines was known. Two informants, //Kabo and ≠Kasin independently identified the same plant sample as *kaauwgoed*, and on this basis the botanical identity was established as Sceletium sp. since no other South African plant has before or since been given this Dutch vernacular name. Indeed, the Afrikaans name for Sceletium to this day is *kougoed*, derived from the older Dutch *kaauwgoed*, meaning "chewing stuff." We finally have the first reports on the uses of Sceletium from indigenous people, in their own words, as well as the original /Xam San name for the plant as *!k"wa:ï* or *!k"wai:n*.

> Bleek's notes documented from //Kabbo *!k"wa:ï* singular and plural. *Kaauwgoed*
>
> A small plant found on the great mountains growing out of crevices in the rocks. It is chewed by Bushmen, and gives strength to their limbs; and takes away pain and makes their memory strong. The two Bushmen from Stuurmansfontein had some with them to enable them to walk till they met the wagon. Is found around the Berg Bushmen.
>
> Lloyd's notes documented from ≠Kasiŋ *!k"wai:n Kaauwgoed*
>
> If a little child that is still being suckled is ill inside, they take a little piece of it, & put it into a spoon of cold water, & rub it about in it, the water becomes yellow (like tobacco water), and they give it to the child to drink. Men and women chew it; and swallow their saliva. The plant is in some cases short, but in others long, like a pumpkin in growth. It grows on the ground. It grows in ≠Kasiŋ's place.

1874

The botanical identity of a sample of *kougoed* was confirmed to be *Mesembryanthemum tortuosum* and the uses of it were described: "The Koegoed [sic], besides being used as stated by Mr. Keyworth as a sedative for cattle, is chewed by the Hottentots as an intoxicating agent, and appears to possess narcotic properties which deserve further attention" (Holmes, 1874).

1876

Twenty-five years after the Great London Exhibition, Sceletium may have become available as a botanical medicine in the United States, evidenced by the inclusion of *Mesembryanthemum tortuosum* in C.E. Hobbs' *Botanical Hand-Book* (Hobbs, 1876) and in J.M. Nicholl's *Botanical Ready Reference* (Nicholl, 1895). These books were lists of botanicals apparently in common use in the United States, and written for apothecaries and pharmacists. In both books, the plant was classified as a narcotic.

1896

The first pharmacological research on Sceletium was reported by Isaac Meiring in the Transactions of the South African Philosophical Society. In this paper, Meiring gives the locality the plant material came from, the vernacular name as "*Hottentot's Kauwgoed*" and had the plant material used in his experiments botanically identified as *Mesembrianthemum tortuosum* L.:

> Like so many Cape plants, it has great medicinal virtues ascribed to it, chief of which are its soporific influence on young children and its curative and quieting effect on them when suffering from acidity. It is alleged that for these purposes the plant is very widely used, the method of procedure being one or two drops of the juice of the green plant is given to the child, who then enjoys a deep, quiet rest for several hours.

Meiring made a crude alkaloid extract from the plant, and noted that when injected into a frog it had a marked hypnotic effect. He then went on to do some "clinical experiments" with a tincture of dry plant material, and found it had marked pain-relieving activity "without concomitant bad effects." Meiring then gave his remaining plant material to a Dr. Rubenstein to take to Germany, where a Dr. Fromm in Freiburg found it contained a compound capable of being crystallised, and which resembled morphine in its action (Meiring, 1896).

1898

In his book Die Heilpflanzen Der Verschiedenen Völker Und Zeiten[1] , Dragendorff lists two species of Sceletium: "*Mesembryanthemum anatomicum* Hav. (*Mesembryanthemum emarcidum* Thbg). Herb is used as a light narcotic (and smoked). Also *Mesembryanthemum tortuosum* L." (Dragendorff, 1898).

1905

Juritz stated that Mesembryantheum tortuosum is soporific, causes dilatation of the pupil, and decreases sensation (Juritz, 1905).

1913

Zwicky isolated a crude alkaloid extract from *Mesembryanthemum tortuosum*, which he called mesembrine, and on testing with various chemical reagents concluded that there was no similarity between cocaine and mesembrine; he further concluded that this active principle, mesembrine, was also found in *Mesembryanthemum expansum*. In the first detailed documentation on self-ingestion of Sceletium plant material and alkaloid extract, Zwicky reported the following observations (Zwicky, 1913):

I. After chewing 5g of Sceletium:

> The taste was bitter, astringent, unpleasant, irritating to the mouth. During the chewing, tingling was noticed on his tongue, later weak anaesthesia in the mouth, which lasted for some time. The pulse remained normal, while the temperature was weakly increased from 36.9 ° to 37.1 °. I noticed nausea, headache, loss of appetite.

II. After taking a decoction of 15g of Sceletium at 14:00:

> Half an hour after taking the decoction I felt blood pressure in the head and slight headache, but it did not last long. I had the feeling that the food was not digested and only at 10:30 in the evening appetite returned. In general, the effects were not very different from the 1st experiment. ; in any case, they were not 3 times as strong as the first.

III. After taking 0.15g of an alkaloid concentrate extracted from Sceletium at 15:00:

> Congestion of the head, noises in the ears, tiredness accompanied by slight tremors in the arms and legs, headache, general depression; loss of appetite until 10 in the evening.

1928

The Khoikhoi chew the leaf for the relief of toothache and pain in the abdomen, "the effect apparently being narcotic" (Laidler, 1928).

---

1 Rough translation: The Medicinal Plants of Different Peoples and Times.

1937

Crystalline pure alkaloid was isolated from Sceletium plant material obtained from Namaqualand (Rimington and Roets, 1937), identified as mesembrine, and assigned the formula $C_{17}H_{23}O_3N$. It was concluded that this formula is identical to hyocyamine and atropine, suggesting that mesembrine is a tropane alkaloid.

1960

All Sceletium species "contain the poisonous principle "mesembrine" a relative of cocaine and other principles" (Jacobsen, 1960). Jacobsen noted that *kougoed* was still being made traditionally and sold, and concluded "perhaps it may give a valuable medicine."

1962

Sceletium tortuosum "is used as a narcotic by the African in the Queenstown district" (Watt & Breyer-Brandwijk, 1962). A geologist and mining engineer observed that "the Nama have a universal addiction to *kougoed*", and it "is also used by the Nama for the relief of all types of pain, and to relieve hunger...A Nama mother chews the root and ejects her saliva into the mouth of her child from an early age" (Watt & Breyer-Brandwijk, 1962).

1971

Herre (1971) stated that while other members of the Aizioaceae also contain mesembrine, it is present in lower concentrations than in Sceletium, which produces mesembrine when grown in North Carolina, but not in Europe and northern countries. He noted that the German pharmaceutical company C.F. Boehringer & Söhne of Mannheim was investigating Sceletium, and also the company S.B. Penick in New York.

Table 1. Summary of historical reports on preparation and uses of *Sceletium* species

SUBJECT	NOTES	REFERENCES
Species	*Mesembryanthemum tortuosum*	Tully, 1858; Pappe, 1868 ; Hobbs, 1876; Nicholl, 1895 ; Meiring, 1896; Juritz, 1905; Zwicky, 1913; Tully, 1858;
	Mesembryanthemum emarcidum	Forbes, 1986; Holmes, 1874
	Mesembryanthemum anatomicum	Dragendorff, 1898
	Mesembryanthemum expansum	Zwicky, 1913
Folk names	Ningin, Ningimm	Purchas 1625; Moreland, 1934
	Kanna, Canna	Tachard, 1686; Kolben, 1731; Moreland, 1934; Serton, 1971; Smith, 1966; Wilson, 2002; Forbes, 1986
	Kauw-goed; *Kaauwgoed; Kauwgoed;* Koegoed, *kougoed*	Holmes, 1874; Meiring, 1896; Marloth, 1917; Smith, 1966; Forbes, 1986
	!k"wa:ï ; !k"wai:n	Prader-Samper, 2007
Preparation	Roots fermented with honey Whole plant fermented Tincture Cold water infusion Drops of freshly squeezed plant Smoked Roots chewed, saliva given to infant	De La Caille, 1763 Forbes, 1986 Pappe, 1868 Prader-Samper, 2007 Meiring, 1896 Forbes, 1986; Dragendorff, 1898 Watt & Breyer-Brandwijk, 1962

SUBJECT	NOTES	REFERENCES
Activities	Intoxicant	Waterhouse et al, 1979; Kolben, 1731; Tully, 1858; Pappe, 1868; Holmes, 1874
	Narcotic, Sedative, Hypnotic	Kolben, 1731; Tully, 1858; Pappe, 1868; Holmes, 1874; Hobbs, 1876; Nicholl, 1895; Meiring, 1896; Dragendorff, 1898; Juritz, 1905; Laidler, 1928; Watt & Breyer-Brandwijk, 1962
	Decrease sensation, local anaesthesia	Juritz, 1905; Zwicky, 1913; Watt & Breyer-Brandwijk, 1962
	Nausea, loss of appetite, decrease hunger	Zwicky, 1913; Laidler, 1928
	Toothache	Laidler, 1928
	Elevate mood	Kolben, 1731
	Analgesic	Meiring, 1896; Laidler, 1928; Watt & Breyer-Brandwijk, 1962
	Pain	Prader-Samper, 2007; Laidler, 1928
	Endurance	Prader-Samper, 2007
	Memory	Prader-Samper, 2007

PART II

ETHNOBOTANY, ETHNOPHARMACOLOGY & PRE-CLINICAL RESEARCH 1995-2017

ETHNOBOTANY

In late 1991, I was given a sample of *kanna* by the ethnobotanist Fiona Archer, who had been documenting local plant uses in Namaqualand for an MSc degree in anthropology at University of Cape Town. At the time, I was searching for South African plants with psychedelic activity. On inquiring if she had encountered possible psychoactive plants from Namaqualand, Fiona told me about a plant called *kougoed*, traditionally used by locals, and that when she had tried some it felt as if her perceptions of time and space had been altered. Fiona gave me a brown paper bag containing about 500g of stringy, brown, traditionally fermented and dried *Sceletium*. I chewed a few grams of the plant material, and after about fifteen minutes, the plant caused a rather sudden rush of euphoria. Over the following hour, this gradually changed to a feeling of deep calm that persisted for some four or five hours. Following from this intriguing initial experience, my wife Olga, myself and Fiona began a period of self-experimentation and gave samples of *kanna* to friends, fellow doctors and psychiatrists, anthropologists, botanists and an African traditional healer. I wrote up some of this early experimentation in Smith et al., 1996:

> Additional information on the effect of *kougoed* has been documented from a dozen individuals who self-experimented with the traditionally prepared plant material, and provided oral anecdotes of these experiences. Most users found that *kougoed* induced a marked anxiolytic effect. One informant used about 5ml of powdered *kougoed* orally before giving a lecture he was anxious about. He reported feeling relaxed throughout the lecture with no cognitive impairment. Many users felt that *kougoed*, on its own or with alcohol, enhanced social intercourse at parties and functions. Users felt considerably less inhibited and self-conscious, and more open than usual in conversation with strangers. One user claimed she felt that *kougoed* was a "truth drug". Of *kougoed*, some claimed there was a synergistic effect with alcohol, and with smoked *dagga* (*Cannabis*

131

sativa). One experimenter, a polysubstance abuser, used *kougoed* in addition to alcohol (whiskey) and smoked *dagga*. He experienced a traumatic flashback to a violent event he had participated in during a regional armed conflict.

A polysubstance abuser, addicted to nicotine and a frequent abuser of alcohol and dagga, reported that after a single dose of *kougoed* he felt no craving for alcohol, dagga or nicotine for 4 days. Some reported euphoria as well as a feeling of meditative tranquility. Several users felt that the relaxation induced by *kougoed* enabled one to focus on inner thoughts and feelings, if one wished, or to concentrate on the beauty of Nature. Some informants reported heightened sensation of skin to fine touch, as well as sexual arousal. A senior traditional healer, not previously exposed to *kougoed*, tried it and announced that it "relaxes the mind" and makes one's body feel "light" the following day.

From 1995 to 1999, I undertook detailed ethnobotanical studies on *Sceletium* in the field to document the local uses of the plant, and to determine whether the plant had addictive potential. The focus of this field work was in the rural hamlets of Paulshoek and Nourivier in the Kamiesberg mountains of Namaqualand, not far from the 1685 trail of the Dutch expedition led by Simon van der Stel. Fieldwork was also undertaken in the vicinity of *Kougoedvlakte* (the area named after the once-abundant wild *Sceletium tortuosum* resource of this arid plain), and interviews and discussions were held with shepherds and goatherds in the western area of what is now the Riemvasmaak Community Conservancy. In rural hamlets, elderly male and female members of the local community, who had themselves used *Sceletium* for many decades, were interviewed. Three key informants, recognized by the communities for their specialist knowledge on medicinal plants, were selected for more detailed interviews: the renowned traditional healer Gert Dirkse or "Oom Gert" (meaning Uncle Gert) living near Paulshoek; a younger healer, Jap-Jap Klaase, living in Nourivier; and the shepherd Lodewyk Mories, living near the farm Ratelkraal situated between the towns Springbok and Pofadder.

Some of this ethnobotanical research has been published in Smith et al., 1996, Gericke & van Wyk, 2000, and in Gericke & Viljoen, 2008. *Sceletium tortuosum* is typically harvested by local people during the dry-season months from October through to January, when the plants have partly died back and become yellowish in colour. The plants are often found growing under woody shrubs, partially shaded and sheltered from the wind and from foraging by animals. The died-back yellowing plants are regarded as having more "power" than the vigorously growing green plants of the June to August winter rainy season. The plant is cut above the ground, leaving the roots and a small portion of stem behind to resprout. While some collectors gather the entire uprooted plant, older healers claim this is not following tradition and will prevent the plants from regenerating. The collected succulent plant material is crushed with a large stone on a flat rock and the resulting dripping wet fibrous pulp is put into a plastic bag. According to local people, traditional sheepskin bags were used in former times. The plastic bag is tied to exclude air, and the material is allowed to macerate in the hot sun for eight days with intermittent mixing. On the eighth or ninth day, the plant material is spread on a flat rock to dry in the sun, resulting in dry clumps of amorphous, light brown plant material with a characteristic musty "old socks" smell. This is the traditional *kougoed* or *kanna* of the Namaqualanders.

ADDICTION POTENTIAL

The following excerpt is taken verbatim from a field report (Gericke, 1995). In order to assess the potential for addiction, I had asked my friend Dr. Greg McCarthy, an academic addictionologist, to accompany me on a field trip to Namaqualand and give me an independent opinion on this. Sadly, Greg passed away in 2016, still working as an academic psychiatrist and addictionologist.

"In order to assess whether *Sceletium* use leads to addiction or dependence, a consultant psychiatrist from the Cape Town Drug Rehabilitation Centre, Dr. Greg McCarthy, accompanied Dr. Gericke on a field trip to Namaqualand to investigate the use of *kougoed* by traditional healers and members of rural communities. Dr. McCarthy is a consultant psychiatrist at Valkenberg Hospital Community Service, and was recently a consultant at Avalon, an alcohol treatment centre. He serves on the Western Cape Alcohol and Drug Forum.

"The DSM-IV criteria for dependence were translated into a questionnaire appropriate to the rural population. Three well-respected traditional healers, and eight long-term regular users of *kougoed* were interviewed. All were cooperative and open. There was clear convergence of the anecdotes and all denied any hallucinogenic or psychotomimetic effects of *kougoed*.

"While *kougoed* is used as a euphoriant or intoxicant, almost solely by elderly men, its medicinal qualities are highly regarded by the entire community. The recognized medicinal uses include use as an hypnotic or sedative, as a mild laxative, as a gripe-water, for abdominal cramps, and for alcohol rehabilitation. All research participants were adamant that *kougoed* was less habit-forming than alcohol, tobacco or *dagga* [*Cannabis sativa*].

"Tolerance was denied by all users except one, who reported "*jy raak gewoond daaraan*" ["you get used to it"]. It was not clear whether he was referring to true tolerance, where increasing doses are required to bring about the same effect, or whether he was referring to the fact that one gets accustomed to the use of *kougoed*, as the naïve user can experience nausea.

"Withdrawal signs or symptoms were not reported by anyone. This significant finding is reliable, because even regular users run out of supplies of *kougoed* due to decreased availability of the material. Mr. Mories (pers. comm.) reported there were no signs or symptoms of withdrawal even if a person ran out of *kougoed* after six months of habitual use. Some regular users would perhaps have a slight feeling as if something was missing, and some would make an effort to contact friends who may have some *kougoed*, but would not run into any difficulties if no more was obtained. All confirmed it would be far easier to give up *kougoed* than alcohol, tobacco or *dagga* [*Cannabis sativa*].

"An idea of the social and occupational functioning of the informants was easy to gauge although formal employment is scarce. The local environment is harsh, and daily living requires hard work, including walking long distances to collect brushwood for firewood, shepherding sheep and goats, and ploughing wheat-fields using donkey-drawn ploughs. There were no reports of "social dropouts" from habitual *kougoed* use, and use in this rural context can be viewed as a socially sanctioned activity. It is not possible to extrapolate what effect habitual use of *kougoed* as an euphoriant would have outside of this context.

"The medicinal use of *kougoed*, administered for specific indications, in lower doses, taken less frequently and for a finite duration must be seen as entirely separate from use as an euphoriant." (Gericke, 1995).

WELL-BEING

Kanna was commonly used by elderly men and women for a sense of calm and well-being. Elderly research participants, some in their eighth and ninth decade of life, were interviewed who had chewed quids of *kanna* daily throughout their adult lives. A small quid of fermented Sceletium is kept in the cheek and sucked, and the resulting saliva is swallowed. For a sense of calm and well-being, the quid is removed about fifteen minutes later. Men in the community then place the wet quid in their hatband to dry out so it can be sucked on or chewed later, a sequence repeated a number of times during the day. The author was cautioned "*Doktor, jy moet leer hoe om dit te gebruik*" – "Doctor, you must learn how to use it" – because once one begins feeling intoxicated by it, one has already chewed far too much. The intention of these users is to enjoy a pleasant sense of well-being, not to get intoxicated.

INTOXICATION

There were convergent reports that some people, invariably older males rather than females, did indeed use *kanna* on occasion as an intoxicant or euphoriant. No visual or auditory hallucinations were associated with the intoxication, and the state was described as being similar to being intoxicated with alcohol: "*dis onse droë drank*" – "it is our dry liquor" (Lodwewyk Mories, pers. comm., 1995). Plants from particular areas are regarded as being more potent intoxicants, and through the traditional "fermenting" process, the *kanna* would give a better "trek" – euphoria or a high. Younger men in the community were not using *kanna* at this time, and it seemed the use of tobacco, alcohol and possibly also *dagga* (marijuana) had displaced the former use of *kanna* by younger people in these rural communities.

INSOMNIA

Kanna is used as a hypnotic, with a small quid kept in the cheek by some users when going to bed. Paradoxically, some participants reported that if too much *kanna* was used, it would in fact cause insomnia.

ALCOHOLISM

Both of the healers, Gert Dirkse and Jap-Jap Klaase, maintained that *kanna* was used to wean alcoholics off of alcohol, but only if the alcoholic was committed to stop drinking. Alcohol was replaced

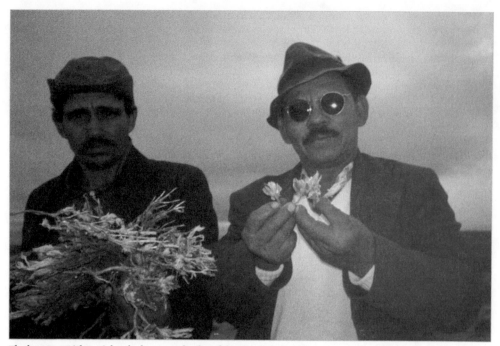

The late Gert Dirkse, right, the last great healer of the Kamiesberg Mountains, with *Sceletium tortuosum*, and Jap-Jap Klaase, left.

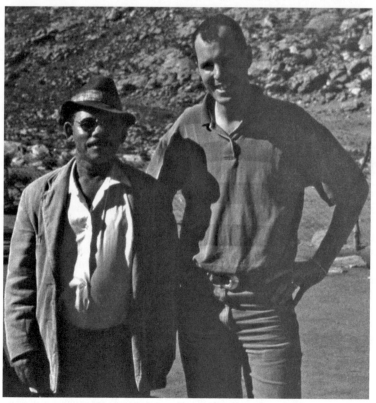

Gert Dirkse with Dr. Nigel Gericke, Paulshoek, Namaqualand, 1995.

by the chewing of *kanna*, and it was not considered to be a problem for the person to subsequently stop using the *kanna*. In some cases, a strong decoction of *kanna* would be added to a bottle of wine, so that if the alcoholic drank this wine it would cause vomiting and an aversion to wine.

CONSCIOUSNESS

The healer Gert Dirkse maintained that using *kanna* "opened the mind", and he used both hands expanding out from his temples to demonstrate this (pers. comm., 1999). He denied that the plant could cause any visions.

PREGNANCY

A quid of *kanna* is commonly chewed by women during pregnancy for treating nausea, indigestion, or for treating constipation in pregnancy. It was noted that if one took too much it had a sedating effect. The plant was not known to cause abortion or congenital defects.

PARTURITION

Infusions of *kanna* are taken to help expel any remaining afterbirth, to help contract the uterus, for abdominal pain after giving birth and for indigestion.

INFANTS

Kanna is commonly administered to infants to treat colic, excessive crying and stomach cramps. A small amount of dried herb (the samples demonstrated were estimated to be ~200-500 mg) or fermented dried herb is wrapped in cloth and dipped in breast milk in a teaspoon until the liquid has turned slightly brown. A few drops of this liquid are given orally to make the infant sleep restfully. Dried fermented herb is also lightly fried in sheep fat taken from the tail of a fat-tail sheep; this is strained through a cloth and kept in a small bottle. One to two drops of this medicated liquid fat are given to an infant with colic. The baby usually falls asleep soon after the administration of the drops. None of the mothers had ever heard of an infant needing to be taken to a doctor after too much *kanna* had been administered; they acknowledged that sometimes too high a dose is inadvertently given, but all that happens is that the baby will sleep for some hours.

CHILDREN

Hot-water infusions or decoctions of *kanna* are given to children for constipation, abdominal pain, winds and also as a "*kalmeermiddel*" or calming medicine. A child suffering from abdominal pain will fall asleep soon after the *kanna* is administered.

OTHER

Kanna is also used in Namaqualand to treat asthma, abdominal cramps, constipation and headache.

RAW MATERIAL SUPPLY

Elderly Namaqualanders confirmed that *kanna* had once been plentiful, but was now very scarce as it had been overharvested for sale to local trading stores and shops in the local towns, including the town of Springbok. Lodewyk Mories (pers. comm., 1995) recalled a time when as a young boy in the 1940s, he had seen wagonloads of *kanna* being transported from Namaqualand, presumably destined for Cape Town. Some local farmers maintained that wild stocks of Sceletium had been eaten by overgrazing sheep; however, indigenous shepherds with more intimate knowledge of the eating habits of stock maintained that sheep would only nibble on Sceletium and then move on, and that it was not the sheep that had depleted wild stocks of Sceletium, but people who had overharvested the plant, who had "run after the money."

It was clear that for the development of a product (at that time, for the South African pharmaceutical company Pharmacare Limited, as I was the Phytomedicines Development Manager), wild-harvesting of plants would not be ecologically sustainable, and that selections of Sceletium would need to be cultivated from scratch as a new crop. For this purpose, plant chemotype studies were started by Professor Ben-Erik van Wyk, and plant propagation and production studies were started by the late Professor Earle Graven and Myke Scott of Grassroots Natural Products. This work was on contract to Pharmacare Ltd., and directed by myself. From 1999 onward, the propagation and production of Sceletium work was continued by Du Roi Nurseries, and in 2004 by Niche Botanicals

Nigel Gericke

(Pty) Ltd., in cooperation with Hannes de Lange, PhD. The first successful large-scale commercial production of a select chemotype of *Sceletium tortuosum*, both under shade-house conditions and open-field conditions, was achieved in 2008 by Du Roi Nurseries and H.L. Hall and Sons Ltd., growing the plants on contract to the South African company HG&H Pharmaceuticals (Pty) Ltd. It had taken more than a decade of investment in research into plant selection, propagation and production studies to demonstrate that Sceletium could be grown successfully on a large scale as a new commercial South African crop. The reliable supply of raw material with a defined alkaloid content and composition finally allowed the development of a standardized and characterized spray-dried extract of the plant, suitable for all subsequent pre-clinical and clinical research.

CHEMISTRY

The literature on the Sceletium alkaloids has recently been thoroughly reviewed (Krstenansky, 2017), and validated analytical methods have been described for quantifying the major mesembrine-type alkaloids including mesembrine, mesembrenol, mesembrenone, mesembranol, Δ7mesembrenone, and epimesembranol (Patnala & Kanfer, 2010; Shikanga et al., 2012).

Based on the alkaloid skeleton, Jeffs et al. (1982) separate Sceletium alkaloids into four structural groups:

I   the 3aaryl-*cis*-octahydroindole class (e.g., mesembrine)

II   the C-seco mesembrine alkaloids (e.g., joubertiamine)

III   alkaloids containing a 2,3-disubstituted pyridine moiety and two nitrogen atoms (e.g., Sceletium alkaloid A4)

IV   a ring C-seco Sceletium alkaloid A4 group (e.g., tortuosamine).

The revision of Gerbaulet (1996) recognizes eight species of Sceletium, of which the alkaloids in *Sceletium strictum*, *Sceletium subvelutum* (=*Sceletium varians*), *Sceletium tortuosum*, *Sceletium joubertii* and *Sceletium namaquense* have been studied in great detail. The latter two species are now considered synonyms of *Sceletium tortuosum*. The local utilization of Sceletium as *kanna*, *kaauwgoed* or *kougoed* has included a number of Sceletium species and a wide range of Sceletium alkaloids. Compounds that have been isolated from the genus Sceletium are presented in Fig 5.

EXTRACT SCELETIUM TORTUOSUM, ZEMBRIN®

The first standardized extract of *Sceletium tortuosum* was made by the German company Gehrlicher GmbH in 1999 on contract to my consulting company, African Natural Health Close Corporation. The first fully standardized and characterized extract of *Sceletium tortuosum*, Zembrin®, was produced to EU-GMP standards by the Spanish company Polifenoles Naturales SL. The company is now renamed Nektium Pharma SL, and continues to manufacture the extract Zembrin® on contract to the company I co-founded, HG&H Pharmaceuticals (Pty) Ltd. This extract was developed and commercialized from a cultivated special selection of plants that are relatively rich in mesembrenol and mesembrenone as the major compounds, and relatively low in mesembrine and mesembranol. Zembrin® is standardized to contain 0.4% total alkaloids by weight, with the relative alkaloid composition of mesembrenone + mesembrenol ≥60%, mesembrine <20%, and mesembranol must be present in the UPLC profile. The structures of these four compounds are given in Figure 6.

PRIOR INFORMED CONSENT
BENEFIT-SHARING AGREEMENT

The development of a product from a medicinal plant used by indigenous people has to take into consideration the contribution that indigenous knowledge – past and present – makes to the foundational ethnobotanical research that gives a preliminary indication of safety, therapeutic indications, and in the case of Sceletium, the apparent lack of potential for dependence. Local participants were able to point out plants that they considered mild in effect in terms of euphoria or intoxication (called *mak* or "tame" plants), and plants which they considered a *trek* variety, which were considered to me far more potent plants than the *mak* variety and which could cause euphoria or intoxication, especially after fermentation.

136

Two years before the launch on the South African market of the standardized Sceletium extract Zembrin®, a prior informed consent benefit-sharing agreement was negotiated and signed between the South African San Council (SASC) and HG&H Pharmaceuticals (Pty) Ltd. (HG&H). The agreement was signed on 21 February 2008, and must be one of the first such agreements entered into with indigenous knowledge holders. This agreement was the result of many months of meetings and discussions with the South African San Council, who were supported in their negotiations by the internationally recognized human rights attorney Roger Chennels, ensuring that the SASC were well informed and that the agreement reached by the two parties was aligned with international best practices.

This benefit-sharing agreement recognized that the San were the primary indigenous knowledge holders of the South African endemic plant *Sceletium tortuosum*. The SASC in turn recognized that the original ethnobotanical research conducted by myself in the Namaqualand communities of Nourivier and Paulshoek contributed important information on the uses of *Sceletium*. In recognition of this contribution to the project, the SASC agreed to share 50% of royalty payments made to SASC with these two communities in an agreement signed on 30 June 2008 (Gericke, 2011). Royalty payments have been made to the SASC by HG&H from 2008 to the present time, at a rate of 5% of royalties on all sales of the extract *Sceletium tortuosum*, Zembrin®, and an additional 1% royalty on the use of the SASC logo on products containing Zembrin®. The payments are based on total invoiced sales, not on "profit" (revenues after costs). The SASC in turn have paid 50% of the royalties to the two communities of Paulshoek and Nourivier, represented by local community organizations established for this purpose. All payments are made into a South African Government trust fund established for this purpose, and are then paid out in full to the SASC, who in turn pay the two Namaqualand community groups. This prior informed consent benefit-sharing agreement has been cited as a positive case study in the commercialization of a product derived from indigenous knowledge (Iatridis and Schroeder, 2016).

PHARMACOLOGY

SEROTONIN REUPTAKE INHIBITION (SRI)

On 25 July 1989, President George Bush, in response to reports by the National Advisory Council of the National Institute of Neurological Disorders and Stroke and the National Institute for Mental Health (NIMH), and the urging of Congress, signed a presidential declaration designating the 1990s as the Decade of the Brain, a national research endeavor to better understand how the brain and nervous system is organized, how it functions, why it fails to function and what can be done to prevent and treat dysfunction. As part of this research, NIMH screened large numbers of compounds through a research agreement with the company Novascreen. In November 1995, I was working as a Visiting Scholar at the US Pharmacopoeia (USP), and not far from USP was the NIMH. I was introduced to Dr. Linda Brady, who was then the chief of the Neuropharmacology and Drug Discovery Program. Dr. Brady kindly agreed to screen an extract of Sceletium as well as isolated pure mesembrine. Both the extract and mesembrine turned out to be exceedingly potent 5-HT uptake inhibitors in the radioligand binding screening and in a subsequent functional assay. This work formed the basis for US Patent 6,288,104 (Gericke and Van Wyk, 1999), which disclosed the use of mesembrine and related compounds, and extracts of Sceletium standardized to these compounds, as serotonin-uptake inhibitors (SRIs), and the use of these compounds in pharmaceutical formulations for the management of depression, anxiety, drug dependence, bulimia and obsessive-compulsive disorder.

Subsequently, the standardized Sceletium extract Zembrin® was confirmed to be an SRI with an IC50 of 4.3µg/ml, and mesembrine was found to be the most active alkaloid against the 5-HT transporter (SERT), with a Ki of 1.4nM (Harvey et al, 2011). See Table 2 below. In fact, mesembrine is a more potent inhibitor on SERT than fluoxetine (Prozac).

PHOSPHODIESTERASE-4 INHIBITION (PDE4 INHIBITION)

I self-experimented with isolated pure mesembrine on a number of occasions from 1996 to 1999, on some occasions with a friend and fellow natural products enthusiast, Dr. George Davidson. Isolated pure mesembrine, taken sublingually in tincture form or on a blotter, resulted in a tangible entactogenic effect with an onset of action some ten to fifteen minutes after taking 100µg. Higher doses at about 500µg gave an experience not dissimilar to MDMA but far more tranquil. It was clear that there had to be additional CNS mechanism/s of action in addition to the SRI activity.

Table 2. The inhibitory constants (Ki in nM) for three mesembrine alkaloids on the serotonin transporter.

Compound	Inhibition of SERT Ki nM
mesembrenone	27
mesembrine	1.4
mesembrenol	63

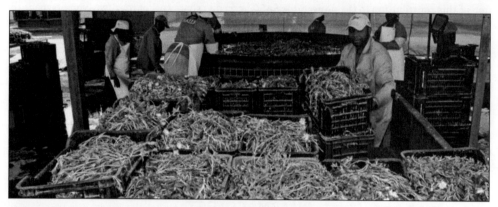

Cultivated Sceletium for the production of the standardized extract Zembrin®.

Table 3. PDE4 inhibition of the prototypical PDE4 inhibitor Rolipram and the Sceletium alkaloids mesembrenone, mesembrine and mesembrenol.

Compound	PDE4B Inhibition IC_{50} µM
Rolipram	0.13
mesembrenone	0.47
mesembrine	7.8
mesembrenol	16

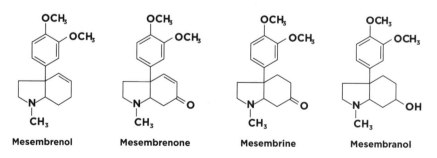

Mesembrenol   Mesembrenone   Mesembrine   Mesembranol

Fig. 1 The four alkaloids quantified in the standardized Sceletium extract Zembrin.

138

The results of the broad *in vitro* screening of the Sceletium extract Zembrin® and some isolated alkaloids is reported in Harvey et al., 2011. Zembrin® was found to be an inhibitor of the phosphodiesterase-4 (PDE4) enzyme in addition to being an SRI (Harvey et al., 2011). The three isolated mesembrine alkaloids tested were all found to be PDE4B inhibitors, with the most potent of the three being mesembrenone, which is about one third as potent as the prototypical research PDE4 inhibitor Rolipram (Harvey et al., 2011; MacKenzie and Houslay, 2000). See Table 3 below. US Patent 8,552, 051 (Harvey et al., 2013) discloses the use of mesembrenone as a dual SRI and PDE4 inhibitor.

While SRIs and selective SRIs (SSRIs) are widely used for the treatment of anxiety disorders and depression, the combination of an SSRI with a PDE4 inhibitor has been argued to have synergistic therapeutic potential. Repeated treatment with SSRIs can upregulate PDE4 (Ye et al., 2000), which in turn reduces sensitivity to SSRIs in response to long-term treatment. The treatment with a dual SSRI and PDE4 inhibitors may thus have a therapeutic advantage (Cashman et al., 2009). Enzymes in the PDE4 family catalyze the hydrolysis of cyclic AMP (cAMP) and have a critical role in controlling the intracellular concentration of cAMP and increasing phosphorylation of cAMP-response element-binding protein. PDE4s are found throughout the brain but their levels are decreased in depressed individuals not on medication, reflecting a downregulation of the cAMP cascade that can potentially be restored using PDE4 inhibitors. The prototypical PDE4 inhibitor Rolipram has been shown in both animal and clinical studies to have antidepressant activity (Terburg et al., 2013).

PRE-CLINICAL RESEARCH

Prior to the development of a standardized extract, I sent samples of milled *Sceletium tortuosum* plant material to colleagues in Japan who were interested in studying the effect of Sceletium in a veterinary clinic setting. The veterinarians reported that the Sceletium reduced cage stress and travel stress in cats, and decreased the excessive nocturnal crying and barking of aged cats and dogs with a clinical diagnosis of dementia. These results have been published in Japanese (Hirabayashi et al., 2002; Hirabayashi et al., 2004; Hirabayashi et al., 2005).

Sceletium extract Zembrin® was studied in a 14-day repeated oral toxicity study conducted at 0, 250, 750, 2500, and 5000 mg/kg body weight/day (equivalent to total mesembrine alkaloids of 0, 1, 3, 10, and 20 mg/kg bw/day). A 90-day subchronic repeated oral toxicity study was conducted on Sceletium extract Zembrin® at 0, 100, 300, 450, and 600 mg/kg bw/day (equivalent to total mesembrine alkaloids of 0, 0.4, 1.2, 1.8, and 2.4 mg/kg bw/day). Since Sceletium species were known to be psychoactive, a functional observation battery, including spontaneous locomotor activity measured using the LabMaster ActiMot light-beam frames system, was employed. Parameters such as locomotion, rearing behavior, spatial parameters and turning behavior were investigated. No mortality or treatment-related adverse effects were observed in the rats in the 14- or 90-day studies. In the 14- and 90-day studies, the No Observed Adverse Effect Levels (NOAEL) for Zembrin® were 5000 and 600 mg/kg bw/d, respectively, the highest dose groups tested (Murbach et al., 2014), equivalent to the NOAEL for total mesembrine alkaloids of 20 and 2.4 mg/kg bw/day.

In a model of restraint-induced psychological stress it was found that a dose of only 5mg/kg of Sceletium extract (although not stated in the paper, this was Lot #8587 of Zembrin®) given by gavage reduced restraint stress-induced self-soothing behavior, as well as decreased stress-induced corticosterone levels (Smith, 2011). This dose is equivalent to a total alkaloid dose of only 20 μg/kg bw/day.

The effect of single doses of Sceletium extract Zembrin® on rat brain electrical activity was studied using wireless EEG recordings in free-living rats. 3 doses of the Sceletium extract Zembrin® and vehicle (0, 2.5, 5.0 and 10.0 mg/kg, equivalent to total mesembrine alkaloids of 0, 10, 20 and 40 μg/kg) were given by gavage. The resulting electropharmacograms (plotted from Fast Fourier Transformation of the analogue EEG recording for each frequency range) of Zembrin® were compared to the databased electropharmacograms of reference herbal extracts, dietary ingredients and the pharmaceutical PDE4-inhibitor Rolipram. Zembrin® had a similar electropharmacogram to the electropharmacograms for extracts of *Ginkgo biloba* and *Rhodiola*. A discriminant analysis confirmed these similarities and also demonstrated that Zembrin® had a similar electropharmacogram to citicoline, a compound originally developed for cognitive enhancement, and to the PDE4-inhibitor Rolipram. These results provide support for future translational clinical studies on Zembrin® to investigate the activity of the extract on cognitive function in Mild Cognitive Impairment, for treating depression and as an analgesic (Dimpfel et al., 2016).

139

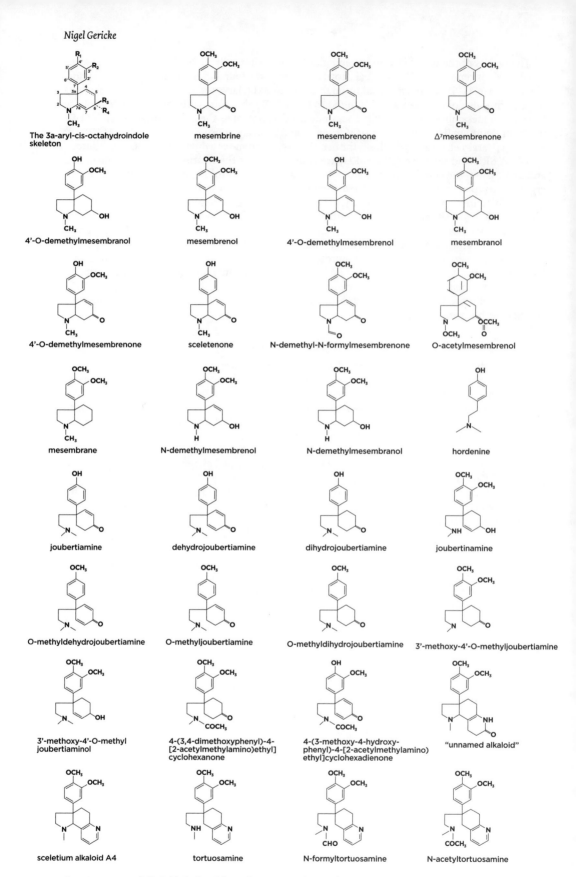

Fig. 2 Structures of alkaloids isolated from the genus Sceletium (Gericke & Viljoen, 2008).

PART III

CLINICAL STUDIES ON SCELETIUM EXTRACT ZEMBRIN®

INTRODUCTION

The following three case reports on the clinical use of Sceletium, presented at the 4th International Conference on Phytotherapeutics on 23-25 February 2001, Kurrajong, NSW Australia, are the first clinical case reports for this plant and demonstrate that the plant has therapeutic potential for anxiety and depression. These historical case reports are given in full from Gericke (2001).

1. PATIENT WITH A FIRST EPISODE OF SEVERE DEPRESSION WITH MARKED ANXIETY

Reported by the author

H.M., a 29-year-old female doctor, presented at my practice asking for a natural treatment for severe depression. She had had no previous psychiatric history, no history of epilepsy, head injury or substance abuse, and had a past medical history of atopic eczema and occasional asthma, not presently on any medication.

MAIN COMPLAINT

A four-month period of depressed mood with diurnal variation: the depression was far worse in mornings, improving somewhat as the day progressed. There was an obvious physiological shift with decrease in appetite, weight loss and insomnia with difficulty initiating sleep and early morning waking. Markedly decreased energy and drive were a significant problem for the patient. The symptoms were accompanied by feelings of anxiety and somatic symptoms of anxiety including palpitations and epigastric discomfort. Other symptoms of note included suicidal ideation, feelings of worthlessness, lack of concentration and motivation, tearfulness, emotional lability and general loss of interest in life.

TREATMENT

The patient requested to be put on *Sceletium*, having heard about it from a colleague who is a psychiatrist, and was started on a low dose of 50mg [milled plant material] as a tablet taken in the mornings.

The patient initially reported a transient increase in anxiety after taking medication, which would last up to three hours. This effect was no longer apparent after a week of continual use. No changes in libido were noted, and libido had not been affected by the depression either. A sustained improvement in mood was reported from somewhere between 1-2 weeks of continual use of 50mg Sceletium taken daily, with a marked decrease in the generalized anxiety. The patient's insomnia improved at the onset of treatment. There was a marked improvement in drive and energy, accompanied with a return of interest in the mundane activities that constitute much of everyday living.

The only side effects elicited were the initial transient increase in anxiety and some initial appetite suppression, neither of which was severe enough to warrant discontinuation of treatment, and both of which were no longer apparent after the first two weeks of treatment.

CONCLUSION

A low dose of *Sceletium* (50mg daily) taken orally as a tablet proved to be a very effective anxiolytic and mood elevator in a first episode of a major depression. The *Sceletium* was discontinued after 4 months of continual use with no signs or symptoms of withdrawal, and there has so far (about 6 months) been no return of symptoms of anxiety or depression.

2. PATIENT WITH POSTNATAL MAJOR DEPRESSIVE DISORDER.

Reported by Dr Olga Gericke MUDR (Vienna) FC Psych. (SA)

A 28-year-old married housewife with two children, aged three and a half and two months old respectively, presented with depressive symptoms that she had had since the seventh month of her second pregnancy. Complaining of depressed mood, increased sleep, overeating, low energy, increased anxiety to the point of perceptual illusions and depersonalization, feelings of worthlessness, psychomotor agitation, thoughts of death, decreased ability to concentrate and forgetfulness. She also complained of inability to bond with her newborn and felt very irritable and aggressive towards her three-year-old. The patient had self-medicated with St John's Wort (*Hypericum perforatum*) over the last two weeks, with minimal effect.

PAST PSYCHIATRIC HISTORY

Severe postnatal depression after her first child, needed hospitalization, was on Aurorix (Moclobemide) for two years with limited success and discontinued it due to side effects. Her first onset of depression was at age 16, which was treated with Amitryptyline and therapy.

PAST MEDICAL HISTORY

Pre-eclampsia with first pregnancy and currently hypertension, obesity.

HABITS: nil.
PRESENT MEDICATION: ACE inhibitor for hypertension.
FAMILY AND SOCIAL: Disruptive upbringing, mother suffered from severe depression and was hospitalized frequently, both sisters suffer from panic disorder.

DIAGNOSIS

- Major depressive disorder, recurrent, severe, postnatal onset
- Borderline personality traits
- Hypertension

TREATMENT

The patient was started on *Sceletium* 50 mg [milled plant material] in the morning and at lunchtime. The immediate effect (the first day of treatment) was mood elevation, significantly decreased sleep (from 14 hours a day to eight hours a day) and increased energy. The patient voluntarily started doing housework again. After four weeks of treatment, symptoms of mild depression and anxiety were present again. After six weeks of treatment with *Sceletium*, and supportive therapy and group sessions with a postnatal depression support group, the patient appeared to be fully recovered and is presently well on a maintenance dose of 50 mg *Sceletium* twice a day.

COMMENT

To date, I have successfully used *Sceletium* in 10 patients with a diagnosis of Major Depressive Disorder according to DSM-IV criteria. My patients are usually more severely depressed or anxious than the clients of psychologists and patients of general practitioners, and most of them have been on various pharmaceutical antidepressants before. Most of the patients had a strong anxiety component to the depression. *Sceletium* alleviates anxiety very quickly, though in sensitive individuals the first dose can actually increase the anxiety for about half an hour, after which it is relaxing. My starting dose is usually 50mg in the morning and most patients increase it to an additional 50mg at lunchtime or early afternoon. If taken later, it can cause insomnia in some patients. In some patients I have had to increase the dose to 100mg/12 hours.

3. CASE REPORT BY CHERYL INGGS

B.A. Honours, MA(Clin. Psych.) Rhodes

The client is a 19-year-old university student who started therapy (once a week) towards the end of her second year (1999). She completed her bachelor's degree at the end of 2000 and has just entered her Honours degree.

THE CLIENT PRESENTED WITH THE FOLLOWING:

Axis I : Dysthymia. She felt despondent and "trapped inside", she isolated herself and "couldn't see a way out", was sometimes tearful, alternating with an emptiness inside and a pervasive sense of sadness; she had low self-esteem, a loss of interest in activities with social withdrawal, loss of motivation, some distractability and short-term memory loss, tiredness, lethargy, hypersomnia and loss of appetite with occasional "comfort eating" mostly of junk food. There was no suicidal ideation.

Axis II : Borderline Personality. Described feeling "out of touch" and depersonalized, with some self-mutilation (scratching her upper arm and wrist). Some impulse binge-drinking when socializing. She had tried "ecstasy" (MDMA) and indulges in marijuana very occasionally. A baseline mood of depression alternating with anxiety and a feeling of tension particularly around her studies and exam performance (sweaty palms, constipation and hair loss). Feelings of emptiness and fear of abandonment. Inappropriate and intense anger. Battling with a sense of self and identity, feeling unsure of who she is, feeling distant, isolated and lonely.

THERAPEUTIC ISSUES

The client clearly presented with long-standing dysthymia and some anxiety. She had also been sexually abused from age 12-15. She is the middle child and only daughter of an emotionally absent father and a career-oriented mother on whom the client is emotionally dependent. She vacillates between idealizing her mother when she is available and feeling abandoned by her when she is unavailable. The client carries a great deal of anger, and has body-image problems coupled with a fear of sexual intimacy.

TREATMENT

The therapeutic approach was from a self-psychology model providing a containing environment with careful intervention and gentle interpretation. The client was able to be very insightful but lacked the capacity to process the insight in any meaningful way. She presented with an ongoing sense of emptiness and depersonalization, with a deep despondency and hopelessness. *Sceletium* was administered as a 50mg tablet daily from October 2000. Within ten days, the patient said that her mood had lifted and that she felt slightly less depersonalized. She was able to feel more focused, more engaged and not so socially "distant." She doubled her dose to two 50-mg tablets daily just prior to her examination (November 2000) and described feeling less anxious and more able to cope with her usual examination anxiety. An interesting development on *Sceletium* was that she described feeling less inclined to overindulge in alcohol (she said that it didn't taste as good).

CONCLUSION

The client clearly has personality problems that require ongoing therapy. However, what is significant is that the *Sceletium* certainly helped her feel more contained, lifted her mood and also helped with anxiety. There is a sense in which the *Sceletium* has stabilized her to the point where we were able to actively engage in some of the more pressing therapeutic issues.

The rapid improvements in mood and anxiety in these initial three patients provided the impetus for the development of the proprietary standardized and characterized *Sceletium* extract Zembrin® for formal clinical research.

SAFETY & TOLERABILITY (Nell et al., 2013)

The safety and tolerability of Sceletium extract Zembrin® was studied in the first formal clinical study of a Sceletium extract. In this randomized, double-blind, placebo-controlled clinical study, two doses of Zembrin® (8mg and 25mg, equivalent to total mesembrine alkaloids of 32µg and 100µg respectively) were taken orally once daily for three months by healthy adult volunteers. No efficacy variables were assessed. The extract was found to be safe and well tolerated. An interesting aspect of the study was unsolicited positive effects on well-being noted in patients' side-effect diaries by some participants taking the extract, including improved coping with stress and improved sleep at night.

PHARMACO-FMRI STUDY (Terburg et al., 2013)

The acute effects of extract Zembrin® were investigated in a pharmaco-fMRI study focused on anxiety-related activity in the amygdala and the connected neuro-circuitry. In a double-blind, placebo-controlled cross-over design, 16 healthy university student participants were scanned during performance of an emotion-matching task under low and high perceptual loads. Amygdala reactivity to fearful faces under low perceptual load conditions was attenuated, with a decreased blood oxygenation level-dependent (BOLD) signal for Zembrin® compared to placebo on low-load exposure to fearful faces compared with neutral challenges in the bilateral amygdala ($P<0.01$) after a single 25mg (equivalent to 100µg total mesembrine alkaloids) dose of Zembrin®. Follow-up connectivity analysis on the emotion-matching task demonstrated that amygdala–hypothalamus coupling was also reduced. These results demonstrated, for the first time, the attenuating effects of an extract of Sceletium on the threat circuitry of the human brain and provided supporting evidence that this extract may have anxiolytic potential by attenuating subcortical threat responsivity. These results are consistent with the *in vitro* dual serotonin reuptake inhibition and PDE4 inhibition reported by Harvey et al., 2011.

COGNITION-ENHANCING ACTIVITY (Chiu et al., 2014).

In a randomized double-blind placebo-controlled cross-over clinical study normal healthy older subjects (total n=21) (mean age: 54.6 years ± 6.0yrs; male/female ratio: 9/12) received either a 25mg capsule of Sceletium extract Zembrin® (equivalent to 100mg total mesembrine-alkaloids) or placebo capsule once daily for 3 weeks. The primary endpoint was to examine the neurocognitive effects of the extract using the CNS Vital Signs battery of tests. Zembrin® at 25mg daily dosage significantly improved executive function (p0.022) and cognitive set flexibility (p0.032) compared with the placebo group. Positive changes in mood and sleep were also found, and the extract was well tolerated. It was concluded that PDE-4 inhibition with the resulting cAMP-CREB cascade may play a role in these cognitive enhancing effects of Zembrin®.

ACTIVITY ON EEG, PSYCHOMETRY, AND ANXIETY
(Dimpfel et al., 2017).

In a randomized, double-blind, placebo-controlled clinical study, the effect of 25mg or 50mg of Zembrin® (equivalent to 100µg and 200µg of total mesembrine alkaloids, respectively) was studied in comparison to placebo after daily repetitive intake for 6 weeks. Sixty healthy male (n = 32) and female (n = 28) subjects between 50 and 80 years old (59.7 ± 5.43 and 56.7 ± 5.88 years, respectively) were recruited. The EEG was recorded bipolarly from 17 surface electrodes. Six cognitive tests were performed: d2-test, memory test, calculation performance test, reaction time test, number identifying test and number connection test. Three questionnaires were included: Profile of Mood States, Hamilton Anxiety Rating Scale (HAM-A) and a sleep questionnaire. Quantitative EEG revealed increases of delta activity during performance of the d2-test, the number identification and number connection tests in the fronto-temporal brain region. Higher theta activity was seen during relaxation and performance of the d2-test after intake of 50mg of Zembrin®. Statistically conspicuous increases of alpha1 spectral power were seen in the relaxed state. With respect to alpha2 spectral power, larger increases were observed in the centro-occipital region. Discriminant analysis of the EEG data revealed a projection of the Zembrin® data into the vicinity of the EEG data plot for a ginkgo-ginseng combination. Statistically significant improvement during performance of the arithmetic calculation test and number connection test was documented. The HAM-A anxiety score revealed a statistically significant decrease (p = 0.03) after six weeks intake within the 50mg Zembrin® group. The results indicate that Zembrin® improves some aspects of cognitive function, and decreases anxiety in healthy older adults.

Part IV
KANNA AND MESEMBRINE-ALKALOIDS: POSSIBLE FUTURES
LEGAL HIGHS

Legal highs are typically sold by online Smart Shops and may be broadly defined psychoactive substances which have not (in some cases not yet) been proscribed by laws or regulations, and are used to elicit a desired state of mind which may be stimulated, euphoric, empathogenic or entactogenic, entheogenic, sedated or a combination. The substances may be isolated natural compounds, synthetic or semi-synthetic compounds, extracts of plants or fungi, or whole or minimally processed plant or fungal material. The first online sales of Sceletium plant material, originally from 40kg of plant material cultivated by Grassroots Natural Products for Pharmacare Ltd., began in 1999 by Om-Chi Herbs in Eugene, Oregon in the USA, and by Conscious Dreams in Amsterdam in the Netherlands, later to be followed by Botanic Art in the Netherlands. These online stores played a major role in introducing *kanna* to a wide international audience. It is now eighteen years later, and there are many online Legal Highs and botanical supply stores selling fermented and unprocessed *kanna* as milled plant material and extracts. From about 2004, there seems to have been a marked increase in the use of *kanna* in the South African trance scene, where powdered *kanna* is used as a snuff, or mixed with marijuana for smoking to induce a "chilled" state of mind and to decrease anxiety in people who get more anxious while smoking marijuana. *Kanna* is used instead of MDMA by some people in the South African trance scene, and to reduce the come-down after an MDMA session by others. By 2017, *kanna* use had become part of the international trance and party scene, with use of *kanna* apparently being well known in Ibiza, Spain.

A recent development of serious concern is the online sale of concentrated to highly concentrated extracts sold as *kanna* which are of uncertain botanical origin, unknown total alkaloid content, unknown relative alkaloid composition and unknown stability. A search of Sceletium extracts on Alibaba.com shows a wide variety of "Sceletium" extracts, many produced in China (some accompanied by photographs of flowers that are definitely not Sceletium flowers). This includes some touted as "100:1" extracts (presumably a raw material to extract ratio, weight/weight) and some purporting to be "98% mesembrine" (Alibaba.com, 2017). There is already nascent legal and regulatory flagging of *kanna*, and overconcentrated extracts carry a potential for serious adverse events. The analysis of Sceletium alkaloids for future forensic toxicology and legislation purposes has already been described (Roscher et al., 2012), and the United Nations Office on Drugs and Crime (UNODC) issued a list of 20 plant-based substances of concern in 2013, including Sceletium. The metabolism of Sceletium alkaloids was investigated in rat urine and pooled human liver preparations (Meyer et al., 2015) because of the increasing popularity of *kanna* as a legal high, and the metabolites, especially in the urine, would be good analytical targets for forensic and legal purposes. Sceletium has already attracted the attention of the Drug Enforcement Agency (DEA) of the United States, featuring in a presentation by a forensic chemist at the DEA Special Testing and Research Laboratory with the title, "Novel Plant Hallucinogens and Plant-Derived Highs" (Dye, undated presentation). Surprisingly, Amazon.com has prohibited the sale of *kanna* and cited it as an example of a plant-derived product that simulates the effect of illegal drugs (Amazon.com, 2017). An additional legal and regulatory threat is the potential for adverse reactions from adulterated *kanna*. During an investigation into the wide phytochemical variability of *kanna* available from online stores, the alarming discovery was made that one of the samples of *kanna* had been adulterated with the stimulant ephedrine (Lesiak et al., 2016).

Notwithstanding the forensic and regulatory flagging, the use of isolated pure mesembrine alkaloids may ultimately become more widely available to the general public via the rapidly growing vaping and electronic cigarettes industries, evidenced by two recent US Patent Applications for electronically heated aerosol systems filed by Philip Morris Products S.A., Neuchatel, Switzerland, with mesembrine given as one of the examples of active ingredients to be vaporized (Schneider J-C. et al., 2016; Thorens and Cochand, 2016).

SUPPLEMENT

The first commercial supplement product containing Sceletium was put on the South African market in 2001 by a South African company I founded, Phyto Nova (Pty) Ltd. This product consisted simply of a low dose of 50mg tablets of milled cultivated *Sceletium tortuosum*, with the traditional uses stated as stress relief and mood elevation. The recommended dose was specified as one to two tablets daily. Tablets containing 25mg of the standardized Sceletium extract Zembrin® were first launched on the South African market in 2010. The recommended dose is 25-50mg taken once a day (containing 100-200 µg total mesembrine alkaloids). The tablets are used for stress, anxiety and mild to moderate depression. In South Africa, these tablets are popular during exam time, used by university students and matriculated school children for improving concentration and reducing stress while studying for exams. The South African National Defence Force has included tablets containing Zembrin® in its code of products that can be prescribed by military psychiatrists and physicians.

A highlight of the Sceletium project was the marketing authorization given to Zembrin® in 2014 by the Natural and Non-Prescription Health Products Directorate of Health Canada, issued as Product Licence number 80052770 on 29 July 2014, for capsules containing 25mg extract, a daily dose of 100µg mesembrine alkaloids.

There are now many brands of tablets, capsules, tinctures and teas of functional food and dietary supplement products containing Sceletium plant material, Zembrin®, and other extracts on the market, mainly in the United States, with lesser sales in much smaller markets including Canada, South Africa, Malaysia and Japan. The cost of formally addressing the diverse national regulatory requirements has limited the international penetration of Sceletium supplements, and it is not clear if companies will be willing to invest in addressing these requirements in the face of increasing competition from what has essentially become a generic botanical dominated by internet sales of these products directly to consumers.

We are living in a fast-paced, highly stressed and uncertain world, challenged with electronic media competing for mindspace, and assaulted daily with news of dramatic geopolitical, economic, social, climatic and environmental changes. Simultaneously, we are on the threshold of the Fourth Industrial Revolution, which is fundamentally changing our lives, our work, our relationships and blurring the boundary between ourselves and our technologies. Low doses of mesembrine alkaloids, probably in the range of only 200µg-400µg and perhaps best in a sustained-release dosage form, have great potential to safely enhance the daily quality of people's lives. More than twenty years of work on this plant has shown me that we have not yet begun to realize the potential that supplements of Sceletium or Sceletium alkaloids hold for:

- reducing stress and situational anxiety
- enhancing well-being
- elevating mood in mild to moderate depression
- enhancing cognitive function
- reducing alcohol and drug abuse
- facilitating psychotherapy
- facilitating meditative and spiritual states

MEDICINE

To date there have been no clinical trials on extracts of Sceletium in a clinical population. Two recent clinical case reports are presented here, where extract *Sceletium tortuosum* Zembrin® was used by my wife Dr. Olga Gericke in her integrative psychiatric practice in Cape Town (Gericke et al., 2017).

CASE REPORT 1.

A 40-year-old married housewife with two children, aged 6 and 9, was referred to Dr. Olga Gericke for medication review. Her history included recurrent major depressive disorder since age 17, postpartum depression and social anxiety disorder. For the previous eight years, she had been on citalopram 20mg per day, which had adequately treated her depression and social anxiety. However, the patient found the side effects difficult to tolerate: loss of libido, emotional blunting and weight gain. Two attempts to discontinue citalopram resulted in recurrence of her depressive symptoms within four months, necessitating resumption of the medication. During consultation, the patient stated she was determined to wean herself off citalopram. After being counseled on pharmaceutical and botanical treatment options, the patient opted for a trial of 25mg extract of *Sceletium tortuosum* (Zembrin®). Citalopram was reduced to 10mg daily for one week and then discontinued while starting 50mg of Sceletium, which was increased to a daily maintenance dose of 75mg. At one-month follow-up, she reported no anxiety/depressive symptoms, though she experienced occasional mild episodes of social anxiety, which she found easy to tolerate. Her libido had returned to normal, she felt much more in touch with her feelings and had lost two kilograms of weight. During the following month, her mood had slightly lowered, but this responded well to an increase of the Sceletium extract to 100mg per day. Eight months after initial assessment, she remained in remission on 100mg per day Sceletium extract Zembrin® with no side effects.

CASE REPORT 2

A 45-year-old married man, visiting South Africa from Europe, was referred to Dr. Olga Gericke by a general practitioner for assessment of depressive symptoms which developed after the birth of the patient's child eighteen months previously. Two prior episodes of depression five years and seven years before were clearly associated with stressors and had resolved without treatment. He had seen a psychotherapist for two years in his country of origin. There was no history of medical illness and routine blood tests were normal. There was a family history of depression but no history of substance abuse. The patient had recently tried self-medicating with a combination product of *Sceletium tortuosum* and *Avena sativa*, but found it too sedating. Treatment was initiated with 50mg per day *Sceletium tortuosum* extract and increased to 100mg a day. In addition, the patient was seen for weekly supportive psychotherapy sessions. Within four weeks, his depressive symptoms remitted and he was discharged from the practice after six weeks when he was returned to his country of origin. He was advised to continue the 100mg *Sceletium tortuosum* extract daily and to seek psychiatric follow-up on his return home.

Standardized and characterized Sceletium extracts clearly have great potential as safe, effective botanical medicines for treating clinical anxiety and depression, and integrating extracts of Sceletium into psychiatric clinical practice has been described based on Olga's fifteen years of experience with Sceletium in her practice in Cape Town, and the clinical experience of Dr. Richard P. Brown, a psychopharmacologist and integrative psychiatrist in New York who has prescribed Sceletium in more than 30 patients during the past 4 years (Gericke et al., 2017).

While standardized Sceletium extracts have great potential to be used as botanical medicine to treat clinical anxiety and depressive states, it is not clear if this potential will ever be realized. The cost of developing the clinical evidence of safety and efficacy to achieve marketing authorization for a botanical medicine is prohibitive, the quality issues of polymolecular botanical medicines continue to be a major challenge, and the regulatory pathway to achieve registration as a botanical medicine is not as clear or as harmonized internationally as for single chemical entities. In the last two decades, the US Food and Drug Administration has only approved two botanical drugs; the first botanical drug approved by the FDA was Veregen®, a treatment for genital and perianal warts that is derived from a green tea extract (*Camellia sinensis* Kuntze), and a number of years later the FDA approved Fulyzaq™, a drug for HIV-associated diarrhea, extracted from the latex of the South American tree (*Croton lechlerii* Müll. Arg) (Ahn, 2017).

Future approved medicines derived from Sceletium are more likely to be developed from isolated pure alkaloids, their metabolites, or from semi-synthetic derivatives. Pathways for the synthesis of mesembrine and related alkaloids have been described from the early 1960s. A review of the synthesis of mesembrine, for example, includes more than thirty described pathways, including isomer-selective synthesis (Zhao et al., 2010). While there is a fairly extensive literature on the chemistry and synthesis of these compounds, the pharmacology of isolated compounds has hardly been explored. The pharmacology of metabolites of these compounds presents a rich field for psychoactive new drug discovery.

Distillation of two decades of experience of indigenous uses, *in vitro* pharmacology, pre-clinical studies, anecdotal reports, clinical case studies and pilot randomized controlled clinical trials suggest that isolated Sceletium alkaloids (and their metabolites and analogues) have enormous potential for the development of rapidly acting psychoactive drugs with a low side-effect profile for:

- Major Depressive Disorder
- Generalised Anxiety Disorder
- Attention Deficit Disorder and Attention Deficit Hyperactivity Disorder
- Post-Traumatic Stress Disorder
- Mild Cognitive Impairment
- Neuroprotection
- Controlling appetite and craving in weight management programs
- Addiction management, including opioid addiction
- Chronic pain
- Schizophrenia

My hope is that this paper will stimulate further academic and pharmaceutical research to realize the potential of Sceletium extracts and mesembrine-type alkaloids for preventing, treating and ameliorating diverse mental health diseases, and for enhancing the quality of life of all people.

ACKNOWLEDGMENTS

Family, friends and colleagues are thanked for their contribution to this Sceletium odyssey: Aaron Santana, Abdulgaseeb Jacobs, Abraham van Rooyen, Alan Gray, Alan Harvey, Alex Schauss, Alison Dyer, Alvaro Viljoen, Andrew Tully, *Mark Tully, *Andries Steenkamp, Antonio Bianchi, Ashley Mashigo, Bani Isaac Mayeng, Barbara Davis, Beatrice Molac, Beatriz Ercilla, Ben-Erik van Wyk, Bruce Gordan, C.C. Kennedy, Carine Smith, Carl Albrecht, Cheryl Inggs, Chris Watson, Christine Tomcheck, Credo Mutwa, Dan Stein, David Terburg, Dennis McKenna, Deon Hofmeyr, Diana-Lee Simon, Dick Doorn, Dierdre Allen, Dorris Schroeder, *Earle Graven, Edda Fiegert, Emmanuel Shikanga, Eric Anderson, Eric Gericke, Fabio Ravanello, Fabio Soldati, Fiona Archer, George Davidson, *Gert Dirkse, *Greg McCarthy, Guy Wertheim-Aymes, Hans van den Hurk, Hannes de Lange, Haylene Nell, *Hibiki Kurono, Holly Bayne, Ingrid Keplinger-Dimpfel, Iris Freie, Isadore Kanfer, Jack van Honk, Jap-Jap Klaasse, Jerry Cott, John Endres, *John Winslow, Julia Wiebe, Kenjiro Shimada, Kenzi Loke, Kia Gericke, Laubi Walters, *Lawrence Penkler, Leana Cloete, Leana Bronkhorst, Linda Brady, Lisa Garson, Lisa Meserole, Lita Cole, Lodewyk Mories, Manuel Lopez-Romero, Marena Manley, Marion Weston, Mark Blumenthal, Maryna Swart, Matt Tripp, Michel Woodbury, Michelle Gericke, Miguel Jimenez del Rio, Myke Scott, Ncindani Maswanganyi, Neal Craft, Nicky Gericke, Nuri Fraile Lopez, Olga Gericke, Patricia Garberg, Paul Flowerman, Paul Jonker, Pete Backwell, Peter Williams-Ashman, Pippa Skotnes, Richard Brown, Roberto Jimenez del Rio, Robb Snaddon, Roger Chennels, Roger Stewart, Roy van Brummelen, Rudi Giger, *Ryo Yonemoto, Satoru Furukawa, Seth Flowerman, Simon Chiu, Sinobu Kurono, Srinivas Patnala, Tanausú Vega, Timothy Murbach, Ulrich Feiter, Veronica Napier, Vladimir Badmaev, Wilfried Dimpfel, William Emboden.
*Deceased.

REFERENCES

Ahn, K., 2017. The worldwide trend of using botanical drugs and strategies for developing global drugs. *BMB reports* 50(3): 111-116.

Alibaba.com, 2017. https://www.alibaba.com/trade/search?fsb=y&IndexArea=product_en&CatId=&SearchText=sceletium+extracts&isGalleryList=G Accessed 20th April 2017.

Amazon.com, 2017. Drugs and drug paraphernalia. Examples of prohibited listings. https://www.amazon.com/gp/help/customer/display.html?ref=hp_rel_topic?ie=UTF8&nodeId=200277220 Accessed 7th April 2017.

Archer, F.M., 1994. *Ethnobotany of Namaqualand: The Richtersveld* (Master of Arts dissertation, University of Cape Town).

Cashman, J.R., et al., 2009. Stereoselective inhibition of serotonin reuptake and phosphodiesterase by dual inhibitors as potential agents for depression. *Bioorganic & Medicinal Chemistry* 17(1), 337-343.

Chiu, S., et al., 2014. Proof-of-concept randomized controlled study of cognition effects of the proprietary extract *Sceletium tortuosum* (Zembrin) targeting phosphodiesterase-4 in cognitively healthy subjects: implications for Alzheimer's Dementia. *Evidence-Based Complementary and Alternative Medicine* Vol. 2014,1-10.

Collot, A.G., 1856. *A New and Improved Standard French and English and English and French Dictionary*. C.G. Henderson and Company, Philadelphia.

De La Caille, M. l'Abbé., 1763. *Journal Historique Du Voyage Fait Au Cap De Bonne Esperance.* Academie Des Sciences, Paris.

Digby, A., 2005. Self-medication and the trade in medicine within a multi-ethnic context: a case study of South Africa from the mid-nineteenth to mid-twentieth centuries. *Social History of Medicine* 18, 439–457.

Digital Bleek & Lloyd. http://lloydbleekcollection.cs.uct.ac.za/xam.html. Accessed 21 June 2017.

Dimpfel, W., et al., 2016. Electropharmacogram of *Sceletium tortuosum* extract based on spectral local field power in conscious freely moving rats. *Journal of Ethnopharmacology* 177, 140-147.

Dimpfel, W., et al., 2017. Effect of Zembrin® on Brain Electrical Activity in 60 Older Subjects after 6 Weeks of Daily Intake. A Prospective, Randomized, Double-Blind, Placebo-Controlled, 3-Armed Study in a Parallel Design. *World Journal of Neuroscience* 7, 140-171.

Dragendorff, G., 1898. *Die Heilpflanzen Der Verschiedenen Völker Und Zeiten.* Verlag Von Ferdinand Enke, Stuttgart.

Dye, E. Undated presentation. Novel hallucinogens and plant-derived highs. Drug Enforcement Agency. https://www.nist.gov/sites/default/files/documents/oles/NIST-Novel-Hallucinogens-and-Plant-Derived-Highs-Final.pdf Accessed 15 April 2017.

Forbes, E.S. (Ed.)., 1986. *Carl Peter Thunberg. Travels at the Cape of Good Hope 1772–1775.* Second Series No. 17, Van Riebeeck Society, Cape Town.

Gerbaulet, M., 1996. Revision of the genus Sceletium N.E. Br. (Aizoaceae). *Botanische Jahrbücher* 118, 9–24.

Gericke, N., 1995. Sceletium Project. Investigation of a Traditional Herbal Sedative. Unpublished research report for South African Druggists Ltd., 30 May 1995.

Gericke, N., 2001. Clinical application of selected South African medicinal plants. *Australian Journal of Medical Herbalism* 13, 3–17.

Gericke, N., 2002. Plants, products and people: southern African perspectives, in: *Advances In Phytomedicine* Volume 1. *Ethnomedicine And Drug Discovery.* Iwu, M.M., Wootton, J.C. (Eds.), Elsevier, Amsterdam.

Gericke, N., 2011. Muthi to medicine. *South African Journal of Botany* 77(4), 850-856.

Gericke, N., 2014. Ethnobotanical records from a corporate expedition in South Africa in 1685. Herbalgram. *Journal of the American Botanical Council* 102, 48-61.

Gericke, N., Van Wyk, B.-E., 1999. Pharmaceutical compositions containing mesembrine and related compounds. US Patent 6,288,104.

Gericke, N., and van Wyk, B.-E., 2000. *People's Plants. A Guide To Useful Plants Of Southern Africa.* Briza, Pretoria.

Gericke, N., and Viljoen, A.M., 2008. Sceletium—a review update. *Journal of Ethnopharmacology* 119(3), 653-663.

Gericke, O., et al., 2017. *Sceletium tortuosum,* in: *Complementary and Integrative Treatments in Psychiatric Practice.* Gerbarg, PL, Muskin PR, Brown RP (Eds.), American Psychiatric Association Publishing, Arlington, VA.

Gordon, D., 1996. From rituals of rapture to dependence: the political economy of khoikhoi narcotic consumption, c.1487–1870. *South African Historical Journal* 35, 62–88.

Gunn, M., Codd, L.E., 1981. *Botanical Exploration of Southern Africa.* A.A. Balkema, Cape Town.

Harvey, A.L., et al., 2011. Pharmacological actions of the South African medicinal and functional food plant *Sceletium tortuosum* and its principal alkaloids. *Journal of Ethnopharmacology* 137(3), 1124-1129.

Harvey, A., et al., 2013. Pharmaceutical compositions containing mesembrenone. U.S. Patent 8,552,051.

Herre, H., 1971. *The Genera Of The Mesembryanthemaceae.* Tafelberg, Cape Town.

Hirabayashi M., et al., 2002. Clinical application of South African tea on dementia dog. *Japanese Journal of Small Animal Practice* 21, 109–113. [Japanese]

Hirabayashi M., et al., 2004. Clinical effects of South African tea for cat. *Japanese Journal of Small Animal Practice* 23, 85–89. [Japanese]

Hirabayashi M., et al., 2005. Clinical effects of South African Tea for dementia animal. *Japanese Journal of Small Animal Practice* 24, 27–31. [Japanese]

Hobbs, C.E., 1876. *C.E. Hobbs' Botanical Hand-Book.* C.E. Hobbs, Boston.

Holmes, E.M., 1874. Materia Medica Notes. *American Journal of Pharmacy* Vol. XlVI (1), 286.

Iatridis, K., Schroeder, D., 2016. *Responsible Research and Innovation in Industry. The Case for Corporate Responsibility Tools.* Springer, Cham, Heidelberg, New York, London.

Jacobsen, H., 1960. *Handbook of Succulent Plants. Vol. III. Mesembryanthemums (Ficoidaceae).* Blandford Press, London.

Jeffs, P.W., et al., 1982. Sceletium alkaloids. Structures of five new bases from Sceletium namaquense. *Journal of Organic Chemistry* 47, 3611–3617.

Juritz, C.F., 1905. *Report of the joint meeting of the British Association for the Advancement of Science and the South African Association for the Advancement of Science* 1, 231.

Klak, C., Bruyns, P.V., 2013. A new infrageneric classification for Mesembryanthemum (Aizoaceae: Mesembryanthemoideae). *Bothalia* 43 (2), 197-206.

Kolben, P., 1731. *The Present State of the Cape of Good Hope.* Translated from German by Mr. Medley. W. Innys, London, 210-213.

Krstenansky, J.L., 2017. Mesembrine Alkaloids: review of their occurrence, chemistry, and pharmacology. *Journal of Ethnopharmacology* 195, 10-19.

Laidler, P.W., 1928. The magic medicine of the Hottentots. *South African Journal of Science* 25, 433–447.

Lesiak, A.D., et al., 2016. Direct analysis in real-time high-resolution mass spectrometry as a tool for rapid characterization of mind-altering plant materials and revelation of supplement adulteration–the case of Kanna. *Forensic science international* 260, 66-73.

MacKenzie, S.J., Houslay, MD, 2000. Action of Rolipram on specific PDE4 cAMP phosphodiesterase isoforms and on the phosphorylation of cAMP-response-element binding protein (CREB) and p38 mitogen-activated protein (MAP) kinase in U937 monocytic cells. *Biochem J.* 347 (Pt 2), 571–578.

Marloth, R., 1917. *The Flora Of South Africa. Dictionary of The Common Names Of Plants.* Specialty Press of South Africa, Cape Town, 105.

Meiring, I., 1896. Notes on some experiments with the active principle of Mesembrianthemum tortuosum, L. *Transactions of the South African Philosophical Society* Volume IX, 48–50.

Meyer, G.M., et al., 2015. GC-MS, LC-MSn, LC-high resolution-MSn, and NMR studies on the metabolism and toxicological detection of mesembrine and mesembrenone, the main alkaloids of the legal high "Kanna" isolated from *Sceletium tortuosum*. *Analytical and bioanalytical chemistry* 407 (3), 761-778.

Moreland, W.H. (Ed.), 1934. *Peter Floris, His Voyage to the East Indies in the Globe, 1611-1615. The Contemporary Translation of His Journal.* Hakluyt Society, London, 4-5.

MSS BC151 006, Manuscript and Archives Department of the Libraries, University of Cape Town.

Murbach, T.S., et al., 2014. A toxicological safety assessment of a standardized extract of Sceletium tortuosum (Zembrin®) in rats. *Food and Chemical Toxicology* 74, 190-199.

Nell, H., et al., 2013. A randomized, double-blind, parallel-group, placebo-controlled trial of extract *Sceletium tortuosum* (Zembrin) in healthy adults. *The Journal of Alternative and Complementary Medicine* 19(11), 898-904.

Nicholl, J.M., 1895. *Botanical Ready Reference.* Murray & Nicholl Manufacturing Company, Chicago.

Nortje, J., 2011. *Medicinal Ethnobotany of the Kamiesberg*, Namaqualand, Northern Cape Province (Doctoral dissertation, MSc thesis), University of Johannesburg.

Nortje, J.M., Van Wyk, B.-E., 2015. Medicinal plants of the Kamiesberg, Namaqualand, *South Africa. Journal of Ethnopharmacology* 171, 205-222.

Pappe, L., 1868. *Florae Capensis Medicae, 3rd ed., Prodromus. An Enumeration of South African Plants used as Remedies by the Colonists of the Cape of Good Hope.* W. Brittain, Cape Town.

Patnala, S., Kanfer, I., 2010. HPLC analysis of mesembrine-type alkaloids in Sceletium plant material used as an African traditional medicine. *Journal of Pharmacy & Pharmaceutical Sciences* 13(4), 558-570.

Prader-Samper, José M. de., 2007. The plant lore of the /Xam San: //Kabbo and ≠Kasiŋ's identification of "Bushman" medicines. Culturas Populares. *Revista Electrónica* 4, 1-17. http://www.culturaspopulares.org/textos4/articulos/deprada.pdf ISSN: 1886-5623.

Purchas, S., 1625. *Purchas His Pilgrimes. In Five Bookes.* Printed by William Stansby for Henrie Fetherstone, London. Book One, 528.

Rimington, C., Roets, C.G.S., 1937. Notes upon the isolation of the alkaloidal constituent of the drug "channa" or "kougoed". *Onderstepoort Journal of Veterinary Science and Animal Industry* 9, 187-191.

Roscher, J., et al., 2012. Forensic analysis of mesembrine alkaloids in *Sceletium tortuosum* by nonaqueous capillary electrophoresis mass spectrometry. *Electrophoresis* 33(11), 1567-1570.

Schneider, J-C, Poljoux, J., Fernando,F., Greim, O. 28 September 2016. Heating assembly for an aerosol generating system. European Patent Application EP20130821804

Scott, G., Hewett, M.L., 2008. Pioneers in ethnopharmacology: the Dutch East India Company (VOC) at the Cape from 1650 to 1800. *Journal of Ethnopharmacology* 115(3), 339-360.

Serton, P., Raven-Hart, W.J. de Kock en E.H. Raidt (Eds.), 1971. *François Valentijn, Beschryvinge van de Kaap der Goede Hoope.* Deel I. Van Riebeeck Society, Cape Town.

Shikanga, E.A., et al., 2012. Validated RP-UHPLC PDA and GC–MS methods for the analysis of psychoactive alkaloids in *Sceletium tortuosum. South African Journal of Botany* 82, 99-107.

Smith, C., 2011. The effects of *Sceletium tortuosum* in an *in vivo* model of psychological stress. *Journal of Ethnopharmacology* 133(1), 31-36.

Smith, C.A., 1966. *Common Names of South African Plants.* Botanical Survey Memoir 35. Government Printer, Pretoria.

Smith, M.T., et al., 1996. Psychoactive constituents of the genus Sceletium NE Br. and other Mesembryanthemaceae: a review. *Journal of Ethnopharmacology* 50(3), 119-130.

Tachard, G., 1686. *Voyage de Siam, Des Pères Jesuites, Envoyez par le Roy aux Indes & à la Chine.* Arnold Seneuze and Daniel Horthemels, Paris, 102.

Terburg, D., et al., 2013. Acute effects of *Sceletium tortuosum* (Zembrin®), a dual 5-HT reuptake and PDE4 inhibitor, in the human amygdala and its connection to the hypothalamus. *Neuropsychopharmacology* 38(13), 2708-2716.

Thorens, M., Cochand, O., 24 March 2016. Electronically heated aerosol delivery system. United States Patent Application 20160081395.

Tully, W., 1858. *Materia Medica or Pharmacology And Therapeutics.* Jefferson Church MD, Springfield, 823.

UNODC, 2013. *The Challenge of New Psychoactive Substances. List of Plant-based Substances, 101-102.*

Waterhouse, G., et al., 1979. *Simon van der Stel's Journey to Namaqualand in 1685.* Human & Rousseau, Cape Town.

Watt, J.M., and Breyer-Brandwijk, M.G., 1962. *The Medicinal and Poisonous Plants of Southern and Eastern Africa*, 2nd ed. Livingstone, London.

Wilson, M.L., 1993. Early records of some flora and fauna used by the Khoisan of the Western Cape. *Southern African Field Archeology* 2, 67-73.

Ye, Y., et al., 2000. Effects of repeated antidepressant treatment of type 4A phosphodiesterase (PDE4A) in rat brain. J *Neurochem* 74, 1257–1262.

Zhao, Y., et al., 2010. *Review of total synthesis of mesembrine.* Youji Huaxue 30 (1), 47–59.

Zwicky, E., 1913. Über Channa, ein Genussmittel der Hottentotten. *Vierteljahrsschr. Naturforsch. Gesell. Zürich* 58, 371-430.

Kratom (*Mitragyna Speciosa*) as a Potential Therapy for Opioid Dependence

Christopher R. McCurdy, PhD, BS Ph, FAAPS

Department of Medicinal Chemistry, College of Pharmacy, University of Florida, Gainesville, Florida

Several psychoactive herbal products are widely available over the Internet with minimal control on their sale. Complicating this availability is the poor understanding of the chemical components and pharmacology of such products. Very little is known about specific chemical entities or combinations of chemicals present in these products. The availability of these products to adolescents and young adults has created a great concern for understanding the chemistry, psychopharmacology, and toxicology of these herbs. Use and abuse of these substances is difficult to measure, other than through anecdotal reports found on websites and through media reports. Particular interest has been generated around kratom (*Mitragyna speciosa* [Korth] Havil.), as it has been on the DEA (United States Drug Enforcement Agency) List of Drugs and Chemicals of Concern for over a decade (DEA, 2016). Kratom has been touted as a "legal high", and the major alkaloid, mitragynine, has been thought to be responsible for its actions at opioid receptors (Babu et al., 2008). In addition, a minor alkaloid and oxidative product of mitragynine, 7-hydroxymitragynine, has also been reported to have potent agonist activity at opioid receptors (Babu et al., 2008). Although 7-hydroxymitragynine occurs in trace amounts in the natural plant, several marketed products are suspected to be adulterated with increased levels of this compound (Lydecker et al., 2016). According to the scientific literature, it is not clear if mitragynine has abuse liability, and has been reported to have mild analgesic properties most similar to codeine or non-steroidal anti-inflammatory drugs (NSAIDs) (Macko et al, 1972). Conversely, 7-hydroxymitragynine (a minor plant constituent), when purified and pharmacologically tested alone, does show a conditioned place preference (drug-seeking behavior) in rodents, as well as potent analgesia (Matsumoto et al., 2008). To complicate matters, it is not entirely known if 7-hydroxymitragynine is produced by the plant, or is an oxidative byproduct of leaf drying, due to the low amounts in which it has been reported to occur in traditional fresh leaf extracts. Synthetic procedures have been published to convert mitragynine to 7-hydroxymitragynine (Takayama et al., 2002), but this involves specialty chemicals that are not commonly available to the public or clandestine laboratories. Nonetheless, from those commercially available products analyzed, it is clear that the levels of 7-hydroxymitragynine are in much greater concentrations than occur in nature (Lydecker et al, 2016).

Kratom has been linked to 16 deaths, although in each case the deceased individuals had multiple substances in their systems. It is important to note that not a single death has been attributed to kratom in Southeast Asia, where it has been traditionally used for over 100 years. In addition, the DEA had rightfully banned synthetic bath salts and synthetic cannabinoids (i.e., K2 or Spice) based on scientific evidence, removing them from the consumer marketplace and providing them a home in the list of Schedule I controlled substances. This void in the consumer market was filled with kratom products in gas stations, herbal shops, and the Internet. The DEA faced pressure from a small but vocal section of the public to ban kratom and place it in Schedule I. Even though very limited scientific information was available on kratom, in the fall of 2016 the DEA nevertheless announced

151

their intention to place kratom, mitragynine, and 7-hydroxymitragynine into Schedule I of the Controlled Substances Act (DEA, 2016). This created a large push from those that have utilized kratom for control of pain and prescription opioid addiction to place pressure on the DEA as well. The result was unprecedented, with the DEA announcing a 30-day open comment period for the public. Over 23,000 written pleas were received by the DEA to reconsider this position (Federal register 2016). These communications came from the general public, legislators, and the scientific community involved in kratom research. In addition, the Botanical Education Alliance published an 8-Factor analysis of kratom by Dr. Jack E. Henningfield that indicated kratom is *not* addictive (Pinney Associates, 2016). Moreover, it stated that the factors that appear important in maintaining kratom use appear more similar to those of normal caffeine intake. This report was submitted to the DEA & FDA in 2016. For the first time in history, the DEA withdrew their intention to place Kratom into Schedule I, though it still has the right to do so at any time (Federal Register, 2016). This manuscript aims to provide the current state of science around kratom.

Kratom is a tree native to Thailand, Malaysia, and other areas of Southeast Asia. The leaves of this tree have been utilized for many years by laborers for their stimulant effects (at low doses), and their ability to invigorate workers in harsh conditions (Jansen et al., 1988). Kratom has also seen much use as a replacement for opium due to its euphoric and sedative effects (at higher doses) (Jansen et al., 1988). Extracts and decoctions have also been noted as a method to alleviate opioid withdrawal. (Jansen et al., 1988; Boyer et al.,2007, 2008). Kratom was outlawed in Thailand through the Kratom Act in 1943; however, it remains a widely popular substance there (DEA, 2017; Jansen et al., 1988). It has been assumed that the ban in Thailand was due to the government's inability to generate tax revenue from the plant, although this is not documented. With the reports of its actions, and the fact that it is not controlled in much of the world, it was introduced to the Western world via the Internet and touted for its stimulant and opium-like effects. Indeed, according to an Internet supplier, sales are very good in the United States[1].

Currently, kratom is not a controlled substance under federal law in the United States, and little information is known on its true pharmacological activities. However, six states have banned kratom as of July 2017: Alabama, Arkansas, Indiana, Tennessee, Vermont, and Wisconsin. It has also been made illegal in Sarasota County, Florida; San Diego, California; and Jerseyville, Illinois. In addition, it is illegal in many countries, including Australia, Burma, Denmark, Lithuania, Malaysia, Myanmar, Poland, Sweden, Thailand, and Vietnam (Kratom Science, 2017).

Extracts of *Mitragyna speciosa* have been used in Thailand and Malaysia for many years for their opium-like effects and coca-like stimulant ability to combat fatigue (Jansen et al., 1988). It is interesting that the plant seems to have these apparently contradictory effects. Some early studies (Wray et al., 1907a; Wray et al., 1907b) indicated a similarity to cocaine in humans, but other studies (Jansen et al., 1988; Takayama 2004; Boyer et al., 2007) have shown opioid-like effects. In fact, kratom has long been promoted in these areas as a substitute for opium, and has also been used to wean addicts off morphine. Some recent clinical reports of kratom being utilized as a self-treatment for opioid withdrawal indicate the medical community is seeing patients who are using kratom (Jansen et al., 1988; Takayama 2004; Babu et al., 2008; DEA Public Affairs, 2016). The plant material and extracts are available on the Internet, making them easily obtainable by those who may want to experiment with such substances. Currently, as mentioned, there are no restrictions on this plant, extracts, or purified compounds in the majority of the United States.

Fortunately, there is some information in the literature about the chemistry and pharmacology of this plant. Some active alkaloids on opioid receptors have been identified from extracts of *Mitragyna speciosa* (Takayama et al., 2002) and are shown in Figure 1. These include: mitragynine (1), 7-hydroxymitragynine (2), and corynantheidine (3).

The studies that have been reported focus on the opioid-like effects of extracts and some of the pure chemicals that have been isolated. Many studies on these substances demonstrate effects that are reversible with naloxone, an opioid-receptor antagonist. It has been reported that extracts of *Mitragyna speciosa* can reduce pain in animal studies. Interestingly, little is known about the mechanism of the reported stimulant actions. A review of the literature demonstrates a wide variety of opioid activity and inconsistency in studies. These inconsistencies range from extraction procedures, binding affinity measurements, and antagonists utilized, as well as *in vivo* reports. These are all detailed below, and underscore the strong need to understand the actions of the extract and isolated natural products in a side-by-side comparison in the same assays to more completely understand the chemistry and pharmacology of this species.

....

1 Salesperson at Naturalorganix.com. Personal communication 8/30/2017

Isolation of some 40 alkaloids from this plant have focused on the most predominant alkaloid, mitragynine (1) (Adkins et al., 2011). Mitragynine, a corynantheidine alkaloid first isolated by Field in 1921 (Field 1921), has demonstrated opioid-receptor affinity and partial agonist activity. Interestingly, opioid-receptor affinities that have been reported in multiple studies are not consistent. In some cases, affinities for some opioid receptor subtypes have been reported by some and not found by others. This may be due to variations in the purity of compounds, receptor preparations, and radioligands utilized in these studies. However, it does lead to an ambiguity of the understanding of these naturally occurring chemical components. Of high interest are the most recent reports that demonstrate mitragynine as a partial agonist that has a G-protein signaling bias (Kruegel et al., 2016). This signaling bias has been hypothesized to result in fewer liabilities from mitragynine than other opioid ligands. Most notably, mitragynine and kratom do not cause significant respiratory depression in rodents, nor presumably in humans. This pharmacology may explain why there have not been any reports of overdose deaths from kratom alone, as unlike traditional morphine-based opioids, there seems to be little to no effect on respiration. If kratom has been listed as a cause of death, it is still suspect, as there are no controls on what products are sold. This lack of control and standardization makes the marketplace a "buyer beware" one. Moreover, it can be almost impossible to analyze a product for an adulterant that is not known. This has been evidenced by the rapidly changing landscape of compounds that are found in synthetic cannabinoid or bath salt preparations.

The first reports of pharmacological studies on mitragynine appeared in the literature in 1972 (Macko et al., 1972). Researchers at Smith, Kline and French (SKF) were interested in finding a novel analgesic that would have less liability than the currently utilized opioids (i.e. morphine). Their studies were the most comprehensive at the time and still remain as one of the more complete in the literature. A battery of animal studies were undertaken to investigate the analgesic potential and opioid actions of mitragynine. These studies did show that mitragynine had analgesic and antitussive properties comparable to codeine. Unlike codeine, mitragynine did not produce emesis or dyspnea, was not blocked by nalorphine, and had much less respiratory depression. Interestingly, it could suppress the opioid withdrawal syndrome. Moreover, it was noted that mitragynine was active only via the oral and intraperitoneal routes of administration (in an equal ratio), and was inactive via the subcutaneous route. It was hypothesized that the analgesic activity may be related to a metabolite, or that the bioavailability of mitragynine is influenced by the acidic conditions of the route of administration. It appeared that SKF decided to abandon further studies on this substance, most likely due to the weak analgesic potency when compared to traditional, marketed opioid pharmaceuticals.

Mitragynine seemed to be discounted for a number of years until the mid-1990s, when researchers in Japan began to study this compound and plant species again. By this time, it had been realized that nalorphine had mixed opioid agonist/antagonist actions, and may have confounded the results previously reported in the study carried out at SKF. The analgesic activity of mitragynine was again investigated in the tail-pinch and hot-plate tests, resulting in antinociceptive activity that was completely abolished by naloxone, a pure opioid receptor antagonist (Matsumoto et al., 1996a). This indicated the involvement of supraspinal opioid receptors in the analgesic actions of mitragynine and sparked a renewed interest in the pharmacology of this molecule.

Shortly thereafter, the same group indicated the contribution of descending noradrenergic and serotonergic systems in the analgesic activities of mitragynine (Matsumoto et al., 1996b). This is similar to what is known with the actions of morphine. Utilizing the same paradigm in their previous study, the involvement of these systems was investigated by employing the a2-adrenoceptor antagonist idazoxan, and the 5-HT receptor antagonist cyproheptadine. Each of these agents significantly antagonized the analgesic effects of mitragynine. This work indicated that mitragynine may stimulate the release of endogenous norepinephrine and serotonin, similar to the actions of other opioid ligands.

Another study to elucidate the mechanism of action of mitragynine involved the 5-methoxy-N, N-dimethyltryptamine-induced head-twitch response in mice (Matsumoto et al., 1997). This study, again from the same researchers in Japan, seemed to echo the findings of the involvement of noradrenergic and serotonergic mechanisms in the actions of mitragynine. Indeed, mitragynine suppressed the effects of head-twitch in this assay, indicating possible agonist actions on adrenergic and antagonist actions on serotonergic systems.

The inhibition of electrically stimulated contraction in the guinea-pig ileum was also demonstrated to work through opioid mechanisms, as it was reversed by naloxone (Watanabe et al., 1997) This study did not employ any subtype-selective antagonists to indicate the possible opioid-recep-

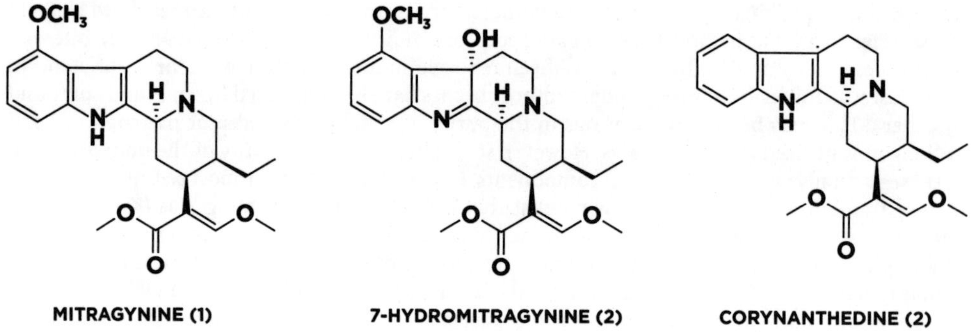

MITRAGYNINE (1)   **7-HYDROMITRAGYNINE (2)**   **CORYNANTHEDINE (2)**

Fig. 1 The opioid-active alkaloids isolated from *Mitragyna speciosa*.

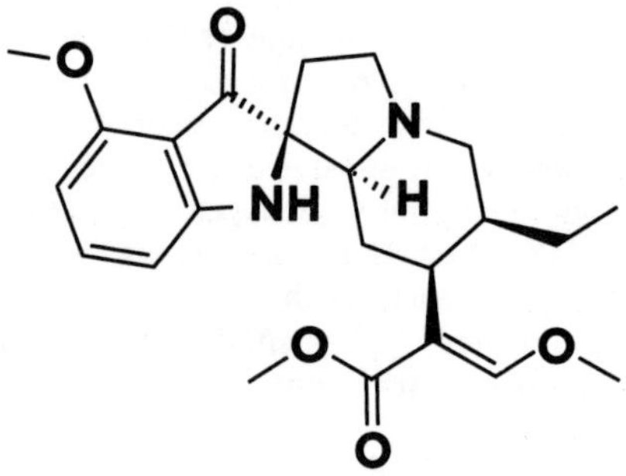

Fig. 2 Structure of the microbial metabolite, mitragynine pseudoindoxyl.

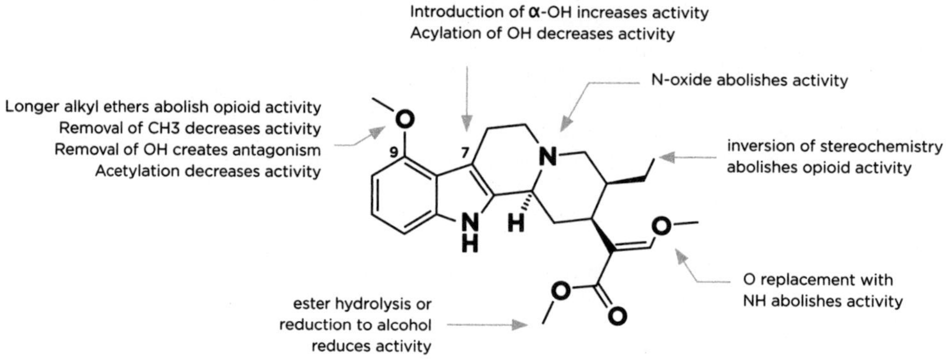

Introduction of α-OH increases activity
Acylation of OH decreases activity

N-oxide abolishes activity

Longer alkyl ethers abolish opioid activity
Removal of CH3 decreases activity
Removal of OH creates antagonism
Acetylation decreases activity

inversion of stereochemistry
abolishes opioid activity

O replacement with
NH abolishes activity

ester hydrolysis or
reduction to alcohol
reduces activity

Fig. 3 Known structure-activity relationships of mitragynine.

tor subtypes involved. Some understanding of the subtypes involved was revealed through a study of antinociception in mice, conducted by the same researchers. Their results indicated the involvement of MOP and DOP (Mu and Delta Opioid) receptors through the use of subtype-selective antagonists. They concluded that mitragynine has different selectivity than morphine for opioid-receptor subtypes, yet no receptor binding data was presented. It was much later that the same group published findings on the inhibitory effects of mitragynine on neurogenic contraction of the guinea-pig vas deferens (Matusumoto et al. 2005). The vas deferens is known to contain high amounts of DOP and MOP receptors. In this study, the effects of mitragynine were unable to be blocked by naloxone, leading to the conclusion that opioid receptors are not involved. The conclusion of these studies indicated that the inhibitory effects of mitragynine in this paradigm were through the blockade of calcium channels. This study was confounded by the fact that morphine could not inhibit electrically induced contraction in this assay, leading a reader to question the validity of the findings.

The first receptor-binding data for mitragynine was presented in 2002 (Takayama et al., 2002). The binding affinities for mitragynine at the three opioid receptors were determined using guinea pig brain membranes and reported as pKi values. The data indicated that mitragynine is a MOP-selective opioid ligand with a pKi value of 8.14 ± 0.28, and a relative affinity of 88.7% for the MOP over the DOP and KOP receptors. The pKi values at the DOP and KOP were 7.22 ± 0.21 and 5.96 ± 0.22, respectively. This report did not include functional data at each of the receptors, so it is difficult to relate it to the previously reported receptor selectivity studies that were conducted in mice. As previously mentioned, the *in vivo* study implicated the roles of the MOP and DOP in the actions of mitragynine. Taken together, these data are a bit inconsistent but still reasonable, since functional activities were not presented in the more recent report. The receptor-binding affinities described in this study also included other naturally occurring alkaloids from *Mitragyna speciosa*, and some semi-synthetic derivatives. Most of the natural products and semi-synthetic analogs had much less affinity than mitragynine. Although most of these compounds had less opioid receptor affinity, 7-hydroxymitragynine was 10 times more potent than morphine, and 40 times more potent than mitragynine in the guinea pig ileum assay. Surprisingly, this compound was not investigated in analgesic studies with mice so it was not determined if the activity was due to opioid receptors. The most interesting finding from this work was the inclusion of a previously reported microbial oxidative metabolite of mitragynine, mitragynine pseudoindoxyl (Zarembo et al., 1974; Takayama et al., 2002) (4, Figure 2).

This compound had a higher affinity for mu-opioid receptors (pKi value 10.06 ± 0.39) and a similar relative affinity to morphine among the other opioid receptors (Takayama et al., 2002). Moreover, mitragynine pseudoindoxyl was 35 times more potent than morphine in the electrically stimulated guinea pig ileum assay. However, when mitragynine pseudoindoxyl was tested *in vivo*, the analgesic activity was less than that of morphine, but greater than mitragynine itself. The effects of mitragynine pseudoindoxyl were completely reversed by naloxone. Studies on this molecule have not appeared in the literature since this report. It may be due to the source of this molecule, as it is a metabolite of *Helminthosporium* sp. and therefore may be difficult to obtain.

This study (Takayama et al., 2002 also provided some insight into the structure-activity relationships of mitragynine, and in two reviews (Takayama 2004; Kruegel et al., 2016) on the chemistry and pharmacology of *Mitragyna speciosa* has included more information on semi-synthetic studies of mitragynine. This structure-activity-relationship information is summarized in Figure 3 (Adkins et al., 2011).

Essentially, all the semi-synthetic derivatives had less activity than mitragynine, indicating some important structural features on the natural product. First, the 9-methoxy seems to be important for agonist activity. When the methyl ether is cleaved to the phenol, a less active agonist is produced. When the oxygen is eliminated to produce the natural product corynantheidine (3), an antagonist is produced. Thus, it is interesting that modulation of functional activity may occur at this position. It is of chemical interest that this small change to the molecule may afford templates for novel opioid antagonists, potentially with superior bioavailability to currently marketed products. Next, it also appears that disruption of the b-acrylate moiety, albeit from a very limited study, leads to less active or inactive products. Finally, loss of the basic character of the tertiary amine abolishes activity. This seems to be consistent with other opioid-based alkaloids that require a protonatable nitrogen to form a salt bridge with a conserved aspartic acid residue in transmembrane III (TM III) of the opioid receptors.

This result may indicate that mitragynine is binding in a similar mode to other known opioid ligands. However, reported comparisons of mitragynine and morphine (Takayama et al., 2002) do not indicate structural similarities, and hypothesize that mitragynine has a different binding mode than classical morphine-based ligands. It could be that some amino acid residues in the receptor are common to the affinity of both classes but some unique epitopes are involved with mitragynine recognition.

Although these studies have indicated some important structural features on mitragynine, detailed studies to elucidate the opioid pharmacophore are lacking. A few other alkaloids that have been isolated from the plant do not appear to have interesting profiles as opioid ligands, but only a few of the over 20 alkaloids have been subjected to receptor-binding studies. The C3 (quinolizidine bridge-head hydrogen) stereoisomer of mitragynine was reported to be 14-fold less active in the guinea pig ileum assay, yet no binding data was reported at opioid receptors (Takayama et al., 2002). Therefore, not all the alkaloids have been investigated nor have other non-alkaloidal ligands been characterized, and it is not entirely clear how important any of the stereochemistry is to the molecule. Moreover, no simplified analogs of mitragynine have been reported in the literature. Thus, there is a great need for a more complete understanding of the chemistry associated with *Mitragyna speciosa*.

From the reports in the literature on the naturally occurring alkaloids from *Mitragyna speciosa*, only a few of the alkaloids have been investigated for activity and some have been reported in separate studies, making them difficult to compare. More recently, the focus of literature studies has shifted to a minor component of the extract, 7-hydroxymitragynine hydroxymitragynine(2) (Ponglux et al., 1994; Matsumoto et al., 2004; Matsumoto et al., 2005). This is simply an oxidized form of mitragynine obtained from *Mitragyna speciosa*. The first report Matsumoto et al. 2004) of the *in vivo* actions of 7-hydroxymitragynine also included receptor-binding data that was obtained under the same conditions as reported for the affinities of mitragynine and 7-hydroxymitragynine. Interestingly, 7-hydroxymitragynine displayed a higher affinity to MOP than previously reported. Affinities for DOP and KOP were consistent with the previous report from the same group (Takayama et al., 2002). In this study, the tail-flick and hot-plate assays were utilized, and 7-hydroxymitragynine showed more potent effects than morphine in both tests. This is interesting since the affinity of 7-hydroxymitragynine is comparable to mitragynine and morphine. An interesting finding from this study was that 7-hydroxymitragynine was orally active and long-acting. It is now hypothesized that most of the opioid actions are a result of this compound and not mitragynine. However, the possibility of an active metabolite cannot be ruled out.

The tolerance and withdrawal symptoms of 7-hydroxymitragynine have also been studied (Matsumoto et al., 2005). In this report, the specific opioid-receptor subtypes responsible for its actions were also investigated. Tolerance developed to 7-hydroxymitragynine over time, as well as cross-tolerance to morphine. Similar to morphine, withdrawal symptoms were equally comparable upon naloxone-induced withdrawal of 7-hydroxymitragynine. It was determined that the analgesic activity of 7-hydroxymitragynine was mediated through MOP and partially through KOP. Attempts to overlay the compound with morphine were not successful, and it was concluded that 7-hydroxymitragynine may be interacting with opioid receptors in a different fashion than morphine. Overall, 7-hydroxymitragynine was shown to be a potent opioid receptor ligand that can potentially cause physical dependence.

An additional study on the effects of 7-hydroxymitragynine on gastrointestinal transit has demonstrated the involvement of MOP receptors in this action (Matsumoto et al., 2006). Interestingly, this study also investigated the receptor subtypes involved in the analgesic activity. This work came from the same group as the previous studies, and was consistent in demonstrating a MOP-selective activity. However, this time the KOP receptor was not shown to be involved. It had been previously reported by other researchers that mitragynine did not inhibit gastrointestinal transit, (Macko et al., 1972) but this study had noted limitations.

Because *Mitragyna speciosa* has been traditionally utilized to combat fatigue and promote the ability to work in harsh conditions, a study was undertaken to determine its effects on working memory (Apryani et al., 2010). This investigation involved the object-location task and the open-field test. In these paradigms, mitragynine was found to impair the cognitive function and decrease locomotion. The authors suggested this finding is similar to other mu-opioid agonists, and they further hypothesized that the memory impairment could be due to decreases in GABA neurotransmission. More studies would need to be carried out in more sophisticated paradigms to learn the effects of chronic use on working memory.

Many users of kratom, both traditional and recreational, have stated that ingestion of the plant material elevates mood and may have potential as an antidepressant. To test this idea, a study was carried out utilizing mitragynine in the mouse forced-swim test and the tail-suspension test (Idayu et al., 2011). It was determined that doses of mitragynine significantly reduced immobility in the forced-swim test and tail-suspension test, demonstrating antidepressant-like effects. Moreover, mitragynine significantly reduced corticosterone release, which is normally elevated in stressful situations. This study showed promising potential for the use of kratom as an antidepressant, and somewhat validated the anecdotal reports of human mood elevation.

Another study was published a few years later looking into the anxiolytic-like effects of mitragynine in the open-field and elevated plus-maze paradigms (Hazim et al., 2014). These studies were done in rats, in contrast to the above study that utilized mice. This work compared the efficacy of mitragynine versus a diazepam control. The findings support the human use of kratom as an anxiolytic, where mitragynine was shown to be effective, although less than diazepam, increasing exploration in both assays. Moreover, the investigators studied three neurological systems with antagonists pre-treatment. All antagonists tested were effective in blocking mitragynine's action. This indicated that the anxiolytic-like effects are possibly due to interactions among opioidergic, GABAergic, and dopaminergic systems in the brain. It was a bit curious that serotonergic systems were not investigated in this study.

Kratom has traditionally been utilized to wean addicts off opium, and two studies have appeared in the literature investigating mitragynine and its ability to attenuate morphine withdrawal syndrome. The first study appeared utilizing zebrafish (Khor et al., 2011). Although not a commonly utilized model in opioid research, this proved to be an interesting study. Morphine was added to the water for a two-week, chronic-exposure paradigm. Mitragynine was shown to attenuate the majority of withdrawal behaviors, and real-time PCR analyses showed that it also reduced the mRNA expression of corticotropin-releasing factor receptors and prodynorphin in the zebrafish. A few years later, a study by researchers in Thailand showed an alkaloid-rich extract from *Mitragyna speciosa* was effective in attenuating naloxone-precipitated morphine withdrawal symptoms in mice (Cheaha; et al., 2017). Interestingly, their study was in direct contrast to the zebrafish study with regard to the effects of purified mitragynine. The study in mice failed to demonstrate efficacy for mitragynine alone in single-dose oral-administration studies. This is most likely due to the design of the study. To habituate the mice to morphine, doses were administered three times (50, 50, 75 mg/kg, respectively) a day for three days, and on the fourth day, mice were given a 50 mg/kg injection of morphine two hours prior to naloxone precipitation of withdrawal. In the studies that looked at ability for the alkaloid-rich extract or purified mitragynine, the mice were given only one dose of extract or mitragynine one hour after a dose of morphine and one hour prior to injection with naloxone. The only behavioral outcome that was considered for withdrawal symptoms was jumping behavior. Although various doses were examined, it is possible that a single dose of either test material would not be enough to attenuate the withdrawal effects. The authors concluded that another constituent of the alkaloid-rich extract may be responsible for the attenuation of effects seen, not mitragynine.

A group of researchers in Malaysia studied morphine-tolerance development in mice with a combination of mitragynine and morphine (Fakurazi et al., 2013). This study looked at a nine-day dosing regimen with both compounds, and evaluated the analgesic effects in the hot-plate test. Not surprisingly, the combination of morphine and mitragynine increased hot-plate latency. However, the combination of these two compounds did produce a significant reduction in morphine tolerance over morphine alone. The investigators looked at CREB-protein expression as well as liver and kidney function tests, but did not see any significant changes in the combination-treated groups. Decreasing opioid-tolerance development is hypothesized to be one way of reducing the abuse or addiction potential of these agents, and certainly a way to avoid some of the side effects that can arise from increasing dosing regimens.

Another way to examine the abuse or addictive potential of opioids is through the conditioned place preference (CPP) paradigm. Two reports have appeared in the literature that are in overall agreement demonstrating that mitragynine causes a place preference, and that indicate a drug-seeking behavior is associated with mitragynine. It is interesting that the first study failed to demonstrate a statistically significant place preference for an extract of *Mitragyna speciosa*, but did show each dose of purified mitragynine to cause a place preference (Sufka et al., 2014). It is important to note that the error bars were quite large in these studies. The second study looked at CPP in a bit more detail, and looked directly at opioid-receptor involvement by the use of antagonists (Yusoff et al., 2017). This study was aimed at investigating whether the reinforcing effects of mitragynine were mediated by opioid receptors. This study demonstrated that naloxone was effective at blocking mitragyine CPP overall. Interestingly, the investigators also showed that the acquisition, but not the expression, of mitragynine place preference is mediated through opioid receptors. These findings add more support to the mu-opioid agonist activity of mitragynine.

Finally, an investigation was carried out to determine the discriminative stimulus properties of mitragynine in rats (Harun et al., 2015). Drug discrimination is a valid paradigm to compare substances, especially psychoactive ones. This work utilized rats that were trained to discriminate morphine from vehicle. Interestingly, the investigators also wanted to examine the stimulant properties (thought to be a result of mitragynine) by using a group trained with cocaine. Rats were able to discriminate between mitragynine and saline, similar to another group that was able to discriminate between morphine and saline. The dose required for mitragynine was 3-fold higher than that of morphine. Both mitragynine and 7-hydroxymitragynine individually substituted completely to morphine discriminative stimulus. This suggests that there is pharmacological similarity between the two compounds. Interestingly, mitragynine also partially generalized to cocaine discriminative stimulus. Thus, both the opioid- and stimulant-like effects of *Mitragyna speciosa* can potentially be due to the major alkaloid, mitragynine.

All of the studies that have been conducted have shown that mitragynine and 7-hydroxymitragynine are opioid-receptor agonists. However, there are inconsistencies (as pointed out above) in these studies, making the interpretation of the entire body of pharmacological literature difficult to fully understand the pharmacology and chemistry associated with these compounds. Mitragynine and 7-hydroxymitragynine have been shown to work through opioid mechanisms *in vivo* and *in vitro* (Babu et al., 2008; Akins et al., 2011). They have also been shown to have activity in the serotonin and adrenergic systems (Matsumoto et al., 1996). This is not surprising upon review of the structure, which contains the tryptamine nucleus. One study that is completely lacking in the literature is the ability of mitragynine or 7-hydroxymitragynine, or extracts of *Mitragyna speciosa*, to be self-administered. Such a study would provide the most solid evidence for the abuse/addiction liability associated with the individual alkaloids or extracts. The fact that mitragynine alone interacts with multiple targets in the CNS, not to mention the full extracts' multiple activities, certainly helps to explain why the pharmacology is complex. However, it may be that this complex pharmacology has provided a natural antidote to opioid addiction. This remains to be seen, at least from a scientifically sound study and carefully controlled human clinical trial. There remains a great deal of scientific work that needs to be carried out on this plant species and its constituents to determine the chemical and pharmacological reasons that it is used traditionally and recreationally, to anticipate potential toxicities and potential therapeutic components. There seems to be great therapeutic promise to kratom.

REFERENCES

Adkins, J.E., Boyer, E.W., McCurdy, C.R., 2011. *Mitragyna speciosa*, a psychoactive tree from Southeast Asia with opioid activity. *Curr. Top. Med. Chem.* 11, 1165-1175.
Apryani, E., Hidayat, M.T., Moklas, MAA., Fakurazi, S., Idayu, N.F., 2010. Effects of mitragynine from *Mitragyna speciosa* Korth leaves on working memory. *J. Ethnopharmacol.* 129, 357-360.
Boyer, E.W., Babu, K.M., Macalino, G.E., Compton, W., 2007. Self-treatment of opioid withdrawal with a dietary supplement, kratom. *Am. J. Addictions* 16, 352-356.
Babu, K.M., McCurdy, C.R., Boyer, E.W., 2008. Opioid receptors and legal highs: *Salvia divinorum* and Kratom. *Clin Toxicol* (Phila). 46, 146-152.
Boyer, E.W., Babu, K.M., Adkins, J.E., McCurdy, C.R., Halpern, J.H., 2008. Self-treatment of opioid withdrawal using kratom (Mitraygna speciosa Korth.). *Addiction* 103, 1048-1050.
Cheaha, D., Chayaporn, R., Nukitram, J., Chittrakarn, S., Phukpattaranot, P., Keawpradub, N., Kumarnsit, E., 2017. Effects of alkaloid-rich extract from *Mitragyna speciosa* (Korth.) Havil. on naloxone-precipitated morphine withdrawal symptoms and local field potential in the nucleus accumbens of mice. *J. Ethnopharmacol.* 208, 129-137.
DEA Diversion Control Division (2016) https://www.deadiversion.usdoj.gov/drug_chem_info/ (accessed 8/03/2017).
DEA Public Affairs (2016) https://www.dea.gov/divisions/hq/2016/hq083016.shtml (accessed 8/03/2017).
Fakurazi, S., Rahman, S.A., Hidayat, M.T., Ithnin, H., Moklas, MAM., Arulselvan, P., 2013. The combination of mitragynine and morphine prevents the development of morphine tolerance in mice. *Molecules* 18, 666-681.
Federal Register (2016) https://www.federalregister.gov/documents/2016/10/13/2016-24659/withdrawal-of-notice-of-intent-to-temporarily-place-mitragynine-and-7-hydroxymitragynine-into (accessed 8/03/2017).
Field, E.J., 1921. Mitragynine and mitraversine, two new alkaloids from species of Mitragyna. *Transactions of the Chemical Society* 119, 887-891.
Grewal, K.S., 1932. Observations on the pharmacology of mitragynine. *J. Pharmacol. Expt. Ther.* 46, 251-271.
Harun, N., Hassan, Z., Navaratnam, V., Mansor, S.M., Shoaib, M., 2015. Discriminative stimulus properties of mitragynine (kratom) in rats. *Psychopharmacol.* 232, 2227-2238.
Hazim, A.I., Ramanathan, S., Parthasarathy, S., Muzaimi, M., Mansor, S.M., 2014. Anxiolytic-like effects of mitragynine in the open-field and elevated plus-maze tests in rats. *J. Physiol. Sci.* 64, 161-169.
Idayu, N.F., Hidayat, M.T., Moklas, MAM., Sharida, F., Raudzah, A.R.N., Shamima, A.R., Apryani, E., 2011. Antidepressant-like effect of mitragynine isolated from *Mitragyna speciosa* Korth in mice model of depression. *Phytomed.* 18, 402-407.

Jansen, K.L.R., Prast, C.J., 1988. Ethnopharmacology of kratom and the Mitragyna alkaloids. *J. Ethnopharm.* 23, 115-119.

Khor, B-S., Jamil, M.F.A., Adenan, M.I., Shu-Chien, A.C., 2011. Mitragynine attenuates withdrawal syndrome in morphine-withdrawn zebrafish. *PLOS One* 6, e28340.

Kratom Science https://www.kratomscience.com/kratom-legality/ (accessed 8/03/2017).

Kruegel, A.C., Gassaway, M.M., Kapoor, A., Varadi, A., Majumdar, S., Filizola, M., Javitch, J.A., Sames, D., 2016. Synthetic and receptor-signaling explorations of the Mitragyna alkaloids: Mitragynine as an atypical molecular framework for opioid receptor modulators. *J. Am. Chem. Soc.* 138, 6754-6764.

Lydecker, A.G., Sharma, A., McCurdy, C.R., Avery, B.A., Babu, K.M., Boyer, E.W., 2016. Suspected adulteration of commercial kratom products with 7-hydroxymitragynine. *J. Med. Toxicol.* 12, 341-349.

Macko, E., Weisbach, J.A., Douglas, B., 1972. Some observations on the pharmacology of mitragynine. *Arch. Int. Pharmacodyn.* 198, 145-161.

Matsumoto, K., Horie, S., Takayama, H., Ishikawa, H., Aimi, N., Ponglux, D., Murayama, T., Watanabe, K., 2005. Antinociception, tolerance and withdrawal symptoms induced by 7-hydroxymitragynine, an alkaloid from the Thai medicinal herb *Mitragyna speciosa*. *Life Sci.* 78, 2-7.

Matsumoto, K., Mizowaki, M., Suchitra, T., Murakami, Y., Takayama, H, Saki, S-I., Aimi, N., Watanabe, H., 1996. Central antinociceptive effects of mitragynine on mice: contribution of descending noradrenergic and serotonergic systems. *Eur. J. Pharmacol.* 317, 75-81.

Matsumoto, K., Mizowaki, M., Suchitra, T., Takayama, H., Sakai, S-I., Aimi, N., Watanabe, H., 1996. Antinociceptive action of mitragynine in mice: Evidence for the involvement of supraspinal opioid receptors. *Life Sci.* 59, 1149-1155.

Matsumoto, K., Mizowaki, M., Takayama, H., Sakai, S-I., Aimi, N., Watanabe, H., 1997. Suppressive effect of mitragynine on the 5-methoxy-N,N-dimethyltryptamine-induced head-twitch response in mice. *Pharmacol. Biochem. Behav.* 57, 319-323.

Matusmoto, K., Horie, S., Ishikawa, H., Takayama, H., Aimi, N., Ponglux, D., Watanabe, K., 2004. Antinociceptive effect of 7-hydroxymitragynine in mice: discovery of an orally active opioid analgesic from Thai medicinal herb *Mitragyna speciosa*. *Life Sci.* 74, 2143-2155.

Matsumoto, K., Yamamoto, L.T., Watanabe, K., Yano, S., Shan, J., Pang, P.K.T., Ponglux, D., Takayama, H., Horie, S., 2005. Inhibitory effect of mitragynine, an analgesic alkaloid from Thai herbal medicine, on neurogenic contraction of the vas deferens. *Life Sci.* 78, 1887-194.

Matsumoto, K., Hatori, Y., Murayama, T., Tashima, K., Wongseripipatana, S., Misawa, K., Kitajima, J., Takayama, H., Horie, S., 2006. Involvement of mu-opioid receptor in antinociception and inhibition of gastrointestinal transit induced by 7-hydroxymitragynine, isolated from Thai herbal medicinal *Mitragyna speciosa*. *Eur. J. Pharmacol.* 549, 63-70.

Matsumoto, K., Takayama, H., Narita, M., Nakamura, A., Suzuki, M., Suzuki, T., Murayama, T., Wongseripipatana, S., Misawa, K., Kitajima, M., Tashima, K., Horie, S., 2008. MGM-9 [(E)-methyl 2-(3-ethyl-7a,12a-(epoxyethanoxy)-9-fluoro-1,2,3,4,6,7,12,12b-octahydro-8-methoxyindolo[2,3-a]quinolizin-2-yo)-3-methoxyacrylate], a derivative of the indole alkaloid mitragynine: a novel dual acting mu- and kappa-opioid agonist with potent antinociceptive and weak rewarding effects in mice. *Neuropharmacology* 55, 154-165.

Pinney Associates 2016. http://mitragenius.com/wp-content/uploads/2017/09/8-point-analysis.pdf (accessed 8/03/2017).

Ponglux, D., Wongseripipatana, S., Takayama, H., Kikuchi, M., Kurihara, M., Kitajima, M., Aimi, H., Saki, S-I., 1994. A new indole alkaloid, 7a-hydroxy-7H-mitragynine, from *Mitragyna speciosa* in Thailand. *Planta Med.* 60, 580-581.

Sufka, K.J., Loria, M.J., Lewellyn, K., Zjawiony, J.K., Ail, Z., Abe, N., Khan, I.A., 2014. The effect of *Salvia divinorum* and *Mitragyna speciosa* extracts, fraction and major constituents on place aversion and place preference in rats. *J. Ethnopharmacol.* 151, 361-364.

Takayama, H., Ishikawa, H., Kurihara, M., Kitajima, M., Aimi, N., Ponglux, D., Koyama, F., Matsumoto, K., Moriyama, T., Yamamoto, L.T., Watanabe, K., Murayama, T., Horie, S., 2002. Studies on the synthesis and opioid agonistic activities of mitragynine-related indole alkaloids: Discovery of opioid agonists structurally different from other opioid ligands. *J. Med. Chem.* 45, 1949-1956.

Takayama, H., 2004. Chemistry and pharmacology of analgesic indole alkaloids from the rubiaceous plant, *Mitragyna speciosa*. *Chem. Pharm. Bull.*, 52, 916-928.

Watanabe, K., Yano, S., Horie, S., Yamamoto, L.T., 1997. Inhibitory effect of mitragynine, an alkaloid with analgesic effect from Thai medicinal plant *Mitragyna speciosa*, on electrically stimulated contraction of isolated guinea-pig ileum through the opioid receptor. *Life Sci.* 60, 933-942.

Wray, L., 1907a. "Biak": An opium substitute. *J. Fed. Malay States Museums*, 2, 53-56.

Wray, L., 1907b. Notes on the anti-opium remedy. *Pharmaceutical Journal*, 78, 453.

Yusoff, N.H.M., Mansor, S.M., Muller, C.P., Hassan, Z., 2017. Opioid receptors mediate the acquisition, but not the expression of mitragynine-induced conditioned place preference in rats. *Behav. Brain Res.* 332, 1-6.

Zarembo, J.E., Douglas, B., Valenta, J., Weisbach, J.A., 1974. Metabolites of mitragynine. *J. Pharm. Sci.* 63, 1407-1415.

The Ibogaine Project: Urban Ethnomedicine for Opioid Use Disorder

■ *Kenneth Alper*, MD ■

*Associate Professor of Psychiatry
and Neurology at the New York
University School of Medicine*

HISTORY

Ibogaine is a monoterpene indole alkaloid that occurs in the root bark of *Tabernanthe iboga* Baill. As a small molecule with apparent clinical effects in the alleviation of opioid withdrawal and diminution of drug self-administration, and an unknown and apparently novel mechanism of action, ibogaine offers an interesting prototype for drug discovery and neurobiological investigation.

In Gabon and elsewhere in West Central Africa, ibogaine is ingested in the form of *eboga*, scrapings of *Tabernanthe iboga* root bark as a psychoactive sacrament in the Bwiti religion for several centuries, and likely among Pygmies in much earlier times (Fernandez, 1982). The ritual aim of eating eboga has been conceptualized as "binding" across time through "the work of the ancestors", and across space, socially on the basis of a common experience of a distinctive consciousness (Fernandez and Fernandez, 2001). In the colonial era, Bwiti offered a dignified realm of spiritual endeavor that supported psychological resistance to the anomie and dislocation imposed by the colonial presence, and became constellated with Gabonese national identity.

Outside of Africa ibogaine has been used most frequently for the treatment of substance use disorders, specifically for detoxification from opioids. Ibogaine has a storied past and an association with controversy, and the medical and nonmedical settings that have been collectively designated as a "vast uncontrolled experiment" (Vastag, 2005), or "medical subculture" (Alper et al., 2008). Ibogaine has been classified as a hallucinogen and illegal in the US since 1967, and is similarly scheduled in 9 of the 28 countries presently in the European Union. As of this writing ibogaine is unregulated, i.e., neither officially approved nor illegal in much of the rest of the world. New Zealand, Canada, Brazil and South Africa have classified ibogaine as a pharmaceutical substance and restrict its use to licensed medical practitioners[1]. A systematic survey and description of the known settings of ibogaine use as of 2006 indicated that approximately 3,400 individuals had taken ibogaine, 68% of whom did so for the treatment of a substance-related disorder, 53% specifically for opioid detoxification (Alper et al., 2008). Now, a decade later the total number treated has likely increased several-fold.

The ethnopharmacological paradigm of drug discovery begins with observational evidence of a clinical effect in an indigenous context of use, followed by subsequent Identification and isolation of the active agent, or possible synthesis of derivatives as candidates for development. With regard to ibogaine in the treatment of addiction, the indigenous context of this urban ethnomedicine is distinct from the use of *T. iboga* as a religious sacrament in Africa. The majority of participants in the ibogaine medical subculture are dependent on opioids. The sacramental alkaloid is used in the hydrochloride form, the ritual aim is opioid detoxification, and ritual space is a clinic outside the US, or an apartment or hotel room.

……………………………………

[1]. Note added in proof by Dennis McKenna, ed.: Canada can be added to this list due to a recent classification of ibogaine as a prescription medicine by Health Canada. http://www.hc-sc.gc.ca/dhp-mps/prodpharma/pdl-ord/pdl-ldo-noa-ad-2017-05-16-eng.php (accessed 09/09/2017).

In June 1962 in Brooklyn (the exact date is not recalled), Howard Lotsof, 19-year-old heroin-dependent lay drug experimenter in an era which hallucinogens had not yet been regulated, serendipitously experienced the resolution of withdrawal following the use of ibogaine (Alper et al., 2001; Lotsof, 1985). Lotsof, an engaging and intrepid provocateur of scientific curiosity, credentialed only with an NYU film degree was eventually able to convince NIDA to support a project of research on ibogaine, with a total of approximately 2 million USD in direct cost support. During its existence from 1991-1996, the NIDA ibogaine project supported preclinical contract work, including toxicology and pharmacokinetics that enabled a privately funded phase 1 study of single dosages of ibogaine for cocaine dependence that was approved by the FDA in 1993. This study ended in contractual and intellectual property disputes (Mash, 1997) and dosages of 1 and 2mg/kg were without reported adverse events (Mash, Kovera, et al., 1998). Data from that study regarding a possible effect of ibogaine on drug use is apparently unavailable. NIDA eventually terminated its ibogaine research program in 1996, and no subsequent clinical research with ibogaine has been conducted in the US.

Beginning in 2012, the National Institute on Drug Abuse (NIDA) has committed a total of over 6 million USD to support preclinical testing and chemical manufacturing and control work intended to enable clinical trials for the development of 18-methoxycoronaridine (18-MC), an apparently safer structural analog discovered by rational design (National Institutes of Health, 2012). 18-MC differs from ibogaine at three of the 21 positions on the ibogamine skeleton that defines the iboga alkaloid class (Figure 1) (Le Men and Taylor, 1965). NIDA has supported preclinical toxicology, pharmacokinetics and chemical manufacturing and control work, which now enables a phase I/II study, the next developmental step that awaits at the present time.

IBOGAINE TREATMENT

DOSING AND MONITORING

Ibogaine is used most frequently for detoxification from opioids, typically administered in the HCl form in a range of approximately 94% to 98% purity according to certificates of analyses. Crude extracts of *T. iboga* root bark vary with regarded to estimated total alkaloid content, which is typically between 15% and 50%, about 25% to 50% of which might be expected to be ibogaine (Alper et al., 2008; Alper et al., 2012). Other iboga alkaloids co-occurring with ibogaine in *T. iboga* root bark include ibogamine, ibogaline, tabernanthine and voacangine (Bartlett et al., 1958), and are present to a variable extent in extracts (see Figure 1).

A.

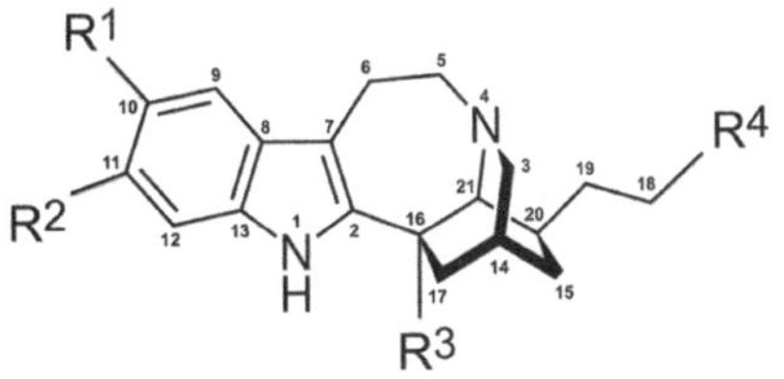

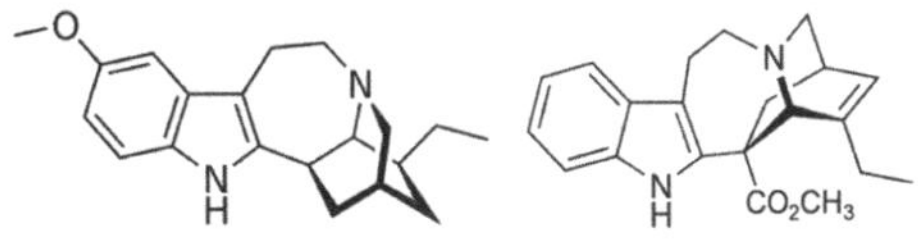

Fig. 1 A. Ibogaine and other iboga alkaloids and structural analogues numbered using the Le Men and Taylor System (Le Men and Taylor, 1965). Ibogamine is the parent iboga alkaloid structural skeleton. Ibogamine, ibogaline, tabernanthine, voacangine co-occur with ibogaine in *T. iboga*. Noribogaine is ibogaine's major metabolite. Coronaridine also occurs naturally. 18-Methoxycoronaridine (18-MC) is a synthetic congener.

B. Ibogaine and catharanthine, another iboga alkaloid of pharmacological importance belonging to an opposite optical series.

Compound	R1	R2	R3	R4
Ibogamine	H	H	H	H
Ibogaine	OCH3	H	H	H
Noribogaine	OH	H	H	H
Ibogaline	OCH3	OCH3	H	H
Tabernanthine	H	OCH3	H	H
Voacangine	OCH3	H	CO2CH3	H
Coronaridine	H	H	CO2CH3	H
18-Methoxycoronaridine	H	H	CO2CH3	OCH3

B.

Ibogaine   Catharanthine

As described in a recent observational study (Brown and Alper, 2017), the "test-flood-booster" opioid detoxification protocol presently in common use begins with a "test" dose of ibogaine on the order of approximately 3 mg/kg, typically administered in the morning after subjects had abstained from opioid use overnight, and begin to exhibit some initial signs of withdrawal. The providers appear to view the response to the test dose, which typically has some effect of reducing withdrawal signs as providing some indication of the degree of physical dependence on opioids. A "flood" ibogaine dose, typically four times the test dose, is given 2 to 12 hours following the test dose. Additional "booster" dosages of ibogaine of 3 to 5 mg/kg may follow the flood dose at intervals in a range from 1 to 16 hours, with the intention of either to alleviate residual or re-emergent withdrawal symptoms, or to increase the intensity of the psychoactive experience.

The total dosages of ibogaine administered in recent observational studies (Brown and Alper, 2017; Noller et al., 2017) are very similar to those used in prior treatments in the US in the 1960s and the Netherlands in the late 1980s (Alper et al., 1999), even though subjects in the present era use larger amounts of heroin that is of substantially greater purity (Drug Enforcement Administration, 2016). In the earlier era, nearly all of the total ibogaine dosage was administered at once. The test-flood-booster approach appears to be an adaptation intended towards maximizing dose efficiency in the face of severe levels of physiological dependence, and suggests that contemporary treatment providers perceive a dose ceiling, possibly due to a greater awareness of medical risk (Alper, Stajic, et al., 2012; Dickinson et al., 2016).

A set of clinical guidelines for detoxification from opioids with ibogaine has been developed by, the Global Ibogaine Therapy alliance (GITA), a group of physician and lay ibogaine treatment providers (Dickinson et al., 2016). Briefly, the guidelines recommend pre-treatment evaluation that includes a medical history, EKG, and electrolyte and liver function tests. Intravenous access, continuous pulse oximetry and three- lead EKG, monitoring of blood pressure are recommended throughout the treatment, with a medical professional (MD, nurse, or paramedic) certified in Advanced Cardiac Life Support (ACLS) present for at least the first 24 hours of the treatment. While the guidelines are unfortunately not followed across all of the varied settings in which ibogaine treatment is available, the emergence of an organized attempt by providers themselves to develop standards for ibogaine treatment is notable. A recent GITA conference in 2016 featured a training course in ACLS certification led by credentialed instructors.

CLINICAL EVIDENCE OF EFFICACY

Ibogaine has been administered most often for opioid detoxification (Alper et al., 2008). A substantive effect ibogaine treatment effect is reported in two early case series. In a series of 33 opioid detoxification treatment episodes in nonmedical settings with single mean dosages of 19.3 mg/kg, full resolution of opioid withdrawal signs and symptoms without drug seeking behavior over a 72-hour posttreatment interval was observed in 25 of 33 patients. Another study of 32 patients treated in a medical setting for the indication of opioid detoxification with fixed dosages of 800 mg reported the resolution of withdrawal of opioid withdrawal signs as indicated by physician-rated structured instruments at 24 hours, with sustained reductions in subjective ratings of withdrawal symptoms during the week following treatment as (Mash et al., 2001).

In two unpublished case series ibogaine appeared effective in opioid detoxification, and about one-third of subjects reported abstinence from opioids for periods of 6 months or longer following treatment. In a series of 52 outcomes assessed by interview following single dosages of ibogaine that became a basis for NIDA's decision to undertake its ibogaine project from 1991 to 1995, individuals reported cessation of use of the substances for which ibogaine treatment had been sought for 2 to 6 months in 30 cases (57%), and over 6 months in 17 cases (32%) (Alper, 2001). The other series, summarized in an academic thesis, is 21 subjects who responded to a Web-based questionnaire adapted from the European Addiction Severity Index at a mean interval of 21.8 months following treatment with ibogaine (Bastiaans, 2004). Of the 17 to 21 patients (81%) who identified opioids as the primary substance for which they had sought treatment, 5 reported abstinence from all substances, and another 9 reported abstinence from their primary substance of dependence while continuing to use alcohol or cannabis after treatment with ibogaine.

A recent prospective observational study reported on one-year follow up of 30 individuals treated with ibogaine for opioid detoxification with mean amount total of 1540 ± 920 mg ibogaine HCl administered according to a test-flood-booster dosing scheme (Brown and Alper, 2017). The subjects in this study were heavy opioid users with histories of failure with conventional treatment. The subjects used mainly oxycodone (n=21; 70%) and/or heroin (n=18; 60%) in respective amounts of 250 ± 180 mg/day and 1.3 ± 0.94 g/day with a mean of 3.1 ± 2.6 prior previous episodes of treatment for opioid dependence. The Subjective Opioid Withdrawal Scale (SOWS) (Handelsman et al., 1987) was used to assess detoxification outcome, and Addiction Severity Index Composite (ASIC) scores (McGahan et al., 1986) were used to assess posttreatment effects at 1, 3, 6, 9, and 12 months.

Assessed just prior to the test ibogaine dose, the pretreatment baseline SOWS score decreased a mean of 17 points from 31.0 to 14.0 at 76.5 ± 30 hours following the initiation of treatment. This clinical effect of ibogaine on acute withdrawal symptoms appeared consistent with prior to be of a comparable order of magnitude to that of methadone reported in the original study that described the development and validation of the SOWS (Handelsman et al., 1987). In that study, subjects were administered the SOWS following two days of methadone stabilization, SOWS decreased by a mean of 18.7 points (from 24.3 to 5.6) in subjects who used opioid exclusively, and 8.7 points (from 23.1 to 14.4) in subjects who additionally abused other, non-opioid substances.

The numbers of subjects who reported no opioid use during the previous 30 days at respective posttreatment time intervals of 1 and 3 months were 15 (50%) and 10 (33%). This appears to be a substantive treatment effect in comparison to those reported in the published literature. For example, recent systematic reviews of studies of opioid detoxification without subsequent maintenance treatment found rates of abstaining from illicit opioid use of 18% at 4 weeks following detoxification with buprenorphine (Bentzley et al., 2015), and 26% at 6 weeks following detoxification with methadone (Amato et al., 2013). Figure 2 plots individual trajectories of the ASIC Drug Use score from pretreatment baseline to 1, 3, 6, 9, and 12 months. The figure indicates an apparently sustained posttreatment effect on opioid use in a subset of subjects. evident as trajectories characterized by large decreases from baseline to 1 month that are sustained at subsequent time points.

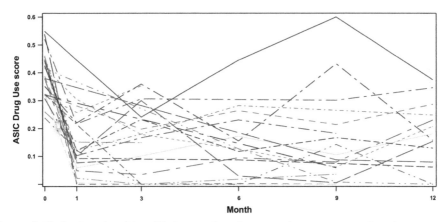

Fig. 2 Individual trajectories of the Addiction Severity Index Composite Drug Use score in patients at 1, 3, 6, 9, and 12 month followup after opioid detoxification with ibogaine (Brown and Alper, 2017) (N= 30).

Other recent work, conducted in New Zealand with a design similar to that discussed immediately above on a smaller subject population (N-14) reported comparable outcomes regarding SOWS ASIC Drug Use scores in subjects followed up for one year (Noller et al., 2017). The study also included assessment with the Beck Depression Inventory that indicated progressive improvement throughout the interval of follow up.

Reported studies on ibogaine as treatment for substance use disorders have been uncontrolled and reliant on self-report without laboratory verification. While laboratory verification will be a necessary feature in future efforts to develop ibogaine or its structural derivatives, self-reporting in clinical research on substance use disorders can be accurate (Darke, 1998), particularly when there are no negative consequences to the subject for reporting use. Reported detoxification outcomes appear valid. The clinical expression of acute opioid withdrawal evolves acutely over a limited time frame, tends to be robust in its expression, and can be assessed accurately by lay providers in the settings in which ibogaine is administered (Alper et al., 2008). Patient self-reports also suggest a substantive, pharmacologically-mediated effect of ibogaine, especially in view of the lack of a significant effect of placebo in opioid detoxification (Amato et al., 2013; Gowing et al., 2017; Gowing et al., 2016).

PRECLINICAL EVIDENCE OF EFFICACY

There are more than 50 published studies of ibogaine or its structural analogs 18-MC or noribogaine in animal models of drug self-administration or opiate withdrawal. Consistent with its apparent effect in opioid detoxification in humans, ibogaine administered intraperitoneally or intracerebrally to animals reduces naloxone- or naltrexone-precipitated opioid withdrawal signs, in rats

(Cappendijk et al., 1994; Dzoljic et al., 1988; Glick et al., 1992; Parker et al., 2002), mice (Frances et al., 1992; Layer et al., 1996; Leal et al., 2003; Popik et al., 1995), and primates (Aceto et al., 1992; Koja et al., 1996). Single dosages of ibogaine administered to rodents diminish self-administration of multiple abused substances including morphine (Belgers et al., 2016; Glick et al., 1994; Glick et al., 1996; Glick et al., 1991), heroin (Dworkin et al., 1995), cocaine (Cappendijk and Dzoljic, 1993; Glick et al., 1994; Glick et al., 1996; Maisonneuve and Glick, 1992; Sershen et al., 1994), amphetamine (Maisonneuve, Keller, et al., 1992), and alcohol (Rezvani et al., 1995), with normal responding for water. A recent meta-analysis of 30 animal studies of the effect of ibogaine on drug self-administration morphine, alcohol, or cocaine found a significant effect on drug self-administration across studies that was greatest at 24 hours but persisted for > 72 hours (Belgers et al., 2016). Sustained effects on morphine self-administration for even longer time intervals have been observed in individual animals (Glick et al., 1991).

Both ibogaine and 18-MC diminish an experimental pharmacological correlate of drug salience, the sensitized response of dopamine efflux in the nucleus accumbens in response to morphine (Maisonneuve and Glick, 1999; Maisonneuve et al., 1991) and nicotine (Glick et al., 1998; Maisonneuve et al., 1997). Ibogaine has had no significant on conditioned place preference, an animal behavioral model of drug craving (Belgers et al., 2016).

SUBJECTIVE EFFECTS: PHENOMENOLOGY, NEUROPHYSIOLOGY, AND IBOGAINE AS A PSYCHOTHERAPEUTIC ADJUNCT

Historically, the use of ibogaine in the medical model began in the 1950s, when clinicians and researchers viewed ibogaine much as they did other compounds classified as hallucinogens. Some, such as Jan Bastiaans, MD (Snelders and Kaplan, 2002), Leo Zeff, PhD (Stolaroff, 2004), and Claudio Naranjo, MD (Naranjo, 1973), were interested in ibogaine as an adjunct to psychotherapy. Ibogaine, like other hallucinogens, was of interest as an experimental model of psychosis (Fabing, 1956; Salmoiraghi and Page, 1957; Schneider and Sigg, 1957; Turner et al., 1955). As with other hallucinogens, ibogaine may have also been investigated for military or intelligence purposes as a "truth serum", or a means of "brainwashing" or incapacitating an adversary which was the focus the US Central Intelligence Agency project MKULTRA (Isbell, 1955; U.S. Senate, 1977).

The French chemist Robert Goutarel hypothesized that ibogaine produces a state with functional aspects shared by the brain states of REM sleep (Goutarel et al., 1993). Descriptions of subjective experiences associated with ibogaine have been designated as "oneiric" and likened to a "waking dream", with interrogatory verbal exchanges involving ancestral and archetypal beings, and movement and navigation within visual landscapes. Another frequently described experience is panoramic memory, the recall of a rapid, dense succession of vivid autobiographical visual memories, which has been termed "the slide show." Mechanistically, these subjective experiences associated with ibogaine possibly suggest functional muscarinic cholinergic effects, which are prominent in the mechanisms of dreaming and memory (Cantero et al., 2003).

Ibogaine is reported to enhance spatial memory retrieval in animals (Helsley et al., 1997; Popik, 1996), and produces an atropine-sensitive EEG rhythm (Depoortere, 1987; Schneider and Sigg, 1957). The atropine-sensitive EEG rhythm is regarded as an animal model of REM sleep and attributed to muscarinic cholinergic input from the ascending reticular activating system (ARAS) (Leung, 1998), and has been suggested to involve the inhibition of acetylcholinesterase (AChE) by ibogaine (Schneider and Sigg, 1957). More recent work indicates that ibogaine does not inhibit AChE (Alper, Reith, et al., 2012), suggesting the possibility that functional muscarinic cholinergic effect may be mediated by modulation of signaling downstream from the receptor itself.

Individuals who have taken ibogaine frequently report that memories and other mental representations which have previously been associated with troubling emotions such as fear, or shame, or anger are experienced with equanimity, allowing a reevaluation and reprocessing of their content (Heink et al., 2017). As memorably expressed by one individual reflecting on her ibogaine treatment for dependence on opioids, *"It's as if all information in your brain file cabinet is shaken out of its drawers on to one big pile, looked at 'objectively' and put back in, untwisted from emotional trauma."* (Lotsof and Alexander, 2001). Equanimity is also a prevalent theme in Bwiti. Ritual outcomes and transactions with ancestors involving the use of eboga are described (utilizing Fernandez's translations) with terms such as "even-handedness", "tranquil-heartedness", or "one-heartedness." The quality of equanimity attributed to ancestral contact is evident in a Fang Bwiti poem (Fernandez, 1982), *"Joy, the ancestors give joyful welcome and hear the news. The troubled life of the born ones is finished.... All the misfortunes are shorn away. They leave. Everything clean. All is new. All is bright. I have seen the dead and I do not fear."*

Narratives of individuals treated with ibogaine subjects appear consonant with themes of "one heartedness", and "binding" to family and ancestors represented in Bwiti. A study that utilized ASIC scores found that Family/Social the most improved ASI composite factor apart from Drug Use (Brown and Alper, 2017). Lotsof provides a descriptive example of the clinical phenomenon of delayed benefit with ibogaine (Lotsof and Alexander, 2001), and suggests the interval of delay might correspond to the ongoing processing and behavioural integration of the psychoactive experience produced by ibogaine.

TOXICOLOGY

CARDIOTOXICITY

Ibogaine has been associated with fatalities (Alper et al., 2012; Koenig and Hilber, 2015). Ibogaine and its major metabolite noribogaine prolong the QT interval of the EKG. The QT interval corresponds to ventricular repolarization between cardiac contractions during which the electrical potential of the cardiac myocyte becomes more negative, inhibiting cell firing. With depolarization the electrical potential in the cardiac myocyte becomes more positive and excitatory, resulting in cell firing and the action potential that underlies ventricular contraction. With prolongation of the QT interval, cardiac myocytes may escape control of the cardiac conduction system and depolarize spontaneously. QT prolongation is viewed as correlate of cardiac instability, a loss of "repolarization reserve" (Roden and Yang, 2005), and is associated with polymorphic ventricular arrhythmias (PVTs) including Torsade de Pointes (TdP), a morphologically distinctive type of PVT that can progress to ventricular fibrillation and death (Kannankeril et al., 2010).

Repolarization of the cardiac myocyte depends importantly on the movement of positively charged potassium ions out of the cell through voltage-gated cardiac potassium channels. The protein that constitutes the pore of the channel is encoded by the human ether-ago-go-related gene (hERG), hence the term hERG channel, and hERG blockade is the major cause of drug-induced QT prolongation and TdP (Kannankeril et al., 2010). Ibogaine and its major metabolite noribogaine block the hERG channel with comparable potency (Alper et al., 2016; Koenig and Hilber, 2015). In a recent study, reported IC50 values for 99.5% ibogaine produced by semisynthesis via voacangine, 95% ibogaine produced from extraction of *T. iboga*, and noribogaine were 4.09 μM, are 3.53 μM, and 2.86 μM respectively. 18-MC produces substantially less hERG blockade (IC50 > 50 μM) (Alper et al., 2016).

The reported values for IC50 for hERG blockade by ibogaine and noribogaine appear clinically relevant. The half-life ($T_{1/2}$) of ibogaine in humans is estimated to be 4 to 7 hours (Kontrimavičiūtė et al., 2006; Mash et al., 2001), and the $T_{1/2}$ of noribogaine is apparently considerably longer than that of the parent compound, possibly on the order of days (Glue et al., 2015). In a sample of 24 subjects that were orally administered ibogaine dosages of 10mg/kg, mean peak blood levels for ibogaine and noribogaine respectively were 2.4 μM and 3.2 μM (Mash et al., 2001). From a postmortem series of 19 fatalities, the subset of 10 cases in which blood ibogaine levels were available, the mean was 7.6 μM (range 0.77 μM to 30 μM), and in the two cases for which they were available, noribogaine levels were 13.4 and 18.8 μM (Alper, Stajic, et al., 2012). Although the interpretation of levels from postmortem studies may be complicated by redistribution, and taking into account that ibogaine is 65% protein bound (Koenig et al., 2013), ibogaine or noribogaine may produce significant hERG channel blockade at clinically relevant concentrations (Koenig et al., 2013).

Bradycardia heightens the risk for fatal cardiac arrhythmia including TdP (Cubeddu, 2009) and has been observed following administration of ibogaine in medical (Mash, Allen-Ferdinand, et al., 1998) and nonmedical (Samorini, 1998) settings and in preclinical studies (Binienda et al., 1998; Dhahir, 1971; Glick et al., 1999; Schneider and Rinehart, 1957). Both laboratory models and multiple clinical case reports indicate that hypokalemia is a particularly important factor in the genesis of arrhythmia associated with ibogaine (Koenig and Hilber, 2015). A case of TdP in the setting of severe depletion of potassium from serum and tissue stores due to the aggressive use of cathartics prior to ibogaine treatment, in which lengthening of the QT interval, bradycardia and ventricular tachydysrhythmias appeared to track potassium levels over an interval of 7 days. illustrates the importance of potassium in ibogaine-related cardiac arrhythmia, as well as the idiosyncratic hazards associated with the unconventional settings in which ibogaine is often administered (Shawn et al., 2012).

Drug-induced TdP is typically multifactorial, involving multiple determinants of cardiac rhythm instability in addition to hERG blockade (Kannankeril et al., 2010), which has been generally been the case with regard to fatalities temporally related to ingestion of ibogaine. Pre-existing cardiovascular medical comorbidities appear to have been particularly prominent in deaths temporally associated with the administration of ibogaine (Alper et al., 2012). The role of preexisting advanced medical comorbidities as contributing causes in ibogaine-related deaths may also be paralleling a general association of risk of fatal overdose with systemic disease (Darke et al., 2006). For example, ibogaine- related fatalities have been associated with cardiac hypertrophy and atherosclerotic disease (Alper et al., 2012), which are associated with chronic methamphetamine and cocaine use (Kaye et al., 2007; Knuepfer, 2003). Additional factors that commonly contribute to cardiac instability in chronic substance-related disorders include various co-ingestants, systemic medical conditions such as liver or respiratory disease, seizures, hypomagnesemia, or withdrawal from cocaine or alcohol (Cubeddu, 2009; Kannankeril et al., 2010; Levin et al., 2008; Otero-Anton et al., 1997).

NEUROTOXICITY

Degeneration of cerebellar Purkinje cells were observed in rats given substantially larger dosages of ibogaine than those used to study drug self-administration and withdrawal (O'Hearn and Molliver, 1993). Ibogaine activates the release of glutamate by neurons in the inferior olive resulting in degeneration of the Purkinje cells in the cerebellum, which are vulnerable to excitotoxic injury due to the redundancy of inputs to cerebellar Purkinje cells, an effect that may be potentiated by ibogaine's s2 agonist activity (Bowen, 2001; O'Hearn and Molliver, 1997). Subsequent research found no evidence of neurotoxicity in the primate (Mash et al., 1998) or mouse (Scallet et al., 1996) at dosages which produced cerebellar degeneration in the rat, or in the rat at dosages used in studies of drug self-administration and withdrawal (Molinari et al., 1996). The FDA was aware of the work that indicated the neurotoxic effect of high dosages of ibogaine in the rat at the time it approved a phase 1 study in which humans received ibogaine (Alper, 2001). Clinical or postmortem evidence does not appear to suggest a characteristic syndrome of neurotoxicity (Alper et al., 2012).

MECHANISM OF ACTION
DISTINCT FROM MEDICATIONS KNOWN TO HAVE CLINICAL EFFECTS IN OUD

The mechanism of action of ibogaine is unknown and apparently novel and unexplained by actions of medications known to have clinical effects in opioid tolerance or withdrawal. Clinical observations suggest that ibogaine is not acting as an MOR agonist. Doses of ibogaine sufficient to detoxify individuals with severe physical dependence do not produce signs of overdose in opioid naïve individuals (Alper et al., 2008). If ibogaine were acting as an opioid agonist, it would not be tolerated by opioid-naïve individuals, because the methadone dosage of 60 to 100 mg per day that is used to stabilize withdrawal symptoms in the maintenance treatment of opioid dependent patients (Fareed et al., 2010) substantially exceeds the estimated the LD50 of 40 to 50 mg in humans who are not pharmacologically tolerant to opioids (Corkery et al., 2004).

Although ibogaine, its major metabolite noribogaine, and 18-MC bind with low micromolar affinity to the MOR, they are neither orthosteric nor allosteric μ opioid receptor agonists assessed by [35S]GTPγS binding in cells expressing the μ opioid receptor (Antonio et al., 2013). The potentiation of morphine analgesia by ibogaine in the animal model, without producing analgesia when administered alone, also suggests that ibogaine may alter signaling through opioid receptors but is not itself an orthosteric agonist (Bagal et al., 1996; Bhargava et al., 1997; Cao and Bhargava, 1997; Frances et al., 1992; Schneider, 1957; Schneider and McArthur, 1956; Sunder Sharma and Bhargava, 1998). Although the potentiation of morphine analgesia without analgesia when administered alone might be consistent with an effect as allosteric MOR agonist, these compounds do not potentiate the activation of G proteins by morphine or DAMGO (Antonio et al., 2013), indicating they do not act as allosteric MOR agonists.

Some evidence suggests that ibogaine might possibly modify neuroadaptations associated with chronic exposure to opioids, such as the apparent reversal of analgesic tolerance to chronic morphine by ibogaine (Pearl et al., 1995; Schneider, 1957; Sunder Sharma and Bhargava, 1998). Ibogaine and noribogaine diminish tolerance in morphine-tolerant mice (Bhargava and Cao, 1997; Cao and Bhargava, 1997; Sunder Sharma and Bhargava, 1998), and dose-dependently potentiate the antinociceptive effect of morphine in morphine-tolerant but not in morphine-naïve mice (Sunder Sharma and Bhargava, 1998). Ibogaine has relatively selective effects on decreasing dopamine efflux in the nucleus accumbens (Pearl et al., 1996) and locomotor activity (Maisonneuve, Rossman, et al., 1992; Pearl et al., 1995) in morphine-tolerant versus non-tolerant rats. Ibogaine's clinical effect of opioid detoxification without causing opioid overdose in non-tolerant individuals also suggests selectivity for neuroadaptations associated with prior exposure.

Ibogaine is an NMDA receptor antagonist (Popik et al., 1995; Skolnick, 2001), and NMDA antagonists such as memantine diminish signs of opioid withdrawal in preclinical models (Trujillo and Akil, 1994) and humans (Bisaga et al., 2001). However 18-MC, which lacks significant affinity for the NMDA receptor, is equally effective as ibogaine in animal models of opioid withdrawal (Cappendijk et al., 1994; Dzoljic et al., 1988; Glick et al., 2001; Glick et al., 1992; Panchal et al., 2005; Parker et al., 2002; Rho and Glick, 1998). Ibogaine has no significant affinity for the α2 adrenergic receptor (Deecher et al., 1992; Sweetnam et al., 1995) or imidazoline I_2 site (MacInnes and Handley, 2002), indicating it does not act as an imidazoline α2 adrenergic receptor agonist such as clonidine.

DISTINCT FROM OTHER COMPOUNDS DESIGNATED AS "PSYCHEDELIC"

Although ibogaine is designated as a hallucinogen, and subsumed under the rubric of "psychedelics" it is pharmacologically distinct from the classical hallucinogens such as LSD, mescaline, or psilocybin, which are thought to act by binding as agonists to the serotonin type 2A (5-HT$_{2A}$) receptor (Nichols, 2016). The 5HT$_{2A}$ receptor is non-essential for recognition of the ibogaine stimulus in drug discrimination studies (Helsley et al., 1998). Serotonin agonist or releasing activity does not appear to explain ibogaine's effects in opioid withdrawal (Glick et al., 2001; Wei et al., 1998). There appears to be no clinical evidence apparent effect of classical hallucinogens in opioid detoxification, and in the animal model ablation of 90% of the raphe, the major serotonergic nucleus of the brain, does not significantly affect the expression of opioid withdrawal (Caille et al., 2002).

Although harmine does have an effect of diminution of antagonist-precipitated opioid withdrawal in rats, this effect is apparently due to its action of imidazoline I_2 receptor agonist (Aricioglu-Kartal et al., 2003). Ibogaine in contrast has no affinity at the I_2 receptor. Ibogaine does not inhibit MAOA (Nelson et al., 1979).

THE α3β4 NICOTINIC ACETYLCHOLINE RECEPTOR (NACHR), NEUROTROPHINS

The enhanced expression of glial-derived neurotrophic factor (GDNF) has been proposed to account for ibogaine's effect on drug self-administration (He et al., 2005). Ibogaine increases GDNF expression *in vivo* and in cultured cells, and 18-MC reportedly does not (Carnicella et al., 2010), but both compounds are equally effective in animal models of drug self-administration (Glick et al., 2001). Ibogaine's action as an allosteric antagonist of the α3β4 nAChR is suggested to mediate its effect on drug self-administration (Glick et al., 2002), but does not appear to readily explain the prolonged effects that appear to persist beyond pharmacokinetic elimination (Pearl et al., 1997). Ibogaine's major metabolite, noribogaine has a longer half-life than the parent compound (Baumann et al., 2001; Glue et al., 2015), and has been suggested to account for persistence of effects on drug self-administration and withdrawal (Mash et al., 2016), although in the animal model the effect of ibogaine in reducing drug self-administration appears to persist beyond the elimination of ibogaine and noribogaine from serum or brain tissue (Pearl et al., 1997).

ADENYLATE CYCLASE

Ibogaine may act downstream from receptor-coupled G protein activation to mediate effects on opioid withdrawal that are unexplained in view of the its lack of agonist activity at the MOR. Adenylate cyclase (AC) is one plausible target of ibogaine. The MOR is negatively coupled to AC via Gαi, and the inhibition of AC is a cardinal opioid agonist signaling effect, as is the AC "superactivation" or "overshoot" of increased production of cyclic adenosine monophosphate (cAMP) in opioid withdrawal (Christie, 2008; Nestler, 2001; Sharma et al., 1975). Ibogaine potentiates the inhibition of AC by morphine (Rabin and Winter, 1996), which may be consistent with its observed clinical effect in opioid withdrawal. The potentiation of morphine analgesia by Ibogaine and noribogaine, without analgesia when administered alone is also consistent with a possible effect of inhibition of AC in view of the upregulation of AC in pain sensitization associated with opioid withdrawal (Bie et al., 2005) and the analgesic effects of drugs that inhibit AC (Pierre et al., 2009; Zhuo, 2012). A hypothesis that iboga alkaloids could inhibit AC might explain why ibogaine does not itself produce signs of opioid overdose but potentiates the toxicity of co-administered opioids (Alper, Stajic, et al., 2012; Bhargava and Cao, 1997; Dhahir, 1971; MPI Research, 1996; Schneider and McArthur, 1956).

WHAT IS IBOGAINE DOING IN THE PLANT?

THE IBOGA CLASS OF MONOTERPENE INDOLE ALKALOIDS

Although there is some discussion among regarding the precise criteria for the term "alkaloid", core attributes are containing a basic nitrogen as an electron donor in a ring or ring system. The term "true alkaloid" has been used to designate those alkaloids that derive from amino acid and share a heterocyclic ring with nitrogen (Aniszewski, 2015). Indole alkaloids are true alkaloids and particularly well-adapted structurally for noncovalent interactions, including cation-π interactions involving the ring system, and hydrogen bonds involving the nitrogen atom. G protein-coupled receptors (GPCRs) are typical targets of alkaloids, often involving aromatic side chains. Receptor binding tends to be diverse, with "off target" and toxic effects.

Alkaloids are formed in plants from pathways of synthesis of amino acids, and extend on amino acid scaffolds, as do neurotransmitters. The monoamine neurotransmitters may be regarded as alkaloids, just as tryptamine is an alkaloid, so is 5-HT (5-hydroxytryptamine, serotonin), as is auxin, an important plant hormone with a close structural relationship to 5-HT. Morphine, nicotine, cocaine, amphetamine, and the major classical hallucinogens are alkaloids.

Alkaloids were historically initially viewed as "secondary metabolites" – chemical detritus, the byproduct of primary metabolic processes such as photosynthesis or energy metabolism. The term secondary metabolites has been retained as generally synonymic with plant natural products, however alkaloids are now recognized as serving ecological aims medicating between the plant and its environment, such as chemical defenses against herbivores or pathogens, or attractants for pollenating insects (Hartmann, 2007). The ecological view is well-validated; however, an emerging view is that alkaloids may also serve functions within the plant itself as modulators of signaling pathways or gene expression (Aniszewski, 2015; Heinze et al., 2015; Neilson et al., 2013).

The phylogenetic lineage of many alkaloids tends to be narrow, as is the case with ibogaine, possibly due to evolutionary selection pressure for chemodiversity. The total number of all plant secondary metabolites is estimated on the order of 200,000 compounds (Neilson et al., 2013), with estimates of total number of alkaloids on the order of 20,000, occurring in quantities ≥ 0.0 I% of the dry plant weight in approximately 20% (Seigler, 1998) of the 405 families of flowering plants (The Plant List, 2013). Ibogaine is a monoterpene indole alkaloid (MIA), a pharmacologically important class of compounds formed by the condensation of the alkaloid tryptamine and the monoterpene secologanin. Estimates of the number of MIAs are in the range of approximately 2000 to 3000 compounds, occurring predominantly in three plant families, Apocynaceae, Loganiaceae, and Rubiacea (O'Connor and Maresh, 2006; Szabó, 2008). The iboga class of MIAs consists of about 100 compounds (Lavaud and Massiot, 2017) apparently limited to 5 of 410 genera within the Apocynaceae family (The Plant List, 2013), *Tabernaemontana*, *Tabernanthe*, *Catharanthus*, *Voacanga* and *Melodinus*.

CROSS-KINGDOM COMMONALITY: PLANT AND ANIMAL HOMOLOGY

Plants lack many of the proteins targeted by drugs that are psychoactive in humans. Most approved psychopharmacological agents in clinical use (e.g., antidepressants, antipsychotics, some anxiolytics), as well as many drugs of abuse target GPCRs or monoamine transporters. Plants lack canonical GPCRs (Urano and Jones, 2014) such as opioid, dopamine, 5-HT or cannabinoid receptors, they lack monoamine transporters (Hoglund et al., 2005) at which cocaine or amphetamine act, and plants do not have pentameric ligand-gated ion channels (Jaiteh et al., 2016) – the targets of nicotine, benzodiazepines or ketamine.

Plants lack canonical GPCRS, but do share remarkable homologies regarding G proteins and effectors that are conserved in plants and metazoans. Figure 3 presents two examples of downstream signaling elements homologously present in plants and linked in humans to GPCRS that activate cardinal signaling pathways of psychoactive substances. In the case of the MOR, the respective transducer, effector, and second messengers present in both plants and animals are Gα, adenylate cyclase, and cyclic AMP. In case of the 5-HT$_2$AR they are Gα, phospholipase A2 and C, and arachidonic acid and inositol 1,4,5-trisphosphate. Clinical psychopharmacology does not generally target transducers and effectors, but plant alkaloids apparently do, and the identification of their targets may provide an interesting paradigm for drug discovery and neurobiological investigation.

A recent study provides an example of an endogenous plant alkaloid as a specific modulator of an effector in the plant itself (Heinze et al., 2015). *Eschscholzia californica* (Papaveraceae) and *Catha-*

Signaling Element	Opioids	Classical hallucinogens
Receptor (GPCR)	μ-opioid receptor (MOR)[*]	Serotonin 2A receptor (5-HT$_{2A}$)[*]
Transducer (G proteins)	Gα[†]	Gα[†]
Effector (enzymes)	Adenylate cyclase[†]	Phospholipase A$_2$[†], C[†]
Second messenger (cyclic nucleotides, lipids/phospholipids)	Cyclic adenosine monophosphate (cAMP)[†]	Arachidonic acid (AA)[†], inositol 1,4,5-trisphosphate (IP3)[†]

[*]*occurs in animals, not in plants*
[†]*occurs in both plants animals*

Fig. 3 Signaling elements linked to two mammalian GPCRs, the MOR and 5-HT$_{2A}$R. Plants lack G-protein coupled receptors, but some downstream G proteins, effectors and second messengers are conserved among plants and metazoans.

ranthus roseus (Apocynaceae) express alkaloids which function as phytoalexins, compounds with antimicrobial activity against fungi and bacteria that are produced and accumulated by plants in response to infection. Microbial elicitors added to cultured cells from either plant increase the production of alkaloids by Gα-dependent activation of phospholipase A2 (PLA2) to generate signaling molecules that code for the induction of biosynthetic enzymes downstream. The respective alkaloids in both of these evolutionary distant plants exert negative feedback to prevent their own overexpression by specifically targeting and inhibiting PLA2. PLA2 is present in metazoans and is an important downstream effector in the action of the classical hallucinogens, linked to the 5-HT$_{2A}$R (Nichols, 2016), suggesting the possibility of a widely conserved, phylogenetically ancient signaling motif. Of note with regard to this present review, catharanthine (Figure 1), which occurs in *C. roseus* and inhibited *C. roseus* PLA2 in the study discussed above (Heinze et al., 2015), is an iboga alkaloid of pharmacological importance (van der Heijden et al., 2004).

PLANT INTELLIGENCE

Plants have extraordinary capacities to sense and respond to their environment, but should they be regarded as intelligent? Intelligence is the capacity for learning, which involves the modification of programs of behavior or thought on the basis of prior experience (Trewavas, 2017). Learning is shaped by reinforcement in individuals within that individual's lifetime. Habituation may be viewed as an elementary form of learning but is limited to adaptations to manage the gain of environmental signals, and is shaped by repeated exposure to a habituating stimulus, such as leaf folding in response to mechanical disturbance (Gagliano et al., 2014). Intelligence differs from instinct, which is reinforced at the level of populations by adaptation and fitness over time spans of generations, and may be exemplified in plants as epigenetic memory in clonal plants (Latzel et al., 2016). Intelligence is distinct from consciousness, which has been defined as "global subjective awareness" (John, 2005), and may only be inferred, and not directly observed by the research investigator.

The example of the climbing behavior of *Passiflora caerulea* L, an experimental paradigm favored by Charles Darwin provides an example of plant intelligence that illustrates the capacity of plants to learn (Baillaud, 1962; Trewavas, 2005). The plant is presented with a support, which the tendril locates by circumnutation, a plant behavioural program of helical movement common in climbing plants that allows triangulation utilizing variations in light intensity registered by the moving tendril. The tendril finds the support each time it is moved to a new location. Locating the support requires some form of memory of the variations in light intensity over the trajectory of the circumnutatory movements (Trewavas, 2017). The tendrils appear to modify their search strategy with the progression of the experiment, and after the support is finally taken away altogether the plant appears to approach the last previous location of the support prior to it being removed.

Not only is the *Passiflora caerulea* plant itself apparently capable spatial learning, but *Passiflora incarnata* L. enhances spatial learning when ingested by rats (Jawna-Zboinska et al., 2016). Both *P. caerulea* and *P. incarnata* contain multiple harmala alkaloids including harmine (Frye and Haustein, 2008). Harmine, as well as ibogaine both enhance spatial learning in the rat (Dos Santos and Hallak, 2017; Helsley et al., 1997; Popik, 1996). Alkaloids frequently accumulate most heavily in the parts of the plant that are growing, such as root tips. This has been viewed as consistent with a hypothesis of alkaloids as chemodefenses which are deployed more extensively in valuable, young growing plant tissue (McCall and Fordyce, 2010). However in the root system, which navigates, senses, and

169

responds to its environment, the accumulation of alkaloids in growing tissue might also reflect a role of alkaloids of endogenous modulators of plant signaling in programs of behavior or growth and development.

CONCLUSION

The iboga alkaloid structural skeleton appears to be a "privileged scaffold", a term of medicinal chemistry for a basic molecular framework prototypic of a class of compounds on which systematic substitutions can be utilized to modulate therapeutic and toxic effects (Welsch et al., 2010). The effect of 18-MC in animal models of drug self-administration and opioid withdrawal is apparently equivalent to that of ibogaine (Maisonneuve and Glick, 2003), although its hERG blockade is much less (Alper et al., 2016), indicating the potential for isolating ibogaine's therapeutic effect from its cardiotoxicity. With an unknown and likely novel mechanism of action, and a structure that evidently accommodates rational drug design, ibogaine may provide an interesting prototype for discovery and development of fundamentally innovative pharmacotherapy.

When a growing root tip meets a rock it cannot move, it revises its behavioral program. In this instance plants may output behavioral responses more intelligently than humans, who are prone to rigidly overdetermined repetitive behavior. It appears possible that possible that a restricted subset of plant alkaloids interacts with an evolutionarily ancient commonality, shared across signaling pathways in both plant and animal kingdoms that may mediate programs of plant adaptive behavior, growth or development in one kingdom, and modify the pathological neuroadaptations of opioid dependence and linkages of motivational states to drug-related memories, representations or environmental cues. True intention, equanimity, distinct from the constraints of obsession and the pathological overattribution of salience, is both a cardinal spiritual goal and a desired outcome of pharmacological treatment of addiction. Recovery from addiction is often, typically, viewed by patients in spiritual terms. It is not entirely unexpected that a plant alkaloid used in an indigenous sacramental context may provide a valuable lead for discovery of pharmacotherapy for addiction.

REFERENCES

Aceto, MD, Bowman, E.R., Harris, L.S., May, E.L., 1992. Dependence studies of new compounds in the rhesus monkey and mouse (1991). *NIDA Res. Monogr.* 119, 513-558.

Alper, K., Bai, R., Liu, N., Fowler, S.J., Huang, X.P., Priori, S.G., Ruan, Y., 2016. hERG Blockade by Iboga Alkaloids. *Cardiovasc. Toxicol.* 16(1), 14-22.

Alper, K., Reith, M.E.A., Sershen, H., 2012. Ibogaine and the inhibition of acetylcholinesterase. *J. Ethnopharmacol.* 139(3), 879-882.

Alper, K.R., 2001. Ibogaine: a review. *Alkaloids Chem. Biol.* 56, 1-38.

Alper, K.R., Beal, D., Kaplan, C.D., 2001. A contemporary history of ibogaine in the United States and Europe. *Alkaloids Chem. Biol.* 56, 249-281.

Alper, K.R., Lotsof, H.S., Frenken, G.M., Luciano, D.J., Bastiaans, J., 1999. Treatment of acute opioid withdrawal with ibogaine. *Am. J. Addict.* 8(3), 234-242.

Alper, K.R., Lotsof, H.S., Kaplan, C.D., 2008. The ibogaine medical subculture. *J. Ethnopharmacol.* 115(1), 9-24.

Alper, K.R., Stajic, M., Gill, J.R., 2012. Fatalities temporally associated with the ingestion of ibogaine. *J. Forensic Sci.* 57(2), 398-412.

Amato, L., Davoli, M., Minozzi, S., Ferroni, E., Ali, R., Ferri, M., 2013. Methadone at tapered doses for the management of opioid withdrawal. *Cochrane Database Syst Rev* 2, CD003409.

Aniszewski, T., 2015. Chapter 1 - Definition, typology, and occurrence of alkaloids. *Alkaloids* (Second Edition). Elsevier, Boston, pp. 1-97.

Antonio, T., Childers, S.R., Rothman, R.B., Dersch, C.M., King, C., Kuehne, M., Bornmann, W.G., Eshleman, A.J., Janowsky, A., Simon, E.R., Reith, M.E., Alper, K., 2013. Effect of iboga alkaloids on μ-opioid receptor-coupled G protein activation. *PLoS One* 8(10), e77262.

Aricioglu-Kartal, F., Kayır, H., Tayfun Uzbay, I., 2003. Effects of harman and harmine on naloxone-precipitated withdrawal syndrome in morphine-dependent rats. *Life Sci.* 73(18), 2363-2371.

Bagal, A.A., Hough, L.B., Nalwalk, J.W., Glick, S.D., 1996. Modulation of morphine-induced antinociception by ibogaine and noribogaine. *Brain Res.* 741(1-2), 258-262.

Baillaud, L., 1962. Mouvements autonomes des tiges, vrilles et autres organes à l'exception des organes volubiles et des feuilles. *Encyclopedia of Plant Physiology / Handbuch der Pflanzenphysiologie* 17/2, 562-634.

Bartlett, M.F., Dickel, D.F., Taylor, W.I., 1958. The alkaloids of *Tabernanthe-Iboga*. Part VI. The Structures of ibogamine, ibogaine, tabernanthine and voacangine. *J. Am. Chem. Soc.* 80(1), 126-136.

Bastiaans, E., 2004. *Life after ibogaine: An exploratory study of the long-term effects of ibogaine treatment on drug addicts.* Doctorandus thesis Faculty of Medicine Vrije Universiteit Amsterdam. https://www.iceers.org/docs/science/iboga/Bastiaans E_Life_After_Ibogaine.pdf. (Accessed 21 September 2017).

Baumann, M.H., Rothman, R.B., Pablo, J.P., Mash, D.C., 2001. *In vivo* neurobiological effects of ibogaine and its

O-desmethyl metabolite, 12-hydroxyibogamine (noribogaine), in rats. *J. Pharmacol. Exp. Ther.* 297(2), 531-539.

Belgers, M., Leenaars, M., Homberg, J.R., Ritskes-Hoitinga, M., Schellekens, A.F., Hooijmans, C.R., 2016. Ibogaine and addiction in the animal model, a systematic review and meta-analysis. *Transl Psychiatry* 6(5), e826.

Bentzley, B.S., Barth, K.S., Back, S.E., Book, S.W., 2015. Discontinuation of buprenorphine maintenance therapy: perspectives and outcomes. *J. Subst. Abuse Treat.* 52, 48-57.

Bhargava, H.N., Cao, Y.J., 1997. Effects of noribogaine on the development of tolerance to antinociceptive action of morphine in mice. *Brain Res.* 771(2), 343-346.

Bhargava, H.N., Cao, Y.J., Zhao, G.M., 1997. Effects of ibogaine and noribogaine on the antinociceptive action of mu-, delta- and kappa-opioid receptor agonists in mice. *Brain Res.* 752(1-2), 234-238.

Bie, B., Peng, Y., Zhang, Y., Pan, Z.Z., 2005. cAMP-mediated mechanisms for pain sensitization during opioid withdrawal. *J. Neurosci.* 25(15), 3824-3832.

Binienda, Z., Beaudoin, MA, Thorn, B.T., Prapurna, D.R., Johnson, J.R., Fogle, C.M., Slikker, W., Jr., Ali, S.F., 1998. Alteration of electroencephalogram and monoamine concentrations in rat brain following ibogaine treatment. *Ann. N. Y. Acad. Sci.* 844, 265-273.

Bisaga, A., Comer, S., Ward, A., Popik, P., Kleber, H., Fischman, M., 2001. The NMDA antagonist memantine attenuates the expression of opioid physical dependence in humans. *Psychopharmacology* (Berl.) 157(1), 1-10.

Bowen, W.D., 2001. Sigma receptors and *iboga* alkaloids. *Alkaloids Chem. Biol.* 56, 173-191.

Brown, T.K., Alper, K., 2017. Treatment of opioid use disorder with ibogaine: detoxification and drug use outcomes. *Am. J. Drug Alcohol Abuse*, 1-13.

Caille, S., Espejo, E.F., Koob, G.F., Stinus, L., 2002. Dorsal and median raphe serotonergic system lesion does not alter the opiate withdrawal syndrome. *Pharmacol. Biochem. Behav.* 72(4), 979-986.

Cantero, J.L., Atienza, M., Stickgold, R., Kahana, M.J., Madsen, J.R., Kocsis, B., 2003. Sleep-dependent theta oscillations in the human hippocampus and neocortex. *J. Neurosci.* 23(34), 10897-10903.

Cao, Y.J., Bhargava, H.N., 1997. Effects of ibogaine on the development of tolerance to antinociceptive action of mu-, delta- and kappa-opioid receptor agonists in mice. *Brain Res.* 752(1-2), 250-254.

Cappendijk, S.L., Dzoljic, M.R., 1993. Inhibitory effects of ibogaine on cocaine self-administration in rats. *Eur. J. Pharmacol.* 241(2-3), 261-265.

Cappendijk, S.L., Fekkes, D., Dzoljic, M.R., 1994. The inhibitory effect of norharman on morphine withdrawal syndrome in rats: comparison with ibogaine. *Behav. Brain Res.* 65(1), 117-119.

Carnicella, S., He, D.Y., Yowell, Q.V., Glick, S.D., Ron, D., 2010. Noribogaine, but not 18-MC, exhibits similar actions as ibogaine on GDNF expression and ethanol self-administration. *Addict. Biol.* 15(4), 424-433.

Christie, M.J., 2008. Cellular neuroadaptations to chronic opioids: tolerance, withdrawal and addiction. *Br. J. Pharmacol.* 154(2), 384-396.

Corkery, J.M., Schifano, F., Ghodse, A.H., Oyefeso, A., 2004. The effects of methadone and its role in fatalities. *Hum Psychopharmacol* 19(8), 565-576.

Cubeddu, L.X., 2009. Iatrogenic QT Abnormalities and Fatal Arrhythmias: Mechanisms and Clinical Significance. *Curr. Cardiol. Rev.* 5(3), 166-176.

Darke, S., 1998. Self-report among injecting drug users: a review. *Drug Alcohol Depend.* 51(3), 253-263.

Darke, S., Kaye, S., Duflou, J., 2006. Systemic disease among cases of fatal opioid toxicity. *Addiction* 101(9), 1299-1305.

Deecher, D.C., Teitler, M., Soderlund, D.M., Bornmann, W.G., Kuehne, M.E., Glick, S.D., 1992. Mechanisms of action of ibogaine and harmaline congeners based on radioligand binding studies. *Brain Res.* 571(2), 242-247.

Depoortere, H., 1987. Neocortical rhythmic slow activity during wakefulness and paradoxical sleep in rats. *Neuropsychobiology* 18(3), 160-168.

Dhahir, H.I., 1971. *A Comparative Study on the Toxicity of Ibogaine and Serotonin*. Doctoral Thesis Department of Pharmacology and Toxicology, Indiana University.

Dickinson, J., McAlpin, J., Wilkins, C., Fitzsimmons, C., Guion, P., Paterson, T., Greene, D., Chaves, B.R., 2016. *Clinical Guidelines for Ibogaine-Assisted Detoxification* 1st Edition, Version 1.1. https://www.ibogainealliance.org/guidelines/. (Accessed 21 September, 2017).

Dos Santos, R.G., Hallak, J.E., 2017. Effects of the Natural beta-Carboline Alkaloid Harmine, a Main Constituent of Ayahuasca, in Memory and in the hippocampus: A systematic literature review of preclinical studies. *J. Psychoactive Drugs* 49(1), 1-10.

Drug Enforcement Administration, 2016. *National Heroin Threat Assessment Summary - Updated*.

Dworkin, S.I., Gleeson, S., Meloni, D., Koves, T.R., Martin, T.J., 1995. Effects of ibogaine on responding maintained by food, cocaine and heroin reinforcement in rats. *Psychopharmacology* (Berl.) 117(3), 257-261.

Dzoljic, E.D., Kaplan, C.D., Dzoljic, M.R., 1988. Effect of ibogaine on naloxone-precipitated withdrawal syndrome in chronic morphine-dependent rats. *Arch. Int. Pharmacodyn. Ther.* 294, 64-70.

Fabing, H., 1956. Trends in biological research in schizophrenia. *J. Nerv. Ment. Dis.* 124(1), 1-7.

Fareed, A., Casarella, J., Amar, R., Vayalapalli, S., Drexler, K., 2010. Methadone maintenance dosing guideline for opioid dependence, a literature review. *J. Addict. Dis.* 29(1), 1-14.

Fernandez, J.W., 1982. *Bwiti: An Ethnography of Religious Imagination in Africa*. Princeton University Press, Princeton, New Jersey.

Fernandez, J.W., Fernandez, R.L., 2001. "Returning to the path": the use of iboga[ine] in an equatorial African ritual context and the binding of time, space, and social relationships. *Alkaloids Chem. Biol.* 56, 235-247.

Frances, B., Gout, R., Cros, J., Zajac, J.M., 1992. Effects of ibogaine on naloxone-precipitated withdrawal in morphine-dependent mice. *Fundam. Clin. Pharmacol.* 6(8-9), 327-332.

Frye, A., Haustein, C., 2008. Extraction, identification, and quantification of harmala alkaloids in three species of Passiflora. *American Journal of Undergraduate Research* 6(3), 19- 26.

Gagliano, M., Renton, M., Depczynski, M., Mancuso, S., 2014. Experience teaches plants to learn faster and forget slower in environments where it matters. *Oecologia* 175(1), 63-72.

Glick, S.D., Kuehne, M.E., Raucci, J., Wilson, T.E., Larson, D., Keller, R.W., Jr., Carlson, J.N., 1994. Effects of iboga alkaloids on morphine and cocaine self-administration in rats: relationship to tremorigenic effects and to effects on dopamine release in nucleus accumbens and striatum. *Brain Res.* 657(1-2), 14-22.

Glick, S.D., Maisonneuve, I.M., Hough, L.B., Kuehne, M.E., Bandarage, U.K., 1999. (±)-18-Methoxycoronaridine: A novel iboga alkaloid congener having potential anti-addictive efficacy. *CNS Drug Reviews* 5(1), 27-42.

Glick, S.D., Maisonneuve, I.M., Kitchen, B.A., Fleck, M.W., 2002. Antagonism of α3β4 nicotinic receptors as a strategy to reduce opioid and stimulant self-administration. *Eur. J. Pharmacol.* 438(1-2), 99-105.

Glick, S.D., Maisonneuve, I.M., Szumlinski, K.K., 2001. Mechanisms of action of ibogaine: relevance to putative therapeutic effects and development of a safer *iboga* alkaloid congener. *Alkaloids Chem. Biol.* 56, 39-53.

Glick, S.D., Maisonneuve, I.M., Visker, K.E., Fritz, K.A., Bandarage, U.K., Kuehne, M.E., 1998. 18-Methoxycoronardine attenuates nicotine-induced dopamine release and nicotine preferences in rats. *Psychopharmacology* (Berl.) 139(3), 274-280.

Glick, S.D., Pearl, S.M., Cai, J., Maisonneuve, I.M., 1996. Ibogaine-like effects of noribogaine in rats. *Brain Res.* 713(1-2), 294-297.

Glick, S.D., Rossman, K., Rao, N.C., Maisonneuve, I.M., Carlson, J.N., 1992. Effects of ibogaine on acute signs of morphine-withdrawal in rats - independence from tremor. *Neuropharmacology* 31(5), 497-500.

Glick, S.D., Rossman, K., Steindorf, S., Maisonneuve, I.M., Carlson, J.N., 1991. Effects and aftereffects of ibogaine on morphine self-administration in rats. *Eur. J. Pharmacol.* 195(3), 341-345.

Glue, P., Lockhart, M., Lam, F., Hung, N., Hung, C.T., Friedhoff, L., 2015. Ascending-dose study of noribogaine in healthy volunteers: pharmacokinetics, pharmacodynamics, safety, and tolerability. *J. Clin. Pharmacol.* 55(2), 189-194.

Goutarel, R., Gollnhofer, O., Sillans, R., 1993. Pharmacodynamics and therapeutic applications of iboga and ibogaine. *Psychedelic Monographs and Essays* 6 6, 71-111.

Gowing, L., Ali, R., White, J.M., Mbewe, D., 2017. Buprenorphine for managing opioid withdrawal. *Cochrane Database Syst Rev* (2), Cd002025.

Gowing, L., Farrell, M., Ali, R., White, J.M., 2016. Alpha(2)-adrenergic agonists for the management of opioid withdrawal. *Cochrane Database Syst Rev*(5), CD002024.

Handelsman, L., Cochrane, K.J., Aronson, M.J., Ness, R., Rubinstein, K.J., Kanof, P.D., 1987. Two new rating-scales for opiate withdrawal. *Am. J. Drug Alcohol Abuse* 13(3), 293-308.

Hartmann, T., 2007. From waste products to ecochemicals: fifty years research of plant secondary metabolism. *Phytochemistry* 68(22-24), 2831-2846.

He, D.Y., McGough, N.N.H., Ravindranathan, A., Jeanblanc, J., Logrip, M.L., Phamluong, K., Janak, P.H., Ron, D., 2005. Glial cell line-derived neurotrophic factor mediates the desirable actions of the anti-addiction drug ibogaine against alcohol consumption. *J. Neurosci.* 25(3), 619-628.

Heink, A., Katsikas, S., Lange-Altman, T., 2017. Examination of the phenomenology of the ibogaine treatment experience: Role of altered states of consciousness and psychedelic experiences. *J. Psychoactive Drugs*, 1-8.

Heinze, M., Brandt, W., Marillonnet, S., Roos, W., 2015. "Self" and "non-self" in the control of phytoalexin biosynthesis: plant phospholipases A2 with alkaloid-specific molecular fingerprints. *Plant Cell* 27(2), 448-462.

Helsley, S., Fiorella, D., Rabin, R.A., Winter, J.C., 1997. Effects of ibogaine on performance in the 8-arm radial maze. *Pharmacol. Biochem. Behav.* 58(1), 37-41.

Helsley, S., Fiorella, D., Rabin, R.A., Winter, J.C., 1998. Behavioral and biochemical evidence for a nonessential 5-HT$_{2A}$ component of the ibogaine-induced discriminative stimulus. *Pharmacology Biochemistry and Behavior* 59(2), 419-425.

Hoglund, P.J., Adzic, D., Scicluna, S.J., Lindblom, J., Fredriksson, R., 2005. The repertoire of solute carriers of family 6: identification of new human and rodent genes. *Biochem. Biophys. Res. Commun.* 336(1), 175-189.

Isbell, H., 1955. Letter from Harris Isbell to Ciba-Geigy Pharmaceutical Products dated 11-29-55, Ciba Document no. AB0491- 492 410.

Jaiteh, M., Taly, A., Henin, J., 2016. Evolution of Pentameric Ligand-Gated Ion Channels: Pro-Loop Receptors. *PLoS One* 11(3), e0151934.

Jawna-Zboinska, K., Blecharz-Klin, K., Joniec-Maciejak, I., Wawer, A., Pyrzanowska, J., Piechal, A., Mirowska-Guzel, D., Widy-Tyszkiewicz, E., 2016. Passiflora incarnata L. Improves Spatial Memory, Reduces Stress, and Affects Neurotransmission in Rats. *Phytother. Res.* 30(5), 781-789.

John, E.R., 2005. From synchronous neuronal discharges to subjective awareness? *Prog. Brain Res.* 150, 143-593.

Kannankeril, P., Roden, D.M., Darbar, D., 2010. Drug-induced long QT syndrome. *Pharmacol. Rev.* 62(4), 760-781.

Kaye, S., McKetin, R., Duflou, J., Darke, S., 2007. Methamphetamine and cardiovascular pathology: a review of the evidence. *Addiction* 102(8), 1204-1211.

Knuepfer, M.M., 2003. Cardiovascular disorders associated with cocaine use: myths and truths. *Pharmacol. Ther.* 97(3), 181-222.

Koenig, X., Hilber, K., 2015. The anti-addiction drug ibogaine and the heart: A delicate relation. *Molecules* 20(2), 2208-2228.

Koenig, X., Kovar, M., Rubi, L., Mike, A.K., Lukacs, P., Gawali, V.S., Todt, H., Hilber, K., Sandtner, W., 2013. Anti-addiction drug ibogaine inhibits voltage-gated ionic currents: a study to assess the drug's cardiac ion channel profile. *Toxicol. Appl. Pharmacol.* 273(2), 259-268.

Koja, T., Fukuzaki, K., Kamenosono, T., Nishimura, A., Nagata, R., Lukas, S.E., 1996. Inhibition of opioid abstinent phenomena by Ibogaine. 69th Annual Meeting of the Japanese Pharmacological Society, March 20-23, 1996. *Jpn. J. Pharmacol.* Volume: 71 Issue: Suppl. 1, 89.

Kontrimavičiūtė, V., Mathieu, O., Mathieu-Daudé, J.C., Vainauskas, P., Casper, T., Baccino, E., Bressolle, F.M., 2006. Distribution of ibogaine and noribogaine in a man following a poisoning involving root bark of the *Tabernanthe iboga* shrub. *J. Anal. Toxicol.* 30(7), 434-440.

Latzel, V., Gonzalez, A.P.R., Rosenthal, J., 2016. Epigenetic Memory as a Basis for Intelligent Behavior in Clonal Plants. *Frontiers in Plant Science* 7.

Lavaud, C., Massiot, G., 2017. The Iboga Alkaloids. *Prog Chem Org Nat Prod* 105, 89-136.

Layer, R.T., Skolnick, P., Bertha, C.M., Bandarage, U.K., Kuehne, M.E., Popik, P., 1996. Structurally modified ibogaine analogs exhibit differing affinities for NMDA receptors. *Eur. J. Pharmacol.* 309(2), 159-165.

Le Men, L., Taylor, W.I., 1965. A uniform numbering system for indole alkaloids. *Experientia* 21(9), 508-510.

Leal, M.B., Michelin, K., Souza, D.O., Elisabetsky, E., 2003. Ibogaine attenuation of morphine withdrawal in mice: role of glutamate N-methyl-D-aspartate receptors. *Prog. Neuropsychopharmacol. Biol. Psychiatry* 27(5), 781-785.

Leung, L.S., 1998. Generation of theta and gamma rhythms in the hippocampus. *Neurosci. Biobehav. Rev.* 22(2), 275-290.

Levin, K.H., Copersino, M.L., Epstein, D., Boyd, S.J., Gorelick, D.A., 2008. Longitudinal ECG changes in cocaine users during extended abstinence. *Drug Alcohol Depend.* 95(1-2), 160-163.

Lotsof, H.S., 1985. Rapid Method for Interrupting the Narcotic Addiction Syndrome. US Patent number 4,499,096.

Lotsof, H.S., Alexander, N.E., 2001. Case studies of ibogaine treatment: implications for patient management strategies. *Alkaloids Chem. Biol.* 56, 293-313.

MacInnes, N., Handley, S.L., 2002. Characterization of the discriminable stimulus produced by 2-BFI: effects of imidazoline I(2)-site ligands, MAOIs, beta-carbolines, agmatine and ibogaine. *Br. J. Pharmacol.* 135(5), 1227-1234.

Maisonneuve, I.M., Glick, S.D., 1992. Interactions between ibogaine and cocaine in rats - invivo microdialysis and motor behavior. *Eur. J. Pharmacol.* 212(2-3), 263-266.

Maisonneuve, I.M., Glick, S.D., 1999. Attenuation of the reinforcing efficacy of morphine by 18-methoxycoronaridine. *Eur. J. Pharmacol.* 383(1), 15-21.

Maisonneuve, I.M., Glick, S.D., 2003. Anti-addictive actions of an iboga alkaloid congener: a novel mechanism for a novel treatment. *Pharmacology Biochemistry and Behavior* 75(3), 607-618.

Maisonneuve, I.M., Keller, R.W., Jr., Glick, S.D., 1991. Interactions between ibogaine, a potential anti-addictive agent, and morphine: an *in vivo* microdialysis study. *Eur. J. Pharmacol.* 199(1), 35-42.

Maisonneuve, I.M., Keller, R.W., Jr., Glick, S.D., 1992. Interactions of ibogaine and D-amphetamine: *in vivo* microdialysis and motor behavior in rats. *Brain Res.* 579(1), 87-92.

Maisonneuve, I.M., Mann, G.L., Deibel, C.R., Glick, S.D., 1997. Ibogaine and the dopaminergic response to nicotine. *Psychopharmacology* (Berl.) 129(3), 249-256.

Maisonneuve, I.M., Rossman, K.L., Keller, R.W., Jr., Glick, S.D., 1992. Acute and prolonged effects of ibogaine on brain dopamine metabolism and morphine-induced locomotor activity in rats. *Brain Res.* 575(1), 69-73.

Mash, D., 1997. Deborah Mash V. NDA International, Inc., Case No.96-3712-CIV-MORENO, Amended Complaint. http://puzzlepiece.org/ibogaine/011198.html. (Accessed 21 September 2017).

Mash, D.C., Allen-Ferdinand, K., Mayor, M., Kovera, C.A., Ayafor, J.F., Williams, I.C., Ervin, F.R., 1998. Ibogaine: clinical observations of safety after single oral dose administrations, in: Harris, L.S. (Ed.) *Problems of Drug Dependence 1998: Proceedings of the 60th Annual Scientific Meeting*. The College on Problems of Drug Dependence, Scottsdale, Arizona, p. 294.

Mash, D.C., Ameer, B., Prou, D., Howes, J.F., Maillet, E.L., 2016. Oral noribogaine shows high brain uptake and anti-withdrawal effects not associated with place preference in rodents. *J Psychopharmacol* 30(7), 688-697.

Mash, D.C., Kovera, C.A., Buck, B.E., Norenberg, MD, Shapshak, P., Hearn, W.L., Sanchez-Ramos, J., 1998. Medication development of ibogaine as a pharmacotherapy for drug dependence. *Ann. N. Y. Acad. Sci.* 844, 274-292.

Mash, D.C., Kovera, C.A., Pablo, J., Tyndale, R., Ervin, F.R., Kamlet, J.D., Hearn, W.L., 2001. Ibogaine in the treatment of heroin withdrawal. *Alkaloids Chem. Biol.* 56, 155-171.

McCall, A.C., Fordyce, J.A., 2010. Can optimal defence theory be used to predict the distribution of plant chemical defences? *J. Ecol.* 98(5), 985-992.

McGahan, P.L., Griffith, J.A., Parente, R., McLellan, A.T., 1986. *Addiction Severity Index Composite Scores Manual*. The University of Pennsylvania/Veterans Administration Center for Studies of Addiction, Philadelphia, PA.

Molinari, H.H., Maisonneuve, I.M., Glick, S.D., 1996. Ibogaine neurotoxicity: a re-evaluation. *Brain Res.* 737(1-2), 255-262.

MPI Research, 1996. Determination of the acute interaction of combined ibogaine and morphine in rats. *MPI Research Identification*: 693-082. Ibogaine Drug Master File Volume 8. National Institute on Drug Abuse (NIDA), Bethesda, MD, pp. 1- 377.

Naranjo, C., 1973. *The Healing Journey: New Approaches to Consciousness*. Pantheon, Random House, New York.

National Institutes of Health, 2012. IND-Enabling Studies and GMP Scale-Up of 18-Methoxycoronaridine Hydrochloride (18 MC) Project Number: 1U01DA034986-01. https://projectreporter.nih.gov/project_info_description.cfm?aid=8448461&icde=16047111&ddparam=&ddvalue=&ddsub=&cr=41&csb=default&cs=ASC. (Accessed 21 September 2017).

Neilson, E.H., Goodger, J.Q., Woodrow, I.E., Moller, B.L., 2013. Plant chemical defense: at what cost? *Trends Plant Sci* 18(5), 250-258.

Nelson, D.L., Herbet, A., Petillot, Y., Pichat, L., Glowinski, J., Hamon, M., 1979. [3H]Harmaline as a specific ligand of MAO-I. Properties of the active site of MAO A from rat and bovine brains. *J. Neurochem.* 32(6), 1817-1827.

Nestler, E.J., 2001. Molecular neurobiology of addiction. *Am. J. Addict.* 10(3), 201-217.

Nichols, D.E., 2016. Psychedelics. *Pharmacol. Rev.* 68(2), 264-355.

Noller, G.E., Frampton, C.M., Yazar-Klosinski, B., 2017. Ibogaine treatment outcomes for opioid dependence from a twelve-month follow-up observational study. *Am. J. Drug Alcohol Abuse*, 1-10.

O'Connor, S.E., Maresh, J.J., 2006. Chemistry and biology of monoterpene indole alkaloid biosynthesis. *Nat. Prod. Rep.* 23(4), 532-547.

O'Hearn, E., Molliver, M.E., 1993. Degeneration of Purkinje cells in parasagittal zones of the cerebellar vermis after treatment with ibogaine or harmaline. *Neuroscience* 55(2), 303-310.

O'Hearn, E., Molliver, M.E., 1997. The olivocerebellar projection mediates ibogaine-induced degeneration of Purkinje cells: a model of indirect, trans-synaptic excitotoxicity. *J. Neurosci.* 17(22), 8828-8841.

Otero-Anton, E., Gonzalez-Quintela, A., Saborido, J., Torre, J.A., Virgos, A., Barrio, E., 1997. Prolongation of the QTc interval during alcohol withdrawal syndrome. *Acta Cardiol.* 52(3), 285-294.

Panchal, V., Taraschenko, O.D., Maisonneuve, I.M., Glick, S.D., 2005. Attenuation of morphine withdrawal signs by intracerebral administration of 18-methoxycoronaridine. *Eur. J. Pharmacol.* 525(1-3), 98-104.

Parker, L.A., Burton, P., McDonald, R.V., Kim, J.A., Siegel, S., 2002. Ibogaine interferes with motivational and somatic effects of naloxone-precipitated withdrawal from acutely administered morphine. *Prog. Neuropsychopharmacol. Biol. Psychiatry* 26(2), 293-297.

Pearl, S.M., Hough, L.B., Boyd, D.L., Glick, S.D., 1997. Sex differences in ibogaine antagonism of morphine-induced locomotor activity and in ibogaine brain levels and metabolism. *Pharmacol. Biochem. Behav.* 57(4), 809-815.

Pearl, S.M., Johnson, D.W., Glick, S.D., 1995. Prior morphine exposure enhances ibogaine antagonism of morphine-induced locomotor stimulation. *Psychopharmacology* (Berl.) 121(4), 470-475.

Pearl, S.M., Maisonneuve, I.M., Glick, S.D., 1996. Prior morphine exposure enhances ibogaine antagonism of morphine-induced dopamine release in rats. *Neuropharmacology* 35(12), 1779-1784.

Pierre, S., Eschenhagen, T., Geisslinger, G., Scholich, K., 2009. Capturing adenylyl cyclases as potential drug targets. *Nat Rev Drug Discov* 8(4), 321-335.

Popik, P., 1996. Facilitation of memory retrieval by the "anti-addictive" alkaloid, ibogaine. *Life Sci.* 59(24), PL379-385.

Popik, P., Layer, R.T., Fossom, L.H., Benveniste, M., Geterdouglass, B., Witkin, J.M., Skolnick, P., 1995. NMDA antagonist properties of the putative antiaddictive drug, ibogaine. *J. Pharmacol. Exp. Ther.* 275(2), 753-760.

Rabin, R.A., Winter, J.C., 1996. Ibogaine and noribogaine potentiate the inhibition of adenylyl cyclase activity by opioid and 5-HT receptors. *Eur. J. Pharmacol.* 316(2-3), 343-348.

Rezvani, A.H., Overstreet, D.H., Lee, Y.W., 1995. Attenuation of alcohol intake by ibogaine in three strains of alcohol-preferring rats. *Pharmacol. Biochem. Behav.* 52(3), 615-620.

Rho, B., Glick, S.D., 1998. Effects of 18-methoxycoronaridine on acute signs of morphine withdrawal in rats. *Neuroreport* 9(7), 1283-1285.

Roden, D.M., Yang, T., 2005. Protecting the heart against arrhythmias: Potassium current physiology and repolarization reserve. *Circulation* 112(10), 1376-1378.

Salmoiraghi, G.C., Page, I.H., 1957. Effects of LSD 25, BOL 148, bufotenine, mescaline and ibogaine on the potentiation of hexobarbital hypnosis produced by serotonin and reserpine. *J. Pharmacol. Exp. Ther.* 120(1), 20-25.

Samorini, G., 1998. The initiation rite in the Bwiti Religion (Ndea Narizanga Sect, Gabon). *Yearbook for Ethnomedicine and the Study of Consciousness* 6-7, 39-56.

Scallet, A.C., Ye, X., Rountree, R., Nony, P., Ali, S.F., 1996. Ibogaine produces neurodegeneration in rat, but not mouse, cerebellum. Neurohistological biomarkers of Purkinje cell loss. *Ann. N. Y. Acad. Sci.* 801, 217-226.

Schneider, J.A., 1957. Tabernanthine, Ibogaine Containing Analgesic Compostions. US Patent no. 2,817,623.

Schneider, J.A., McArthur, M., 1956. Potentiation action of ibogaine (bogadin TM) on morphine analgesia. *Experientia* 12(8), 323-324.

Schneider, J.A., Rinehart, R.K., 1957. Analysis of the cardiovascular action of ibogaine hydrochloride. *Arch. Int. Pharmacodyn. Ther.* 110(1), 92-102.

Schneider, J.A., Sigg, E.B., 1957. Neuropharmacological studies on ibogaine, an indole alkaloid with central-stimulant properties. *Ann. N. Y. Acad. Sci.* 66(3), 765-776.

Seigler, D.S., 1998. *Plant Secondary Metabolism.* Springer Science+ Business Media, New York.

Sershen, H., Hashim, A., Lajtha, A., 1994. Ibogaine reduces preference for cocaine consumption in C57BL/6By mice. *Pharmacol. Biochem. Behav.* 47(1), 13-19.

Sharma, S.K., Klee, W.A., Nirenberg, M., 1975. Dual regulation of adenylate cyclase accounts for narcotic dependence and tolerance. *Proc. Natl. Acad. Sci. U. S. A.* 72(8), 3092-3096.

Shawn, L.K., Alper, K., Desai, S.P., Stephenson, K., Olgun, A.M., Nelson, L.S., Hoffman, R.S., 2012. Pause-dependent ventricular tachycardia and torsades de pointes after ibogaine ingestion [2012 Annual Meeting of the North American Congress of Clinical Toxicology (NACCT)]. *Clin. Toxicol.* 50, 654.

Skolnick, P., 2001. Ibogaine as a glutamate antagonist: relevance to its putative antiaddictive properties. Alkaloids *Chem. Biol.* 56, 55-62.

Snelders, S., Kaplan, C., 2002. LSD therapy in Dutch psychiatry: changing socio-political settings and medical sets. *Med. Hist.* 46(2), 221-240.

Stolaroff, M., 2004. *The Secret Chief Revealed.* Multidisciplinary Association for Psychedelic Studies (MAPS), Sarasota, FL.

Sunder Sharma, S., Bhargava, H.N., 1998. Enhancement of morphine antinociception by ibogaine and noribogaine in morphine-tolerant mice. *Pharmacology* 57(5), 229-232.

Sweetnam, P.M., Lancaster, J., Snowman, A., Collins, J.L., Perschke, S., Bauer, C., Ferkany, J., 1995. Receptor binding profile suggests multiple mechanisms of action are responsible for ibogaine's putative anti-addictive activity. *Psychopharmacology* (Berl.) 118(4), 369-376.

Szabó, L.F., 2008. Rigorous biogenetic network for a group of indole alkaloids derived from strictosidine. *Molecules* 13(8), 1875-1896.

The Plant List, 2013. Version 1.1. http://www.theplantlist.org/. (Accessed 21 September 2017).

Trewavas, A., 2005. Green plants as intelligent organisms. *Trends Plant Sci* 10(9), 413-419.

Trewavas, A., 2017. The foundations of plant intelligence. *Interface Focus* 7(3), 20160098.

Trujillo, K.A., Akil, H., 1994. Inhibition of opiate tolerance by non-competitive N-methyl-D-aspartate receptor antagonists. *Brain Res.* 633(1-2), 178-188.

Turner, W.J., Merlis, S., Carl, A., 1955. Concerning theories of indoles in schizophrenigenesis. *Am. J. Psychiatry* 112(6), 466-467.

U.S. Senate, 1977. *Project MKULTRA, The CIA's Program Of Research In Behavioral Modification,* Joint Hearing Before the U.S. Senate Select Committee on Intelligence and the Subcommittee on Health and Scientific Research of the Committee on Human Resources. U.S. Government Printing Office, Washington, D.C., p. 244.

Urano, D., Jones, A.M., 2014. Heterotrimeric G protein-coupled signaling in plants. *Annu. Rev. Plant Biol.* 65, 365-384.

van der Heijden, R., Jacobs, D.I., Snoeijer, W., Hallared, D., Verpoorte, R., 2004. The Catharanthus alkaloids: Pharmacognosy and biotechnology. *Curr. Med. Chem.* 11(5), 607-628.

Vastag, B., 2005. Addiction research. Ibogaine therapy: A 'vast, uncontrolled experiment'. *Science* 308(5720), 345-346.

Wei, D., Maisonneuve, I.M., Kuehne, M.E., Glick, S.D., 1998. Acute *iboga* alkaloid effects on extracellular serotonin (5-HT) levels in nucleus accumbens and striatum in rats. *Brain Res.* 800(2), 260-268.

Welsch, M.E., Snyder, S.A., Stockwell, B.R., 2010. Privileged Scaffolds for Library Design and Drug Discovery. *Curr. Opin. Chem. Biol.* 14(3), 347-361.

Zhuo, M., 2012. Targeting neuronal adenylyl cyclase for the treatment of chronic pain. *Drug Discovery Today* 17(11-12), 573-582.

Psychoactive Initiation Plant Medicines: Their Role in the Healing and Learning Process of South African and Upper Amazonian Traditional Healers

Jean-Francois Sobiecki, BSc Hons

Research Associate,
Univ. of Johannesburg;
Founder, Khanyisa Healing
Gardens Project,
Johannesburg, South Africa

ABSTRACT

There is an accelerating interest in strong acting psychoactive plants such as *ayahuasca* for healing and personal development. However, what has become apparent with initiating into South African traditional healing, and key literature sources from South America, is the importance not only of the strong mind 'opening' visionary plants but the equally significant utilization of subtle acting psychoactive plants that cleanse and strengthen the initiate healers, that are used in a sequence of initiation plant medicines both in the South African and South American traditional medicine systems. This paper explores and describes a cross cultural technology of healing with psychoactive initiation plants that are used in a sequential manner in order to take the initiate traditional healer through a process of self enquiry, growth and potential self-mastery. Understanding this sequential use of traditional initiation plant medicines and their physiological and psychological correlates could elucidate possible therapeutic mechanisms involved with the use of psychoactive traditional medicines and their potential applications in future medicine and healing. The connection is also made between the role of perturbation in the learning process healers engage and how psychoactive plants produce perturbation in the nervous system and what adaptive benefit this may have.

INTRODUCTION

Little academic attention has been paid to the subject of psychoactive plants and their role in the initiation process of southern African traditional healers. Mentions of psychoactive plant use from the southern African anthropological and ethnobotanical literature are scant and anecdotal. One rare, early paper highlights the significance of plants used in the initiation and religious practices of the Sotho speaking people and their potential psychoactive properties (Laydevant, 1932). This lack of data on African psychoactive plant use in general, encouraged the author to conduct anthropological fieldwork from 1998 onwards, to document the role of psychoactive plants in the spiritual healing practices of the South African diviners (*Izangoma*) and herbalists (*Izinyanga*).

Some findings from conducting a literature review and long standing fieldwork included a preliminary inventory being published indicating over 300 species of plants being used for psychoactive purposes in southern African healing traditions (Sobiecki, 2002). A review of plants used in divination in southern Africa and their psychoactive effects was also conducted, that indicated that

175

approximately 45% of the plants reported with uses in divination have other psychoactive uses (Sobiecki, 2008). Much of the traditional meanings and therapeutic significance of these plants remain undocumented and is in urgent need of study.

Having experienced a category of South African plant medicines called *ubulawu* and Ayurvedic *vamana* emesis therapy in Dharamsala in 2011, indicated that there is a common mechanism of action of using plant medicines to vomit and cleanse with in both the Ayurvedic and South African traditional medicine systems that has a corresponding psychoactive healing effect on the mind (Note: these are not emetics, but medicines that one manually cleanses with) (Sobiecki, 2012).

Thereafter, having completed my initiation using South African plant medicines with a masterful Northern Sotho African healer Mrs. Letty Maponya in 2012, provided valuable insights that what I had experienced through the use of initiation plants in South Africa paralleled what I had subsequently read about the *curandero* (shaman's) use of initiation plants in South America (Jauregui et al. 2011). In this paper they describe plants that were administered as part of a particular sequence during the initiation process namely: (I) purification and cleansing (II) sensitivity and intuition; (III) strengthening; and (IV) protection and defence. I recognized this same sequence of plant medicines as what I had gone through with the African initiation plant medicine process.

The aim of this paper is to put forward the hypothesis that this same sequential use of initiation plant medicine categories in both the South American and South African traditional medicine systems indicates a cross cultural therapeutic technology of healing and self development by traditional healers from both South America and South Africa.

METHODS

My training and initiation followed a long-time friendship and apprenticeship with a Northern Sotho healer and diviner Mrs. Letty Mamonyai Maponya. Having met Mrs. Maponya during my initial fieldwork in Johannesburg in 1998, to answer whether the *Izangoma* (South African diviners) were using psychoactive plants as part of their spiritual practices to induce trance states, Mrs. Maponya immediately offered to assist me where she could. This initiated a 15 year friendship and mentorship with her. It was only later towards the end of our relationship in 2012 (Mrs. Maponya passed over in 2013), that Mrs. Maponya finally agreed to facilitate a formal process of initiation with plant medicines for me during which time (approximately 3 months) I would come to realize the importance of the stages of medicine used in the initiation. I rented a cottage in Jeppestown, Johannesburg, so as to be close to my teacher to receive instruction. It was a time of introspection and isolation focusing on the self knowledge facilitated by the use of the initiation medicines.

THE SOUTH AFRICAN TRADITIONAL MEDICINE INITIATION PROCESS

CLEANSING MEDICINES

I started the initiation process using cleansing medicines, the purpose of which was to ritually let go of the past while preparing for the new to emerge. One key medicine I used to cleanse myself with was *Elaeodendron transvaalense* (Burtt Davy) R.H. Archer, or *Ingwavuma* (Zulu). I used the bark of this medicine, which is ground finely into a powder, to steam with, as well as a small quantity that is consumed as a decoction to vomit with. *Ingwavuma* is rich in tannins and flavonoids that not only cleans ritual pollution but is very effective in clearing diarrhea, impurities and pathogenic or toxic heat conditions from the body. Having cleansed myself sufficiently with this and other medicines for around two weeks made me feel energized and more confident. Mrs. Maponya advised me from the start of the 3 month period on behavioural and dietary restrictions: to not have sex or intimate relationships and to restrict social engagement (the energetic relationships with people would disturb my process of introspection and self-enquiry), as well as keeping a clean simple diet without stimulants. These restrictions are important in helping the initiate familiarize with the enhanced states of consciousness experienced and to help anchor new learnings. Jauregui et al., 2011, describes the significance of cleansing plants in the initiation of *curanderos*: "The first plants ingested during the diets are species that are well-known by the Amazonian societies and highly utilized in their traditional medicine due to their purgative, laxative, anthelmintic, and emetic properties. These plants are ingested by the apprentices at the start of the process so that they can purify themselves and prepare their bodies for meeting with the spirit of the vegetables or mothers of the plants." From my experience, I learnt that strict monitoring by my teacher was essential throughout the initiation period to ensure correct dosages and administration methods of the medicines are used - too much *Ingwavuma* can negatively affect digestion because of its high tannin content, for example.

MIND OPENING MEDICINES

The next stage of the initiation required that I use one species of *ubulawu* medicines that I call the 'mirror *ubulawu*', that is an initiation secret. *Ubulawu* is a preparation form of Southern African traditional medicine made from a number of different plant species that are all used to open the mind and that are described as "lucky medicines" by the indigenous people of Southern Africa (Sobiecki, 2012). The term *ubulawu* refers mostly to the roots of a variety of plants that are ground and made into a cold water infusion that is churned with a forked stick to produce foam. The foam is eaten at night and the infusion is drank on an empty stomach first thing in the morning and vomited with to cleanse the person. The foam is said to indicate saponins some of which are reported to be psychoactive. *Ubulawu* is used in traditional South African healing to open luck, and as my teacher said "all *ubulawu* opens luck." I describe the term "lucky medicines" as an example of a metaphorical indicator of physiological actions from using psychoactive medicinal plants (Sobiecki, 2014), that is, using *ubulawu* medicines enhances dreaming, produces clearer thinking and produces more energy, and all of which are effects that are lucky to be experienced, which is why they are called "lucky medicines." In the Nguni speaking groups of South Africa dreams are considered to belong to the domain of the ancestors (Sobiecki, 2008). A fundamental use of *ubulawu* in African healing traditions is to facilitate connection and communication with ones ancestors (deceased ancestral relatives) through dreams and/or intuitive feelings, that the medicines can help to access. Thus, these medicines are believed to be important tools to connect with one's deceased ancestral spirits, (that incidentally my teacher equated with angels). Manton Hirst (1990, 1997), comprehensively describes the importance of *ubulawu* in the initiation of South African Xhosa diviners and the medicines' role in their dreaming and ancestral connection. Having used the "mirror *ubulawu*", I was expecting my dreams to be clearer but disappointingly this did not happen. However, what did happen was my intuition and sensitivity increased to the point I felt overwhelmed to be in any place with a lot of stimuli, e.g., shopping malls. I describe in Sobiecki (2012) how the cleansing action of vomiting with the *ubulawu* plant medicines, together with the psychoactive properties of the species used that are absorbed in the body, results in these effects. The importance of being clean in ones body so as to have good mental well-being and connection cannot be overstated in African traditional society and should be more utilized in western society. The culmination of using this medicine at twelve days was the feeling of being forced to face the deepest personal question of my life. I felt the intensity of emotions reaching a crescendo to the point that I wanted to run away from my home I was renting close to my teacher for the initiation period. I stopped the medicine at this point after consultation with my teacher. Some of the *ubulawu* species used by various ethnic groups in southern Africa are described in a previous paper (Sobiecki, 2008). While the role of strong visionary medicines like *ayahuasca* used by the *curandero* healers to open the mind appears to predominate, there are also a number of plants that are also used to vomit with such as *Aristolochia cauliflora* Ule., to cleanse and open the initiate (Jauregui et al., 2011).

STRENGTHENING MEDICINES

To help ground myself after this intense introspective stage of the process I was introduced to using a red strengthening mixture containing a plant called *Maytenus undata* (Thunb.) Blakelock, or *Dabulovalo* (Zulu). This medicines name connotes "shock" and is used to relax a person. This and another tree that I cannot name at this stage, is used together as a strengthening medicine in order to help the initiates stabilize and strengthen after the intense opening period. This is similar to the use of tree medicines by the *curanderos* where Jauregui et al. 2011, explains: "The initiates need to strengthen themselves both physically and spiritually in order to move forward in the learning process, and therefore the diet should consist mainly of palos, the large rainforest trees, the jainoa onanti jihui, which means "tree that teaches" in the Shipibo-Konibo language." I also used during the initiation a powder made from Licorice (*Glycyrrhiza gabra* L.) that is eaten off the palm of the hand (to *kotha-Zulu*). The licorice medicine is called 'sweet mouth' and works as a tonic to calm and boost ones energy (Sobiecki, 2014). While the name "sweet mouth" and its traditional use to talk nicely may sound superstitious, its quick uplifting affects allows one to be calm and to speak easily and such behaviour is easily reflected by others through communicating owing to the well known mirror neuron phenomenon. Thus the name "sweet mouth" is not magical at all, but a metaphorical indicator of the physiological and psychological effects (Sobiecki, 2014), resulting from the tonic actions of the medicines. Together these medicines are used to assist in grounding the initiate after what can be an intense opening, and to help anchor the new insights into possible new learning's and behaviour. It is worthwhile to note that some of the medicines used in the initiation process are considered a secret that requires a proper research project platform with ABS agreements in place for the local communities involved, in order to study these plants and their applications correctly.

INITIATION PLANTS AS
PERTURBATORY LEARNING TOOLS

In retrospect, this period of initiation involved a pragmatic approach to self growth and development through firstly; letting go of ones past through cleansing medicines, then opening to new knowledge through using *ubulawu* that encourages dreaming and enhanced intuition and sensitivity, and then finally absorbing and anchoring the new insights with red strengthening medicines. The hypothesis I make here is that this initiation medicine process is a pragmatic technology used to interrupt old patterns of behaviour and familiarize the initiate with enhanced states of awareness, self-enquiry, growth and potential self-mastery afforded by the psychoactive plant medicines and the ritual context. Other traditional healers have affirmed that the use of initiation plant medicines in this way is to achieve self-growth and mastery (Dr. Hlati, pers. comm, 2015).

At present, it appears that many westerners are focusing entirely on the opening class of medicines such as *Ayahuasca*, and are not familiar with the equally important cleansing and grounding medicines used in Amazonian and South African traditional healing systems demonstrated here. While *ayahuasca* has cleansing and purgative actions there are many other plants used in both traditions whose primary indication is to cleanse the body, thereby opening the mind through a gradual process of enhanced sensitivity and intuition. Thus, the subtle psychoactive affects of initiation plant medicines plays a significant role in psychological and spiritual healing in shamanic and other tribal societies.

What further significance may there be regarding the use of initiation plants in this sequence in terms of healing?

What I understood as part of my training and what my teacher Mrs. Maponya explained is "that too much power is not good for a *twasa* (initiate), they must also relax." I experienced this, in that following the power and intensity from the opening *ubulawu* medicines, one can ground and balance oneself with the relaxing red medicines that gives time for the insights and teachings to be absorbed and anchored.

This destabilizing (opening with *ubulawu* medicines) and then stabilizing (grounding with red medicines) reminds me of a number of other examples in the neuroscience field where perturbation has potential adaptive and therapeutic value.

For example, Dr. Froese proposes the possible selective benefits of mind alteration that he terms as the *interruption mechanism* as part of a self-optimizing spiking neural network model. In this study they found if the model 'brain' is subjected to occasional perturbations that profoundly alter its normal state of activity, in this case via the randomisation of its activity, synaptic plasticity spontaneously starts to reshape the network's connectivity in a way that enhances coordination of neural activity (Froese, 2015). He goes on to say "This result is only based on an artificial model, but it is nevertheless suggestive: neuroscientists investigating the psychedelic state have found it to be associated with a similar disruption of normal activity, including cortical desynchronisation (Muthukumaraswamy et al. 2013) and increased disorder of neural activity (Carhart-Harris et al., 2014), and that these modified states of consciousness may have positive adaptive consequences by increasing integration between brain areas (Winkelman, 2010), providing users with functional adaptation of cognition (Müller and Schumann, 2011), and as influencing creativity (Dobkin de Rios and Janiger, 2003). Furthermore, Dr Carhart-Harris describes what he terms as elevated entropy with the use of psychedelic medicine that results in the breakdown of brain networks and that this is beneficial in interrupting familiarized conditioned learning (Carhart-Harris et al., 2014). These examples demonstrate that perturbation resulting from the action of psychoactive medicines and other stimuli can be advantageous in interrupting old behaviours while providing opportunities to initiate new behaviours.

From my experience, I propose that the ritual sequential use of psychoactive opening and grounding initiation plant medicines as part of the South African traditional healers initiation provides such a perturbative process that fosters the disruption of old conditioned behaviours and offers the opportunity to familiarize with new insights that can translate, under certain conditions, into new learnings and behaviours with attendant personal growth and maturation, which is one desired outcome of a successful and completed initiation process of African traditional healers.

Thus, in summary, the perturbatory affects catalyzed by psychoactive initiation plant medicines is positively and pragmatically utilized in the initiation process of the traditional healers in Southern Africa and in South America towards healing ends.

FUTURE RESEARCH

Much on the African traditional initiation plants and their cultural and corresponding scientific understandings is yet to be documented and investigated, and is one key reason for the inception of the Khanyisa Healing Garden Project, that aims to create a network of healing and research gardens between South America and South Africa to study these psychoactive plants and their application in medicine, healing and community health promotion through multidisciplinary collaborative projects.

Many of the plants in question are over-harvested and face eradication, without having been researched. Therefore, there is an urgent need for such documentation of this eroding knowledge and for new conservation strategies to be developed, which is a further objective of the Khanyisa project. The Khanyisa Project aims to establish sustainable working relationships with the local communities involved in the research through generating viable ethnobotanical tourism related to the African plant knowledge and establishing Access Benefit Sharing (ABS) agreements with research interest groups. This innovative project has much to offer in terms of integrating research, health promotion, conservation and community development relating to the use of psychoactive plants and furthering our understanding of healing consciousness with traditional plant medicine.

ACKNOWLEDGEMENTS

I would like to thank Dr. Dennis McKenna and the other organizers of the Ethnopharmacological Search for Psychoactive Drugs II conference for their support and inclusion of this work in the proceedings, Mrs. Maponya for her teaching and sharing of the knowledge of African Healing Plants, Dr. Nigel Gericke for his valuable inputs and Dr. Froese for his correspondence.

REFERENCES

Carhart-Harris, R. L., Leech, R., Hellyer, P.J., Shanahan, M., Feilding, A., Tagliazucchi, E., Chialvo, D.R., & Nutt, D. 2014. The entropic brain: A theory of conscious states informed by neuroi aging research with psychedelic drugs. *Frontiers in Human Neuroscience* 8(20): 1-22.

Dobkin de Rios, M. & Janiger, O. 2003. *LSD, Spirituality, and the Creative Process*. Rochester, VT: Park Street Press.

Froese, T. Pre-Print. 2015. The ritualised mind alteration hypothesis of the origins and evolution of the symbolic human mind. *Rock Art Research*. 32.

Hirst, M. 1990. *The healers Art: Cape Nguni Diviners in the Township of Grahamstown*. PhD Thesis, Rhodes University.

Hirst, M. 1997. A river of metaphors: Interpreting the Xhosa diviner's myth. In: McAllister, P., ed., *Culture and The Commonplace: Anthropological Essays in Honour of David Hammond-Took*. Johannesburg: Witwatersrand University Press.

Jauregui, X., Clavo, Z.M., Jovel, E.M., & Pardo-de-Santayana M. 2011. "Plantas con madre": Plants that teach and guide in the shamanic initiation process in the east-central Peruvian Amazon. *Journal of Ethnopharmacology*.134: 739-752.

Khanyisa Healing Garden. 2013. http://www. khanyisagarden.co.za.

Laydevant, F. 1932. Religious or sacred plants of Basutoland. *Bantu Studies* 6: 65-9.

Müller, C. P. & Schumann, G. 2011. Drugs as instruments: A new framework for non-addictive psychoactive drug use. *Behavioral and Brain Sciences* 34: 293-347.

Muthukumaraswamy, S. D., Carhart-Harris, R.L., Moran, R.J., Brookes, M.J., Williams, T.M., Errtizoe, D., Sessa, B., Papadopoulos, A., Bolstridge, M., Singh, KD., Feilding, A., Friston, K.J., & Nutt, D. 2013. Broadband cortical desynchronization underlies the human psychedelic state. *The Journal of Neuroscience* 33(38): 15171-15183.

Sobiecki, J.F. 2002. A preliminary inventory of plants used for psychoactive purposes in southern African healing traditions. *Transactions of the Royal Society of South Africa*, 57(1 and 2): 1-24.

Sobiecki, J.F. 2008. A review of plants used in divination in southern Africa and their psychoactive effects. *South African Humanities* 20: 333–351.

Sobiecki, J.F. 2012. Psychoactive *Ubulawu* spiritual medicines and healing dynamics in the initiation process of southern Bantu diviners. *Journal of Psychoactive Drugs*, 44(3): 1-8.

Sobiecki, J.F. 2014. The intersection of culture and science in South African traditional medicine. *Indo Pacific Journal of Phenomenology*, 14(1): 1-11.

Winkelman, M. 2010. *Shamanism: A Biopsychosocial Paradigm of Consciousness and Healing* (Second Edition) Santa Barbara, CA: Praeger.

Psychoactive Australian Acacia Species and their Alkaloids

Snu Voogelbreinder

Ethnobotanist, author of *The Garden of Eden: Shamanic Use of Psychoactive Flora and Fauna and the Study of Consciousness*

INTRODUCTION

The genus Acacia *sensu lato* (Fabaceae, subfamily Mimosoideae) is one of the largest in the plant kingdom, with over 1,000 species native to Africa, the Middle East, Asia, Australia, the Pacific Islands and the Americas. Recent taxonomy has split the genus Acacia into several genera (*Acacia, Senegalia, Vachellia, Faidherbia, Mariosousa* and *Acaciella*), with Acacia controversially being retained for the Australian species[1] and their close relatives from Oceania, Southeast Asia, and the Mascarene Islands. Some *Acacia* spp. which are native to Australia have also been introduced in many parts of the world, either for erosion control, timber, tannin production, or ornamental purposes, and in some cases they have become invasive weeds following naturalisation.

In Australia, the genus is numerous and widespread, with over 900 recognised species, known commonly as wattles. At certain times of year when there are mass-flowerings, these plants are such a noticeable feature of life in Australia that one species (*A. pycnantha* Benth., the golden wattle) became the national floral emblem, and the "green and gold" colours of the flowering plant have been used as national colours for sporting events. There is even a Wattle Day (1st of September), though for most people today this is a quaint artefact of the recent past. Since the early years of European colonisation, new Australians have exploited several species for tannin production and timber, and only relatively recently have they begun to appreciate the food potential of wattle seeds. It is even less known that many *Acacia* spp. have properties which transcend the utilitarian.

HISTORICAL USE OF AUSTRALIAN ACACIAS AS PSYCHOACTIVE AGENTS

Historical use of Acacia spp. *sensu lato* as psychoactive agents has been previously reported from Africa (Lehmann & Mihalyi, 1982; Watt & Breyer-Brandwijk, 1962) and possibly the Americas (e.g., Pendleton & Pendleton, 2008; Taylor, 1979, 1996). Certain species also have ancient traditions of sacred significance in Egypt, the Middle East, and India, and some scholars believe they may have once played an entheogenic-sacramental role in early religions (e.g., Dannaway, 2007; Graves, 1961; Newman, 2015; Shannon, 2008). This paper will focus on the psychoactive properties and related uses of native Acacia spp. *sensu lato* in Australia.

---

1. A small group of Vachellia spp. are also native to Australia.

The first Australians and their indigenous descendants have made extensive use of Acacias, presumably for tens of thousands of years. Various species have been utilised for food (from the nutritious seeds, and sometimes the gum), medicine, and the manufacture of tools and ritual objects. These uses have been well documented (eg. Clarke, 2007; Cribb & Cribb, 1982; Latz 1995), but any traditional use of these plants as psychoactive agents in Australia remains obscure.

Since the colonisation of Australia by Europeans, Australian indigenous people have, in general, been quite open in sharing their plant knowledge with anthropologists, ethnobotanists, and other interested parties. However, they have withheld their knowledge of sacred ceremonial plant use to a large extent, as this is reserved for fully initiated men and women, who have their own gender-separate rituals and knowledge. Where such knowledge has been at least partly disclosed to an outsider, that person is generally sworn to secrecy, which has resulted in a paucity of public knowledge of indigenous Australian plant shamanism. In addition, many traditions have been abandoned and forgotten following more than 200 years of colonial settlement and subsequent massacres, breaking up of families, and forced assimilation. Despite this, in some parts of the country these traditions have not been lost. Whilst there has been good work done to document any surviving knowledge of indigenous plant use in a number of publications, details regarding sacred ceremonial plants are at best only ever hinted at ambiguously in print, and are reserved for private oral communication. However, some other traditional uses of Acacias are suggestive of central nervous system (CNS) activity.

SMOKING MEDICINES

Many plants have been (and still are) used medicinally and ritually in Australia by what is called "smoking", but this is not smoking in the usual sense. It involves spreading fresh branches and foliage (and sometimes pieces of termite mound) on hot coals in a pit, with the patient or subject of the ceremony lying on a temporary bed frame constructed over the top, or sometimes lying directly on or next to the fuming foliage. Sometimes a wooden vessel is used to hold the coals and foliage, so that the smoke can be moved around and directed, as with "smudging". Alternately, a person can simply stand by the pit, bathed in thick smoke. Smoking ceremonies are conducted in order to purify an area for ritual, or to cleanse a person before a long journey or important undertaking. Babies are traditionally exposed to smoke from various Acacia spp. or other plants after birth; in that case, they may be held and wafted briefly through the smoke, although sometimes mother and child may sleep overnight next to the fuming foliage. The purpose of this is to make the newborn child and its mother strong; in the case of the mother, squatting over the smoke and fumes of some species also serves to alleviate postpartum bleeding.

A. ligulata A. Cunn. ex Benth. is of ritual and spiritual importance to Warlpiri women, and the phyllodes are used in smoking ceremonies to treat a wide variety of illnesses. *A. dictyophleba* F. Muell.[2], *A. pruinocarpa* Tindale, and *A. lysiphloia* F. Muell. phyllodes are used as smoking medicines in northern Australia for newborn babies and their mothers (Aboriginal Communities, 1988; Bindon, 1996; Clarke, 2007; Latz, 1995; Low, 1990; Smith, 1991). Probable sedative or narcotic activity is suggested by a different use of smoke on Groote Eylant: "excited and uncontrollable" children are sometimes held head-down in smoke from the phyllodes of (what is probably) *A. pellita* O. Schwarz, to quieten them (Levitt, 1981). Although not known to be a smoking medicine, *A. acuminata* Benth. has been used as a sedative inhalant – the Noongar of s.w. Western Australia sometimes inhale the vapours from crushed flowers "to relax the mind for a good night's sleep" (Hansen & Horsfall, 2016).

In southeast South Australia, the Tangane used to rub emu fat over their bodies and smoke themselves with fresh branches of an Acacia spp. before fighting. The context in which this anecdote was related gives the impression that this preparation helped make a warrior strong, brave, and calm in the face of angry (and therefore unbalanced) foes. Another more interesting ritual use of "smoked" Acacia can be mentioned here, as it has previously been published, is presumably no longer practiced, and the species used was not identified. Some Tangane men could reputedly vanish and travel large distances in one night for secret purposes – sometimes malicious sorcery – by means of a practice translated as "walking with magic shoes". For the Tangane, this involved wearing shoes made from bark of a Leptospermum sp. and human hair, with the feet and insides of the shoes smeared with a mixture containing death adder (*Acanthophis antarcticus* Loveridge) venom, as well as skin and hair from a corpse, whilst "standing in the dense smoke of a fire made of green

---

2. This use of *A. dictyophleba* might instead refer to *A. melleodora* Pedley (Butcher et al., 2001).

wattle branches" (Tindale, 1937). Known in central Australia as "kurdaitja", such "magic shoes" are well known, although they were made of emu feathers stuck together with blood and hair, and were generally written about as being worn when literally sneaking up on a sleeping victim at night to ritually murder them (Spencer & Gillen, 1899). Less commonly, such shoes have reportedly been "used by the "Doctors" when seeking out the evil being who has swallowed the rain, and thus caused droughts" (A.W. Howitt, in Etheridge, 1894). Tindale's report appears to be unique in mentioning an associated use of plants and snake venom, shoes made from bark and not feathers, and explicitly stating that the practitioner vanishes and travels impossible distances rather than sneaking about physically.

PAIN MEDICINES

Some species have also been applied topically to relieve pain. In northern Australia, the Ngariny-man heat phyllodes and branches of *A. lysiphloia* on hot coals, and apply them to sore muscles or joints as an analgesic (Aboriginal Communities, 1988; Smith, 1991; Smith et al., 1993). The Gurindji heat the phyllodes in water and use them as a wash to treat muscle pain and stomach ache (Wightman et al., 1994). The Mudburra use the same species "to ward off spirits who are annoying people." For this, the branches are heated and held on the temples and forehead. *A. monticola* J.M. Black may be used in the same way (Wightman et al., 1992). An infusion of the phyllodes and pods of *A. auriculiformis* A. Cunn. ex Benth. is used as an analgesic wash to relieve body pains (Low, 1990). Seeds of *A. pruinocarpa* are used to treat headaches (Latz, 1995). On Groote Eylandt, a species which is probably *A. pellita* is used for the same purpose. Phyllodes and seeds are used externally to relieve body pains, and heated phyllodes are also applied to the forehead for headaches (Levitt, 1981). *A. difficilis* Maiden phyllodes are heated and "applied to chest, back, or ears to relieve pain" (Brock, 1988). Bark strips from *A. holosericea* A. Cunn. ex G. Don are tied around the head with the inner bark against the skin to relieve headache (Aboriginal Communities, 1988). In the Pilbara region of Western Australia, phyllodes and twigs of *A. ancistrocarpa* Maiden & Blakely and *A. trachycarpa* E. Pritz. are used as a wash to treat headaches, and heated and applied externally to treat internal pain (Reid, 1977). Phyllodes and twigs of *A. translucens* A. Cunn. ex Hook. are also made into a wash to relieve headaches. A tea of *A. dictyophleba* phyllodes is drunk to treat headaches, coughs and colds. A decoction of *A. ligulata* bark has been used to treat "dizziness, nerves and fits" (Bindon, 1996). It remains to be seen if any of these uses indicate narcotic effects. At least some of the analgesic applications may be effective due to anti-inflammatory rather than neurological activity. The uses of *A. lysiphloia* and *A. monticola* by the Mudburra in the Northern Territory, and *A. ligulata* in Western Australia certainly suggest some kind of CNS activity is involved. These species may prove useful in the search for more effective psychiatric medicines.

FISH POISONS

Numerous species have been used as fish poisons, which temporarily stun freshwater fish without rendering them inedible. For this purpose, plant parts are crushed, thrown into a water hole and agitated, or placed in a mesh bag made from plant fibres and used like an oversized toxic tea bag. After a short time, stunned or asphyxiated fish rise to the surface where they are easily caught. Species used in Australia as fish poisons include *A. auriculiformis* (phyllodes), *A. binervata* DC. (phyllodes), *A. colei* Maslin & L.A.J. Thomson (bark, phyllodes), *A. decurrens* Willd., *A. falcata* Willd. (bark), *A. hemignosta* F. Muell. (bark, phyllodes), *A. holosericea* (branches, phyllodes, pods, seeds), *A. longifolia* (Andrews) Willd. (phyllodes), *A. melanoxylon* R. Br. (bark, twigs), *A. oncinocarpa* Benth. (bark, phyllodes), *A. pellita* (pods, seeds), *A. penninervis* Sieber ex DC. (bark, phyllodes), *A. pulchella* R. Br., *A. salicina* Lindl. (bark, twigs, phyllodes), *A. tumida* F. Muell. ex Benth. (pods, seeds) and *A. verniciflua* A. Cunn. (Brock, 1988; Cribb & Cribb, 1982; Hamlyn-Harris & Smith, 1916; Hurst, 1942; Maiden, 1889, 1913; Marrfurra et al., 1995; Sadgrove, 2009; Smith, 1991; Webb, 1948; Wightman et al., 1994). The ichthyotoxic pharmacology of Acacia spp. is poorly understood, but is presumed to involve tannins and saponins reducing the amount of oxygen available to the fish (Sadgrove, 2009); any alkaloids present might also affect the central nervous system (pers. obs.). Tannic acid in water has been found to cause "marked physiological disturbance" and death in fish at concentrations of 1:10,000 (Hamlyn-Harris & Smith, 1916). Saponins extracted from "*A. cunninghamii*" pods (note: this may no longer be an accepted name; see comments below under *A. concurrens* Pedley) "produced total insensibility of the leg" and muscle paralysis when injected into the leg of a frog. Injection of an extract of one pod into the arm of a human resulted in pain, swelling, nausea, and shivering; an extract of two pods also resulted in headache, mydriasis, and paralysis of the eye muscles (Lauterer, 1897). Applied topically to mucous membranes, saponins from *A. delibrata* A. Cunn. ex Benth. pods act as an irritant, and applied to the heart, muscle, or nerves of a frog, they resulted in paralysis of those parts (Bancroft, 1887).

ALKALINE ASH SOURCES FOR CHEWING WITH TOBACCO AND PITURI

Selected Acacia spp. (such as *A. auriculiformis*, *A. aneura* F. Muell. ex Benth., *A. beauverdiana* Ewart & Sharman, *A. calcicola* Forde & Ising, *A. coriacea* DC., *A. estrophiolata* F. Muell., *A. hakeoides* A. Cunn. ex Benth., *A. kempeana* F. Muell., *A. ligulata*, *A. omalophylla* A. Cunn. ex Benth. or *A. cambagei* R.T. Baker, *A. pruinocarpa*, and *A. salicina*) are burned to produce a fine, alkaline ash for chewing with tobacco or pituri/pitcheri (*Nicotiana* spp., *Duboisia hopwoodii* F. Muell.), to aid in alkaloid release. The part used is usually the phyllodes, bark, or twigs, varying from species to species (Aiston, 1937; Johnston & Cleland, 1933; Latz, 1995; Maiden, 1922; Marrfurra et al., 1995; Meggitt 1966; Reid, 1977; Smith, 1991). In the Lake Eyre district, *A. salicina* used for ash production is itself called "pitcheri". In the case of this species, the young branch tips were cleaned of damaged and diseased growth. To make the ash, the tips "were tied in bundles, ignited over the fire, and then allowed to burn out while held over a wooden bowl" (Aiston, 1937). One report claimed that in Woorabinda, Queensland, *A. salicina* ash is "smoked to produce "drunkenness, drowsiness, or dopiness, and finally deep and lengthy sleep"", but this is most likely a confusion with the drug the ash is mixed with (Webb, 1969). Nevertheless, pituri is rarely if ever smoked, and would not require alkaline ash to be added when doing so. Furthermore, attempting to smoke ash by itself would be a futile exercise. This strange report is intriguing despite its apparent inaccuracies.

COFFEE AND TEA SUBSTITUTES

Acacia spp. were experimented with by early colonial settlers as substitutes for coffee and tea, due to local shortages of those imported stimulants. However, it appears that these plant parts were used not because of any caffeine- or theophylline-like effects, but simply because they could be used to prepare beverages that looked, tasted, and/or smelled a little like the real thing in the absence of anything better. Certainly, some wattle seeds have a coffee-like aroma when roasted. Ludwig Leichhardt and his "convict companion" Mr. Phillips trialled numerous plants as coffee substitutes in Australia's early colonial days. Their experience with the bushfire-roasted seeds of an Acacia sp. in Expedition Range, Queensland, is worth quoting:

> "Mr. Phillips (who was always desirous of discovering substitutes for coffee[...]) collected these seeds, and pounded and boiled them, and gave me the fluid to taste, which I found so peculiarly bitter that I cautioned him against drinking it; his natural desire, however, for warm beverage, which had been increased by a whole day's travelling, induced him to swallow about a pint of it, which made him very sick, and produced violent vomiting and purging during the whole afternoon and night. The little I had tasted acted on me as a lenient purgative, but Mr. Calvert, who had taken rather more than I did, felt very sick."

The species used was not recorded (Leichhardt, 1847), but was possibly *A. bidwillii* Benth. (*Vachellia bidwilli* (Benth.) Kodela) (Fensham et al., 2006). Mature seeds of *A. murrayana* F. Muell. ex Benth. were roasted and used as a coffee substitute by early European settlers (Latz, 1995), and seeds of *A. victoriae* Benth. are currently used as such (Ariati et al., 2007), although a stimulant effect has not been noted.

Leaves of *A. decurrens* and phyllodes of *A. suaveolens* (Sm.) Willd. were used as tea substitutes by early settlers (Low, 1989). No stimulant effect has been mentioned, although the phyllodes of *A. suaveolens* contain phenethylamine (White, 1944a, 1951, 1954). *A. iteaphylla* F. Muell. ex Benth., which is very close to *A. suaveolens*, has a bitter taste at some times of the year and may also prove to contain phenethylamines. The phyllodes (harvested in March) make a reasonable substitute for Japanese green tea, in a dose of 1 tablespoon finely chopped and dried phyllodes steeped in just-boiled water. A higher dose (2 tab.) decocted for 10 minutes had a less agreeable taste. This tea appears to have some mild stimulant activity, but further experimentation is required to eliminate the placebo effect (personal observations, 2017). Root shavings of *A. georginae* F.M. Bailey are said to be used as a tea substitute in modern times (Latz, 1995), but again, no stimulant effects have been reported. As some specimens of *A. georginae* can produce dangerous levels of sodium fluoroacetate (see below), drinking tea made from this species is not recommended.

MODERN NON-TRADITIONAL USE OF ACACIAS AS PSYCHOACTIVE DRUGS

In 1965, the first report of the isolation of N,N-dimethyltryptamine (DMT) and N-methyltryptamine (NMT) from an Acacia species – *A. maidenii* F. Muell. – was published in a scientific journal (Fitzgerald & Sioumis, 1965), followed shortly by another which reported the isolation of DMT from *A. phlebophylla* H.B. Will. (Rovelli & Vaughan, 1967), both Australian species. Several other journal papers followed over the next decade, reporting the finding of these alkaloids in other Acacia species from Africa, Asia, and Oceania. These reports arrived at a time in Western history that saw a large increase in public curiosity about psychedelic drugs, yet they remained obscure footnotes in the phytochemical literature for more than 20 years, apparently unnoticed by anyone who might wish to make use of the information by extracting the alkaloids for human use. This may be due to the fact that DMT itself remained an obscure and unpopular psychedelic agent until at least the late 1980s, but despite the information being published in science journals rather than popular books or articles, it is still surprising that it took so long for academically-inclined drug enthusiasts to notice these papers and spread the information into the wider culture, as would occur rapidly today.

Several publications which emerged in the early 1990s raised awareness of the fact that some Acacias contain DMT. The first was a scientific text book (Collins et al., 1990), followed by popular nonfiction books more specifically about psychoactive plants and drugs (eg. Ott, 1993). Around the same time, several university students in Australia had stumbled across this information in the journal papers by Fitzgerald & Sioumis (1965) and Rovelli & Vaughn (1967), and the work of Collins et al. (1990). In 1992, one of these anonymous researchers published a report on successful experiments in extracting and smoking the alkaloids from *Acacia maidenii* bark. The investigator had first tried smoking the bark itself, with very mild effects (Anonymous, 1992). Early the following year, another researcher posted a report to an internet newsgroup detailing the first documented use of a decoction of *Acacia phlebophylla* phyllodes, drunk after having swallowed ground *Peganum harmala* L. seeds. This produced powerful psychedelic effects in two human subjects (C.G., 1993). Later that year, another anonymous person consumed the same combination with one of the original bioassayists, and this was written up and posted to an internet newsgroup (Anonymous, 1993). All of these reports were soon reproduced on various websites as the Internet grew over the 1990s (e.g., Michael from Melbourne, 1992). At this time, experimentation with what have become known as "ayahuasca analogues" – the combining of plants not traditionally used in *ayahuasca*, but which contain monoamine oxidase (MAO)-inhibiting β-carboline alkaloids (such as harmine and harmaline), and DMT – was in its infancy. In the United States, a small number of people had been experimenting with *Desmanthus spp.* root and *Phalaris spp.* leaves in combination with *Peganum harmala* seeds prior to 1993 (Appleseed, 1993; J.G., 1992), but this was not widely known until Jonathan Ott published his book *Ayahuasca Analogues*, by which time he had performed his own bioassays with the *A. phlebophylla/P. harmala* combination (Ott, 1994).

In the mid-1990s, a period of intense investigation into the psychoactive properties of Acacia species began, not by sanctioned academics, but by interested amateurs in many parts of the world, particularly Australia. Initially, much of the focus by drug enthusiasts was on *Acacia phlebophylla* – which has a fairly reliable DMT content with few other alkaloids present, if any – and *Acacia maidenii*, which has proven to be a less reliable source of DMT due to variation within the species, and with an NMT content often higher than that of DMT. This limited focus quickly led to some negative impacts on both species in the wild. *Acacia phlebophylla* is found only on Mt. Buffalo in Victoria, Australia, and the population has suffered both from overharvesting, and widespread galling caused primarily by a rust fungus, Uromycladium sp., which was adversely affecting the health of much of the population by the late 1990s (Heinze et al., 1998). Since then, an extensive bushfire at Mt. Buffalo appears to have destroyed the infected material, and the species is currently regenerating well. This granite-loving species has also proven difficult to cultivate to maturity outside of its natural habitat; however, this author is aware of several successes.

Acacia maidenii suffered partly due to ignorance – as the initial report by Fitzgerald & Sioumis

(1965) detailed extraction of alkaloids from the bark, many people assumed that this was the only part of the plant to contain alkaloids. Subsequently, wild and cultivated plants were crudely decorticated by people hoping to extract tryptamine alkaloids, and many trees were killed outright by this treatment, not all of them even correctly identified. To this day, similar episodes continue to occur, and are documented and discussed by concerned "Acaciaphiles" on internet discussion forums and in private. This has most often been the case with *Acacia obtusifolia* A. Cunn. (the first "new" species to have been discovered as a source of tryptamine alkaloids by the underground researcher then known as E, and later publicised by Mulga (1996a)), and more recently, *Acacia acuminata* Benth., plus a very rare species which will not be named here. Unfortunately, the financial profit and peer-group status that can be derived from a plentiful supply of DMT or mixed Acacia alkaloids have been seized upon by a small minority of people, and those who buy these alkaloid extracts are apparently mostly unaware of the ecological destruction that may be associated with their production.

Due to these issues, some Australian underground researchers decided to begin to share some of what they had learned about Acacias. These people hoped to encourage others to learn sustainable harvesting techniques; to shun commercial trade in Acacia alkaloids; and to explore a variety of other species in order to take the pressure away from threatened species such as *Acacia phlebophylla*. These efforts appear to have been somewhat successful, although there are still incidences of over-harvesting in the wild and death of plants due to bark removal. Also, the discovery that root bark of some species can contain high levels of alkaloids has sometimes led to trees being killed by root bark harvesting from living plants *in situ*, or whole plants being uprooted and ground up for alkaloid extraction (Kelly, 2012; Nen & Nickles, 2014; personal communications).

METHODS OF INVESTIGATION AND USE

Amateur researchers have investigated species which had no previously published chemical analysis, and species which had been reported as alkaloid-positive in published chemical screenings but not explored further. Some have approached this by performing acid/base or straight-to-base alkaloid extractions, and/or thin-layer chromatography and spot tests on all species they can obtain. Some have learned to narrow down the field of inquiry by taste, chewing a small sample of the plant and comparing it to samples known to contain tryptamines. Another method used is the "burn test", lighting a dried phyllode or leaf briefly and smelling the smoke for traces of indolic aromas associated with the presence of tryptamines. Some other researchers who believe they have a kind of sensitive spiritual connection to these plants select species to assay based on intuitive feelings, allegedly with a high degree of success. Amateur researchers have been hindered by lack of affordable access to laboratory equipment used to identify alkaloids with a high degree of certainty. Due to this, with much of the early amateur work in particular, identification of any alkaloids present in a sample was subjective guesswork following autoingestion – generally as a smoked or vapourised crude alkaloid extract – and basic, preliminary analysis with thin-layer chromatography and spot tests using plant samples with known alkaloid content for comparative reference. Occasionally, some researchers have been able to get alkaloid samples analysed by professionals using GC-MS equipment. Through all of these approaches, amateur researchers working in a legal grey area have vastly increased the knowledge of Acacia alkaloids, in a period where such work has almost disappeared from mainstream academia. The risks involved have been not only of a legal nature, but include the potential dangers of experimenting with human ingestion of plants or plant extracts of poorly known or unknown chemical content.

Acacia alkaloid extracts are usually vapourised in a glass pipe, or mixed with other herbs – sometimes Cannabis – and smoked in a water pipe or cigarette, in the same manner as DMT has been used in the last fifty years worldwide. DMT has been evaporated from a solvent solution onto carrier herbs (usually parsley) for smoking since the 1960s. However, since the early 2000s, herbal blends for smoking Acacia alkaloids, with the novel inclusion of *Banisteriopsis caapi* (Spruce ex Grisebach) Mort. leaves (with their MAO-inhibiting β-carboline alkaloid content), have become a popular means of consumption, and are known as "changa" (pronounced with a hard "g"). The addition of *B. caapi* leaves boosts the effectiveness of the Acacia alkaloids, and makes it easier to inhale an effective dose by extending the window of administration time. Mullein herb (Verbascum spp.) added to the blend also makes the smoke milder and easier to inhale and hold in the lungs. A variety of other herbs may also be included to modify the flavour and perhaps the effects (Palmer, 2015). This approach has been taken on in other parts of the world, using tryptamine-containing source plants other than *Acacia spp.*, such as *Mimosa tenuiflora* (Willd.) Poir. non Benth.

The oral ingestion of Acacia decoctions (or alkaloid extracts) in combination with an MAO-inhibitor (usually *Peganum harmala* seeds, *Banisteriopsis caapi*, or *Passiflora* spp.) is much less common than smoking, but does occur in Australia (Cakic et al, 2010; personal communications and observations). As already stated, *A. phlebophylla* has been used in this way by a small number of people since at least 1993 (C.G., 1993; Ott, 1994). In addition, *A. obtusifolia* has been used in this way since 1993; *A. maidenii* has been used in this way since the mid-1990s; *A. acuminata* has been used in this way since the late 1990s/early 2000s; and in more recent years, *A. floribunda* (Vent.) Willd. and other species have been occasionally used as well. *Ayahuasca* ceremonies held with small groups of people in Australia now frequently use DMT-containing Acacias or their alkaloid extracts in place of more traditional DMT-containing additives such as *Psychotria* spp. However, because of their high tannin content[3], brews using Acacia spp. (rather than an alkaloid extract thereof) are often very astringent and more difficult to keep down for long compared to brews using *Psychotria* spp. They can also result in particularly powerful and challenging experiences – physically and mentally – depending on the alkaloid composition. In some cases with *A. obtusifolia*, this has led to speculation of the presence of 5-MeO-DMT, which has not been confirmed. The alkaloid/s responsible for the unpleasant physical effects of some Acacias when consumed with an MAO-inhibitor (MAOI) has not been determined. Caution is advised in casually boiling up unknown Acacia spp. and ingesting them orally with or without an MAOI. Not all species contain DMT, and many contain non-tryptamine alkaloids of unknown pharmacology, as well as unidentified alkaloids which might be toxic, or dangerous in combination with an MAOI.

GENERAL SUMMARY OF
RECENT DISCOVERIES

Underground researchers in Australia have made a number of significant discoveries (not including the specifics of alkaloid content in different species):

* Foliage and twiggy branches can be used instead of stripping bark from the main stem or main branches. These parts generally may contain useful concentrations of similar or identical alkaloids to the bark, and represent a much more sustainable source of alkaloids. Fallen phyllodes collected from beneath a plant can also retain significant alkaloid content if they have not begun to degrade (nen888, 2011-2013). This is also highly sustainable, but care should be taken to leave some on the ground to feed the plant and soil biota.

* Alkaloid content may be highly variable even amongst plants growing in the same wild population, and at different times of year. Some species have been found to contain alkaloids only in an occasional individual specimen; some individuals may be more or less alkaloid free for most of the year, yet produce high concentrations of alkaloids occasionally. Even at that time, another specimen of the same species growing nearby may still contain no detectable alkaloids. Heavy rain appears to minimise alkaloid content for a short period afterwards, but this is not always the case (personal communications).

* Acacia alkaloid extracts comprised of a mix of indole alkaloids have transitioned from being regarded as "impure" by those seeking DMT, to being appreciated in their own right, and sometimes preferred to pure or near-pure DMT. Many users have reported that such alkaloid mixtures have subjective effects that are gentler and longer-lasting than DMT alone while still being very powerful, and may bring about an experience that is easier to assimilate and learn from (personal communications and observations).

* One researcher investigated non-DMT fractions from some such alkaloid mixtures and found that NMT (tentatively identified) is psychoactive when smoked or vapourised and inhaled (60 mg+), with psychedelic effects that are much less visual than those of DMT, and with a longer duration of 45-70 minutes. The researcher has described this alkaloid as a "spatial entheogen" (nen888, 2011a).

* Some Acacia alkaloid extracts containing mainly tryptamines and a smaller proportion of phenethylamines can result in a greatly extended duration of psychedelic effects when smoked/vapourised (nen888 pers. comm., 2017).

* Some Acacia spp. have been found to be mildly psychoactive when chewed, or drunk as a de-

---

3. Some people have found that adding an egg white to an unreduced, acidic decoction attracts many of the tannins – as well as a small proportion of the alkaloids present – and after the egg white congeals, it can be filtered out through a cloth or decanted.

coction, with no further MAO-inhibitor required (personal communications). In some cases, this is likely to be due to samples containing both tryptamines and β-carbolines (endlessness & nen888, 2011-2012), although the possible role of flavonoids or other non-alkaloidal constituents in MAO-inhibition (e.g., Dixon-Clarke & Ramsay, 2011) should be explored. It must be noted that chewing large amounts of fresh plant matter is potentially risky due to the cyanogenic compounds present in many species, which might occasionally occur at levels toxic to humans. However, many species probably only contain these compounds at levels problematic to ruminants eating large quantities, and even then, some species appear not to contain the enzymes necessary for the liberation of hydrocyanic acid (Everist, 1981; Hurst, 1942).

* Seeds of some species (*A. acuminata ssp. burkittii* (F. Muell. ex Benth.) Kodela et Tindale, *A. maidenii*, *A. pendula* A. Cunn. ex G. Don., *A. podalyriaefolia* A. Cunn. ex G. Don) have been bioassayed via smoking, and are claimed to be mildly psychoactive (t st tantra et al., 2009).

ALKALOIDS IN THE GENUS ACACIA

Alkaloids are common in the genus Acacia, and where they occur, several different classes of alkaloids have been identified. Simple phenethylamines are well represented, such as phenethylamine, N-methyl-phenethylamine, tyramine, and hordenine. Claims of the presence of mescaline, amphetamine derivatives and tetrahydroisoquinolines in some North American species (*A. berlandieri* Benth. (Clement et al., 1997), *A. rigidula* Benth. (Clement et al., 1998)) remain controversial and unproven, although the tetrahydroisoquinoline calycotomine has been found in the Indian species *A. concinna* (Willd.) DC. (Gupta & Nigam, 1971). Less common alkaloids include pyridines such as nicotine (which requires further confirmation), histamine derivatives, and the spermidine alkaloid (-)-acacine, so far found only in *A. myrtifolia* (Sm.) Willd. (Nichols, 1983). The most attention has recently been focused on species which contain indole alkaloids, including N,N-dimethyltryptamine and other tryptamines, and a variety of β-carboline derivatives. It is these species which are most sought after by neo-shamans and other modern sacramental drug users, although species containing mainly phenethylamines may also prove to have psychoactivity in humans.

Other phytochemicals found in Acacia spp. include tannins/flavonoids, terpenes/saponins, cyanogenic glycosides, imino acids, and polysaccharides (Clarke-Lewis & Dainis, 1967; Everist, 1981; Kunii et al., 1996; Maslin et al., 1998; Seigler, 2003; Tindale & Roux, 1969, 1974). At least one species (*A. georginae*) can contain dangerous levels of the toxin sodium fluoroacetate (Everist, 1981; McEwan, 1978; Peters et al., 1965). Seeds of Acacia spp. contain carbohydrates, fatty acids, proteins, amino acids, non-protein amino acids, and imino acids (such as albizziine, djenkolic acid, pipecolic acid, and others), and sometimes alkaloids, saponins, and oxalates. Some of the proteins present are protease inhibitors with anti-nutritional effects, which are greatly diminished by brief roasting, along with any saponins and oxalates present (Ee & Yates, 2013; Evans et al., 1977; Kunii et al., 1996).

ALKALOIDS IN AUSTRALIAN NATIVE ACACIA SPP.

In general, the presence of indole alkaloids is concentrated in the section *Juliflorae*, species of which bear multi-nerved phyllodes and spike inflorescences on mature plants. However this class of alkaloids is also encountered less commonly in other sections of the genus. Only a small portion of the 900+ Acacia spp. in Australia have been investigated chemically. Below is presented a summary of investigations into the alkaloids of Acacia spp. native to Australia. Introduced species that have become naturalised, such as *A. farnesiana* L. (*Vachellia farnesiana* (L.) Wight & Arn.) and *A. nilotica spp. indica* (Benth.) Brenan (*Vachellia nilotica ssp. indica* (Benth.) Kyal. & Boatwr.), are not included. Several native species that contain tryptamines have been excluded for conservation reasons, due to their rarity. One of these species is not only rare but has a high concentration of alkaloids, and has already been subject to much exploitation in the space of a few years. The rare *A. phlebophylla* has been included because it is now firmly established in the literature.

Note: all species analysed by E.P. White were growing in New Zealand, unless stated otherwise. It is uncertain if a nonnative environment can influence the alkaloid content of Acacias, which are known to form symbiotic relationships with Rhizobium spp. bacteria to fix nitrogen. Also, White's identification of alkaloids should be taken as inconclusive, because he failed to identify DMT in several species which are now known to often contain it as a major alkaloid. Some of White's yields of tryptamine may have actually consisted of a mixture of indoles, including DMT.

Acacia acinacea Lindl. (gold-dust wattle) – Stems and phyllodes yielded 0.04-0.07% alkaloids in Feb., 0.79-0.82% in Dec.; ripe seed pods yielded 0.08% alkaloids; seeds contained 0 traces of alkaloids. The alkaloid mixture consisted largely of phenethylamine (White, 1951).

Acacia acuminata Benth. **ssp. *acuminata*** (mungart, raspberry jam wattle) – Yielded 0.72% alkaloids from stems and phyllodes of a "broad-leaf" form (harv. Oct.), consisting mostly of tryptamine. A "narrow-leaf" form (either of ssp. acuminata or ssp. burkittii – see below) yielded 1.5% alkaloids from stems and phyllodes (harv. Oct.), consisting mostly of tryptamine, as well as smaller amounts of phenethylamine, and another unidentifed non-volatile base (White, 1957). In an alkaloid screening, phyllodes of a plant from a nursery in Victoria gave strong positive results (Collins et al., 1990). TLC/GC-MS analysis of the "narrow-leaf" and "small-seed" varieties found phyllodes to contain 0.6-0.8% DMT, and up to 1.6% in bark; young phyllodes contained almost entirely tryptamine (J.J., 2007). Another phyllode sample of the "narrow-leaf" variety (harv. Feb.) yielded 0.9-1% alkaloids, found by GC-MS to consist mainly of DMT, with traces of 2-methyl-1,2,3,4-tetrahydro-β-carboline (2-methyl-THβC) and an unidentified peak. Phyllodes from the "broad-leaf" variety (harv. Jun.) yielded c.1% alkaloids, found by GC-MS to consist of mainly tetrahydroharman, as well as (in decreasing concentration) DMT, tryptamine, 3-methyl-quinoline (tentative), harman, N-methyl-phenethylamine, and phenethylamine. Preliminary TLC assay tentatively showed DMT, NMT, and 4 unidentified spots, although NMT did not show up in the GC-MS analysis (endlessness & nen888, 2011-2012). A decoction of 50 g phyllodes from this same specimen had mild psychedelic activity lasting c.90 minutes, taken orally with no additional MAOI (nen888, 2011-2013).

Acacia acuminata spp. burkittii (F. Muell. ex Benth.) Kodela et Tindale (*A. burkittii* F. Muell. ex Benth.) (gunderbluey, Burkitt's wattle, fine leaf jam wattle, sandhill wattle) – See ssp. acuminata above for an analysis on an indeterminate specimen which might have been ssp. *burkittii* (White, 1957). TLC/GC-MS analysis found ssp. *burkittii* to be very variable in content, with the bark of wild plants yielding 0.2-1.2% DMT, and phyllodes yielding under 0.1% alkaloids, mostly NMT (J.J., 2007).

Acacia adunca A. Cunn. ex G. Don. (*A. accola* Maiden & Betche) (Wallangarra wattle, cascade wattle) – Stems, phyllodes, and flowers (harv. Aug.) yielded 3.2% alkaloids, which appeared to consist of c.70% N-methyl-phenethylamine, with smaller amounts of phenethylamine (White, 1957); phyllodes from Queensland yielded 2.4% N-methyl-phenethylamine (Fitzgerald, 1964a).

Acacia alpina F. Muell. (alpine wattle) – Suspected of containing DMT based on human bioassay of 30-40 g dry phyllodes with 4 g *Peganum harmala* seeds (nen888, 2011-2013). Rovelli (1967) detected no alkaloids.

Acacia auriculiformis A. Cunn. ex Benth. (marra, northern black wattle, ear-pod wattle) – Phyllodes have tested positive for alkaloids (Aboriginal Communities, 1988); others have tentatively identified 5-MeO-DMT in stem bark (harv. Apr.) by TLC (Trout ed., 1997). Phyllodes were found to contain small amounts of 2-OH-pyridine, 3-OH-pyridine, 4-OH-pyridine, 2-MeO-pyrazine, 6-methyl-3-pyridazinone, 1,1,3,3-tetramethylbutylamine, 2-methyliminoperhydro-1,3-ozazine, and 4-methyl-2-oxopentanenitrile, as well as numerous non-nitrogenous compounds (GC-MS) (Ibrahim et al., 2015). Aerial parts have also yielded 0.01% auriculoside, a flavan glycoside with mild CNS-depressant activity (Sahai et al., 1980). An ethanol extract of fresh phyllodes from Indian plants (harv. Jun.) improved memory and inhibited brain acetylcholinesterase in rats (Sharma et al., 2014).

Acacia baileyana F. Muell. (Cootamundra wattle) – Leaves from plants growing in California yielded 0.02% alkaloids in late March [80% tetrahydroharman, 20% tryptamine], and 0.028% in early October [tryptamine only]; July collections yielded no alkaloids (Repke et al., 1973). Stems, leaves, flowers, and seeds from plants growing in New Zealand (harv. Mar., Aug.) were shown to contain small amounts of alkaloids (White, 1944a). Ripe and unripe pods have yielded c.0.02% unidentified alkaloids, with ripe and unripe seeds showing only traces (White, 1951). Seeds might contain DMT and 2 other indoles (all tentative) in small amounts (TLC) (Trout ed., 1997). One amateur researcher claimed to have extracted DMT from the bark (EsKaTaRi, 2010), but based on descriptions of the psychoactive effects of the smoked alkaloid/s at a reported dose of 200-300 mg, there is no reason to think DMT was present in the extract unless the dose was actually 20-30 mg or less. Several people have experimented with smoking the leaves, the effect of which has been described by one person as "somewhere in between tobacco and weed" (Cannabis) (maxzar100, 2009; personal observations).

Acacia binervata DC. (two-veined hickory) – Phyllodes yielded c.0.2-0.3% alkaloids; may contain DMT based on reagent-positive reactions, compared with *Psychotria viridis* Ruíz et Pav. leaf as a reference standard (nen888, 2011-2013). Another researcher obtained no alkaloid yield from the bark, despite it having an alkaloidal taste (chocobeastie, 2011-2012). One screening detected no alkaloids in phyllodes (harv. Jun.) (Smolenski et al., 1973).

Acacia buxifolia A. Cunn. (box-leaf wattle) – Stems and phyllodes (harv. Dec.) from a variety slightly different than the norm yielded 0.65% alkaloids; seeds yielded 0.09% alkaloids; pods yielded 0.58% alkaloids. The alkaloid mixture appeared to consist largely of phenethylamine (White, 1951).

Acacia cardiophylla A. Cunn. ex Benth. – Stems, leaves, and flowers (harv. Oct.) yielded 0.03% alkaloids; stems and leaves yielded 0.02-0.06% alkaloids (highest in Mar.). The alkaloid mixture appeared to contain tryptamine and phenethylamine (White, 1957). In an alkaloid screening, leaves and stems from Mitcham, Victoria gave negative results (Collins et al., 1990).

Acacia caroleae Pedley (narrow-leaf currawang) – Phyllodes have yielded alkaloids, mainly DMT (subjective identification from vapourisation) (nen888, 2011-2013; nen888 pers. comm., 2017).

Acacia colei Maslin & L.A.J. Thomson (Cole's wattle) – Has been claimed to contain high concentrations of DMT (Kruszelnicki, 2005), but it is unclear where Kruszelnicki obtained this information, which may be based on misidentification of the closely related A. neurocarpa (see below), or simply false. Plants believed to be true *A. colei* have not yet yielded alkaloids (Palmer pers. comm., 2011).

Acacia complanata A. Cunn. ex Benth. (flat-stemmed wattle, weeping wattle) – Phyllodes and stems from south Queensland yielded 0.3% N-methyl-tetrahydroharman, and traces of tetrahydroharman (Johns et al., 1966). Another sample yielded 0.22% alkaloids from phyllode and stem (Collins et al., 1990). Bark has been claimed to contain DMT based on at least one reported successful extraction. Attempts have been made to utilise A. *complanata* alkaloids as an oral MAOI, in order to allow for the activity of orally consumed tryptamine alkaloids from A. *obtusifolia*. 100 mg of alkaloids in HCl salt form extracted from the foliage did not activate tryptamine alkaloids taken orally, but did seem to potentiate and lengthen the effects of smoked A. *obtusifolia* alkaloids (Mulga, 1996b). Another person found no oral activation of DMT using up to 1000 mg of A. *complanata* alkaloids (Torsten, 2008). A decoction of 20 phyllodes from a bitter-tasting specimen had sedative effects in one person (nen888, 2011-2013).

Acacia concurrens Pedley (curracabah) – Evaporated ethanol tincture of branch bark was reported to be psychoactive when taken orally with an MAOI (seldom, 2012); identification of the plants needs to be confirmed, as this species is readily confused with the closely related A. *crassa* Pedley, A. *leiocalyx* (Domin) Pedley, and A. *longispicata* Benth., which all used to be grouped under A. *cunninghamii* Hook. f., now an invalid name (Butcher et al., 2001). As such, it is not known which species under that name was found to contain saponins in the unripe seed pods, described as "a strong poison for the muscles and nerves and producing local anaesthesia very much like cocaine", as well as having irritant properties (Lauterer, 1897). It is also unclear whether Lauterer's cocaine comparison was in reference specifically to the saponins isolated from this plant, or to "saponin" in general, as the diversity of saponins was poorly known at that time, and Lauterer's writing style was imprecise in this case.

Acacia cultriformis A. Cunn. ex G. Don (knife-leaf wattle) – Phyllodes and stems yielded 0.07% alkaloids in Feb., 0.06% in Apr.; an August assay found 0.02% alkaloids in stems, 0.02% in phyllodes, and 0.04% in seeds. The alkaloids appeared to include phenethylamine (White, 1944a). Stems and phyllodes from two separate plants (harv. Dec.) yielded, respectively, traces and 0.02% alkaloids, and unripe seed pods yielded 0.04% alkaloids; this appeared to consist mainly of tryptamine (White, 1951). Stems and phyllodes (harv. Jul.) yielded 0.02% alkaloids, consisting partly of tryptamine, and a phenethylamine-like base (White, 1957). TLC analysis showed tentative presence of 5-MeO-DMT in phyllodes, twigs, and flowers (Trout, ed., 1997).

Acacia cyclops A. Cunn. ex G. Don (western coastal wattle) – Bark and phyllodes from a specimen growing in South Africa yielded a small amount of unidentified alkaloids, which were psychoactive on vapourisation, with a slow onset (roughly two minutes) and lasting about twenty minutes. Effects were psychedelic in character but not as visual as DMT, and the extract possibly consists of NMT and other alkaloids. Bark from a different specimen harvested after heavy rain yielded no alkaloids (PrimalWisdom, 2011). In Australia, people have had variable results, with low or absent yields of what seem to be tryptamine alkaloids (subjective i.d., plus TLC assay of unspecified plant parts in one case) (nen888, 2011-2013; shanedudddy2, 2013).

Acacia dallachiana F. Muell. (catkin wattle) – Phyllodes may contain DMT based on limited human bioassays of vapourised alkaloid extracts (nen888, 2011-2013; nen888 pers. comm., 2017), although some attempts at extraction obtained no alkaloids (chocobeastie, 2011-2012).

Acacia dealbata Link (silver wattle) – Leaf from Queensland plants (harv. Jun.) gave weak positive results in alkaloid screening (Webb, 1949). Stems, leaves (harv. Nov.), and seeds were found to contain <0.01% alkaloids which were not identified (White, 1944a). Plants growing in Portugal yielded 0.58-1.9% unidentified alkaloids from aerial parts, with highest yields from acetone extracts and lowest from ethanol extracts (Luís et al., 2012). Has been claimed to contain DMT (EsKaTaRi, 2010)[4] in some specimens, not others (Palmer pers. comm., 2011).

Acacia difformis R.T. Baker (wyalong wattle, drooping wattle) – Tryptamines including 5-MeO-DMT were tentatively detected (TLC) in young plants initially misidentified as *A. implexa* Benth. (Trout, ed., 1997), though specifics are currently under review due to discovery of a data mix-up (Trout pers. comm., 2017).

Acacia effusifolia Maslin & Buscumb (*A. coolgardiensis ssp. effusa* R.S. Cowan & Maslin) – Bark yielded 0.4-0.5% alkaloids, phyllodes yielded 0.2% alkaloids, consisting mainly of NMT, as well as DMT; exposed plants seem to contain more NMT, as well as norharman (TLC) (J.J., 2009).

Acacia elata A. Cunn. ex Benth. (mountain cedar wattle) – Branches and bark yielded c.0.3% alkaloids, consisting of DMT, 5-MeO-DMT, NMT, N-formyltryptamine (tentative), and β-carbolines (GC-MS). The alkaloids were strongly psychedelic when vapourised in doses of 30-50 mg, lasting up to 45 minutes. An alkaloid extract from a flowering specimen had much milder, non-visionary effects with a meditative quality (nen888, 2011-2013). An early analysis found <0.01% alkaloids in stems, leaves (harv. Mar. & Nov.), and seeds, which were not identified (White, 1944a); unripe pods were found to contain traces of alkaloids, with none in the bark or unripe seeds (White, 1951).

Acacia excelsa Benth. (ironwood, rosewood) – Phyllodes and stems gave positive tests for alkaloids (Collins et al., 1990); TLC analysis of unspecified parts found 5-MeO-DMT and unidentified tryptamines (J.J., 2009).

Acacia falcata Willd. (burra, hickory wattle) – Phyllodes and twigs from young, flowering trees yielded 0.025% alkaloids, which were psychoactive on vapourisation, but with unusual non-psychedelic effects that lasted up to 45-60 minutes. The dose (c.20mg) consisted of the entire crude alkaloid extract, so effects of higher doses are unknown (nen888, 2011-2013). An early analysis found <0.01% alkaloids in phyllodes and stems (harv. May), which were not identified (White, 1944a); "insignificant" alkaloid concentrations were found in stems/phyllodes (harv. Apr., Dec.), stems/phyllodes/flowers (harv. Jul.), and ripe seeds/pods. One sample of phyllodes (harv. Jul.) contained no alkaloids (White, 1957).

Acacia fimbriata A. Cunn. ex G. Don. (fringed wattle, Brisbane golden wattle) – Phyllodes and bark (harv. Mar.) tested positive for alkaloids (Webb, 1949); in a later screening, phyllodes (harv. time unspecified) also tested positive for alkaloids (Collins et al., 1990); phyllodes and twigs appear to contain phenethylamines, based on reagent colour reactions, and compared with similar colour reactions with A. harpophylla (see below) (nen888, 2011-2013).

Acacia flavescens A. Cunn. ex Benth. (yellow wattle, red wattle) – Bark has been claimed to have "strongly psychoactive" properties (Anonymous, 2015), with no reference or supporting information.

Acacia floribunda (Vent.) Willd. (gossamer wattle, sally wattle) – Phyllodes yielded 0.07-0.08% alkaloids; stems yielded 0.04-0.19% alkaloids; stems/phyllodes combined yielded 0.06-0.16% alkaloids; and flowers yielded 0.15-0.98% alkaloids. Phenethylamine was isolated as a minor component (White, 1944a). In follow-up work, tops (harv. Apr.) yielded 0.18% alkaloids, consisting mostly of tryptamine, with traces of phenethylamine; flowers (harv. Sep.) yielded 1.18% alkaloids (0.82% from an undated harvest), consisting of +/- equal quantities of tryptamine and phenethylamine (White, 1944b); bark has yielded traces of an alkaloid that was not identified (White, 1951). Using TLC/GC-MS, phyllodes were found to contain mostly DMT (usually less than 0.1%); bark yielded up to c.1% alkaloids, with 0.3-0.5% DMT, slightly less NMT, and small amounts of tryptamine, harman, and norharman (J.J., 2007). A specimen infected with galls gave particularly good yields of tryptamines (personal communication, 2011).

Acacia harpophylla F. Muell. ex Benth. (brigalow) – Phyllodes and twigs from Queensland yielded 0.6% alkaloids (phenethylamine and hordenine in a 2:3 ratio) (Fitzgerald, 1964b); another screening found 0.1% alkaloids in phyllodes and 0.3% in bark (Collins et al., 1990). Bark from branchlets (harv. Jun.) tested strongly positive for alkaloids, though bark of the stems tested negative (Webb, 1949). One screening detected no alkaloids in phyllodes and stem bark (harv. Apr.) (Smolenski et al., 1973). An alkaloid extract from phyllodes taken orally (dose not recorded) was reported to have sedative effects (nen888, 2011-2013; nen888 pers. comm., 2017).

Acacia holosericea A. Cunn. ex G. Don (soap bush, silver-leaved wattle) – Bark from Queensland has yielded 1.2% hordenine (Fitzgerald, 1964b); plants from another Queensland location yielded 1.22% alkaloids from the bark, and phyllodes and stems gave weak positive reactions for the pres-

---

4. See comments for *A. baileyana* by this source regarding the questionable subjective identification of DMT.

ence of alkaloids (Collins et al., 1990). Two other screenings detected no alkaloids in phyllodes and stem bark (harv. Jul.) (Smolenski et al., 1973), or in phyllodes, bark, and root (harv. time not specified) (Aboriginal Communities, 1988). The identity of the plants assayed in all cases may be in question, as this species has often been confused with the similar *A. colei*, *A. neurocarpa* (both of which were only distinguished from *A. holosericea* after these reports), and *A. cowleana* (Maslin & Thomson, 1992).

Acacia kettlewelliae Maiden (buffalo wattle) – Phyllodes and stems yielded 1.3% alkaloids in Apr. and 1.88% in Oct., which appeared to consist of more than 92% phenethylamine, with no tryptamine (White, 1957); phyllodes from central Victoria yielded 0.9% N-methyl-phenethylamine (Fitzgerald, 1964a).

Acacia latior (R.S. Cowan & Maslin) Maslin & Buscumb (*A. coolgardiensis ssp. latior* R.S. Cowan & Maslin) – Found to contain roughly equal amounts of NMT and DMT in phyllodes in some samples, though many samples had no observable tryptamines (TLC). Very variable in morphology and alkaloids. (J.J., 2011).

Acacia leiocalyx (Domin.) Pedley ***ssp. leiocalyx*** (curracabah, early flowering black wattle) – Stem bark yielded 0.3-0.4% unspecified tryptamine alkaloids (nen888, 2011-2013). Others have had no success in extracting alkaloids from this subspecies (seldom, 2014). Alkaloid content appears to fluctuate greatly, possibly depending on weather (Borris, 2012-2013).

Acacia leptostachya Benth. (*A. argentea* Maiden) (slender wattle, Townsville wattle) – Phyllodes have yielded 0.03-0.6% N-cinnamoyl-histamine (Fitzgerald, 1964b).

Acacia linifolia (Vent.) Willd. (*A. linearis* (J.C. Wendl.) J.F. Macbr.) (flax-leaved wattle, white wattle) – Stems and phyllodes were reported to contain phenethylamine (White, 1944a), but the plants analysed were later found to have been *A. prominens* (see below). Stems, phyllodes, and flowers of genuine *A. linifolia* (harv. Apr., Sydney) yielded 0.03% of an alkaloid that was not identified (White, 1951). Stems and phyllodes from Sydney plants contained "insignificant concentrations of alkaloid" in Oct. (White, 1957).

Acacia longifolia (Andrews) Willd. *ssp. longifolia* (sallow wattle, Sydney golden wattle) – Tops from plants growing in New Zealand (harv. Nov.) yielded 0.12% alkaloids; c.1% was obtained from tops with an unspecified harvest time; flowers (harv. Sep.) yielded 0.186% alkaloids. In both, phenethylamine was identified as a minor constituent, and though tryptamine-like bases seemed to be present, tryptamine itself was not detected (White, 1944b), except in some samples of flower spikes (White, 1951). Tops and flowers combined have yielded up to 0.01% phenethylamine; in one sample, it only comprised 9.2% of the total alkaloids. Stems and phyllodes collected at various times in New Zealand yielded 0.02-0.29% alkaloids; there was no clear correlation between yield and month of harvest. From an Oct. harvest, stems yielded 0.15% alkaloids, phyllodes 0.06%, and flowers 0.14-0.29% (White, 1944a). Bark (harv. Apr.) yielded 0.03% alkaloids; seeds yielded 0.01% alkaloids (White, 1951). Material from Australia (location not specified) was found to contain N-cinnamoyl-histamine, 3-OH-dec-2-enoyl-histamine, and other histamine-amides in the phyllodes (from 0.2% total crude alkaloids) (Rovelli, 1967). Plants growing naturalised in California yielded N-cinnamoyl-histamine and N-decadienoyl-histamine. Respectively, phyllodes (harv. late Jan.) yielded 0.0038-0.004%/0.0225-0.024%, phyllodes (harv. Mar.) yielded 0.0067%/0.027%, bark (harv. late Jan.) yielded 0.015%/0.0175%, and pods (harv. at maturity in Jul.) yielded 0.09-0.17%/0.06-0.112%. Seeds (harv. Jul.) and flower spikes (harv. in Mar., fresh) contained traces of these two compounds (Repke, 1975). However, independent psychonauts have verified that at least some examples of this species can produce DMT and other alkaloids. Up to 0.3% DMT (as well as what may be tryptamine) has reportedly been obtained from aerial parts, with highest yields in winter (E, 1996; nen888, 2011-2013). Also, in 1995, a friend succeeded in obtaining DMT (subjective i.d.) from the bark of *A. longifolia ssp. longifolia* from Victoria. This was successfully smoked by six people (pers. comms.). Phyllodes have also rarely been used in *ayahuasca* analogues in New South Wales, although caution is advised when consuming decoctions of specimens of unknown alkaloid content (nen888, 2011c; nen888 pers. comm., 2017). Although heavy rain is often associated with low alkaloid yields, with this species one person obtained higher yields of alkaloids, including DMT, from material harvesting during heavy rain, and lower yields with proportionally less DMT present from material harvested 2 weeks after the last rain (acacian, 2014).

Acacia longifolia ssp. sophorae (Labill.) Court (*A. sophorae* (Labill.) R. Br.) (coast sallow wattle) – Alkaloid screening in Australia revealed strong presence of alkaloids in the phyllodes (Collins et al., 1990). Specimens from Mentone, Victoria, were found to contain N-cinnamoyl-histamine, 3-OH-dec-2-enoyl-histamine, and other histamine-amides in phyllodes (from 0.1% crude bases in May, 0.03% in Jan.) (Rovelli, 1967). A form of *A. longifolia* close to ssp. *sophorae* yielded 0.15% crude alkaloids from unripe pods, 0.07% from stems and phyllodes (harv. May), and none from seeds; the alkaloids apparently included phenethylamine (White, 1944a). In the "informal" literature, some forms have been reported to contain tryptamine alkaloids. One specimen was claimed to have yielded DMT, 5-MeO-DMT, gramine, and histamine derivatives at levels of 0.6% in bark, and 0.15% in phyllodes, in an elusive unpublished analysis (E pers. comms., 1999-2001; E 1996). Alkaloids extracted from plants growing in California were found to contain DMT as a minor alkaloid in both bark and phyllodes, a faint spot possibly corresponding to NMT, and a major component that was not identified (TLC). GC-MS follow up of the same extract confirmed the presence of DMT and NMT (as well as numerous unidentified peaks), but could not identify the major alkaloid, which was possibly a phenethylamine (Siebert, 2017). Branch bark from one specimen of a more erect, tree-like variety from NSW yielded c.0.5% alkaloids, including mainly DMT (subjective i.d.). Seed pods have also yielded alkaloids including tryptamines (nen888, 2011-2013). Success in obtaining tryptamine alkaloids from this subspecies has been highly variable, from many attempts by different people over the last two decades (pers. comms.).

Acacia longissima Hort. ex H.L. Wendl. (*A. linearis* Sims) (narrow-leaf wattle) – Phyllodes yielded 0.2-0.3% alkaloids, including DMT (subjective i.d.) (nen888, 2011-2013). Plants from Springbrook, Queensland, yielded 0.25% alkaloids from phyllodes and 0.02% from bark; the identity of the alkaloid/s was not reported. As *A. linearis* Sims, phyllodes gave positive results in alkaloid screening; however these plants were from the same source as the plants analysed as *A. longissima* (Collins et al., 1990), suggesting that the *A. linearis* analysis was on *A. linifolia* (syn. *A. linearis* non Sims, see above). Less than 0.01% alkaloids were detected in stems and phyllodes (harv. Jul., Oct.), and seeds (White, 1944a). One screening detected no alkaloids in phyllodes and stem bark (harv. May) (Smolenski et al., 1972).

Acacia mabellae Maiden (Mabel's wattle, black wattle) – Phyllodes and twigs from a tree in east NSW yielded unidentified psychoactive tryptamines (subjective i.d. from vapourisation) (timeloop, 2012).

Acacia macradenia Benth. (zig-zag wattle) – Claimed to have "tested positive for tryptamine content" (translated from Polish – http://herbarium.0-700.pl/Akacje.html), but no details were given for the source of this information, and it is yet to be publicly verified.

Acacia maidenii F. Muell. (Maiden's wattle) – Bark yielded 0.36% DMT, and 0.24% NMT (Fitzgerald & Sioumis, 1965), though a later screening found a slightly higher yield of 0.71% total alkaloids. Bark extracted for pharmacological testing yielded 0.13% alkaloids, consisting of DMT and NMT (Collins et al., 1990). Younger trees are said to give the best yields (E, 1996). Others have had little success with obtaining DMT from this plant, due to quite variable yields. The common form with broader, more falcate phyllodes appears to be +/- deficient in alkaloids. The phyllodes of useful varieties are said to sometimes contain greater levels of alkaloids than bark (Mulga, 1996a; nen888, 2011-2013; pers. comms.); in an early alkaloid screening, the phyllodes gave a strong-positive reaction (Rovelli, 1967). Phyllodes and bark from Tamborine, Queensland (harv. Jun.) tested strongly positive for alkaloids (Webb, 1949). 5-MeO-DMT was tentatively detected in wood (weak positive) and twigs (TLC) (Trout, ed., 1997).

Acacia mangium Willd. (hickory wattle, black wattle) – Rumoured to contain psychoactive alkaloids, though documented extraction attempts by amateur researchers have been inconclusive so far (nen888, 2011-2013). Phyllodes and bark gave weak positive test for alkaloids (Collins et al., 1990), although one screening detected no alkaloids in stem bark (harv. Jul.) (Smolenski et al., 1973).

Acacia mearnsii De Wild. (*A. decurrens var. mollis* Lindl.) (black wattle) – Yielded <0.01% unidentified alkaloids from seeds (White, 1944a), 0.02% from stem, leaf, and flower (harv. Oct.), and none in galls (White, 1951); leaf and stem of one sample from Healesville, Victoria, gave negative results in alkaloid screening (Collins et al., 1990). However, bark from one specimen in northern Victoria (harv. Dec.) yielded 1.2% alkaloids including DMT (subjective i.d. following vapourisation), though the same tree yielded no alkaloids four months later (chocobeastie, 2011-2012). Branch bark from another specimen in central Victoria (harv. Dec.) yielded c.0.4-0.5% unidentified tryptamines (nen888, 2011-2013; nen888 pers. comm., 2017).

Acacia melanoxylon R. Br. (mugerabah, blackwood) – Phyllodes and stems (harv. Apr., Aug.) were found to contain <0.01% alkaloids (White, 1944a); phyllodes and stems from one Victorian location gave negative tests for alkaloids, though young phyllodes from another Victorian location gave strong positive results (Collins et al., 1990). Bark and seeds in one sample were alkaloid free, but pods yielded 0.03% unidentified alkaloids (White, 1951). Many people have attempted to extract tryptamine alkaloids from this variable species, mostly without success. However, one large fallen tree in NSW, growing near *A. maidenii*, yielded 0.6-0.7% tryptamine alkaloids (subjective i.d.) (nen888, 2011-2013). Plants growing in Portugal yielded 0.41-1.8% unidentified alkaloids from aerial parts, with highest yields from methanol extracts and lowest from hydroalcoholic extracts (Luís et al., 2012).

Acacia mucronata ssp. longifolia (Benth.) Court (*A. mucronata var. dissitiflora* Benth.) (narrow-leaf wattle) – Alkaloids were detected in the phyllodes (Collins et al., 1990), and also in an unspecified variety of the species, which gave a slightly stronger reaction (Rovelli, 1967). Young plants 6-8 months old yielded c.0.3-0.4% crude alkaloids from phyllodes and stems; phyllode alkaloids consisted of tryptamine, NMT, and 2-methyl-THβC as the main alkaloids, with lesser amounts of harmine, possibly N-formyl-NMT, and 6 unidentified peaks; twig alkaloids contained mainly tryptamine, with (in decreasing concentration) harmine, NMT, possibly N-formyl-NMT, oleamide, 2-methyl-THβC, tetrahydroharman, indole, harman, tryptophol, and several unidentified peaks and possible solvent contaminants (TLC/GC-MS) (endlessness & nen888, 2011-2012). A decoction of 50-60 g phyllodes from the same specimen had mild psychedelic effects when taken orally with no additional MAOI. Stem bark from another specimen yielded 0.4-0.6% alkaloids, including DMT, NMT, tryptamine, and β-carbolines (GC-MS) (nen888, 2011-2013). Phyllodes of some specimens appear to sometimes contain DMT and other alkaloids (E pers. comms., 1999-2001).

Acacia multisiliqua (Benth.) Maconochie – Low amounts of DMT & NMT were detected in bark of one specimen, with no tryptamines detected in other samples (TLC) (J.J., 2011).

Acacia myrtifolia (Sm.) Willd. (myrtle wattle, red-stemmed wattle) – Phyllodes and stems yielded 0.76% crude bases, including (-)-acacine (a new spermidine alkaloid), and traces of unidentified alkaloids (Nichols, 1983). Alkaloid yield did not vary seasonally in plants from the Dandenong Ranges (Vic.) (Rovelli, 1967). Stems and phyllodes from Sydney, Australia (harv. Apr.) did not yield any alkaloids (White, 1951). Another screening detected no alkaloids in phyllodes (harv. Jun.) (Smolenski et al., 1973).

Acacia neurocarpa A. Cunn. ex Hook. (*A. holosericea var. neurocarpa* (A. Cunn. ex Hook.) Domin) – Claimed to be a good source of DMT (subjective i.d.) (Palmer pers. comm., 2011). Has been confused with *A. pellita* (Maslin & Thomson, 1992).

Acacia neurophylla W. Fitzg. – Hybridises with *A. acuminata*, and is represented by two subspecies – ssp. *neurophylla* and ssp. *erugata* R.S. Cowan & Maslin. The former is very variable, and some specimens may represent new species or subspecies. Plants from the *A. neurophylla* complex were found to contain mostly DMT in the bark, with phyllodes containing mostly harman and norharman, with only traces of DMT or no DMT (TLC/GC-MS) (J.J., 2007).

Acacia obtusifolia A. Cunn. (blunt leaf wattle) – A variable species which has sometimes been confused with *A. maidenii*, *A. longifolia ssp. longifolia*, and *A. orites* in the field (pers. comms.). Bark has yielded 0.15% alkaloids, though their identities were not reported (Collins et al., 1990); in northeast NSW, 0.15-0.2% has typically been isolated (E pers. comms., 1999-2001), though others have achieved higher yields of 0.4-0.5%. Fresh young phyllodes yielded c.0.07% alkaloids (Mulga, 1996a). Dried phyllodes from different locations have yielded 0.15-0.3% alkaloids, consisting mostly of NMT with lesser amounts of DMT and traces of β-carbolines, according to two commissioned analyses (GC-MS) (E pers. comms., 1999-2001; nen888 pers. comm., 2017), although TLC performed on an extract of another phyllode sample (using pure reference standards) observed mostly DMT with lesser amounts of NMT (Siebert, 2017). Preliminary TLC analysis of one bark extract revealed the presence of at least five alkaloids, including what were very tentatively identified as DMT, 5-MeO-DMT, and bufotenine. At some times of year, plants from the same patch yielded an extract seemingly comprised of DMT and a larger quantity of NMT (E pers. comms., 1999-2001). In one array of extracts, initial analysis by GC-MS found all to contain mainly DMT, with traces of bufotenine in an orange-coloured summer extract, and higher levels of bufotenine in darker-coloured extracts; a second analysis of the darkest sample found no bufotenine, but did find 1,2-dimethyl-THβC (Trout, 2005). Any bufotenine present might not have been detected in this second analysis due to technical issues (Trout, pers. comm., 2017). Another analysis of stem bark extract by HPLC-MS found DMT as the major alkaloid by far, with traces of tryptamine, possibly NMT, and unidentified β-carbolines; no 5-MeO-DMT or bufotenine was observed (Mulga, 2005). Another analysis (TLC/GC-MS) using plants from various sources also found no 5-MeO-DMT or bufotenine. In general, bark contained mostly DMT, with lesser amounts of NMT, tryptamine, harman and norharman; phyllodes contained mostly NMT, with lesser amounts of DMT (J.J., 2007). A form from south NSW (harv. Mar.) yielded 0.6-0.7% alkaloids from twigs, 0.4-0.5% from phyllodes, and 0.5-0.6% from bark; alkaloids appeared to consist almost entirely of DMT, with traces of 2-methyl-THβC, and possibly 3-methylquinoline; traces of DMT N-oxide were also detected in the twig extract. The phyllode and bark extracts indicated the presence of small levels of NMT (TLC) which appear to be co-chromatographing with DMT in the GC-MS analysis of these samples due to its low concentration. Another south NSW specimen (harv. Mar.)

yielded 0.3-0.4% alkaloids from twigs, consisting mostly of DMT, with traces of 2-methyl-THβC, harmine, and possibly 3-methylquinoline (TLC/GC-MS) (endlessness & nen888, 2011-2013).

Acacia orites Pedley (mountain wattle) – Has on occasion been confused with *A. obtusifolia* and *A. longissima* (see above). Some underground researchers have reported obtaining alkaloids that might be β-carbolines (E pers. comms., 1999-2001).

Acacia oxycedrus Sieber ex DC. (spike wattle) – Phyllodes and stems from Victoria gave positive tests for alkaloids in a screening; another sample yielded 0.16% unidentified alkaloids (Collins et al., 1990; Rovelli, 1967). Some samples have yielded useful quantities of tryptamine alkaloids including DMT (subjective i.d.), although others have yielded no alkaloids. Branch and stem bark of a naturally occurring hybrid (possibly x with *A. longifolia ssp. longifolia*, or *A. mucronata*) has yielded 0.3-0.7% alkaloids, including DMT (subjective i.d.) (nen888, 2011b, 2011-2013).

Acacia phlebophylla H.B. Will. (Buffalo sallow wattle) – Phyllodes (harv. May) gave a strongly positive result in alkaloid screening; "leaves and tops" harvested later (Aug.) yielded 0.3% DMT as apparently the sole alkaloid (or at least the major alkaloid by far) (Rovelli, 1967; Rovelli & Vaughan, 1967). A recent TLC/GC-MS analysis estimated phyllodes to contain up to 0.6% DMT, though the youngest growth was much less potent (J.J., 2007). Young phyllodes contain mostly tryptamine (TLC) (J.J., 2009).

Acacia podalyriaefolia A. Cunn. ex G. Don (Queensland silver wattle) – Bark from Ipswich, Queensland, yielded 0.12% alkaloids; stems and phyllodes yielded 0.28% alkaloids (Collins et al., 1990); stems and phyllodes (harv. Feb.) yielded 0.11% alkaloids, which appeared to contain phenethylamine (White, 1944a); stems and phyllodes (harv. Nov.) yielded 0.29% alkaloids, which appeared to consist mainly of tryptamine, with smaller amounts of phenethylamine (White, 1957); stems and phyllodes collected after flowering yielded 0.11% alkaloids, consisting mostly of tryptamine, with no phenethylamine (White, 1951); seeds and pods yielded 0.11% alkaloids, also consisting mainly of tryptamine, with smaller amounts of phenethylamine (White, 1957). Phyllodes harvested at an unspecified time yielded (w/w) 0.06% tryptamine (Balandrin et al., 1978). One screening detected no alkaloids in phyllodes and stem bark (harv. Sep.) (Smolenski et al., 1973).

Acacia polystachya A. Cunn. ex Benth. – Bark yielded 0.35% N-cinnamoyl-histamine (Fitzgerald, 1964b).

Acacia pravissima F. Muell. (Oven's wattle, wedge-leaf wattle) – Stems (harv. Aug.) yielded 0.13% alkaloids; phyllodes (harv. Aug.) yielded 0.31% alkaloids; stems/phyllodes combined (harv. Mar.) yielded 0.44% alkaloids. This appeared to consist largely of phenethylamine (White, 1944a). Tops (harv. Jan.) yielded 0.69% crude alkaloids, consisting mostly of phenethylamine (White, 1954).

Acacia prominens A. Cunn. ex G. Don (*A. praetervisa* Domin) (Gosford wattle, golden rain wattle) – Stems/phyllodes yielded 0.2-0.65% alkaloids (highest found in Aug. and Dec.); stems and phyllodes separately (harv. Aug.) yielded 0.17% alkaloids each; seeds yielded 0.04% alkaloids. Phenethylamine appeared to be the major alkaloid (White, 1944a, 1951). Stems and phyllodes from both a small and a large tree yielded 0.23% and 0.25% alkaloids, respectively (harv. Aug.); this consisted of c.50% phenethylamine and c.20% N-methyl-phenethylamine (White, 1957). Flowering tops of a horticultural variety yielded 1.8% alkaloids, consisting mostly of what was tentatively identified as phenethylamine and N-methyl-phenethylamine. Other samples of tops yielded 1.11-2.38% crude alkaloids. Both types varied in which alkaloid was predominant at different times, though no definite correlations could be determined (White, 1954). *A. hakeoides* A. Cunn. ex Benth. was reported to contain phenethylamine (White, 1944a), but the plants analysed were later determined to have been *A. prominens* (White, 1951).

Acacia provincialis A. Camus (wirilda, swamp wattle) – Bark and phyllodes of plants growing in Bolivia yielded varying quantities of unidentified alkaloid/s, not DMT but apparently a tryptamine or tryptamines (subjective i.d.). The effects of the alkaloid/s were psychedelic when vapourised or snuffed, with a slow onset peaking after 20-30 minutes and lasting up to an hour (yatiqiri, 2011). A very variable species, formerly classified under *A. retinodes* (see below) (O'Leary, 2007).

Acacia pruinosa A. Cunn. ex Benth. (frosty wattle) – Tops have yielded 0.04% alkaloids, consisting mostly of tryptamine, with small amounts of phenethylamine (White, 1944b); stems and leaves (harv. Feb.) yielded 0.03% alkaloids; (harv. May) 0.09% alkaloids; and (harv. Oct.) 0.02% alkaloids (White, 1944a); stems, leaves, and flowers (harv. Aug., Dec.) yielded 0.02% alkaloids from both samples; no alkaloids were found in seeds or unripe pods (White, 1951, 1957).

Acacia pycnantha Benth. (golden wattle) – Less than 0.01% alkaloids were detected in phyllodes and stems (harv. Apr.), and stems, phyllodes, and flowers (harv. Sep.) (White, 1944a). An alkaloid screening did not reveal the presence of alkaloids in the phyllodes of the "weeping variety" (Rovelli, 1967). A small amount of what may have been DMT (subjective i.d.) was extracted from phyllodes, but the small quantity was only sufficient for mild threshold effects (pers. obs., 1996). Attempts at extracting alkaloids from this species by amateurs have had variable results, usually with low or absent yields, but occasional plants have given good yields of alkaloids including DMT (subjective i.d.) (nen888, 2011-2013). Small stems of one specimen yielded c.0.1% alkaloids which were described as an "easy smoke with meteorically intense effects" (seldom, 2014). Phyllodes have shown acetyl-cholinesterase-inhibiting activity (Subhan et al, 2014).

Acacia retinodes Schltdl. (wirilda) – Phyllodes and green twigs from 3-year-old plants cultivated in the Netherlands yielded 0.01% nicotine. However, the identity of the plants was not certain, as they had not flowered (Fikenscher, 1960). Phyllodes of plants from Melbourne gave a small yield of a single major alkaloid which did not correspond with nicotine; also, phyllodes of plants from Mornington Peninsula [Vic.] gave a very low yield of an alkaloid that could not be identified in comparison to the reference standards (which were phenethylamine, hordenine, NMT, DMT, tetrahydrohar-man, and N-methyl-tetrahydroharman) (Rovelli, 1967). Stems and phyllodes (harv. Apr.) and seeds were found to contain <0.01% alkaloids (White, 1944a); in another assay, stems, phyllodes, bark, ripe and unripe seeds, and unripe pods contained no alkaloids (White, 1951). The identities of the plants used in all of these assays remains uncertain, as the very variable *A. retinodes* has now been split into *A. retinodes*, *A. provincialis* (see above), and *A. uncifolia* O'Leary (O'Leary, 2007).

Acacia spectabilis A. Cunn. ex Benth. (mudgee wattle, pilliga wattle) – Leaf and bark (harv. Jun.) gave strong positive results in some alkaloid screening tests (Webb, 1949); leaves and stems yielded 0.21-0.35% alkaloids, consisting of 60-72% phenethylamine, with traces of a non-volatile base and no tryptamine; leaves and bark (harv. Jun.) were rich in alkaloids (White, 1957).

Acacia suaveolens (Sm.) Willd. (sweet wattle) – Stems and phyllodes yielded 0.7-0.89% alkaloids; stems (harv. Sep.) yielded 0.07% alkaloids, phyllodes 0.69%, seeds 0.01%, and unripe seed pods 0.05-0.17%. Stems, phyllodes, and flowers (harv. Apr., Sydney) yielded 0.97% alkaloids. The alkaloid mixture in all cases appeared to consist mainly of phenethylamine (White, 1944a, 1951). Tops (harv. Nov.) yielded 1.1% crude alkaloids, consisting mostly of phenethylamine (White, 1954).

Acacia vestita Ker Gawl. (hairy wattle, weeping boree) – Stems and phyllodes gave different alkaloid yields at different times – 0.03-0.04% (Jan.), 0.28% (May), 0.08% (Jul.-Aug.), and 0.12% (Oct.); this consisted of up to 83% tryptamine, with traces of a non-volatile base (White, 1957).

Acacia victoriae Benth. (gundabluie, narran, arlep, bramble wattle) – Alkaloid screening of phyllodes and stems was negative in spot tests (Collins et al., 1990), though Rovelli (1967) obtained a weak-positive reaction with the phyllodes (Rovelli, 1967). Young plants were tentatively found to contain DMT in aerial parts (1-year-old seedling), and 5-MeO-DMT in roots (2-year-old seedling) (TLC) (Trout, ed., 1997). Stem bark from specimens in South Australia yielded tryptamine alkaloids consisting mainly of DMT, possibly with some 5-MeO-DMT (subjective i.d. from vapourisation) (nen888, 2011-2013).

In broad alkaloid screenings, a number of other Australian *Acacia* spp. were found to contain alkaloids which were not identified – *A. amblygona* A. Cunn. ex Benth. (phyllodes and stems; only detected in some tests), *A. aneura* F. Muell. ex Benth. (0.009% in phyllodes), *A. angusta* Maiden & Blakely (0.08% in phyllodes and stems) (Collins et al., 1990), *A. aulacocarpa* R.S. Cowan & Maslin (phyllodes harv. Jul., weak-positive; none in Jan.) (Webb, 1949), *A. beauverdiana* Ewart & Sharman (phyllodes and stems) (Collins et al., 1990; Rovelli, 1967), *A. cedroides* Benth. (Aplin & Cannon, 1971), *A. conferta* A. Cunn. ex Benth. (phyllodes harv. Jun., weak-positive) (Webb, 1949), *A. cowleana* Tate (phyllodes), *A. deanei* (R.T. Baker) Welch, Coombs & McGlynn (leaves and stems) (Collins et al., 1990), *A. decora* Rchb. (phyllodes harv. Jun.; traces in stems and phyllodes harv. Mar., Apr., & Oct.) (Webb, 1949; White, 1957), *A. decurrens* Willd. (<0.01% in stems and leaves harv. May; 0.02% in Feb.; none in Dec.; weak-positive in leaves harv. Jun.) (Webb, 1949; White, 1944a, 1951), *A. doratoxylon* A. Cunn. (0.06% in phyllodes and stems) (Collins et al., 1990), *A. drumondii* Lindl. (<0.01% in leaves and stems harv. Feb., none in Aug., or in flowers) (White, 1944a, 1951), *A. estrophiolata* F. Muell. (phyllodes) (Aboriginal Communities, 1988; Collins et al., 1990), *A. filifolia* Benth. *var. pedunculata* C.A. Gardn. (Aplin & Cannon, 1971), *A. flexifolia* A. Cunn. ex Benth. (traces in stems, phyllodes and flowers harv. Jul.) (White, 1957), *A. fragilis* Maiden & Blakely (Aplin & Cannon, 1971), *A. gilbertii* Meisn. (leaves), *A. gono-phylla* Benth. (phyllodes) (Collins et al., 1990; Rovelli, 1967), *A. heteroclita* Meisn. (phyllode) (Rovelli, 1967), *A. howittii* F. Muell. (reported incorrectly as *A. vestita* Ker Gawl.; <0.01% in stems and phyllodes harv. Feb.-May; no alkaloid in other assays of stems, phyllodes, ripe seeds, and pods) (White, 1944a, 1951), *A. implexa* Benth. (moderate to strong positives in phyllodes and unripe pods, negative in bark, harv. Nov.; weak positive in phyllodes, in some tests, harv. Dec., and unspecified) (Rovelli, 1967; Webb, 1949), *A. iteaphylla* F. Muell. ex Benth. (phyllodes positive in one assay, negative in others) (Rovelli, 1967), *A. ixiophylla* Benth. (phyllodes, harv. Jun.) (Webb, 1949), *A. juncifolia* Benth. (0.008%

in phyllodes), *A. kybeanensis* Maiden & Blakely (phyllodes), *A. latipes* Benth. (phyllodes), *A. leichhardtii* Benth. (0.007% in phyllodes and stems), *A. leiophylla* Benth. (phyllodes) (Collins et al., 1990), *A. leprosa* Sieber ex DC. (<0.01% in stems and phyllodes harv. Feb., stems/phyllodes/flowers harv. Sep.) (White, 1944a), *A. leptocarpa* A. Cunn. ex Benth. (0.09% in phyllodes; some tests negative) (Collins et al., 1990), *A. lineolata* Benth. (Aplin & Cannon, 1971), *A. loxophylla* Benth. (phyllodes) (Rovelli, 1967), *A. lunata* G. Lodd. (phyllodes harv. Jun., strong-positive) (Webb, 1949), *A. lysiphloia* F. Muell. (phyllodes; some tests negative) (Aboriginal Communities, 1988), *A. maitlandii* F. Muell. (phyllodes), *A. neriifolia* A. Cunn. ex Benth. (1.3% in phyllodes, 1.2% in bark) (Collins et al., 1990), *A. nervosa* DC. (phyllodes) (Collins et al., 1990; Rovelli 1967), *A. paradoxa* DC. (0.01% in tops; as *A. armata* R. Br., plants in New Zealand gave no alkaloid from stems and phyllodes harv. Mar., or stem, phyllodes, and flowers harv. Oct., though ripe pods contained traces) (Collins et al., 1990; White, 1951), *A. pendula* A. Cunn. ex G. Don. (phyllodes, bark), *A. penninervis* Sieber ex DC. (phyllodes and bark harv. Jun.; phyllodes gave stronger reaction) (Webb, 1949), *A. rhodoxylon* Maiden (phyllodes and stems) (Collins et al., 1990), *A. rupicola* F. Muell. ex Benth. (traces in stems, phyllodes, and flowers harv. Jul.) (White, 1957), *A. salicina* Lindl. (phyllodes harv. Nov., weak-positive; has also given negative results) (Aplin & Cannon, 1971; Collins et al., 1990; Webb, 1949), *A. saligna* (Labill.) H.L. Wendl. (<0.01% in stems and phyllodes harv. Feb.; traces in stems and phyllodes harv. Apr., as *A. cyanophylla* Lindl.) (White, 1944a, 1957), *A. semilunata* Maiden & Blakely (phyllodes; some tests negative) (Collins et al., 1990; Rovelli, 1967), *A. shirleyi* Maiden (identity uncertain; phyllodes harv. Jun.) (Webb, 1949), *A. simsii* A. Cunn. ex Benth. (0.03% in phyllodes), *A. stenoptera* Benth. (phyllodes) (Collins et al., 1990), *A. stricta* (Andrews) Willd. (<0.01% in stems and phyllodes harv. Feb. & Aug., also in seeds; another assay found none in stem, phyllodes, flowers, ripe seeds, or pods) (Collins et al., 1990; White, 1944a, 1951), *A. subcaerulea* Lindl. (Aplin & Cannon, 1971), *A. terminalis* (Salisb.) J.F. Macbr. (as *A. discolor* (Andrews) Willd.; 0.03% in stems, leaves and flowers harv. Feb.; traces in stems and leaves harv. Apr.-May, traces in flower spikes) (White, 1951), *A. tetragonophylla* F. Muell. (root bark; phyllodes negative) (Aboriginal Communities, 1988; Collins et al., 1990), *A. torulosa* Benth. (phyllodes, not in bark) (Collins et al., 1990), *A. triptera* Benth. (phyllodes and branches harv. Jun.), *A. ulicifolia* (Salisb.) Court (as *A. juniperina* nom. illeg.; phyllodes and stems harv. Nov., strong-positive) (Webb, 1949), *A. umbellata* A. Cunn. ex Benth. (0.013% in phyllodes) (Collins et al., 1990), *A. urophylla* Benth. (phyllodes) (Aplin & Cannon, 1971; Collins et al., 1990), *A. verniciflua* A. Cunn. (traces in stems and phyllodes harv. Feb.; another Feb. harv. gave no alkaloids, as have others from unspecified harv. times) (Collins et al., 1990; Rovelli, 1967; White, 1951), *A. verticillata* (L'Hér.) Willd. (<0.01% in phyllodes and stems harv. Sep., as well as in seeds and flowers; other assays of stems, phyllodes, seeds, and pods yielded no alkaloids; moderate positive in phyllodes in another assay, none detected in bark) (Collins et al., 1990; White, 1944a, 1951), *A. viscidula* Benth. (phyllodes and stems harv. Nov.) (Webb, 1949), and *A. xiphophylla* E. Pritz. (Aplin & Cannon, 1971).

CLOSING REMARKS

The recent growth of interest in Acacia spp. as a source of DMT reflects a growing interest in consciousness expansion and direct spiritual experience that has been occurring globally for some time. However, this increased interest has also brought with it greed and commercial exploitation. Many users of Acacia alkaloid extracts have no idea of the source, or whether it was produced sustainably. To them it is just DMT (even when it is a mix of alkaloids), and they may not even know what an Acacia is. Some of the species being commercially (and illegally) exploited are extremely rare and may be threatened with extinction in the wild if current practices continue or increase. Regardless of legality, the use of these plants will continue, but it is hoped that all people doing so can learn to tread lightly and discreetly. If these substances are shared respectfully through friends with no profit motive, and people cultivate plants and use sustainable harvesting methods, scenes of trees killed by bark-stripping could be a thing of the past. This author calls for DMT users to boycott the sale and purchase of Acacia alkaloid extracts, as well as non-propagative plant parts, and to show respect to the plants from which they are trying to learn.

ACKNOWLEDGMENTS

I would like to dedicate this paper to Nick Tree (aka nen888, aka E), whose work with and for the plants has been inspiring. Thanks to Nick for sharing his knowledge over many years. I would also like to thank Keeper Trout, endlessness, J.J., Daniel Siebert, C.G., and my learned botanist friends (for identifying yatiqiri's mystery wattle), who will remain anonymous in this context – you know who you are!

REFERENCES

Aboriginal Communities of the Northern Territory of Australia, 1988. *Traditional Bush Medicines: An Aboriginal Pharma-copoeia*. Greenhouse Publications, Victoria.

acacian, 2014. Posts in *Trying to Improve Acacia Information*. https://www.dmt-nexus.me/forum/default.aspx-?g=posts&t=23472

Aiston, G, 1937. The Aboriginal narcotic pituri. *Oceania* 7, 372-377.

Anonymous, 1992. Obtaining DMT from *Acacia maidenii*. First published in University of Sydney student newspaper *Honi Soit* [issue # unknown], subsequently reprinted in abridged and expanded forms on the alt.drugs newsgroup, in the Australian supplement for the Natural Highs FAQ (Michael from Melbourne, 1992) and various websites. Currently at http://www.erowid.org/plants/acacia/acacia_extract1.shtml as *Extracting DMT from Acacia maidenii*.

Anonymous, 1993. *Dr D.M.T. (or how I learned to stop reality and love psychadelics* [sic]. Posted by Jeremy [not the author] to alt.drugs newsgroup 29/6/1993 as Ayahuasca report (long). Currently at http://www.lycaeum.org/leda/docs/8446.shtml?ID=8446 with corrected spelling.

Anonymous, 2015. *List of psychoactive plants*. http://www.lycaeum.org/wiki/List_of_psychoactive_plants [Note: numerous other Acacia spp. listed here as psychoactive are erroneously referred to a work which does not support the claims. These are not discussed further in this current paper.]

Aplin, T.E.H., Cannon, J.R., 1971. Distribution of alkaloids in some Western Australian plants. *Economic Botany* 25(4), 366-380.

Appleseed, J., 1993. Ayahuasca analog experiences. *The Entheogen Review* 2(2), 27-28. [Refers to experiments performed in late 1992.]

Ariati, S.R. et al., 2007. Morphological and genetic variation within the widespread species *Acacia victoriae* (Mimosaceae). *Australian Systematic Botany* 20, 54-62.

Balandrin, M.F. et al., 1978. Reversed-phase high-pressure liquid chromatography of some tryptamine derivatives. *J. Chromatog.* 157, 365-370.

Bancroft, T.L., 1887. On the discovery of *saponin* in *Acacia delibrata, A. Cunn. Proceedings of the Royal Society of Queensland* 4, 10-11.

Bindon, P., 1996. *Useful Bush Plants*. Western Australian Museum, Perth.

Borris, 2012-2013. Posts in *Trying to Improve Acacia Information*. https://www.dmt-nexus.me/forum/default.aspx-?g=posts&t=23472

Brock, J., 1988. *Top End Native Plants*. Darwin, Australia.

Butcher, P.A. et al., 2001. *Flora of Australia* Vol. 11A & 11B – Mimosaceae, Acacia. CSIRO Publ., Melbourne.

Cakic, V. et al., 2010. Dimethyltryptamine (DMT): subjective effects and patterns of use among Australian recreational users. *Drug and Alcohol Dependence* 111, 30-37.

C.G., 1993. 2 ayahuasca experiences. Post to Usenet alt.drugs newsgroup, 14/1/1993. Reprinted as Twin perspectives on Ayahuasca Australis at http://www.lycaeum.org/leda/docs/8443.shtml?ID=8443

chocobeastie, 2011-2012. Posts in *Trying to Improve Acacia Information*. https://www.dmt-nexus.me/forum/default.aspx-?g=posts&t=23472

Clarke, P.A., 2007. *Aboriginal People and Their Plants*. Rosenberg, NSW, Australia.

Clarke-Lewis, J.W., Dainis, I., 1967. Flavan derivatives XIX. Teracacidin and isoteracacidin from *Acacia obtusifolia* and *Acacia maidenii* heartwoods; phenolic hydroxylation patterns of heartwood flavonoids characteristic of sections and subsections of the genus Acacia. *Aust. J. Chem.* 20, 2191-2198.

Clement, B.A. et al., 1997. Toxic amines and alkaloids from *Acacia berlandieri*. *Phytochem.* 46(2), 249-254.

Clement, B.A. et al., 1998. Toxic amines and alkaloids from *Acacia rigidula*. *Phytochem.* 49(5), 1377-1380.

Collins, D.J et al., 1990. *Plants For Medicines: A Chemical and Pharmacological Survey of Plants in the Australian Region*. CSIRO, Australia.

Cribb, A.B., Cribb, J.W., 1982. *Useful Wild Plants in Australia*. Collins Publ., Sydney.

Dannaway, F.R., 2007. *Celestial botany: entheogenic traces in Islamic mysticism*. www.scribd.com/doc/15744793/Celestial-Botany-Entheogenic-Traces-in-Islamic-Mysticism

Dixon-Clarke, S.E., Ramsay, R.R., 2011. Dietary inhibitors of monoamine oxidase A. *J. Neural Transm.* 118, 1031-1041.

E, 1996. Urgent report on the Australian Acacia situation. *The Entheogen Review* 5(4), 10.

Ee, K.Y., Yates, P., 2013. Nutritional and antinutritional evaluation of raw and processed Australian wattle (*Acacia saligna*) seeds. *Food Chemistry* 138, 762-769.

endlessness & nen888, 2011-2012. *Acacia analysis thread*. https://www.dmt-nexus.me/forum/default.aspx-?g=posts&t=27722

EsKaTaRi, 2010. Post 29/9/2011 in *Acacia's alkaloid content based on weather*. www.shaman-australis.com/forum/index.php?/topic/25586-acacias-alkaloid-content-based-on-weather/

Etheridge, R. (Jr.), 1894. The kūditcha shoes of Central Australia. *Proc. Linn. Soc. NSW* 19, 544-550.

Evans, W.C. et al., 1977. Free amino acids in the seeds of Acacia species. *Phytochem.* 16, 565-570.

Everist, S.L., 1981. *Poisonous Plants of Australia*. [Revised edition; originally published 1974] Angus & Robertson.

Fensham, R.J. et al., 2006. This disastrous event staggered me: Reconstructing the botany of Ludwig Leichhardt on the expedition from Moreton Bay to Port Essington, 1844-45. *Cunninghamia* 9(4), 451-506.

Fikenscher, L.H., 1960. Het voorkomen van nicotine in het genus Acacia. *Pharm. Weekblad* 95, 233-235.

Fitzgerald, J.S., 1964a. Alkaloids of the Australian Leguminosae. III. The occurrence of phenylethylamine derivatives in Acacia species. *Aust. J. Chem.* 17, 160-162.

Fitzgerald, J.S., 1964b. Alkaloids of the Australian Leguminosae. IV. Cinnamoylhistamine, the alkaloid of *Acacia argentea* and *A. polystachya*. *Aust. J. Chem.* 17, 375-378.

Fitzgerald, J.S., Sioumis, A.A., 1965. Alkaloids of the Australian Leguminosae. V. The occurrence of methylated tryptamines in *Acacia maidenii* F. Muell. *Aust. J. Chem.* 18, 433-434.

Graves, R., 1961. *The White Goddess: A Historical Grammar of Poetic Myth*. Faber & Faber, London.

Gupta, G.L., Nigam, S.S., 1971. Chemical examination of the leaves of *Acacia concinna*. *Planta Medica* 19, 55-62.

Hamlyn-Harris, R., Smith, F., 1916. On fish poisoning and poisons employed among the Aborigines of Queensland. *Memoirs of the Queensland Museum* 5, 1-22.

Hansen, V., Horsfall, J. 2016. *Noongar Bush Medicine – Medicinal Plants of the South-West of Western Australia*. UWA Publishing, Crawley, WA.

Heinze, D. et al., 1998. Buffalo sallow wattle *Acacia phlebophylla* of Mount Buffalo. *The Victorian Naturalist* 115(5), 205-209.

Hurst, E., 1942. *The Poison Plants of New South Wales*. Poison Plants Committee of NSW.

Ibrahim, H. et al., 2015. Potential of earleaf Acacia (*Acacia auriculiformis*) leaves for industrial raw materials. *Int. J. Scientific Engineering and Applied Science* 1(4), 1-6.

J.G., 1992. Preliminary report on two ayahuasca analogues. *The Entheogen Review* 1(2), 15.

J.J., 2007. *Entheogenic Acacias of Australia: an introduction to several previously unreported active species*. Presentation at EGA (Entheogenesis Australis) Conference.

J.J., 2009. *Entheogenic Acacias of Australia: A review of known active species and an introduction to more previously unreported species*. Presentation at EGA (Entheogenesis Australis) Conference.

J.J., 2011. *Wattles you want to know*. Presentation at EGA (Entheogenesis Australis) Conference.

Johns, S.R. et al., 1966. Alkaloids of the Australian Leguminosae. VII. N-methyltetrahydroharman from *Acacia complanata* A. Cunn. ex. Benth. *Aust. J. Chem.* 19, 1539-1540.

Johnston, T.H., Cleland, J.B., 1933. The history of the Aboriginal narcotic, pituri. *Oceania* 4, 201-223, continued 268-289.

Kelly, J., 2012. Trees stripped of bark to produce hallucinogenic drug. *Avon Valley Gazette* (Western Australia), issue and pages unknown. http://www.communitynews.com.au/news-and-views/local-news/Trees-stripped-of-bark-to-produce-hallucinogencic-drug/7623598/ [sic] No longer online; text reproduced at https://www.shroomery.org/forums/showflat.php/Number/16310699

Kruszelnicki, K.S., 2005. Mike wants to know if there's any kind of shamanism associated with petrol sniffing in the Northern Territory. *Dr Karl's Q&A forum*. http://www.abc.net.au/science/k2/stn/q&a/notes/051027-9.htm

Kunii, Y. et al., 1996. 4-Hydroxypipecolic acid and pipecolic acid in Acacia species: their determination by high-performance liquid chromatography, its application to leguminous plants, and configuration of 4-hydroxypipecolic acid. *J. Agric. Food Chem.* 44(2), 483-487.

Latz, P., 1995. *Bushfires & Bushtucker: Aboriginal plant use in Central Australia*. IAD Press, Northern Territory.

Lauterer, J., 1897. Occurrence of saponin in Australian Acacias and Albizzias. *Proceedings of the Royal Society of Queensland* 12, 103-107.

Lehmann, A.C., Mihalyi, L.J., 1982. Aggression, bravery, endurance, and drugs: a radical re-evaluation and analysis of the Masai warrior complex. *Ethnology* 21(4), 335-347.

Leichhardt, L., 1847. *Journal of an overland expedition in Australia - From Moreton Bay to Port Essington, a distance of upwards of 3000 miles, during the years 1844-1845*. T. & W. Boone, London.

Levitt, D., 1981. *Plants and People – Aboriginal uses of plants on Groote Eylandt*. Australian Institute of Aboriginal Studies, Canberra.

Low, T., 1989. *Bush Tucker: Australia's wild food harvest*. Angus & Robertson, Australia.

Low, T., 1990. *Bush Medicine: a pharmacopoeia of natural remedies*. Angus & Robertson, Australia.

Luís, Â. et al., 2012. Antioxidant activities of extracts from *Acacia melanoxylon*, *Acacia dealbata* and *Olea europaea* and alkaloids estimation. *Int. J. Pharmacy and Pharmaceutical Sciences* 4(suppl. 1), 225-233.

Maiden, J.H., 1889. *The Useful Native Plants of Australia (Including Tasmania)*. Turner & Henderson, Sydney.

Maiden, J.H., 1913. *The Forest Flora of New South Wales* Vol. VI, Appendix Part LII: Fish-Poisons of the Australian Aborigines. Govt. Printer, Sydney.

Maiden, J.H., 1922. *The Forest Flora of New South Wales* Vol. VII Parts 61-70. Govt. Printer, Sydney.

Marrfurra, P. et al., 1995. *Ngan'gikurunggurr and Ngan'giwumirri Ethnobotany – Aboriginal Plant Use From the Daly River Area Northern Australia*. Northern Territory Botanical Bulletin No. 22. Conservation Commission of the Northern Territory, Darwin.

Maslin, B.R., Thomson, L.A.J., 1992. Re-appraisal of the taxonomy of *Acacia holosericea*, including the description of a new species, *A. colei*, and the reinstatement of *A. neurocarpa*. *Australian Systematic Botany* 5, 729-743.

Maslin, B.R. et al., 1988. Cyanogenesis in Australian species of Acacia. *Phytochem.* 27(2), 421-428.

maxzar100, 2009. Post 17/12/2009 in *Acacia Baileyana THH in phyloids!!!* [sic] https://www.dmt-nexus.me/forum/default.aspx?g=posts&t=8498

McEwan, T., 1978. Organo-fluorine compounds in plants, in Keeler, R.F. (Ed.), *Effects of Poisonous Plants on Livestock*. Academic Press, NY.

Meggitt, M.J. 1966. Gadjari among the Walbiri Aborigines of Central Australia (continued). *Oceania* 37(2), 124-147. Part 4, beginning in Oceania 36(3), 173-213.

Michael from Melbourne, 1992. *Australian supplement for the Natural Highs* FAQ. Document originally posted to alt.drugs newsgroup and occasionally updated; currently at https://erowid.org/psychoactives/faqs/faq_natural_high_australia.shtml

Mulga, 1996a. *The genus Acacia and entheogenic tryptamines*. www.lycaeum.org//~mulga/ (later at www.mulga.yage.net; both appear to be currently offline).

Mulga, 1996b. *Acacia complanata – phytochemical studies.* http://www.lycaeum.org/~mulga/acacia/comphy.html

Mulga, 2005. HPLC-MS analysis of Acacia obtusifolia. *The Entheogen Review* 14(1), 113-115.

nen888, 2011a. *Entheogenic effects of NMT (monomethyltryptamine).* https://www.dmt-nexus.me/forum/default.aspx-?g=posts&t=23544 [note: nen888 is Nick Tree, formerly known also as E in some publications]

nen888, 2011b. *Acacia oxycedrus (more reports needed) Active!* https://www.dmt-nexus.me/forum/default.aspx-?g=posts&m=256760

nen888, 2011c. Post 11/11/2011 in *Passifloras of interest.* https://www.dmt-nexus.me/forum/default.aspx?g=posts&t=26892

nen888, 2011-2013. *Trying to improve Acacia information.* https://www.dmt-nexus.me/forum/default.aspx-?g=posts&t=23472

Nen [nen888], Nickles, D., 2014. *When DMT equals killing the environment.* http://the-nexian.me/home/knowledge/131-when-dmt-equals-killing-the-environment

Newman, P.D., 2015. The use of DMT in early Masonic ritual. *Dragibus* 3(2), 16-18.

Nichols, J.K., 1983. *Alkaloids of the Hovea and Acacia Genera.* Master Thesis. Victorian College of Pharmacy, Melbourne.

O'Leary, M.C., 2007. Review of *Acacia retinodes* and closely related species, *A. uncifolia* and *A. provincialis* (Leguminosae: Mimosoideae: sect. Phyllodineae). *J. Adelaide Bot. Gard.* 21, 95-109.

Ott, J., 1993. *Pharmacotheon – Entheogenic drugs, their plant sources and history.* Natural Products Co., Wa.

Ott, J., 1994. *Ayahuasca Analogues – Pangaean Entheogens.* Natural Products Co., Wa.

Palmer, J., 2015. Explaining the smoking blend changa. *Dragibus* 3(2), 11-13.

Pendleton, M.W., Pendleton, B.B., 2008. Psychotropic or ritual use of Acacia flowers prior to abandonment of a prehistoric Mimbres-Mogollon archeological site. *The Internet Journal of Biological Anthropology* 1(2) doi:10.5580/1ab5

Peters, R.A. et al., 1965. Fluoride metabolism in *Acacia georginae* gidyea. *Biochem. J.* 95, 724-730.

PrimalWisdom, 2011. Posts in *Trying to Improve Acacia Information.* https://www.dmt-nexus.me/forum/default.aspx-?g=posts&t=23472

Reid, E., 1977. *The Records of Western Australian Plants Used By Aboriginals As Medicinal Agents.* W.A. Institute of Technology, Pharmacy Dept. Bentley, W.A.

Repke, D.P., 1975. The histamine amides of *Acacia longifolia. Lloydia* 38(1), 101-105.

Repke, D.P. et al., 1973. Alkaloids of *Acacia baileyana. Lloydia* 36(2), 211-213.

Rovelli, B., 1967. *Alkaloids of the Acacia Species.* M. Sc. Thesis, University of Sydney.

Rovelli, B., Vaughan, G.N., 1967. Alkaloids of Acacia I. NbNb-Dimethyltryptamine in *Acacia phlebophylla* F. Muell. *Aust. J. Chem.* 20, 1299-1300.

Sadgrove, N.J., 2009. The influence of indigenous food procurement techniques on populations of cyanobacteria in pre-European Australia: a potential small-scale water amelioration tool. *EcoHealth* 6, 390-403.

Sahai, R. et al., 1980. Auriculoside, a new flavan glycoside from *Acacia auriculiformis. Phytochem.* 19, 1560-1562.

Seigler, D.S., 2003. Phytochemistry of Acacia - sensu lato. *Biochem. Syst. Ecol.* 31, 845-873.

seldom, 2012. Post 25/7/2012 in *Trying to Improve Acacia Information.* https://www.dmt-nexus.me/forum/default.aspx-?g=posts&t=23472

seldom, 2014. Posts in *Trying to Improve Acacia Information.* https://www.dmt-nexus.me/forum/default.aspx-?g=posts&t=23472

shanedudddy2, 2013. Post 22/5/2013 in *Trying to Improve Acacia Information.* https://www.dmt-nexus.me/forum/default.aspx?g=posts&t=23472

Shannon, B., 2008. Biblical entheogens: a speculative hypothesis. *Time and Mind: The Journal of Archaeology Consciousness and Culture* 1(1), 51-74.

Sharma, A. et al., 2014. Effect of ethanolic extract of *Acacia auriculiformis* leaves on learning and memory in rats. *Pharmacognosy Research* 6(3), 246-250.

Siebert, D., 2017. Personal communications. The *A. longifolia ssp. sophorae* analysis was done in 1995; the GC-MS portion of this analysis was done by A.T. Shulgin. The *A. obtusifolia* analysis referred to was done in 1998.

Smith, N.M., 1991. Ethnobotanical field notes from the Northern Territory, Australia. *J. Adelaide Bot. Gard.* 14(1), 1-65.

Smith, N. et al., 1993. *Ngarinyman Ethnobotany – Aboriginal Plant Use from the Victoria River Area, Northern Australia.* N.T. Bot. Bull. 16. Conservation Commission of the Northern Territory.

Smolenski, S.J. et al., 1972. Alkaloid screening. I. *Lloydia* 35(1), 1-34.

Smolenski, S.J. et al., 1973. Alkaloid screening. III. *Lloydia* 36(4), 359-389.

Spencer, B., Gillen, F.J., 1899. *The Native Tribes of Central Australia.* MacMillan, London.

Subhan, N. et al., 2014. Antioxidant, anti-diabetic and neuroprotective activities of four Australian Acacia species. Abstract of paper presented at *Royal Australian Chemical Institute Natural Products Chemistry Group [RACI NPG] One Day Symposium 2014,* Wagga Wagga, NSW.

Taylor, W.B., 1979. *Drinking, Homicide and Rebellion in Colonial Mexican Villages.* Stanford Univ. Press.

Taylor, W.B., 1996. *Magistrates of the sacred: priests and parishioners in eighteenth-century Mexico.* Stanford Univ. Press.

timeloop, 2012. Posts in *Trying to Improve Acacia Information.* https://www.dmt-nexus.me/forum/default.aspx-?g=posts&t=23472

Tindale, M.D., Roux, D.G., 1969. A phytochemical survey of the Australian species of Acacia. *Phytochem.* 8, 1713-1727.

Tindale, M.D., Roux, D.G., 1974. An extended phytochemical survey of Australian species of Acacia: chemotaxonomic and phylogenetic aspects. *Phytochem.* 13, 829-839.

Tindale, N.B., 1937. Native songs of the south-east of South Australia. *Transactions of the Royal Society of South Australia* 61, 107-120.

Torsten, 2008. Quoted by shruman 13/11/2008 in *AUSSIE Ayahuasca.* http://www.shaman-australis.com/forum/index.php?/topic/19133-aussie-ayahuasca

Trout, K., ed. 1997. *Acacia Species Reported to Contain Tryptamines and/or β-Carbolines.* Trout's Notes.

Trout, K., 2005. Some thoughts on analysis and comparisons of extracts and synthetic DMT. *The Entheogen Review* 14(1), 116-118.

t st tantra et al., 2009. *Ozopo!* www.shaman-australis.com/forum/index.php?/topic/20188-ozopo

Watt, J.M., Breyer-Brandwijk, M.G., 1962. *Medicinal and Poisonous Plants of Southern and Eastern Africa*. E&S Livingstone Ltd., Edinburgh.

Webb, L.J., 1948. *Guide to the Medicinal and Poisonous Plants of Queensland*. Council for Scientific and Industrial Research Bulletin No. 232. CSIR, Melbourne.

Webb, L.J., 1949. *An Australian Phytochemical Survey 1. Alkaloids and cyanogenetic compounds in Queensland plants*. CSIRO Bulletin 241. CSIRO, Melbourne.

Webb, L.J., 1969. The use of plant medicines and poisons by Australian Aborigines. *Mankind* 7(2), 137-146.

White, E.P., 1944a. Isolation of β-phenethylamine from Acacia species. *New Zealand J. Sci. & Tech.* 25B, 139-142.

White, E.P., 1944b. Isolation of tryptamine from some Acacia species. *New Zealand J. Sci. & Tech.* 25B, 157-162.

White, E.P., 1951. Legumes examined for alkaloids – additions and corrections. *New Zealand J. Sci. & Tech.* 33B, 54-60.

White, E.P., 1954. The occurrence of N-methyl-β-phenylethylamine in *Acacia prominens* A. Cunn. *New Zealand J. Sci. & Tech.* 35B, 451-455.

White, E.P., 1957. Evaluation of further legumes, mainly Lupinus and Acacia species for alkaloids. *New Zealand J. Sci. & Tech.* 38B, 718-725.

Wightman, G. et al., 1992. *Mudburra Ethnobotany: Aboriginal Plant Use From Kulumindini (Elliott) Northern Australia*. Northern Territory Botanical Bulletin No. 14. Conservation Commission of the Northern Territory, Palmerston.

Wightman, G. et al., 1994. *Gurindji Ethnobotany: Aboriginal Plant Use From Daguragu Northern Australia*. N.T. Bot. Bull. No. 18. Conservation Commission of the Northern Territory, Darwin.

yatiqiri, 2011. *Question about my acacia spice*. https://www.dmt-nexus.me/forum/default.aspx?g=posts&t=23532

From 'There' to 'Here': Psychedelic Natural Products and Their Contributions to Medicinal Chemistry [Keynote]

David E. Nichols, PhD

Division of Chemical Biology
and Medicinal Chemistry,
Eshelman School of Pharmacy,
University of North Carolina,
Chapel Hill, NC

ABSTRACT

This review will be an excursion that considers each of the major types of psychedelic agents: tryptamines, ergolines, and phenethylamines. The review will feature natural product templates ("there"), and show how each template evolved through chemical structural modification that led either to optimized potency or unique psychopharmacology ("here"). Each chemotype has at some point in time been the focus of attention by medicinal or natural products chemists. For example, in the "modern" era, Western attention to psychedelics was first directed to mescaline, a simple trimethoxy-substituted phenethylamine produced by the peyote cactus, *Lophophora wiliamsii*. Anthropological studies have indicated the use of peyote by Native North Americans was ongoing as long as 5700 years ago. Following the identification of mescaline as the active component in peyote by Heffter in 1897, it was then synthesized in 1919 by Späth. More than four decades would then pass before the prodigious efforts of Alexander Shulgin led to a variety of ring-substituted analogues of mescaline. Part of Shulgin's inspiration derived from his knowledge of the structures of essential oils. Additional medicinal chemistry efforts led to extremely potent congeners of mescaline. Similar, although less productive, studies occurred with simple tryptamines, and with the tetracyclic ergolines. Each of these chemotypes will be discussed, and it will be seen how natural products played a significant role in bringing psychedelics of various types to the present moment ("here").

INTRODUCTION

Although the focus of this symposium is on the "ethnographic search" for psychoactive drugs, what I plan to show in this presentation is what medicinal chemists do once a lead compound has been identified from a natural source. My talk will highlight the development of the classic (serotonergic) psychedelics, beginning with tryptamines, proceeding to phenethylamines, and ending with ergolines. I will note which portions of the molecule are essential for activity, and which can be modified to effect changes in its qualitative and/or quantitative actions. This review will not be an encyclopedic compendium, which would probably take an entire book, but will highlight some of the more important structural elements and approaches to understanding the medicinal chemistry of psychedelics.

TRYPTAMINES

Tryptamines are naturally occurring compounds that have been employed in religious and sha-manic practices for millennia. There are three basic types of tryptamines that are psychoactive, and they are all *N,N*-dimethylated tryptamines, either with no substitution on the indole ring, with a 4-hydroxy substituent, or with a 5-oxygen substituent.

The simplest psychoactive tryptamine is *N,N*-dimethyltryptamine, or DMT. It occurs widely throughout nature and is produced by many plants. Several species of *Mimosa* are native to east-ern Brazil, and are known as Jurema or Jurema Preta. The dried root bark of *Mimosa tenuiflora* has been shown to contain 1-1.7% DMT, and is referred to as "Black Jurema" (Jurema Preta) (Schultes and Hofmann, 1979). DMT is not orally active, but was employed as a snuff. When ingested orally, DMT is deaminated by monoamine oxidase enzymes in the liver. However, it is rendered orally active when administered with inhibitors of monoamine oxidase. The most well-known example is that of *aya-huasca*, which is a decoction prepared by boiling pounded vines of *Banisteriopsis caapi* with leaves of *Psychotria viridis*. The latter contain DMT, whereas *Banisteriopsis caapi* contains beta-carbolines that inhibit monoamine oxidase. *Ayahuasca* was incorporated as a sacrament by two syncretic churches, the *União do Vegetal* (UDV), and the *Santo Daime*, and has become popular in recent years for those wishing to have a legal psychedelic experience by traveling to various sites in South America, pri-marily Peru, where *ayahuasca* is administered in various rituals.

Perhaps next in structural complexity is 5-hydroxy-*N,N*-dimethyltryptamine (bufotenine). Bu-fotenine is likewise not orally active. Seeds and pods of *Anadenanthera peregrina* served as the basis of one of the most widely used shamanic inebriants in South American Andean cultures. Evidence for this use has been recovered from archeological sites at least four millennia old. Seeds were roasted, pulverized, and inhaled through the nose as cohoba or *yopo* snuff, or were smoked in pipes or as ci-gars (Torres and Repke, 2006). Seeds contain up to 7.4% bufotenine (5-hydroxy-*N,N*-dimethyltrypt-amine), 0.16% DMT, and 0.04% 5-MeODMT. Based on the amounts of snuff used, bufotenine was likely the most active component, although its psychoactivity still remains controversial.

Whereas the hallucinogenic activity of bufotenine is still controversial, its *O*-methyl derivative, 5-methoxy-*N,N*-dimethyltryptamine (5-MeODMT) is extremely potent, although again lacking oral activity. This tryptamine is found in the red bark resin of *Virola theiodora* or *Virola elongata* and is used by the Yanomamo to make a potent snuff known as Epená (Schultes and Hofmann, 1980). Re-cently, a fad has developed for smoking the venom of *Bufo alvarius* (the psychedelic toad of the So-noran desert). This toad secretes a toxin in its parotid gland that contains significant concentrations of 5-MeODMT. In fact, the dry weight of the parotid and tibial glands may include as much as 15% 5-MeODMT (Weil and Davis, 1994). Although the secretion of the parotid gland is quite toxic if in-gested orally, when smoked, the toxic components are evidently destroyed.

Whereas DMT and 5-MeODMT are not active orally, substitution with a 4-oxygen substituent confers oral activity on the molecule. Although Richard Evans Schultes clarified the correct botan-ical identity of psychedelic (hallucinogenic) mushrooms used for various rituals in ancient Mexi-co (Schultes, 1940), Western attention on these natural products was heightened by a May 13, 1957 *Life Magazine* article titled "Seeking the Magic Mushroom", by banker and amateur mycologist R. Gordon Wasson. In this story, he recounts travel to Southern Mexico and meeting with a *curandera* named Maria Sabina and her daughter, who allowed him to participate in a ceremony where *Psilo-cybe* mushrooms were ingested. They emerged from the experience "awestruck," having "expected nothing so staggering as the ... astonishing effects of the mushrooms" (Wasson, 1957).

These remarkable mushrooms had been named *teonanacatl* by the Aztecs, which roughly trans-lates to "divine flesh." Although Spanish missionaries had made concerted efforts to destroy all traces of "pagan" worship involving these mushrooms, nonetheless, more than 200 mushroom stone effigies had escaped destruction and were discovered by later explorers. Chemical investiga-tions by Dr. Albert Hofmann at the Sandoz laboratories revealed that the active component of *Psi-locybe* mushrooms was psilocybin, with lesser amounts of psilocin, its dephosphorylated analogue (Hofmann et al., 1958), as shown below:

Although most of the literature published on the so-called magic mushrooms has largely dealt with their use by indigenous South American peoples, there is some evidence that their use may go much further back into history. For example, the ancient ritual in Eleusis, Greece, which was part of that culture for about 2000 years, employed a drink known as *kykeon*, whose important ingredients have been lost to history. There have been many debates as to what type of psychoactive material might have been in the beverage, and some have speculated, based on barley being one of the com-ponents, that some form of psychoactive ergot may have been included in the drink (Wasson et al.,

H3C
N–CH3
N
H
HO
H3CO
N,N-dimethyltryptamine
Bufotenine
5-Methoxy-DMT

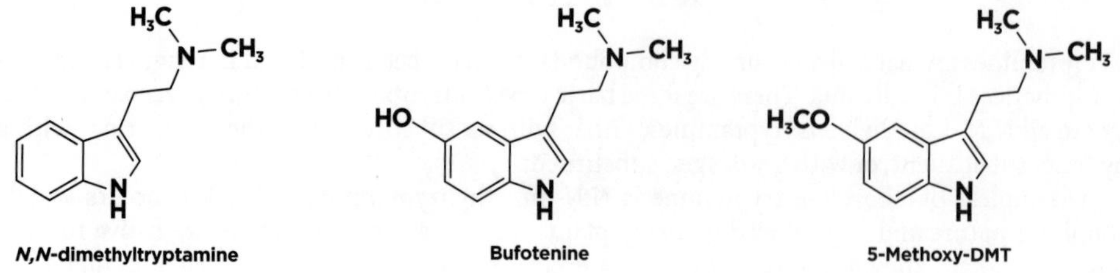

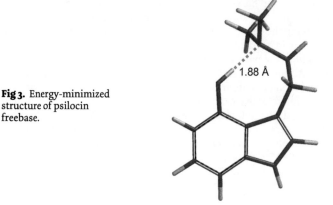

Fig 1. Three naturally occurring tryptamine chemotypes that are not orally active.

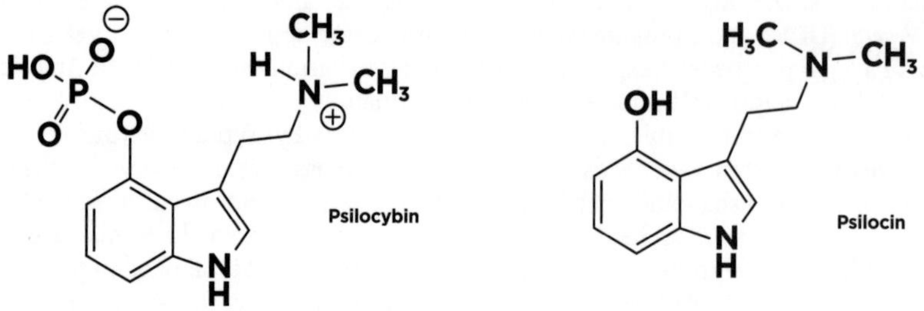

HO
P
O
CH3
H
N
CH3
N
H
Psilocybin
H3C
N–CH3
OH
Psilocin

Fig 2. The chemical structures of orally active psilocybin and psilocin.

Fig 3. Energy-minimized structure of psilocin freebase.

1.88 Å

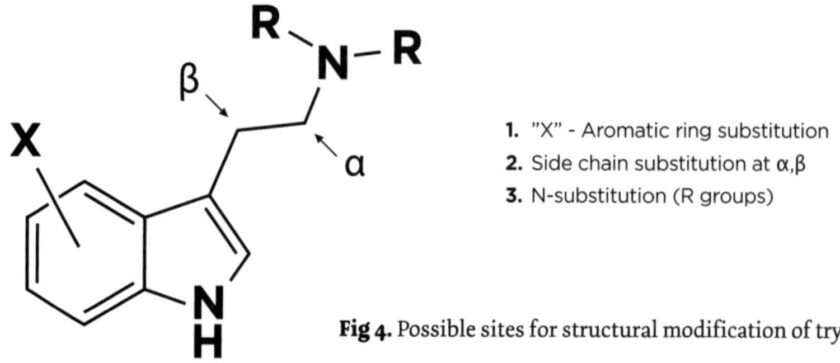

R
N–R
β
α
X
N
H
1. "X" - Aromatic ring substitution
2. Side chain substitution at α,β
3. N-substitution (R groups)

Fig 4. Possible sites for structural modification of tryptamines.

1978). By contrast, Berlant (2005) has argued that a type of psilocybe mushroom may have been the key ingredient in *kykeon*.

The identification of the ancient Vedic Soma, praised for its effects in the Rig-Vedas, also remains elusive. Although Wasson has argued persuasively that only the mushroom *Amanita muscaria* fits the physical description of the central component of Soma (Wasson, 1968; Wasson and Ingalls, 1971), there is no solid evidence that ingestion of this mushroom actually has the sort of psychoactive properties that would be expected of Soma. Recently, however, diggings were carried out in 2009 by an expedition of the Institute of Archaeography and Ethnography, Siberian Branch of the Russian Academy of Sciences, at 31 Xiongnu tumuli dated from the late 1st century B.C.E. to the early 1st century A.D. of the Noin-Ula burial ground in Mongolia (Polosmak, 2010). The expedition discovered preserved embroidered woolen textiles that filled a narrow space between the chamber's wooden walls and the coffin. The partially restored textiles depict an altar scene, with men in it who are speculated, from their style of clothing, to be Indo-Scythians or Indo-Parthians, performing a ritual indicating that they acknowledge a form of Zoroastrianism, with the symbol of a sacred fire altar. A king or possibly the priest is shown holding a mushroom in his hands that appears to belong to the family *Strophariaceae*, with an external appearance similar to *Psilocybe cubensis*.

An interesting feature of psilocybin and psilocin is the fact that they are orally active, whereas the other tryptamines discussed earlier are only active by insufflation, or if combined with a monoamine oxidase inhibitor. Psilocybin is dephosphorylated in the body to psilocin, so the latter molecule is the one of most interest. We addressed this issue in a study published in 1981, where we compared the solution side chain conformations of bufotenine with psilocin, as well as experimentally measuring their octanol-water Log P values, and the pKa values of their amines (Migliaccio et al., 1981). 360 MHz ^{1}H NMR spectra were recorded in $CDCl_3$ for bufotenine and psilocin freebases. Whereas spectral analysis indicated that the side chain of bufotenine preferred to exist in the *trans* conformation, the side chain of psilocin freebase highly favored the *gauche* conformation, indicating that the adjacent 4-hydroxy group was somehow influencing the side chain conformation. If the effect was purely a nonbonded steric one, the side chain would not be expected to favor conformations where it was folded closer to the 4-OH substituent.

The nature of this stabilization was therefore of some interest; it was speculated that it might result from an intramolecular hydrogen bond. Energy minimization using Hartree-Fock 6-31G* potentials (freebase in vacuum) revealed that intramolecular hydrogen bonding is likely in one gauche side-chain conformer of psilocin. The side-chain amino to 4-oxygen hydroxyl distance is 1.88 Å, with other bond angles and distances nearly ideal. The minimized structure is shown in figure 2.

The consequences of this intramolecular hydrogen bond are manifested as reduced basicity for the amino nitrogen of psilocin (pKa 8.47) compared to bufotenine (pKa 9.67), as well as increased hydrophobicity for psilocin (Log P 1.45) compared to bufotenine (Log P 1.19) (Migliaccio et al., 1981). At a physiological pH of 7.4, only about 0.5% of bufotenine will exist in the unprotonated (unionized) form, whereas about 8% of psilocin will exist in the unprotonated form. Recognizing that it is the unprotonated form of a base that is transported across membranes, psilocin therefore will more readily penetrate into the brain. The experimental Log P value of psilocin also indicates a more favorable lipid solubility than bufotenine. That may reflect the fact that to cross membranes, not only will the amine have to be unionized, but it must also undergo loss of solvation, and the intramolecular hydrogen bond will partially compensate for that in psilocin.

A final factor that is also likely important for the oral activity of psilocin relates to the mechanism of action for monoamine oxidase, which deaminates other tryptamines, such as DMT and 5-MeODMT, in the liver. Possible mechanisms in the first step of the deamination reaction are: 1. a single-electron transfer mechanism, and 2. a nucleophilic mechanism (Gaweska and Fitzpatrick, 2011). Importantly, with either mechanism, the first step involves access of the enzyme's flavin cofactor to the electrons of the basic amino group. In psilocin, however, the electrons are engaged in the intramolecular hydrogen bond with the phenolic 4-OH group, and would be less available for donation to the flavin cofactor of MAO.

STRUCTURAL MODIFICATIONS OF TRYPTAMINES

Conceivably, tryptamines could be modified on the aromatic portion, in the side chain, or on the nitrogen atom. It has been found that no substitutions on the aromatic portion of the molecule other than hydrogen (DMT), or 4-OH, or 5-OCH3 lead to active molecules. Thus, medicinal chemists have explored the effect of small alkyl groups on the side chain and a variety of different alkyl groups on the nitrogen.

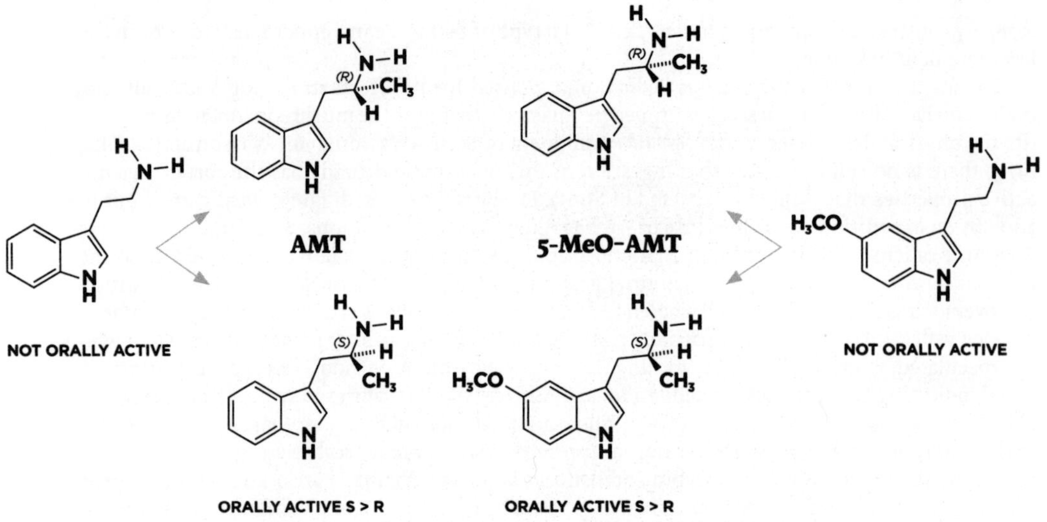

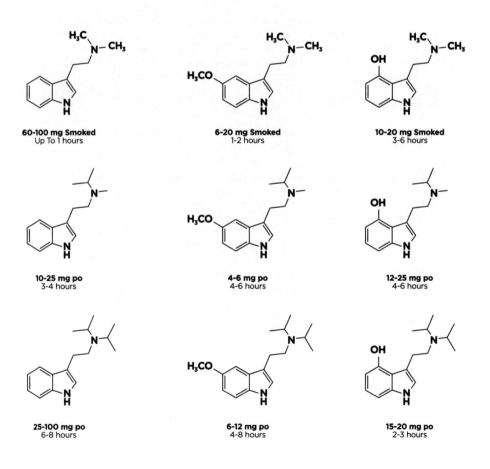

Fig. 5 Tryptamines with an alpha-methyl in the side chain.

Fig. 6 Tryptamine structures with approximate oral doses and durations of action. (Shulgin and Shulgin, 1997)

A methyl group attached to the alpha side chain position has proven to give the most active compounds, with the enantiomer having the S configuration being more potent than the R isomer. 5-methoxy-AMT is the most potent simple tryptamine that has been reported (Shulgin and Shulgin, 1997).

Although simple N-methylated tryptamines (DMT and 5-MeODMT) are not orally active, introduction of larger N-alkyl groups on the basic nitrogen leads to oral activity. In particular, an N-isopropyl group confers good oral activity. Figure 6 illustrates dosages and approximate duration of action for a variety of N-substituted tryptamines (Shulgin and Shulgin, 1997)

PHENETHYLAMINES

Although several naturally occurring tryptamines serve as templates for structural modification, only a single phenethylamine was available as a natural psychedelic. Dr. Arthur Heffter first identified mescaline, a simple phenethylamine, as the active component of the peyote cactus, *Lophophora williamsii* (Heffter, 1898). He isolated the various alkaloids present in the cactus, and in self-experiments found mescaline to be the compound that produced the psychoactive effects and colored visions characteristic of peyote. This cactus is native to the American Southwest and Northern Mexico and has been used for millennia by the indigenous peoples in that region. Analysis and radiocarbon dating of two peyote samples from a cave on the Rio Grande River, in Texas, were found to date between 3780–3660 B.C.E (El Seedi et al., 2005). This evidence supports the use of peyote by Native North Americans as long as 5700 years ago (Bruhn et al., 2002). Today, peyote is a sacrament used by the Native American Church in its all-night religious services.

MESCALINE

Although mescaline has relatively low potency, requiring a dose of about 250-400 mg of the sulfate salt, it served as the prototype for the phenethylamine-type psychedelics. Several hundred phenethylamines have been synthesized and tested as of today. As with the tryptamines, there are several sites for structural modification. Although the tryptamines are active psychedelics when they are tertiary amines, the phenethylamines generally do not tolerate N-substitution. Thus, the modifications can be carried out on the ring substituents as well as the side chain.

The earliest modifications were to change the orientations of the methoxy groups. Those changes led to inactive compounds, such as 2,3,4-trimethoxyphenethylamine (Slotta and Heller, 1930), and 2,4,5-trimethoxyphenethylamine (Dittrich, 1971)(Fig. 8). At least in the case of 2,3,4-trimethoxyphenethylamine, it was found to be very quickly metabolized *in vivo* compared with mescaline, and that could be the explanation for its lack of activity (Demisch and Seiler, 1975). Similar studies of 2,4,5-trimethoxyphenethylamine have not been carried out, but rapid deamination *in vivo* might also account for its lack of activity.

Interestingly, however, replacing the 4-methoxy of mescaline with higher-order alkoxy groups such as ethoxy, propoxy, and isopropoxy, led to compounds substantially more active than mescaline. In addition, 4-alkylthio substituents also led to highly active compounds (Fig. 9) (Shulgin and Shulgin, 1991).

Larger alkoxy groups replacing the 3-methoxy of mescaline did not lead to active compounds, although certain compounds with an alkylthio replacing the 3-methoxy did retain activity. Although 2,4,5-trimethoxyphenethylamine was not orally active, when the 4-methoxy was replaced by alkyl, halogen, or alkylthio groups (Fig. 10), surprisingly, the compounds were orally active and quite potent (Shulgin and Shulgin, 1991).

These compounds are all active within dose ranges averaging between 6-30 mg, depending on the substituent. Although it has not been studied, it seems possible that the enzyme that deaminates the side chain readily attacks a molecule with a 4-methoxy, whereas compounds with a hydrophobic 4-substituent may not be substrates for the enzyme. Many of these phenethylamines also have a fairly long duration of action (e.g., 12-15 hours).

A number of essential oils provided ideas for a variety of ring substitution patterns, as illustrated in figure 11.

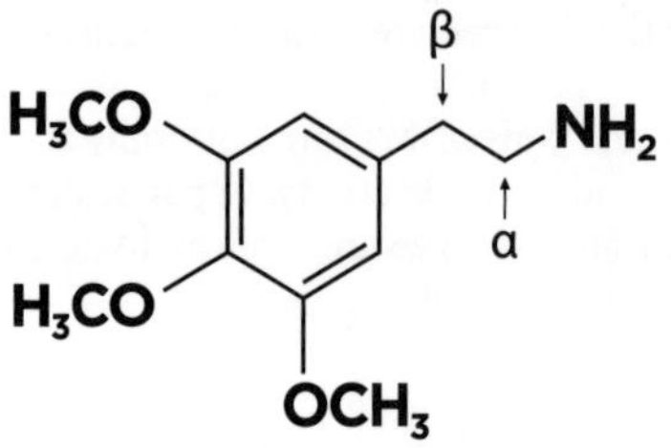

1. Aromatic ring substitution
2. Side chain substitution at α,β

Fig. 7 Mescaline, with locations where structural variation has been studied.

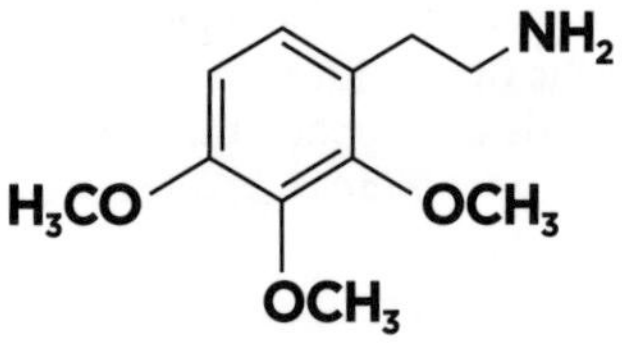

2,3,4-trimethoxyphenethylamine

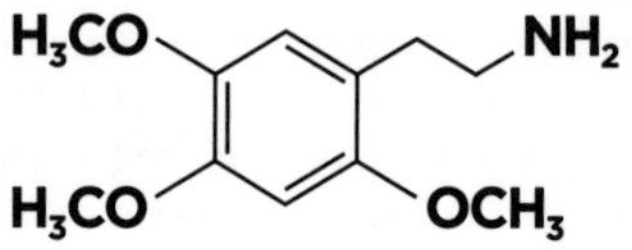

2,4,5-trimethoxyphenethylamine

Fig. 8 Inactive mescaline isomers.

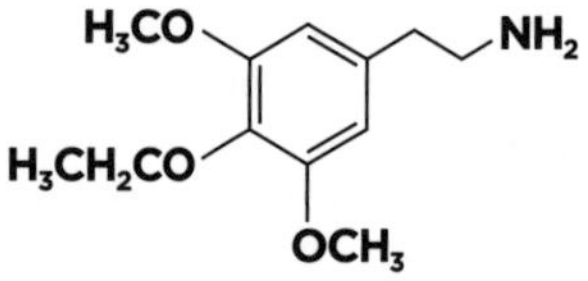

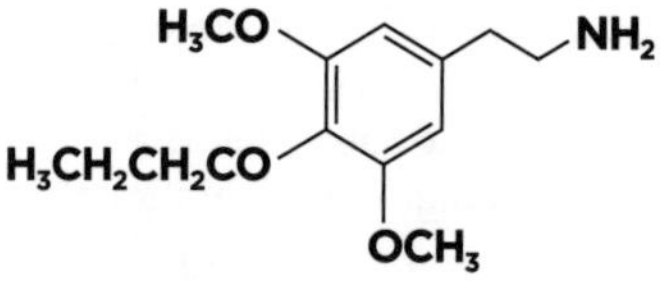

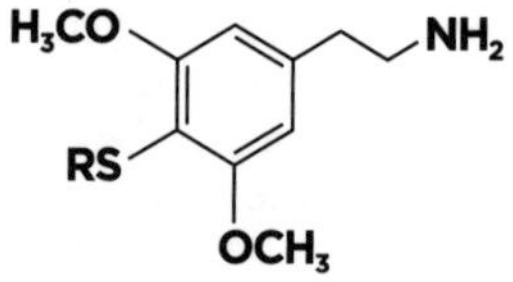

Fig. 9 Mescaline analogues with higher potency than mescaline.

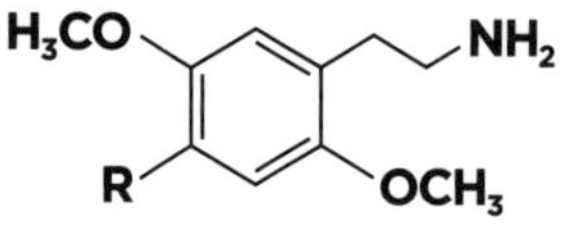

R = CH₃; 2C-D
R = Et; 2C-T2

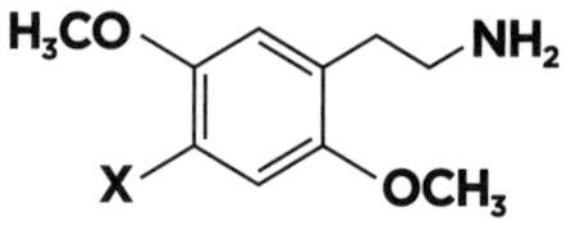

X = Br; 2C-B
X = I; 2C-I

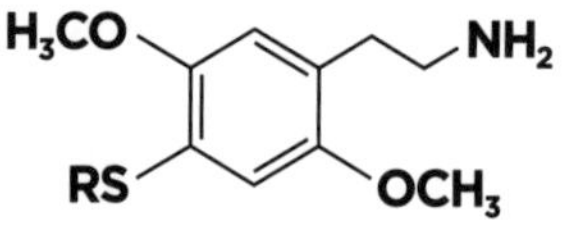

R = Et; 2C-E
R = nPr; 2C-T7

Fig. 10 Potent, orally active 2,4,5-substiuted phenethylamine psychedelics.

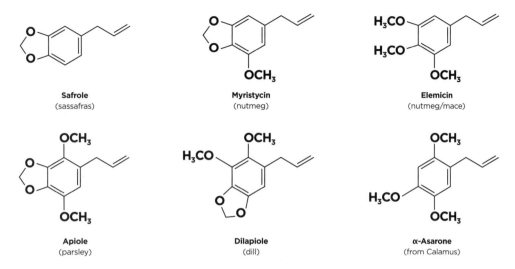

Fig. 11 Essential oils with substitution patterns that inspired novel psychedelics.

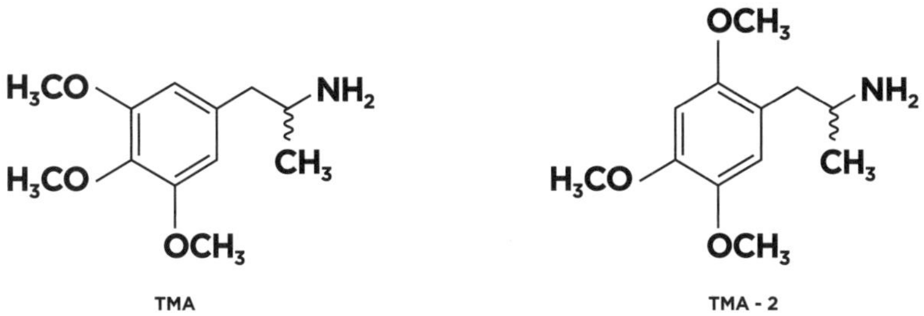

TMA

TMA - 2

Fig. 12 Structures of phenethylamines with an alpha-methyl in the side chain.

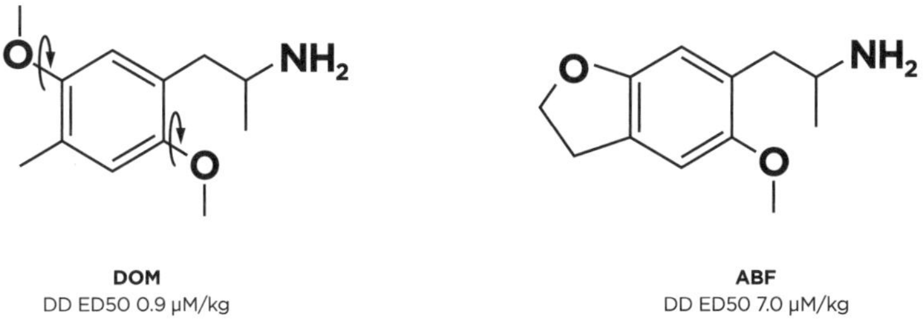

DOM
DD ED50 0.9 µM/kg

ABF
DD ED50 7.0 µM/kg

Fig. 13 The DOM molecule, with flexible methoxy groups, and the first benzofuran molecule with a constrained "methoxy." ED50 values are from the two-lever rat drug discrimination assay in rats trained to discriminate LSD from saline. ABF can be seen to be much less potent.

In addition to changes in ring-substitution patterns, it was also found that placing a methyl group at the alpha side-chain position gave active compounds (Fig. 12). These compounds are often referred to as substituted amphetamines, based on the fact that amphetamine itself has an alpha-methyl, which prevents rapid deamination by monoamine oxidases. The first such compound was 3,4,5-trimethoxyamphetamine (TMA), shown in figure 12. TMA has about twice the potency of mescaline (Peretz et al., 1955). TMA-2 has more than ten times the potency of mescaline, in spite of the fact that the non-methylated 2,4,5-trimethoxyphenethylamine is inactive! A large number of substituted amphetamine psychedelics have now been prepared and tested, and those experiments and testing results are detailed in the Shulgins' book, *PIHKAL* (Shulgin and Shulgin, 1991). It is also known that it is the R-(-)-enantiomers of the substituted amphetamines that are most potent, as contrasted with amphetamine or methamphetamine, where it is the S-(+)-enantiomer that is most potent as a stimulant (Dyer et al., 1973; Nichols et al., 1973; Shulgin, 1973).

Although the addition of the alpha-methyl to the side chain likely prevents metabolic deamination, it also enhances the efficacy of the molecules. That is, the unsubstituted phenethylamines are partial agonists, but their alpha-methyl congeners have significantly higher intrinsic activity at the PLC signaling pathway (Parrish et al., 2005).

Extension of the alpha-methyl to an alpha-ethyl abolishes activity (Standridge et al., 1976). Incorporation of the side chain into a trans-cyclopropylamine also leads to active compounds (Aldous et al., 1974; Cooper and Walters, 1972; Nichols et al., 1979; Pigott et al., 2012), but the corresponding cyclobutylamines are inactive (Nichols et al., 1984).

In addition to studies of the ring substituents and substitutions on the side chain, several studies have indicated that the methoxy groups must have a particular orientation, presumably to interact with polar residues within the receptor. Early on, we prepared a compound we called ABF, shown in figure 13, and found that in a rat drug discrimination assay, it had very little activity when compared with DOM, a congener with freely rotating methoxy groups.

This led us to prepare several series of compounds where the methoxy groups were tethered in an orientation that was "anti" with respect to the 4-substituent. To that end, we made the series of compounds in figure 14 to illustrate the active orientation of the methoxy groups, and that the oxygen at the 2-position fits into a more sterically restricted location in the receptor. Activities listed below each compound represent the ED50 value in rats trained to discriminate 0.08 mg of LSD tartrate from saline in the two-lever drug discrimination assay (Monte et al., 1996; Nichols et al., 1991; Schultz et al., 2008; Whiteside et al., 2002).

When either the 3- or 5-methoxy groups of mescaline were similarly tethered, the resulting compounds were inactive (Monte et al., 1997). They had higher affinity at the 5-HT2A receptor than mescaline, but their efficacy was markedly diminished. When the compound "bromofly" was made fully aromatic (i.e., double bonds were introduced into both of the furan rings) the molecule was even more potent, comparable to LSD in the rat drug discrimination assay (Parker et al., 1998).

Based on extensive design of rigid analogues of psychedelic amphetamine-type molecules in this author's laboratory over many years, it may be concluded that the active binding conformation of these molecules at the 5-HT2A receptor can be represented by Figure 15 (see, for example McLean et al., 2006). The side chain is proposed to reside in a plane nearly perpendicular to the plane of the aromatic ring. The 5-methoxy oxygen may be a hydrogen-bond acceptor from serine 5.42 in the receptor.

ERGOLINES

Ergolines have a tetracyclic nucleus with an indole aromatic system as its key pharmacophore. Naturally occurring ergot alkaloids have the R stereochemistry at the 5-position, as shown in figure 16, and the R configuration at the 8-position.

The substituents at the 8-position can vary, but most typically are complex cyclic peptoid-like moieties, such as in ergotamine. Ergotamine and similar ergot alkaloids are produced by the ergot fungus, most notably *Claviceps purpurea*, which can parasitize rye and barley, and is visible as dark curved and enlarged black growths, known as sclerotia, emerging from the grain stalk. The ergot alkaloids are very potent vasoconstrictors, and ingestion of breads containing significant amounts of ergot can cause prolonged peripheral vasospasms and vasoconstriction, ultimately leading to gangrene. Symptoms of ergot poisoning include burning sensations in the fingers and toes, and hallucinations. Once gangrene sets in, the fingers and toes become necrotic, and take on a black, charred appearance. More than 40,000 people died from an epidemic of ergotism during the Middle

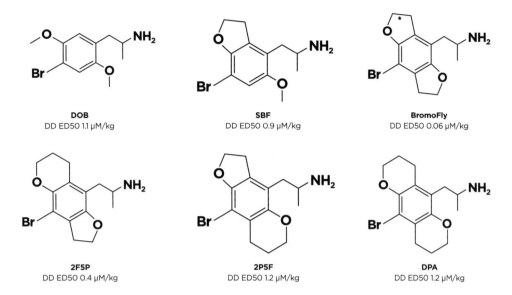

DOB
DD ED50 1.1 µM/kg

SBF
DD ED50 0.9 µM/kg

BromoFly
DD ED50 0.06 µM/kg

2F5P
DD ED50 0.4 µM/kg

2P5F
DD ED50 1.2 µM/kg

DPA
DD ED50 1.2 µM/kg

Fig. 14 Phenethylamines with constrained "methoxy" groups, comparing their potency to the flexible molecule DOB. Five-membered furan congeners were more potent than the corresponding six-membered pyran compounds.

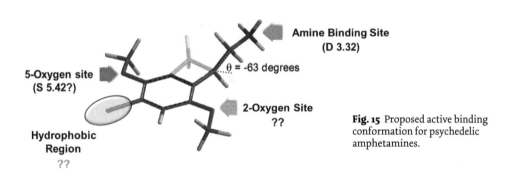

Fig. 15 Proposed active binding conformation for psychedelic amphetamines.

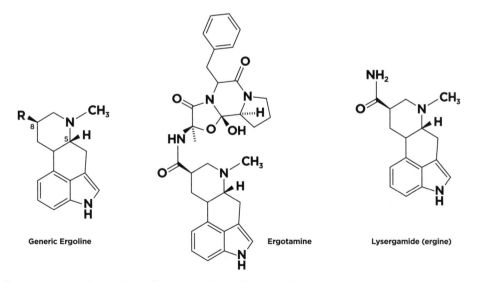

Generic Ergoline

Ergotamine

Lysergamide (ergine)

Fig. 16 Structures of a generic ergoline, ergotamine, and lysergamide.

211

Ages. Ergotism was referred to as St. Anthony's fire, due to the intense burning sensations in the limbs and the charred appearance of gangrenous fingers and toes. St. Anthony was the patron saint of ergotism victims.

In spite of the toxicity of ergot alkaloids, if the substituent at the 8-position is a simple amide, as in lysergamide (ergine), the vasoconstrictor pharmacology is markedly reduced, and instead, ergine can produce a mild hallucinogenic intoxication. Indeed, *Rivea corymbosa (Turbina corymbosa)* is a species of morning glory native throughout Latin America, from Mexico as far south as Peru. Their seeds contain ergine, were employed by the Aztecs for their intoxicant effect, and were known as *Ololuiqui*.

Ipomoea violaceae and *Ipomoea tricolor* are other species of morning glory whose seeds contain ergine. The former have white flowers that open at night, and the latter are commonly known as heavenly blue morning glories.

Knowledge of the psychoactive properties of the seeds from these flowers and the nature of their chemistry was unknown when Albert Hofmann first synthesized the diethylamide of lysergic acid, LSD-25, in 1938, but he later determined that the active principle was ergine (Hofmann and Tscherter, 1960), and was thus chemically related to LSD.

Research on lysergic acid derivatives has focused on three areas of the molecule, as shown in figure 17.

Although in theory, substituents could be introduced into the aromatic system, in practice the synthesis of such analogues is extremely difficult. The total synthesis of lysergic acid itself was considered by natural products chemists to be a sort of "Mount Everest" of chemistry. The first total synthesis, by Kornfeld et al., in 1956, was a tour de force at the time, and was not amenable to the synthesis of derivatives substituted in the aromatic ring(s) (Kornfeld et al., 1956).

One productive approach was to examine the effect of various alkyl groups attached at N(6) of LSD. Hashimoto et al. (1977) had previously studied the anti-serotonin and oxytocic activities of several of these compounds in rat uterus. The N(6) ethyl, propyl, and allyl compounds were more potent in that regard. We resynthesized a series of these analogues, and tested them in the two-lever drug discrimination assay in rats trained to discriminate saline from 0.08 mg/kg of LSD tartrate. In this assay, the ethyl, propyl, and allyl analogues were all more potent than LSD (table 1) (Hoffman and Nichols, 1985). These three compounds were subsequently reported to be at least as potent as LSD in humans, with the N(6) ethyl being somewhat more active then LSD itself (Shulgin and Shulgin, 1997).

A large number of different amides of lysergic acid have been studied over the years. Generally, any structural change from the *N,N*-diethyl, no matter how minor, leads to a dramatic loss in potency (e.g., see Pfaff et al., 1994). The high potency of LSD thus seems to depend specifically on the *N,N*-diethylamide moiety. We hypothesized that there might be a particular region of the receptor that was highly complementary to the diethylamide moiety. Our first simple experiment asked the question, "Is this region of the receptor stereochemically defined?" If the amide binding region was within the orthosteric binding site, and given that the receptor is made exclusively of L-amino acids, we predicted that a lysergic acid amide with a chiral substituent might show stereoselective effects. We thus prepared lysergic acid amides of R and S-2-aminobutane (Oberlender et al., 1992), shown in figure 18.

Shown below the two stereoisomers are the ED50 values in the two-lever drug discrimination assay in LSD-trained rats. Clearly, the stereoisomer with the 2-butyl substituent having the R configuration is approximately four times more potent than the stereoisomer with the S configuration in the 2-butyl substituent. This finding clearly indicated that the amide substituent engaged stereoselective elements of the receptor.

We next rigidified the diethylamide moiety of LSD to provide the cis-meso, trans-S,S-, and trans R,R-dimethylazetidines, shown in figure 19 (Nichols et al., 2002). Testing in the rat two-lever drug discrimination assay revealed that the stereoisomer with the S,S-dimethylazetidine had activity most similar to LSD itself.

Virtual docking of LSD into a homology model of the human 5-HT2A receptor indicated that the diethylamide likely interacted with a portion of extracellular loop 2 (EL2), which connects the extracellular end of transmembrane helix 4 to the extracellular end of helix 5. John McCorvy, a senior graduate student working in my laboratory, then prepared receptors with mutations in EL2: L228A, L228V, L229A, L229S, L229I, A230L, and A230N (McCorvy, 2012). Comparing their affinities to displace [³H]LSD in each of the receptors showed that LSD and the S,S-azetidide most closely resembled each other, and also that the polar mutation L229S had the most dramatic effect on each azetidide stereoisomer. Thus, we proposed that the S,S-azetidide represented the binding conformation

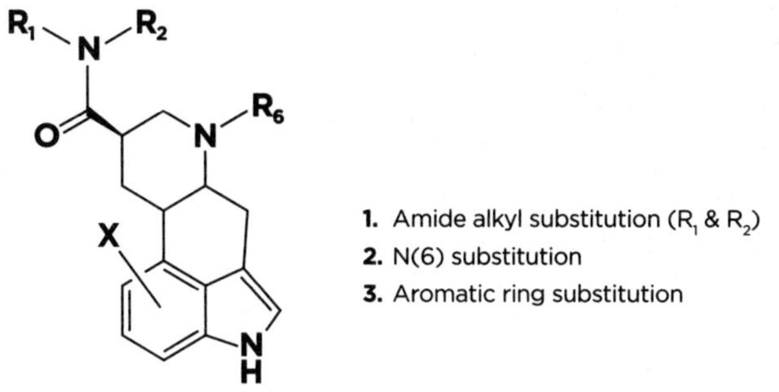

1. Amide alkyl substitution (R₁ & R₂)
2. N(6) substitution
3. Aromatic ring substitution

Fig. 17 Areas for structural modification in lysergic acid amides.

Table 1. Potency comparison of N(6)-alkyl-norLSD derivatives in the rat two-lever drug discrimination in rats trained to discriminate LSD from saline. ED50 values are in mM/kg.

R	ED50	Potency *
H	No Sub	NA
CH_3 (LSD)	0.046	1.00
CH_2CH_3 (Ethlad)	0.020	2.30
C_3H_7 (ProLad)	0.037	1.24
CH_2CHCH_2 (ALLAD)	0.013	3.54
$CH(CH_3)_2$ (iPrLAD)	0.10	0.46
C_4H_9 (BuLAD)	0.357	0.13
CH_2CH_2Ph	No sub	NA

* Relative to LSD; Based on ED50s.

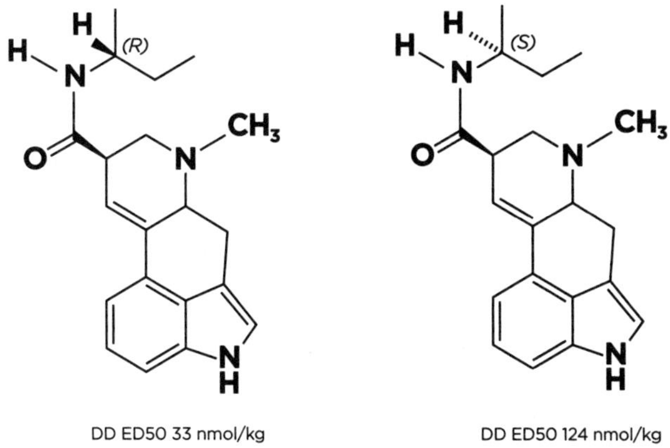

DD ED50 33 nmol/kg

DD ED50 124 nmol/kg

Fig. 18 Comparison of the behavioral potency of the lysergic acid amides of R and S 2-butylamine. ED50 values are from the two-lever drug discrimination assay in rats trained to discriminate LSD from saline.

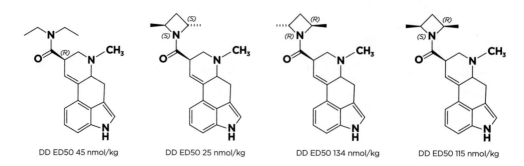

DD ED50 45 nmol/kg   DD ED50 25 nmol/kg   DD ED50 134 nmol/kg   DD ED50 115 nmol/kg

Fig. 19 Comparative potencies of LSD and the stereoisomers of lysergic acid amides prepared from the three possible 2,4-dimethylazetidines. Values are from two-lever drug discrimination assays in LSD-trained rats.

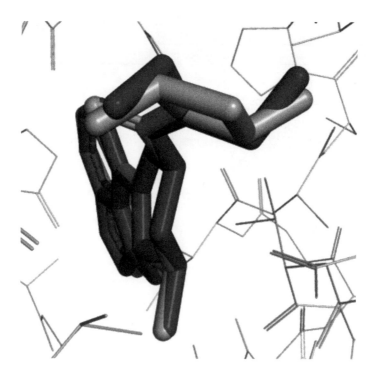

Fig. 20 Superposition of lysergic acid S,S-azetidide onto the crystal structure conformation of LSD bound in the serotonin 5-HT2B receptor (Wacker et al., 2017).

of the more flexible diethylamide groups of LSD, and further, that residue L229 in EL2 directly inter-acted with the diethylamide moiety of LSD.

In 2017, it was possible to obtain the x-ray crystal structure of LSD bound within the serotonin 5-HT2B receptor (Wacker et al., 2017). The *S,S*-azetidide stereoisomer could essentially be superim-posed on the LSD molecule in the crystal structure, where the dark structure in figure 20 is LSD, and the grey structure that of the *S,S*-azetidide.

In the same report, it was experimentally observed using cloned human 5-HT2A receptors that LSD had a very slow association rate with the 5-HT2A receptor at 37 °C, and an even slower dissocia-tion rate, requiring several hours for the LSD molecule to be completely dissociated from the recep-tor. It was seen that EL2 folds over the bound LSD molecule, essentially "trapping" it in the receptor so that it only dissociates with great difficulty. Furthermore, LSD was found to be a highly biased ligand, markedly recruiting β-arrestin2 relative to G protein-mediated signaling.

Molecular dynamics simulations in the same report indicated that EL2 was not very mobile, consistent with the receptor-binding experiments. However, when L229 was mutated to L229A, the receptor kinetics of LSD were changed dramatically, with a rapid on and off rate. In addition, β-ar-restin2 recruitment was also markedly attenuated in the L229A mutant, suggesting that the long residence time of LSD in the receptor was correlated with its bias for β-arrestin2 recruitment.

CONCLUSIONS

Natural products of the tryptamine, phenethylamine, and ergoline types are exemplified in na-ture. Medicinal chemists have exploited these natural product chemotypes to develop structure-ac-tivity relationships. Active tryptamines have largely been confined to ring-unsubstituted or 4- or 5-oxygenated molecules, with most of the structural variation being in larger alkyl groups attached to the basic nitrogen atom, comprising a relatively small number of new molecules. By contrast, following mescaline as the single prototype for psychedelic phenethylamines, literally hundreds of novel molecules have been synthesized. A large variety of ring substituents have been examined, with some compounds approaching the potency of LSD. The binding orientations of the methoxy groups have been determined, and the active side-chain conformation has been proposed. Finally, starting with lysergic acid amide and lysergic acid diethylamide, it has been found that replacing the N(6)-methyl of LSD with ethyl, allyl, or propyl leads to compounds with potency in humans sim-ilar to LSD. The diethyl groups of LSD have been rigidified as stereoisomeric 2,4-dimethylazetidines to map their binding orientations at the receptor. In addition, the crystal structure of LSD bound within the serotonin 5-HT2B receptor has recently been determined, which validated the prediction that the lysergic acid amide of the S,S-dimethylazetidine would be the active conformation. It was also discovered that extracellular loop 2 of the receptor folds over LSD after it binds, resulting in a very long receptor occupancy, as well as a bias for beta-arrestin 2 signaling relative to signaling via G proteins.

REFERENCES

Aldous, F.A., Barrass, B.C., Brewster, K., Buxton, D.A., Green, D.M., Pinder, R.M., Rich, P., Skeels, M., Tutt, K.J., 1974. Structure-activity relationships in psychotomimetic phenylalkylamines. *J. Med. Chem* 17(10), 1100-1111.

Berlant, S.R., 2005. The entheomycological origin of Egyptian crowns and the esoteric underpinnings of Egyptian religion. *J. Ethnopharmacol* 102(2), 275-288.

Bruhn, J.G., et al., De Smet, P.A., El Seedi, H.R., Beck, O., 2002. Mescaline use for 5700 years. *Lancet* 359(9320), 1866.

Cooper, P.D., Walters, G.C., 1972. Stereochemical Requirements of the Mescaline Receptor. *Nature* 238(5359), 96-98.

Demisch, L., Seiler, N., 1975. Oxidative metabolism of mescaline in the central nervous system--V. In- vitro deamination of mescaline to 3,4,5-trimethoxy-benzoic acid. *Biochem Pharmacol* 24(5), 575-580.

Dittrich, A., 1971. Alteration of behavioural changes induced by 3,4,5-trimethoxyphenethylamine (mescaline) by pre-treatment with 2,4,5-trimethoxyphenethylamine. A self-experiment. *Psychopharmacologia* 21(3), 229-237.

Dyer, D.C., et al., Nichols, D.E., Rusterholz, D.B., Barfknecht, C.F., 1973. Comparative effects of stereoisomers of psychot-omimetic phenylisopropylamines. *Life Sci* 13(7), 885-896.

El Seedi, H.R., et al., Smet, P.A., Beck, O., Possnert, G., Bruhn, J.G., 2005. Prehistoric peyote use: alkaloid analysis and radiocarbon dating of archaeological specimens of Lophophora from Texas. *J. Ethnopharmacol* 101(1-3), 238-242.

Gaweska, H., Fitzpatrick, P.F., 2011. Structures and Mechanism of the Monoamine Oxidase Family. *Biomol Concepts* 2(5), 365-377.

Hashimoto, H., et al., Hayashi, M., Nakahara, Y., Niwaguchi, T., Ishii, H., 1977. Actions of D-lysergic acid diethylamide

(LSD) and its derivatives on 5-hydroxytryptamine receptors in the isolated uterine smooth muscle of the rat. *Eur J. Pharmacol* 45(4), 341-348.

Heffter, A., 1898. Ueber pellote. Beitrag zur chemischen und pharmakologischen kenntnis der cacteen. *Naunyn Schmiedebergs Arch Exp Path Pharmacol* 40, 385-429.

Hoffman, A.J., Nichols, D.E., 1985. Synthesis and LSD-like discriminative stimulus properties in a series of N(6)-alkyl norlysergic acid N,N-diethylamide derivatives. *J. Med Chem* 28(9), 1252-1255.

Hofmann, A., et al., Frey, A., Ott, H., PETR, Z.T., Troxler, F., 1958. [Elucidation of the structure and the synthesis of psilocybin]. *Experientia* 14(11), 397-399.

Hofmann, A., Tscherter, H., 1960. [Isolation of lysergic acid alkaloids from the Mexican drug ololiuqui (Rivea corymbosa (L.) Hall.f.)]. *Experientia* 16, 414.

Kornfeld, E.C., et al., Fornefeld, E.J., Kline, G.B., Mann, M.J., Morrison, D.E., Jones, R.G., Woodward, R.B., 1956. The Total Synthesis of Lysergic Acid. *Journal of the American Chemical Society* 78(13), 3087-3114.

McCorvy, J.D., 2012. *Mapping the binding site of the 5-HT2A receptor using mutagenesis and ligand libraries: insights into the molecular actions of psychedelics, medicinal chemistry and molecular pharmacology.* Purdue, West Lafayette, IN.

McLean, T.H., et al., Parrish, J.C., Braden, M.R., Marona-Lewicka, D., Gallardo-Godoy, A., Nichols, D.E., 2006. 1-Aminomethylbenzocycloalkanes: conformationally restricted hallucinogenic phenethylamine analogues as functionally selective 5-HT2A receptor agonists. *J. Med. Chem* 49(19), 5794-5803.

Migliaccio, G.P., et al., Shieh, T.L., Byrn, S.R., Hathaway, B.A., Nichols, D.E., 1981. Comparison of solution conformational preferences for the hallucinogens bufotenine and psilocin using 360-MHz proton NMR spectroscopy. *J. Med Chem* 24(2), 206-209.

Monte, A.P., et al., Marona-Lewicka, D., Parker, MA, Wainscott, D.B., Nelson, D.L., Nichols, D.E., 1996. Dihydrobenzofuran analogues of hallucinogens. 3. Models of 4-substituted (2,5-dimethoxyphenyl)alkylamine derivatives with rigidified methoxy groups. *J. Med. Chem* 39(15), 2953-2961.

Monte, A.P., et al., Waldman, S.R., Marona-Lewicka, D., Wainscott, D.B., Nelson, D.L., Sanders-Bush, E., Nichols, D.E., 1997. Dihydrobenzofuran analogues of hallucinogens. 4. Mescaline derivatives. *J. Med. Chem* 40(19), 2997-3008.

Nichols, D.E., et al., Barfknecht, C.F., Rusterholz, D.B., Benington, F., Morin, R.D., 1973. Asymmetric synthesis of psychotomimetic phenylisopropylamines. *J. Med Chem* 16(5), 480-483.

Nichols, D.E., et al., , 1979. Resolution and absolute configuration of trans-2-(2,5-dimethoxy-4- methylphenyl)cyclopropylamine, a potent hallucinogen analogue. *J. Med Chem* 22(4), 458-460.

Nichols, D.E., et al., 1984. Synthesis and evaluation of substituted 2-phenylcyclobutylamines as analogues of hallucinogenic phenethylamines: lack of LSD-like biological activity. *J. Med. Chem* 27(9), 1108-1111.

Nichols, D.E., et al., 1991. 2,3-Dihydrobenzofuran analogues of hallucinogenic phenethylamines. *J. Med Chem* 34(1), 276-281.

Nichols, D.E., et al., 2002. Lysergamides of isomeric 2,4-dimethylazetidines map the binding orientation of the diethylamide moiety in the potent hallucinogenic agent N,N-diethyllysergamide (LSD). *J. Med. Chem* 45(19), 4344-4349.

Nichols, D.E., Frescas, S., Marona-Lewicka, D., Kurrasch-Orbaugh, D.M., 2002. Lysergamides of isomeric 2,4-dimethylazetidines map the binding orientation of the diethylamide moiety in the potent hallucinogenic agent N,N-diethyllysergamide (LSD). *J. Med. Chem* 45(19), 4344-4349.

Nichols, D.E., Jadhav, K.P., Oberlender, R.A., Zabik, J.E., Bossart, J.F., Hamada, A., Miller, D.D., 1984. Synthesis and evaluation of substituted 2-phenylcyclobutylamines as analogues of hallucinogenic phenethylamines: lack of LSD-like biological activity. *J. Med. Chem* 27(9), 1108-1111.

Nichols, D.E., Snyder, S.E., Oberlender, R., Johnson, M.P., Huang, X.M., 1991. 2,3-Dihydrobenzofuran analogues of hallucinogenic phenethylamines. *J. Med Chem* 34(1), 276-281.

Nichols, D.E., Woodard, R., Hathaway, B.A., Lowy, M.T., Yom, K.W., 1979. Resolution and absolute configuration of trans-2-(2,5-dimethoxy-4- methylphenyl)cyclopropylamine, a potent hallucinogen analogue. *J. Med Chem* 22(4), 458-460.

Oberlender, R., et al., Pfaff, R.C., Johnson, M.P., Huang, X.M., Nichols, D.E., 1992. Stereoselective LSD-like activity in d-lysergic acid amides of (R)- and (S)-2-aminobutane. *J. Med Chem* 35(2), 203-211.

Parker, MA, et al., Marona-Lewicka, D., Lucaites, V.L., Nelson, D.L., Nichols, D.E., 1998. A novel (benzodifuranyl)aminoalkane with extremely potent activity at the 5-HT2A receptor. *J. Med. Chem* 41(26), 5148-5149.

Parrish, J.C., et al., Braden, M.R., Gundy, E., Nichols, D.E., 2005. Differential phospholipase C activation by phenylalkylamine serotonin 5-HT2A receptor agonists. *J Neurochem* 95(6), 1575-1584.

Peretz, D.I., et al., Smythies, J.R., Gibson, W.C., 1955. A new hallucinogen: 3,4,5-trimethoxyphenyl-beta-aminopropane (with notes on a stroboscopic phenomenon). *J. Mental. Sci* 101, 317-329.

Pfaff, R.C., et al., Huang, X., Marona-Lewicka, D., Oberlender, R., Nichols, D.E., 1994. Lysergamides revisited. *NIDA Res. Monogr* 146, 52-73.

Pigott, A., et al., Frescas, S., McCorvy, J.D., Huang, X.P., Roth, B.L., Nichols, D.E., 2012. Trans-2-(2,5-Dimethoxy-4-iodophenyl)cyclopropylamine and trans-2-(2,5-dimethoxy-4-bromophenyl)cyclopropylamine as potent agonists for the 5-HT(2) receptor family. *Beilstein J Org Chem* 8, 1705-1709.

Polosmak, N.V., 2010. We drank soma, we became immortal. *Science Firsthand* 2 (26), 62-71.

Schultes, R.E., 1940. Teonanacatl: The Narcotic Mushroom of the Aztecs. *American Anthropologist* 42(3), 429-443.

Schultes, R.E., Hofmann, A., 1979. *Plants of the Gods. Origins of Hallucinogenic Use.* Alfred van der Marck Editions, New York.

Schultes, R.E., Hofmann, A., 1980. *The botany and chemistry of hallucinogens*, Rev. and enl. 2d ed. Thomas, Springfield, Illinois.

Schultz, D.M., et al., Prescher, J.A., Kidd, S., Marona-Lewicka, D., Nichols, D.E., Monte, A., 2008. 'Hybrid' benzofuran-benzopyran congeners as rigid analogs of hallucinogenic phenethylamines. *Bioorg. Med Chem* 16(11), 6242-6251.

Shulgin, A., Shulgin, A., 1991. *PIHKAL: A chemical love story*. Transform Press, Berkeley, CA.

Shulgin, A.T., 1973. Stereospecific requirements for hallucinogenesis. *J. Pharm. Pharmacol* 25(3), 271-272.

Shulgin, A.T., Shulgin, A., 1997. *TIHKAL: The continuation.* Transform Press, Berkeley, CA.

Slotta, K.H., Heller, H., 1930. Uber beta-Phenethylamine. I. Mezcalin-ahnlicher Substanzen. *Chem. Ber.* 63, 3029-3044.

Späth, E 1919. Monatsch. *Chem.* 40, 129.

Standridge, R.T., et al., Howell, H.G., Gylys, J.A., Partyka, R.A., Shulgin, A.T., 1976. Phenylakylamines with potential psychotherapeutic utility. 1. 2-Amino-1- (2,5-dimethoxy-4-methylphenyl)butane. *J. Med. Chem* 19(12), 1400-1404.

Torres, C.M., Repke, D.B., 2006. *Anadenanthera. Visionary Plant of Ancient South America.* The Haworth Press, Inc., New York.

Wacker, D., et al., Wang, S., McCorvy, J.D., Betz, R.M., Venkatakrishnan, A.J., Levit, A., Lansu, K., Schools, Z.L., Che, T., Nichols, D.E., Shoichet, B.K., Dror, R.O., Roth, B.L., 2017. Crystal Structure of an LSD-Bound Human Serotonin Receptor. *Cell* 168(3), 377-389, e312.

Wasson, R.G., 1957. Seeking the Magic Mushroom. *Life Magazine,* May 13 1957: 100-120

Wasson, R.G., 1968. *Soma: divine mushroom of immortality.* Harcourt Brace, New York.

Wasson, R.G., et al., Hofmann, A., Ruck, C.A.P., 1978. *The Road to Eleusis. Unveiling the Secret of the Mysteries.* Harcourt Brace Jovanovich, Inc., New York.

Wasson, R.G., Ingalls, D.H., 1971. The soma of the Rig Veda: what was it? *J. Am. Orient. Soc* 91, 169-187.

Weil, A.T., Davis, W., 1994. Bufo alvarius: a potent hallucinogen of animal origin. *J. Ethnopharmacol* 41(1-2), 1-8.

Whiteside, M.S., et al., Kurrasch-Orbaugh, D., Marona-Lewicka, D., Nichols, D.E., Monte, A., 2002. Substituted hexahydrobenzodipyrans as 5-HT2A/2C receptor probes. Bioorg. *Med. Chem* 10(10), 3301-3306.

SESSION II

MEXICO & CENTRAL AMERICA

Fertile Grounds? – Peyote and the Human Reproductive System

Stacy B. Schaefer, PhD

Professor Emerita
Department of Anthropology,
California State University,
Chico, California

ABSTRACT

This paper examines the ingestion of the mind-altering peyote cactus, (*Lophophora williamsii*, endemic from the borderlands of Texas to Central Mexico), its medicinal properties, and how it may interact with the human reproductive system, specifically in women. The influence of peyote on pregnancy will be discussed through scientific studies involving peyote alkaloids such as mescaline, as well as qualitative data collected through ethnographic interviews with indigenous women from the Huichol Indian culture in Mexico and members of the Native American Church (NAC) in the United States. The paper will briefly compare the practice of peyote consumption by pregnant Huichol women, and ayahuasca tea consumption by pregnant ayahuasca church members. From personal perspectives informed through bioassays and participant/observation in Huichol and NAC peyote ceremonies, the topics of menstruation and fertility will be examined. Information grounded in biomedical and fertility research will be presented to hypothesize the interplay that may occur between peyote alkaloids, the nervous and endocrine systems, and the human reproductive system. Peyote, its medicinal qualities, and the interrelationship between peyote and women, specifically through pregnancy and the female reproductive system, are the themes highlighted in this paper. This report may have broader implications for other serotonergic entheogens.

INTRODUCTION

In 1967, the first Ethnopharmacologic Search for Psychoactive Drugs conference served as a landmark in the multidisciplinary quest to discover and explore novel psychoactive plants and drugs. Just one year later, American anthropologists Peter T. Furst and Barbara G. Myerhoff were the first outsiders to participate in and document a Huichol peyote pilgrimage to Wirikuta, the sacred desert in the Mexican state of San Luis Potosí, led by the Huichol Indian shaman apprentice, Ramón Medina Silva. The Norwegian explorer and anthropologist Carl Lumholtz was the first to note this annual pilgrimage in the 1890's (Lumholtz, 1900, 1902). However, although he never had the opportunity to join Huichols on their sacred journey to the peyote desert, he did have an opportunity to eat peyote when trekking with some Huichol companions in their sierra homelands, where native shrines, sacred caves, and god-houses dot the countryside. He writes:

> Under ordinary circumstances the plant (peyote) was nauseating to me; but now, when I was thirsty and tired, I could, rather to my surprise, swallow the cool, slightly acid cuts (sections of peyote) without difficulty. I found them not only refreshing, quenching my thirst and allaying hunger, but also capable...of taking away any sense of fa-

tigue, and I felt stimulated, as if I had had some strong drink. ... during the night I suffered from the after effects of the drug, which when my eyes were closed, showed themselves in colour visions consisting of beautiful purple and green flashes and zig-zags... (Lumholtz, 1902: 178-179)

Barbara Myerhoff also shared her narrative of the first time she consumed peyote. She writes:

.......after an inestimable period of time I began to be aware of a growing euphoria; I was flooded with feelings of goodwill. With great delight I began to notice sounds... Time and space evaporated as I floated about in the darkness and vague images be-gan to develop...I sat concentrating on a mythical little animal...the little fellow and I had entered a yarn painting and he sat precisely in the middle of the composition. I watched him fade and finally disappear into a hole ... (Myerhoff, 1974: 43-44)

This event took place prior to the pilgrimage she and Furst would take with Ramón and his ex-tended family to "hunt", harvest, and consume this mind-altering cactus that enables Huichols to intimately commune with their gods. This pioneering work resulted in Myerhoff's 1974 ethnograph-ic book *Peyote Hunt: The Sacred Journey of the Huichol Indians*, and Furst's 1969 documentary movie *To Find Our Life: The Peyote Hunt of the Huichols of Mexico*.

Now let's fast forward to 1987. I was a doctoral student in anthropology at UCLA working under the guidance of Johannes Wilbert, the same mentor who had supervised the research of Furst and Myerhoff. That year, I myself participated in the peyote pilgrimage with a large group of Huichols from the San José temple. Participating in this pilgrimage was a transformative experience, for not only did I gain a much more intimate understanding of my companions and their peyote traditions and beliefs, but the experience was an important event in my own personal development. It was challenging to participate in as well as document the journey. The authorities of the temple group had granted me permission to photograph the journey, and I was even instructed at times by the leading shaman as to what subjects would be important for me to include.

Weeks later, when I returned to the community to share copies of the photographs, one of my Huichol companions abruptly walked up to me, obviously disturbed, and in an assertive manner told me: "You *tewaris* (outsiders), you come on the pilgrimage, take photos, you even eat the peyote. But you never ask 'why" to the peyote. You never ask 'why'. Well, I am going to tell you why: Peyote is everything. It is the crossing of the souls. It is everything that is. Without peyote, nothing would exist."

Initially, I was taken aback by this confrontation, but in retrospect, I welcomed it because his challenge motivated me to learn everything I could about this innocuous-looking, yet powerful, entheogenic cactus. Since then, I have participated in three more peyote pilgrimages to Wirikuta, and in many peyote ceremonies in the Sierra. For over eight years, beginning in 1993, I also learned about peyote from the Mexican-American "dealers" in South Texas, who are federally licensed to sell peyote to members of the Native American Church (NAC), and from NAC members. I have partici-pated in more than two dozen NAC meetings in the "Peyote Gardens" of South Texas. Over the years since that first remarkable peyote pilgrimage, I am reminded that there will always be more to learn about this enigmatic plant.

In 1996, I began initial research on the topic of pregnancy and peyote, providing Huichol and Western scientific perspectives, and I published a seminal article on this subject (Schaefer, 1996b). At that time, I learned about the origin and spread of ayahuasca churches in Brazil and beyond, which led me to a preliminary inquiry into the use of ayahuasca during pregnancy, and to a compar-ison with peyote. This paper summarizes what is known to date on this topic, and provides an in-teresting comparison between two major entheogenic families, the phenethylamines (peyote) and tryptamines (ayahuasca), relative to women's health.

METHODOLOGY

It may be useful to the reader to provide an overview of the methodologies of cultural anthro-pology. As a cultural anthropologist, I have been trained to carry out qualitative ethnographic field-work. For me, this has involved living with Huichol family members on their ranches, learning from the women to become a master weaver on the Huichol back-strap loom, forming kinship ties as a godmother to various children in the family, and accompanying the family in their domestic and religious traditions. These activities have spanned the years from 1977 to the present.

My research approach is called participant/observation; it includes partaking of peyote within this cultural context, and conducting formal and informal interviews with my many Huichol consultants. This kind of fieldwork is an immersive experience; learning the language of Huichol ideas, concepts, and metaphors is necessary to decoding the information they have shared with me. This is to discern the emic perspective, the cultural viewpoint of the group being studied.

Another component to my research methodology brings an etic perspective to the study, and incorporates the knowledge and information that Western science can provide about the world, nature, humans, life, and even death. Scientific inquiries can bring meaningful explanations along Western ideological lines to the questions addressed. In my research, I incorporate the etic approach primarily through the scholarly literature and in consulting with experts in pertinent fields of study.

Both the objective and the subjective perspectives can be integrated to provide a holistic understanding of the world, and in many ways explain the same phenomena; perhaps the only difference is in the language by which these phenomena are conveyed. This is what has been termed "natural modeling" by Johannes Wilbert in his discussion of tobacco shamanism (Wilbert, 1987). I have utilized the methodologies described above to understand the peyote plant from various levels. These include ethnobotanical knowledge held by botanists, chemists, and Huichol shamans; the preparation and consumption of peyote as it was observed and discussed by Huichol consultants; the integration of tobacco and other desert-dwelling plants as experienced by shamans and understood by medical doctors and botanists; peyote visions expressed by Huichol pilgrims and explained by neurobiologists; and cultural traditions and the meaning attributed to the peyote experience as seen by Huichol participants and Western psychologists (Schaefer, 1996a, 2004, 2005, 2011).

PEYOTE: THE PLANT

Peyote is a low, grey-green, spineless cactus that naturally occurs in harsh landscapes which include both the Tamaulipan thorn scrub habitat from South Texas across the Mexican border, as well as the Chihuahuan Desert from West Texas south to San Luis Potosí, Mexico (Fig. 1). The oldest evidence of peyote and its importance to prehistoric peoples comes from ancient sites from Coahuila, Mexico, to the Lower Pecos region of Texas. Necklaces of dried peyote strung beadlike on fiber cord have been found associated with burials in rock shelters that date from 800 A.D. to as far back as 6000 B.C. (El-Seedi et al., 2005). Along the Pecos River in West Texas, peyote sam-

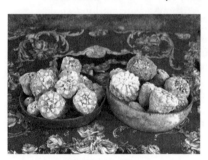

Fig. 1 Peyote (*Lophophora williamsii*) collected in Wirikuta and placed in votive bowls. Photo by Stacy B. Schaefer

ples dating to around 5000 B.C. were discovered in the Shumla Caves. After careful analysis, researcher Martin Terry and his team were intrigued when they discovered that these samples were composed of a mixture of peyote and other plant material, and appear to have been intentionally created as plant effigies (Terry et. al., 2006). This region is filled with spectacular rock art; the artists appear to have most likely been proto-Uto-Aztecan speakers. Some of the themes in the rock art along the Rio Grande River north of Eagle Pass, Texas, may include renderings of powerful peyote-related experiences and beliefs (Boyd and Dering, 1996, Boyd, 2003, 2016). Light, compact, and potent, peyote could very well have been a trade item along with other precious goods, such as salt and obsidian, that were carried along the pre-Columbian trade networks (Weigand, 1981).

Through the centuries, this precious psychoactive cactus was considered to be sacred by many indigenous people, and called the "devil's root" by Spanish missionaries and other Christian officials. Known by the Aztecs as "peyotl" in the Nahuatl language, "hikuri" by the Huichol Indians, and "medicine" by many Native American tribe members, its botanical name is *Lophophora williamsii* (Lem. Ex Salm-Dyk) J. M. Coult.[1] Peyote contains more than 60 alkaloids, yet little is known about the effects many of these have on the human body. Phenylethylamines and tetrahydroisoquinolines make up more than half of the naturally occurring chemical compounds in the plant. Mescaline (3,4,5-trimethoxyphenethylamine) was identified by chemist Arthur Heffter in 1897 as the principal alkaloid responsible for peyote's mind-altering effects. Research on isoquinoline alkaloids indicates that they, or other monoamine oxidase inhibitors (MAOIs) in the tissue of peyote, may enable normally orally inactive compounds to become orally active (Shulgin & Perry, 2002; Bruhn et. al., 1978).

---

1. Most indigenous groups that use peyote have a name for this revered plant in their own language.

PEYOTE AS MEDICINE

With its abundance of alkaloids, peyote is like a virtual pharmacy. It is no wonder that this plant is also used for medicinal purposes. Richard Evans Schultes, who became renowned for his research and publications on psychoactive plants, began his lifelong career in the 1930s with his field study of peyote among the Kiowa Indians. In his groundbreaking article, "The appeal of peyote (*Lophophora willliamsii*) as medicine", he wrote of the therapeutic value of peyote that he learned from Native Americans (Schultes, 1938). Peyote is said to provide relief from pain and fevers, and it is used to treat scorpion stings and snake bites. Poultices made from peyote are applied externally to arthritic joints, cuts, and bruises. Juice from the peyote has been used as eye drops to treat cataracts. It is taken as a tonic to stimulate energy, allay hunger, and promote feelings of well-being (Schultes, 1938, Anderson, 1996, Schaefer, 2015b). Another salubrious benefit of peyote is as a treatment for intestinal problems. Scientific studies have discovered that some of the peyote alkaloids (ex., hordenine) have antibiotic qualities, inhibiting the growth of penicillin-resistant strains of the bacterium *Staphylococcus aureus* (McCleary et al., 1960; Rao, 1970).

Laboratory research also indicates that peyote appears to increase immune response to cancerous tumors (Franco-Molino et. al., 2003). In this study, 50 g of *Lophophora williamsii* was macerated, treated with 50 mL of methanol, and filtered. This methanol extraction of peyote was added to *in vitro* murine lymphocytes and macrophages, and human peripheral blood mononuclear cells (HPBMCs), and applied directly to murine and human tumor cell growth. The results showed that "a methanol extract of peyote cannot only potentiate some immune parameters, but also directly kill tumor cells" (Franco-Molino et al., 2003). Citing research by Sissors and Voss (1978), which indicated that mescaline inhibits *in vitro* murine lymphocyte proliferation, Franco-Molino et al (2003) suggest from the results of their study that there "might be some immunostimulatory compounds in peyote's extract whose concentration might exceed that of a potential inhibitor of lympho-proliferation, such as mescaline." The authors also noted that the peyote extract activated murine leukocytes as well, and increased signals to proteins in human mononuclear cells that are known to be "extremely potent inflammatory molecules" that are "involved in acute and chronic inflammation" (ibid).

Indeed, the term "medicine" used by Native Americans for peyote is most appropriate. It has medicinal qualities, but it is not a "drug" that some fear can be abused. Numerous studies have demonstrated that it is not addictive. In fact, peyote consumption, especially within a religious context such as NAC ceremonies, can be beneficial in the rehabilitation of individuals from alcohol and drug abuse (Halpern et al., 2005, Calabrese, 1997, Schultes, 1938). Also, one must not overlook the positive influence that peyote experiences may have on individuals, which in turn can lead to greater spiritual awareness and meaning in their lives.

PEYOTE AND PREGNANCY

The Huichol pilgrimage to the peyote desert is a formidable journey that enables pilgrims to "find their lives." There are many layers of meaning for this trip, some formalized in traditional myths. My female consultants recounted to me an origin myth of the first peyote pilgrimage, and one of my companions drew a picture to visually tell the story, which involves three women, the Earth Goddess (Utüanaka), the Goddess of Peyote (Wiri'uwi), and the Blue Corn Goddess (Yuawime) (Fig. 2). One day, while Utüanaka was weaving on her loom, the design of the path to Wirikuta appeared, and the road manifested before them. These women traveled to the entrance of the peyote desert. The Deer Messenger, Kauyumarie, accompanied them. Utüanaka and Wiri'uwi were allowed to enter this sacred place, where they encountered peyote and consumed it. Yuawime stayed behind. The two goddesses who entered became pregnant while in Wirikuta. Utüanaka returned to share the wonders of peyote with her community, and showed them how to make the pilgrimage to Wirikuta. Wiri'uwi remained in Wirikuta and became the Mother of Peyote.

This theme of peyote and pregnancy is also ever present in the daily lives of Huichol women. Some Huichol women may be pregnant and consume peyote while on the pilgrimage or in ceremonies in their communities. On my first peyote pilgrimage with the San José temple group, I noticed that various women were pregnant. One woman, who was the wife of the leading shaman, was eight months pregnant. Another woman was six months along, and a third woman was two months into her pregnancy. All of these women ate large quantities of peyote because, as I later learned, they

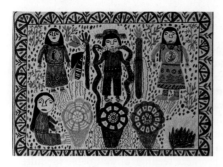

Fig. 2 Drawing of the myth of the original pilgrimage to Wirikuta by Estela Hernandez. The two women on top are the goddesses Wiri'uwi, and Utüanaka with babies in their wombs. The seated woman below is the goddess Yuawime, who was not fertile and could not enter the sacred peyote desert. Photo by Stacy B. Schaefer

were either shamans or learning to become shamans. I found out that these mothers did not experience any complications when giving birth, and that by all appearances their babies were healthy and well adjusted. I continued to be involved in the ceremonies of this temple group, and I came to know these babies and watch them grow from childhood to adulthood. They are active members in the community and beyond, and have their own families. During their reproductive years, many Huichol women are pregnant on average every other year. For Huichol women, as it is for the men, following cultural traditions inevitably involves consuming peyote in ritual contexts. Peyote may be consumed fresh, dried, or powdered and mixed into a beverage. Women, like their male counterparts, consume peyote throughout their lifetimes, even when pregnant.

I spoke with various Huichol women about the practice of ingesting peyote during pregnancy. One said that it was best to wait until the second trimester to do so, because in the first three months the baby was in a very delicate state and could abort. Several others commented that they consumed peyote during all stages of their pregnancy, and they and their babies did not experience any ill effects. Another explained that to ensure that there will be no problems or complications, the shaman provides prenatal care throughout the pregnancy by palpating the woman's stomach, healing with power wands, dreams, prayers and offerings to the gods for the mother and the baby in her womb.

The Huichol women whom I interviewed about their peyote experiences while pregnant all agreed that the babies in their wombs felt the effects of the peyote. One female shaman who specializes in fertility and childbirth told me:

> The baby is naturally much purer than others, the gods are helping it, like the fire and the deer, like the shaman who blesses the fire and blesses the sun…for this reason when the mother eats peyote she knows everything that is happening and the baby knows too…the baby feels the same as the mother…when a woman is pregnant even the baby inside receives messages from the deer, messages from the peyote…the baby always feels the same as a person…the baby cannot talk, it communicates without words, only with its 'iyari', heart memory (a kind of genetic memory of the soul).

A second woman described that first there is a quiet period. Her husband, speaking for her, said yes, her baby was "drunk" with the peyote and the two could communicate their thoughts telepathically. "My wife said that when this happened to her, that the baby remained in the womb, but their 'iyaris' went up to the sky to Niwetüka (the goddess who cares for the souls to be born). When the effects of the peyote wore off, her heart memory returned to her body, and that of her fetus returned to its place in the womb."

After this quiet period, the fetus can become very active and move in the womb; some women say the baby is "dancing" inside. One other female shaman described her sister's peyote experience in the eighth month of her pregnancy:

> At first it hurts. Then the baby inside is real quiet. Then it moves around a lot. The baby is 'inebriated' with the peyote also but does not know how to communicate well. My sister said that when she was pregnant and "traveling with the peyote", that although the baby was inside of her, she saw it right in front of her eyes. She didn't talk with the baby. She communicated with the gods to see that everything was all right, that the baby was formed well and there was nothing wrong with it.

Female shamans, because of their spiritual calling, may consume more peyote than other Huichol women; consequently, their children, while *in utero*, are more likely to experience peyote's effects than others' babies in the womb. A female shaman shared with me her thoughts, "I always like to eat peyote. It doesn't matter if I am pregnant ... If I feel well I like to eat it. There in Wirikuta, the people pray to the gods, and for some the gods give them the prize (a child) that has the design of a shaman...a clearer of fields...or a deer hunter ... that's how they are born. I think it happens like this because it is a custom that will never be lost."

This female shaman recounted her peyote experience in Wirikuta when she was two months pregnant with her son:

> (In Wirikuta) I thought we would eat a lot of peyote, to see what we could encounter to learn more about our customs. So I ate eight large peyotes, and the peyote was strong. I got dizzy and then 'inebriated with the peyote.' I never thought I was pregnant. Kauyu-marie (the deer messenger) appeared like a person, and told me how I was feeling ... he was talking to me from his heart. ... I think that Kauyumarie was talking (to my son in my womb). ... Afterwards, the shamans said that he was given to me in Wirikuta by the gods, with our goddess Wiri'uwi, the mother of peyote, so that our customs will not be lost...That is why he was born, why they gave him to me in Wirikuta, with me eating peyote, that's why he is peyote. I think he is peyote. He likes to eat peyote a lot ... that's how (some) are born.

Let us turn from the emic perspective of Huichol women to scientific studies and neurobiology. Research shows that when peyote is ingested, the mescaline in the plant functions like naturally occurring transmitters in the brain. Depending on the dosage, mescaline can inhibit, or block, the chemical transmission of impulses between nerve cells at synaptic receptor sites in the central nervous system. This affects the manner in which impulses are transmitted in the brain, and how the brain processes these signals. Mescaline has the same basic monoamine structure as the neurotransmitters norepinephrine, serotonin, and dopamine. Norepinephrine is abundantly concentrated in the limbic system of the brain, the site where emotions such as love, hate, joy, and sadness are stimulated. Greater clarity of thought can be induced by the release of norepinephrine. As norepinephrine neurons descend to the spinal cord, they play an important role in regulating behavioral responses to sensory stimuli influencing the muscles in the arms and legs (Snyder, 1996). The serotonin system affects sleep, mood, appetite, and depression, as well as sensorimotor processes. The release of serotonin causes the secretion of growth hormones, and it acts as a vasoconstrictor, stimulating the smooth muscles. Dopamine pathways are related to reward-behavior responses and hormonal release. Dopamine neurons are linked to motor abilities, and serve to maintain thoughts and perceptions in accord with the reality of one's mundane environment (Snyder, 1996: 209).

So how does ingestion of peyote by a pregnant woman affect her fetus? Laboratory research in the 1960s and 1970s was carried out to determine the risks of taking psychedelic substances during pregnancy. This was at a time when propaganda circulated widely, prompting public concern that verged on hysteria. For example, unfounded claims were disseminated about the health dangers of "psychedelic drugs", especially LSD, and the alleged chromosomal damage that could influence future generations. During this time and in this social climate, laboratory studies were conducted on mescaline and fetal development (Gerber, 1967; Maickel and Snodgras, 1973; Shah, 1973; Taska and Schoolar, 1972) using pregnant laboratory rats, mice, hamsters, and monkeys, which were injected with varying doses of mescaline and then euthanized to examine the results. In some cases, a radioactive carbon isotope was incorporated in the injected mescaline to trace where it traveled in the body. The animals used in the various experiments ranged in their pregnancies from the eighth day of gestation, as in one study with hamsters, to the fifteenth day of gestation in the study of mice, to the third semester in the monkey study. The amount of mescaline injected into the animals also varied among the studies.

This research demonstrated that mescaline could cross the placental barrier in each case. Some restrictions in the passage of mescaline to the fetus were noted, indicating that the fetus did not receive as high a dose of mescaline as the mother. However, once the mescaline entered the fetus, its distribution to the central nervous system did not appear to be restricted, and the brain tissue rapidly accumulated mescaline in high concentrations. The action, it was suggested, may have been due to the partially developed blood-brain barrier in the fetus. The younger the fetus was in its development, the greater the amount of mescaline that passed to the brain. The metabolism of mescaline in the fetal brain was slower than in the brain of the mother. Upon examination of the maternal tissues, mescaline was found in high concentrations in the kidney, liver, and spleen, with relatively low amounts in the brain. This result was attributed to the well-developed protective blood-brain barrier of the mother. Also noteworthy was that among the maternal tissues, the uterus was capable of storing mescaline for longer periods of time than other tissues studied, and the uterine smooth muscle had a great affinity for mescaline. Congenital malformations of the fetus were found only in one study, on hamsters on the eighth day of pregnancy that were injected with 0.45 to 3.25 mg/kg of mescaline.

While these laboratory studies ascertained that mescaline can cross the mother's placental barrier and the blood-brain barrier of the fetus, these animal experiments did not precisely replicate the dose/response of peyote consumption or its effects on a human mother and her fetus (Fig. 3). In addition to mescaline, there are an abundance of other alkaloids in peyote, and little is known about how they interact in the human body. The manner in which mescaline was administered to the animals by injection does not replicate typical human ingestion of peyote. Likewise, there are physiological differences between people and these research animals. The dosage of mescaline administered, the stage of fetal development, and the marked differences that exist in the gestation periods of mice, rats, hamsters, monkeys, and human beings are all important considerations.

ANIMALS	STUDY	DOSE AMMOUNT	EQ. DOSE FOR 55KG. WOMAN
hamsters	Greber 1967	0.45 mg	24.75 mg
hamsters	Greber 1967	1.33 mg	73.15 mg
hamsters	Greber 1967	3.25 mg	178.75 mg
monkeys	Taska 1972	5 mg/kg ^{14}C-mesc.	231.4 mg
mice	Shah 1973	μmol/kg ^{14}C-mesc.	96.8 mg
rats	Maickel 1973	0.50 μmol/kg ^{14}C-mesc.	27.5 mg

Fig. 3 Dosages of mescaline given to the laboratory animals in the various reports and how these correspond to equivalent dosage for a 55 kg. woman. I am grateful to Jonathan Ott for helping calculate these dosages.

To date, the only scientific study that examined human subjects who consumed peyote and its effects on their offspring was conducted by Dorrance et. al. (1975). The research compared lymphocyte chromosomes of 57 Huichol Indians with a lifelong and generational history of peyote ingestion to 50 peyote-naïve Huichol control subjects and ten laboratory control animals. The results indicated that no association could be made between multigenerational consumption of peyote and abnormalities in lymphocyte chromosomes (Dorrance et. al, 1975: 301-302). Also noteworthy in this report was the clinical opinion of the physician responsible for the treatment of the Huichols in the study, who stated that despite the common use of peyote by pregnant Huichol women, there was no evidence for any increase in congenital malformations among their offspring (ibid: 302).

If some Huichol women ingest peyote during their pregnancy, and scientific studies on mescaline show that it can cross the placental and blood-brain barriers, it is worth contemplating what effects this may have on the baby's cognitive development while in the womb. Beginning at three months and onward, the primary sensory areas in the neocortex of the fetus' brain begins to develop. The tactile senses, followed by the visual and then auditory centers begin to develop. At twenty-four weeks of development, many of the neurons in the brain are present. At this stage, the eyes are light sensitive and the fetus reacts to sound. By the third trimester, the brain of the fetus develops rapidly, causing sensory and behavioral capacities to expand (Berk, 2006: 86).

Due to the nature of such research, we have a limited understanding of the processes of cognitive development in a fetus. Researchers turn to the cognitive development of infants and newborns to try to assess what may be occurring while *in utero*. Theoretically, internal and/or external stimulation of the neocortex of the fetus may help with the connection of neurons in the brain. Along these lines, it is also theorized that the reason newborns sleep so much, and that 50% of this is REM sleep, is because they do not get the stimulation they need from the environment in the waking state. REM provides the stimulation necessary in young infants for development of the central nervous system that they do not get in an alert state (Berk, 2006: 130; DiPetro et. al., 1996; de Weerd and van den Bossche, 2003). Professionals believe that the earlier in its life a baby receives ongoing stimulation, the better its nervous system will develop; this includes cognitive and reflex abilities, etc. (Gary Montgomery, 1996, personal communications).[2] (Fig. 4). Laboratory studies indicate that the

2. I have consulted over the years about this topic with Gary Montgomery, PhD, Professor of Psychology, who has for several

younger the fetus, the greater the amount of mescaline that can cross the partially developed blood-brain barrier. Could that mean that two-month-old babies in the womb are exceptionally stimulated from the peyote the mother ingested? Could such episodes at various stages in development influence the cognitive development, even the neurological networking, of the fetus to the point where the baby literally perceives the world differently than those who have not had this experience? Huichols say that babies who have received peyote while in the womb are more predisposed to becoming shamans.

Peyote is also ingested by women in smaller doses during childbirth. Women I have interviewed say that it helps alleviate the pain of childbirth, quickens the delivery, and results in less blood loss in the birthing process.

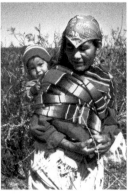

Fig. 4 Mother and child in the peyote desert. Photo by Stacy B. Schaefer

PARALLELS WITH AYAHUASCA AND PREGNANCY

Some pregnant members of ayahuasca churches drink the entheogenic brew of ayahuasca (*Banisteriopsis caapi* and *Psychotria viridis*), also known as *daime*, as a sacramental tea. One Brazilian woman who was a devout member of the *Santo Daime* Church, Yatra W. da Silveira Barbosa, spoke with me (personal communication, 1996) about pregnancy and the ritual use of ayahuasca. She explains:

> [Ayahuasca] doesn't affect the physical development of the fetus. The children in the forest who were born with *daime* and received *daime* from their mother throughout her whole pregnancy, they have a very special character, they are more observant, they are very wise ...

Yatra also conveyed that during childbirth the mother drinks ayahuasca, and other women who are present for the delivery also partake.

> During the labor, they invoke the entities to come and do the labor, deliver the child. When the baby is delivered, it is under these circumstances and it is already around these entities and these people around them. And the child, the first thing they put in its mouth, even before the mother's milk, is a drop of *daime*. That means that they are born in this other dimension ... [3]

Anthropologists Marlo Eakes Meyers and Matt Meyers, who carried out fieldwork in Brazil and participated in the Universal Light Christian Illumination Center - Alto Santo, discuss ayahuasca and pregnancy. They report that pregnant women are supervised, as are other special members, by the Godmother of the church.[4] Some women may take smaller amounts of ayahuasca during their

....

decades focused his research on child development at the University of Texas-Pan American (now University of Texas-Rio Grande Valley).
It should also be noted that Huichol children consume peyote, first via their mothers' milk, and then by eating small amounts. Some children show an affinity for peyote and seek it out. It is never forced upon children. Upon reaching adolescence, they are given specific peyote plants selected by family members to ingest as a kind of "rite of passage."

3. Yatra da Silveira Barbosa was instrumental in bringing ayahuasca and the *Santo Daime* Church to Amsterdam. While living in Amsterdam, she founded the organization Friends of the Forest, dedicated to conservation of the Brazilian rainforest, the indigenous people, and the scientific study of ayahuasca. When I interviewed her in 1996, she related that women in Amsterdam who were initiated into using ayahuasca for religious purposes were also drinking ayahuasca throughout their pregnancies. She described the first baby that received ayahuasca *in utero* and at birth in the Netherlands. During the mother's labor in the hospital, up to five women from this group were present. Clandestinely, they gave ayahuasca to the mother during the delivery, and they all sang as the baby was born. A small amount of ayahuasca was put on a piece of cotton that was then put on the tongue of the newborn. The women called this baby "Star Baby", because it was the first baby born in this way in the Netherlands.
Also, according to Silveira Barbosa, in Brazil and the Netherlands, Church babies are baptized two or three weeks after birth with salty water, honey water, and ayahuasca on their tongues. Henceforth, they drink ayahuasca during meetings. The mothers give their babies ayahuasca - the amount is determined by their size - and then the mothers drink it.

4. Marlo Eakes Meyer and Matt Meyer are former students of mine at California State University, Chico. We had numerous conversations about entheogens, including peyote among the Huichols, my research on pregnancy and peyote, and what I had learned about pregnancy and ayahuasca as presented in this paper. Upon completing their MA degrees in Anthropology, Matt Meyer continued in the PhD program at the University of Virginia, conducting fieldwork in Brazil on ayahuasca religion for 15 pregnancy than they normally would (Eakes Meyer and Meyer, 2013: 197). Brazilian anthropologist Beatrice Labate (2011) interviewed one woman who was a member of the *Santo Daime* Church, and her consultant also stated that smaller doses of ayahuasca are ingested by pregnant women. She reported:

> *Daime* gives women a profound experience of pregnancy and a strong contact with the baby in her womb ... And children who take *Daime* are normal, healthy, and intelligent. At this point, there are many families who have used *Daime* in the church for several generations, and in general they are healthy, happy, prosperous, and well balanced.

Another woman, Vera Fróes, who is a Brazilian historian and member of the *Daime* church Colônia Cinco Mil, wrote about her own experience taking *daime* during childbirth. Her description of the event, as discussed and translated from Portuguese to English by Eakes Meyer and Meyer (2013, in Fróes, 1988) is as follows:

> I started to ingest the liquid at 7 in the morning, and from there took another dose every half hour ... I felt the contractions accelerate quickly; I had never felt that before, and by two in the afternoon, already suffering a lot, the mirações (visions) gave me relief [from pain] ...
>
> At that moment I had a vision of Our Lady giving me the cup and saying:
>
> 'Take it, my daughter, it is your last dose.'
>
> Believing what I saw and heard, I grabbed the cup and drank. Right afterwards I entered into labor, and the baby began to 'crown.' The time had arrived, and Marco, who was singing the hymn 'Sol, Lua, Estrela,' wanted to help me, but it depended all on me...the Daime achieved true miracles in women's childbirth. I saw that all the spirits who were helping me turned and looked at the spirit that would incarnate in the baby, a burst of light lit up everything and the baby cried, I felt an indescribable happiness, was in harmony with all the world, floating on clouds of light.

Eakes Meyer and Meyer relate that church members look favorably upon pregnant women who ingest *daime*. This same sentiment is held for infants and older ones. Having intimately experienced *daime* in the womb or as babies, they are sometimes considered by church members to be enlightened, for they truly are children of the Queen, meaning the Virgin Mary who is "Queen of the Forest" (Eakes Meyer and Meyer, 2013; Froes, 1988: 198).

Cultural practices allow pregnant Huichol women and ayahuasca church members to ingest peyote or the ayahuasca brew, respectively. This is viewed by some as a special kind of initiation and a favorable way to bring a child into the world.[5] It would appear that this is not a maladaptive practice. Care is taken in these situations to safeguard the health and development of the fetus. Likewise, the mothers are consciously aware that their actions enable the babies in their wombs to experience the effects of the sacramental plants and commune with the spirit world as they understand and perceive it to be. In both practices, these plants are intentionally taken during childbirth to quicken the delivery and assuage the pain. Some Huichol women relate that consuming peyote also reduces the blood involved in childbirth. In the case of some female ayahuasca church members, drinking this tea during childbirth also opens a doorway for their own direct communication, as well as that of their newborns, with spiritual beings, such as the Virgin Mary.

In scientific terms, both peyote and ayahuasca interact with the same serotonergic system. Stimulation of serotonin receptors, particularly 5HT2, induces vasoconstriction in the uterus, which causes blood vessels to constrict the flow of blood; hence, a lesser amount of blood is shed during the delivery process. Serotonin also interfaces with the smooth muscle in the uterus and can induce contractions (Pharmacorama.com Drug Knowledge, accessed 07/12/2017). Peyote or ayahuasca taken during childbirth, or to induce it, interact with the 5HT2 serotonin receptors, which in turn can enable greater ease in parturition.

....

months from 2002-2007 (Meyer, 2014). Marlo accompanied him in the field with their children. Together, they became interested in the use of ayahuasca by pregnant women, and summarized their preliminary findings in the article by Eakes Meyer and Meyer (2013). I received a draft copy of this article written in English; later it was translated into Spanish for publication.

5. This paper does not advocate for or against the ingestion of entheogens during pregnancy. It is important to not only note that the practice does exist, but also to understand the processes at work on many levels.

MENSTRUATION, FERTILITY, AND PEYOTE

Having examined the topic of peyote consumption during pregnancy and at childbirth, let us turn to peyote and fertility and revisit the Huichol myth of the origin of the pilgrimage to Wirikuta, the peyote desert, with the three women who made the journey – Utüanaka, Wiri'uwi, and Yuawime. Before entering Wirikuta, they stopped at a lake to leave offerings. Kauyumarie, the deer messenger, looked to see if they had fertile wombs. Utüanaka and Wiri'uwi were menstruating. They washed themselves in the lake and the water turned red from their menstrual blood. To this day, this sacred place is called Haa Xuretü Mayema, "where there is red water." Utüanaka and Wiri'uwi were allowed to enter Wirikuta. Yuawime was infertile, and so she stayed behind and became a mountain in the western part of the Sierra.

Interestingly, Huichol couples that go on the pilgrimage may do so in hopes of having children. I have observed some women receiving healings by shamans in Wirikuta in order to become pregnant and bear children.[6] One Huichol woman I know told me with great excitement that she and her husband had wanted to have another child, but were unsuccessful until they went on the pilgrimage to Wirikuta. During one pilgrimage on which I participated, a couple was desperately seeking to have a child. Upon entering Wirikuta and after ingesting peyote, the woman began to menstruate. The shaman who was overseeing the healing of this couple told me that this was a good sign for preparing the woman to become pregnant. I also began to bleed in Wirikuta earlier than anticipated in my menstrual cycle, and participated with this woman in a ritual in which a lock of hair at the crown of the head was cut by the shaman to "calm the heat from the menstrual blood." Otherwise, it is believed that the blood will spoil the peyote.[7] This was not the first time I discovered that consuming peyote on the pilgrimage, or during peyote ceremonies in the Huichol Sierra, often caused me to bleed, even when it was out of sync with my cycle.

Later on in South Texas, when I began to participate in peyote ceremonies conducted by members of the NAC, I had the same experience. According to NAC traditions, menstruating women should not enter the tipi to participate in the meeting. Being very respectful, I made a point of adhering to this taboo. Despite my vigilance, at times I discovered that in the middle of the night or the early morning hours of the ceremony, I would unexpectedly begin to bleed. Afterwards, other women who had been in the meeting also commented that they, too, had begun to bleed. I was puzzled by my response and that of other women of reproductive age, and sought to find a cause and effect between consuming peyote and the monthly cycle.

THE INFLUENCE OF PEYOTE
ON REPRODUCTIVE HORMONES
PROGESTERONE

I contacted various specialists in women's reproductive health. First, I spoke with Dr. Erica T. Wang, MD and OB/GYN reproductive specialist at Cedars Sinai Medical Center in Los Angeles, California. She was not well-versed about peyote or mescaline, but she told me that, if she had to guess what was occurring, she would say that peyote is stimulating the release of progesterone. Progesterone is a female hormone that prepares the uterus for pregnancy and helps maintain a fertilized egg. It causes the uterine lining to thicken and is essential before and during pregnancy (Healthline.com, accessed 7/02/2017).

I also spoke with Nurse Practitioner and Advanced Practice Midwife Maria Victoria Mangini, who practices in the San Francisco Bay area of California and is knowledgeable about peyote. She responded to my inquiry by mentioning the work of Russell Marker, a chemist who discovered that local people in Orizaba, Veracruz, Mexico, used a wild yam in the genus *Dioscorea* as a gynecological medicine. Marker was able to extract the compound diosgenin from the yam and further synthesize

---

6. There is a scene in Furst's 1969 documentary video, *To Find Our Life: The Peyote Hunt of the Huichols of Mexico*, in which the leading shaman, Ramón Medina Silva, is curing a Huichol woman on the pilgrimage so that she may become pregnant.

7. In Huichol culture, menstrual blood is perceived as "hot," and menstruating women are seen as very powerful yet dangerous. There are various taboos forbidding menstruating women from carrying out certain kinds of tasks, such as preparation of ceremonial foods and drink, or working in the cornfield. On the peyote pilgrimage, menstruating women must tell the shaman so that he or she can perform the hair-cutting ritual to "neutralize" the "heat" they emit. Otherwise, it is believed that the pilgrims are put into grave danger, because the peyote will spoil because of their blood.

it into progesterone. Progesterone has been used to treat menstrual problems, difficult pregnancies, and gynecological cancers (Redig, 2003, Hahn et al., 2009). Ms. Mangini emphasized the fact that Russell Marker took indigenous people's folk medicine seriously.

Juanita Nelson, another certified professional midwife who is director of Community Midwives in Durango, Colorado, has been involved with the NAC for more than 20 years, during many of which she was the wife of a prominent roadman (religious specialist of the NAC). In her response to my questions, she concurred with what the other two specialists had told me by saying that she believes peyote alkaloids activate the release of progesterone. Ms. Nelson explained that she can empirically validate what I related above; she has seen it happen over and over again. If a woman is close to menstruating and she eats peyote, then she will get her period. If a woman is off cycle, she will also bleed. However, if a woman is ovulating or just finished with her period, she will not bleed. Ms. Nelson went on to say that in her experiences and observations at NAC meetings, pregnant women who eat peyote have very little problem with miscarriage, and that it helps establish the placenta and maturation of the fetus.

ESTROGEN

Estrogen is another essential hormone in the reproductive endocrine system. It has multifaceted effects on the hypothalamus and can rapidly alter the firing of neurons (Kelly et al., 2005). Estrogen and serotonin receptors are found to coexist in a variety of tissues. The activation of estradiol at E2 beta receptor sites stimulates an increase in serotonin receptor 5HT2a (Getz, 2013; Rybaczyk et al., 2005). Serotonin also functions as a hormone that can physiologically affect systems outside the central nervous system. It would seem that estrogen could also be triggered in response to ingestion of mescaline and other peyote alkaloids.[8]

OXYTOCIN

Oxytocin, a hormone produced in the hypothalamus and stored in the posterior lobe of the pituitary gland, plays a role in sexual reproduction, childbirth, and breastfeeding (Smith, accessed 7/20/17; Yang et al., 2013). Studies have shown that serotonergic transmission via 5-HT2a receptors stimulates the release of oxytocin into the bloodstream (Saydoff et. al., 1991). Mescaline and MDMA are both molecules in the phenethylamine family. Research points to the interaction MDMA has with the release of oxytocin (Kirkpatrick et al., 2014a, 2014b). The same release of oxytocin secretions in the body may also occur with mescaline. Perhaps the "heart-opening" emotions numerous people attribute to eating peyote could mean, in scientific terms, the release of oxytocin into the body's system.

PROLACTIN

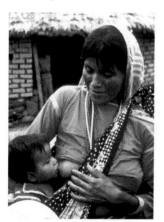

Prolactin is a hormone in the anterior lobe of the pituitary gland that also promotes the production of breast milk (Smith, accessed 7/20/17). Oral administration of mescaline has been found to affect 5-HT2a receptors and trigger the secretion of prolactin more than fourfold above baseline level. Human Growth Hormone (HGH) secretion was also stimulated (Demisch and Neubauer, 1979). It is interesting to point out that mescaline and other peyote alkaloids can be transmitted to babies and children via their mothers' milk. Huichol women are well aware of this, and have remarked to me that they will, at times, notice that their babies appear to be affected (Fig. 5). In one case, the nursing child on his mother's lap contentedly quieted down, and after a while tried to grasp at things in the air that were not visible to his mother or to me.

Fig. 5 At a Huichol temple peyote ceremony (Hikuri Neixa) the mother, who has consumed peyote for the last couple of days, nurses her baby. Photo by Stacy B. Schaefer

DISCUSSION

As we have seen, the ingestion of peyote alkaloids may influence the production of hormones in the endocrine system via the neurons in the

8. An interesting variable to consider is the age of a woman. Pre-menopausal women will have an abundance of estrogen and serotonin in circulation. As women age past their reproductive years, estrogen levels decline. This, in turn, leads to a decline in serotonin receptors, and may also lessen the amount of serotonin stored in the body (https://neuroendoimmune.wordpress.com/2013/10/29/thought-you-knew-everything-about-estrogen-what-about-its-effects-on-the-nervous-system/).

nervous system. The endocrine and nervous systems are linked via the hypothalamus and adjacent pituitary gland. Together, they are responsible for producing hormones, directly or indirectly, that are released and transported throughout the body (Sargis, 2015).

Progesterone- and estrogen-binding neurons are concentrated in the hypothalamus, and along the ascending monoamine neuron systems that innervate the hypothalamus and adjacent areas. Dopamine and norepinephrine systems, as well as the Raphe Serotonin System, are interlinked with the hypothalamus region (Moore, 1986: 13)(Fig. 6).

Seeking possible explanations for the association I observed between peyote consumption and the unexpected onset of bleeding within hours, I contacted neurobiologist Adam Haberstadt, an adjunct professor in the Department of Psychiatry at UCSD. His response was as follows: "Such an effect isn't surprising – there are 5-HT2a receptors in the hypothalamus that regulate hormonal secretion, so the effects that you observed are likely occurring as a consequence of this action..." (personal communication via email April 20, 2017). Another idea offered by pharmacologist and medicinal chemist David E. Nichols, PhD, (personal communication, June

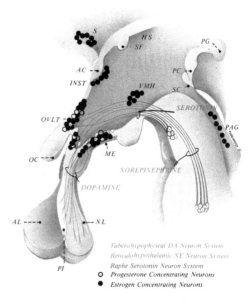

Fig. 6 Estrogen and progesterone-binding neurons in the hypothalamus and surrounding areas (Moore 1986:13).

8, 2017) was to examine the modulation of neurotransmitter release, that is "the process by which a given neuron uses one or more chemicals to regulate diverse populations of neurons.." See also https://en.wikipedia.org/wiki/Neuromodulation

Along this line of reasoning, perhaps neurotransmitters from neurons potentiated by mescaline and/or other peyote alkaloids at 5-HT2a receptor sites can diffuse to nearby hypothalamus areas. In response, this action could possibly potentiate the process discussed by Hoffman et al. (2016), in which neurotransmitters enter into the circulatory system and travel to reach distant target organs such as a woman's ovaries.

In addition to activity in the brain, one can look to other leads to understanding peyote's effects on the body. It is worth revisiting the results of animal studies that showed that the uterus is capable of storing mescaline for longer periods of time than other tissues studied, and that the uterine smooth muscle has a great affinity for mescaline both before and during pregnancy (Shah et al., 1973). In fact, 5-HT2a receptors have been documented in the uterus (Sonier, 2005). Research has shown that many hallucinogens can cause constriction in the umbilical veins of humans (Gant, 1970; Dyer & Gant, 1973). Nair (1974) documented contraction of umbilical arteries by mescaline, and mescaline was found to stimulate uterine contractions (Jacques, 1976). Although dated as a result of legal and political realities in the intervening years, in the future such research might lead us to alternate avenues to understanding the observed effects that peyote and ayahuasca have on the female reproductive system.

CONCLUSION

The integration of Western science and indigenous empirical knowledge is crucial to advancing our understanding of the world. We have much to learn from cultures such as the Huichol that are wise and experienced in the use of entheogenic plants. We need to listen closer to their myths, and strive to more deeply understand their perspectives, their rituals, and their practices. People such as the Huichols have acquired intimate knowledge of peyote and its effects. They have developed and fine-tuned a complex, elaborate worldview that provides members with tools and traditions to heal their bodies, promote fertility, manage healthy pregnancies, and raise their babies. In all of these actions they expand their understanding of consciousness and human existence.

Clearly, there is much to learn about the interactions of mescaline and other entheogens on the human neuroendocrine system. The activation of 5-HT2a and other receptor sites can stimulate the endocrine system via the hypothalamus/pituitary complex in the brain as well as in the reproductive system, including the uterus. Hopefully, this paper will inspire further thought and study in this fertile field of research with entheogenic plants, including peyote, and contribute to our understanding of the complex nature of "being human."

ACKNOWLEDGEMENTS

First and foremost, I want to sincerely thank Dennis McKenna for making the ESPD 50 conference a reality and for inviting me to participate in this momentous event. I am also grateful to Annette Badenhorst for her amazing organizational powers, and Rory Spowers, Anton Bilton, and the conference sponsors for their grand contributions. Thanks also go out to my friends and colleagues with whom I have brainstormed over the years about peyote and entheogens in culture: Manolo and Donna Torres, Luis Eduardo Luna, Keeper Trout, Martin Terry and the Cactus Conference bioneers, Jonathon Ott, Bia Labate, and Marlo and Matt Meyer. I am also extremely grateful to my Huichol and NAC consultants, whose names I have not disclosed in respect for their privacy, and to the experts and practitioners cited in this paper. My deepest heartfelt appreciation goes out to my husband, compañero, and fellow adventurer Jim Bauml for his contributions and editing wizardry, and for the many experiences and conversations he has shared with me in this work.

FUNDING

Support for the long-term fieldwork that has led to this paper has come from a Fulbright-Garcia Robles Fellowship; numerous Faculty Research Council Grants from the University of Texas-Pan American; several travel and professional development grants from the College of Behavioral and Social Sciences at California State University, Chico; a Research Grant from the Foundation for the Advancement of Mesoamerican Studies; an Organization of American States Fellowship; and a Fulbright Fellowship for Graduate Studies.

REFERENCES

Anderson, E., 1996. *Peyote: The Divine Cactus*. University of Arizona Press, Tucson.

Berk, L.E., 2006. *Child Development*. Pearson Education, Boston.

Boyd, C.E., 2003. *Rock Art of the Lower Pecos*. Texas A&M University Press, College Station.

Boyd, C.E., 2016. *The White Shaman Panel: An Enduring Creation Narrative in the Rock Art of the Lower Pecos*. University of Texas Press, Austin.

Boyd, C. E. & Dering, P. J., 1996. Medicinal and hallucinogenic plants identified in the sediments and pictographs of the Lower Pecos, Texas archaic. *Antiquity* 70 (268), 256-275.

Bruhn, J.G. et al., 1978. Peyote Alkaloids: Identification in a Prehistoric Specimen of *Lophophora* from Coahuila, Mexico. *Science* 199 (4336), 1437-1438.

Calabrese, J.D., 1997. Spiritual healing and human development in the Native American Church: Toward a cultural psychiatry of peyote. *Psychoanalytic Review* 84 (2), 237–255.

De Weerd, A.W., van den Bossche, A.S., 2003. The development of sleep during the first months of life. *Sleep Medicine* 7, 179-191.

Demisch L., M. Neubauer, 1979. Stimulation of human prolactin secretion by mescaline. *Psychopharmacology* 64, 361-363.

DiPetro, J.A. et al., 1996. Fetal neurobehavioral development. *Child Development*, 67, 2553-2567.

Dorrance, D.L. et al., 1975. Effect of peyote on human chromosomes: Cytogenetic study of the Huichol Indians of Northern Mexico. *JAMA* 234(3), 299-302.

Dyer, D.C., & Gant, D.W., 1973. Vasoconstriction produced by hallucinogens on isolated human and sheep umbilical vasculature. *Journal of Pharmacology and Experimental Therapeutics* 184(2), 366-375.

El-Seedi, H. et al., 2005. Pre-historic peyote use: Alkaloid analysis and radiocarbon dating of archaeological specimens of *Lophophora* from Texas. *Journal of Ethnopharmacology* 101, 238–242.

Franco-Molino, M. et al., 2003. *In vitro* Immunopotentiating properties and tumour cell toxicity induced by *Lophophora williamsii* (peyote) cactus methanolic extract. *Phytotherapy Research* 17, 1076-1081.

Eakes Meyer, M., Meyer, MDS, 2013. Los ninos de la reina yahuasca y embarazo: Un informe preliminar, in: Labate, B. C., & Bouso, J.C. (Eds.), *Ayahuasca y Salud*, Los Libros de La Liebre de Marzo, España.

Fróes, V., 1988. *Santo Daime* Cultura Amazônica. História do povo juramidam, 2nd ed., Manaus, Brazil: SUFRAMA.

Furst, P.T., 1969. *To Find Our Life: The Peyote Hunt of the Huichols of Mexicon*(documentary video). Latin American Studies Center, UCLA, 1 hr. 3 min.

Gerber, W., 1967. Congenital malformations induced by mescaline, lysergic acid diethylamide, and bromolysergic acid in hamster. *Science* 157: 265-266.

Getz, M., 2013. Thought you knew everything about estrogen? What about its effects on the central nervous system?, *The NEI Connection*. https://neuroendoimmune.wordpress.com/2013/10/29/thought-you-knew-everything-about-estrogen-what-about-its-effects-on-the-nervous-system. (accessed 07/10/17).

Gant, D.W., 1970. *Pharmacologial studies on isolated human umbilical veins*. M.S. Thesis, University of Washington, Seattle.

Hahn, H.S., MD, et al., 2009. Conservative Treatment with Progesterone and Pregnancy Outcomes in Endometrial Cancer. *International Journal of Gynecological Cancer* 19 (6), 1068-1073. http://journals.lww.com/ijgc/Abstract/2009/08000/Conservative_Treatment_WithProgestin_and.14.aspx. (accessed 07/12/17).

Halpern, J.H., et al., 2005. Psychological and cognitive effects of long-term peyote use among Native Americans. *Biological Psychiatry* 58(8), 624–631.

Healthline. *Low Progesterone: Complications, Causes, and More*.http://www.healthline.com/health/womens-health/low-progesterone#overview1/ (accessed 07/02/17).

Hoffman, B.L., et al., 2016. Chapter 15: Reproductive endocrinology, in: *Williams Gynecology*, 3E, McGraw Hill.

Jacques, R., 1976. Beta-adrenergic blocking agents as potent antagonists of mescaline-induced contractions in the rat uterus. *Experientia* 32(8), 1038-1039.

Kelly, M.J., et al., 2005. Estrogen signaling in the hypothalamus. *Vitamins & Hormones* 71, 123-45.

Kirkpatrick, M.G., et al., 2014a. Effects of MDMA and intranasal oxytocin on social and emotional processing. *Neuropsychopharmacology* 39(7), 1654-1663. Published online 2/12/2014.

Kirkpatrick, M.G., et al., 2014b. Plasma oxytocin concentrations following MDMA or intranasal oxytocin in humans. *Psychoneuroendocrinology* 46, 23-31. Published online 4/19/2014.

Labate, B.C., 2011. Consumption of *ayahuasca* by children and pregnant women: Medical controversies and religious perspectives. *Journal of Psychoactive Drugs* 43(1), 27-35.

Lumholtz, C., 1900. Symbolism of the Huichol Indians. *Memoirs of the American Museum of Natural History* 3(1), New York.

Lumholtz, C., 1902. *Unknown Mexico, Vol. 2.* Scribner's and Sons, New York.

Maickel, R.P., Snodgras, W.R., 1973. Psychochemical factors in maternal-fetal distribution of drugs. *Toxicology and Applied Pharmacology* 26, 218-230.

McCleary, J.A., et al., 1960. Antibiotic activity of an extract of peyote [*Lophophora williamsii* (Lemaire) Coulter]. *Economic Botany* 14(3), 247–249.

Meyer, MDS., 2014. *"In the Master's House": History, Discourse, and Ritual in Acre, Brazil.* PhD dissertation, University of Virginia, Department of Anthropology.

Myerhoff, B.G., 1974. *Peyote Hunt: The Sacred Journey of the Huichol Indians.* Cornell University Press, Ithaca, New York.

Moore, R.T., 1986. Neuroendocrine mechanisms: Cells and Systems, in: Yen, S.C., MD, Jaffe, R.B., MD, (Eds.) *Reproductive Endocrinology: Physiology, Pathophysiology, and Clinical Management*, W.B. Saunders Co., Philadelphia, Pp. 3-31.

Nair, X, 1974. Contractile responses of guinea pig umbilical arteries to various hallucinogenic agents. *Research Communications in Chemical Pathology and Pharmacology* 9 (3), 535-542.

Neuromodulation. Wikipedia.com https://en.wikipedia.org/wiki/Neuromodulation (accessed 08/29/17).

Pharmacorama drug knowledge. *Serotonin – Receptors and Effects.* http://www.pharmacorama.com/en/Sections/Serotonin_2_2.php/ (accessed 07/12/17).

Rao, G.S., 1970. Identity of peyocactin, an antibiotic from peyote (*Lophophora williamsii*), and hordenine. *Journal of Pharm. Pharmacol.* 22, 544-545.

Redig, M., 2003. Yams of fortune: The (uncontrolled) birth of oral contraception, *Journal of Young Investigators* 6 (7). http://legacy.jyi.org/volumes/volume6/issue7/features/redig.html)

Rybaczyk. L.A., et al., 2005. An overlooked connection: Serotonergic mediation of estrogen-related physiology and pathology. *BMC Women's Health* 2005, 5-12. https://www.researchgate.net/publication/7402877_An_overlooked_connection_Serotonergic_mediation_of_estrogen-related_physiology_and_pathology (accessed 07/11/17).

Sargis, R.M., MD, 2015. An overview of the hypothalamus: The endocrine system's link to the nervous system. *Endocrineweb.* https://www.endocrineweb.com/endocrinology/overview-hypothalamus (accessed 07/12/17).

Saydoff, J.A, et al., 1991. Enhanced serotonergic transmission stimulates oxytocin secretin in conscious male rats. *Journal of Pharmacology and Experimental Therapeutics* 257 (1), 95-99.

Schaefer, S.B., 1996a. The crossing of the souls: Peyote, perception and meaning, in: Schaefer, S.B., Furst, P.T. (Eds.), *People of the Peyote: Huichol Indian History, Religion and Survival*, University of New Mexico Press, Albuquerque, pp.138-168.

Schaefer S.B., 1996b. Pregnancy and peyote among the Huichol Indians of Mexico: A Preliminary Report. *Yearbook for Ethnomedicine and the Study of Consciousness/Jahrbuch für Ethnomedizin und Bewußtseinsforschung* 7, 205-221.

Schaefer, S.B., 2004. In search of the divine: Wixárika (Huichol) peyote traditions in Mexico, in: Coomber, R., South, N. (Eds.), *Drug Use and Cultural Contexts 'Beyond the West'*, Free Association Books, England.

Schaefer, S.B., 2005. Plants and healing on the Wixárika (Huichol) peyote pilgrimage, in: Dubisch, J., Winkelman, M. (Eds.), *Pilgrimage and Healing*, The University of Arizona Press, Tucson.

Schaefer, S.B., 2011. Peyote and meaning, in: Cardeña, E.,Winkleman, M. (Eds.), *Altering Consciousness: A Multidisciplinary Perspective*, Praeger Publishers, Santa Barbara, California.

Schaefer, S.B., 2015a. *Huichol Women, Weavers, and Shamans*, University of New Mexico Press, Albuquerque.

Schaefer, S.B., 2015b. *Amada's Blessings from the Peyote Gardens of South Texas*, University of New Mexico Press, Albuquerque.

Schultes, R.E., 1938. The appeal of peyote (*Lophophora williamsii*) as medicine. *American Anthropologist* 40, 698–725.

Shah, N.S., et al., 1973. Placental transfer and tissue distribution of Mescaline-14C in the mouse. *Journal of Pharmacology and Experimental Therapeutics* 182, 489-493.

Shulgin, A.T., Perry W.E., 2002. *The Simple Plant Isoquinolines*, Transform Press, Berkeley, California.

Sissors, D.L., Voss, E.W., 1978. Inhibition of lectin stimulation of murine lymphocytes by mescaline. Biochem. *Pharmacology* 27, 2705-2711.

Smith, C. The endocrine system: Hypothalamus and pituitary, *Visible Body* Blog, https://www.visiblebody.com/blog/endocrine-system-hypothalamus-and-pituitary (accessed 7/20/17)

Snyder, S., 1996. *Drugs and the Brain*, Scientific American Library, New York.

Sonier, B., et al., 2005. Expression of the 5-HT2A serotoninergic receptor in human placenta and choriocarcinoma cells: mitogenic implications of serotonin. *Placenta* 26(6), 484-90.

Taska, R.J., Schoolar, J.C., 1972. Placental transfer and fetal distribution of Mescaline-14C in monkeys. *Journal of Pharmacology and Experimental Therapeutics* 182, 427-432.

Terry, M.K, et al., 2006. Lower Pecos and Coahuila peyote: new radiocarbon dates. *Journal of Archaeological Science* 22, 1017-1021.

Weigand, P.C., 1981. Differential acculturation among the Huichol Indians, in: Hinton, T.B., Weigand, P.C. (Eds.), Themes of indigenous acculturation in northwest Mexico. *Anthropological Papers* 38, University of Arizona Press, Tucson, pp. 9–21.

Wilbert, J., 1987. *Tobacco and Shamanism in South America*, Yale University Press, New Haven, CT.

Yang H.P., et al., 2013. Nonsocial functions of hypothalamic oxytocin. *Neuroscience.* Article ID 179271, 13 pages, http://dx.doi.10.1155/2013/179272. (accessed 07/09/2017).

Mescal, Peyote and the Red Bean: A Peculiar Conceptual Collision in Early Modern Ethnobotany

■ *Keeper Trout* ■

Self-taught ethnobotanist, scholar and author of *Trout's Notes*; active with Cactus Conservation Institute and Shulgin Archives Project

ABSTRACT

Most people think of a fiery alcohol rich drink when they hear the word mescal/mezcal. That thought is correct but there is a larger picture, as the name "'mescal" has been applied to three quite different plants. Scientific carelessness, puritanical propaganda, and government overreach have confused peyote and the frijolillo with each other and with agave, all under the name "'mescal." This paper employs extensive archival research of newspapers, scientific publications, and government documents to identify the sources of these confusions and, where possible, to draw a more disentangled history of these plants, so that they may be more easily understood on their own terms and in relation to each other.

1. Our three "mescal" plants, will be presented in the order of their appearance in the historical record:

2. Maguey: *Agave* spp. (Agavaceae)

3. Peyote: *Lophophora williamsii* (Lem. ex Salm-Dyck) J.M. Coult. (Cactaceae)

4. Texas mountain laurel AKA the red bean: *Dermatophyllum secundiflora* (Ortega) Ghandi & Reveal (Leguminosae) (This is the presently accepted synonym. *Calia secundiflora* (Ortega) Yakovlev, *Sophora secundiflora* (Ortega) DC, and *Sophora speciosa* Benth. have also appeared in pertinent published phytochemical or toxicological accounts.)

5. For reasons that will become clear, the name "'mescal" came to be applied to the latter two of these plants only by virtue of their reputation as intoxicants and, in the case of *Lophophora williamsii*, also known as peyote, accompanied an 'education' effort meant to establish such a reputation.

AGAVE SPP. AS "MESCAL"

The first candidates referred to as 'mescal' and 'the mescal plant' were the *Agave* species that now go by the common name "maguey" and, in English, "century plant."

This is the original mescal.

Since antiquity, the hearts of the maguey (i.e. the bases of the stems) have been roasted in earth ovens to prepare an important sugary food (Castetter, 1935). In addition to being a foodstuff, cooked agave hearts serve as a sugar source enabling production of fermented drinks and the distilling of a liquor named mezcal (Bruman 2000). In fact, the word "mescal" derives from the Nahuatl word "mexcalli", a word that combines "metl" (agave) with either "ixcalli" (stew) or "ixca" (to bake) to mean "cooked agave" (*Random House Dictionary 2017*). In early occurrences of the name 'mescal' in Hispanophone literature, its loanword status was indicated through its spelling. As the name gained wider acceptance and use, the spelling shifted to the current "mezcal."

It was a common practice among the Spaniards to assign names to indigenous peoples based on common foods, practices or geographic features, rather than by the names those peoples already used to describe themselves. Several different groups found themselves indicated by their practice of roasting and eating the mescal plant.[1]

It is important not to confuse mescal as is associated with *Agave* spp. with mescal beans. *Agaves* do not possess beans. The 2017 *Random House Dictionary* describes the phrase "mescal bean" as an "Americanism" that first appeared in use during 1855-1860, but did not include a reference. The only point of publication we could locate around that time frame was in a 1854 Grand River Times account of a peculiar musical review, penned by George Horatio Derby (writing as "John Phoenix"), of a symphony titled *The Plains*. This piece of prose appears to have coined the phrase "'mescal beans." His satirical "review" continued to be re-run in newspapers for many years (example, the 1875 *Helena Weekly Herald*), and was eventually published in Stedman & Hutchinson 1891.

A small excerpt:

> The symphonie [sic] opens upon the wide and boundless plains in longitude 115° W., latitude 35° 21' 03" N., and about sixty miles from the west bank of Pitt River. These data are beautifully and clearly expressed by a long (topographically) drawn note from an E flat clarionet. The sandy nature of the soil, sparsely dotted with bunches of cactus and artemisia, the extended view, flat and unbroken to the horizon, save by the rising smoke in the extreme verge, denoting the vicinity of a Pi Utah village, are represented by the bass drum. A few notes on the piccolo call the attention to a solitary antelope, picking up mescal beans in the foreground. The sun, having an altitude of 36° 27', blazes down upon the scene in indescribable majesty.

Ignore, for a moment, the glaring problems with those "'mescal beans": plugging those coordinates into Google Maps generated something that is worth noticing.

Derby's coordinates place his fictional mescal bean-eating antelope less than fifty miles away from the Mescal Range. The Mescal Range in eastern San Bernardino County are named after cooked hearts of the locally abundant *Yucca mohavensis* (Gudde & Bright 2004), in the aforementioned Hispanophone tradition.

A short review of the aforementioned troubling details can help illuminate what Derby meant, and, for our discussion more importantly, what Derby did not mean when creating the phrase "mescal beans":

- Derby certainly can't be speaking of beans from an *Agave* spp or a *Yucca* spp. Only leguminous plants produce beans.

- Peyote can be ruled out as it is not referred to as mescal beans in print until several decades later, in 1888.

- The red-bean can also be removed from consideration as it is not recorded with the name mescal beans until a few years after peyote.

- Which leads us to the conclusion that the "antelope, picking up mescal beans in the foreground" does not clearly refer to anything real.

Stedman & Hutchinson (1891) claimed that the symphony *The Plains* was first performed at San Diego's Odeon theatre in 1855. Derby lived in California, so, while the name choice may be a coinci-

---

1. For example:
The Mescales were noted to be in Coahuila in 1760 by García.
The Mescal [a singular or plural noun] were encountered by Massanet in 1688 about fifty miles north of the Rio Grande in South Texas (see Massanet 1691 or Portillo 1888).
Mescale/Mescales were recorded as being on both sides of the Rio Grande in the 17th century (de Leon 1689 (1905) and National Park Service (NPS) 2002, citing Wade 1999).
A Coahuiltecan-language group in south Texas was known as the Mescalero in 1691 (Hodge 1912 citing Terán 1691-1692).
Mescalero apaches were recorded with that name by 1724 (NPS 2002, citing Rivera 1945:6).

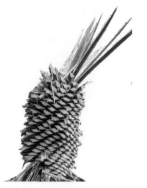

Image 1 Agave heart with most leaves removed.

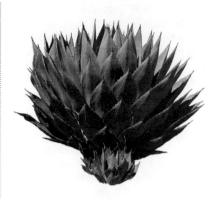

Image 2 Agave parryi. Images from Creative Commons. Agave parryi was a favorite food of some of the Apache groups including the Mescalero according to Castetter, 1935.

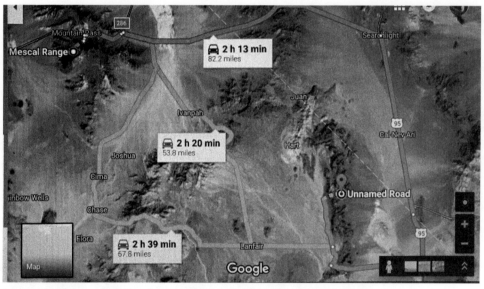

Image 3 Google map of the Mescal range in Eastern San Bernardino County, California.

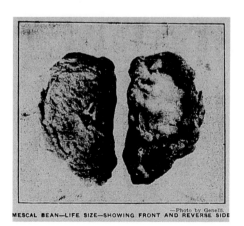

Image 4 Mescal buttons, Anon., *The Mitchell Capital*, 1906.

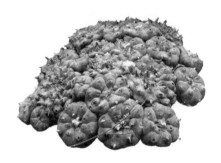

Image 5 *Lophophora williamsii* in the Peyote Gardens.

236

dence, it is at least plausible he was familiar with the Mescal Range and that his "mescal beans" were coined based on that name.

Despite those problems concerning the phrase mescal beans, our next mescal was somehow ascribed as actually having beans but it is unknown how or why the word beans came to be applied to something that does not look anything like beans.

LOPHOPHORA WILLIAMSII AS "MESCAL"

In 1888, E.E. White referred to our second mescal designate, *Lophophora williamsii* (Peyote), as the "mescal bean," and James Mooney called it "the mescal plant" in 1891. These two names create a particularly problematic point of shared identity, which we will examine in some detail. White (1888) sources his term from "white people" in Oklahoma, whereas Mooney appears to have gotten his information from one of his Kiowa friends in 1891, while engaged in field research on their calendar history. The Smithsonian Bureau of Ethnology later assigned him to specifically study the peyote religion (Owen, 1921).

Something very peculiar happened here.

The peyote plant had been known in print by the name peiotl or peyotl (the ancient name in the Nahuatl language) and then peyote (the Spanish derivative of the Nahuatl name), ever since the Spanish invaders of Mexico began writing about the plant (examples: de Cárdenas, 1591, Hernandez 1651). Despite their widespread and common use in print for both the plant and the drug up to and through the 1800s (a few examples: de León, 1611; Massanet, 1691; Morfi, 1778; Orozco y Berra, 1864), for a few decades in the USA starting in the 1880s, peyote became known as mescal, the mescal plant, mescal beans and mescal buttons (in various spellings):

SUMMARY OF EARLY APPLICATIONS OF THE TERM "MESCAL" TO LOPHOPHORA WILLIAMSII.

1. (1885 is given as the date of first use, but no reference has included details of that use. We presently suspect this date may be erroneous.)

2. 1887 Briggs – Muscale buttons. (This was also used by Lewin and by Hennings in 1888, and by Rusby in 1894.)

3. 1888 White – Mescal bean.

4. 1891-1893 Mooney – Mescal and as the Mescal plant. Mooney's first use of "Mescal" appears to have been in a presentation and in a personal letter during 1891.

5. 1894 Heffter – Mezcal. (Heffter "corrected" muscale to mezcal on the basis both of 'muscale' not being a proper Spanish word and of the term's reference to an intoxicant. Heffter then coined mezcaline. Mescaline was thus derived from mezcal, and reflects Heffter's belief that peyote was intoxicating.)

6. 1895 Prentiss & Morgan – Mescal buttons. (Prentiss & Morgan obtained their material from Mooney, as did Weir Mitchell, Wylie and Ewell.)

It is valuable to consider why the particular name "'mescal" rather abruptly appeared, as the history of this name illuminates an enduring part of peyote's story. Sources such as Turner (2010) claim that "the term [mescal] came to be applied indiscriminately to other intoxicants, or perceived intoxicants." However, as far as we can determine, "mescal" appears to have been applied to just three "intoxicants": peyote, the red bean and, as a misspelling of mezcal, the distilled alcoholic beverage.

"Mescal buttons" are more understandable than "mescal beans," but dense levels of confusion almost typify this small area of study.

Whether buttons or beans, some clarity can be obtained through historical context and that era's political environment.

Despite the fact that peyote had been known to botanists for almost half a century, confusion about the plant's identity was abundant when it first came to the attention of medical, chemical, and pharmaceutical science. Parke, Davis & Company's documented distribution of dried peyote to several prominent researchers as "muscale buttons" was only part of this confusion: Parke, Davis & Company was initially unaware that it was a dried cactus (See Bender, 1968; Bruhn & Holmstedt, 1978; and Stewart, 1987).

Those opposing indigenous use of peyote also added to the confusion. Missionaries and religious organizations vehemently condemned peyote as it compounded their universal opposition to alcohol and other intoxicants with their vilification of quasi-pagan and indigenous religious ceremonies and dances. These organizations campaigned for legislation against the mescal bean, despite often not knowing what it was they opposed.[2] How much of their confusion was genuine and how much was disingenuous is anyone's guess.

A surprising degree of confusion about peyote still persists today. Mescal's "Definition 5" at Memidex.com, for example, offers that "The button-shaped top of the mescal cactus [is] a source of psilocybin" (Accessed in 2017). Likewise, the University of Maryland's CESAR tells us that "Peyote (*Lophophora williamsii* or *Lophophora diffusa*) is a spineless cactus with small protrusions called "buttons" that are used for psychoactive hallucinogenic purposes. Mescaline, an amphetamine, is the principal active psychedelic compound in peyote" (Accessed in 2017, last updated in 2013).

There are at least two leading possibilities for how peyote became known as mescal. These are not mutually exclusive, nor do they preclude the existence of additional reasons, including a speaker or writer's deliberate attempt to cause confusion:

Possibility 1: This may have been an instance of the "tastes like chicken" phenomenon, where people choose a "best fit" drawn from a limited range of experience and belief to describe something novel.

Example: "The fact that a wild state of intoxication can be produced by chewing a few of the beans and swallowing the juice causes them to be called 'mescal' beans by many Mexicans" (Anon. 1909 *The Yakima Herald*). Likewise, Safford (1922) offered a variant, proposing that the name referred to the beverage mezcal fortified with peyote.

Possibility 2: During their rise to power, prohibitionists saw political value in peyote being perceived as an intoxicant. Many of these prohibitionists were Christian reformers who wished to eliminate all traditional religions, and saw similar political value in its ceremonial use. Missionaries of this time actively tried to obliterate indigenous cultures and their religious practices as a matter of policy: the assimilation and transformation of all Native Americans into hard-working and prosperous Christian farmers was a core plank in their political and religious platform (Keller, 1983). This neatly dovetailed with the campaign against alcohol and all intoxicants: peyote found itself referred to as Indian dope, Indian cocaine, the dope bean, the jag bean, the drunk bean, the bean drunk, the booze bean, whiskey root and dry whisky in addition to the common misnomer 'mescal bean.' We will look at a number of instances in which peyote was deliberately confused with alcohol and other drugs, as well as where it was linked variously with a sinister and spurious religion, violence, immorality, and insanity for this specific purpose.

Examples: "The craze for mescal has been growing rapidly on the reservations, being identified with the development of a secret cult which is half religion and half a sort of freemasonry" (Anon. 1912, *The Continent*). Gertude Bonnin made the accusation that an "unscrupulous organization, through its agents, is promoting the Peyote cult, under a religious guise, solely for the easy money gotten from their superstitious victims" (1917: 39).

Consider some comments from that period and overlay them onto the ongoing effort to eliminate the use of all intoxicants worldwide. The goal was not just to ban alcohol – it included everything from coca to cocoa. While national Prohibition never saw a large majority of support (McGirr 2015), this was a popular and well-funded campaign that operated on a national level through several different religious organizations, and which was financed both by some of the leading capitalists and, what are mistakenly referred to as, the "idle rich"of the day, such as Herbert Walsh, so it proved to be highly effective. (The prohibition movement is too complex for adequate treatment

---

2. For example:

"A new narcotic to tempt mankind. Mescal a drug which surpasses hashish and furnishes devotees dreams more entrancing than De Quincey's" (Anon. 1904 *The Washington Times*).

"A rare variety of the plant [*Agave*] called "Button Mescal" is found in the Rio Grande valley which is a powerful narcotic, and is now being investigated by the agricultural department at Washington, D. C." (Anon. 1895 *Arizona Republican*).

"The mescal bean is not a bean at all. It is a small circular blossom from a plant in Mexico. The blossom is dried" (Anon. 1898 *Wichita Daily Eagle*).

"The buttons are the seed pods of a variety of the century plant called bayote" (Anon. 1916 *The Topeka State Journal*).

"It is related by federal officials [...] the Indians succeeded for many years in concealing the true quality of the beans. They led the white people to believe that they used the beans to season certain kinds of stews which they made" (Anon. 1909 *The Yakima Herald*).

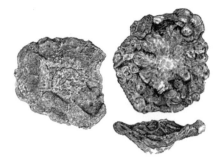

Image 6 Prentiss & Morgan's Mescal buttons

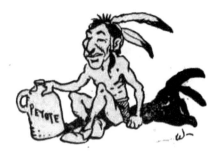

Image 7 Columbus Commercial, Anon. 1913.

here, beyond touching upon its relevance to peyote and mescal. See the afore cited McGirr (2015) for an in-depth and well-referenced discussion of prohibition's larger scope and history.) Efforts to ban peyote were inseparable from alcohol and other addictive drugs in the minds of the prohibitionists.

Activities intended to educate the public that peyote was a dangerous intoxicant persisted during the decades that followed and the opposition to peyotism[3] has not stopped[4] [see endnote 1]. Early comments that its effects were the same as or stronger than alcohol were common (ex. *Yakima Herald*, 1909). Some accounts such as the 1909 *Brownsville Daily Herald* confusedly asserted, "These beans ... are not only a strong intoxicant but contain opium and cocoaine [sic] as well." while *The Spokane Press* (1909) claimed, "The bean, chewed, results in an exaltation of spirits similar to that action that follows a combination highball of cocaine and whisky with a dash of champagne." Other sources such as the 1913 *El Paso Herald* referred it as being akin to hasheesh, "with visions which make a strong appeal to the aboriginal sense of the supernatural." The Medical World (1907:201) invoked opium, digitalis and strychnine in their description of its effects.

In his 1911 annual report Commissioner of Indian Affairs Robert G. Valentine asserted "The physiological and toxic action of peyote places it in the same general class with opium, cocaine, Indian hemp and chloral hydrate. ... It is needless to say that peyote is a greater enemy to civilization, especially to the Indian race, than whiskey." It is not coincidental that Valentine was a committed prohibitionist.

Peyote use was purported by Agent McShoridge to first drive the user insane and then kill them. Unsubstantiated claims of actual deaths can be found in the testimony presented to Congress (see the 1918 peyote hearings for many examples) as well as in the media. Some of the claims pushed the limits of belief considering that insanity and death seem at odds with something gaining in popularity.

Interestingly a couple of the errors appearing in prohibitionist news copy during that period persisted into modern times forming the basis of urban legends about smoking peyote or the hairs being active or toxic.[5]

The 1911 report of Commissioner of Indian Affairs Robert G. Valentine also contained a telling spot of honesty concerning the motivations being religious in basis. "Even if the physiological effects of this drug were not serious, its use would have to be prohibited for the same sociological reasons as have led the Government strongly but tactfully to modify Indian dances. As is well known, exercises which the Indian consider of a religious nature are made the occasion of taking the drug. These meetings are held as often as once a week."

Spaulding (1915) spoke similarly when commenting that efforts to prevent the use of peyote existed "chiefly because it is believed by some of those interested in the Christianizing of the Indians that it has a tendency to make them revert to their primitive condition and to their heathen beliefs."

James Mooney captured the dilemma nicely in a 26 October 1920 letter to Joseph Thoburn, "This is the native Indian religion ... which I have defended before Congress committees and other bodies,

---

3. Peyotism: A religious practice that is based on the sacramental use of peyote.
Peyotist: A person using peyote within a religious context and regarding it as sacrament.

4. As examples, see Bromberg, 1942; Bromberg & Tranter, 1943; Tranter, 1942; Davis, 1961; ProjectKnow 2017.

5. From Anon. 1918 *Free Trader Journal*: "In the center is a little tuft of cotton. This cotton is more highly charged with the stuff that makes users wild than any other part of the plant, ... Its effect is more like insanity than intoxication. The mescal buttons are also smoked. ... A few whiffs of mescal smoke and the smoker becomes completely insane. The drug works more quickly when smoked than in any other way, and the effects last longer."

for such defense and stand have been recalled from Oklahoma by Dr. Fowkes on demand of Cato Sells and the local agent. ... They are oppressed, persecuted and vilified by interested missionaries and officials who fear the development of Indian initiative as a danger to their own monopoly of religious and economic control."

The rejection of the validity of the peyote faith for being just a form of deviant drug taking wearing a spurious mantle of religious respectability was quite commonplace.[6]

Herbert Walsh (1920:53-54) made an often repeated claim that if a peyote church could legally exist surely so could a "whiskey church", Mabel Luhan compared peyotism with the religious defense of hashish, cocaine or morphine (Stewart, 1987), while the Indian Leader (1917) took this a step further with their comment averring that "there would be nothing to prevent setting up in any of our cities a pagan temple, with prostitutes offering themselves under the name of religion as ministers to lust." Perhaps the most incredulous dismissal appeared on page 4688 of the 1921 Congressional Record where the peyote debate included a particularly interesting comment by Representative Chalmers on the subject of the conscientious practice of the peyote religion. "I would remind the gentleman that some mothers conscientiously and religiously believe that they are doing the right thing when they sacrifice their offspring to the alligators, religiously." It is difficult to argue with anyone who is willing to make a statement like that.

The dire prediction that the Winnebagos were facing actual extinction, due to their use of peyote, appeared in many newspapers across the USA during 1906. The accompanying media barrage coincided with several Protestant womens' groups coming together to declare that they were waging a "War on Mescal" (example: 1906, *Norfolk Weekly News Journal*).

It is difficult to imagine any other outcome considering that the story headlines were then declaring: "Drug killing off Winnebago Indians – Victims of Mexican Bean dying at startling rate – ... Will be extinct in few years – Introduced but a year ago habit has seized men and women alike – 700 in an orgie [sic]."

It is worth reflecting on how any average American with no better information would have received the news accounts including this sort of content. That headline was drawn from *Abbeville Press & Banner* in 1906 but this was a popular news story that year and versions appeared in many newspapers over a period of a few months.

A larger account in *The Mitchell Capital* (1906) added the absurd claims that: "Fearless of the horrors of insanity; resolutely facing racial extinction; conscious of inevitable physical decline; courting death itself in the practice of strange and weird religion ... Men and women who were among the brightest and most intelligent Indians on the reservation ... are now dull of comprehension, driveling idiots who chatter like monkeys, speaking neither English nor their native tongue intelligently."

This included only a minute sampling from the era of the "mescal bean" to illustrate the consistency of the overall message about peyote that was intended.

Charges of wanton behavior, loss of morality, and sexual inappropriateness were abundant and persisted in the media for many years. In 1961 an article by Davis appeared damning peyote to be "America's baffling sex buttons" and purported it to be used in "Indian sex rites."

Similarly, the 1909 *Rural New Yorker* ran the headline "Getting Drunk on Beans - The demoralizing Mescal and its Effects," whose article read: "A friend who observed one of these ceremonies in Indian Territory told me that the Indians divide themselves into two squads during this part of their ceremony, one-half of them remaining sober to restrain those who eat the mescal buttons from killing themselves or each other. This gives a good idea of the excitement produced by this intoxicant."

Despite the period's leading anthropologists' and ethnobotanists' work to defend peyotism's religious legitimacy, the opposition continued unabated. In his 1920 annual report, Commissioner of Indian Affairs Cato Sells commented, "Scientific investigation of the nature of this narcotic drug shows conclusively its dangerous effects. ... [Medical] scientists say that peyote has no medicinal value and if habitually used results in the derangement of both mental and physical structure. Its defense as a religious rite is largely fictitious, the promoters of its use having seized upon this idea in an attempt to prevent or delay prohibiting legislation." Dissenting scientists and laypeople were generally dismissed, belittled, or simply ignored. This has remained the case. The presence of such

---

6. Examples:

Becker, 1921, "The evil effects of this drug cannot be questioned, although there is much propaganda to allow the Indians to retain this drug."

Daiker, 1914 "The great cry of those in favor of its use is that the Office is attempting to interfere with their religious liberties, but in my opinion the religious feature is being used as a cloak to cover its general use by the Indians."

Valentine, 1908:14, "Apparently for the purpose of justifying the use of this narcotic, a religious cult has been built up based on its use."

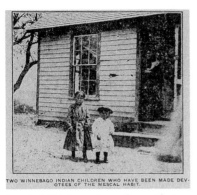

TWO WINNEBAGO INDIAN CHILDREN WHO HAVE BEEN MADE DEV-
OTEES OF THE MESCAL HABIT.

Image 8 This image is worth considering as a
potential hook for the intended audience.

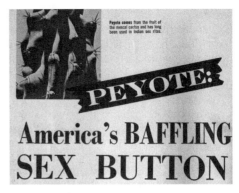

Image 9 Davis 1961

commentary in religious publications is scarcely surprising but trivializing and even contemptuous comments were and still are casually included in mainstream publications and peer review journals, contemporary or bygone.

As examples, an image of Frank Takes Gun appearing in *TIME* (1959) holding a depiction of a peyote ceremony was entitled "For some a hangover after the service."

Similarly a 1975 issue of the journal *Human Behavior* included an article concerning peyote being evaluated in the treatment of alcoholism. Notice the density of pejorative and trigger wording contained within the brief excerpt below.

"Hair-of-the-Dog is an alcoholic. But as with other American Indians who receive treatment for problem drinking in a program by the US Public Health Service Indian Hospital, Clinton, Oklahoma, he is learning to get his buzz from peyote instead of a bottle of Ripple."

Participants were said to "pop an average dozen mescaline-packed peyote buttons apiece" (Anon. 1975).

Their wording might be anticipated if this was a religious tract rather than a peer review journal.

Dismissive and antithetical comments were not limited to written articles, James Mooney's recognition of the legitimacy of the peyote religion led anti-peyotists to successfully demand his removal.

Herbert Walsh 1919 expressed a sentiment, then common to this camp, suggesting that Mooney was "anxious to see the Indians retain their old ways and be regarded as interesting ethnological specimens for the study of scientists. It does not look well for a representative of one branch of the Government (Ethnological Bureau) to try to interfere with the work of the Indian Bureau in its endeavor to advance the cause of civilization among these Indians."

After first being banned from two reservations, followed by a request for his recall by Agent Stinchecum at Anadarko, Mooney was recalled to Washington. Senator Robert L. Owen (Oklahoma) wrote letter protesting Mooney's removal and defending his integrity, but it likely fell on deaf ears when it reached Commissioner Sells. Becker (1921) included a comment illuminating how Mooney was regarded by those forces. "... [They] waged a losing fight for their religion [and] had no legal protection as a religion, until a representative of the Smithsonian Institution at Washington, for reasons not yet clear, started active propaganda among the various tribes to arouse a new enthusiasm in peyote and the Indian dance. ... The harm of reviving the pagan practice became so apparent that the United States Government sent officers out to investigate and ordered white agitators from the reservation." It is worth reflecting that during this period Mooney had specifically been assigned by the Bureau of Ethnology to study the peyote religion (Owen, 1921).

While the religious use of peyote was clearly part of anti-peyotist objections, the prejudices held against peyote were also based on the erroneous assumption that peyote was no different from alcohol or other addictive drugs.

The so-called third "Great Awakening," following the 1859-1860 revivalist craze, stimulated a lasting activist imperative whose core goals included achieving the prohibition of all intoxicants

241

worldwide. In a syndicated news flash extolling the progress of the Women's Christian Temperance Union (WCTU), Clarence True Wilson clarified their intentions that "Prohibition is a World Movement. The evil it aims to remove is worldwide in extent and as old as the human race. ... [The] downward tendency of human nature is to seek excitement in the sub-cellar of its being, and the biggest task we have is to get folks to move upstairs. ... For people of every clime and age have found methods of gratifying this lower propensity with intoxicants" (Wilson, 1910).

Wilson listed opium, coca, cocaine, alcohol, hashish, Datura, fly-agaric, betel, tobacco and mescal beans as well as yaupon [*Ilex vomitoria* Aiton], tea and cocoa as pernicious influences from which humans needed compulsory liberation. The sentiment was captured nicely in a quip from R.G. Watermulder in 1914: "[Peyote] then appeals to his craving for leadership and to the lust of the flesh. And today we have a new semi-religious movement among our Indian people, with peyote as a fetish that is worshipped, as something extra ordinarily supernatural. ... I stand appalled and cry, 'O God, we will fail in all our work unless thou dost set these men free-and then they shall be free indeed-and use us to set them free.'"

One prohibitionist summed it up simply: "When we know we're right, the trouble comes in convincing the other fellow and the other fellow's fellows" (*American Advance*, 1911). As this quote demonstrates the speakers are clearly of a mindset that lack of agreement is only an indication that more convincing or coercion is required.

And there's the rub. While temperance refers to the use of personal self-control to limit intoxicant ingestion, the goal of a prohibitionist is instead achieving legislation to implement their religious ideology through force of law by declaring what they consider sins to be crimes. This line of thought was captured succinctly in a comment appearing in Kinney (1922) "... the only right way to deal with an evil is to outlaw it."

Their contemporary H.L. Mencken (1914) offered some lucid observations about what was then occurring: "The new Puritanism is not ascetic but militant. Its aim is not to lift up the saint but to knock down the sinner. ... Differing widely in their targets and working methods, these various Puritan enterprises have had one character in common: they are all efforts to combat immorality with the weapons designed for crime." It was not a casual word choice when the biographer of Special Agent William E. Johnson complimented his dedication to the 'temperance' cause with the comment, "He is a good soldier of Jesus Christ" (McKenzie, 1920). The personally-held Christian militant imperative may well have remained the strongest driving force of anti-intoxicant activity even after perception of the subject matter had been transformed into one of public health and safety.

Lisa McGirr (2015) produced a very well researched study of prohibition that largely served as the basis for the following analysis.

The Prohibitionists' decades-long campaign to eradicate the nation's then-legal drug and alcohol sales, production, and distribution finally succeeded, despite the actual population being very divided on this subject. A majority of the country did not actually favor Prohibition but the contest was close enough that a good showing at the polls could take a majority of the votes; especially if the naturalized immigrant turnout was low. Achieving Prohibition required many years of persistent effort accompanied by having success with getting their supporters elected or appointed into positions of influence and policy making. An under-appreciated part of those successes was the huge increase in the ranks of enforcement personnel and support staff, creating a large body of professional enforcers and enablers. A dramatic expansion of the federal government's power in national law enforcement accompanied this and led directly to the creation of the modern federal legal machinery (McGirr, 2015).

After establishing legislative dominance at the end of the 19th century, the Prohibitionists implemented a number of policies over the course of the next three decades that not only gave birth to the modern federal legal system but turned mass incarceration and prison building into a boom industry, setting the conditions and providing the impetus for the modern war on drugs. By 1930 over half of the federal prison population was there for drug or alcohol offenses, and by 1935 half of that same population was there specifically on narcotics violations (McGirr, 2015).

Special courts, overcrowding in prisons (some states reported having two prisoners for every bed), armed vigilante goon squads (sometimes comprised of the Ku Klux Klan) assisting law enforcers, and the shooting of unarmed suspects all became commonplace in the aftermath of the Volstead Act, commonly known as the National Prohibition Act (See US Congress, 1919). Prohibitionists ran roughshod over basic civil rights in their zeal to shut down alcohol production and distribution, conducting door to door warrantless searches in immigrant and minority neighborhoods. At law enforcement's behest, President Hoover set the tone for a "tough on crime" approach that has never disappeared from favor. (McGirr, 2015).

Kinney quoted President Warren G. Harding from 1922: "In another generation I believe that liquor will have disappeared not only from our politics but from our memories." Echoing this unrealistic view (or, perhaps, statement of intent?), a 1922 article in The Evening World described the word 'whiskey' as "obsolete" in American English. It added that a cactus known as whiskey root was "also obsolete," adding, despite that "it still grows" (Anon., 1922, *The Evening World*).

During Prohibition, as now, unrealistic expectations were the norm. Sound bites that are still familiar today began appearing during this era: "We hope and believe the raids by Federal and local officers mark the definite beginning of the end of the dope traffic in the United States." Harry J. Anslinger, 8 December 1934. Other headlines from 1929 to 1935, also gleaned from the Dope Chronicles which sadly omits the venues and most of the dates: "Federal machinery limited in combatting drug traffic declared Anslinger," "Victory in War on Dope," "Situation is well in hand" – Dr. Mott, "Drastic Rules to Curb Trade in Narcotics," "Drastic Jail Terms Urged in Dope Evil," and "Congress Will Rush Dope Bill" (Silver, 1979).

Enforcement laid heaviest on small producers and operators in urban poor, minority, and immigrant communities, who could not afford to pay for protection like the larger producers and distributors for whom Prohibition often proved a highly lucrative period. (McGirr, 2015) It is also clear that in some cases the laws were sought less as a ban on the drugs and more as a tool to control people who used those drugs: laws targeting cannabis were enforced in Mexican communities, cocaine in African-American communities, and peyote in Native American reservations.

Peyote drew malicious attention from multiple directions. Opposition to peyote and peyotists was organized on a national basis by several prohibitionist societies and related organizations, including the Indian Rights Association, whose spear-fronts were active at both the state and federal level. They enjoyed an almost seamless working relationship with the various agencies involved in the 'welfare' of indigenous people, which lasted until John Collier entered the picture in the 1930s (see *Daily* 2004). As was also true of law enforcers such as Johnson and Anslinger, each of those groups lobbied, issued press releases, wrote articles for popular magazines and news syndicates[7], and, through assorted (often rural) Protestant churches, conducted national letter writing campaigns to garner public sentiment and pass legislation. (See *American Advance*, 1911; Bonnin, 1917; Bromberg, 1942; Bromberg & Tranter, 1943; *Daily*, 2004; Ellis, 1918; Friends of the Indian, 1914; Home-Missions-Council, 1920[8]; Indian Rights Association, 1918; McGirr, 2015; McKenzie, 1920; Tranter, 1942; Wilson, 1910.) Valentine (1912) complained that the amount of mail received by his office had nearly tripled in the prior decade. In addition to letter writing campaigns, appearance of news items and submissions of articles to popular magazines, some stand-alone publications were also produced and distributed. Gertrude Bonnin published a booklet "The Menace of Peyote" which was widely read and promoted. Bonnin was an active peyote opponent who moved to Washington for several years so as to be able to devote adequate time to congressional lobbying. Another active lobbying force on capitol hill, Herbert Walsh and the Indian Rights Association, produced a similar but larger work in 1918 entitled "Peyote; An Insidious Evil." The Outlook 1917 described that book as having been prepared to spare busy congress people the need to spend time reading through the voluminous submissions in the peyote hearings of that year (US Congress, 1918). State laws most commonly appeared in the wake of perceived failures by the federal authorities to suppress peyotism. An underappreciated part of this picture was the federal mandate to convert the Indian nations to Christianity combined with the Bureau of Indian Affairs, the Board of Indian Commissioners and the employees of all reservations being largely comprised of a membership drawn from the missionary ranks who shared a common belief that traditional Native American religious practices, including the use of peyote, impeded the acceptance of Christianity. [Becker, 1921; Valentine, 1911] The "Indian Nations" were governed by the Board of Indian Commissioners who, since their inception, had been drawn entirely from the ranks of missionaries and religious leaders (Keller, 1983) with the following well-defined understanding of their duties and obligations to their "wards."

"... the duty of the [government] being to protect them, to educate them in industry, the arts of civilization, and the principles of Christianity; ..." (Board of Indian Commissioners, 1869).

---

7. Then, as now, the domestic syndicated press organizations were owned by conservative Christians.

8. Robert D. Hall, commented in the report from the thirteenth annual meeting of the Home Missions Council, "... it rests with the Christian citizens of this country to see that Congress votes right on this matter. The women of America are largely responsible for prohibition.. American Christian womanhood is asked to bring all pressure possible to bear upon the members of Congress to vote for the suppression of peyote at the present session of Congress." (1920:89). See also comments therein by G.A. Watermulder on page 159).

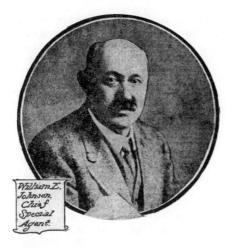

Image 10 Chief Special Agent
William E. "Pussyfoot" Johnson.
Image from Anon., 1912, *Sunday Oregonian*.

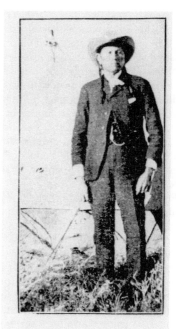

Image 11 Quanah Parker dressed
appropriately in Brownell 1907.

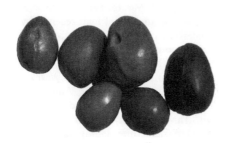

Image 12 The Red Beans.

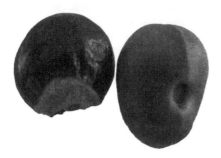

Image 13 *Dermatophyllum secundiflorum.*

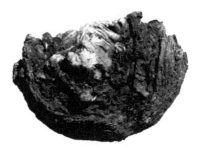

Image 14 Dried *Lophophora williamsii.*

When John Collier tried to introduce a sense of moderation and respect for indigenous culture[9], the attacks were expanded both by the missionary groups and by BIA employees in an attempt to remove him from office or at least negate his influence (*Daily* 2004).

That Collier's shift in policy would cause problems for him seems unsurprising as his opposition included the people in charge of the reservations.

The results of that mandate to Christianize Native Americans created a long-lasting legacy of misguided efforts aimed at the destruction of indigenous culture and religion in general, not just peyote.

DERMATOPHYLLUM SECUNDIFLORUM AS "MESCAL"

To round up the last member of our trio, another mescal bean appeared on the scene. Mescal beans became applied to *Dermatophyllum secundiflorum* at some point after the name was associated with peyote.

The Oklahoma Session Laws of 1899 that illegalized the activity of "Medicine men" also outlawed Mescal beans in Section 2: "That it shall be unlawful for any person to introduce on any Indian reservation or Indian allotment situated within this Territory, or to have in possession, barter, sell, give, or otherwise dispose of, any "Mescal Bean," or the product of any such drug, to any allotted Indian in this Territory: Provided, That nothing in this Act shall prevent its use by any physician authorized under existing laws to practice his profession in this Territory." These laws did not provide an appropriate definition of the phrase "'mescal bean," and contributed to the existing confusion between the red bean and peyote. Definitional complaints along these lines in 1907–1908 left the ban unrenewed.

The exact point of appearance of the common name "'mescal bean" might be unclear but it is demonstrable that the red bean was being called by that name by 1907 as the following comment from Stewart 1987 illustrates. "After August 21, 1907, [Special Agents] Shell and Johnson had no excuse for confusing the terms "peyote" and "'mescal," for Special Agent R.S. Connell, then at Rosebud, South Dakota, brought to their attention the difference between the mescal bean, *Sophora secundiflora*, ... and peyote, *Lophophora williamsii*". During the 1907 struggle against the ongoing anti-peyotist activity, Quanah Parker testified to the Medical Committee of the Constitutional Convention (in Oklahoma) "that mescal beans were poison and peyote is an herb learned from the Mexican Indians to the Lipan Apache, then Comanche, Kiowa, etc." (Stewart, 1987). Nevertheless, a number of authorities ignored this clarification and continued to call peyote "mescal," "the mescal bean" and "the mescal button."

Undaunted by the continuing confusion, Kansas state legislators seized the bull by both horns. Legislation sailed through both the State House and Senate under the following title: "An act relating to *Lophophora williamsii* or Peyote (Pellote) and *Agava* [sic] *americana* (commonly known among the Kansas Indians as mescal); prohibiting the use or possession thereof, traffic therein, and providing penalties for the violation of this act." This act was made state law in 1920, and Arizona and South Dakota enacted almost identical laws in 1923. Evidence that bad laws die hard can be found in modern-day Dodge City Code 2014 (Dodge City, Kansas), which echoes Kansas' precedent: "11-404. PEYOTE; MESCAL BUTTON; INDIAN HEMP; CANNABIS. It shall be unlawful for any person to plant, cultivate, protect, harvest, cure, prepare, barter, sell, give away or use, or offer to sell, furnish or give away, or to have in his or its possession peyote (pellote), botanically known as *Lophophora williamsii*; or *Agave americana*, commonly known as mescal button; ... or any compound, derivative or preparation of the above-mentioned plants. (K.S.A. 65-4127a; 65-4127b; Code 1983, 20-137)" page 11-6. At least this one spelled *Agave* correctly.

Now that we have gotten to an actual red bean, it seems like a good time to clear up some related misconceptions. An influential 1976 paper by Adovasio & Fry further contorted the conceptual relationship between peyote and the red bean. Based on archeological finds, they speculated that psychotropic drug use had followed a logical and sequential path from more toxic to safer choices. They proposed that the Mexican buckeye, *Ungnadia speciosa* Endl. (Sapindaceae), had been succeeded by the red bean, *Dermatophyllum secundiflora* (Leguminosae), which was then eventually replaced

---

9. John Collier's act that drew the most furor was Circular 2970, in which it said, "No interference with Indian religious life or ceremonial expression will hereafter be tolerated. The cultural liberty of Indians is in all respects to be considered equal to that of any non-Indian group."

by peyote, *Lophophora williamsii* (Cactaceae). This hypothesis has somehow become accepted as fact, despite it including a number of disturbing deficiencies which have not been previously addressed and must be considered:

1. The data presented in Adovasio & Fry's paper appear to be inadequate to support its conclusion. If there was more data, they did not mention it; in any case, it is not possible to consider what may have been omitted.

2. Their oldest reported find apparently yielded only the red bean: they said its presence in the strata was continuous from 8440 BC – 1040 AD. *Ungnadia* was not mentioned.

3. Most of the other sites listed had both the red bean and buckeye. No reported site showed only the *Ungnadia* seeds, and neither empirical data nor any indication of relative proportions were given, outside of a single inadequate comment that the proportion was higher in the older finds.

4. The only example of *Lophophora* was reported at their youngest date. Other ancient peyotes were known to exist, but none were slated for dating. Mardith Schuetz (1963) commented that the Pecos River Focus represented the most archaic culture known in Texas, estimating their age to be "at least" 5000 years, and possibly up to 7000 years. Schuetz added that both peyote and the red bean had been found together in the Shumla Caves, "suggesting contemporaneity or overlapping of mescal and peyote cults." Adovasio & Fry, who were familiar with her paper, omitted this overlap. We will return to the significance of the Shumla cave excavations in a moment.

5. Use of buckeye as a drug is, at best, implausible. We will return to this below.

Details of the evidence presented in Adovasio & Fry:
Some facts concerning this ancient peyote:

1. Taylor (1956) determined the age of the Cuatro Ciénegas (CM79) peyote indirectly, based on pieces of matting that was believed to be in the same context.

2. Taylor and Adovasio & Fry both reported the Cuatro Ciénegas site to date from 810–1070 AD. Terry et al., (2006) corrected these dates to 1070–1280 AD, reflecting direct radiocarbon dating of the peyote.

3. The peyote buttons strung on a cord clearly show that 'best' harvesting practices were already known and being employed by this date.

4. Bruhn, et al., (1978) reported a chemical analysis of the material.

5. In more recent times there has been investigation into an even older discovery of ancient "peyote."

Members of the 1933 G.C. Martin Expedition from the Witte Museum in San Antonio reportedly found the specimens in the Shumla Caves of Val Verde County in Texas. It is believed that the specimens came from Cave #5, but the excavation details were inadequately documented. For sake of context, all of the Shumla Caves sites are located within the same few miles as the Val Verde County sites mentioned in Adovasio & Fry (see map in Story & Bryant, 1966), and date to the same time frame.

Several dates have been given for the Shumla Caves peyotes. Peter Furst slipped an estimated date of 7000 BC for the specimens into a 1989 book review (not mentioning how many were sacrificed or how many remained). The full data from the UCLA Radiocarbon Lab on the Shumla Caves specimen(s) were never retrieved, due to the fatal illness of the technician who did the work and the laboratory's subsequent closing. El-Seedi et al., (2005) and Bruhn et al., (2002) reported two of the remaining Shumla Caves peyote artifacts to average 5700 years old. In both of those cases the published values could be extrapolated as representing the age for all of the artifacts. Radiocarbon dating destroys what it evaluates so it can be a stretch of faith when applying the results to additional materials found in archaeological excavations, even when not inadequately documented as was the case with the Witte expedition to the Shumla Caves.

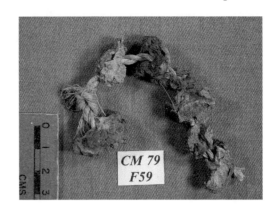

Image 15
This string of buttons was
recovered from a burial site.
Photograph by Martin Terry

Table 1. Summary of the archeological evidence discussed in Adovasio & Fry (1976).

8440–8120 BC (continuous to —1040 AD)	BONFIRE SHELTER Val Verde County, Texas	ONLY *Dermatophyllum*
7500 BC—570 AD	FRIGHTFUL CAVE Val Verde County, Texas	*Dermatophyllum & Ungnadia*
7000 BC—1000 AD	EAGLE CAVE Val Verde County, Texas	*Dermatophyllum & Ungnadia*
7000 BC -1000 AD	COONTAIL SPIN Val Verde County, Texas	*Dermatophyllum & Ungnadia*
4000 BC—1000 AD	FAT BURRO CAVE Coahuila, Mexico	*Dermatophyllum & Ungnadia*
2500—200 BC	ZOPILOTE CAVE Coahuila, Mexico	*Dermatophyllum & Ungnadia*
420—1040 AD	BONFIRE SHELTER Val Verde County, Texas	ONLY *Dermatophyllum*
810—1070 AD (corrected 1070–1280 AD)	CUATRO CIENÉGAS (CM79) Coahuila, Mexico	ONLY *Lophophora*

Image 16
Shumla peyote effigy
Believed to have come from a residential
site rather than accompanying a burial.
Photograph by Martin Terry

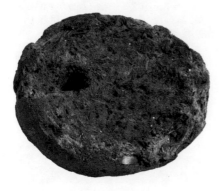

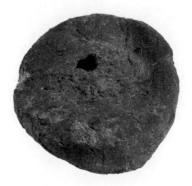

Image 17 Back of one of the Shumla effigies. Photograph by Geoffrey Brune; courtesy of Martin Terry

Image 18 Front of the same Shumla effigy. Photograph by Geoffrey Brune; courtesy of Martin Terry

Terry et al., (2006) established that the three remaining Shumla Caves peyote artifacts were made in two different time periods, each in the range of 4200–3950 BC.

You might have noticed the word artifacts. The most amazing observation in the study by Terry et al., (2006) was that these specimens were not specimens of whole peyote crowns, contrary to reports by Bruhn et al., (2002). There are no signs of ribs, areoles, or any evidence of any vascular structures as are normally present on peyote buttons.

When examined under magnification, these were discovered to have been manufactured; incorporating what is assumed to be peyote but showing a random fibrous internal composition that looks a lot like the wood in chip-board.

Was this an archaic pharmacist's preparation? That would seem to strain credibility and is probably more than a little controvertible.

What is known without any controversy is that these were artifactual items (Terry et al., 2006) incorporating what is assumed to be peyote , based on the reported presence of mescaline (Bruhn et al., 2002; El-Seedi et al., 2005), along with a fibrous plant material binder (Terry et al., 2006). These archaeological artifacts were shaped from some sort of dough to represent a peyote crown that had been cut at ground level. The oldest two of the three remaining artifacts were partially made with non-cactaceous C3 plant material, and the third was made entirely from CAM plants (Terry et al., 2006; with added elements from unpublished data of Martin Terry, Karen L. Steelman, Tom Guilderson and Phil Dering 2003).

As far as learning anything more, the obstacles appear nearly insurmountable. There are no more specimens of this type known and the likelihood of anyone recovering any additional specimens seems remote even if they exist.

All went unrecognized as artifacts, rather than actual peyote buttons, until the Terry et al., examinations. Even El-Seedi et al., referred to the Witte artifacts as "peyote buttons, i.e. the dried tops of the cactus." It is worth noting, though, that El-Seedi's odd comment describing Carolyn Boyd as being someone "who also accepted this identification," as well as Furst's reference to them as "shriveled" (in a 2003 conversation with Jon Hanna) and the peculiar descriptor of "mummified" in Martin (1933) suggests that many may have noticed that something seemed odd.

Of the effigies once at the Witte Museum, two were completely consumed during Furst's inadequately published dating attempt (Hanna 2003). Bruhn's group hollowed out the backs of two of the remaining three.

The latest radiocarbon dates obtained by the Texas A&M group determined at least two different makers created the three surviving effigies of peyote at times separated by several human generations, and using different binder choices (Terry et al., 2006). Nothing further can be known about the other two peyote artifacts. It is also unknown how many there may once have been: there appear to have been at least five, yet Martin (1933) mentioned just one. Schuetz (1963) said that the Shumla Caves peyote was commonly encountered with the red bean. What is also known is that out of all of the specimens reported to have been recovered in a handful or so of archaeological excavations only these two examples appear still to be in the possession of their respective museums. (We refer to the eight whole buttons, originally nine, recovered by Taylor from CM79 and which are housed in the Smithsonian, and to the three ancient manufactured specimens from the Shumla Caves still housed by the Witte Museum.) Peyote specimens were historically common targets of thefts from museum holdings and from herbaria, seriously hampering historical research concerning the plant (Martin Terry, pers. comm., 2012).

The most peculiar datum of all was made by El-Seedi et al.: they report observing 2% mescaline, with no other identifiable alkaloid. To still have 2% mescaline left after six millennia would require a far higher original level, especially as a large percentage of the artifact is the inert fibrous binder. We have many questions without answers in that area.

El-Seedi et al., (2005) suggested that the presence of only mescaline was the result of mescaline's relative stability, compared to other alkaloids. Bruhn et al. (1978) reported 2.25% total alkaloid content in the almost thousand year old peyote from Cuatro Ciénegas. They observed mescaline and four isoquinolines. Bruhn & Holmstedt (1974) analyzed peyote buttons from Rusby in 1887 and compared them to newer material. They found that the material from 1887 contained slightly more alkaloid content overall than the new peyote contained (8.86% vs 8.41%), but that the mescaline content, specifically, was lower in the eighty-seven year old buttons. Nothing conclusive was determined, but they did comment that "the mescaline content of the 'old mescal buttons' was found to be much lower than that of the "new mescal buttons." Only minor discrepancies could be observed regarding the other alkaloids. It is not possible to say whether the relatively lower amount of mescaline in the old material is due to degradation of mescaline with time, or is just a natural variation."

Despite their questions, this material and its associated data are highly significant to the claims in Adovasio & Fry as these are by far the oldest known archaeological finds of peyote or peyote objects, falling deep into the same Archaic period and occurring in the very same 'neighborhood' as Adovasio & Fry's Val Verde County archaeological references, a context where Schuetz (1963) mentioned peyote and the red bean co-occur.

The simple use of the peyote plant itself would surely have preceded processing and reforming it into high potency effigies, so it makes no sense to place peyote consumption at a later date based on a dearth of specimens. A much simpler explanation than a sequential replacement of *Dermatophyllum* by *Lophophora* could be that botanical materials from *Lophophora* does not persist as well as the red bean or those effigies, or perhaps that peyote buttons are more readily eaten by rodents.

There are three points that are worthy of closer examination.

1. The plaited and twilled basketry in the finds was woven closed. Because it would be necessary to tear them open to access the large quantities of seeds inside, Adovasio & Fry suggested that they were used for drug storage. There were quite a lot of *Ungnadia* seeds inside: Adovasio & Fry report eleven pounds in a single basket, and Martin similarly reports finding half a bushel stored in one badly deteriorated basket at Shumla. However, Adovasio & Fry closed their paper by saying that "[the] enormous quantities found in some of the sites seems much more than ritual alone would require, particularly given the small amount needed to become crazed. The incidental use of such agents as simple intoxicants is therefore not to be discounted." In fact, non-drug uses for the seeds can more readily explain the presence of seeds in those large amounts.

Two alternative scenarios come to mind. Martin (1933) speculated that the large quantities may have meant that they were eaten as food. The people at Shumla may have found some method to detoxify them prior to consumption, as the toxicity of *Ungnadia* seems quite likely to involve the high levels of cyanogenic lipids mentioned in Seigler et al. (1971). If so, and if the detoxification process involved prolonged leaching, perhaps the closed baskets were used to enclose the seeds.

They could also have been sound producers. The sound that such a container would produce whether shaken, tilted or rotated would be amazing to a person in a peyote-induced state.

2. A larger problem concerning assertions of relative toxicity enters the picture, as *Ungnadia* and *Dermatophyllum* do not appear to be as toxic as some literature suggests. Neither *Ungnadia* nor *Dermatophyllum* have a locatable report of a human lethality: we have been unable to verify any human death resulting from the ingestion of either type of seed. At least, there is no such report in either medical or morbidity literature: only early anecdotal comments exist for *Dermatophyllum*, and nothing has been located for *Ungnadia*. A direct question voiced to Ronald Siegel in late May 2017 was dodged, casting doubts on his published statement that *Dermatophyllum* had killed a child. It seems that, unlike the red bean, one or two *Ungnadia* seeds can be eaten with impunity.

Curiously, both plants share a reputation of being terribly dangerous; careful reading of those claims' origins is recommended.

3. Let's examine more closely why Adovasio & Fry proposed that *Ungnadia speciosa* may be used as an intoxicant. Their original comment: "*Ungnadia speciosa* is a suspected psychotropic agent because it is invariably associated with the red bean" (1976: 94). That is to say, the primary reason they suspected the seed to possess psychoactivity was its common abundance accompanying the red bean.

Adovasio & Fry had referenced the account of a poisoning event in a child that was described in Havard (1885: 507–508): "These, although pleasant to the taste, are quite poisonous; cooking does not render them innocuous. An adult can eat one or two with impunity; three or four soon produce giddiness and a sensation of heat and discomfort at the pit of the stomach." Havard then discussed a child who, after eating two or three seeds, "[...] grew very giddy, staggered up to his mother, asked for water and then fell." The child recovered in a few hours. Havard's short account of the child's giddiness and collapse seems to be the only example suggesting human "intoxication" and was the only piece of evidence for *Ungnadia's* psychotropic use that was offered in support by Adovasio & Fry. There is no indication in either the scientific or drug culture literature that anyone has deliberately experienced, or sought, intoxication from *Ungnadia*. Accordingly nothing that is known of its reported chemistry suggests this plant to possess psychoactivity.

We mentioned that Martin (1933) proposed there may have been archaic food use of *Ungnadia* seeds. That might seem far-fetched considering what we are discussing but humans, such as Havard (1885), Stanford (1981) and Andés (1902), have all mentioned eating limited numbers, sometimes one, of the seeds without adverse effects. The seeds have long been known to be sweet tasting but causing nausea and vomiting if too many are eaten (one or two can be fine according to Havard 1885). The induction of vomiting early in the toxic syndrome may be why a report of a human fatality has remained elusive for *Ungnadia*?

For unclear reasons, a physician named Geoffrey Stanford, and some friends, evaluated the potential of the seeds as a food and reported eating up to twenty without any ill effects. They apparently asserted that an animal study caused them to abandon their evaluation. They claimed that "Rats which had ingested Mexican buckeye seeds soon exhibited numerous signs of both neurological and organ damage and most died within 3 weeks." Wildflower Center webpage citing Stanford 1981. Clearly Stanford and his associates did not die from eating twenty seeds, however no actual meaningful details were included about those rats and we are unable to locate any publication of their results, so it is not possible to say much more.

Havard (1885) appears to be the only source to mention any effect beyond nausea and vomiting.

All poisonings may correctly be called intoxications, but it is misleading to refer to all poisons as intoxicants: users most often actively choose intoxicants for their effects, whereas the actions of poisons are commonly experienced only through accident or other mishap.

As for the mountain-laurel, Dayton (1931) may be the source of later claims (e.g., Siegel, 1989) of children dying from the red bean: "Children have been known to die as a result of eating the seeds, one of which is said to be sufficient to kill an adult human being." Dayton here references Havard (1896: 39–40), whose account was actually a misquote of an anecdote in Wood (1877) about a single frijolillo (mescal-bean). Wood's account did not mention children.

According to Merrill (1977), more than 30 tribes and groups were familiar with the red bean, and possibly as many as 47. Less than half (13-15) actually ingested them. Four to six of those groups are believed to have combined the red beans with peyote tea. Two added red beans to their sprouted-corn beer. Six had medicine societies which restricted red bean use to members during ceremony, sometimes limiting ingestion to a single time during their initiation (always men). Other groups allowed free use of the red bean to both men and women.

Reported human employment spans a diverse and contradictory spectrum, including use as an intoxicant (with common names of the "big drunk bean," "whiskey bean" and "mescal bean"), as a stimulant for dancing, as a purgative, as a soporific variously claimed to last for 1-3 days, for unclear purposes by secret societies, and sometimes for magical purposes in which it was not ingested. It is commonly assumed to be a hallucinogen, but this claim has been disputed. It was used topically as a war medicine. It also was employed in horse medicine, including both oral and external use. It has occassionally been used for seeking visions or seeing the future. It has been burned inside of homes for 'good luck,' and been attached to the fringe of clothing to provide protection against menstrual blood. Beans were often used as beads and for charms. Bandoliers of beans were highly prized, including by peyote leaders (Merrill, 1977).

The first recorded use of "mescal beans" in reference to this plant seems to be in Hugh Lennox Scott's Ft. Sill ledger notes, from 1889-1897. However, as far as I am aware, these were not published until much later in Meadows, 2015.

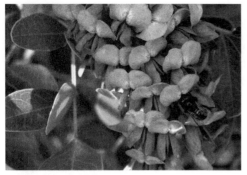
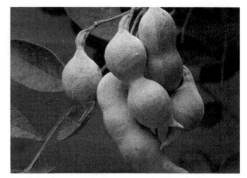

Image 19 *Dermatophyllum secundiflorum*: flowers.   **Image 20** *Dermatophyllum secundiflorum*: pods.

Earlier workers who were familiar with the bean did not refer to it as mescal, instead choosing names such as coral bean, poison bean, frijolillo, frixolillo, or frijolito.' This new and unusual name for the ancient red bean seems to have appeared around or during the same time period as Scott's original notes.

Comments in Garcia's famous 1760 bilingual confessional include two points that are applicable to our discussion of the red bean's intoxicant qualities:

Has comido carne de gente?	Have you eaten people's flesh?
Has comido el peyote?	Have you eaten the peyote?
Te emborrachaste?	Did you get drunk?
Has comida frixolillo?	Have you eaten the 'little bean'?
Te emborrachaste?	Did you get drunk?
Has baylado mitote?	Have you danced the mitote?

Garcia was 1) familiar with the use both of the red bean and of peyote, and 2) does not refer to either as mescal. He uses the familiar names peyote for the cactus and frixolillo for the bean. Based on the lines subsequent to each, he also clearly regards both as for intoxication.

The 'vanished' tribes and groups of south Texas did not actually disappear into oblivion. Instead they 'melted' together, their descendants still prominently represented among the people who live there today (Logan, 2001). Coahuiltecan is a catch-all name including many peoples in South Texas. One of Logan's informants voiced a comment suggesting a continuity of use for both peyote and the red bean. "We come from indigenous people who were hunters and gatherers, and then they build the missions, and then they embrace Catholicism, they become farmers. ... The sun would go down, they would sneak out, they would go do their *mitotes*, and they would have their mescal bean ceremony and the peyote ceremonies, and then they would get caught and they would get beat by the priests or by the Spanish soldiers who went to hunt them down. ... To this day we still do the same type of ceremonies" (Cohen, 2001).

Clearly the red bean had some value to people, but there are many unknowns. It is probable that the red bean and peyote were never considered interchangeable by the cultures using them but instead had separate applications and rituals.

Woods (1877) anecdotally "asserted" that one seed was potentially fatal; this has echoed onward to today and has transformed into established fact. Schultes (1937) commented "the red bean drink was highly toxic, often resulting in death from overdoses." (Schultes did not indicate how "often" or include a reference.) Adam Gottlieb (1973) similarly urged caution: "Extremely toxic. Even just a little too much (½ bean for some) may cause convulsions and death". He suggested a quarter bean as a dose.

It is curious that this perception of extreme danger is so common, given the absence of any credible report of a human death. There are only the historical anecdotes mentioned above, or those involving another cytisine source such as *Laburnum* spp. (Cytisine, a partial nicotinic agonist is the primary alkaloid in the red-bean and there is no question that it could potentially be fatal with a large enough dosage.) There are very few published bioassay reports. However, I know two people who have undertaken a bioassay, one of whom ate three beans. It seems reasonable to wonder how many additional unpublished bioassays have occurred, as there is no venue where those type of accounts could find an outlet. The trip reports at Erowid (Anon 1997, Anon 2006) are the closest resource of that type. The largest amount claimed to have been eaten by a human was fourteen seeds, (Howard, 1957).

The published accounts sound overall uninteresting and rather unpleasant. The most intriguing element, in light of those accounts, is that people have historically used it. That alone seems a likely stimulus for new people to try the red bean.

There is one comment that caught my attention: "One fatal case was reported after ingesting 34 to 50 mg of cytisine. One chewed seed of *Sophora secundiflora* has been reported to be lethal to humans, but supporting evidence is unavailable. ... A lethal dose of seed pods of cytisine-containing *Laburnum anagyroides* Medik. for large animals is estimated as 0.5 g/kg." (*ToxNet*, 2017)

I have not yet been able to learn anything about the particulars of the "one fatal case," whose quoted dose falls within a range of what could in fact be obtained from a few beans. This stands at odds with the oral LD50 numbers for mice (50mg/kg in Hatfield et al., 1977, and 100mg/kg in Dale & Laidlaw, 1912) and also with the results of the two failed suicide attempts by a German pharmacist discussed at ToxNet.nlm.nih.gov under cytisine.

Cytisine is available in pure form to help nicotine addicts quit smoking. *ToxNet* (2017) offers the following adverse reactions: "Pallor, dilated pupils, incoordination, drowsiness, headache, delirium, and hallucinations have been reported. ... Numbness of the hands, muscle weakness, and incoordination can occur. ... Primary effects of toxic doses include: profuse vomiting (which may persist for several hours), abdominal pain, hypotension, tachycardia, confusion, agitation, tremor, and fatigue with an onset time of 15-60 minutes." Outside of stimulation, intoxication and purging appear to be the most commonly reported applications among the few groups who actually used them. In light of all of that, it is not clear why some people are attracted to the bean.

One reason the beans might still be sought by the occasional bioassayist is the rare account of their visionary use. The Ponca reported receiving visions on occasion, while any visionary use that the Pawnee and the Wichita may have associated with red bean was limited to medicine society novitiates at the time of their initiation. Swanton (1942) suggested there was a visionary or divinatory component for the Hasinai Caddo, who used both the red bean and peyote for "intoxication."

Merrill (1977) attributed any visions to set, setting, cultural beliefs, and expectations. "[There] is no evidence that any of these alkaloids, ingested either in isolation or in combination with the others, are capable of inducing hallucinations." The primary use of the red bean, per Merrill, was for "emesis, purging, and perhaps stimulation."

Delirium, agitation and hallucinations have been mentioned in cytisine overdoses and in some Laburnum poisonings (*ToxNet,* 2017). Wiegand (2007) did not mention "hallucinations" in their red bean case but did describe an "agitated delirium" with a "fluctuating consciousness." Oral or high doses of tobacco can be hallucinogenic albeit physically distressing (Janiger & Dobkin de Rios, 1973 & 1976). Cytisine feels somewhat similar to nicotine but has been more relaxed and less euphoriant in our bioassays.

Perhaps the confounding point in the debate about whether the red bean is a hallucinogen or not involves simply how one chooses to define 'hallucinogen.' Is a 'hallucinogen' necessarily limited to something that most people are willing to experience or deliberately repeat? Clearly nicotine can be regarded to possess hallucinogenic properties despite how few people use it for that purpose. The red bean may be prove to be similar if an adequate dosage is employed.

Evaluating the red bean holds some challenges: Hatfield et al. (1977) reported 0.25% cytisine in the beans, while Husemann (1896) found 3.23% and 3.37%. Greshoff (1900) gave 3.5%. Tabex, on the other hand, is derived from *Laburnum anagyroides* seeds, and contains 1.5 mg of pure cytisine per tablet. Furthermore, it has been approved for human use since 1965. For someone who is bent on tasting the bean that seems like a saner starting place than the red bean itself. This is clearly an area in need of much more study, even 140 years after Wood's work.

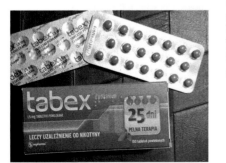

Image 21 Tabex from Bulgaria; ordered online in April 2017.

ENDNOTE

After more than a dozen failures to pass a federal peyote law, often by attempting to sneak a ban into the rewording of an appropriations bill involving liquor traffic, Congress successfully included a provision for admission of peyote addicts when it created the two federal Narcotic Farms in 1929 (US Congress, 1929). It was confirmed by the US Public Health Service in 1945, and again in 1955, that no peyote addicts ever entered either facility (Slotkin, 1975).

As of 2017, it is still possible to find services offering to help break peyote addiction; one need only google "peyote addiction treatment." One of these services, "ProjectKnow," comments that "[some] people can use peyote religiously for years, and then one day stop cold turkey. Others need help and support to break their addiction." Their material suggests that sedatives, professional supervision and "spiritual support" may be needed to offset the hallucinations and other withdrawal symptoms of peyote addiction. Medical doctors have never been in short supply on the anti-peyote bandwagon.

ACKNOWLEDGEMENTS

With special thanks to Dr. Martin Terry for providing valuable comments, corrections and input on this manuscript, and for sharing images and data including access to the partially unpublished work of Terry, Steelman, Guilderson & Dering. Thanks are also extended to both of our reviewers. Their comments and suggestions have substantially improved this work.

REFERENCES

Adovasio, J.M., Fry G.F., 1976. Prehistoric psychotropic drug use in northeastern Mexico and Trans-Pecos Texas. *Economic Botany*, 30: 94–96.

Anderson, E.F. 1980. Peyote. *The Divine Cactus*. The University of Arizona Press, Tucson.

Andés, L.E. 1902. *Vegetable Fats and Oils: Their Practical Preparation, Purification, Properties, Adulteration and Examination.* Scott, Greenwood & Company, London.

Anon. 1854. John Phoenix — a musical critic. *Grand River Times* (Grand Haven, MI), 27 September, page 1.

Anon. 1875. The Plains — Oratio by John Phoenix. *Helena Weekly Herald*, 24 June, page 1.

Anon. 1895. Arizona's Desert Flora. *Arizona Republican* (Phoenix, AZ), 12 December, page 1.

Anon. 1898. Does it really cure — Indian discovers new remedy for consumption — Famous mescal bean — Brings about some remarkable changes. *Wichita Daily Eagle*, 5 October, page 6.

Anon. 1904. A new narcotic to tempt mankind. Mescal a drug which surpasses hashish and furnishes devotees dreams more entrancing than De Quincey's. *The Washington Times*, Magazine Features, 23 October, page 7 .

Anon. 1906. Drug killing off Winnebago Indians — Victims of Mexican Bean dying at startling rate — Rich but degraded tribe — Will be extinct in few years — Introduced but a year ago habit has seized men and women alike — 700 in an orgie [sic]. *The Abbeville Press and Banner* (Abbeville, SC), 20 June, page 2.

Anon. 1906. Insidious Mescal Fatal to Indians — Juice of Mexican Plant Has Succeeded Bad Whisky Among Winnebagos — Men, Women and Children Become Idiotic Under Its influence-Drink Poisonous Drug So They May See Savior. *The Mitchell Capital*, 22 June, page 11.

Anon. 1906. Women Will Fight the 'Mescal.' *The Norfolk Weekly News Journal*, 23 February, page 1.

Anon. 1906. Comment. *The Vinita Daily Chieftain*, 8 February, page 4. Editorial section.

Anon. 1907. Mescal. *The Medical World*, 25: page 201.

Anon. 1909. Mescal bean condemned — Strong intoxicant — Government will prosecute for selling. *The Brownsville Daily Herald*, 13 May, page 4.

Anon. 1909. Getting Drunk on Beans — The demoralizing Mescal and its Effects. *The Rural New Yorker*, 68, 29 May, page 551.

Anon. 1909. Won't Even Let Poor Indians Chew the Joyous Bean That Jags Him Fine. *The Spokane Press*, 17 May, Page 5.

Anon. 1909. Trade in Jag Beans Ends — Juice produces effect like that of strong alcoholic drinks. *The Yakima Herald*, 16 June, page 2.

Anon. 1911. Yankton Indians Use Mescal Beans — Three Men Are Arrested on Complaint of Major Runke and Taken to Sioux Falls for Trial. *Omaha Daily Bee*, 13 April, page 5.

Anon. 1912. Comment. *The Continent*, 10 April, page 489. Editorial section.

Anon. 1913. Indians Chew Up Cactus Buttons and Then See Wonderful Visions and have Peculiar Sensations — Doctor chews it and has visions that best ordinary DTs. El Paso Herald, 16 November, *Comic Section*, page 4.

Anon. 1913. The Senator from New Mexico Had to Explain. *The Newport Plain Talk* (Newport, TN), 6 November, page 4. .

Anon. 1917. Peyote. *The Indian Leader*, 21(13): 18–19.

Anon. 1918. Makes Indians Wild — Terribly ruinous drug introduced on reservation by Mexicans discovered by government agent. *Free Trader Journal*, 28 October, page 3.

Anon. 1922. Where did you get that word? *The Evening World*, (New York, NY), 3 July, *Wall Street* final-edition, page 14.

Bass, A. 1962. James Mooney in Oklahoma. *Chronicles of Oklahoma*, 44(1): 246–262.

Becker, D.A. 1921. Comanche Civilization with History of Quanah Parker. *Chronicles of Oklahoma*, 1(3): 243–252.

Bender, G.A. 1968. Rough and Ready Research — 1887 style. *Journal of the History of Medicine and Allied Sciences*, 23(2):159–166.

Board of Indian Commissioners 1869. *Annual Report of the Board of Indian Commissioners for 1869*, page 10. Government Printing Office, Washington.

Bonnin, G. 1917. Comments on page 39. *34th Annual Report of the Executive Committee of the Indian Rights Association*, Office of the Indian Rights Association, Philadelphia.

Bonnin, G. 1918. *The Menace of Peyote*. Privately printed booklet.

Briggs, J.R. 1887. Muscale buttons — Physiological action — Personal experiences. *Medical Register*, 1: 276–277.

Bromberg, W. 1942. The Storm Over Peyote. *Nature Magazine*, 35(8): 410–412, 444.

Bromberg, W., Tranter, C.L. 1943. Peyote Intoxication — Some Psychological Aspects of the Peyote Rite. *Journal of Nervous and Mental Disease*, 97: 518–527.

Brownell, A. 1906. Chief Quanah Parker — Home of the Comanche Half-Breed in Oklahoma. *New York Tribune*, 2 December, page 20.

Bruhn, J.G., Holmstedt, B. 1974. Early Peyote Research. An Interdisciplinary Study. *Economic Botany*, 28(4): 353–390.

Bruhn, J.G., Lindgren, J.-E., Holmstedt, B. 1978. Peyote alkaloids: Identification in a Prehistoric Specimen of *Lophophora* from Coahuila, Mexico. *Science*, 199: 1437–1438.

Bruhn, J.G., De Smet, P.A.G.M., El-Seedi, H.R., Beck, O. 2002. Mescaline use for 5700 years. *Lancet* (correspondence) 359(9320): page 1866.

Bruman, H.J. 2000. *Alcohol in Ancient Mexico*. University of Utah Press, Salt Lake City.

Burlin, N.C. 1907. *The Indian's Book*, page 162. Harper and Bros, New York.

Castetter, E. 1935. The use of plants for foods, beverages and narcotics. Ethnobiological Studies in the American Southwest I . *Uncultivated Native Plants Used as Sources of Food*. The University of New Mexico. Biological Series, 4(1): 48-61.

CESAR 2006. *Peyote/Mescaline*. http://www.cesar.umd.edu/cesar/drugs/peyote.pdf (accessed 24 April, 2017). CESAR is the Center for Substance Abuse Research at the University of Maryland.

Cohen, J. 2001. Interview Transcripts. Transcription of Dr. Jeff Cohen's (JC) interview with Rick Mendoza (RM) and Rey Ríos (RR), San Juan Mission, San Antonio, TX, 8/25/99. Appendix E, pages 227 — 302, in Thoms, A.V. *Reassessing Cultural Extinction: Change and Survival at Mission San Juan Capistrano, Texas*. Texas A & M University Press, College Station, TX.

Daiker, F.H. 1914. Liquor and Peyote — A Menace to the Indian. *Friends of the Indian 1914*, 62–68.

Daily, D.W. 2004. *Battle for the BIA — G.E.E. Lindquist and the missionary crusade against John Collier*. The University of Arizona Press, Tucson.

Dale, H.H., Laidlaw, P.P. 1912. The physiological action of cytisine the active alkaloid of laburnum (Cytisus laburnum). *Journal of Pharmacology and experimental Therapeutics*, 3: 205–221.

Davis, J.H. 1961. Peyote — America's Baffling Sex Button. *Escape to Adventure*, May 14–15, 60: 62–64.

Dayton, W.A. 1931. *Important Western Browse Plants*. Misc. Publ. 101. U.S. Department of Agriculture, Government Printing Office, Washington.

Dodge City Code 2014. 11-404. *Peyote; Mescal button; Indian hemp; Cannabis*. (Dodge City, Kansas) page 11-6.

Ellis, MD 1918. Our Washington Letter. *The Union Signal*, 46(7): 2–3. National Women's Temperance Union, Washington, DC.

El-Seedi, H.R., De Smet, P.A.G.M., Beck, O., Possnert, G., Bruhn, J.G., 2005. Prehistoric peyote use: Alkaloid analysis and radiocarbon dating of archaeological specimens of *Lophophora* from Texas. *Journal of Ethnopharmacology*, 101: 238–242.

Erowid bioassay reports: 1997 (Atom: 6 seeds) https://erowid.org/experiences/exp.php?ID=50931; 2006 (Pedro: 1.5 seeds) https://erowid.org/experiences/exp.php?ID=50546 (accessed 2 April 2017).

Friends of the Indian 1914. Comment by R.D. Hall on page 74. *Report of the 32nd Annual Lake Mohonk Conference*, 1914. Government Printing Office, Washington.

Furst, P. 1989. Book Review of Peyote Religion: A History, by Omer C. Stewart. *American Ethnologist*, 16: 386–387.

Garcia, Fr. B. 1760. *Manual para Administrar los Santos Sacramentos de Penitencia, Eucharistia, Extreme-Uncion, y Matrimonio*. Herederos de Dona Maria de Rivera, México.

Gottlieb, A. 1973. Legal Highs, *Twentieth Century Alchemist*. [Given elsewhere as Manhattan Beach, CA but this detail is not printed in the actual book.]

Greshoff, M. 1900. Monographia de plantis venenatis et sopientibus quae pisces capiendos adhiheri solent. part II. *Mededeelingen uit 'S Lands Plantentuin*, vol. 29, Landsdrukkerij, Batavia, page 44.

Gudde, E.G., Bright, W. 2004. *California Place Names: The Origin and Etymology of Current Geographical Names*, page 200. University of California Press, Berkeley.

Hanna, J. 2003. Correspondence concerning a conversation with Peter Furst that same year.

Hatfield, G.M., Valdes, L.J., Keller, W.J., Merrill, W.L., Jones, V.H. 1977. An investigation of *Sophora secundiflora* seeds (Mescal Beans). *Lloydia*, 40(4): 374–383.

Havard, V. 1885. *Report on the Flora of Western and Southern Texas*. Proceedings of the US National Museum, 8(29): 449–533.

Havard, V. 1896. Drink plants of the North American Indians. *Bulletin of the Torrey Botanical Club*, 23(2): 33–46.

Heffter, A. 1894. Ueber Pellote. Ein Beitrag zur pharmakologischen Kenntnis der Cacteen. *Naunyn-Schmiedeberg's Archiv für Experimentelle Pathologie und Pharmakologie*, 34: 65–86.

Hennings, P. 1888. *Eine giftige Kaktee, Anhalonium Lewinii N. Sp. Gartenflora*, 37: 410–412. (Figures 92–93).

Hernandez, N.A.O. 2015. La prohibición de lo sagrado. *Edictos y amparos del peyote*. http://www.animalpolitico.com/blogueros-el-dispensario-dialogo-sobre-drogas/2015/11/16/la-prohibicion-de-lo-sagrado-edictos-y-amparos-del-peyote/ (accessed 15 March 2015).

Hodge, F.W. 1912. *Handbook of American Indians North of Mexico*, volume 2, page 106. Government Printing Office, Washington.

Home Missions Council, 1920. Comments by R.D. Hall: pages 75 and 89; G.A. Watermulder: page 159. *Thirteenth Annual Meeting of the Home Missions Council*, Home Missions Council, New York.

Howard, J.H. 1957. The mescal bean cult of the Central and Southern Plains: an ancestor of the peyote cult? *American Anthropologist*, 59: 75–87.

Husemann, T. 1896. Pharmacologie und Toxicologie. *Jahresbericht ueber die Leistungen und Fortschritte in der Gesamten Medicin*, 30: 335–407.

Indian Rights Association 1918. *Peyote an Insidious Evil*. Indian Rights Association, Philadelphia.

Janiger, O., Dobkin de Rios, M. 1973. Suggestive hallucinogenic properties of tobacco. *Medical Anthropology Quarterly*, 4(4): 6–11.

Janiger, O., Dobkin de Rios, M. 1976. Nicotiana an hallucinogen? *Economic Botany*, 30(3): 295—297.

Keller, R.H. jr. 1983. *American Protestantism and United States Indian Policy 1869–82*. University of Nebraska Press.

Kinney, N.J. 1922. *Prohibition a success*. Washington Herald, 8 April, page 4.

León, A. de 1689. see in *West* 1905.

León, Fr. M. (N.) de 1611. *Camino del Cielo en Lengua Mexicana*. Diego Lopez Daualos, México.

Lewin, L. 1888a. XXVII. Ueber *Anhalonium Lewinii*. *Naunyn-Schmiedeberg's Archiv für Experimentelle Pathologie und Pharmakologie*, 24: 401–411.

Lewin, L. 1888b. *Anhalonium Lewinii*. *Therapeutic Gazette*, 3rd. Ser., 4: 231–237.

Logan, J. 2001. Linguistics, pages 95—100, in Thoms, A.V. *Reassessing Cultural Extinction: Change and Survival at Mission San Juan Capistrano*, Texas. Texas A & M University Press, College Station, TX.

Martin, G.C. 1933. *Archaeological exploration of the Shumla Caves*. Southwest Texas Archaeological Society — Witte Memorial Museum, Bulletin 3. Big Bend basket maker papers No. 3.

Massanet, D. 1691. Diario que hicieron los padres misioneros. Reproduced and translated in Lilia M. Casis 1899. Carta de Don Damian Manzanet a Don Carlos de Siguenza sobre el descubrimiento de la Bahia de Espiritu Santo. *The Quarterly of the Texas State Historical Association*, 2(4): 253–312. Also discussed in Portillo 1888.

McGirr, L. 2015. *The War on Alcohol. Prohibition and the rise of the American state*. W.W. Norton, NY & London.

McKenzie, F.A. 1920. *"Pussyfoot" Johnson, Crusader — Reformer — A man Among Men*. Fleming H. Revell Company, London.

Meadows, W.K. 2015. *Through Indian Sign Language: The Fort Sill Ledgers of Hugh Lenox Scott and Iseeo, 1889–1897*. University of Oklahoma Press, Norman.

Memidex. nd. *Mescal*. http://www.memidex.com/mescal (accessed 17 April 2017).

Mencken, H.L. 1914. The American-His new Puritanism. *The Smart Set*, February, 87–94.

Merrill, W.L. 1977. *An investigation of ethnographic and archaeological specimens of mescal bean* Sophora secundiflora *in American museums*. Museum of Anthropology, University of Michigan, Technical report 6. University of Michigan Press, Ann Arbor.

Mooney, J. 1891. Correspondence to Major Charles E. Adams at Anadarko was mentioned in *Bass 1962*.

Mooney, J. 1892. Eating the Mescal. *The Augusta Chronicle* (Augusta, Ga), January 24, page 11.

Mooney, J. 1893. The mescal plant and ceremony. *The Therapeutic Gazette*, 7–11.

Mooney, J. 1920. *October 26 correspondence sent to Joseph Thoburn*. [2 pages; retrieved from the Shulgin Archive, Lafayette, California on 1 March 2017.]

Morfi, Fr. J.A. 1778 (1856). *Documentos para la Historia de Mexico*, 3rd series, book 1. J. M. Andrade, México.

National Park Service (NPS) 2002. *Amistad Tribal Affiliation Study-Annotated Bibliography*. https://www.nps.gov/parkhistory/online_books/amis/aspr-34/contents.htm (accessed 24 April 2017).

Orozco y Berra, M. 1864. *Coahuila*. *Geografía de las lenguas y carta etnográfica de México*, pages 301–309. J.M. Andrade y F. Escalante, México.

The Outlook 1917. Peyote. *The Indian-Leader*, 21(13): 18–19. The Outlook Company, New York

Owen, R.L. 1921. *Correspondence of 21 February sent to Cato Sells*, cc'd with a cover letter to Charles D. Walcott, Secretary, Smithsonian Institution. [2 pages; retrieved from the Shulgin Archive, Lafayette, California on 1 March 2017.]

Portillo, E.L. 1888. *Apuntes para la Historia Antigua de Coahuila y Texas*. Amado Prado, Saltillo, México.

Prentiss, D.W., Morgan, F.P. 1895. *Anhalonium Lewinii* (Mescal Buttons). A Study of the Drug with Special Reference to its Physiological Action upon Man. *Therapeutic Gazette*, 19: 577–585.

ProjectKnow, 2017: *Peyote addiction*. http://www.projectknow.com/research/peyote/ and Mescaline addiction.http://www.projectknow.com/research/mescaline/ (both accessed 12 May 2017),

Random House Dictionary 2017. *Mescal-bean*. http://www.dictionary.com/browse/mescal-bean?s=t (accessed 22 March 2017).

Rivera, P. de 1945. Diario y Derrotero de lo Caminado, Visto y Obcervado en el Discurso de la Visita General de Precidios, Situados en las Provincias Ynternas de Nueva Espana. B. Costa-AMIC, México (original 1736) From *NPS 2002*.

Rusby, H.H. 1894. Mescal Buttons. *Bulletin of Pharmacy*, 8: page 306.

Safford, W.E. 1917. *Narcotic Plants and Stimulants of the Ancient Americans*. Annual Report. Smithsonian Institution, 1916: 387–424, plus 17 plates. Government Printing Office, Washington.

Safford, W.E. 1922. Peyote, the Narcotic Mescal Button of the Indians. *Journal of Pharmaceutical Sciences*, 11(2): 93–96.

Schuetz, M.K. 1963. An analysis of Val Verde County cave material: Part III. *Bulletin of the Archeological Society*, 131–165.

Schultes, R.E. 1937. *Peyote and Plants Used in the Peyote Ceremony*. Botanical Museum Leaflets. Harvard University, 4(8): 129–152.

Schumann, K. 1895. Ueber giftige Kakteen. *Pharmazeutische Zeitung*, 40(175): 577–585.

Scott, H.L., see as *Meadows* 2015.

Seigler, D. et al., 1971. New cyanogenetic lipids from *Ungnadia speciosa*. *Phytochemistry*, 10(2): 485–487.

Sells, C. 1920. Peyote. *Annual Report of the Commissioner of Indian Affairs*, page 20. Government Printing Office, Washington.

Siegel, R.K. 1989. *Intoxication. Life in pursuit of artificial paradise*. Pocket books.

Silver, G. (ed.) 1979. *The Dope Chronicles 1850—1950*. Harper & Row, San Francisco. The unattributed news items drawn from this source lacked bibliographic details.

Slotkin, J.S. 1975. *The Peyote Religion*, Octagon, New York, p. 124.

Stanford, G. 1981 (also found as 1982). *Ungnadia speciosa* (Mexican buckeye). *Plant Propagator*. 28(2): 5–6. This reference has proven inaccessible. It contains an error in the year and/or volume number.

State of Kansas 1920. *Proceedings of the House of Representatives*, 5 January to 27 January 1920, page 111. Kansas State Printing Plant, Topeka.

State of Kansas 1920. *Senate Journal*, page 142. Kansas State Printing Plant, Topeka.

State of Oklahoma 1899. *Article 2 — Medicine Men and Mescal Beans*. Oklahoma Session Laws, page 122. State Capital [sic] Printing Company, Guthrie.

Stedman, E.C., Hutchinson, E.M. 1891. Musical Review Extraordinary. By George Horatio Derby (1823–1861). A Library of American Literature. Vols. VI–VIII: *Literature of the Republic*, Part III., 1835–1860. C.L. Webster, New York.

Stewart, O. 1987. *The Peyote Religion*. University of Oklahoma Press, Norman.

Story, D.A., Bryant, V.M., 1966. *A Preliminary Study of the Paleoecology on the Amistad Reservoir Area*. University of Texas, Austin.

Swanton, J.R. 1942. *Material on the History and Ethnology of the Caddo Indians*. Smithsonian Institution, Bureau of American Ethnology, Bulletin 132. Government Printing Office, Washington.

Tabex product literature, Sopharma, Sofia, Bulgaria. [Purchased online in March of 2017]

Taylor, W.R. 1956. Some implications of the carbon-14 dates from a cave in Coahuila, Mexico. *Bulletin of the Texas Archeological Society*, 27: 215–234.

Terán de los Rios, D. 1691-1692. Descripción y Diario Demarcatión. *Mem. de Nueva España*, xxvii, 25, MS. [cited in Hodge 1912]

Terry, M.K., Steelman, K.L., Guilderson, T., Dering, P., Rowe, M.W. 2006. Lower Pecos and Coahuila peyote: new radiocarbon dates. *Journal of Archaeological Science*, 20: 1–5.

ToxNet.nlm.nih.gov (Toxicology Data Network) NIH; U.S. National Library of Medicine, *HSDB: Cytisine*. https://toxnet.nlm.nih.gov/cgi-bin/sis/search2/f?./temp/~abQ7i1:3. (accessed 1 June 2017)

Tranter, C.L. 1942. Peyote — New Dope Menace. *PIC Magazine*, 8 December, pages 6–9.

Turner, M.W. 2010. *Remarkable plants of Texas: Uncommon accounts of our common natives*. University of Texas Press, Austin.

U.S. Congress 1918. Peyote H.R. 2614. *Hearings before a Subcommittee on Indian Affairs*. Government Printing Office, Washington.

U.S. Congress 1918. Prohibition of Use of Peyote. *65th Congress House Reports*, volume 2, report number 560, pages 1–26. Government Printing Office, Washington.

U.S. Congress 1919. National Prohibition Act (P.L. 66) *Congressional Record*, pages 305–323. Government Printing Office, Washington.

U.S. Congress 1921. Comment. *Congressional Record*, page 4688. Government Printing Office, Washington.

U.S. Congress 1929. *Porter Narcotic Farm Act* (P.L. 70–672, 45 Stat. 1085) [See chapter 82.] Government Printing Office, Washington.

Valentine, R.G. 1909. Suppression of the liquor traffic. *Annual Report of the Commissioner of Indian Affairs*, 1908–1909, pages 11–14. Government Printing Office, Washington.

Valentine, R.G. 1911. Comments made on page 35. *Annual Report of the Commissioner of Indian Affairs*, 1911. Government Printing Office, Washington.

Valentine, R.G. 1912. Comments made on pages 5–6. *Annual Report of the Commissioner of Indian Affairs*, 1912 Government Printing Office, Washington.

Wade, M. 1999. Unfolding Native American History: The Entrada of Fr. Manuel de la Cruz and the Bosque Larios Expedition. *Bulletin of the Texas Archeological Society*, 70: 29–48.

Walsh, H. 1920. Comments made on pages 53–54. *37th Annual Report of the Executive Committee of the Indian Rights Association*. Office of the Indian Rights Association, Philadelphia.

Watermulder, Rev. G.A. 1914. Mescal. *Friends of the Indian* 1914: 67–74.

West, E.H. 1905. De Leon's Expedition of 1689. *Quarterly of the Texas Historical Association*, 8(3): 199 — 205. (Details are also discussed in Portillo 1888.)

White, E.E. 1888. Report of Kiowa, Comanche, and Wichita Agency. in *Fifty-Seventh Annual Report of the Commissioner of Indian Affairs for 1888*, See pages 95, 98 & 99. Government Printing Office, Washington.

Wiegand, T.J., Smollin, C.G. 2007. Ingestion of Mescal Beans *Sophora secundiflora* Causing Agitation in an Adolescent — A New Intoxicant. *Clinical Toxicology*, 45: 333–390. EAPCCT Abstracts, page 344.

Wildflower Center 2017. *Mr Smarty Plants column*. http://www.wildflower.org/expert/show.php?id=7496&frontpage=true, (accessed 2 April 2017).

Wilson, C.T. 1910. Poisons charms. *American Prohibition Year-Book for 1910*, pages 67–68.

Wood, H.C., jr. 1877. Preliminary note on a new medicinal plant and its alkaloid. *Philadelphia Medical Times*, 7(258) 4 August: 510–511.

Reflections on the Peyote Road with the Native American Church – Visions & Cosmology

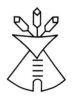

Jerry Patchen

Attorney and trial lawyer;
Represented the Native
American Church to preserve
religious freedoms.
Houston, Texas

ABSTRACT

The historical courageous struggle of the Native American Church (NAC) to use their sacrament Peyote is unprecedented in American culture. Without the Native Americans' indomitable spirit and arduous legal battles extending over four centuries, there would be no legal use of Schedule 1 controlled substances in the United States, except for cannabis in various states. As an attorney representing the NAC for four decades, the author was integrally involved in protecting and advancing the religious freedom rights of Indians and the legal status of Peyote. In 2005, he was awarded the distinguished Lifetime Achievement Award by the State Bar of Texas for this service. He chronicles his extensive knowledge of Peyote, its history, some important individuals, legal proceedings, law, and the contributions by ethnologists, ethnobotanists, anthropologists, and academics from related fields, to the victory of the NAC. Having served as an officer in the NAC and participated in many NAC Peyote prayer services, the author shares some of his personal visions and life-shaping experiences with Peyote.

WHY WOULD AN ATTORNEY ADDRESS AN ETHNOPHARMACOLOGICAL SYMPOSIUM?

It is the case that the law has a dramatic impact on the ethnopharmacological search for and use of psychoactive drugs. There has been an interplay between law and psychoactive drugs in the Americas since the 1600s. The courageous and historical struggle of Native Americans to use their sacrament Peyote, *Lophophora williamsii*, blazed the trail securing the legal right to use psychoactive Schedule I controlled substances in the United States. The Native American Church (NAC), assisted by ethnologists, ethnobotanists, anthropologists, pharmacologists, and psychiatrists, was the spear point that established the court precedents and legislation that resulted in the legal use of Peyote and *ayahuasca* as sacraments for religious purposes in the U.S.

Serving as an attorney for the NAC over four decades, I provided *pro bono* representation to protect and secure the legal status of Peyote for use by Native Americans in NAC prayer services (Peyote meetings). I also represented the Texas Peyote dealers, who are licensed by the Drug Enforcement Administration and the Texas Department of Public Safety to harvest and sell Peyote to Indian members of the NAC. I fought many legal battles for Indians arrested for possession of Peyote in courts throughout the U.S., along with advancing Native American religious freedom rights in the U.S. Congress. I will present a survey of historical and contemporary law regarding Peyote. There is extensive literature on Peyote which covers scientific and academic studies. There is a void in the literature describing Peyote visions, which are varied and unique to time, person, place, and events. I discuss visions I experienced in NAC Peyote meetings and some Indian cosmology.

My wife Linda and I participated in Peyote meetings with the fabled, fearless, horse-riding Indian warriors of the Southern Plains (Fig. 1). With their buffalo food supply purposefully decimated, their numbers annihilated through massacre and disease, conquered and removed from their homelands, the Plains Indians were restricted to reservations by the U.S. Cavalry parading under the banner of God-ordained Manifest Destiny. We were privileged and fortunate to join in Peyote meetings with Indian elders of the NAC whose grandfathers and grandmothers had survived the Indian genocide[1], and who were removed from the Southern Plains to Oklahoma (Fig. 2). Plains Indian wisdom and traditions were orally passed on from grandparents to grandchildren. We were in direct contact with the lineage, experiences, and wisdom of the free-spirited Indians, specifically the Apache, Comanche, Kiowa, Cheyenne, and Arapaho, the Southern Plains Indians who pioneered and developed the Peyote ceremony in its present-day form, and who were instrumental in establishing the NAC in Oklahoma in 1918 (Fig. 3).

THE ESTABLISHMENT OF THE NATIVE AMERICAN CHURCH IN OKLAHOMA

The Carizzo, Lipan Apache, Mescalero Apache, and Tonkawa ranged south into what is now Texas and Mexico. They were in contact with Mexican Indian Tribes. The Apaches brought Peyote to their Comanche allies. It was then spread to other Southern Plains tribes. Ultimately, Peyote spread to the Northern Plains Indians and later to the Navajo. A number of the elements found in the 19th-century Peyote ritual of the Southern Plains Indians were present in their Mexican precursors, including drums, rattles, tobacco, fire, and ceremonial foods such as corn and meat, and of course Peyote.[2]

The NAC is a syncretic religion. Indians readily adopted Christian concepts and combined them with their own cosmology. Article II of the Charter of Incorporation of the NAC of 1918 states:

> The purpose for which this corporation is formed is to foster and promote the religious beliefs of the several tribes of Indians in the state of Oklahoma, in the Christian religion with the practice of the Peyote Sacrament . . . and to teach the Christian religion with morality, sobriety, industry, kindly charity, and right living and to cultivate a spirit of self-respect and brotherly union among the members of the Native race of Indians. . . .[3]

Indians honored the "Great Spirit" and the "Great Mystery" long before the voyage of Columbus. Indians steadfastly honored a Spirit greater than themselves. The Indians were not attached to labels. If the dominant culture insisted that the Great Spirit was God, the Indians' attitude was the Great Spirit by any name is just as powerful and mysterious. Likewise, accepting Christ as the Son of God was in rhythm with the Indian experience that we are all God's children. Indian people are very spiritual and traditionally monotheistic. The Catholic Church has archangels, similarly Indians have spirits. Like Christians, Native Americans have earnestly and humbly used prayer for thousands of years. It was easy for Indians to accept prayer since it had always been a part of their spiritual practice.

Indians honor and respect Mother Earth and all of Nature and are free of the Christian hubris of dominating all forms of life. Indians insist that we are not separate and apart from Nature, we are

---

1. Author's comment: The Cherokee Trail of Tears is well known, as is the Wounded Knee Massacre. Every tribe experienced its own genocide, land seizure, displacement, and removal to reservations. By way of example, the Pawnee tribe had a population over 10,000 before the Indian Wars. By the time of their removal, they numbered approximately 1,500. The proud Cheyenne, fierce warriors, victims of the Sand Creek massacre, came near to total extinction. The Wichita tribe, which numbered in the thousands, was reduced to 572 when they were removed to an Oklahoma reservation. Dee Brown's bestselling book *Bury My Heart at Wounded Knee* is an excellent treatise on the American Indian Genocide.

2. Swan, Daniel C., 1999. *Peyote Religious Art – Symbols of Faith and Belief*. Univ. Press of Mississippi, 3.

3. Stewart, Omer C., 1987. *Peyote Religion: A History*. U of Oklahoma Pr., Norman, Okla., 224. Author's note: Omer Stewart, longtime anthropologist at the University of Colorado, dedicated his life's work to the study of Peyote. Stewart's book *Peyote Religion* is the seminal treatise on Peyote. Stacy Schaefer's definitive study, *Peyotism: Amada's Blessings from the Peyote Gardens of South Texas* (Univ. of New Mexico Press, 2015), is a remarkable contemporary book lovingly focused on Amada Cardenas. See also: La Barre, Weston, 1938. *The Peyote Cult*, Yale Univ. Publications in Anthropology – Number 19. Yale Univ. Press; Aberle, David, 1966, revised 1982. *The Peyote Religion Among the Navaho*. The Univ. of Chicago Press. Omer Stewart's student George Morgan produced an outstanding thesis on Peyote: Morgan, George R., 1976. *Man, Plant and Religion – Peyote Trade on the Mustang Plains of Texas*. PhD Thesis, Univ. of Colorado.

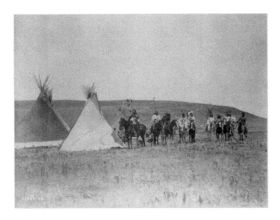

Fig. 1 Gathering War Party
Courtesy of the Library of Congress,
LC-USZ62-103068.

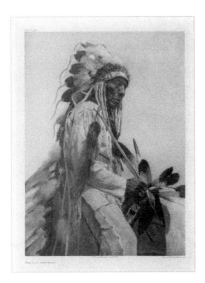

Fig. 2 The Old Cheyenne – Edward Curtis
Courtesy of McCracken Research Library.

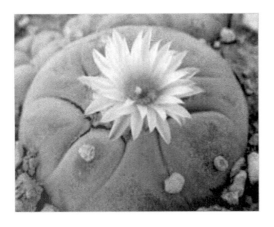

Fig. 3 Peyote cactus in bloom.

part of Nature. Before Darwin, Indians realized that all birds, animals, plants, trees, insects, wind, water, and elements are our "relations", and they, along with all life forms, are an inseparable part of Nature. A fundamental distinction between Christianity and Indian cosmology was the Christian belief that humans uniquely possess a spirit or soul, while Indians believe that all life forms have a spirit that ultimately transcends the earth.

Native Americans take the cosmology a step further. All birds, animals, and other life have a spirit, and our spirit can communicate with the spirit of all life. They grew up immersed in Nature, communicating with the spirits of birds, animals, and all life. When this life view is embraced, one learns to perceive a language beyond words that is just as real as the spoken word. The sounds, sights, movements, patterns, intuitions, and feelings that are communicated by birds, animals, plants, trees, and all other life provide inspiration, direction, and omens that become important guide posts in our lives.

THE SUMMER OF LOVE AND THE BIG BANG!

Linda and I met at the University of Houston in 1967, the Summer of Love (Fig. 4). I was in law school and serving as the Student Association's Attorney General. Linda served as the secretary. The counterculture came into public awareness as a mass movement. A huge shift and transformation of the social paradigm was occurring, which involved creative expression, art, music, dress, grooming, sexual freedom, civil rights, antiwar politics, Eastern spirituality, yoga, meditation, marijuana, psilocybin, LSD, mescaline, and Peyote. We were young, healthy, and curious college students. So what did we do? We tuned into the zeitgeist – the spirit of the times.

I happenstance secured some mescaline, which I ingested during yoga and breathing exercises. I was totally unprepared for what occurred. It was the classic kundalini experience. Suddenly, a bolt of lightning coursed up my spine and ignited a thermonuclear explosion. The simultaneous ignition of every atomic bomb on the planet would have been a hummingbird's whisper compared to the magnitude of that explosion.

I experienced the Big Bang. I was instantaneously transported to the moment of creation – the center point of all consciousness – which contained peace, radiance, and ecstatic wonder beyond comprehension. My ego was completely annihilated. I experienced eternal boundlessness, unity beyond time and space. I merged with the Divine. I had a profound sense of knowing that my essence always was, always is, and always will be. I am not suggesting that my personality will survive bodily death, but that my essence will reunite with the Divine Life Force.

Forty-five years later, this remains one of the most influential experiences of my lifetime. My understanding of reality was totally and permanently transformed. We are limited human beings on the planet Earth, and yet paradoxically we are the Universe.

As a young attorney, I was determined to stay within the bounds of the law. I was aware that mescaline was the psychoactive compound in Peyote. Linda and I learned there was a tradition of Indians annually coming to Texas to the home and property of Amada Cardenas, a legendary Peyote dealer (Peyotera) near Laredo, erecting a tipi, and legally conducting a Peyote prayer service (Fig. 5).

In the U.S., Peyote is only abundant and indigenous near Laredo. It occurs in a narrow band east of Laredo that extends down into Mexico. Indians consider it a very special privilege to experience a Peyote meeting where it grows, and where their ancestors pilgrimaged to harvest Peyote and to pray.

MEETING AMADA CARDENAS AND THE INDIANS

Having learned of the annual Peyote meeting with Amada Cardenas, Linda and I traveled to south Texas in 1972 and found Amada's home, which was located a little south of Mirando City. We shyly tapped on the door of Amada's small, humble casa. Amada opened the door and gave us the most wonderful open-hearted welcome that we have ever experienced. She saw us and emphatically said, "Come in! I am so glad you are here! Can I get you some coffee or something to eat?"

Our experience was not unique. Amada was legendary for her open heart, and open hearth. It did not matter who arrived at her door. She was delighted with every visitor that came to her home. It did not matter to her what color you were. It did not matter whether you were poor. Your position in life was not important to her. She was glad to welcome you. She would busy herself scurrying around providing coffee and food, and taking care of her visitors.

Upon meeting Amada Cardenas, she invited us to come visit the Indians when they came to her home for the annual NAC Peyote meeting in February. We were hesitant to do so because, as we told her, "We do not know any Indians." She responded emphatically, "That is okay, you can be my guest." The following February in 1973, we returned to Amada's home. Arriving mid-afternoon, we parked outside the fence, and saw numerous Indians around her property. There was a tipi erected near the back center of the property. Almost hesitantly, we got out of our car and slowly began walking up her driveway. A striking Indian with a big smile walked toward us and greeted us in a most friendly way. His name was Rutherford Loneman. He invited us to briefly go inside the tipi. We then hung around Amada's home and property observing the activities.

As the sun went down, the Indians entered the tipi and had a NAC prayer service. It was a cold and rather windy February night. Linda and I sat outside all night on a railroad tie on the north side of the tipi. We listened to the singing, drumming, and humble, even pleading prayers of the Indians. The next morning after the meeting, Rutherford Loneman approached us. Rutherford said to us, "I could feel you outside all night. You are looking for something good. Come back next year. I want you to go in the tipi with us."

RUTHERFORD "WHITE STAR" LONEMAN, NAC PEYOTE ROAD CHIEF

After the invitation from Rutherford Loneman to return, Linda and I made our own pilgrimage to the annual meeting place on the property of Amada Cardenas outside of Mirando City, Texas. We attended our first Peyote prayer service accompanied by Rutherford Loneman (Fig. 6 & 7).

An amazing Southern Arapaho Indian Road Chief[4], Rutherford was the grandson of Old Man Loneman, who escaped the genocide, was removed to Oklahoma, and passed on his Plains Indian wisdom to Rutherford. During Rutherford's birth, Rutherford's mother consumed Peyote in an old frame house near Concho, Oklahoma, in a practice sometimes used by Indian women during labor. Old Man Loneman, Rutherford's grandfather, erected a tipi near the house. Old Arapaho Chiefs gathered with Old Man Loneman in a Peyote meeting. Immediately after Rutherford was born, he was taken inside the tipi and was passed around to the old Chiefs. Rutherford told me, "Each of them put something in me."

Linda and I began an annual pilgrimage, returning every February for decades to the annual meeting at Amada's. Pilgrimage, in and of itself, is a powerful process. We had many glorious experiences and developed many close and loving relationships with Indians from many tribes, most especially Rutherford Loneman, who adopted me in the Indian way as his son.

In addition to an annual meeting in Texas, we began traveling and rendezvousing with Rutherford, other Road Chiefs, and Indian friends, going to Peyote meetings on many different reservations and in many different states, including Oklahoma, Arkansas, New Mexico, Arizona, Colorado, Utah, Nevada, Wyoming, California, and South Dakota. Rutherford could create an atmosphere of love in the tipi that was palpable. Love is an important principle in the NAC. Peyote produces a profound connection with and appreciation for those around you, Nature, all life, and the environment. Peyote produces an astonishing mental clarity and elevated conscious awareness. Peyote can produce powerful and clear visions through all our senses. Peyote fosters deep and meaningful self-examination and a sincere motivation for self-correction and improvement. Peyote is a mirror to your soul. Ecstatic experiences reliably occur in Peyote meetings, fostered by the drumming, the gourd, the singing, the colors, the fire, aromatic cedar, and the whole sacred process.

Linda and I attended a beautiful Peyote Meeting outside of Santa Fe that Rutherford led. He doctored a sick elderly Asian lady with his red-tailed hawk fan during the meeting. She was brought in and laid in the tipi. Rutherford told me that he removed things from people with his feathers. The next morning at early light, Rutherford held the staff and gourd and sat silent. He looked at the fire and held his hand out toward the fire and said, "From where I sit this morning, it is all right there. It is very simple. It is all right there. Those who have gone on and those that are coming. It is all very simple, and it is all right there." It was a profound moment for me. Rutherford transmitted something ineffable about life. Rutherford always told me, "In the tipi we talk about life, this process of life." Peyote meetings must be approached in a serious and reverent way.

Sometimes during Peyote meetings, the old people would solemnly reach out with tears rolling down their faces, as if they were embracing and touching someone wonderful standing before them, though no one was there. I asked Rutherford why that occasionally occurred. He told me, "Some-

---

4. A Road Chief is the NAC functional equivalent of a Catholic Priest, Jewish Rabbi, or Zen Roshi. The term Road Man is used interchangeably with Road Chief.

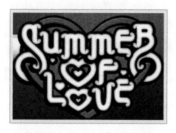

Fig. 4 Summer of Love.

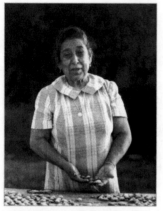

Fig. 5 Amada Cardenas, age 68
Courtesy of Linda Patchen,
Nov. 1972.

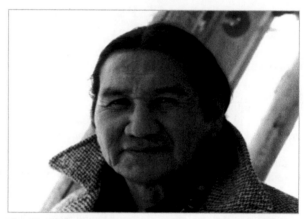

Fig. 6 Rutherford Loneman, Southern Arapaho, NAC Road Chief.
Courtesy of Linda Patchen.

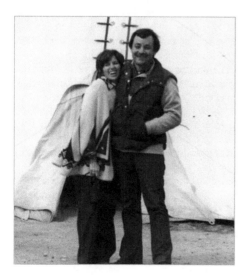

Fig. 7 Jerry & Linda Patchen at Peyote Meeting.
Courtesy of Linda Patchen.

times a Friend of mine comes in here at a special time. I sure want you to meet my Friend. I sure want you to meet my Friend." It was fifteen years later that I experienced the phenomenon he was describing, the appearance of a Spirit image.

ANCIENT USE OF PEYOTE IN THE AMERICAS

The use of Peyote is the oldest religious practice on the North American continent. Its ancient roots are lost in time. The Witte Museum of San Antonio, Texas, possesses three archaeological specimens of Peyote radiocarbon dated between 3660 and 3780 BCE[5], the Middle Archaic Period. These Peyote specimens were discovered in a hunter-gatherer context in the Shumla Cave in the lower Pecos Region of Texas, near the confluence of the Rio Grande and Pecos Rivers. Rock art petroglyphs with Peyote motifs in the area have been dated to the same period. 56[6]

Gas chromatography-mass spectrometry identified mescaline in the Shumla Cave Peyote specimens, which identification establishes that Native Americans recognized the psychopharmacological properties of Peyote 6,000 years ago. it is reasonable to suggest that Native American use of Peyote is even more ancient; perhaps over 10,000 years, from the era of late Pleistocene Paleo-Indian hunters of mastodons to the present day. The Spanish Franciscan missionary and ethnographer Bernardino de Sahagún, who traveled to Mexico in 1529, chronicled the earliest historical reference to Peyote in his Historia General de las Cosas de Nueva España, published in Mexico City in 1591[7]. In 1577, Fernando Hernandez studied plants used by the Aztecs which included Peyotl, the Aztec word for Peyote[8]. When the Spanish Conquistadors arrived in Mexico in the 15th and 16th centuries, the Aztec, Huichol, Tarahumara, Zacateco, and other Indian tribes had ceremonies that centered around the use of Peyote.[9]

THE PROSECUTION OF NATIVE AMERICANS FOR PEYOTE IN NEW SPAIN

Spanish imperialism included supplanting native religions with Catholicism. Mexico and Peyote did not escape the Inquisition. Christianization was forced at the point of the sword under the authority of the Inquisitor General. Plants used in native rituals were condemned. In 1620, the Inquisitors issued an edict declaring Peyote a "heretical perversity . . . opposed to the purity and integrity of our Holy Catholic Faith." Further, Peyote was characterized as the "[I]ntervention of the Devil, the real author of this vice . . . ." The inquisitors proclaimed, "[O]ur duty imposes on us the obligation to stop this vice and to repair the harm and great offense to our God and Lord resulting from this practice . . . ."[10] Consequently, Peyote was the first ethnobotanical psychoactive substance prohibited by law and punished by imprisonment in the Americas. The Catholic Church enforced this edict for over two centuries. In historical Church archives, there are records of 90 prosecutions in 45 locations in North America. [11]

THE PROSECUTION OF NATIVE AMERICANS FOR PEYOTE IN THE UNITED STATES

Indians in the United States were also prosecuted. The Bureau of Indian Affairs (BIA), from its formation in 1824 through the 1930s, was very strongly influenced by missionary societies. For five decades, federal officials on reservations and in Washington D.C. were appointed by Christian mis-

5. Terry, Martin, et al., 2006. *"Lower Pecos and Coahuila Peyote: New Radiocarbon Dates."* Journal of Archaeological Science 33 (7), 1017- 1021.

6. Ibid. See also: Boyd, Carolyn, 2003. *Rock Art of the Lower Pecos.* Texas A&M University Press.

7. Stewart, Omer, 1987. *Peyote Religion*, 18.

8. Ibid, 19.

9. Swan, Daniel C., 1999. *Peyote Religious Art*, 3.

10. Ramo de inquisicion, tomo 289, Archivo General de la Nacion Mexico City, cited in Leonard, Irving A., 1942. *"Peyote and the Mexican Inquisition, 1620."* American Anthropologist 44(2), 324-26.

11. Stewart, Omer, 1987. *Peyote Religion*, 21-22.

sionary groups. Although the Peyote religion has Christian theology combined with Indian spiritual practices, Christian missionaries began to seek legislation to prohibit the use of Peyote. The first such law criminalizing Peyote was enacted in Oklahoma in 1899. Many other states followed suit, including Nevada in 1913, and Utah and Colorado in 1917.[12]

The Oklahoma anti-Peyote law was repealed in 1908 after a delegation of Indian Chiefs, including the famous and eloquent Comanche Chief Quanah Parker (Fig. 8), testified before the Medical Committee of the Oklahoma Constitutional Convention in 1907 (Fig. 9). Quanah was the most influential and instrumental Indian in the creation, development, and spread of the Peyote ritual and ceremony in Oklahoma. [13]

The era of prohibition was raging through American culture. The suppression of Peyote became closely involved with the prohibition against the Indian use of alcohol. In 1906, Congress passed a law against the sale of intoxicating liquor to Indians, with a special appropriation to prosecute violators. President Theodore Roosevelt commissioned a well-known prohibitionist zealot, William "Pussyfoot" Johnson, as a special officer to enforce prohibition in Indian country, and armed Johnson with 100 deputies. Johnson considered Peyote "dry whiskey" and fanatically raided Peyote meetings, arrested and caused the prosecution of Indians for Peyote[14]. Some of the prosecutions were unsuccessful because the law was only intended to apply to alcohol intoxicants. Other cases were defeated as a result of the confusion of Peyote with mescal beans[15]. Nevertheless, many Peyotists were prosecuted and punished for their religious devotion.

ROLE OF ETHNOLOGISTS, ETHNOBOTANISTS, AND ANTHROPOLOGISTS IN PROTECTING THE RIGHTS OF NATIVE AMERICANS TO USE PEYOTE

A BIA commission began in 1912 to lobby for a federal law against Peyote. In 1918, the U.S. House of Representatives held extensive committee hearings. James Mooney, an ethnologist with the Bureau of American Ethnology of the Smithsonian Institution, led the defense of Peyote. (Fig. 10) Mooney studied the Kiowa pictorial calendar in the late 1800s. Between 1891 and 1918, Mooney spent many months with Southern Plains Indians on reservations in Oklahoma. He observed and participated in several Peyote meetings. Mooney, Francis La Flesch (also an ethnologist), and William Safford, a botanist, along with many other supporters of Peyote including eloquent Indians, testified that Peyote had done much good and was a sincere and genuine religion. Naturally, there was fierce opposing testimony from prohibitionists. The bill to outlaw Peyote was passed by the House of Representatives, but rejected in the Senate when a senator from Oklahoma, under pressure from his Indian constituency, persuaded his colleagues to vote against it.[16]

A bitter conflict occurred between the BIA and Bureau of American Ethnology as a result of Mooney supporting Indians during the 1918 hearings. The BIA accused the ethnologists of "encouraging Indians to maintain old, heathenish, unhealthy, uncivilized customs so that scientists could write books, take pictures, and thus exploit the Indians with cheap publicity while doing nothing to help them become civilized."[17] Mooney defended himself and ethnologists, and denounced the accusation as an "absolute falsehood." He returned to the Kiowa reservation in Oklahoma. The commissioner of Indian Affairs requested that the director of the Smithsonian recall Mooney, on the grounds that he was interfering with the administration of the BIA, had participated in Peyote ceremonies, and had assisted the Indians in incorporating their religion as the Native American Church. To the shame of the Bureau of American Ethnology and the Smithsonian, Mooney was recalled and never again allowed to return to Oklahoma to continue his study of Peyote. He died a few years later of a heart attack.[18]

....

12. Stewart, Omer, 1956. *"Peyote and Colorado Inquisition Law."* The Colorado Quarterly 5 (1), 79-90.

13. Quanah Parker's mother, Cynthia Ann Parker, was an Anglo who was kidnapped as a child by the Comanches and reared as a Comanche.

14. Stewart, Omer, 1987. *Peyote Religion* Chapter 6, Early Efforts to Suppress Peyote, 128-147.

15. See: Trout, Keeper. *"Mescal, Peyote, and the Red Bean; A Peculiar Conceptual Collision in Early Modern Ethnobotany"*, ESPD 50 Book.

16. Stewart, Omer, 1987. *Peyote Religion* Chapter 8, Efforts to Pass a Federal Law, 213-238, at 216.

17. Ibid, 221.

18. Ibid, 219-222.

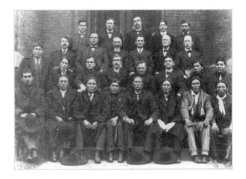

Fig. 8 Indian Delegation testifying to Oklahoma Constitutional Convention, 1907 (Quanah Parker, left to right #5). Courtesy of Fort Sill, Oklahoma Museum # P-4868.

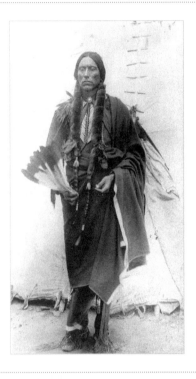

Fig. 9 Quanah Parker. Courtesy of the Library of Congress, LC-USZ62-98166.

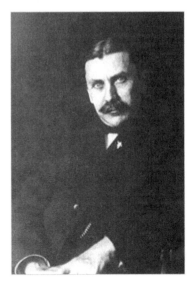

Fig. 10 James Mooney (1861-1921). U.S. Bureau of Ethnology Courtesy of Smithsonian Institute – Bureau of American Ethnology Collection

The first attempt to pass a federal anti-Peyote law was in 1937, during Franklin D. Roosevelt's administration. Frank Takes Gun, a Crow Indian from Montana and President of the Native American Church, rallied the support of seven anthropologists[19]. The group included Richard Evans Schultes, then a Harvard graduate student with the Harvard Botanical Museum. Schultes presented a bibliography of 383 references regarding research on Peyote, and related his field research in Oklahoma. Schultes and the other anthropologists concluded that Peyote is not a "habit-forming drug" and is used as a "religious sacrament"[20]. The United States Senate Committee accepted their conclusion. By this time, the Christian missionaries had been supplanted in the Bureau of Indian Affairs by administrators more protective of the religious rights of Indians. The efforts to prohibit Peyote on a federal level ended for three decades, until the 1960s.

In 1965, the Drug Abuse Control Amendments were proposed. Again, NAC President Frank Takes Gun marshalled evidence from five anthropologists[21] who signed and submitted a joint "Statement on Peyote" to Congress through the Department of Health Education and Welfare. The Statement included in part:

> "In connection with the current national campaign against narcotics, there has been some propaganda to declare illegal the peyote used by many Indian tribes. We are professional anthropologists who have made extensive studies of Peyotism in various tribes. We have participated in the rites and partaken of the sacramental peyote. We therefore feel it our duty to protest against a campaign which only reveals the ignorance of the propagandists concerned.
>
> . . . [T]he Native American Church is a legitimate religious organization deserving of the same right to religious freedom as other churches . . . ."[22]

W.B. Rankin, Deputy Commissioner of the Department, wrote Frank Takes Gun in January 1966 that Peyote was to be added to the Drug Abuse Controlled Amendment of 1965. However:

> "I am writing to state that on the basis of the evidence you have submitted, we recognize that Peyote has a non-drug use in bona fide religious ceremonies of the Native American Church. It is not our purpose to bring regulatory action based on the shipment, possession, or use of Peyote in connection with such ceremonies."[23]

The 1965 Amendment was not enforced against the NAC. Ultimately, in 1971, the Federal Code of Regulations Section 1307.31 incorporated a specific exemption for the NAC, declaring in part, "The listing of peyote as a controlled substance in Schedule I does not apply to the nondrug use of peyote in bona fide religious ceremonies of the Native American Church."

THE JURISPRUDENCE OF PEYOTE IN THE UNITED STATES FROM 1970 ONWARD

The First Amendment to the United States Constitution provides, "Congress shall make no law respecting an establishment of religion, or prohibiting the free exercise thereof." In 1963, in the case of *Sherbert vs. Verner*, 374 U.S. 398, the United States Supreme Court, in an elegantly written opinion by Justice Brennan, declared, "The door of the Free Exercise Clause stands tightly closed against any governmental regulation of religious beliefs. . . . In this highly sensitive constitutional area, only the gravest abuses, endangering paramount interests, give occasion for permissible limitation." The

---

19. Franz Boas, PhD, Columbia, A.L. Kroever, PhD University of California Berkeley, Ales Hrdlicka, PhD Smithsonian Institution (anthropologist and MD), John P. Harrington Smithsonian Institution, M.R. Harrington, PhD, Curator Southwest Museum, Los Angeles, California, Weston La Barre, PhD Yale, Vince Petrullo, PhD, Works Progress Administration, Washington, D.C.; Personal Archives of author from Frank Takes Gun.

20. Personal Archives of author from Frank Takes Gun.

21. Weston La Barre, PhD Duke Univ., David McAllester PhD Wesleyan Univ., J.S. Slotkin, PhD Univ. of Chicago, Omer Stewart, PhD Univ. of Colorado, and Sol Tax, PhD Univ. of Chicago - Personal Archives of author from Frank Takes Gun.

22. Personal Archives of author from Frank Takes Gun.

23. Ibid.

Court established the "compelling interest" test, which required the States and the federal government to balance the right of the free exercise of religion against government restriction, while giving great weight to religious freedom. The Court concluded that the regulated conduct must pose "some substantial threat to public safety, peace or order", even when the religious practice is "abhorrent to the authorities."[24]

In a shocking decision in 1990, Justice Scalia, speaking for the U.S. Supreme Court, overruled the 30-year compelling interest test of *Sherbert* in the case of *Oregon vs. Smith*, 494 U.S. 872. The U.S. Supreme Court held that the Oregon state criminal law prohibiting the possession of Peyote was paramount to the Free Exercise Clause of the First Amendment of the United States Constitution. The Supreme Court held that police power is superior to freedom of religion. With the stroke of his pen, Justice Scalia transformed the nation's "first liberty" into a constitutional step-child.

A dark cloud hung over the continued religious use of Peyote by the Native American Church. The NAC had no remedy in the courts and was forced to turn to the United States Congress as the last resort. The use of Peyote is central to the religious practice of the NAC. The existence of the NAC was threatened. To ensure the continued religious use of Peyote by the NAC, I helped create and draft the strategy of petitioning the U.S. Congress to enact the Religious Freedom Restoration Act (RFRA), and to amend the American Indian Religious Freedom Act of 1978 (AIRFA) to specifically include Peyote.

Outstanding and respected Native American leaders, such as Reuben Snake, Jr., a Winnebago, descended on Congress. Native American rights' attorneys such as James Botsford and attorneys with the Native American Rights Fund went to the halls of Congress and ardently advocated for the passage of RFRA and AIRFA. Botsford was one of the primary authors of AIRFA and his advocacy was vital. The NAC, joined by a large coalition of religious institutions from many faiths, including Baptist, Methodist, Jewish, Mormon, Unitarian, and other associations, lobbied Congress for the passage of RFRA. The strategy was successful: RFRA[25] was passed in late 1993 and the Amendment to AIRFA[26] was passed in 1994 as a result of the Native American Church initiative.

This legislation, fostered by the arduous efforts of the NAC, was foundational in the favorable decision involving *ayahuasca* by the U.S. Supreme Court, *Gonzales v. UDV*[27], which relied on RFRA & AIRFA. The same is true for the *Santo Daime* decision in a U.S. District Court in *Holy Light of the Queen v. Mukasey*[28]. Without the tenacious commitment of the NAC, there would be no legal use of Peyote or *ayahuasca* in the U.S. today.

Richard Glen Boire, attorney and editor of the 1990s Entheogen Law Review, and I determined that 17 states provide various levels of protection for religious use of Peyote, in addition to protection by the federal government. If the state does not appear below, there were no explicit legislative exemptions found concerning Peyote.

---

24. Sherbert vs. Verner, 374 US 398 (1963) , p. 402, 403.

25. Title 42 USC 2000bb-1 RELIGIOUS FREEDOM RESTORATION ACT of 1993
Sec. 3, Free exercise of religion protected
(a) In general - Government shall not substantially burden a person's exercise of religion even if the burden results from a rule of general applicability, except as provided in subsection (b).
(b) Exception - Government may substantially burden a person's exercise of religion only if it demonstrates that application of the burden to the person— (1) is in furtherance of a compelling governmental interest; and (2) is the least restrictive means of furthering that compelling governmental interest.

26. American Indian Religious Freedom Act (AIRFA) Amendment, 42 USC § 1996a
Sec. 2 - Traditional Indian Religious Use of Peyote (b)(1) Notwithstanding any other provision of law, the use, possession, or transportation or peyote by an Indian for bona fide traditional ceremonial purposes in connection with the practice of a traditional Indian religious practice is lawful, and shall not be prohibited by the United States or any State. No Indian shall be penalized or discriminated against on the basis of such use, possession or transportation, including, but not limited to, denial of otherwise applicable benefits under public assistance programs.
(2) This section does not prohibit such reasonable regulation and registration by the Drug Enforcement Administration of those persons who cultivate, harvest, or distribute peyote as may be consistent with the purposes of this section and section 1996 of this title.

27. Gonzales v. O Centro Espirita Beneficiente Uniao do Vegetal (UDV) 546 U.S. 418 (2006). Author's comment: Working with Jeffrey Brofman, as an attorney representing the UDV, I found Jeffrey to be courageous, caring, and unyieldingly dedicated to his stewardship of the UDV. Brofman is the Quanah Parker of the UDV.

28. Oregon Church of the Holy Light of the Queen v. Mukasey 615 F.Supp.2d 1210 (D. Or., 2009).

	Religious intent, good faith practice or ceremony	With a bonafide religious organization	Within NAC ceremony	NAC membership required	Native American descent or tribal enrollment required	On reservation only
FEDERAL [29]		X	X	X		
AK [30]		X	X	X		
AZ [31]	X					
CA [32]	X	X				
CO [33]		X				
ID [34]	X	X			X	X
IA [35]	X		X			
KS [36]			X	X		
MN [37]	X		X	X		
NV [38]	X	X				
NM [39]	X	X				
OK [40]				X		
OR [41]	X					
SD [42]			X			
TX [43]		X	X	X	X	
UT [44]	X				X	
WI [45]	X		X			
WY [46]	X			X		

....

29. 21 C.F.R. § 1307.31 (1985)

30. Alaska Stat. § 11.71.195 (2017)

31. A.R.S. § 13-3402 (2017)

32. People v. Woody (1964) 394 P2d 813 (1964)

33. C.R.S. 27-80-209 (2016)

34. Idaho Code § 37-2732A (2017)

35. Iowa Code § 124.204 (2016)

36. K.S.A. § 65-4116 (2017)

37. Minn. Stat. § 152.02 (2017)

38. Nev. Rev. Stat. Ann. § 453.541 (2017)

39. N.M. Stat. Ann. § 30-31-6 (2017)

40. Whitehorn v. State, 561 P.2d 539 (1977)

41. ORS § 475.752 (4) (2017)

42. S.D. Codified Laws § 34-20B-14 (2016)

43. Tex. Health & Safety Code § 481.111 (2017)

44. Utah Code Ann. § 58-37-8 (12)(b) (2016)

45. Wis. Stat. § 961.115 (2017)

46. Wyo. Stat. § 35-7-1044 (2017)

THE RITUAL FORM OF THE PEYOTE MEETING

Many authors have detailed the ritual form of the Peyote meeting. Omer Stewart provides very detailed descriptors of the Peyote ritual.[47] As there is abundant literature easily available on the form of the Peyote meeting, I will only briefly describe the Peyote meeting ritual in general terms.

The exquisite beauty and ambience of the NAC Peyote ceremony is beyond words. This ineffable experience cannot be adequately described in language. A tipi is erected immediately before the meeting. The door of the tipi always faces east. The participants enter the meeting at sundown, single file and clockwise, and sit in a circle on blankets and small cushions on the ground. There is something very special about sitting together with a group in a circle. Even more so, there is something extraordinary about sitting on the ground and connecting with the earth. A small meeting might have only 10 to 15; an average meeting has 20 to 30 participants; a large meeting perhaps as many as 40 (Fig. 11).

An altar is constructed from sand and clay in the shape of a crescent moon immediately before the meeting. The Road Chief sits on the west side of the tipi facing east, the Drummer sits to the right, and the Cedar Chief to the left of the Road Chief. The Fire Chief sits next to the door and feeds the fire with hand-split links of wood throughout the night. A Chief Peyote, which is a large dried Peyote, often passed down through a family lineage, is placed at the center of the crescent moon. There are many purposes for meetings, such as a birthday, appreciation, wedding, healing, education, departing soldier, honoring someone, or memorial for a deceased. The focus of all minds and prayers is on the purpose of the meeting. This is a powerful process.

The Road Chief Frank Takes Gun is holding the instruments used in the meeting – staff, feather fan, and gourd rattler. He is standing in front of the crescent moon altar on which sits the small Chief Peyote (Fig. 12). The Drummer is sitting behind the drum, and the Cedar Chief sits to the left. As the Road Chief sings, Peyote is passed around the circle clockwise. After the Road Chief sings four songs, the instruments, including the drum, are passed around the circle; each individual sings Peyote songs if they wish to do so, or they may simply pass the instruments on. The instruments circulate around the tipi for various rounds. At midnight, the Fire Chief brings in water. After several more rounds, in the morning a woman brings a water bucket into the meeting, and prays over the water. The water is then circulated to all the participants. Ultimately, there is a conclusion song sung by the Road Chief.

During the conclusion, a small ceremonial breakfast consisting of corn, dried meat, fruit, and water is passed around the tipi circle, clockwise, after someone prays blessings on the food. This is a glorious time. There is conversation, laughter, and expressions of love and gratitude. Stories are exchanged. With their oral tradition, Indians are gifted and spellbinding storytellers. Traditionally, everyone stays at the meeting place and visits until the noon meal. This is a time of visiting, meeting new friends, exchanging information, and experiencing satisfaction and conviviality prior to leaving for home. Many participants have driven long distances. I have found the Peyote meeting form that was established by the Comanches and Kiowas to be inspirational and brilliant.

THE ORIGIN OF THE PEYOTE TRADE
IN TEXAS AT LOS OJUELOS

The tradition of Indians making long pilgrimages to Texas to harvest and trade for Peyote with Hispanics occurred as early as 1870 in the small Rancheria Settlement of Los Ojuelos,[48] the birthplace in 1904 of Amada Cardenas and her husband Claudio Cardenas. The Peyote traders were known as Peyoteros. Indians would come to Los Ojuelos by horseback or wagon, and later in Model T's, to secure dried Peyote. Dry Peyote is ideal for transport. It is lightweight, small in volume, and can be preserved indefinitely. Green Peyote is bulky and subject to spoiling on the long trip back to Indian country.

Hispanics living in Los Ojuelos began to harvest and dry Peyote for Indians that traveled there. Esiquio Sanchez, Amada Cardenas's father, was a Peyotero. She related that her brothers would go out with her father and harvest Peyote to take back to their home in Los Ojuelos. At age four, Amada and her sisters would turn each Peyote button over on caliche beds daily as part of the drying process.

---

47. Stewart, Omer, 1987. Peyote Religion, 339-375.

48. Morgan, George R., 1976. Man Plan and Religion, iv.

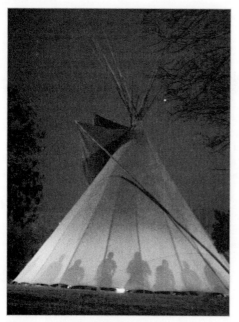

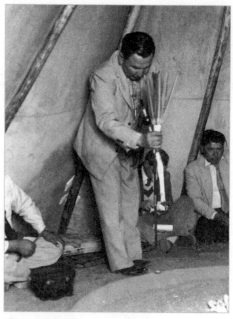

Fig.11 Peyote Meeting at Mirando City, Texas
Courtesy of Robert Black, Mirandocity.com.

Fig. 12 Frank Takes Gun, 1956
Original photo. Author's archives from Frank
Takes Gun.

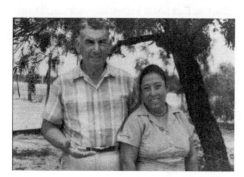

Fig. 13 Claudio, Sr. and Amada Cardenas
Courtesy of Linda Patchen, gift from Amada. (Note:
Chief Peyote in Claudio's hand).

Fig. 14 Rare Snake
Peyote in bucket on
Amada Cardenas' porch;
Courtesy of Linda
Patchen.

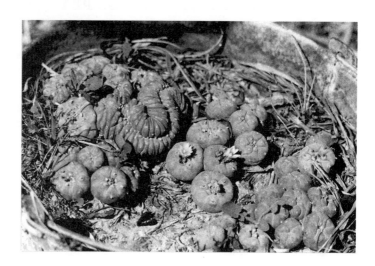

In 1932, Amada married Claudio Cardenas, Sr., who was also from Los Ojuelos (Fig. 13). They worked together and carried on the Amada family's tradition of harvesting, drying and trading Peyote with the Indians at Los Ojuelos. In 1942, they moved five miles north of Los Ojuelos to the outskirts of Mirando City, a small town with a population of around 300, and continued their Peyote trade. It was said of Claudio, Sr. that he would give up his bed for Indians that had traveled a long, exhausting distance, and sleep in his truck. Claudio, Sr. passed away in 1967, and Amada continued in the Peyote trade.

The annual NAC Peyote meeting at Amada's home in Mirando City has continued through 2018. Amada was the Mother Teresa of the Native American Church. She was love in action. Her home became the national home for all Native American Churches. Amada was loved and is still revered throughout Indian country as a saint. Tens of thousands of Indians and individuals of all races have visited Amada. Amada passed away in 2005, one month prior to her 101st birthday. I was honored to deliver the eulogy at Amada's funeral (Fig. 14).

FRANK TAKES GUN
– THE JOHNNY APPLESEED OF THE NAC

No single individual achieved as much for the NAC as Frank Takes Gun (1908-1988), a Crow Indian from the Crow Reservation in Montana. His skill in creating organizational structure, chartering NAC chapters in many states, bringing court cases, and leading the passage of legislation in Indian states and the U.S. Congress, was amazing and unmatched.

The long odyssey of Frank Takes Gun fighting for the rights of Indians to use Peyote began when he was sixteen years old. In 1924, he was with his family on the Crow reservation at a Peyote meeting. After the meeting, U.S. Marshals arrived and arrested the Road Chief, Big Sheep. The women were crying, "Holy Creator, we prayed all night to you for something good in our lives. Then these men came and took Big Sheep away. We do not understand. What can we do?" The old men gathered. Frank Takes Gun was the only person there who could speak English. They instructed him to get in a horse-drawn buckboard with Big Sheep's wife, go where they had taken Big Sheep, and bring him back home. As if by miracle, when the teenager Takes Gun talked to the Marshals, they released Big Sheep. Takes Gun and Big Sheep's wife brought him home.[49] Big Sheep was ultimately charged with possessing Peyote.[50]

I was privileged to know Frank Takes Gun in his later years. In the 1980s, I arranged for him to fly from Montana to Laredo so he and Amada could have a reunion after many years of being apart. I picked him up at the airport. As we drove 45 miles east to Amada's, Takes Gun related to me that the two-lane asphalt highway we traveled on had been an old single-lane dirt wagon and vehicle trail when he was first on the roadway. He explained that some fifty years earlier, Big Sheep had taken him down to the Peyote area around Los Ojuelos as a reward for Takes Gun having secured Big Sheep's release from jail.

I asked Takes Gun if they had put up a tipi and had a Peyote meeting on the trip with Big Sheep. He told me they had brought some tarps, cleared an area of the chaparral and simply strung some tarps in a circle as a wind break. They gathered mesquite wood and had a Peyote meeting with a fire in the center of the open-air tarps. As he related this story, I was suddenly at that Peyote meeting he was describing, even though it had occurred fifty years earlier. My visual, aural, somatic, tactile, and olfactory senses were all keenly experiencing the Peyote meeting, the same as if I was present. I seemingly was not driving the vehicle on the highway. After being present at the meeting for several minutes, I came back from this impactful vision in perplexed amazement. I told Takes Gun what had occurred, that I was there observing the meeting and totally unaware of driving the vehicle. Takes Gun simply looked at me, pointed to his temple with his right index finger, and said, "This mind is a powerful thing."

Takes Gun was a truly great man. In 1944, at age 36 (Fig. 15 – back row, third from left) he was elected Vice President of the Native American Church of the United States (NAC U.S.). Mack Haag (Fig. 15 - front left). Haag was the first signatory on the NAC Oklahoma 1918 Charter, and served as Vice President and later President.

Though he was not an attorney and had no legal training, Takes Gun was a brilliant legal strategist. Very few attorneys in any area of law achieved in their careers the success with state and federal

---

49. Oral history told by Frank Takes Gun to author.

50. Montana v. Big Sheep, 243.P.1.1067, 75 Mont. p. 219 (1926).

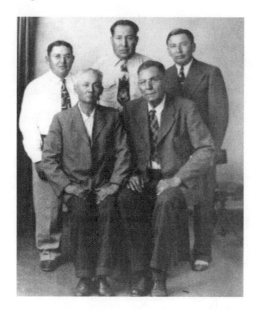

Fig. 15 First Officers of the NAC of the U.S. Front row: Mack Haag (Southern Cheyenne), Alfred Wilson (Southern Cheyenne). Back row, left-right: Joe Kaulity (Kiowa), Truman Dailey (Oto), Frank Takes Gun (Crow). Courtesy of Author, gift from Takes Gun.

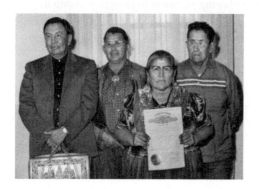

Fig. 16 Frank Takes Gun, Sam Captain, Dela Oliver, James Oliver with Utah NAC Charter – The Olivers were placed in jail several times and fined heavily. Courtesy of Author, gift from Frank Takes Gun.

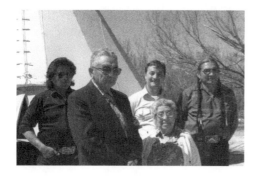

Fig. 17 Officers of NAC U.S. - Feb. 1988 Front left to right: Frank Takes Gun, age 80, Amada Cardenas, age 84; back left to right: Jerry Ettcity, Jerry Patchen, Rutherford Loneman) Courtesy of Linda Patchen.

legislation, and the court victories, of Frank Takes Gun. During the decades that he served the NAC, he defeated attempted federal anti-Peyote legislation in 1937, and convinced the Federal Bureau of Indian Affairs (BIA) to recognize the NAC in 1945. His successful advocacy resulted in the following state legislatures legalizing Peyote in Colorado, New Mexico, Utah, North Dakota, Montana, Nevada, and Wyoming[51] (Fig. 16) Various other Indian country states, such as Texas, had no anti-Peyote law in this time period.

Takes Gun organized, chartered, and served as an officer in Native American Churches throughout Indian country, including Colorado, Texas, California, Nevada, Wyoming, and New Mexico. The term NAC is a generic term for all of the churches that operated in various states. Schisms occurred and in some cases the names of specific churches were changed. The NAC U.S. remains only in Texas[52]. I was honored to serve as an officer in the NAC U.S. with Frank Takes Gun and Amada Cardenas in the 1980s and 1990s (Fig. 17). In 1965, his advocacy caused the exemption of Peyote from the Drug Abuse Control Amendment. In 1967 he was instrumental in the Navajo Tribal Council repealing their anti-Peyote ordinance.[53]

ARIZONA - A master of litigation, Frank Takes Gun directed significant precedent-setting Peyote cases in several courts. His first major success was in *Arizona v. Mary Attakai*[54]. In July 1960, Judge Yale McFate ruled that the state of Arizona has police power to prohibit the use of substances, even in religious rites, if necessary to protect public health and safety. Holding that liberty of conscience secured by the Constitution may not be construed to justify practices within the peace and safety of the public, Judge McFate ruled:

> The use of Peyote is essential to the existence of the Peyote religion. Without it, the practice of the religion would be effectively prevented. From the foregoing, it follows:
> First, the only significant use made of Peyote is in connection with Indian rites of a bona fide religious nature, or for medicinal purposes.
> Second, there are no harmful after-effects from the use of peyote.
> Third, it is not a narcotic, nor is it habit-forming.
> Fourth, the practical effect of the statute outlawing its use is to prevent worship by members of the Native American Church, who believe the Peyote plant to be of divine origin and to bear a similar relation to the Indians –most of whom cannot read – as does the Holy Bible to the white man.[55]

CALIFORNIA - In April 1962, three Navajo men, Jack Woody, Leon Anderson and Dan D. Nez, were arrested and charged in San Bernardino County with illegal possession of Peyote (Fig. 18). Frank Takes Gun masterminded the defense. Working with attorneys, he marshalled evidence from anthropologists and psychiatrists, and ensured that the attorneys raised Constitutional objections. Nonetheless, Judge Hillard of the Superior Court convicted all three defendants. Takes Gun mobilized an appeal to the California Supreme Court, maintaining that California could not constitutionally apply a statute proscribing the use of Peyote so as to prevent Indians from using Peyote as a sacrament similar to the bread and wine used in Christian churches. Justice Tobriner's opinion held that an examination of the evidence compelled the conclusion that the statutory prohibition most seriously interfered upon the observation of the religion:

....

51. Personal archives of author from Frank Takes Gun.

52. The Native American Church is not a monolith. Since the formation of the Native American Church in Oklahoma in 1918, the NAC divided into various official organizations. The original NAC in Oklahoma was the mother church. It advised and aided the incorporation of NAC churches in other states, and in 1934 amended its charter accepting NAC churches from many states as legal affiliates. In 1944 the NAC of Oklahoma nationalized its name and amended its charter to the name of the Native American Church of the United States. A few years later, because some Oklahoma leaders preferred the old traditional state organization without national focus the NAC of Oklahoma reinstated its original name, the Native American Church. In 1950, a new charter was obtained for the NAC US without replacing the Oklahoma State Church. In 1955, the NAC US changed its name to the NAC of North America as a result of expansion into Canada. In 1946, because Texas was vital to the Peyote supply, a NAC US was also established in Texas of which Frank Takes Gun and four prominent NAC leaders from Oklahoma were the Trustees. Claudio Cardenas and Amada Cardenas were added as Trustees to the Texas NAC US in 1957. The only remaining NAC US is in Texas. Today, three primary National Native American Churches are the NAC of Oklahoma, the NAC of North America and the NAC of Navajoland. There are many small independent NAC churches without any national organizational affiliation.

53. Stewart, Omer, 1987. Peyote Religion, 310-311.

54. Decision of the Honorable Yale McFate.

55. State of Arizona vs. Mary Attakai, Superior Court, Coconino County, Flagstaff, Arizona, No. 4098 July 26, 1960.

Jerry Patchen

Three Arrested For Possession Of Peyote Drug

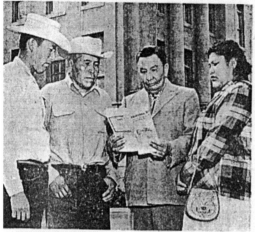

NO PEACE PIPE — Ready for attle are Navajo Indians charged with ossession of peyote. Two of the deendants, Jack Woody and Leon Anlerson (from left) discuss the case rith Frank Takes Gun, president of Native American Church, and their. Interpreter, Mrs. Howard Yazzie, outside the county courthouse yesterday. A third defendant, Dan Dee Nez, is not shown. (Sun-Telegram photo)

Fig. 18 The San Bernardino Daily Sun Article – Author's personal archives from Frank Takes Gun.

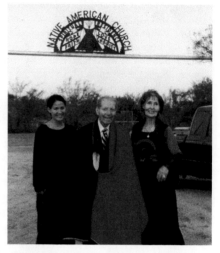

Fig. 19 Judge E. J. Kazen (center) Reunion Peyote Meeting at Amada's in late 1990's Drusilla Kazen, Wife (right); Lisl Kazen Friday grand-daughter (left) – note eagle feather and Peyote robe presented to Judge Kazen at Amada's in 1969 – Courtesy of Linda Patchen.

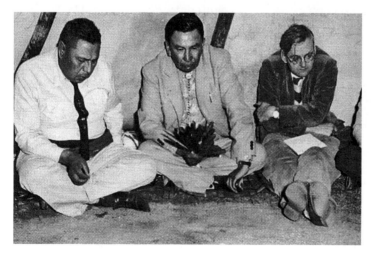

Fig. 20 (left to right) William Russell - President NAC Montana, Frank Takes Gun and Humphry Osmond, M.D. (psychiatrist) who coined the word psychedelic - Original photo. Author's archives from Frank Takes Gun.

Although Peyote serves as a sacramental symbol similar to bread and wine in certain Christian churches, it is more than a sacrament. Peyote constitutes in itself an object of worship; prayers are directed to it much as prayers are devoted to the Holy Ghost. On the other hand, to use Peyote for nonreligious purposes is sacrilegious. Members of the church regard Peyote also as a 'teacher' because it induces a feeling of brotherhood with other members; indeed, it enables the participant to experience the Deity. Finally, devotees treat Peyote as a 'protector'. Much as a Catholic carries his medallion, an Indian G.I. often wears around his neck a beautifully beaded pouch containing one large Peyote button. [56]

The California Supreme Court accepted the opinion of scientists, including anthropologist Omer Stewart and pharmacologist Gordon Alles,[57] that Peyote has no deleterious effect on the Native Americans and that the moral standards of members of the NAC were higher than those outside of the church. The court rejected the Attorney General's argument that "Peyote . . . obstructs enlightenment and shackles the Indian to primitive conditions." In persuasive language reversing the convictions of the three defendants, the court concluded:

> [T]he right to free religious expression embodies a precious heritage of our history. In a mass society, which presses at every point toward conformity, the protection of a self-expression, however unique, of the individual and the group becomes important. The varying currents of the subcultures that flow into the mainstream of our national life give it depth and beauty. We preserve a greater value than an ancient tradition when we protect the rights of the Indians who honestly practiced an old religion in using Peyote one night at a meeting in a desert Hogan near Needles, California.[58]

TEXAS - In August of 1967, Texas passed a total ban on Peyote. The new Texas law placed severe criminal penalties on the growing or distribution of Peyote, mescaline, and other hallucinogens. There was no exemption for the use of Peyote for Indians or religious purposes. Texas was the only source of Peyote for the Native American Church. The NAC was in a state of deep distress over the loss of their sole source of Peyote.

Takes Gun swung into action. He arranged for a test case. Sam Houston Clinton, Jr., an attorney in Austin, Texas who worked with the ACLU, agreed to assist. Takes Gun enlisted the aid of David Clark, a brave Navajo. [59] There were five male Peyote dealers in south Texas. One by one Takes Gun requested each of them to provide Peyote. They all refused, fearing arrest. He then went to Amada Cardenas. Amada was courageous and readily agreed to provide Peyote. She and her husband, Claudio, Sr., had previously been arrested in 1953 for Peyote and prevailed in the case.

David Clark drove out of Amada Cardenas' driveway in Takes Gun's Ford with Peyote. The Texas Highway Patrol had been alerted by Takes Gun of his intention. The vehicle was stopped and David Clark was arrested, placed in jail, and charged with possession of Peyote. In April of 1968, David Clark's case went to trial before Judge E. James Kazen in the Webb County, 49th District Court in Laredo. Judge Kazen, citing the *Mary Attakai* case and the *Jack Woody* case, found the Texas law unconstitutional (Fig. 19).

After the decision, the Native American Church conducted a Peyote meeting in honor of Judge Kazen at Amada Cardenas' home in October 1969. Judge Kazen attended the Peyote meeting. He was presented with an eagle feather and given the name "Eagle Feather, symbolizing wisdom and justice." He ate some Peyote and "found it bitter and unpalatable." [60]

Upon learning of Takes Gun's victory in the David Clark case, the area director of the BIA, Graham Holmes, wrote a congratulatory letter to Takes Gun, stating:

> Your management of the Native American Church has been amazingly successful. The winning of the recent case in Texas is the last step in the long battle for the right of the members of the Church. Many years ago when you first started this crusade, no one

....

56. The People v. Jack Woody, et al. 394 P. 2d. 831 (1964).

57. Stewart, Omer, 1987. Peyote Religion, 308.

58. The People v. Jack Woody, et al. Ibid.

59. David Clark became the first president of the Native American Church of Navajoland.

60. The Laredo Times, October 13, 1969. "Judge Kazen Honored by Indian Tribes In All Night Ceremony." No. 103.

could have predicted that you would win every battle, and that the Native American Church would finally reach its rightful place and receive its rightful recognition in this country. [61]

Humphrey Osmond of New Jersey's Bureau of Research of Neurology and Psychology likewise wrote a congratulatory letter stating:

Congratulations on once again steering your church through the rapids. You have undoubtedly been a fine pilot for them. I still think of that remarkable time, or perhaps one should call it out of time, that we enjoyed together almost twelve years ago in the tepee on the bluffs of North Battleford. It remains one of the most vivid and remarkable experiences of my life [62] (Fig. 20).

Until he drew his last breath, Frank Takes Gun remained an ardent advocate for the religious freedom of Native Americans. On September 18, 1988, I delivered the eulogy at his funeral in Lodge Grass, Montana overlooking the Little Bighorn River, near the site where U.S. Cavalry Commander George Custer met his fate.

RUTHERFORD LONEMAN'S FUNERAL MEETING

On August 8, 1988, while coincidentally visiting Amada, I received a phone call that Rutherford Loneman had passed away early that morning. I was heartbroken. I remember crying. Rutherford had led a Peyote meeting for our oldest child, Maya, when she was fourteen, and gave her the name "Morning Star." I had always envisioned that Rutherford would lead a meeting for all three of our children. Ultimately, Anthony "White Thunder" Davis, a Pawnee, led a meeting for our daughter, Michelle, whom he named "White Star", and for our son, Justin, whom he named "White Wolf." After receiving the call, I was sitting beside Amada and mourning Rutherford's passing. I began to see and feel an energy field radiating soft purple light from Amada's left side into my right side. I felt a tremendous amount of strength and energy being directly transmitted to me by Amada, who just sat silently beside me. I said gently, "Amada, I am sure getting a lot of strength from you." She continued to look straight ahead and nodded her head, acknowledging the process that was occurring.

Funeral arrangements were immediately undertaken for a service and burial of Rutherford on the Arapaho reservation at Concho, Oklahoma. Rutherford's wife, Wanada Loneman, a who belonged to the Sac and Fox Tribe, planned a NAC funeral Peyote meeting. I knew what that meant and somewhat felt a sense of dread, although I knew I must be there. The Sac and Fox bring the body of the deceased in the tipi and lay the body on the ground inside the tipi throughout the Peyote funeral meeting.

Linda and I traveled to Oklahoma for the funeral. The Peyote funeral meeting was led by a Sac and Fox Road Chief. Rutherford was laid out on the ground along the north side, with blankets around his body up to his shoulders. Wanada sat next to Rutherford. Linda sat next to Wanada with me sitting on Linda's right. I was sad and having a difficult time throughout the beginning hours of the meeting. My Indian father, closest friend, and teacher lay deceased a few feet from me. I had a container of small, strong, specially dried Peyote buttons. I ate a lot of Peyote. I would eat two or three Peyote buttons often. Rutherford always told me, "If you are in a meeting, eat Peyote. If you cannot sit comfortable, eat Peyote. If your mind is spinning and agitated, eat Peyote. If something is bothering you, eat Peyote. You are in the tipi to eat Peyote."

Suddenly, Rutherford appeared bigger than life. His physical body was laid out a few feet to my left, yet he simultaneously appeared in the center of the tipi above the fire before me. He had a big smile on his face. Rutherford said to me, "Son, don't be upset. Don't be sad. This is just another lesson that I am teaching you about life, this process of life." As he completed this communication, a ray of tremendously powerful energy about 8 inches in diameter streamed down from his chest into my chest. It was the most joyful and exhilarating moment of my life. I completely understood the process of life. This life wisdom was radiated into every dimension of my being. I experienced a sure knowing that we are all an interconnected, inseparable, and eternal unity of all that is, was, or ever will be. We are all part of an inseparable whole. I was elated. I was at the funeral of my dearest and closest friend, and I was experiencing ecstatic joy and appreciation for life. It was an unimaginable divine paradox.

....

61. Personal Archives of author from Frank Takes Gun.

62. Ibid.

The next morning, we came out of the tipi and proceeded to the grave site at the Arapaho cemetery for a traditional burial. I was filled with an afterglow and still in contact with the incredible Divine Universal Life Force transmitted to me from Rutherford's image. The next day, the essence experience was still with me, but beginning to fade. As the days and weeks passed, it gradually became fainter and fainter. Ultimately, it vanished. The memory of the experience was still intellectually there, but not the direct connection with it.

ANTHONY "WHITE THUNDER" DAVIS, PAWNEE

My close friend Denny Sandoval, a Navajo, sensed that with Rutherford Loneman's passing, I had lost my mooring, my anchor with the NAC. Denny committed to sponsor a meeting for Linda and me at Dzit Na Ooditii, on the Navajo reservation. Denny selected his close friend, Marcellus "Bear Heart" Williams, a Creek Indian Road Chief from Oklahoma, to lead the meeting for us. Marcellus requested Anthony "White Thunder" Davis (1911-2003) (Fig. 21), a Pawnee Road Chief, to be the Cedar Chief at our Peyote meeting. A wise elder is generally designated to be the Cedar Chief. The Peyote meeting went well. I keenly paid attention to everything that was occurring during the meeting. At midnight, Anthony Davis gave the traditional Cedar Chief prayer with cedar. The meeting continued for several hours, then Marcellus called for his wife Edna to bring in morning water an hour before dawn. Again, it was Anthony's duty as Cedar Chief to give a prayer with cedar. He said words and then gave a short prayer in the Pawnee language. Linda and I were sitting on the northwest side very close to where Marcellus and Anthony were sitting. As Anthony began the cedar prayer, I took special notice. Somehow, there was a time warp. There was no time between Anthony's midnight prayer and his morning prayer. It was as if he had reversed time from his midnight prayer, and somehow linked it with his morning prayer. That caught my attention. I had experienced Rutherford seemingly reversing time in a meeting on a prior occasion.

Anthony completed his prayer. He then stood erect with the cedar and an eagle feather in his hand, stepped close to the altar, and cast the cedar on the coals. Bending forward and reaching down, he touched the Chief Peyote on the crescent moon altar with the tip of the eagle feather. Anthony then raised the eagle feather up in an arc, ending with his arm fully extended with the eagle feather pointing straight up. He opened another dimension with the eagle feather. Christ was standing in the arc. I was astonished. Simultaneously with the appearance of this Christ image, I heard Marcellus softly cry, "weihai" acknowledging that he saw the Spirit. The image of Christ vanished after a few timeless seconds. I looked toward Marcellus, who had formerly been a Presbyterian ordained Minister. Marcellus, looking directly at me, softly quoted Biblical scripture: "At first we see through a glass darkly, then face to face" (1 Corinthians 13:12). I knew that Marcellus had seen what I had seen. Linda saw a bright transcendent light that filled the entire tipi. She recognized the light as the divine. I am convinced that the three of us, Marcellus, Linda, and I, were the only individuals that had seen the vision.

I am not asserting that Jesus Christ was actually standing in the arc, although I did view a clear vision of Christ standing before me. I have a Christian heritage. I was reared in the Southern Baptist Church as a child. I received an eight-year pin for not missing a Sunday. My three sisters and I were marched to the Baptist Church every time the doors opened. As a young teenager, I developed serious questions about Christianity concerning the proposition that a wonderfully good and helpful person, reared in a foreign culture, who had never heard the name of Jesus Christ, was damned to eternal hellfire. I resisted worshiping such a cruel and punishing God. Yet, because of my long cultural history with Christianity and years of Bible study, the image of the divine necessarily appeared to me in Christian form. I had no other model for Divinity. As Richard Schultes suggested, had I been Jewish, the image of Divinity would appear as Abraham; to a Buddhist as the Buddha; to a Hindu as Lord Krishna; to a physicist as patterns of energy; and to an Amazonian Indian as an image of a Jaguar. In fact, while visiting in South America our daughter Michelle had a profound vision of Divinity as a female Jaguar embracing around her and melding into her with protection and Divine love (Fig. 22). Interestingly, an image of Divinity appeared to Dennis McKenna as the process of photosynthesis. Anthony Davis had an experience where he saw a bright light that he referred to as Christ. He also had two different visions where a white wolf appeared to him as Divinity, and on another occasion a scissor-tailed fly catcher. I once asked Anthony why I experienced seeing Jesus Christ. He told me, "I don't know. Sometimes things like that just happen around me." It was clear to me that it was not something that he consciously caused or willed. One must understand the role of the imagination - the imaginal. My simple way of expressing the imaginal is, "Spirit communicates with image, but spirit is not the image." The 5th-century Neoplatonist, Proclus, writing on Plato, penned:

277

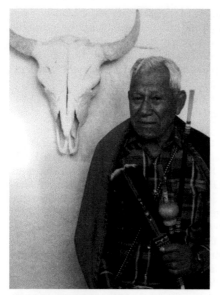

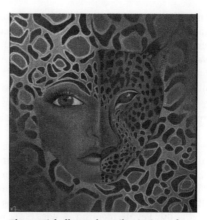

Fig.22 Michelle Mackey oil painting of jaguar vision Courtesy of Michelle Mackey.

Fig. 21 Anthony "White Thunder" Davis holding anhinga fan he made Courtesy of John Running.

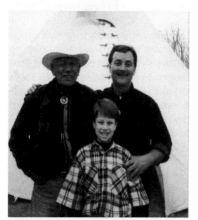

Fig.23 Anthony "White Thunder" Davis, Justin Patchen and Jerry Patchen Courtesy of Linda Patchen.

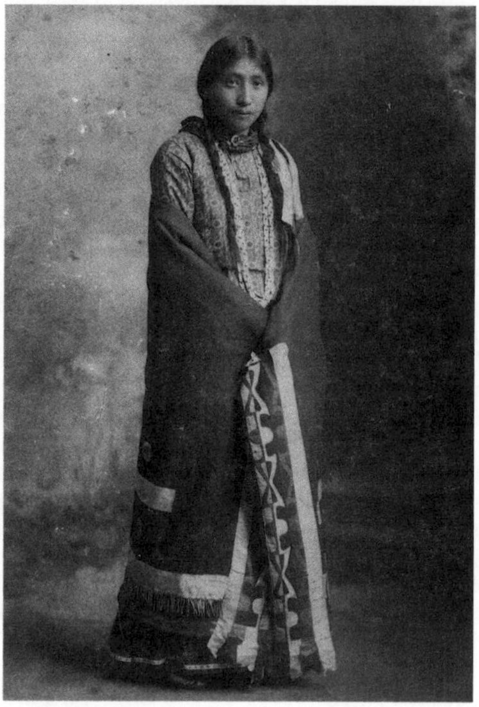

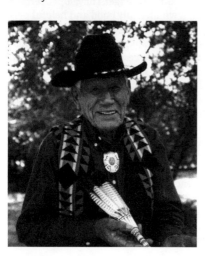

Fig. 24 White Star – Mother of Anthony "White Thunder" Davis.

Fig. 25 Anthony "White Thunder" Davis holding Mexican eagle "Totachi" – cara cara Peyote Fan that he made for Michelle Mackey and presented at her Peyote meeting. Courtesy of Linda Patchen.

Self-realization of the Gods necessarily happens in such a way that the formless take form, and the shapeless take shape, with each soul receiving a firm and simple vision of the Gods according to that soul's particular nature, with imagination providing shape and form to these visions.[63]

In this respect, I depart from the fundamentalist view that understands psychedelic visions literally. Our beliefs are limitations. The Tao that can be spoken is not the Tao.

Naturally, after the vision I had in the tipi with Anthony, I pursued a relationship with him. A few months later in a Peyote meeting, Anthony accepted me as his son. Not long after making that relationship with me, Anthony became very ill, and was admitted to the Indian hospital in Santa Fe with sepsis. He almost died. He was very weak, thin, and frail. It was very cold in Santa Fe, so my son Justin, aged five, who adored Anthony, and I went to Santa Fe, bundled Anthony up, and brought him to our home in the temperate Houston climate. Linda lovingly nursed Anthony back to health. It was a long and slow process, but he gradually regained his health. He was determined. He struggled to move around, saying, "I want to walk good on this Mother Earth." (Fig. 23, 24 & 25).

By late spring, Anthony had regained his health and strength. He wanted to take me to Oklahoma for a special annual Mother's Day meeting. Anthony and I traveled from Houston to Kiowa country at Hog Creek, Oklahoma. We were well greeted and the meeting started in a nice way. It was a stormy night in May. It was raining, thundering, and lightning some during the meeting, but that was of no concern. Everyone had a good feeling. After midnight water, the staff and gourd reached Anthony around 2:00 am. We were sitting together on the south side of the tipi, with me on his right. Anthony handed me the gourd that was being passed with the staff, and opened his Peyote box, which was sitting between us. He took out a gourd that his wife Julia, an Arapaho, had beaded for him. She had passed away two years before, after 49 years of marriage. He said to me, "Son, I do not get this gourd out often anymore, but I am going to use it tonight."

Anthony began singing old Comanche songs he favored. As he was singing, a phenomenon occurred that was awe-inspiring. Simultaneously with his songs, continuous lightning began to occur all around. There was constant thunder. It was not rolling thunder, but continuous thunder and lightning. It was a very dark night, but suddenly the sky was as bright as the noonday sun. It was "White Thunder." Anthony sang two songs, then stopped and spoke a few words. When he stopped singing and spoke, the lightning and thunder ceased. When he began singing again, the same constant thunder and lightning occurred again. I sat there astounded. Witnessing this phenomenon, I understood the origin of his name, "White Thunder." Anthony completed his turn singing, and the thunder and lightning again stopped. He passed the instruments to his left. I opened his Peyote box so that he could place his gourd back into the box. I looked at Anthony and our eyes locked. I said, "Damn! That's powerful." With an austere gaze at me, he momentarily shook the gourd in his hand. Simultaneously, there was a quick burst of thunder and lightning. Anthony then placed his gourd back in his Peyote box. I treasure the experience of Anthony introducing me to "White Thunder."

Anthony lived with Linda and me for several months a year for the next twelve years. We had marvelous experiences together until he passed on. The three of us went down to Amada's every year for the annual meeting. He was in high demand to lead Peyote meetings throughout Indian country. I traveled with him to many Peyote meetings. We sure enjoyed ourselves together.

Like all Indians, he was a great storyteller, but Anthony's presence communicated something beyond words. Anthony always taught me, "Whatever happens, take it in a good way. It's all good." Anthony "White Thunder" Davis was a blessing in our lives.

We can experience the Mystery, yet ultimately we are confronted with a Great Mystery that our small minds can never grasp.

---

63. Proclus, On the Republic of Plato, Vol I.39.5-11. Author's note: The 3rd-century Neoplatonist philosopher Iamblichus advances the same idea.

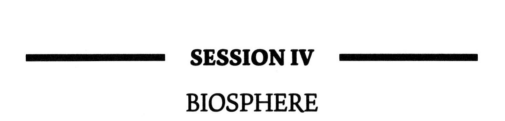

SESSION IV

BIOSPHERE

Phylogenetic Analysis of Traditional Medicinal Plants: Discovering New Drug Sources from Patterns of Cultural Convergence

■■■ *Jeanmaire Molina, PhD* ■■■

Long Island University
Brooklyn, New York

ABSTRACT

Medicinal and psychoactive plants have long been used by different cultures worldwide, inspiring the development of modern pharmaceutical drugs. Phylogenetic investigation of these traditional plants may shed light on which plant groups are used similarly by various cultures (cultural convergence), and which may be evolutionarily important pharmacologically. New York City (NYC) is a microcosm of global cultural diversity, which makes it convenient as a location to survey and phylogenetically analyze traditionally important medicinal plants. In a separate study, culturally diverse psychoactive plant genera and their effects were also phylogenetically analyzed. In both studies, medicinal and psychoactive plants were found to be phylogenetically clustered within certain groups or clades, suggesting evolutionarily conserved bioactivity independently discovered by different cultures through generations of trial and error. The phylogenetic scaffold also allows us to make predictions about unstudied taxa within a clade, to prioritize assays that test for bioactivity known to exist in other members of that clade. Phylogenetic ethnopharmacology, as evidenced in these studies, offers a refreshing perspective to the process of drug discovery, and facilitates scientific validation of traditional therapies through patterns of cultural convergence.

INTRODUCTION

Traditional medicine encompasses culturally transmitted forms of medicine, including the use of plants and other natural products, outside conventional medicine (World Health Organization, 2013). Traditional medicine is the primary form of health care system for 80% of the world's population (Alves and Rosa, 2005). Given its long history of use, safety and efficacy (Gu et al., 2014), the demand for this alternative form of medicine has been growing even in developed nations where conventional medicine is well established. More than 80% of plant-derived pharmaceuticals have been developed from plants used traditionally, including common analgesics such as aspirin and morphine, antimalarials like quinine and artemisinin, and even the anticancer drug irinoctan (Farnsworth, 1988; Fabricant and Farnsworth, 2001). Thus, it is not surprising that the US National Cancer Institute's strategy of random collection and evaluation of 12,000 plant species in the 1960s only resulted in the development of two pharmaceutical drugs, taxol & camptothecin (Atanasov et al., 2015). This suggests that the process of drug discovery could greatly benefit from ethnobotanical leads and would allow us to prioritize screening among the >300,000 species of plants, of which only 15% have been systematically investigated phytochemically (Atanasov et al., 2015). Furthermore, analysis of traditionally important medicinal plants and their medicinal uses within a phylogenetic framework would allow us to determine plant groups that have evolved medicinal attributes based on their ubiquitous use for similar applications by diverse cultures.

Previous studies (Saslis-Lagoudakis et al., 2012; Xavier and Molina, 2016; Alrashedy and Molina, 2016) have shown that traditional medicinal plants across different cultures are phylogenetically clustered, with different cultures using related but geographically disjunct plants for similar therapeutic applications, a pattern of cultural convergence (Xavier and Molina, 2016; Alrashedy and Molina, 2016). The traditional uses can be viewed as traits; common occurrence of these traits within a group may be assumed to be a conserved character purportedly inherited by all members of that group. This signifies that these plant groups, or clades, possess evolutionarily conserved phytochemicals and bioactivity that have been independently discovered by different cultures through repeated trial and error over time (Gupta et al., 2005), and their record of safety and efficacy has allowed these plants to persist through generations of use. Though previous studies (Xavier and Molina, 2016; Alrashedy and Molina, 2016) were limited in the plant taxa included in the phylogeny, and may have missed other pertinent phylogenetic patterns, this is easily rectified through the addition of more plants and their traditional uses. This could corroborate the therapeutic importance of previously identified plant clades (Xavier and Molina, 2016; Alrashedy and Molina, 2016) and highlight other plant groups and taxa that may be pharmacologically important.

Xavier and Molina (2016) presented a phylogeny of 95 medicinal plant species used by various immigrant cultures in New York City (NYC). NYC is a microcosm of global cultural diversity, which makes it convenient to study cross-cultural ethnobotanical patterns. In their study, Xavier and Molina (2016) found that certain families showed disproportionate importance as traditional therapies for gastrointestinal (e.g., Lauraceae, Zingiberaceae), respiratory (e.g., Lamiaceae) and musculoskeletal ailments (Burseraceae), and even as antibiotics (e.g., Meliaceae). Surveyed immigrant cultures included Indian (Ayurvedic), African, Latin/Caribbean, Islamic/Middle Eastern and Chinese. Here, I add plants used by Native Americans and immigrant Europeans to uncover additional phylogenetic patterns. In a separate study, psychoactive plants were also analyzed phylogenetically by Alrashedy and Molina (2016). Similarly, certain plant families emerged as cross-culturally important, as hallucinogens (e.g., Myristicaceae, Convolvulaceae, Solanaceae), anxiolytics (Lamiaceae), antidepressants (Apocynaceae), analgesics (Papaveraceae), and as aphrodisiacs (asterids). Within these families, similar phytochemicals mediate similar psychoactive effects via the same neurological mechanisms, yet interestingly, unrelated families promoting the same psychoactive effect were also found to sometimes modulate similar neurological pathways. This mechanistic convergence is exemplified in the unrelated Myristicaceae and Convolvulaceae, whose members are often used as hallucinogens by different cultures, yet which have evolved distinct phytochemicals similarly acting as serotonin agonists. To highlight other psychoactive groups that may be cross-culturally important, additional psychoactive plants from Australia and Africa were added to the phylogeny. In both cases, new phylogenetic patterns emerged in the updated phylogenies. This emphasizes the utility of phylogenies in finding pharmacologically important medicinal plant sources from patterns of cultural convergence.

MATERIALS & METHODS

To update the medicinal plant phylogeny in Xavier and Molina (2016), 21 genera used in Native American traditional medicine and 43 genera used in Western/European herbalism were added (for a total of 139 genera), with their medicinal uses mapped on the phylogeny (Table 1). Plant names were obtained from online catalogs of NYC herbal stores, and scientific names, if unavailable on the product label, were retrieved from Internet searches based on the common name on the label. rbcL sequences for respective genera were downloaded from Genbank (https://www.ncbi.nlm.nih.gov/genbank/), aligned and phylogenetically analyzed to reconstruct a genus-level phylogeny following methods in Alrashedy and Molina (2016). If the majority (>60%) of the genera within a clade is used for the same medicinal application by different cultures, then presumably this is a conserved "trait" for members of that clade, and this medicinal application is indicated on the ancestral node (e.g., in Lamiaceae, 6 were used for gastrointestinal concerns out of 9 genera, so 6/9=67%, and the "gastrointestinal trait" is placed by the node in Figure 1). Medicinal applications were categorized as follows: gastrointestinal, cardiovascular, respiratory/immunostimulant, nervous, musculoskeletal and antiparasitic/antibiotic, and were primarily obtained from Moerman (2003), Alshamrani (2016) and UMMC (2017).

To update the psychoactive plant phylogeny (Alrashedy and Molina, 2016), a total of 25 psychoactive genera – 10 used multiculturally, 5 from Australia, and 10 from Africa – (Table 2; Sobiecki, 2008; Voogelbreinder, 2009) were added to the psychoactive phylogeny published in Alrashedy & Molina (2016) for a total of 151 genera. rbcL sequences were downloaded from Genbank, aligned and phylogenetically analyzed. Psychoactive effects (hallucinogen, stimulant, sedative, anxiolytic, antidepressant, aphrodisiac, analgesic) from the said references were also superimposed on the phylogeny.

RESULTS & DISCUSSION

PHYLOGENY OF PLANTS USED IN NYC HERBAL MEDICINE

Figure 1 presents the genus-level phylogeny of traditional medicinal plants used by immigrants in NYC (Xavier and Molina, 2016), updated with plants and their uses from Native American and Western/European herbalism (Moerman, 2003; Alshamrani , 2016; UMMC, 2017). In this phylogeny that conforms to expected relationships from the Angiosperm Phylogeny Group (2016), 3 new clades were identified to be cross-culturally important (i.e., 3 or more genera were used cross-culturally): the family Asteraceae and orders Dipsacales and Fagales, in addition to the 10 families that were previously identified (Xavier and Molina, 2016)—Lauraceae, Zingiberaceae, Malvaceae, Meliaceae, Combretaceae, Burseraceae, Fabaceae, Apiaceae, Rubiaceae, Lamiaceae). However, some of these clades are inherently diverse, and their identification here may be an artifact of this diversity. For example, Asteraceae has >1600 genera, while Burseraceae only has 19. To account for this disparity, Figure 2 shows the relative proportion of medicinally important genera within the family, obtained by dividing the number of traditional medicinal genera included here by the overall generic diversity within the family (from Christenhusz and Byng, 2016). Though Fagales and Dipsacales are ordinal classifications, they only have 19 and 33 genera, respectively. Plant groups with the highest relative medicinal importance, in ascending order, include Lamiaceae (used for gastrointestinal and respiratory ailments, represented at c. 5%), Zingiberaceae (8%, gastrointestinal), Lauraceae (9%, gastrointestinal/antibiotic), Meliaceae (10%, antibiotic), Dipsacales (16%, nervous system applications), Fagales (20%, gastrointestinal/antibiotic), and Burseraceae (27%, musculoskeletal ailments). These plant families are disproportionately used medicinally by various cultures in NYC.

Gastrointestinal, respiratory and antibiotic plants. As discussed in Xavier and Molina (2016), the presence of essential oils rich in terpenes, terpenoids and phenolics in members of Lamiaceae (Kumari et al., 2014), Zingiberaceae (Kumari et al., 2014), and Lauraceae (Ahmad et al., 2013) contribute to their therapeutic applications for gastrointestinal ailments. These phytochemicals exhibit carminative, antispasmodic and anti-inflammatory effects (Lewis and Elvin-Lewis, 2003; Heinrich et al., 2012). They also possess antimicrobial properties, explaining the use of Lauraceae members as antibiotics (Joshi et al., 2010). In Lamiaceae, the volatile oils also exert respiratory activity as an expectorant and antitussive, and for mitigating bronchial infections (Mamadalieva et al., 2017).

In the order Fagales, which overall only has 19 genera, phenolics (e.g., ellagic acid) as well as tannins are described to be gastroprotective (Polya, 2003; European Medicines Agency, 2011). Flavonols that characterize Fagales (Giannasi, 1986) like galangin (Polya, 2003), kaempferol (Calderon-Montano et al., 2011), and quercetin (Cushnie and Lamb, 2005) are also antibacterial. However, in the unrelated Meliaceae, limonoids are the primary antimicrobial constituents (Roy and Saraf, 2006).

Nervous system plants. The order Dipsacales, with only 33 genera, has been highlighted as a medicinally important group for nervous system complaints, particularly for the sedative action of its members. The popular herbal valerian (*Valeriana officinalis*), widely used to alleviate insomnia and anxiety in folk medicine (Shi et al., 2014), contains the sesquiterpene valerenic acid which stimulates the GABAergic system, the main inhibitory neurotransmitter system, resulting in its sedative and muscle-relaxing effects (Yuan et al., 2004). Iridoids and related valepotriates in valerian may also contribute to its tranquilizing effects (Polya, 2003). GABA-stimulating sesquiterpenes were also identified in *Nardostachys* spp. (Takemoto et al., 2009) used as a sedative in Ayurvedic/Indian culture (Chaudhary et al., 2015), as well as in *Viburnum* spp. used in Native American (Moerman, 2003) and traditional Chinese medicine (Wang and Wang, 2013). There was no ethnobotanical use for the Dipsacales member *Sambucus nigra* as a sedative, but experimental evidence was found that suggest extracts of the plant have anticonvulsant activity by increasing the inhibitory neurotransmitter GABA

(Ataee et al., 2016). These studies suggest that Dipsacales may be an important evolutionary group to explore for tranquilizing/sedating drugs.

Plants for musculoskeletal applications. Relative to its diversity, many members of Burseraceae have been employed in various cultures as treatments for musculoskeletal problems such as pain and arthritis (Xavier and Molina, 2016), making up 27% of the medicinal plant genera (Figure 2). Triterpene acids such as boswellic acids and mansumbinoic acid have been found to promote its anti-inflammatory effects (Duwiejua et al., 1993). The sesquiterpenoid furanoedesma-1,3-diene has also been found to bind to opioid receptors, promoting analgesia, similar to morphine (Spinella, 2001). Thus, newly discovered species within this family should first be explored for such antinociceptive molecules.

PHYLOGENY OF CULTURALLY IMPORTANT PSYCHOACTIVE PLANTS

Psychoactive plant taxa were also phylogenetically clustered (Figure 3) in certain families. The families Aizoaceae, Ranunculaceae, Malpighiaceae, Apiaceae and Caprifoliaceae were not in Alrashedy & Molina (2016) and emerged as cross-culturally important in the updated phylogeny (Figure 3) after addition of new genera. However, after correcting again for the disparities in generic diversity, as in Figure 2, plant families that remain disproportionately important include, in ascending order, Malpighiaceae (4%, hallucinogen, Figure 4), Ranunculaceae (7%, analgesic), Convolvulaceae (11%, hallucinogen), Papaveraceae (10%, sedative/analgesic), Caprifoliaceae (11%, sedative), Solanaceae (16%, hallucinogen/sedative) and Myristicaceae (19%, hallucinogen). These families are discussed here and the reader is referred to Alrashedy and Molina (2016) for a discussion of the phytochemistry and pharmacology of the other families.

Hallucinogenic plants. The presence of serotonin-mimicking alkaloids, e.g., harmaline, harmine, beta-carboline and dimethyltryptamine (DMT) in members of Malpighiaceae (Callaway et al., 1999) may mediate their hallucinogenic effects by acting as 5HT receptor agonists (Aghajanian and Marek, 1999). This is true for *Banisteriopsis caapi* and *Diplopterys cabrerana* (Ratsch, 2005). The confamilial *Sphedamnocarpus* is used in African divination practices (Sobiecki, 2008), and phytochemical and pharmacological studies would likely confirm the presence of 5HT ligands. The same serotonergic mechanism is exerted by hallucinogenic members of the unrelated families Myristicaceae and Convolvulaceae (Polya, 2003; Schiff, 2006), each possessing serotonin-mimicking compounds such as DMT and ergot alkaloids, respectively. Though phylogenetically related to Convolvulaceae, Solanaceae surprisingly modulates its psychoactive effects through tropane alkaloids (e.g., atropine, scopolamine) that work via anticholinergic mechanisms, resulting in sedation and deliriant hallucinations characterized by confusion and stupor (Duncan and Gold, 1982), in contrast to the higher-level cognitive and perceptual changes in serotonergic hallucinogens (Aghajanian and Marek, 1999).

Plants for sedation and analgesia. The closely related Papaveraceae and Ranunculaceae, of the order Ranunculales, both promote analgesia, but current experimental studies seem to suggest different mechanisms. Morphine and codeine are benzylisoquinoline alkaloids (BIAs) characteristic of Ranunculales (Hagel and Facchini, 2013), and they bind to opioid receptors to relieve pain (Spinella, 2001; Polya, 2003). Phylogenetically, it is expected that BIAs would also mediate analgesia in Ranunculaceae. The BIA berberine in *Hydrastis canadensis* does work this way (Chen et al., 2015; Mikołajczak et al., 2015). However, in *Aconitum ssp.*, anesthesia is mediated by the diterpenoid alkaloid aconitine, which targets Na+ channels (Polya, 2003), while in *Clematis*, flavonoids seem to be antinociceptive (Mostafa et al., 2010). It is possible that other pain-relieving BIAs exist in Ranunculaceae. Apart from analgesia, sedation in Papaveraceae is also mediated via the opioid pathway (Spinella, 2001). In contrast, sedative members of the unrelated Caprifoliaceae mediate their effects via the GABAergic pathway, as discussed previously (see Dipsacales above).

Caprifoliaceae (Dipsacales) is highlighted in both phylogenies (Figs. 1 and 3), which underscores the neuropharmacological importance of this clade. The families Apiaceae, Apocynaceae, Asteraceae, Fabaceae, Malvaceae and Rubiaceae were also redundant in both phylogenies, but this is perhaps a function of their generic diversity that made them easily accessible, hence their ubiquitous ethnobotanical uses. Nonetheless, pharmacological studies of these families would still be interesting to understand certain trends, such as the prominent use of Apiaceae members as stimulants, or the use of Apocynaceae members as antidepressants.

CONCLUSION

Traditionally important medicinal and psychoactive plants are phylogenetically clustered within certain groups or clades, whose members have been independently discovered by different cultures through generations of trial and error. This implies an evolutionarily conserved phytochemistry that should be pharmacologically investigated. Though the identification of certain commonly used plant groups may be a function of their innate diversity, investigation of their phytochemistry is still worthwhile. The phylogenetic scaffold allows us to make predictions about unexplored taxa within a plant family and prioritize assays that test for bioactivity known to exist in other members. For instance, anti-inflammatory assays could be explored for newly discovered species in Burseraceae, which was highlighted here as a plant family cross-culturally important in alleviating musculoskeletal pain and inflammation. Phylogenetic ethnopharmacology, as evidenced in these studies, offers a refreshing perspective to the process of drug discovery and facilitates scientific validation of traditional therapies through patterns of cultural convergence.

ACKNOWLEDGMENTS

I am indebted to my former graduate students Camilla Xavier, Nashmiah Alrashedy and Maryam Alshamrani, whose theses inspired this work. I am also grateful to Dennis McKenna, Annette Badenhorst, Snu Voogelbreinder, Jean-Francois Sobiecki and other ESPD participants.

REFERENCES

Aghajanian, G.K., Marek G.J., 1999. Serotonin and hallucinogens. *Neuropsychopharmacology* 21, 16S–23S.

Ahmad, S., et al., 2013. Phytochemical analysis and growth inhibiting effects of *Cinnamomum cassia* bark on some pathogenic fungal isolates. *J. Chem. Pharm. Res.* 5, 25–32.

Alrashedy N.A., Molina J., 2016. The ethnobotany of psychoactive plant use: a phylogenetic perspective. *PeerJ* 4: e2546 https://doi.org/10.7717/peerj.2546.

Alshamrani, M., 2016. *An eye for an eye: phylogenetic evaluation of the medicinal uses of plants with "healing signatures."* Master's thesis submitted to Long Island University, Brooklyn, New York.

Alves, R.R.N., Rosa, I.L., 2005. Why study the use of animal products in traditional medicines? *J. Ethnobiol. Ethnomed.* 1, 1–5.

Ataee, R., et al., 2016. Anticonvulsant activities of *Sambucus nigra*. *Eur. Rev. Med. Pharmacol. Sci.* 20, 3123-3126.

Atanasov A.G., et al., 2015. Discovery and resupply of pharmacologically active plant-derived natural products: A review. *Biotechnol Adv.* 33, 1582-1614.

Calderon-Montano, J.M., et al., 2011. A review on the dietary flavonoid kaempferol. *Mini Rev. Med. Chem.* 11, 298-344.

Callaway, J.C., et al., 1999. Pharmacokinetics of Hoasca alkaloids in healthy humans. *J. Ethnopharm.* 65, 243–256.

Chaudhary, S., et al., 2015. Evaluation of antioxidant and anticancer activity of extract and fractions of *Nardostachys jatamansi* DC in breast carcinoma. *BMC Complement Altern Med* 15, 50.

Chen, C., et al., 2015. Berberine improves intestinal motility and visceral pain in the mouse models mimicking diarrhea-predominant irritable bowel syndrome (ibs-d) symptoms in an opioid-receptor dependent manner. *PLoS ONE* 10, e0145556. http://doi.org/10.1371/journal.pone.0145556

Cushnie, T.P., Lamb, A.J., 2005. Antimicrobial activity of flavonoids. *Int. J. Antimicrob Agents* 26, 343-356.

Christenhusz, M.J., Byng, J.W., 2016. The number of known plant species in the world and its annual increase. *Phytotaxa* 261, 201-217.

Duncan, D.F., Gold, R.S., 1982. *Drugs and the Whole Person.* John Wiley & Sons, New York.

Duwiejua, M., et al., 1993. Anti-inflammatory activity of resins from some species of the plant family Burseraceae. *Planta Med.* 59, 12-16.

European Medicines Agency, 2011. Assessment report on *Quercus robur* L., *Quercus petraea* (Matt.) Liebl., *Quercus pubescens* Willd. cortex. http://www.ema.europa.eu/docs/en_GB/document_library/Herbal_HMPC_assessment_report/2011/05/WC500106476.pdf (accessed 10.07.17).

Fabricant, D.S., Farnsworth, N.R., 2001. The value of plants used in traditional medicine for drug discovery. *Environ. Health Perspect.* 109 (Suppl. 1), 69–75.

Farnsworth, N., 1988. Chapter 9, Screening Plants for New Medicines, in: Wilson, E.O., Peter, F.M., (Eds.), *Biodiversity.* National Academies Press, Washington, DC. Available from: https://www.ncbi.nlm.nih.gov/books/NBK219315/

Giannasi, D.E., 1986. Phytochemical Aspects of Phylogeny in Hamamelidae. *Ann. Mo. Bot. Gard.* 73, 417-437.

Gu, R., et al., 2014. Prospecting for bioactive constituents from traditional medicinal plants through ethnobotanical approaches. *Biol. Pharm. Bull.* 37, 903-915.

Gupta, R., et al., 2005. Nature's medicines: traditional knowledge and intellectual property management. Case studies from the National Institutes of Health (NIH), USA. *Curr. Drug Discov. Technol.* 2, 203–219.

Hagel, J.M., Facchini, P.J., 2013. Benzylisoquinoline alkaloid metabolism: a century of discovery and a brave new world. *Plant Cell Physiol.* 54, 647-672.

Heinrich, M., et al., 2012. *Fundamentals of Pharmacognosy and Phytotherapy*, 2nd ed., Churchill Livingstone, New York.

Joshi, S.C., et al., 2010. Antioxidant and antibacterial activities of the leaf essential oils of Himalayan Lauraceae species. *Food Chem Toxicol.* 48, 37-40.

Kumari, S., et al., 2014. EssOilDB: a database of essential oils reflecting terpene composition and variability in the plant kingdom. *Database* doi:http://dx.doi.org/10.1093/ database/bau120.

Lewis, W.H., Elvin-Lewis, M.P.F., 2003. *Medical Botany: Plants Affecting Human Health*, 2nd ed., John Wiley and Sons, New Jersey.

Mamadalieva, N.Z., et al., 2017. Aromatic medicinal plants of the Lamiaceae Family from Uzbekistan: ethnopharmacology, essential oils composition, and biological activities. *Medicines* 4, 8.

Mikołajczak, P.L., et al., 2015. Evaluation of anti-inflammatory and analgesic activities of extracts from herb of *Chelidonium majus* L. *Cent. Eur. J. Immunol.* 40, 400–410.

Moerman, D., 2003. *Native American Ethnobotany: a database of foods, drugs, dyes and fibers of Native American peoples, derived from plants.* http://naeb.brit.org/ (accessed 17.07.11)

Mostafa M., et al., 2010. Anti-inflammatory, antinociceptive and antipyretic properties of the aqueous extract of *Clematis brachiata* leaf in male rats. *Pharm Biol.* 48, 682-689.

Polya, G., 2003. *Biochemical targets of plant bioactive compounds: a pharmacological reference guide to sites of action and biological effects.* CRC Press, Boca Raton.

Ratsch, C 2005. *The Encyclopedia of Psychoactive Plants: Ethnopharmacology and Its Applications.* Park Street Press.

Roy, A., Saraf, S., 2006. Limonoids: overview of significant bioactive triterpenes distributed in plants kingdom. *Biol. Pharm. Bull.* 29, 191–201.

Sobiecki, J.F., 2008. A review of plants used in divination in southern Africa and their psychoactive effects. *S. Afr. Hum.* 20, 333–351.

Saslis-Lagoudakis, C.H., et al., 2012. Phylogenies reveal predictive power of traditional medicine in bioprospecting. *Proc. Nat. Acad. Sci. USA* 109, 15835-15840.

Schiff, P.L., 2016. Ergot and its alkaloids. *Am J Pharm Educ.* 70, 98.

Shi, Y., et al., 2014. Herbal insomnia medications that target GABAergic systems: a review of the psychopharmacological evidence. *Curr. Neuropharm.*, 12, 289–302.

Spinella, M., 2001. *The psychopharmacology of herbal medicine: plant drugs that alter mind, brain, and behavior.* MIT Press, London.

Takemoto, H., et al., 2009. Inhalation administration of the sesquiterpenoid aristolen-1(10)-en-9-ol from *Nardostachys chinensis* has a sedative effect via the GABAergic system. *J Nat Med.* 63, 380-385.

The Angiosperm Phylogeny Group, 2016. An update of the Angiosperm Phylogeny Group classification for the orders and families of flowering plants: APG IV. *Bot. J. Linn. Soc.* 181, 1-20.

University of Maryland Medical Center (UMMC), 2017. *Complementary and Alternative Medicine Guide.* http://www.umm.edu/health/medical/altmed (accessed 10.07.17).

Voogelbreinder, S., 2009. *Garden of Eden: The Shamanic Use of Psychoactive Flora and Fauna, and the Study of Consciousness.* Black Rainbow Press, Australia.

Wang, X., Wang, W., 2013. Cytotoxic and radical scavenging nor-dammarane triterpenoids from *Viburnum mongolicum*. *Molecules* 18, 1405-1417.

World Health Organization (WHO), 2013. *WHO traditional medicine strategy: 2014-2023* http://who.int/medicines/publications/traditional/trm_strategy14_23/en/ (accessed 17.07.12)

Xavier, C., Molina, J., 2016. Phylogeny of medicinal plants depicts cultural convergence among immigrant groups in New York City. *J. Herb. Med.* 6, 1-11.

Yuan, C.S., et al., 2004. The gamma-aminobutyric acidergic effects of valerian and valerenic acid on rat brainstem neuronal activity. *Anesth Analg.* 98, 353-358.

Table 1 List of medicinal plants used in Native American and European/Western traditional medicine and added to the NYC herbal phylogeny published in Xavier and Molina (2016). Medicinal uses were obtained primarily from Moerman (2003), Alshamrani (2016) and University of Maryland Medical Center (2017).

Family	Scientific Name	Common Name	Predominant Culture	Traditional Medicinal Uses
Adoxaceae	Sambucus nigra	elderberry	European/Western	Respiratory/immune support, antibiotic
Adoxaceae	Viburnum prunifolium	stagberry	Native American	Nervous; female reproductive
Apocynaceae	Apocynum androsaemifolium	bitterroot	Native American	Gastrointestinal, respiratory/immune support, cardiovascular, antibiotic, nervous, urinary
Aristolochiaceae	Asarum canadense	snake root	Native American	Gastrointestinal, respiratory/immune support, cardiovascular, female reproductive, urinary, stimulant
Asteraceae	Arctium lappa	great burdock	European/Western	Gastrointestinal, respiratory/immune support, cardiovascular
Asteraceae	Arnica montana	arnica	European/Western	Musculoskeletal
Asteraceae	Calendula officinalis	pot marigold	European/Western	Gastrointestinal
Asteraceae	Echinacea spp.	coneflower	Native American	Gastrointestinal, respiratory/immune support, cardiovascular, musculoskeletal
Asteraceae	Lactuca serriola	prickly lettuce	European/Western	Gastrointestinal, respiratory/immune support, cardiovascular
Asteraceae	Silybum marianum	milk thistle	European/Western	Gastrointestinal
Asteraceae	Tussilago farfara	coltsfoot	European/Western	Respiratory/immune support
Asteraceae	Rudbeckia hirta	coneflower	Native American	Respiratory/immune support, antibiotic
Berberidaceae	Berberis vulgaris	European barberry	European/Western	Gastrointestinal, musculoskeletal, antibiotic
Betulaceae	Alnus rubra	red alder	Native American	Gastrointestinal, respiratory/immune support, musculoskeletal, antibiotic
Betulaceae	Betula papyrifera	paper birch	Native American	Gastrointestinal, respiratory/immune support, cardiovascular, female reproductive, musculoskeletal, antibiotic
Caprifoliaceae	Valeriana officinalis	valerian	European/Western	Nervous
Caryophyllaceae	Stellaria media	chickweed	European/Western	Musculoskeletal
Cupressaceae	Juniperus scopulorum	rocky mountain juniper	Native American	Gastrointestinal, respiratory/immune support, cardiovascular, musculoskeletal, antibiotic, urinary, cosmetic
Fabaceae	Trifolium pratense	red clover	European/Western	Gastrointestinal, respiratory/immune support, cardiovascular, female reproductive
Fagaceae	Quercus robur	oak	European/Western	Gastrointestinal, antibiotic
Gentianaceae	Gentiana lutea	yellow gentian	European/Western	Gastrointestinal

Family	Scientific Name	Common Name	Predominant Culture	Traditional Medicinal Uses
Hamamelidaceae	*Hamamelis virginiana*	witch hazel	Native American	Gastrointestinal, respiratory/immune support, cardiovascular, musculoskeletal, urinary
Hypericaceae	*Hypericum perforatum*	St. John's wort	European/Western	Gastrointestinal, nervous
Iridaceae	*Iris missouriensis*	rocky mountain iris	Native American	Gastrointestinal, musculoskeletal, urinary
Juglandaceae	*Juglans cinerea*	walnut	Native American	Gastrointestinal, cardiovascular, female reproductive, antibiotic
Lamiaceae	*Glechoma hederacea*	ground ivy	European/Western	Gastrointestinal, respiratory/immune support, urinary
Lamiaceae	*Marrubium vulgare*	white horehound	European/Western	Gastrointestinal, respiratory/immune support
Lamiaceae	*Melissa officinalis*	lemon balm	European/Western	Gastrointestinal, nervous
Lamiaceae	*Thymus vulgaris*	common thyme	European/Western	Gastrointestinal, respiratory/immune support, antibiotic
Lamiaceae	*Vitex agnus-castus*	chaste berry	European/Western	Female reproductive
Lauraceae	*Sassafras albidum*	sassafras	Native American	Gastrointestinal, respiratory/immune support, cardiovascular, antibiotic, urinary
Loganiaceae	*Spigelia marilandica*	pink root	Native American	Gastrointestinal
Melanthiaceae	*Trillium erectum*	red trillium	Native American	Gastrointestinal, respiratory/immune support
Myricaceae	*Myrica cerifera*	wax myrtle	Native American	Gastrointestinal, musculoskeletal, antibiotic
Onagraceae	*Oenothera biennis*	evening primrose	Native American	Gastrointestinal, musculoskeletal
Papaveraceae	*Sanguinaria canadensis*	blood root	Native American	Gastrointestinal, respiratory/immune support, cardiovascular, female reproductive, urinary, stimulant
Polygonaceae	*Polygonum pennsylvanicum*	pinkweed	Native American	Gastrointestinal, cardiovascular, female reproductive
Polygonaceae	*Rumex crispus*	curled dock	European/Western	Gastrointestinal, cardiovascular, antibiotic
Portulacaceae	*Portulaca oleracea*	purslane	European/Western	Gastrointestinal, respiratory/immune support, cardiovascular, musculoskeletal, urinary
Ranunculaceae	*Actaea racemosa*	black cohosh	Native American	Respiratory/immune support, female reproductive, musculoskeletal
Rosaceae	*Agrimonia eupatoria*	agrimony	European/Western	Gastrointestinal
Salicaceae	*Populus tremuloides*	quaking aspen	Native American	Gastrointestinal, respiratory/immune support, nervous, female reproductive, musculoskeletal, antibiotic
Scrophulariaceae	*Verbascum thapsus*	great mullein	European/Western	Respiratory/immune support
Vitaceae	*Vitis aestivalis*	summer grape	Native American	Gastrointestinal, respiratory/immune support, cardiovascular, musculoskeletal

Family	Scientific Name	Common Name	Predominant Culture	Traditional Medicinal Uses
Aizoaceae	*Aptenia cordifolia*	ibohlololo	African	analgesic
Aizoaceae	*Carpobrotus spp.*	pigface	Australian	analgesic
Apiaceae	*Anethum graveolens*	dill	Multicultural	sedative, aphrodisiac
Apiaceae	*Conium maculatum*	hemlock	Multicultural	sedative, aphrodisiac
Apiaceae	*Daucus carota*	wild carrot	Multicultural	stimulant, aphrodisiac
Apiaceae	*Ferula spp.*	giant fennel	Multicultural	stimulant, aphrodisiac
Apiaceae	*Foeniculum vulgare*	fennel	Multicultural	stimulant
Apiaceae	*Heracleum spp.*	cow parsnip	Multicultural	sedative, aphrodisiac
Apocynaceae	*Vinca spp.*	periwinkle	Multicultural	anxiolytic, sedative
Apocynaceae	*Xysmalobium undulatum*	leshokhoa	African	anxiolytic/sedative? (= anti-hysteria)
Caprifoliaceae	*Centranthus spp.*	centranthes	African	sedative
Convolvulaceae	*Cuscuta spp.*	dodder	Multicultural	stimulant, aphrodisiac
Convolvulaceae	*Evolvulus alsinoides*	sky convolvulus	Multicultural	sedative
Fabaceae	*Albizia adianthifolia*	muvhadangoma	African	hallucinogen (= induces dreams)
Fabaceae	*Bauhinia bowkeri*	umlandlovu	African	hallucinogen
Fabaceae	*Canavalia maritima*	coastal jack bean	Australian	sedative, analgesic
Fabaceae	*Chamaecrista mimosoides*	umbonisela	African	sedative
Fabaceae	*Erythrophleum lasianthum*	umkhwangu	African	analgesic
Fabaceae	*Indigofera flavicans*	naiego	African	hallucinogen (= induces trance)
Lamiaceae	*Clerodendrum floribundum*	buwatanganing	Australian	stimulant, analgesic
Lamiaceae	*Stachys aethiopica*	bolao ba litaolla	African	anxiolytic (= soothing)
Malpighiaceae	*Sphedamnorcarpus pruriens*	pupuma	African	hallucinogen?
Malvaceae	*Brachychiton diversifolius*	nanungguwa	Australian	stimulant
Ranunculaceae	*Clematis glycinoides*	headache vine	Australian	analgesic
Rubiaceae	*Galium spp.*	bedstraw	Multicultural	stimulant

←

Table 2 List of psychoactive plants added to the phylogeny published in Alrashedy and Molina (2016). Psychoactive effects were obtained primarily from Sobiecki (2008) and Voogelbreinder (2009).

→

Fig. 1 Phylogeny of traditionally important medicinal plants (139 genera) used by various immigrant cultures in NYC. Branches in black (bold) represent genera of ethnopharmacologically important plant groups/clades with their corresponding taxon names (family/order). Symbols on nodes represent the primary therapeutic application of that clade. "*" indicates clades that are disproportionately important even after correcting for generic diversity (cf. Fig. 2).

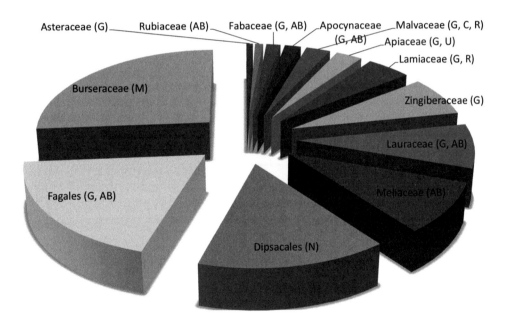

Fig. 2 Relative medicinal importance of each clade identified in the NYC herbal phylogeny (Fig. 1). Proportions were standardized according to generic diversity within the clade, e.g., Asteraceae is represented by 9 medicinal genera here but has 1623 genera total, so its medicinal importance here is relatively nil (9/1623=0.0055). Cross-culturally important medicinal clades include Lamiaceae, Zingiberaceae, Lauraceae, Meliaceae, Dipsacales, Fagales and Burseraceae in ascending sequence and are discussed in text. AB: antibiotic; C: cardiovascular; G: gastrointestinal; M: musculoskeletal; N: nervous; R: respiratory; U: urinary.

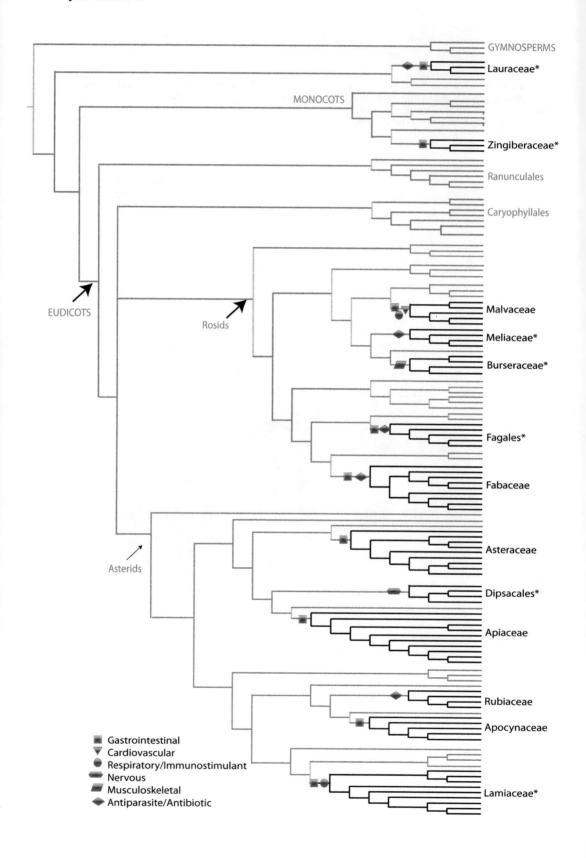

Jeanmaire Molina

GYMNOSPERMS
Lauraceae*
MONOCOTS
Zingiberaceae*
Ranunculales
Caryophyllales
EUDICOTS
Rosids
Malvaceae
Meliaceae*
Burseraceae*
Fagales*
Fabaceae
Asteraceae
Dipsacales*
Asterids
Apiaceae
Rubiaceae
Apocynaceae
Lamiaceae*

Gastrointestinal
Cardiovascular
Respiratory/Immunostimulant
Nervous
Musculoskeletal
Antiparasite/Antibiotic

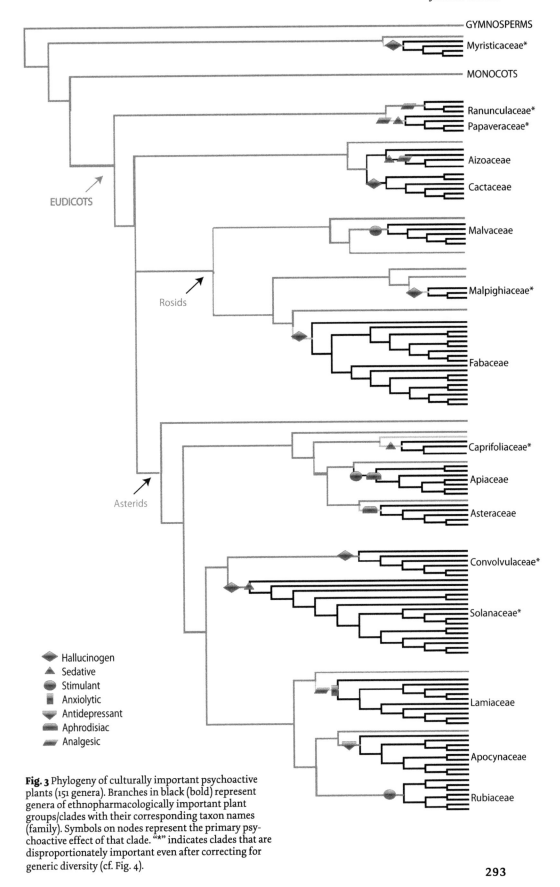

GYMNOSPERMS

Myristicaceae*

MONOCOTS

Ranunculaceae*

Papaveraceae*

Aizoaceae

Cactaceae

EUDICOTS

Malvaceae

Malpighiaceae*

Rosids

Fabaceae

Caprifoliaceae*

Apiaceae

Asteraceae

Asterids

Convolvulaceae*

Solanaceae*

◆ Hallucinogen
▲ Sedative
⬭ Stimulant
▯ Anxiolytic
▼ Antidepressant
⬬ Aphrodisiac
▰ Analgesic

Lamiaceae

Apocynaceae

Rubiaceae

Fig. 3 Phylogeny of culturally important psychoactive plants (151 genera). Branches in black (bold) represent genera of ethnopharmacologically important plant groups/clades with their corresponding taxon names (family). Symbols on nodes represent the primary psychoactive effect of that clade. "*" indicates clades that are disproportionately important even after correcting for generic diversity (cf. Fig. 4).

293

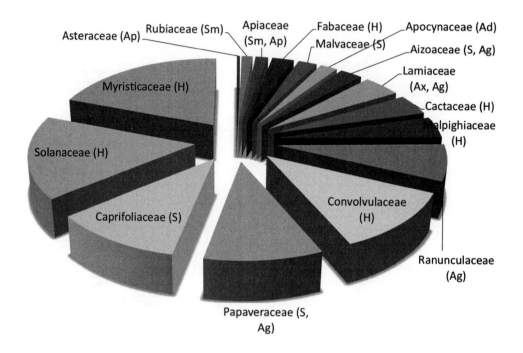

Fig. 4 Relative psychoactive importance of each clade in the psychoactive plant phylogeny (Fig. 3). Proportions were standardized according to generic diversity within the clade. Cross-culturally important psychoactive clades include Malpighiaceae, Ranunculaceae, Convolvulaceae, Papaveraceae, Caprifoliaceae (Dipsacales), Solanaceae and Myristicaceae in ascending order. Ag: analgesic; Ad: antidepressant; Ap: aphrodisiac; Ax: anxiolytic; H: hallucinogen; S: sedative; Sm: stimulant.

Ethnopharmacology Meets the Receptorome: Bioprospecting for Psychotherapeutic Medicines in the Amazon Rainforest

■ *Dennis J. McKenna*, PhD ■

Director, Ethnopharmacology,
Heffter Research Institute;
Assistant Professor, Center for
Spirituality and Healing,
University of Minnesota,
Minneapolis, MN

Note: This paper consists of a subset of the data presented in the multi-author publication in the *Journal of Ethnopharmacology*: McKenna, D.J., Ruiz, J.M., Hoye, T.R., Roth, B.R., Shoemaker, A.P., 2011. Receptor screening technologies in the evaluation of Amazonian ethnomedicines with potential applications to cognitive deficits. *Journal of Ethnopharmacology* 134, 475-492. I am grateful to my co-authors for their contributions to this work, and thank them for permission to present sections of it in this paper.

ABSTRACT

Ethnopharmacological relevance: Amazonian peoples utilize a variety of psychoactive plants that may contain novel biologically active compounds. Efforts to investigate such remedies in terms of neuropharmacology have been limited. Aim of this study: This study identified Amazonian ethnomedicines with potential for the treatment of cognitive deficits in schizophrenia and dementias, and characterized their interactions with CNS neurotransmitter receptors *in vitro*. Materials and Methods: Approximately 300 Amazonian species with folk uses or constituents indicative of central nervous system activity were incorporated into a database constructed from literature searches, herbarium surveys, and interviews with traditional practitioners. Approximately 130 of these targeted species were collected in Loreto province, Peru, and 228 fractions derived from them were screened in 31 radioligand receptor assays via the resources of the NIMH Psychoactive Drug Screening Program (PDSP). Results: 91 samples displayed ≥ 60% inhibition of radioligand-binding activity in receptor assays. Conclusions: Potential CNS activity was detected in about 40% of the samples screened, with some correlations to both folk uses and phytochemical constituents. These results may point to novel and potentially therapeutic CNS-active compounds.

INTRODUCTION

Advances in psychopharmacology have resulted in the development of medications that are effective for the treatment of overt psychotic symptoms of schizophrenia, sometimes characterized as positive symptoms of the disease. By contrast, the negative symptoms of schizophrenia are associated with neurocognitive deficits in functions such as attention, executive functions, short- and long-term memory, and verbal ability (Lysaker and Buck, 2007; Peuskens et al., 2005). Treatment of the neurocognitive deficits in schizophrenia is likely key to eventual long-term recovery and productive reintegration of individuals with schizophrenia into social, educational, and employment contexts. While "atypical" antipsychotics such as clozapine have shown some promise for the treatment of neurocognitive deficits in schizophrenia, there remains a continued need for the identification of structurally novel compounds that are more effective, and have more acceptable side-effect profiles (Hill et al., 2010). Similar considerations also inform the search for effective medications to treat neurocognitive deficits in Alzheimer's disease and other dementias (Mangialasche et al., 2010).

Ethnopharmacology – the interdisciplinary investigation of biologically active substances used by indigenous cultures – has repeatedly demonstrated utility for the discovery of natural compounds that eventually find medical applications. In the field of psychopharmacology, ethnopharmacological research has uncovered a wide spectrum of CNS-active compounds, ranging from sedatives to anxiolytics to analgesics to hallucinogens. Receptor-binding methodologies – in which isotopically labeled compounds are employed to selectively label neurotransmitters or other receptors – have been widely utilized in drug discovery. The technique enables rapid screening of compound "libraries" or crude extracts derived from plants or other natural sources. The application of ethnopharmacology to identify potentially therapeutic psychotropic medicines with a history of human use, combined with receptor-binding and functional receptor assays to identify activity in crude extracts, is a productive approach to the discovery and evaluation of psychotropic ethnomedicines that may be suitable for development into clinically applicable psychotherapeutic agents.

ETHNOPHARMACOLOGY APPLIED TO CNS DRUG DISCOVERY

The search for new psychotropic medications for the treatment of diseases of the nervous system and mental illnesses has benefited enormously from ethnopharmacology. The history of CNS drug discovery is inextricably intertwined with ethnopharmacology, due to the considerable ingenuity displayed by human societies in identifying and utilizing diverse psychotropic plants. A plethora of psychotropic plant-derived natural substances has resulted. The alkaloid reserpine, for example, from the plant *Rauvolfia serpentina* L. Benth ex Kurz (Apocynaceae), was used in treating psychosis in Ayurvedic medicine, and provided the prototype of modern antipsychotics (Curzon, 1990); the hallucinogens LSD and psilocybin were regarded as possible pharmacological models of psychosis, and basic research with these compounds led to insights into the function of serotonin in the central nervous system (Geyer and Vollenweider, 2008). Some have been a mixed blessing, as their pharmacological properties render them prone to abuse; others, even though abused, also have therapeutic properties that have been a boon to modern medicine; almost all, abused or not, have proven to be valuable tools for basic researchers investigating the neuropharmacology of brain functions and dysfunctions (Duke, 1995; Vortherms and Roth, 2006).

NATURAL PRODUCTS IN THE TREATMENT OF SCHIZOPHRENIA AND NEUROCOGNITIVE DEFICITS

Ethnopharmacology has led to the discovery of botanical medicines or natural products useful in psychiatric disorders such as anxiety and depression, sleep disorders, and dementias. The identification of natural products effective for the treatment of psychosis has met with less success. The alkaloid reserpine, from the Ayurvedic medicine *Rauvolfia serpentina*, is the prototype antipsychotic; its discovery resulted from ethnopharmacology, but it was quickly supplanted by synthetic neuroleptics such as chlorpromazine (Marder et al., 1993), although it still finds occasional use in the treatment of tardive syndromes (Fernandez and Friedman, 2003). Recent research has resulted in the identification of traditional medicines with promise for the treatment of a range of psychiatric/neurological disorders including seizures, anxiety, substance abuse, depression, psychosis, and dementias; with few exceptions, most of these studies are in the early stages (Lake, 2000). In a few instances, e.g., *Ginkgo biloba* L. (Ginkgoaceae) for dementia and memory deficits, and St. John's Wort (*Hypericum perforatum* L. (Hypericaceae) for depression, these natural medicines have been commercialized as popular dietary supplements (Fugh-Berman and Cott, 1999). There has been considerable interest in recent years in the investigation of botanical remedies for dementia and cognitive disorders (Howes et al., 2003; Kidd, 1999; Ott and Owens, 1998), but almost all of the interest has been focused on cognitive deficits of dementias rather than those associated with schizophrenia. The influence of botanical medicines on schizophrenia, either on the exacerbation of symptoms by patients self-medicating with St. John's Wort in combination with antidepressants (Lal and Iskandar, 2000; Parker et al., 2001), exacerbation of extrapyramidal symptoms by betel nut (*Areca catechu* L. (Arecaceae) (Deahl, 1989), or the incidental amelioration of symptoms by betel nut (Wilson, 1979; Sullivan et al., 2000), or in adjunct treatment with *Ginkgo biloba* (Zhang et al., 2001), has been noted, but systematic clinical studies are rare. Many of these reports are case studies related to one or at most a few patients (Hanes, 2001). Most published clinical studies have been conducted by Chinese researchers, and are often published in Chinese in journals not readily accessible to Western investigators; moreover, many of these studies have focused on herbal adjunct treatments to conventional antipsychotic therapies, and not on the positive or negative symptoms of schizophrenia (Zhu et al., 1996; Yamada et al., 1997; Zhang et al., 1987; Wang, 1986; Hu, 1984; Yuan, 1979). Thus the clinical literature on botanical therapies for schizophrenia is both disappointing and tantalizing; there are promising leads, but the information is sketchy, clinical studies are lacking, and those that do exist are almost all within the context of Chinese Traditional Medicine. Other than the sparse reports on betel nut, there is little published on cognition-enhancing ethnomedicines in schizophrenia. The Amazon basin represents another geographic area with a high biodiversity index and numerous indigenous ethnomedical traditions (Schultes and Raffauf, 1990). Ethnomedical practices in the region incorporate shamanic elements in which the use of psychotropic plants, such as the hallucinogen *ayahuasca* (Coe and McKenna, 2017) is the rule rather than the exception. Amazonian traditional healers are often familiar with the psychotropic properties of many botanical remedies, but ethnopharmacologists have paid disproportionate attention to hallucinogens; those with nootropic, or cognition-enhancing, properties are poorly investigated. Nonetheless, intriguing leads to cognition enhancers have been noted (Schultes, 1993, 1994; McKenna et al., 1995).

RADIOLIGAND-BINDING METHODOLOGIES
IN DRUG DISCOVERY

The development of radioligand receptor-binding methodologies, pioneered by Solomon Snyder and colleagues in the early 1970s, was a significant breakthrough that has been particularly important for the neurosciences (Pert and Snyder, 1973). The technique gave molecular pharmacologists the means to selectively label specific receptors, enzymes, or other cellular targets using isotope-labeled compounds. Such methodologies have been invaluable for the elucidation of the sites and mechanisms of action of a vast array of drugs and other bioactive substances. Receptor-binding methodologies have also been an important tool in drug discovery, enabling the rapid, cost-effective screening of compound libraries for activity against a variety of molecular targets, including neurotransmitter receptors (Phillipson, 1999). The application of these methodologies to the detection and bioassay-directed isolation of psychotropic or neuroactive compounds in plant extracts has been successful in the identification of constituents with analgesic activity (Phillipson, 1999; Sampson et al., 2000), anti-epileptic activity (Jäger et al., 2004), serotonin-reuptake inhibition activity (Nielsen et al., 2004), and Ayurvedic medicines with memory-enhancing activities (Misra, 1998). More recently, functional assays have emerged as high-throughput approaches to screen for the activities of compounds at CNS targets (Armbruster and Roth, 2005).

OBJECTIVES OF THE PRESENT STUDY

In the present study, we utilized a combination of screening approaches to evaluate a selected sample of Amazonian ethnomedicines for indications of CNS activities that may have therapeutic applications for the treatment of cognitive deficits. We used literature reviews, databases, surveys of herbarium collections, and field interviews with traditional healers to compile a database of approximately 311 candidate species. Approximately 130 species from this original list were collected, and crude extracts and fractions were screened in a broad spectrum of *in vitro* radioligand receptor-binding assays.

METHODS AND MATERIALS

IDENTIFICATION AND PRE-SELECTION OF TARGETED SPECIES

We relied on a variety of resources to partially pre-select candidate species for collection and follow-up investigation. Because of the lack of extensive published data on the use of Amazonian ethnomedicines specifically for schizophrenia or cognitive deficits, and due to the lack of exact correspondence between Western diagnostic categories and cultural conceptualizations of mental disease, we elected to develop a list of species targeted for collection that conformed to a broad set of inclusion criteria. The rationale for this approach was that initial, broadly defined inclusion criteria would be less likely to overlook candidates of potential interest compared to inclusion criteria that were more narrowly defined. Our reasoning was that fractionation and *in vitro* screening of a set defined using broad criteria would rapidly result in the identification of a subset of collections inviting more extensive evaluation.

LITERATURE SURVEY

We initially relied on literature searches in PubMed, supplemented by published ethnobotanical references on Amazonian ethnomedical species and on searches in the NAPRALERTsm database to identify targeted species. Four published volumes were key to our literature survey, viz. Duke and Vasquez, 1994; Schultes and Raffauf, 1990; Von Reis and Lipp, 1982; Von Reis, 1973.

In addition to published volumes, targeted species were selected based on peer-reviewed journal articles accessed through Pubmed. Three of these were key references for the identification of promising leads (Schultes, 1993; Schultes, 1981; Russo, 1992).

NAPRALERT[SM] SURVEYS

NAPRALERT[sm] and Pubmed were primary online resources used in conducting the literature survey. The NAPRALERT[sm] database (http://www.napralert.org) is a natural products database maintained and administered by the Program for Collaborative Research in the Pharmaceutical Sciences in the College of Pharmacy, University of Illinois at Chicago (Loub et al., 1985; Farnsworth, 1993). It contains information on the ethnomedical uses, chemical constituents, and pharmacological and biological activities of natural products from plant, animal, microbial, and marine sources. The information is compiled from a variety of sources including published abstracts, journals, government reports, newsletters, patents, and books. Approximately 50% of the data is derived from a systematic survey of the literature from 1975 to the present, but includes some data from older sources, some as old as 1650. NAPRALERT[sm] is the most comprehensive collection of data on natural products and ethnomedicine in existence. Of particular relevance to this project, NAPRALERT[sm] contains over 3600 biological/pharmacological activity codes related to compounds and extracts. For example, there are approximately 98 codes related to central nervous system activity; more than 50 codes related to autonomic nervous system activity; over 126 codes related to receptor-binding or receptor-mediated activity. Initially, NAPRALERT[sm] was searched for references to plants or extracts having one or more pharmacological codes related to CNS activity, with the additional constraint that the plants were native to South America (Table 1). Plants indigenous to South America that were identified in searches of the NAPRALERT[sm] pharmacological activity codes were parsed for occurrence in Peru, then the genus and species (or the genus if the species was not listed) was searched again in NAPRALERT[sm] using its "3-part" search protocol, which retrieves information on ethnomedical uses, biological activities detected in extracts evaluated *in vitro* and in animal models (including humans), lists secondary compounds isolated, and presents a consolidated citation summary. Genera and species retrieved from the NAPRALERT[sm] searches were further parsed to omit well-known and well-studied species (e.g., *Nicotiana tabacum* L. (Solanaceae), *Banisteriopsis caapi* Spruce ex. Griseb Morton (Malpighiaceae). Additionally, species with relatively well-studied secondary chemistry (as evidenced by the existence of extensive phytochemical studies in published literature) were not included as candidates, or were assigned a lower priority than species with relatively unstudied phytochemistry, on the rationale that species with limited phytochemical data were more likely to yield novel compounds.

COLLECTIONS DATABASE

The information acquired through NAPRALERT[sm], PubMed, published books, and later through herbarium surveys and field interviews with local informants, was incorporated into a database using the program Filemaker Pro™ (Filemaker, Inc., Santa Clara, CA). Filemaker is a relational database that accommodates the incorporation of large text blocks into data fields, and that permits simultaneous searches on numerous text and numerical parameters. It is easily customized for specific uses, is cross-platform compatible (Macintosh™ and Microsoft Windows™ PCs) and can be published on the World Wide Web using HTML formats. Filemaker Pro™ was thus ideal for the purposes of this project, as it enables data to be shared among all investigators and is suitable for eventual publication of the data on the Internet. The initial database was constructed using Filemaker Pro 5™, but the software was periodically upgraded over the course of the project, and the current version now runs under Filemaker Pro 9™. The Filemaker database was initially constructed as a repository for the data collected on targeted species in the literature surveys, but over the course of the project lifetime, this database was expanded to include the collection data on the acquired specimens (including herbarium voucher labels), digitized scans of targeted species and associated herbarium labels from the Herbarium Amazonense at UNAP, and records of the fractions generated by chemical-fractionation protocols and the summarized results of radioligand binding.

Based on the data extracted from NAPRALERT[sm], PubMed, and other data sources, searchable database fields were defined for probable CNS activities (including all of the searched NAPRALERT[sm] activity codes, plus additional activity definitions based on folk uses). Additional fields included information on the plant parts used, modes of preparation, routes of administration, presence/absence of classes of secondary compounds, and results of radioligand receptor assays (Table 2).

HERBARIUM SURVEY

Species that were targeted for collection based on the data collected from NAPRALERT[sm] and the other literature searches specified were cross-referenced with the genera on file in the Herbarium Amazonense at the Universidad Nacional de la Amazonía Peruana (UNAP) in Iquitos. In some cases, the identical species were found in the herbarium, while in others only related species were found, and in still others, there were no specimens on deposit. If the genus and species of interest was found in the herbarium, or if related species belonging to the same genus were found, the specimens were digitally photographed, and these images, along with the data recorded on the herbarium labels, were incorporated into the database. The herbarium labels in most cases contained information on the location of the collection, the collector(s), date of collection, and, rarely, information on ethnobotanical and/or ethnomedical uses. All of this information was also incorporated into the database.

SPECIMEN COLLECTIONS

Specimen collections were carried out in the Loreto province of Peru on several different expeditions between November 2004 and July 2006. The initial focus of the collections was on the acquisition of targeted species that had been identified in the literature surveys and for which location data was available. In addition, other species, not originally on the target-acquisition list, came to our attention in the course of fieldwork, usually as a result of information shared by local informants, and these were also collected when possible. Other targeted species were not collected either because no location data was available, the location of the populations was inaccessible, or the species were not known from the area of collections. Herbarium voucher specimens for each collection were prepared and assigned a unique collection number. Duplicate vouchers were deposited in the Herbarium Amazonense and in the Herbarium of the Bell Museum of Natural History, University of Minnesota. In addition to the vouchers, small samples (~100 – 500 g) of plant materials were also collected for each specimen to provide material for chemical analysis and bioassay. The bulk collections were ground in a ball mill, dried at ~60° C in a forced-convection plant drying room at Gracia Ethnobotanicals, and stored in heat-sealed polyethylene-lined storage pouches (4.5 mil, 10 x 12" or 9.5 x 16", Fisher Scientific catalog # 01-812F series) until shipment.

Table 1 Selected NAPRALERTsm Activity codes relevant to Neuropsychiatry (Modified from Lake, 2000)

CNS activity (NAPRALERT code)	Number of Cumulative Citations as of 2009
Anticonvulsant activity (11006)	783
Narcotic antagonist activity (11020)	45
Antipsychotic activity (11081)	24
Tranquilizing effect (11041)	225
Memory-enhancing effect (11044)	263
Antiaggressive effect (11052)	24
Antidepressant activity (11062)	254
Antianxiety activity (11094)	29
Psychotropic activity (11032)	45
Hallucinogenic activity (11012)	162
Monoamine oxidase inhibition (16005)	127

Table 2 Searchable categories defined in the Filemaker™ Collections Database.

CNS Activities	analgesic; anxiolytic; stimulant; sedative; sudorific; antipyretic; tranquilizer; smoke-d[a]; snuffa; epilepsy; tremorogenic; paralytic; memory; geriatric; dementia; depressant; intoxicant; hallucinogen; anticonvulsant; convulsant; headache; narcotic; antitussive; hysteria; insomnia; insanity; nervousness; "susto"[b]; tremors; vertigo; depression; magical[c]; tonic; spasmolytic; aphrodisiac; nervous disorders.
Preparation methods	Decoction; Infusion; Poultice; Topical Application; Baths; *Ayahuasca* Admixture; Not Specified; Not Processed; Squeezed Juice; Macerate; Powder; Alcoholic Extract.
Plant parts utilized	Wp – whole plant; Ap – aerial parts; Lv – leaves; Bk – bark; Rt – roots; Br – branches; St – stems; Wd – wood; Sd – seeds; Fl – flowers; Ft – fruits; Sp – sap; Lx – latex; Rz – rhizomes; Co – corms; Eo – essential oil; Ns – not specified.
Secondary compound occurrence	acetogenins; acyclics; alkaloids (any type); benzenoids; betaines; cardenolide glycosides; chromones; coumarins; diterpenes; essential oil; flavonoids; glycosides; indole alkaloids; iridoids; isoflavonoids; isoquinoline alkaloids; lactones; lignans; lipids; monoterpenes; nitrogen heterocycles; non-protein amino acids; phenylpropanoids; polyacetylenes; pyrrolizidine alkaloids; quinoids; quinoline alkaloids; saponins; sesquiterpenes; β-carbolines; steroids; triterpenes; unknown; xanthones.
Binding profiles[d]	5HT1A; 5HT1B; 5HT1D; 5HT1E; 5HT2A; 5HT2C; 5HT3; 5HT5A; 5HT6; 5HT7; α1A; α1B; α2A; α2B; α2C; D1; D2; D3; D4; D5; DOR; MOR; H2; M1; M2; M3; M4; M5; DAT; NET; SERT.

a Preparations that were commonly smoked or snuffed were interpreted as likely to display psychoactive effects.
b "Susto" is a folk disease commonly recognized in Amazonian ethnomedicine that is similar to generalized anxiety disorder (cf. Logan, 1993).
c "Magical" indicates the plant is used in the context of ritual, witchcraft, or sorcery rather than for a specific pharmacological action. It is included here because plants used in this context are often psychoactive or have other CNS activities.
d 5HT – 5-hydroxytryptamine, (serotonin) receptor subtypes; α – alpha adrenergic receptor subtypes; D – dopamine receptor subtypes; DOR, MOR – delta-opiate and mu-opiate receptors; H2 – histamine-2 receptor; M – muscarinic acetylcholine receptor subtypes; DAT – dopamine reuptake transporter; NET – norepinephrine reuptake transporter; SERT- serotonin reuptake transporter.

COLLECTION DATA AND HERBARIUM LABELS

The Filemaker™ database program was used to design collection labels, and each collection was assigned a unique collection number. Collection data included the family, genus, species, and taxonomic authority of the collected specimen, the GPS coordinates and other location data, the date of collection, the name of the collectors, the elevation in meters (where known), common names, the plant parts collected, any pertinent data on the specimen derived from the literature and NAPRA-LERT^{sm} searches (and incorporated from the targeted species in the database), and a cross-reference to NAPRALERT^{sm} profiles, if they existed. By designing the labels as a layout in the Filemaker™ database, it enabled collection data to be easily revised, updated, and selectively searched and sorted. A complete list of all collected specimens is available as supplementary data, posted online at: http://www.sciencedirect.com/science/article/pii/S037887411000913X

COLLECTION AND EXPORT AUTHORIZATIONS

Collections in the Loreto region and the export of dried plant biomass and herbarium voucher specimens were carried out under joint authorization from UNAP, Department of Biosciences, and INRENA (Instituto Nacional Recursos Naturales), the Peruvian Department of Natural Resources that has jurisdiction over bioprospecting, export of plant specimens, and scientific investigations of Peruvian biota. Bulk dried samples were shipped to the Department of Chemistry at the University of Minnesota and stored at room temperature until extractions could be carried out. Herbarium voucher specimens were hand-carried to the University of Minnesota and released into the care of Dr. George Weiblen, vascular plant curator of the Herbarium at the Bell Museum of Natural History. A full set of duplicate voucher specimens was deposited in the Herbarium Amazonense at UNAP in Iquitos.

SCREENING OF EXTRACTS AND FRACTIONS IN

RADIOLIGAND ASSAYS

Bulk dried plant specimens were processed into crude extracts in preparation for screening. 20 to 50 grams of the powdered, dried plant material were placed in a 250 mL screw-capped rotary shaker flask, and covered with ca. 150 mL of 1:1 CH_2Cl_2:MeOH. The flask was gently agitated on a rotary shaker table for 24 hours. The solvent was decanted, additional solvent was added, and the extraction procedure was repeated for an additional 24 hours. The extracts were combined, and the solvent was removed under vacuum by rotary evaporation. Other investigators have reported yields ranging from 2 to 16% of the dry weight using a similar strategy (Zhu et al., 1996), so extraction of 50 grams of plant material yields between 1 and 8 g of crude extract. The combined extracts were reduced in volume to ca. 5% of the original volume by rotary evaporation. The concentrated extracts from each collection were transferred to 30 mL screw-capped Nalgene™ vials for storage. Vials were labeled with a collection number keyed to the collection data in the project database, plant part, weight of plant material extracted, and final volume of the concentrated extract. In instances where multiple plant parts were collected (e.g., bark and leaves), each part was extracted and processed separately. Excess dried plant material was resealed in the heat-sealable plastic pouches, labeled, and stored until needed for further extractions.

PREPARATION OF CRUDE EXTRACTS

FOR SCREENING

Samples were screened using the resources of the NIMH Psychoactive Drug Screening Program (PDSP), first at Case Western University Medical School and, later, after the program relocated, at the Department of Pharmacology in the School of Medicine at the University of North Carolina at Chapel Hill. Samples were submitted to the program in two batches, and preparation procedures were modified for the second batch to address some of the difficulties encountered in screening of the initial batch, in order to improve the reliability of the results. Full details of the sample preparation can be found in the original reference, online at: http://www.sciencedirect.com/science/article/pii/S037887411000913X?via%3Dihub

RADIOLIGAND RECEPTOR-BINDING
AND FUNCTIONAL ASSAYS

The NIMH Psychoactive Drug Screening Program (PDSP) has published standardized methods for radioligand-binding assays and functional assays (for example see Roth et al., 2002; Shapiro et al., 2003; Keiser et al., 2009). Assays are conducted according to standardized methods, but the details of each assay vary according to the receptor being analyzed. Full details of the methods used in the radioligand receptor assays and the functional assays are described in the PDSP Assay Protocol Book (https://pdspdb.unc.edu/pdspWeb/?site=assays).

RESULTS

ETHNOBOTANICAL CHARACTERISTICS
TARGETED VS. ACQUIRED COLLECTIONS

Initial literature and database surveys resulted in the compilation of 258 species targeted for acquisition. Subsequent herbarium surveys and interviews with traditional practitioners resulted in an expanded list of 311 species. 80 species and 62 genera on the original list were collected, and a total of 121 species and 90 genera were collected. The family distribution of the targeted and acquired collections is shown in Figure 1. In general, the most represented families in the targeted list were also the most represented in the acquired collections, with the Apocynaceae, Fabaceae, Rubiaceae, and Solanaceae being the most frequently represented families on both lists.

FOLK USE CATEGORIES

36 categories of folk use deemed to be indicative of CNS activity were defined in the Filemaker database (Table 2). Of these, the five most frequently represented categories in both the targeted collections and the acquired collections were intoxicants, hallucinogens, analgesics, stimulants, and those used for geriatric purposes (Table 3).

PHYTOCHEMICAL DISTRIBUTION

Based on published literature, the phytochemical distribution of targeted and acquired collections (Figure 2), show a parallel distribution, with the most frequently represented phytochemical categories being 1. Unknown constituents; 2. Alkaloids of any type; 3. Triterpenes; 4. Sesquiterpenes; 5. Flavonoids; 6. Isoquinoline alkaloids; and 7. Indole alkaloids. The distribution of collections in these categories show approximately the same frequencies with some discrepancies (Figure 2). For example, flavonoids were more frequent in the acquired species than in the targeted species (16.5% vs 12.9%), while species reported to have isoquinoline alkaloids and indole alkaloids were somewhat more frequent in the acquired species than in the targeted collections (12.4% of acquired species contained isoquinolines vs. 9% of targeted species; 9.9% of acquired species were reported to contain indole alkaloids, vs. 7.4% of targeted species).

RECEPTOR-BINDING ASSAYS

A total of 228 crude extracts and fractions were screened in the radioligand receptor assays. Of these, 91 samples displayed "hits" in one or more receptor assays, with a "hit" being defined as $\geq$ 60% inhibition of the radioactive ligand (Table 4). Table 5[1] presents the data according to the receptor subtypes screened. A total of 39 genera displayed "hits"; Table 6 displays the genera displaying "hits" ranked by the number of active fractions for each genus.

----

1. Table 5 has been omitted for brevity, but can be accessed online in the full paper at: http://www.sciencedirect.com/science/article/pii/S037887411000913X?via%3Dihub

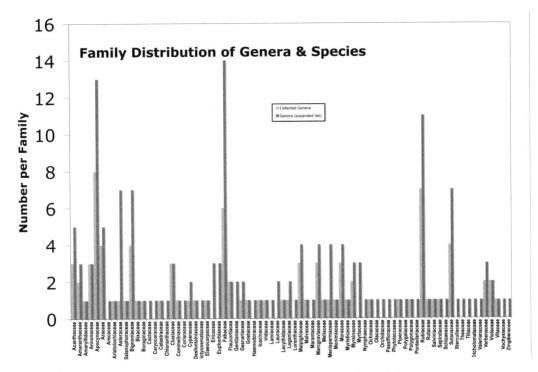

Fig. 1 Family distribution of targeted genera, compared to family distribution of collected genera.

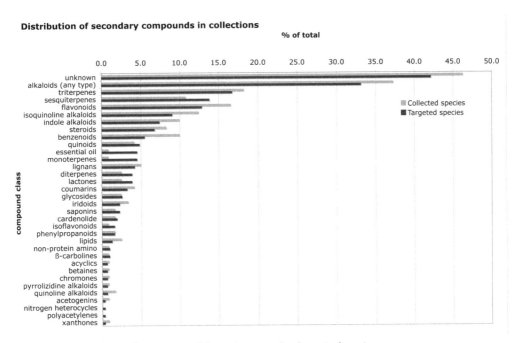

Fig. 2 Distribution of secondary compound classes in targeted and acquired species.

Table 3 Frequency of folk use categories in targeted and acquired collections

Folk Use	Targeted (number)	Targeted (%)	Collected (number)	Collected (%)
intoxicant	84	27.0	29	24.0
hallucinogen	76	24.4	31	25.6
analgesic	61	19.6	35	28.9
stimulant	51	16.4	21	17.4
geriatric	47	15.1	16	13.2
nervousness	41	13.2	10	8.3
magical	40	12.9	20	16.5
antipyretic	38	12.2	22	18.2
tranquilizer	35	11.3	9	7.4
insanity	35	11.3	19	15.7
anxiolytic	34	10.9	9	7.4
sedative	34	10.9	9	7.4
headache	33	10.6	16	13.2
spasmolytic	28	9.0	8	6.6
dementia	26	8.4	7	5.8
narcotic	23	7.4	5	4.1
tonic	23	7.4	8	6.6
anticonvulsant	22	7.1	9	7.4
insomnia	21	6.8	4	3.3
susto	20	6.4	5	4.1
memory	18	5.8	6	5.0
depressant	16	5.1	4	3.3
hysteria	16	5.1	3	2.5
paralytic	15	4.8	3	2.5
depression	15	4.8	9	7.4
snuff	12	3.9	12	9.9
aphrodisiac	12	3.9	6	5.0
nerv. disorders	11	3.5	5	4.1
tremors	10	3.2	5	4.1
sudorific	9	2.9	5	4.1
epilepsy	9	2.9	9	7.4
smoked	8	2.6	8	6.6
vertigo	6	1.9	1	0.8
tremorogenic	5	1.6	2	1.7
antitussive	4	1.3	2	1.7
convulsant	2	0.6	1	0.8

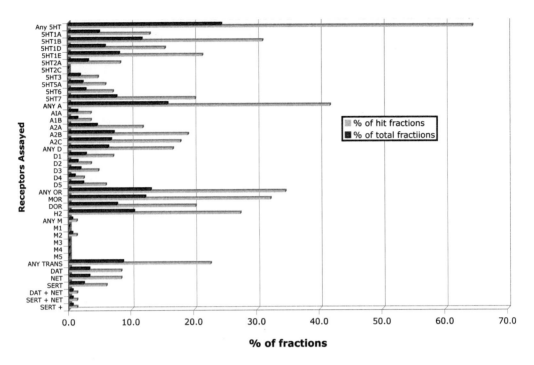

Fig. 3 Receptor-binding profiles of extracts and fractions.

DISCUSSION

A major finding of this study is that the largest number of receptor "hits" were concentrated in those genera that characteristically contain indole alkaloids (Table 6); secondarily, the greatest number of "hits" overall were with one or more 5HT receptors (Figure 3). The taxonomic distribution of the collected species corresponded in most respects to that of the species on the expanded list of targeted species. From an expanded list of 311 species and 172 genera, we were able to acquire 121 species in 90 genera. 80 species in 62 genera were on the original list of targeted collections, while 38 species and 34 genera collected were on the expanded target list, but not on the original list. 116 genera, representing 178 species, were on the original list but were not collected. 40 genera and 70 species were collected that were related, but not identical, to species on the original or expanded target list.

Examination of the family distribution of collected and targeted species and genera indicates a fairly good correspondence in both categories, i.e., those families that were most represented in the target list were also most frequent in the acquired collections (Figure 1). The Apocynaceae, Araceae, Bignoniaceae, Fabaceae, Rubiaceae, and Solanaceae were among the most frequently represented families in both the target list and the acquired list. The distribution of the genera and species on the lists appears to be determined by the criteria for folk use (CNS activity) more than the natural distribution of genera and species in the Amazonian biome. Although the families cited above contain some of the largest numbers of species and genera in Amazonian flora, other families are underrepresented in the sample compared to their abundance in the Amazonian flora (Ayala, 2003). Underrepresented families in the target and collection lists include the Asteraceae, Cucurbitaceae, Cyperaceae, Euphorbiaceae, Melastomataceae, Orchidaceae, and Poaceae.

The most frequently encountered categories of folk use based on published reports were similar in both the targeted collections and the acquired collections (Table 3). The most frequent categories in both were intoxicants or hallucinogens, followed by analgesics, stimulants, and those used in geriatrics. The acquired collections contained a greater percentage of analgesics than the targeted collections (28.9% vs. 19.6% in the targeted collections). The acquired collections also contained relatively greater proportions of "magical" plants, antipyretics, plants used for insanity, and headache remedies than the targeted species, and a smaller proportion of plants used for nervousness,

Table 4 Distribution of samples showing "hits" in receptor assays

Receptors assayed	Number of Samples Displaying "Hits" in Binding Assays	
	≥ 60% inhibition	≥ 75% inhibition
5HT1A	11	7
5HT1B	25	10
5HT1D	13	12
5HT1E	18	9
5HT2A	7	1
5HT2C	0	0
5HT3	4	3
5HT5A	5	4
5HT6	6	2
5HT7	18	10
D1	6	4
D2	3	2
D3	4	1
D4	2	1
D5	5	2
α1A	3	2
α1B	3	2
α2A	8	7
α2B	16	4
α2C	15	10
DOR	17	12
MOR	29	17
H2	24	17
M2	1	0
DAT	8	7
NET	6	0
SERT	2	1

a Abbreviations for binding sites assayed are listed in Table 2.

tranquilizers, anxiolytics, or dementia than the proportions represented in the targeted collections. Some folk categories do not have any correspondence to Western diagnostic criteria, for example "susto", which resembles chronic depression but is not classified as such (Logan, 1993).

The phytochemical distribution of secondary compounds, based on published literature, in the targeted and acquired collections shows approximately the same frequencies, with the most frequent phytochemical categories being 1. Unknown constituents; 2. Alkaloids of any type; 3. Triterpenes; 4. Sesquiterpenes; 5. Flavonoids; 6. Isoquinoline alkaloids; 7. Indole alkaloids (Figure 2). These similarities are probably a reflection of our limited knowledge of the overall abundance of secondary compounds in the Amazonian flora, and are an indication of what has been reported in published literature rather than the actual distribution. There are some discrepancies; for example, flavonoids were more frequent in the acquired species than in the targeted species (16.5% vs 12.9%), while species reported to have isoquinoline alkaloids and indole alkaloids were somewhat more frequent in the acquired species than in the targeted collections (12.4% of acquired species contained isoquinolines vs. 9% of targeted species; 9.9% of acquired species were reported to contain indole

Table 6 Genera displaying "hits" in receptor assays, ranked by the number of active fractions

Genera	Family	Fractions displaying "hits"	No. of species collected
Tabernaemontana	Apocynaceae	8	2
Hamelia	Rubiaceae	7	1
Potalia	Gentianaceae	7	1
Ambelania	Apocynaceae	6	1
Aspidosperma	Apocynaceae	5	1
Erythrina	Fabaceae	4	1
Gloeospermum	Violaceae	3	1
Gnetum	Gnetaceae	3	1
Sloanea	Elaeocarpaceae	3	2
Byrsonima	Malpighiaceae	2	1
Cybianthus	Myrsinaceae	2	1
Eucharis	Amaryllidaceae	2	1
Lantana	Verbenaceae	2	1
Mimosa	Fabaceae	2	1
Siparuna	Monimiaceae	2	2
Teliostachya	Acanthaceae	2	1
Xylopia	Annonaceae	2	2
Abuta	Menispermaceae	1	1
Alternanthera	Amaranthaceae	1	1
Annona	Annonaceae	1	1
Bixa	Bixaceae	1	1
Duroia	Rubiaceae	1	1
Guarea	Meliaceae	1	1
Indigofera	Fabaceae	1	1
Justicia	Acanthaceae	1	1
Lippia	Verbenaceae	1	1
Mansoa	Bignoniaceae	1	1
Mayna	Flaucortiacea	1	1
Memora	Bignoniaceae	1	1
Norantea	Marcgraviaceae	1	1
Philodendron	Araceae	1	1
Psychotria	Rubiaceae	1	1
Remijia	Rubiaceae	1	1
Schlegelia	Bignoniaceae	1	1
Sida	Malvaceae	1	1
Tovomita	Clusiaceae	1	1
Triplaris	Polygonaceae	1	1
Witheringia	Solanaceae	1	1
Zanthoxylum	Rutaceae	1	1

Table 7 Summary of receptor-binding profiles vs. categories of folk use

Folk Uses	5HT	ALPHA	DA	DOR/MOR	H2	M2	TRANS	Total
analgesic	25	17	5	13	9	1	4	74
antipyretic	15	13	5	6	10	1	4	54
headache	11	10	5	6	6	0	1	39
stimulant	13	5	3	7	4	0	3	35
hallucinogen	11	5	2	9	4	0	1	32
intoxicant	11	5	1	9	4	0	1	31
geriatric	9	5	0	6	4	0	2	26
magical	11	4	1	5	4	0	0	25
sedative	6	6	2	3	1	0	3	21
anxiolytic	6	5	2	3	1	0	1	18
nervousness	7	5	1	3	1	0	1	18
insanity	7	2	2	2	2	0	0	15
tonic	5	2	1	4	3	0	0	15
tremors	2	3	1	4	2	0	2	14
narcotic	2	3	1	4	2	0	1	13
memory	5	3	0	2	1	0	1	12
depression	3	1	1	3	2	0	0	10
spasmolytic	6	1	1	1	0	0	1	10
aphrodisiac	3	1	2	1	0	0	2	9
anticonvulsant	2	1	2	2	0	0	1	8
sudorific	3	1	0	1	1	0	1	7
epilepsy	1	1	0	1	0	0	1	4
tranquilizer	2	2	0	0	0	0	0	4
dementia	2	0	1	0	0	0	0	3
insomnia	1	0	1	1	0	0	0	3
nervous disorders	0	1	0	0	0	0	2	3
antitussive	1	0	0	1	0	0	0	2
paralytic	1	1	0	0	0	0	0	2
susto	1	0	1	0	0	0	0	2
convulsant	0	0	0	1	0	0	0	1
hysteria	1	0	0	0	0	0	0	1
depressant	0	0	0	0	0	0	0	0

Table 8 Receptor profiles of anti-dementia plants reported by Schultes (1993)

Collection #	Genus & species	Receptor "hits"
106	*Abuta rufescens*	5HT1B, 5HT1E, 5HT7, D3, D4, D5
067	*Gnetum leyboldii*	5HT7, MOR, DOR, H2, α2C
105	*Schlegelia macrophylla*	5HT1B, 5HT1E
087	*Tabernaemontana heterophylla*	5HT1A, 5HT1B, 5HT1D, 5HT2A, 5HT6, 5HT7, α2A, α2B, α2C, DOR, MOR, H2, NET
097	*Tabernaemontana sananho*	5HT1A, 5HT1B, 5HT1D, 5HT1E, 5HT7

alkaloids, vs. 7.4% of targeted species). It is noteworthy that the largest category of secondary compounds in both the acquired and targeted collections is "unknown", which is a reflection of the paucity of phytochemical investigations in this subset of Amazonian flora, and of the Amazonian flora as a whole. There are some indications of clustering with respect to the phytochemical profiles, in that the largest numbers of overall receptor interactions were samples from characteristically alkaloidal families (Table 6). However, these results should not be over interpreted, since alkaloids were the second most abundant category of secondary constituents in this sample, after "unknown" constituents (2). Since the sample contains such a large proportion for which the phytochemical profiles are "unknown", it is difficult to gain an accurate picture of the correlations that may exist between phytochemical profiles and receptor interactions.

A total of 228 crude extracts and fractions were generated from the acquired collections, and of these, 91 generated "hits" in one or more receptor-binding assays, with a "hit" being defined as ≥60% inhibition of radioligand binding. This data is summarized and presented in various ways in Tables 4-6[2]. Perhaps unsurprisingly, the greatest number of active fractions ("hits") was clustered in genera in families that are known to be rich in alkaloids, since these secondary products frequently affect the central nervous system. The 6 top-ranked genera in Table 6 are from alkaloid-rich families, and of these, 3 of the 6 belong to the Apocynaceae, a family that is well known for its abundance of indole alkaloids.

The overall distribution of "hits" at all receptors screened is graphed in Figure 3. 91 active fractions displayed inhibition in receptor-binding assays of ≥60%; over 60% of "hit" fractions (vs. approximately 25% of total fractions) were at one or more 5HT receptor subtypes. Of the 5HT subtypes screened, none of the samples displayed ≥60% inhibition at $5HT_{2C}$ receptors. The most frequent 5HT receptors displaying "hits" were $5HT_{1B}$, $5HT_{1D}$, $5HT_{1E}$, $5HT_7$, and $5HT_{1A}$, respectively, with all other 5HT receptors screened showing less than 10 "hits" out of the 91 samples screened (Table 4, Figure. 3). More than 10% of samples displayed "hits" at α_{2A}, α_{2B} and α_{2C} receptors, while less than 5% showed activity at α_{1A} and α_{1B}-adrenergic receptors. Only about 5% of the sample showed activity at any dopamine (D) receptors; the most frequent dopaminergic receptor showing activity was D_1, at which 6 out of 91 samples displayed more than 60% inhibition. Over 30% of samples displayed "hits" at μ-opiate receptors, and about 20% inhibited binding at δ-opioid receptors; altogether, 46 samples gave "hits" at one or both opiate receptors. Histamine H_2 receptors also gave relatively large percentages of "hits" (28%). Surprisingly, only one sample yielded a "hit" on any muscarinic cholinergic receptor (M_2) (Table 4).

Table 7 shows the distribution of receptor activities with respect to folk classification of the CNS activities of the collections. Analgesia was the most frequent folk use of the collections indicative of probable CNS activity, followed by antipyretics and headache remedies. There does not appear to be any clear correlation between receptor binding and folk uses. The receptor "hits" are distributed in about the same proportions in all folk categories, with 5HT, α-adrenergic, and opiate-receptor inhibition the most common, with lower levels of activity at the remaining receptors assayed.

CONCLUSIONS

The study has shown that interactions with serotonin receptor subtypes were the most common activity detected, followed by α-adrenergic receptors, opiate receptors, and histamine H_2 receptors. In contrast, fewer than 10% of samples showed any interaction with dopamine receptors or monoamine transporters, and only one sample displayed any inhibition of muscarinic receptors (Figure 3 and Table 4). Although inhibition of 5HT receptors was the most common, there were anomalies in this data as well; at the criteria level defined as a "hit" (≥60% inhibition), none of the samples yielded "hits" at $5HT_{2C}$ receptors, while 7 samples yielded "hits" at the homologous $5HT_{2A}$ receptor, although only one of these (*Potalia resinifera* Mart. (syn. *Potalia amara* var. *resinifera* (Mart.) Progel) (Loganiaceae) had an inhibitory value greater than 70%. The factors contributing to this distribution of receptor interactions in this sample may be both co-evolutionary (in the sense that plants evolve biologically active constituents to mediate their interactions with other organisms) and ethnobotanical (in the sense that indigenous populations will introduce an unconscious bias into their selection of plants with CNS activity). Since all of the plants screened have one or more folk uses related to CNS activity, it is unsurprising that there is a spectrum of receptor interactions;

---

2 Note that Table 5 is omitted from this paper but available online (vide supra).

what is perhaps more surprising is that there appears to be little correlation between folk uses and receptor interactions; the relative proportions of receptor inhibitions is about the same regardless of the folk use. Analgesics, for example, are not overrepresented by opiate receptor interactions; this category contains nearly twice as many 5HT receptor interactions, although this may be misleading because serotonin is also involved in analgesia. There are also indications of correlations in some cases; nearly 50% of the plants used for "insanity" show inhibition at 5HT receptors; similarly, 41% of plants used for "memory" and 35% used for "geriatric" show 5HT interactions. Plants used as "hallucinogens" or "intoxicants" have a high proportion of 5HT interactions (~35%), as might be expected since the actions of hallucinogens are known to be mediated through 5HT receptors (Nichols, 2004).

Roth (Roth et al., 2000, 2004a; Gray and Roth, 2007a, 2007b) reviewed serotonin receptor subtypes that show promise for the development of medications to treat cognitive deficits in schizophrenia. These investigators highlight $5HT_{1A}$ partial agonists, $5HT_{2A}$ antagonists, $5HT_4$ partial agonists, and $5HT_6$ antagonists as likely targets for improving cognition in schizophrenia. On these criteria, 6 species in our collections displayed $5HT_{1A}$ receptor interactions, 5 species displayed $5HT_{2A}$ interactions, and 3 species displayed interactions at $5HT_6$ receptors. $5HT_4$ receptors were not included among the receptors assayed in this study. The species that displayed inhibition of binding at the receptors mentioned may represent candidates for further investigation.

A review by Gray and Roth (2007b) discusses other receptors that bear investigation as potential targets for cognition enhancers, in addition to the 5HT receptors mentioned above. These include D_1 agonists, D_4 agonists and antagonists, nicotinic α_7 and nicotinic $\alpha_4\beta_2$ agonists, M_1 and M_4 agonists, M_5 antagonists, NMDA enhancers, glycine transport inhibitors, AMPA/kainite receptors, mGluR2/3 and mGluR5 agonists, α-adrenergic agonists, sigma agonists, and GABA-A agonists and antagonists. Of the receptors mentioned, our collections included 6 fractions that showed inhibition at D_1 sites, and 2 at D_4 sites. 35 samples showed inhibition at one or more A_2 subtypes in binding assays. Only 1 sample was active at any muscarinic site (M_2) in binding assays; no other samples inhibited binding at other muscarinic sites.

Schultes (1993) reported on 28 species that are used in the Northwest Amazon to treat dementia-like disorders in the elderly. Of the species cited by Schultes, 18 were represented in our collections and 4 displayed inhibition at various receptors, including 5HT, dopamine subtypes, opiate subtypes, and adrenergic subtypes (Table 8). Of the samples screened, various fractions from *Tabernaemontana heterophylla* Vahl (Apocynaceae) (collection # 87) displayed activity at 6 5HT subtypes, 3 adrenergic subtypes, both opiate subtypes, the histamine H_2 receptor, and the norepinephrine transporter (NET). *Tabernaemontana* is a chemically well-studied genus, known to contain indole alkaloids and with numerous folk uses in Amazonian ethnomedicine (Van Beek et al., 1984). 6 of 8 fractions derived from this species were active in the receptor assays. Another species, *Tabernaemontana sananho* Ruiz & Pavon (Apocynaceae) is not mentioned by Schultes, but fractions showed an inhibition profile similar to *T. heterophylla* at several 5HT receptor subtypes. These results suggest that future investigations should focus on a more complete characterization of *Tabernaemontana* alkaloids at receptor subtypes relevant to cognitive functions.

Other investigators have applied radioligand receptor-binding assays as tools to detect potentially therapeutic activity in medicinal plant extracts (Phillipson, 1999; Sampson et al., 2000; Jäger et al., 2004; Nielsen et al., 2004; Misra, 1998; Zhu et al., 1996), but none have been applied to the investigation of Amazonian ethnomedicines. Moreover, most previous studies have utilized a restricted battery of receptor screens applied to a relatively small number of extracts. The present study is the first to apply an extended battery of receptor assays to a large number (>228) of extracts and fractions derived from 121 species in 90 genera. The data reported here must be considered incomplete, or at least as a work in progress. The results reported highlight both the promise and the limitations of such an approach. It has provided, for example, a picture of the distribution of CNS activity (to the extent that this is reflected in receptor interactions) in a subset of Amazonian flora, sampled according to both ethnobotanical and phytochemical criteria. It has not succeeded in definitively identifying one or more Amazonian species that are certain to lead to the development of medications that will find clinical use for the treatment of cognitive deficits in schizophrenia or dementias. It has, however, identified a subset of species that are promising candidates for further investigation.

ACKNOWLEDGEMENTS

This work was supported under Grant # 04T-505 from the Stanley Medical Research Institute and the NIMH Psychoactive Drug Screening Program, Contract # N01MH32004 (NIMH PDSP).

REFERENCES

Armbruster, B.N., Roth, B.L., 2005. Mining the receptorome. *Journal of Biological Chemistry* 280, 5129-32.

Ayala, F., 2003. *Taxonomia Vegetal: Gymnospermae y Angiospermae de la Amazonía Peruana.* Centro de Estudios Teológicos de la Amazonía (CETA), Iquitos, Peru.

Coe, MA, McKenna, D.J., 2017. Therapeutic Potential of *Ayahuasca*. Chapter 7, in: Camfield, David A., McIntyre, Erica, Sarris, Jerome (Eds.), *Evidence-based herbal and nutritional treatments for anxiety disorders.* Springer Publishing Co.

Curzon, G., 1990. How reserpine and chlorpromazine act: the impact of key discoveries on the history of psychophar-macology. *Trends in Pharmacological Sciences* 11, 61-3.

Deahl, M., 1989. Betel nut-induced extrapyramidal syndrome: an unusual drug interaction. *Movement Disorders* 4, 330-2.

Duke, J.A., 1995. Commentary – novel psychotherapeutic drugs: a role for ethnobotany. *Psychopharmacological Bulletin* 31, 177-84.

Duke, J.A., Vasquez, R., 1994. *Amazonian Ethnobotanical Dictionary.* CRC Press, Boca Raton, FL.

Farnsworth, N.R., 1993. Ethnopharmacology and future drug development: the North American experience. *Journal of Ethnopharmacology* 38, 145-52.

Fernandez, H.H., Friedman, J.H., 2003. Classification and treatment of tardive syndromes. *Neurologist* 9, 16-27.

Fugh-Berman, A., Cott, J.M., 1999. Dietary supplements and natural products as psychotherapeutic agents. *Psychoso-matic Medicine* 61, 712-28.

Geyer, MA, Vollenweider, F.X., 2008. Serotonin research: contributions to understanding psychoses. *Trends in Pharma-cological Sciences* 29, 445-53.

Gray, J.A., Roth, B.L., 2007a. The pipeline and future of drug development in schizophrenia. *Molecular Psychiatry* 12, 904-22.

Gray, J.A., Roth, B.L., 2007b. Molecular targets for treating cognitive dysfunctions in schizophrenia. *Schizophrenia Bulletin* 33, 1100-1119.

Hanes, K.R., 2001. Antidepressant effects of the herb *Salvia divinorum*: a case report. *Journal of Clinical Psychopharmacol-ogy* 21, 634-35.

Hill, S.K., Bishop, J.R., Palumbo, D., Sweeney, J.A., 2010. Effect of second-generation antipsychotics on cognition: current issues and future challenges. *Expert Review of Neurotherapeutics* 10, 43-57.

Howes, M.J., Perry, N.S., Houghton, P.J., 2003. Plants with traditional uses and activities relevant to the management of Alzheimer's disease and other cognitive disorders. *Phytotherapy Research* 17, 1-18.

Hu, G.C., 1984. [*Anticonvulsants used for controlling induced seizures during the treatment of schizophrenia with lactoni Coriari-ae*] Zhong Xi Yi Jie He Za Zhi 4, 675-8, 644.

Jäger, A.K., Mohoto, S.P., van Heerden, F.R., Viljoen, A.M., 2004. Activity of a traditional South African epilepsy remedy in the GABA-benzodiazepine receptor assay. *Journal of Ethnopharmacology* 96, 603-6.

Keiser, M.J., Setola, V., Irwin, J.J., Laggner, C., Abbas, A.I., Hufeisen, S.J., Jensen, N.H., Kuijer, M.B., Matos, R.C., Tran, T.B., Whaley, R., Glennon, R.A., Hert, J., Thomas, K.L., Edwards, D.D., Shoichet, B.K., Roth, B.L., 2009. Predicting new molecular targets for known drugs. *Nature* 462, 175-81.

Kidd, P.M., 1999. A review of nutrients and botanicals in the integrative management of cognitive dysfunction. *Alterna-tive Medicine Review* 4, 144-61.

Lake, J., 2000. Psychotropic medications from natural products: A review of promising research and recommenda-tions. *Alternative Therapies in Health and Medicine* 6, 36-60.

Lal, S., Iskandar, H., 2000. St. John's Wort and schizophrenia. *Canadian Medical Association Journal* 163, 262-3.

Logan, M.H., 1993. New lines of inquiry on the illness of susto. *Medical Anthropology* 15, 189-200.

Loub, W.D., Farnsworth, N.R., Soejarto, D.D., Quinn, M.L., 1985. NAPRALERT, computer handling of natural product research data. *Journal of Chemical Information and Computer Sciences* 25, 99-103.

Lysaker, P.H., Buck, K.D., 2007. Neurocognitive deficits as a barrier to psychosocial function in schizophrenia: effects on learning, coping, and self-concept. *Journal of Psychosocial Nursing and Mental Health Services* 45, 24-30.

Mangialasche, F., Solomon, A., Winblad, B., Mecocci, P., Kivipelto, M., 2010. Alzheimer's disease: clinical trials and drug development. *Lancet Neurology* 9, 702-16.

Marder, S.R., Ames, D., Wirshing, W.C., Van Putten, T., 1993. Schizophrenia. *The Psychiatric Clinics of North America* 16, 567-87.

McKenna, D.J., Towers, G.H.N., Luna, L.E., 1995. Biodynamic constituents in *Ayahuasca* admixture plants: an unin-vestigated folk pharmacopoeia, in: von Reis, S., and Schultes, R.E. (Eds.), *Ethnobotany: Evolution of a Discipline.* Dioscorides Press, Portland, OR, pp. 349-361.

Misra, R., 1998. Modern drug development from traditional medicinal plants using radioligand receptor-binding assays. *Medicinal Research Reviews* 18, 383-402.

Nichols, D.E., 2004. Hallucinogens. *Pharmacology and Therapeutics* 101, 131-181.

Nielsen, N.D., Sandager, M., Stafford, G.I., van Staden, J., Jäger, A.K., 2004. Screening of indigenous plants from South Africa for affinity to the serotonin reuptake transport protein. *Journal of Ethnopharmacology* 94, 159-6.

Ott, B.R., Owens, N.J., 1998. Complementary and alternative medicines for Alzheimer's disease. *Journal of Geriatric*

Psychiatry and Neurology 11, 163-73.

Parker, V., Wong, A.H., Boon, H.S., Seeman, M.V., 2001. Adverse reactions to St John's Wort. *Canadian Journal of Psychiatry* 46, 77-9.

Pert, C.B., Snyder, S.H., 1973. Opiate receptor: demonstration in nervous tissue. *Science* 179, 1011-4.

Peuskens, J., Demily, C., Thibaut, F., 2005. Treatment of cognitive dysfunction in schizophrenia. *Clinical Therapeutics* 27 Suppl. A, S25-37.

Phillipson, J.D., 1999. Radioligand receptor-binding assays in the search for bioactive principles from plants. *The Journal of Pharmacy and Pharmacology* 51, 493-503.

Roth, B.L., Baner, K., Westkaemper, R., Siebert, D., Rice, K.C., Steinberg, S., Ernsberger, P., Rothman, R.B., 2002. Salvinorin A: a potent naturally occurring nonnitrogenous kappa opioid selective agonist. *Proceedings of the National Academy of Sciences of the United States of America* 99, 11934-9.

Roth, B.L., Hanizavareh, S.M., Blum, A.E., 2004b. Serotonin receptors represent highly favorable molecular targets for cognitive enhancement in schizophrenia and other disorders. *Psychopharmacology* (Berlin) 174, 17-24.

Roth, B.L., Lopez, E., Patel, S., Kroeze, W., 2000. Multiplicity of serotonin receptors: useless diverse molecules or an embarrassment of riches? *The Neuroscientist* 6, 252-262.

Roth, B.L., Sheffler, D.J., Kroeze, W.K., 2004a. Magic shotguns versus magic bullets: selectively non-selective drugs for mood disorders and schizophrenia. Nature Reviews. *Drug Discovery* 3, 353-9.

Russo, E.B., 1992. Headache treatments by native peoples of the Ecuadorian Amazon: a preliminary cross-disciplinary assessment. *Journal of Ethnopharmacology* 36, 193-206.

Sampson, J.H., Phillipson, J.D., Bowery, N.G., O'Neill, M.J., Houston, J.G., Lewis, J.A., 2000. Ethnomedicinally selected plants as sources of potential analgesic compounds: indication of *in vitro* biological activity in receptor-binding assays. *Phytotherapy Research* 14, 24-9.

Schultes, R.E., 1981. Phytochemical gaps in our knowledge of hallucinogens, in: Reinhold, L., Harbourne, J. B., and Swain, T. (Eds.), *Progress in Phytochemistry Vol. 7*. Pergamon Press, Oxford, U.K., pp 301-331.

Schultes, R.E., 1993. Plants in treating senile dementia in the northwest Amazon. *Journal of Ethnopharmacology* 38, 129-35.

Schultes, R.E., 1994. Amazonian ethnobotany and the search for new drugs. *Ciba Foundation symposium* 185, 106-12.

Schultes, R.E., Raffauff, R., 1990. *The Healing Forest: Medicinal and Toxic Plants of the Northwest Amazon*. Timber Press, Portland, OR.

Shapiro, D.A., Renock, S., Arrington, E., Chiodo, L.A., Liu, L.X., Sibley, D.R., Roth, B.L., Mailman, R., 2003. Aripiprazole, a novel atypical antipsychotic drug with a unique androbust pharmacology. *Neuropsychopharmacology* 28, 1400-11.

Sullivan, R.J., Allen, J.S., Otto, C., Tiobech, J., Nero, K., 2000. Effects of chewing betel nut (Areca catechu) on the symptoms of people with schizophrenia in Palau, Micronesia. *British Journal of Psychiatry* 177, 174-8.

Van Beek, T.A., Verpoorte, R., Svendsen, A.B., Leeuwenberg, A.J., Bisset, N.G., 1984. *Tabernaemontana L. (Apocynaceae):* a review of its taxonomy, phytochemistry, ethnobotany and pharmacology. *Journal of Ethnopharmacology* 10, 1-156.

Von Reis, S., 1973. Drugs and foods from little-known plants: *Notes in Harvard University Herbaria*. Harvard University Press, Cambridge, MA.

Von Reis, S., Lipp, F.J., 1982. *New plant sources for drugs and foods from the New York Botanical Garden herbarium*. Harvard University Press, Cambridge, MA.

Vortherms, T.A., Roth, B.L., 2006. Salvinorin A: from natural product to human therapeutics. *Molecular Interventions* 6, 257-65.

Wang B. [Observations on the effects of traditional Chinese medicine to invigorate blood and relieve stasis in treating schizophrenia]. Zhonghua Shen Jing Jing Shen Ke Za Zhi. 1986 Feb;19(1):44-6.

Wilson, L.G., 1979. Cross-cultural differences in indicators of improvement from psychosis: the case of betel nut chewing. *The Journal of Nervous and Mental Disease* 167, 250-1.

Yamada, K., Kanba, S., Yagi, G., Asai, M., 1997. Effectiveness of herbal medicine shakuyaku-kanzo-to) for neuroleptic-induced hyperprolactinemia. *Journal of Clinical Psychopharmacology* 17, 234-5.

Yuan DJ. [Clinical observations on the effects of Lactoni Coriariae and Tutin in the treatment of schizophrenia (report of 140 cases) (author's transl)]. Zhonghua Shen Jing Jing Shen Ke Za Zhi. 1979. 12, 196-200

Zhang, L.D., Tang, Y.H., Zhu, W.B., Xu, S.H., 1987. Comparative study of schizophrenia treatment with electroacupuncture, herbs and chlorpromazine. *Chinese Medical Journal* (Engl.) 100, 152-7.

Zhang. X.Y., Zhou, D.F., Su, J.M., Zhang, P.Y., 2001. The effect of extract of *Ginkgo biloba* added to haloperidol on superoxide dismutase in inpatients with chronic schizophrenia. *Journal of Clinical Psychopharmacology* 21, 85-8.

Zhu, M., Bowery, N.G., Greengrass, P.M., Phillipson, J.D., 1996. Applications of radioligand receptor-binding assays in the search for CNS-active principles from Chinese medicinal plants. *Journal of Ethnopharmacology* 54, 153-164.

A Preliminary Report on Two Novel Psychoactive Medicines from Northern Mozambique

Dale Millard

Wasiwaska, Research
Center for the Study
of Psychointegrator
Plants, Visionary Art and
Consciousness,
Florianópolis, Brazil

ABSTRACT

This communication seeks to report, for the first time on the use of a medicinal plant *Aeschynomene cristata* Vlakte for psychoactive purposes. Although several species of *Aeschynomene* are used medicinally in various parts of the world, this is the first report of a member of this genus being used for psychoactive or visionary purposes.

INTRODUCTION

In February of 2017, the author was asked to join a team of scientists on an exploration trip to Mount Mabu which only became known to the scientific community as recently as twelve years ago. Mount Mabu is the largest of several granitic inselbergs, extending east of Lake Malawi, and north of the Zambezi River into Northern Mozambique. The mountain itself consists of a relatively rare type of wet forest, surrounded by vast *Brachystegia* woodlands. This means that the species of the wet forest have been in isolation for long evolutionary periods [Bayliss et al, 2014]. This forest has been described as possibly the largest tract of unbroken medium altitude forest in Southern Africa, and is situated at 900 -1400 meters. In the recent past this forest type used to be more common, though due to deforestation largely to support a highly destructive charcoal industry, much has been cleared. The region has received little scientific investigation, probably due to its remoteness and fact that Mozambique endured civil war from 1977 - 1992. Then in 2013, after 20 years of peace, fighting resumed and is ongoing, making the area potentially unsafe for travel. Since the first trip in December 2005, there have only been ten trips to the region which have revealed both high levels of biodiversity and well as numerous new endemic species of plants and animals. Due to the war, it is believed that many people withdrew into this forest seeking safety. Currently, the people living in villages around the forest are mostly Makua, from the larger Lomwe group. Lomwe, which is also the name of the spoken language, is believed to have originated out of the Congo basin about a thousand years ago. Virtually all inhabitants of this region rely on subsistence farming. The Lomwe are Mozambique's largest matriarchal tribe and are still strongly animist to this day, maintaining their ancestral belief system. Many of the Lomwe believe they originated from a cave on nearby sacred Mount Namuli from where all animals and humans were born. A female foot is said to be imprinted outside the cave. Hence the matriarchal family structure.

MATERIALS AND METHOD

The author's role in the expedition was to perform the first preliminary ethnobotanical survey of the region, and particularly the wet forest, as virtually nothing is known about the use of the plants from this biome. The study was conducted over a period of 9 days and consisted of formal interviews with healers from the surrounding communities. In addition walks were conducted into the forest where the healers were asked to point out medicines and explain how they are used. Both Lomwe and Portuguese interpreters were present. In total six healers were interviewed regarding approximately 60 plant species used as medicine. It was during these interviews that psychoactive properties of *Aeschynomene cristata* were mentioned by one of the informants. It was decided to devote a two day period specifically to explore the knowledge of this healer, who is the main focus of this communication. Of all the plant medicines observed in the survey, about 25% are ascribed to having magico-medicinal properties, that is, plants that are used in conjunction with a particular ritual or belief system. Due to this, extra care was taken to exclude other phenomena such as dreams, when questioning healers specifically about possible psychoactive roles of medicines. Plant specimens were collected and positively identified by Hassam Patel of the Zomba Herbarium, Malawi. Samples of *Aeschynomene cristata* root bark were collected and are awaiting chemical analysis.

RESULTS AND DISCUSSION

The history of this particular healer is worth mentioning. He is an African male, currently 42 years old. At age 20 he began developing psychological problems, which in a western model may be associated with schizophrenia. He described hearing voices and seeing visions. Unable to face his community he escaped to live in the forest. It was here where his deceased grandfather appeared to him, and proceeded to show him which plants to use to heal himself. This kind of initiation whereby a healer receives knowledge or training directly from their ancestral spirits is not a rare phenomenon in Africa. This is significant as it often involves the use of new or different species of plants, as well as unique ways in which the plants are employed.

This healer described the use of two plants species used for visionary or psychoactive purposes. The first being a well known medicinal plant, *Myrothamnus flabellifolius* Welw. also known as the Resurrection plant. This plant is capable of virtual total desiccation, returning to a green vegetative state within an hour of receiving water. This common name is derived from this habit. Locally the plant is known as Thriabe. The young leaves of this plant are smoked by several African tribes for asthma and other chest complaints [Gechev et al, 2014]. Smoking the leaves is reported to have a mild sedative effect which this healer described as being similar to smoking cannabis. This plant has a wide distribution and its use in this way is known to the author to be widespread throughout Southern Africa.

The second plant reported as being used to induce visionary phenomena is known locally as Mwecheche and botanically as *Aeschynomene cristata*. Not much is known of the chemistry of this genus, though several species of *Aeshynomene* are used medicinally throughout the tropics. *Aeschynomene abyssinica* Vatke is a well known anti-cancer plant in Kenya[Ochwang'i et al, 2014] *Aeschynomene fascicularis* Schltdl. & Cham is used in Mayan traditional medicine to treat cancer [Caamal-Fuentes et al, 2011]. The Buddha Pea *Aeschynomene indica* is a famous herb both in Chinese and Ayurvedic medicine used to treat kidney stones and urinary tract infections. This plant has demonstrated potent antimicrobial activity [Aruna et al, 2012]. The seeds of this plant are known to contain Rotenoids, neurotoxic to pigs and rodents [Haraguchi et al, 2003]. However the benzene and alcoholic extracts of roots of the Asian *Aeschynomene aspera* L. were found to have significant hepatoprotective properties similar to silymarin in a study using using carbon tetrachloride to induce hepatotoxicity in rats [Thirupathy Kumaresan and Pandae,2011].

The plant is vetch-like in its growth habits and reaches from 1 – 3 meters in height. The specimens observed were growing in rich, black loam soils on the border between the two vegetations types. The *Aeschynomene* genus consists of about 60 species occurring throughout the world in tropical and sub tropical regions. *A cristata* is found in Africa and Madagascar. Original distribution of this and several species of *Aeschynomene* is difficult to determine as they are believed to be introduced so widely.

The roots are first washed in water to remove soil. Then the root bark is scraped from the roots, dried and pounded to a fine powder. Small quantities (an estimated ¼ teaspoon) of this powder are insufflated into the nose, causing immediate burning and sneezing. The onset is said to begin within 2 minutes, characterised by a buzzing in the ears and difference in visual and colour perception, resolving in approximately ten minutes. When questioned about dosage and safety of this plant, the informant stipulated that is was not dangerous, and if one did this several times the effects would last longer, and if one increased the dosage, it was relayed by direct translation "that one sees small people", and specifically "not the tall ones!" These little people were described as being at about knee height. Though when questioned further about these little people, it was also stated that "one can see anything according to his own spirit."

The informant said he did not use this medicine in patients, unless they specifically requested it. He explained that he took this medicine personally in order to receive answers, to diagnose illness, and to learn which medicine to use for a particular patient. He also mentioned that sometimes he would take it before praying, or before ritual dancing which amongst the Makua is often associated with trance states. It was later confirmed with the hunters who together with the healers are the only people who venture deep into the forest, that they use the powdered root bark blown into the noses of their hunting dogs in order to sharpen their senses. A similar practice has been reported in the Amazon amongst the Ecuadorian Shuar [Bennett and Alarcon, 2015].

Unfortunately due to limited time and bad weather, the author was unable to confirm these psychoactive effects with any other healers of the area. To the author's knowledge, this the first time a member of this genus has been reported to elicit psychoactive effects.

At present the samples collected are awaiting analysis to see if perhaps they contain known or new psychoactive chemistry.

ACKNOWLEDGMENTS

The author would to thank the following people for their support, the invitation to participate in the expedition to Northern Mozambique, and also for their assistance in the field. B Linton, Proff. J Bayliss, J Barbee, C Borgstein, A Lyman and H Patel.

REFERENCES

Aruna, C., Chaithra, C., Alekhy, C., Yasodamma, N. 2012. Pharmacognostic studies of Aeschynomene indica L. *International Journal of Pharmacy and Pharmaceutical Sciences*. Vol 4, Suppl 4. 393-405.

Bayliss, J., Timberlake, J., Branch, W., Bruessow, C., Collins, S., Congdon, C., Smith, P. (2014). The discovery, biodiversity and conservation of Mabu fores – the largest medium-altitude rainforest in southern Africa. *Oryx*, 48(2), 177-185.

Bennett BC, Alarcón R. 2015. Hunting and hallucinogens: The use of psychoactive and other plants to improve the hunting ability of dogs. *J. Ethnopharmacology*, 171:171-83

Caamal-Fuentes E, Torres-Tapia LW, Simá-Polanco P, Peraza-Sánchez SR, Moo-Puc R. 2011. Screening of plants used in Mayan traditional medicine to treat cancer-like symptoms. *J. of Ethnopharmacology* 2011 135:719-24.

Gechev TS, Hille J, Woerdenbag HJ, Benina M, Mehterov N, Toneva V, Fernie AR, Mueller-Roeber B. 2014. Natural products from resurrection plants: Potential for medical applications. *Biotechnology Advances*, 32:1091-1101.

Thirupathy Kumaresan , Pandae 2, 2011. Hepatoprotective Activity of Aeschynomene Aspera. *Pharmacologyonline* 3: 297-304

Ethnopharmacology – From Mexican Hallucinogens to a Global Transdisciplinary Science

[Keynote]

■■■■■ *Michael Heinrich* [I,III*] &
Ivan Casselman [II,III]

I. Research Cluster 'Biodiversity and Medicines' / Research Group 'Pharmacognosy and Phytotherapy', UCL School of Pharmacy, University of London, England

II. Rubia Solutions Inc. Vancouver, Canada

III. Environmental Sciences, Southern Cross University, Lismore, Australia

ABSTRACT

Psychoactive natural substances have been reported from practically all regions of the world, but Mexican indigenous cultures have played a crucial role having influenced medical, toxicological, biological, chemical, pharmaceutical, and, of course, anthropological research.

Especially in the 1950's and 1960's peyotl, teonanacatl and other psychoactives came to the attention of researchers and revelers alike. In this overview we highlight the developments of ethnopharmacology from the initial development of the term until today using one psychoactive species as an example - *Salvia divinorum*. In 1962 "ethnopharmacologists", Albert Hofmann and R. Gordon Wasson, documented and collected a flowering specimen of *Ska María Pastora* allowing the species botanical description as *Salvia divinorum* Epling & Játiva. Five years later Efron et al. (1967) organised a symposium "Ethnopharmacologic search for psychoactive drugs" which over the next decades would give its name to a discipline which today is much more broadly defined, dealing with local and traditional medicines, their biological activities and chemistry. Globalisation has resulted in a world-wide commodification of many traditional medicines and psychoactives, as exemplified by *S. divinorum*. This fascinating Lamiaceae has become globally recognized for its best known active constituent salvinorin A, a kappa-opioid antagonist which has a unique effect on human physiology.

While today ethnopharmacology is a thriving discipline, the interest in psychoactive substances is no longer central to the discipline. The search for anti-cancer agents (which also started in earnest in the 1960's) had been of particular relevance and today includes among its many foci:

- The scientific study of local and traditional knowledge not only in remote regions, but for example, also in urban immigrant communities

- Research linking ethnopharmacology to biodiversity research both in terms of a sustainable use of natural resources (ecosystems)

- Pharmacological studies with the aim of understanding the effects of complex mixtures on specific diseases or disease targets

- The safety of herbal medicines

- Anthropological and historical approaches on the use of medicinal and food plants and the link between food and medical uses of plants and fungi.

50 years on ethnopharmacology is very different from what D. Efron and colleagues had envisioned.

INTRODUCTION

To the best of our knowledge, the term "ethnopharmacology" was first published in 1967 by Efron and colleagues who used it in the title of a book on hallucinogens: *Ethnopharmacological Search for Psychoactive Drugs* (Efron, et al., 1970; Holmstedt, 1967). Thus with this book, we celebrate both 50 years of a ground-breaking symposium and the introduction of a new term. This introduction is much later than, for example, the term ethnobotany which in 1896 was coined by the US-American botanists William Harshberger describing the study of human's plant use. Both ethnopharmacology and ethnobotany investigate the relationship between humans and plants in all its complexity. "Ethnopharmacology" also replaced the many other terms which had been used previously like "Pharmakoëthnologie" used already by Tschirch (1910) in his classic *Handbuch der Pharmakognosie* or pharmacoetnologia or Aboriginal botany. (cf. Heinrich, 2014).

However, there is considerable variation in terms for what constitutes ethnopharmacology. In a book edited in 2015 by the first author and Prof. Anna Jaeger (Heinrich and Jaeger, 2015), we compiled definitions of ethnopharmacology as they were given by the contributors to this book. The range from definitions which are very much embedded in the:

- Sociocultural sciences [e.g. Dan Moerman (USA): Ethnopharmacology is the study of the way people use plants, informing us about the varying ways people create meaning about these living objects.];

- Biomedical research [eg. Pravit Akarasereenont (Thailand): "A science dealing with the study of the pharmacology of traditional medicine and focusing on the active substances and their pharmacological action." or Thomas Efferth (Germany): "Ethnopharmacology focuses on research on efficacy, safety, and modes of actions of traditional medicines with pharmacological methods."]

In general the multidisciplinary of the field is highlighted very well clearly recognized by [e.g. Tony Booker (UK): The study of the historical and modern interactions between humans and flora, fauna and minerals and how these substances, their extracts and the chemical compounds derived from them, may be utilised to prevent and treat ill-health in people and their dependent animals]. Others stress the link between local and traditional knowledge with research conducted by academically trained investigators, with – in our view – Graham Jones (Australia) expressing it most eloquently and clearly: "Ethnopharmacology constituting a respectful marriage between modern science and ancient wisdom with much to be gained in both directions."[1]

Consequently, ethnopharmacology is not a very sharply circumscribed field of research and is heavily influenced by the academic, cultural and political background of a researcher.

In the beginning, the discipline of ethnopharmacology was focused primarily on the study of the traditional use psychoactive substances. However, the trajectory of this discipline has expanded in to an array of studies. We explore one of the early ethnopharmalogical studies, the discovery, description and chemical elucidation of the Mexican Lamiacea *Salvia divinorum*. While this species is not as famous as other Mexican psychoactives such as *Psilocybe* mushrooms, it does demonstrates one of the earliest ethnopharmacological studies, as well as a 50 year trajectory of discovery, from the description of the plant to its genetic profiling.

There can be no doubt that in 2018 ethnopharmacology is a thriving discipline, embedded in a range of larger disciplinary contexts like botany, pharmacy, anthropology, and medicine. Estab-

1. Note added by Editor, Dennis McKenna. My personal favourite definition is that proposed by Holmstedt and Bruhn (1983): "The interdisciplinary scientific exploration of biologically active agents traditionally employed or observed by humans." In my opinion this definition is succinct, specific and sufficient, in that it notes that ethnopharmacology is not restricted to medicines, nor to plants, or to substances ingested, but also correctly restricts the discussion to "traditional use."

lished journals now publish thousands of articles in this field of research and while there are not many institutes that have the term in their name, many groups based in the pharmaceutical, biological, chemical and other schools publish in the field. This is impressive for a field that has had a surprisingly short history.

THE EARLY YEARS

While research on local and traditional plants dates back many centuries and includes, for example, the many explorers "discovering" exotic treatments, the modern history is a post-World-War II development. The 1950's and 1960's saw a dramatic socio-cultural change in "Western" societies. As part of the opening up of the rigid post-WW2 societies, numerous new developments in the cultures including music, the performing, and visual arts, but also tremendous socio-cultural conflicts formed new societal perspective. A key element of this was a fast developing interest in psychedelic substances, most importantly hallucinogenic plants. For example, in the 1960's and 1970's the psychologist and prolific writer Timothy Leary (1920 - 1996) impacted on the political and societal thinking on mind-altering drugs including most notably LSD and those which were derived from traditional and local knowledge (especially *Psilocybe* spp.). With the group's experiments on psychedelic substances during his "Harvard Years" (1960 – 1963), Timothy Leary may have had more impact on what later one was called ethnopharmacology, than we are aware of.

Cannabis and products derived from it became an important element of this (counter-)culture. A key role in this context played research on and experiences with hallucinogenic plants and fungi from modern day Mexico, The highly toxic *Toloatzin* or Jimson weed *Datura stramonium* L. (Solanaceae) is one of the main and widely distributed hallucinogenic plants and fungi of Mesoamerica (together with peyotl - *Lophophora williamsii* (Lem. ex Salm-Dyck) J.M. Coult., ololiuhqui – *Turbina corymbosa* (L.) Raf.and the mushrooms teonanacatl – *Psilocybe* spp.); all have long traditions of use as hallucinogens. The following example, however, was only discovered by Western societies in 1962 - *Salvia divinorum*. It sparked great interest both in scientific terms and by those interested in its use. While no detailed historical information is available, it is clear that this discovery also contributed to the interest in holding the symposium at the University of California, San Francisco Medical Center (January 28-30 1967) and, therefore, to the book by Efron et al (1967, republished 1970)

Salvia Divinorum

In 1962, ethnopharmacologists, Albert Hofmann and R. Gordon Wasson, undertook an expedition to Oaxaca, México (Hofmann, 1980; Wasson, 1962). Their main informants in the region became a curandera – Maria Sabina – who later became first persecuted and then famous. She provided the essential link between Mazatec traditional culture and the 'explorers'. On this trip, they recorded several different plants and their use by Mazatec healers. As well as recording the cultural uses, they attended ceremonies, which incorporated the use of *S. divinorum* Epling & Jativa, a member of the Lamiaceae (Labiatae). This expedition contributed much to the early understanding of the cultural role and use of this species. Wasson and Hofmann were also able to obtain a flowering specimen of this plant, making the scientific description of *S. divinorum* possible (Epling and Jativa 1962; Casselman et al 2014). This "discovery" was met with great excitement and led to a flurry of research in ethnopharmacology, phytochemistry, neuropharmacology and other disciplines.

Many years later, in 1982, Ortega and his team (Ortega, Blount, and Manchand, 1982) isolated and identified the main active compound in *S. divinorum*, salvinorin A. In the early 1990s, the psychoactive properties of salvinorin A were elucidated (Siebert, 1994). With the confirmation of its psychoactivity, the cultural adoption of *S. divinorum* as a "new" psychoactive, outside of Mexico, gained considerable momentum.

THE BOTANY OF *Salvia Divinorum*

All recorded native populations of *S. divinorum* are in Oaxaca, southern Mexico. This state is bordered by the Pacific Ocean to the west and, in the north, the Sierra Mazateca mountain range. Much of this mountain range is covered by tropical montane cloud forest (Ott, 1995, 1996; Reisfield, 1993), an ecosystem typified by high humidity and persistent cloud cover. Growing in the understory of the forest, *S. divinorum* has been found in several locations between 500 and 1500 meters altitude (Ott, 1995, 1996). Populations of this plant are mostly found near water courses in partial or full shade and grow in moist, nutrient-rich soil. In these conditions, *S. divinorum* grows and reproduces primarily vegetatively, flowering sporadically when enough sun penetrates the forest canopy (Reisfield, 1993).

S. divinorum grows up to 1.5 m in height and has a hollow, quadrangular stem, which is green, translucent and crisp (Ott, 1996; Reisfield ,1993). The leaves are 10–25cm long, 5–10 cm wide, and are opposite on the stem, elliptic in shape and have serrated margins (Epling and Jativa 1962; Ott 1996; Reisfield 1993). Numerous glandular and non-glandular trichomes are present on the leaf surface (Kowalczuk, et al., 2013; Siebert, 2004). The flowers have white corollas with purple calices. The flowers are three to four centimeters in length and grow on panicles of 20 to 30 flowers. According to reports on wild populations, as well as laboratory experiments, *S. divinorum* does not produce flowers on a regular, seasonal basis (Reisfield, 1993; Valdés, et al., 1987). In Oaxaca, this plant is observed to flower between October and June (Reisfield, 1993). Flowering is initiated by set durations of uninterrupted darkness greater than 12 hours (Reisfield, 1993). In laboratory experiments, it has been found that if plants are exposed to light during a dark period, flowering is aborted and the plant returns to vegetative growth (Reisfield, 1993).

There is limited information on the sexual reproduction of *S. divinorum*, however, it is very adept at clonal propagation both naturally and anthropogenically. On the basis of the reported reproductive behaviour of *S. divinorum*, it has been suggested that the more recent evolutionary trajectory of this plant may have been influenced by humans (Reisfield, 1993). It is hypothesized that *S. divinorum* may have been translocated from its original environment at some point in history, however, this has not been confirmed nor have other populations of *S. divinorum* been discovered in the Americas (Reisfield, 1993). The pollination vector for *S. divinorum* is also uncertain. It has been suggested that the pollination may be ornithophilous (Reisfield, 1993). This is corroborated by the dimensions of the corolla as well as the sugar content and the volume of nectar produced (Reisfield ,1993).

HISTORY OF *Salvia Divinorum*

Until 1964, the use of *S. divinorum* appears to have been confined to the Mazatecs, an indigenous Mexican group located in northeast Oaxaca. The name Mazatec or Mazateca is said to mean "Lords of the Deer," and was the name given to this group by the Aztec (Mooney, 1911). After Spanish colonization in the 1500s, the Dominicans and Jesuits began to convert indigenous peoples to Catholicism (Mooney, 1911). Although Spanish attempts at conversion were largely successful, the Mazatec also maintained their traditional beliefs, which are still practiced today (Hofmann, 1990, 1980; Mooney, 1911; Ott, 1996). The Mazatec employ three main plants with psychoactive properties as part of their spiritual practices. These include *Psilocybe* spp. mushrooms, the seeds from *Ipomoea violacea* L. (morning glory) and the leaves of *S. divinorum* (Allen, 1994, 1997; Foster, 1984; Schultes, 1969). Mazatec use of *S. divinorum* takes place primarily during healing and divination ceremonies, as well as in the training of medical practitioners (Giovannini and Heinrich, 2009).

There are four illnesses for which Mazatecs are known to have used *S. divinorum* (Johnson, 1939; Ott, 1996; Prisinzano, 2005; Valdés, Diaz, and Paul, 1983). First, this plant is often employed to cure eliminatory dysfunction such as diarrhoea. Secondly, people who are near death can be given an infusion of the plant's juices as a palliative, after which it is reported that the patient often recuperates for a short time. Thirdly, *S. divinorum*, in small doses, is used to cure headaches and rheumatism. Finally, it is given to cure a Mazatec illness known as *panzón de arrego* or a swollen belly. This Mazatec illness is believed to be caused by a curse from a brujo, (male witch) someone who practices black or evil magic (Prisinzano, 2005; Ott, 1996; Valdés, Diaz, and Paul, 1983; Johnson, 1939).

S. divinorum is tended in secret groves, deep within the forest, by medicinal practitioners known as a *curandero* (male) or *curandera* (female) (Reisfield, 1993). It is planted in rich, black soil at the bottom of a gully, usually in close proximity to a stream (Diaz, 2013). Cuttings can be taken from the mother plant and planted directly into the moist soil, however, this plant will also root itself, if a branch breaks off and falls on the ground (Beifuss, 1997). Although these *S. divinorum* groves may be natural, it is difficult to determine the extent of human influence (Ott, 1996; Reisfield, 1993). The locations are well-protected by each individual *curandero* or *curandera* to avoid theft, and more importantly, contamination by malicious magic (Johnson, 1939). The large, mature leaves of *S. divinorum* are harvested by pinching the petiole of the leaves close to the main stem of the plant. The leaves are either eaten or crushed into a fine pulp using a mortar and pestle, and then infused in water (Campbell, 1997; Valdés, 2001).

Mazatec *curanderos* and *curanderas* are trained through an informal apprenticeship, during which they are led through a series of progressive visions by an experienced teacher (Valdés, Diaz, and Paul, 1983; Diaz 1979). These visions are initiated by the three psychoactive plants mentioned previously and are an integral part of training. Over a period of two years, *curanderos* and *curanderas* ingest these plants at regular intervals to integrate the knowledge from their experiences into their practice (Valdés, Diaz, and Paul, 1983). Initially, trainees ingest increasingly larger doses of *S. divinorum* leaves, which show them the way to heaven, where the initiated learn from the tree of knowledge (Valdés, Diaz, and Paul, 1983).

During consumption of *S. divinorum*, either the leaves are chewed or the juice from crushed leaves is infused in water and ingested as a liquid (Diaz, 2013, 1979; Valdés, 2001). These ceremonies are led by a *curandero* or *curandera*, and last approximately two to three hours, during which time the participants, who ingested the plant, are guided through different states of consciousness (Schultes, Hofmann, and Rätsch, 2001; Ott, 1996; Valdés, Diaz, and Paul, 1983; Hofmann, 1980, 1990; Estrada, 1977; Schultes, 1976). These ceremonies take place at night in a dark and remote location to prevent disruptions (Valdés, 2001; Valdés, Diaz, and Paul, 1983; Diaz, 1979), as absolute quiet is considered essential to the success of the ceremony. Several leaves are rolled into cigar-shaped tubes, chewed and swallowed. If the participant is unable to chew the leaves or manage the bitter taste, he or she is permitted to drink juice-infused water instead (Estrada, 1977). During each ceremony, there is one person present who does not ingest *S. divinorum*. It is the role of this person to watch over the ceremony and prevent any harm to participants (Diaz, 1979; Valdés, Diaz, and Paul, 1983). After the effects of *S. divinorum* have worn off, the *curandero* or *curandera* will often bathe the participant in the juice of the leaves (Valdés, 2001), which is said to end the effects of the experience (Valdés, Diaz, and Paul, 1983). After the ceremony, participants are "debriefed"; this dialogue helps to explain the meaning of their visions and ensure the success of the ceremony (Diaz, 1979; Estrada, 1977; Hofmann, 1990; Valdés, Diaz, and Paul, 1983).

The Spanish chronicled many of the rituals, which employed psychoactive plants, but very little about *S. divinorum* was recorded. One reason for this could be that the Mazatecs have several names for *S. divinorum*. In their native language it is referred to as Ska Maria Pastora, Ska Maria, Ska Pastora, and in Spanish it is called Hojas de Maria Pastora, Hojas de la Pastora, Hoja de adivinación, Hierba Maria or La Maria (Valdés, 2001; Valdés, Diaz, and Paul, 1983; Schultes, 1972; Wasson, 1962). The Mazatecs associate this plant with the Christian saint, Mary (Valdés, Diaz, and Paul, 1983), however, the reference to her as a shepherdess is not consistent with Christian mythology (Wasson, 1962). This name may reflect an interpretation of a pre-contact description of the plant that was later incorporated into Christian beliefs (Ott, 1995).

In the scientific literature, *S. divinorum* has not received as much attention as the other plants used by the Mexican indigenous peoples including the Mazatec; the seeds of the morning glory *Ipomoea violacea* and hallucinogenic mushrooms *Psilocybe* spp. (Valdés, 2001; Valdés, Diaz, and Paul, 1983; Schultes, 1970). *S. divinorum* was first mentioned in western academic literature in 1939 by anthropologist J. Johnson (Johnson, 1939). In 1945, B. Reko reported a "magic plant" used by the Mazatecs called "hoja de adivinación" or "the leaf of the prophecy", indicating that the indigenous people used this plant to produce visions (Valdés, Diaz, and Paul, 1983; Diaz, 1979; Schultes, 1967). Seven years later in 1952, R. Weitlander reported "yerba de Maria" used by *curanderos* in Oaxaca (Weitlander, 1952). The first botanical specimen of *S. divinorum* was collected by A. Pompa, a Mexican botanist. He described this plant as "xka [sic] Pastora" however, he was unable to collect a flowering specimen at the time leaving his collection only identified to the genus level (Pompa, 1957).

R. Gordon Wasson was a very important ethnopharmacologist and chronicler of psychoactive plants, especially those used by the Mazatec people. Wasson is best known for his research on the traditional Mexican use of *Psilocybe* spp. mushrooms. In July 1961, during his second expedition to Mexico, Wasson participated in an *S. divinorum* ceremony along with Albert Hoffman, known for his discovery of lysergic acid diethylamide or LSD (Reisfield, 1993; Hofmann, 1980; Wasson, 1962). In doing so, Wasson and Hoffman were the first western academics to participate in, and record, this ceremony. In December 1962, Wasson and Hoffman successfully collected a flowering sample of *S. divinorum*, which was classified by Carl Epling as a new species (Epling and Jativa, 1962). Contrary to popular belief, the first living *S. divinorum* specimen to be propagated outside Mexico was not collected by Wasson and Hoffman, but by psychiatrist and ecologist, Sterling Bunnell, who, in 1962, brought back a living *S. divinorum* specimen to UCLA Davis from an expedition to Oaxaca (Siebert, 2003).

Research on the effects of salvinorin A on its molecular target, the kappa-opioid receptor, has been extensive since it represents the only known non-nitrogenous kappa-opioid receptor selective agonist (Casselman, et al., 2014).

In conclusion, *S. divinorum* was "discovered" just five years prior to the symposium on ethnopharmacology. We have no information on the links between these "discoveries" and the developing plans for such a symposium. It may well be timely, to start a historical project on academic and social developments in the USA and beyond driven by the ethnopharmacologic search for psychoactive substances .

ETHNOPHARMACOLOGY 50 YEARS ON

Returning to the ethnopharmacology at the end of the 2nd decade of the third millennium, ethnopharmacology today has a very different focus and interest. In the years after the symposium, it seems that only limited research was going on, aside from studies on psychoactive plants and fungi as exemplified by *S. divinorum*.

The next key event was the launch of the *Journal of Ethnopharmacology* in1979, which was founded by Laurent Rivier and Jan G. Bruhn. Here the scope shifted to "a multidisciplinary area of research concerned with the observation, description, and experimental investigation of indigenous drugs and their biological activity" (Rivier and Bruhn, 1979). Eleven years later the 1st International Congress on Ethnopharmacology was held in Strasbourg, France (5-9 June 1990) and since then 18 conferences have been held on four continents, all organized by the International Society for Ethnopharmacology (ISE - http://www.ethnopharmacology.org/), which was originally founded in 1990 in Strasbourg. In 2013 the Society for Ethnopharmacology, India was founded affiliated to the ISE.

Research is conducted in numerous institutions and most active are many of the fast emerging economies especially in Asia (most notably China, but also India, South Korea, Thailand, and other ASEAN countries, some African (South Africa) and American countries (esp. Brazil). Clearly, the *Journal of Ethnopharmacology* is the leading journal in the field today. In its first year (1979) 29 articles were published, ten years later (1989) this had risen to 85, in 1999 to 205, and in 2009 to 465, with 2016 seeing 649 published articles. Overall, at the time of writing (August 2017) just over 9600 articles have been published in the *Journal of Ethnopharmacology* alone.

The main areas of research today are on antioxidant, anti-inflammatory and anticancer agents (Table 1). The vast majority of these are *in vitro* or *in vivo* studies. In recent years more clinical studies on traditional preparations (often small and not well designed) have also been conducted. Studies describing the use of medicinal and other useful plants are another element of research in the field of ethnopharmacology, and these are often conducted with the goal that they lead to an experimental study of some of these botanical drugs (cf. Heinrich, et al., 2017). At the same time, it is noteworthy that psychoactive and other effects on the CNS have not been of that much importance (Yeung et al 2018). However, one must also acknowledge that this measure (i.e. keywords used in Medline) is a relatively crude one, most importantly, because research which later on focuses on pure compounds or well-defined extracts may not be coded in such a way that it is visible in this comparison.

Antioxidant	2057	Malaria		588
Inflammation	2054	Urinary		411
Cancer	2026	Central nervous system		310
Infecti$	1971		CNS	165
Food	1600		psychoactive	62
Diabetes	1546		hallucinogen$	64
Skin	1089	Cosmetic$		188
Gastrointestinal	826	Fertility		156
Respiratory	638	aphrodia$		111

Table 1 Main topics covered in ethnopharmacological research (number of hits): Medline database search (13/05/2017) combing "Ethnopharmacology or traditional medicine" with specific therapeutic areas as specified. (Ethnopharmacology or traditional medicine): 21,697 [Ethnopharmacology only: 11,607] and .....:

CORE CHALLENGES

Plants (and animal) based medicines are an integral part of indigenous medical systems in many regions of the world, and form a part of the traditional knowledge of a culture. While the focus of the symposium which gave ethnopharmacology its "modern" name and the current areas of research differ, it is the conviction of the authors of this paper, that the commonality is in the hope that this research will not only provide scientific evidence both in socio-cultural as well as in biomedical terms but that it will help in empowering people, recognising their autochthonous traditions and enabling them to make the best use of such knowledge.

A key criticism the field had to engage with is the accusation of exploiting local and traditional knowledge without fair and appropriate benefits to the regions of origin and the original keepers of this knowledge and practice. However, scientists have been the first to highlight the inextricable link between cultural and biological diversity. In 1988 a group of dedicated scientists involved in research on local and traditional uses of plants and biodiversity conservation and with strong interest in supporting indigenous and local peoples called for the recognition of indigenous rights and for increased support for research on ethnobiological inventories, on conservation and management programmes – resulting in the *Declaration of Belem* (Posey and Dutfield, 1996). Four years later, in 1992, the Convention on Biological Diversity (Rio Convention) was signed and has since been amended in numerous treaties and protocols, most recently (2010) the Nagoya Protocol (*Nagoya Protocol on Access to Genetic Resources and the Fair and Equitable Sharing of Benefits Arising from their Utilization (ABS) to the Convention on Biological Diversity*). This development is both driven by the historical experience of many countries, and as importantly, indigenous peoples in exploitative extractions of biodiversity. Ethnopharmacology was one of the disciplines both involved the debate and affected by the resulting legal changes. 25 years after the Convention on Biological Diversity and 50 years after San Francisco conference that led to a named new field of research, there are still no examples where research and the requirements for benefit sharing have resulted in concrete and long term benefits to the regions or countries of origin.

In the last 25 years, numerous efforts have focused on translating the principles of this treatise into best practice. However, examples of problematic or poor practice also abound. We continue to have a very complex and critical debate about who benefits from this research and on how we best follow the ethical guidelines which in this field are most prominently, based on the Convention on Biological Diversity (the Rio Convention, 1992) and subsequent agreements. An understanding of these efforts needs to be based on the fast changing framework, and for example, the Sustainable Development Goals directly impact on the research and development needs globally. Consequently, modern ethnopharmacological research provides new evidence for old preparations and contributes to primary health care (Heinrich 2010). How to best achieve this is still in its infancy and we – as scientists – have still not achieved large scale contributions to improving healthcare globally.

In this regard ethnopharmacology is embedded in a wider debate about the historical and future role of traditional medicines and medical systems globally. In 2016 some systems of traditional medicine (TM) were included in the 11th edition of the International Classification of Diseases (ICD-11), providing a strong impetus both for closer links between traditional medicines and biomedicine, but also adding new responsibilities to practitioners of TM and to those who investigate such medical systems

Ongoing debates relate to best practice in the field (e.g. Cos, et al., 2006, Heinrich, et al., 2017). Here concerns about what constitutes best practice in terms of concepts and methods are addressed and clearly, there is a need to improve the methods we use in data acquisition and analysis. These debates are shared with many other fields of research, and, for example, best practice in pharmacological research is an important concern in many areas of the discipline. Biomedical research that cannot be reproduced or which is of poor quality or which is poorly reported will ultimately undermine the credibility, relevance, and sustainability of the research process in general (e.g. Mullane, et al., 2015).

CONCLUSION

This volume celebrates the fiftieth anniversary of a very important conference, and in this paper, we have looked beyond the scope "ethnopharmacology" covered at its start. While one must acknowledge that psychoactive natural substances are no longer at the center, the detailed look at the history of the discovery of *Salvia divinorum* by Western science and society has been an important driving force not only leading the conference (Schultes, 1967), but has continued with a flurry of neuropharmacological research on the species and its active metabolites. As such it exemplifies how ethnopharmacology links the study of local knowledge and practices and bio-scientific and biomedical investigations. Today's research is thriving but also the conflict exemplified in the history of "discovering" and researching *Salvia divinorum* are a part of the current scenario. Research in ethnopharmacology must, by definition be interdisciplinary, or preferably transdisciplinary, and applying these findings in prevention and treatment should be an element of such research.

ACKNOWLEDGEMENT

This work has benefitted from numerous discussions with students and colleagues and the ideas expressed here evolved over many years with earlier "reincarnations" of these ideas presented at conferences and in various peer-reviewed papers especially Heinrich 2014.

REFERENCES

Allen, J.W. 1994. Chasing the Ghost of Maria Sabina, Saint Mother of the Sacred Mushroom. *Psychedelic Illuminations* 6 (28).

Allen, J.W. 1997. *Maria Sabina, Saint Mother of the Sacred Mushroom: Ethnomycological Journals Sacred Mushrooms Studies.* Psilly Publications / Raver-Books.

Beifuss, W. 1997. Cultivating Diviner's Sage: A Step by Step Guide to Cultivation, Propagation, and Keeping Your Salvia Plants Happy. *The Resonance Project* 1 (32).

Campbell, R. 1997. Sage Wisdom. *The Resonance Project* 1: 27–31.

Casselman, I. et al. 2014. From Local to Global – Fifty Years of Research on *Salvia divinorum. Journal of Ethnopharmacology* 151: 768 – 783.

Cos, P., Vlietinck, A.J., Van den Berghe, D., Maes, L. 2006. Anti-infectivepotential of natural products: how to develop a stronger *in vitro* "proof-of-concept". *Journal of Ethnopharmacology.* 106, 290–302.

Diaz. 1979. Ethnopharmacology and Taxonomy of Mexican Psychodysleptic Plants. *Journal of Psychedelic Drugs* 11: 71–101.

Diaz, J.L. 2013. *Salvia Divinorum*: A Psychopharmacological Riddle and a Mind-Body Prospect. *Current Drug Abuse Reviews* 6 (1): 43–53.

Efron D., Farber S.M., Holmstedt, B., et al. 1970. *Ethnopharmacologic Search for Psychoactive Drugs.* Public Health Service Publications no. 1645. Government Printing Office, Washington, DC (reprint, orig. 1967)

Epling, C., and C.D. Jativa. 1962. *A New Species of Salvia from Mexico.* Botanical Museum Leaflets, Harvard University 20 (3): 297–99.

Estrada, A. 1977. *La Vida de Maria Sabina: La Sabia de Los Hongos.* Mexico: Ross-Erikson.

Foster, S. 1984. *Herbal Bounty! The Gentle Art of Herb Culture.* Gibbs Smith.

Giovannini, P. and M. Heinrich. 2009. Xki Yoma' (Our Medicine) and Xki Tienda (Patent Medicine). Interface between Traditional and Modern Medicine among the Mazatecs of Oaxaca, Mexico. *Journal of Ethnopharmacology* 121 (3): 383–99.

Heinrich, M. 2014. Ethnopharmacology – quo vadis? Challenges for the future. *Revista Brasileira de Farmacognosia* 24: 99-102

Heinrich, M. and A.K. Jaeger, eds. 2015. *Ethnopharmacology.* Wiley, Chichester. ISBN: 978-1-118-93074-8.

Heinrich, M.; Lardos, A.; Leonti, M.; Weckerle, C.; Willcox, M. with the ConSEFS advisory group. 2017. Best Practice in Research: Consensus Statement on Ethnopharmacological Field Studies – ConSEFS. *Journal of Ethnopharmacology* http://dx.doi.org/10.1016/j.jep.2017.08.015

Heinrich, M., Leonti, M., Frei Haller, B. 2014. A perspective on natural products research and ethnopharmacology in México. The eagle and the serpent on the prickly pear cactus. *Journal of Natural Products* 77: 678–689. dx.doi.org/10.1021/np4009927

Hesketh 2015. Ethnopharmacology and Intellectual Property Rights. Pp 87 – 96. In: Heinrich, M. and A.K. Jaeger (eds.) *Ethnopharmacology.* Wiley, Chichester. ISBN: 978-1-118-93074-8.

Hofmann, A. 1980. *LSD: My Problem Child.* McGraw-Hill.

Hofmann, A. 1990. Ride through the Sierra Mazateca in Search of the Magic Plant "Ska Maria Pastora." In *The Sacred Mushrooms Seeker: Essays for R. Gordon Wasson,* edited by T. J. Riedlinger, 115–27. Dioscorides Press / Timber Press.

Holmstedt, B., Bruhn, J.G. 1983. Ethnopharmacology – A Challenge. *Journal of Ethnopharmacology,* 8(3) 251-256.

Johnson. 1939. The Elements of Mazatec Witchcraft. *Goteborgs Etnografiska Museum Etnologiska Studier* 9, 119–49.

Kowalczuk, A.P., Raman, V., Galal, A.M., Khan, I.A., Siebert, D.J., Zjawiony, J.K. 2013. Vegetative Anatomy and Micromorphology of Salvia Divinorum (Lamiaceae) from Mexico, Combined with Chromatographic Analysis of Salvinorin A. *Journal of Natural Medicines,* April, 1–11.

Mooney, J. 1911. *Mixe Indians.* New York: Robert Appleton Company.

Mullane, K., Enna, S.J., Piette, J., Williams, M. 2015. Guidelines for manuscript submission in the peer-reviewed pharmacological literature, *Biochemical Pharmacology* 97(3): 225-235,

Ortega, Alfredo, John F. Blount, and Percy S. Manchand. 1982. Salvinorin, a New Trans-Neoclerodane Diterpene from Salvia Divinorum (Labiatae). *Journal of the Chemical Society* Perkins Transactions 1: 2505–8.

Ott, Jonathan. 1995. Ethnopharmacognosy and Human Pharmacology of Salvia Divinorum and Salvinorin A. *Curare* 18 (1): 103–29.

Ott, Jonathan 1996. Psychoactive Card IV. *Eleusis* 4: 31–39.

Penner, J (ed.). 2014. *Timothy Leary – The Harvard Years* Park Street Press. Rochester, VT, USA and Toronto, Canada.

Pompa, G. 1957. *Salvia divinorum Herbarium Sheets:* 87556 & 93216. Mexico City: Mexican National Herbarium (UNAM).

Posey, DA and G. Dutfield. 1996. *Beyond Intellectual Property: Traditional Resource Rights for Indigenous Peoples and Local*

Communities. International Development Research Centre. Ottawa, Canada

Prisinzano, T. E. 2005. Psychopharmacology of the Hallucinogenic Sage Salvia Divinorum. *Life Sciences* 78 (5): 527–31.

Reisfield, A. S. 1993. The Botany of *Salvia divinorum* (Labiatae). *SIDA* 15 (3): 349–66.

Schultes. R. E. 1967. The Place of Ethnobotany in the Ethnpharmacologic Search for Psychotomimetic Drugs. In *Ethnpharmacologic Search for Psychotomimetic Drugs*, edited by D. H. Efron et al, 37–57. US Government Printing Office.

Schultes. R. E. 1969. Hallucinogens of Plant Origin. *Science* 163: 245–54.

Schultes. R. E. 1970. The Botanical and Chemical Distribution of Hallucinogens. *Annual Review of Plant Physiology* 21: 571–98.

Schultes. R. E. 1972. An Overview of Hallucinogens in the Western Hemisphere. In *Flesh of the Gods: The Ritual Use of Hallucinogens*, edited by P. T. Furst, 3–54.

Schultes. R. E. 1976. *Hallucinogenic Plants*. A Golden Guide. Golden Press.

Schultes, R.E., Hofmann, A, Rätsch, C. 2001. *Plants of the Gods - Their Sacred, Healing, and Hallucinogenic Powers*. Rochester: Healing Arts Press.

Siebert. D. 2003. The History of the First *Salvia divinorum* Plants Cultivated Outside of Mexico. *The Entheogen Review* 12 (4): 117–18.

Siebert. D. 2004. Localization of Salvinorin A and Related Compounds in Glandular Trichomes of the Psychoactive Sage, Salvia Divinorum. *Annals of Botany* 93 (6): 763–71. doi:Doi 10.1093/Aob/Mch089.

Siebert, D. 1994. *Salvia divinorum* and Salvinorin A: New Pharmacological Findings. *Journal of Ethnopharmacology* 43: 53–56.

Valdés, Jose Luis Diaz, Ara G. Paul. 1983. Ethnopharmacology of Ska Maria Pastora (Salvia Divinorum, Epling and Jativa-M.). *Journal of Ethnopharmacology* 7: 287–312.

Valdés, G., Hatheld, M. Koreeda, A. Paul. 1987. Studies of *Salvia Divinorum* (Lamiaceae), an Hallucinogenic Mint from the Sierra Mazateca in Oaxaca, Central Mexico. *Economic Botany* 41 (2): 283–91.

Valdés, L. J. 2001. The Early History of *Salvia divinorum*. *The Etheogen Review* X: 73–75.

Wasson, R. G. 1962. A New Psychotropic Drug from the Mint Family. *Botanical Museum Leaflets, Harvard University* 20 (3).

Weitlander, R. J. 1952. Curaciones Mazatecas. *Anales del Instituto Nacional de Antropologia e Historica* 4: 279–85.

Yeung, A.W.K., Heinrich, M., Atanasov, A.G. 2018. Ethnopharmacology - A bibliometric analysis of a field of research meandering between medicine and food science? *Frontiers in Pharmacology* (Section Ethnopharmacology) 8 doi: 10.3389/fphar.2018.00215

Afterword

An oft-quoted aphorism attributed to the anthropologist Margaret Mead proposes that "one should never hesitate to follow a small group of individuals committed to change as that is the only way in which most change actually happens."

The scientists who attended and spoke at the first "Ethnopharmacological Search for Psychoactive Drugs" (ESPD) symposium at the UC Medical Center were one such group. They had all been inspired and enlightened by sacred plant potions and other magical chemicals they had imbibed over the years. These researchers knew that there were other ways of knowing; they knew that indigenous peoples understood plants in ways they themselves did not. These scientists knew that there were enchanted plants and animals and fungi still waiting to be discovered; and they knew that hallucinogenic plants, in particular, were vegetal scalpels that shamans employed to dissect, analyze, diagnose, treat, and often cure the ailing human mind and spirit.

These beliefs were well outside the mainstream of western science and medicine in 1967, but have stood the test of time. Psychedelic plants are increasingly accepted as legitimate objects of study and wonder, with the understanding that some of these "new" mind-altering compounds may well soon take a position of honor alongside Mother Nature's other greatest healing gifts such as ACE inhibitors, antibiotics, aspirin, beta blockers, and statins.

The 2017 ESPD 50 Symposium marked the 50th anniversary of this historic gathering — scientists and researchers traveled from the far corners of the earth to historic Tyringham Hall, Buckinghamshire, to compare notes, discuss results and honor our predecessors. As in the first meeting, the primacy of indigenous wisdom regarding plants and their potential healing benefits were featured or mentioned in almost every presentation. Of particular note this time were rich and detailed accounts of "new" bioactive compounds that were little known or appreciated outside traditional societies in 1967: iboga, kratom, hallucinogenic frog peptides, and ayahuasca admixtures.

Much of the discussion at the recent conference centered not only on the historical use of plants like ayahuasca and peyote, but how the entheogenic compounds they produce are now being employed in clinical settings to treat intractable or even "incurable" afflictions like depression, drug addiction, end of life anxiety, infertility, PTSD, and others – sometimes with promising results.

We discussed the great irony that, at the same time that the world awakens to these biological wonders, the forests and the cultures that know them best are being obliterated at an ever-increasing pace. Speakers at ESPD50 and other attendees departed Tyringham with a redoubled sense of purpose: to further spread the "ethnopharmacological gospel" about the healing power of these plants, animals and fungi; to encourage further scientific research and documentation of these therapeutic experiments and successes; and to fight against the destruction of these species and the forced homogenization of these tribal cultures just as we come to appreciate this healing wizardry as never before.

Mark J. Plotkin
Amazon Conservation Team
Kwamalasamutu, Suriname

Index

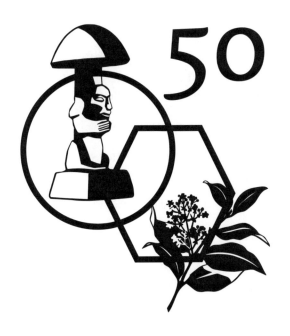

also from SYNERGETIC PRESS

VINE OF THE SOUL:
MEDICINE MEN, THEIR PLANTS AND RITUALS IN THE COLOMBIAN AMAZONIA
by Richard Evans Schultes and Robert F. Raffauf
Foreword by Sir Ghillean Prance
Preface by Wade Davis

CHANGING OUR MINDS:
PSYCHEDELIC SACRAMENTS AND THE NEW PSYCHOTHERAPY
by Don Lattin

AYAHUASCA READER:
ENCOUNTERS WITH THE AMAZON'S SACRED VINE
(New Expanded Edition) Edited by Luis Eduardo Luna and Steven F. White

ZIG ZAG ZEN: BUDDHISM AND PSYCHEDELICS
(New Expanded Edition)
by Allan Badiner and Alex Grey
Foreword by Stephen Batchelor, Preface by Huston Smith

MYSTIC CHEMIST:
THE LIFE OF ALBERT HOFMANN AND HIS DISCOVERY OF LSD
by Dieter Hagenbach and Lucius Werthmüller
Foreword by Stanislav Grof

BIRTH OF A PSYCHEDELIC CULTURE:
CONVERSATIONS ABOUT LEARY, THE HARVARD EXPERIMENTS, MILLBROOK AND THE SIXTIES
by Ram Dass and Ralph Metzner with Gary Bravo
Foreword by John Perry Barlow

WHAT HAS NATURE EVER DONE FOR US?:
HOW MONEY REALLY DOES GROW ON TREES
by Tony Juniper
Foreword by HRH Prince Charles

Synergetic Press is pleased to print this book with Bang Printing, a green initiative company, which is FSC, SFI, and PEFC certified. Bang works with publishers, printers, paper manufacturers and others in the book industry to minimize social and environmental impacts, including on endangered forests, climate change, and communities where paper fiber is sourced. This book is printed on paper certified by the Sustainable Forestry Initiative. www.sfiprogram.org

Find us at www.synergeticpress.com

Published in association with the HEFFTER RESEARCH INSTITUTE.
For more information on their ground-breaking medical research with psychedelics, visit heffter.org.

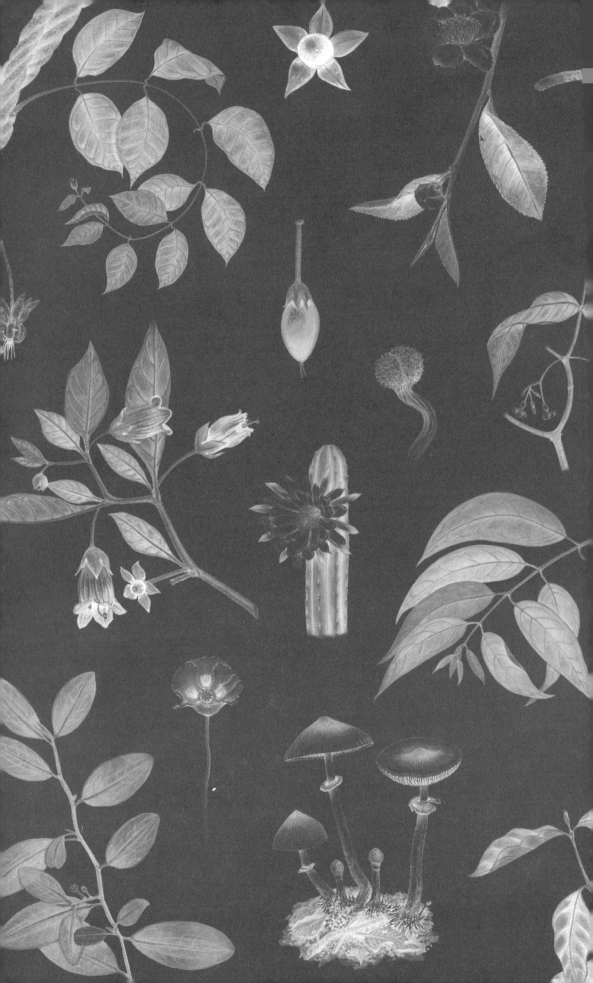